D1327806
MEDWAY
LIBRARY

Modern Pharmaceutics

DRUGS AND THE PHARMACEUTICAL SCIENCES

A Series of Textbooks and Monographs

1. Pharmacokinetics, *Milo Gibaldi and Donald Perrier*
2. Good Manufacturing Practices for Pharmaceuticals: A Plan for Total Quality Control, *Sidney H. Willig, Murray M. Tuckerman, and William S. Hitchings IV*
3. Microencapsulation, *edited by J. R. Nixon*
4. Drug Metabolism: Chemical and Biochemical Aspects, *Bernard Testa and Peter Jenner*
5. New Drugs: Discovery and Development, *edited by Alan A. Rubin*
6. Sustained and Controlled Release Drug Delivery Systems, *edited by Joseph R. Robinson*
7. Modern Pharmaceutics, *edited by Gilbert S. Banker and Christopher T. Rhodes*
8. Prescription Drugs in Short Supply: Case Histories, *Michael A. Schwartz*
9. Activated Charcoal: Antidotal and Other Medical Uses, *David O. Cooney*
10. Concepts in Drug Metabolism (in two parts), *edited by Peter Jenner and Bernard Testa*
11. Pharmaceutical Analysis: Modern Methods (in two parts), *edited by James W. Munson*
12. Techniques of Solubilization of Drugs, *edited by Samuel H. Yalkowsky*
13. Orphan Drugs, *edited by Fred E. Karch*
14. Novel Drug Delivery Systems: Fundamentals, Developmental Concepts, Biomedical Assessments, *Yie W. Chien*
15. Pharmacokinetics: Second Edition, Revised and Expanded, *Milo Gibaldi and Donald Perrier*
16. Good Manufacturing Practices for Pharmaceuticals: A Plan for Total Quality Control, Second Edition, Revised and Expanded, *Sidney H. Willig, Murray M. Tuckerman, and William S. Hitchings IV*
17. Formulation of Veterinary Dosage Forms, *edited by Jack Blodinger*
18. Dermatological Formulations: Percutaneous Absorption, *Brian W. Barry*
19. The Clinical Research Process in the Pharmaceutical Industry, *edited by Gary M. Matoren*
20. Microencapsulation and Related Drug Processes, *Patrick B. Deasy*
21. Drugs and Nutrients: The Interactive Effects, *edited by Daphne A. Roe and T. Colin Campbell*
22. Biotechnology of Industrial Antibiotics, *Erick J. Vandamme*
23. Pharmaceutical Process Validation, *edited by Bernard T. Loftus and Robert A. Nash*
24. Anticancer and Interferon Agents: Synthesis and Properties, *edited by Raphael M. Ottenbrite and George B. Butler*
25. Pharmaceutical Statistics: Practical and Clinical Applications, *Sanford Bolton*
26. Drug Dynamics for Analytical, Clinical, and Biological Chemists, *Benjamin J. Gudzinowicz, Burrows T. Younkin, Jr., and Michael J. Gudzinowicz*
27. Modern Analysis of Antibiotics, *edited by Adjoran Aszalos*
28. Solubility and Related Properties, *Kenneth C. James*
29. Controlled Drug Delivery: Fundamentals and Applications, Second Edition, Revised and Expanded, *edited by Joseph R. Robinson and Vincent H. Lee*
30. New Drug Approval Process: Clinical and Regulatory Management, *edited by Richard A. Guarino*
31. Transdermal Controlled Systemic Medications, *edited by Yie W. Chien*
32. Drug Delivery Devices: Fundamentals and Applications, *edited by Praveen Tyle*
33. Pharmacokinetics: Regulatory • Industrial • Academic Perspectives, *edited by Peter G. Welling and Francis L. S. Tse*
34. Clinical Drug Trials and Tribulations, *edited by Allen E. Cato*
35. Transdermal Drug Delivery: Developmental Issues and Research Initiatives, *edited by Jonathan Hadgraft and Richard H. Guy*
36. Aqueous Polymeric Coatings for Pharmaceutical Dosage Forms, *edited by James W. McGinity*
37. Pharmaceutical Pelletization Technology, *edited by Isaac Ghebre-Sellassie*
38. Good Laboratory Practice Regulations, *edited by Allen F. Hirsch*
39. Nasal Systemic Drug Delivery, *Yie W. Chien, Kenneth S. E. Su, and Shyi-Feu Chang*
40. Modern Pharmaceutics: Second Edition, Revised and Expanded, *edited by Gilbert S. Banker and Christopher T. Rhodes*
41. Specialized Drug Delivery Systems: Manufacturing and Production Technology, *edited by Praveen Tyle*
42. Topical Drug Delivery Formulations, *edited by David W. Osborne and Anton H. Amann*
43. Drug Stability: Principles and Practices, *Jens T. Carstensen*

44. Pharmaceutical Statistics: Practical and Clinical Applications, Second Edition, Revised and Expanded, *Sanford Bolton*
45. Biodegradable Polymers as Drug Delivery Systems, *edited by Mark Chasin and Robert Langer*
46. Preclinical Drug Disposition: A Laboratory Handbook, *Francis L. S. Tse and James J. Jaffe*
47. HPLC in the Pharmaceutical Industry, *edited by Godwin W. Fong and Stanley K. Lam*
48. Pharmaceutical Bioequivalence, *edited by Peter G. Welling, Francis L. S. Tse, and Shrikant V. Dinghe*
49. Pharmaceutical Dissolution Testing, *Umesh V. Banakar*
50. Novel Drug Delivery Systems: Second Edition, Revised and Expanded, *Yie W. Chien*
51. Managing the Clinical Drug Development Process, *David M. Cocchetto and Ronald V. Nardi*
52. Good Manufacturing Practices for Pharmaceuticals: A Plan for Total Quality Control, Third Edition, *edited by Sidney H. Willig and James R. Stoker*
53. Prodrugs: Topical and Ocular Drug Delivery, *edited by Kenneth B. Sloan*
54. Pharmaceutical Inhalation Aerosol Technology, *edited by Anthony J. Hickey*
55. Radiopharmaceuticals: Chemistry and Pharmacology, *edited by Adrian D. Nunn*
56. New Drug Approval Process: Second Edition, Revised and Expanded, *edited by Richard A. Guarino*
57. Pharmaceutical Process Validation: Second Edition, Revised and Expanded, *edited by Ira R. Berry and Robert A. Nash*
58. Ophthalmic Drug Delivery Systems, *edited by Ashim K. Mitra*
59. Pharmaceutical Skin Penetration Enhancement, *edited by Kenneth A. Walters and Jonathan Hadgraft*
60. Colonic Drug Absorption and Metabolism, *edited by Peter R. Bieck*
61. Pharmaceutical Particulate Carriers: Therapeutic Applications, *edited by Alain Rolland*
62. Drug Permeation Enhancement: Theory and Applications, *edited by Dean S. Hsieh*
63. Glycopeptide Antibiotics, *edited by Ramakrishnan Nagarajan*
64. Achieving Sterility in Medical and Pharmaceutical Products, *Nigel A. Halls*
65. Multiparticulate Oral Drug Delivery, *edited by Isaac Ghebre-Sellassie*
66. Colloidal Drug Delivery Systems, *edited by Jörg Kreuter*
67. Pharmacokinetics: Regulatory • Industrial • Academic Perspectives, Second Edition, *edited by Peter G. Welling and Francis L. S. Tse*
68. Drug Stability: Principles and Practices, Second Edition, Revised and Expanded, *Jens T. Carstensen*
69. Good Laboratory Practice Regulations: Second Edition, Revised and Expanded, *edited by Sandy Weinberg*
70. Physical Characterization of Pharmaceutical Solids, *edited by Harry G. Brittain*
71. Pharmaceutical Powder Compaction Technology, *edited by Göran Alderborn and Christer Nyström*
72. Modern Pharmaceutics: Third Edition, Revised and Expanded, *edited by Gilbert S. Banker and Christopher T. Rhodes*
73. Microencapsulation: Methods and Industrial Applications, *edited by Simon Benita*
74. Oral Mucosal Drug Delivery, *edited by Michael J. Rathbone*
75. Clinical Research in Pharmaceutical Development, *edited by Barry Bleidt and Michael Montagne*
76. The Drug Development Process: Increasing Efficiency and Cost-Effectiveness, *edited by Peter G. Welling, Louis Lasagna, and Umesh V. Banakar*
77. Microparticulate Systems for the Delivery of Proteins and Vaccines, *edited by Smadar Cohen and Howard Bernstein*
78. Good Manufacturing Practices for Pharmaceuticals: A Plan for Total Quality Control, Fourth Edition, Revised and Expanded, *Sidney H. Willig and James R. Stoker*
79. Aqueous Polymeric Coatings for Pharmaceutical Dosage Forms: Second Edition, Revised and Expanded, *edited by James W. McGinity*
80. Pharmaceutical Statistics: Practical and Clinical Applications, Third Edition, *Sanford Bolton*
81. Handbook of Pharmaceutical Granulation Technology, *edited by Dilip M. Parikh*
82. Biotechnology of Antibiotics: Second Edition, Revised and Expanded, *edited by William R. Strohl*
83. Mechanisms of Transdermal Drug Delivery, *edited by Russell O. Potts and Richard H. Guy*
84. Pharmaceutical Enzymes, *edited by Albert Lauwers and Simon Scharpé*
85. Development of Biopharmaceutical Parenteral Dosage Forms, *edited by John A. Bontempo*
86. Pharmaceutical Project Management, *edited by Tony Kennedy*
87. Drug Products for Clinical Trials: An International Guide to Formulation • Production • Quality Control, *edited by Donald C. Monkhouse and Christopher T. Rhodes*
88. Development and Formulation of Veterinary Dosage Forms: Second Edition, Revised and Expanded, *edited by Gregory E. Hardee and J. Desmond Baggot*
89. Receptor-Based Drug Design, *edited by Paul Leff*
90. Automation and Validation of Information in Pharmaceutical Processing, *edited by Joseph F. deSpautz*
91. Dermal Absorption and Toxicity Assessment, *edited by Michael S. Roberts and Kenneth A. Walters*

92. Pharmaceutical Experimental Design, *Gareth A. Lewis, Didier Mathieu, and Roger Phan-Tan-Luu*
93. Preparing for FDA Pre-Approval Inspections, *edited by Martin D. Hynes III*
94. Pharmaceutical Excipients: Characterization by IR, Raman, and NMR Spectroscopy, *David E. Bugay and W. Paul Findlay*
95. Polymorphism in Pharmaceutical Solids, *edited by Harry G. Brittain*
96. Freeze-Drying/Lyophilization of Pharmaceutical and Biological Products, *edited by Louis Rey and Joan C. May*
97. Percutaneous Absorption: Drugs—Cosmetics—Mechanisms—Methodology, Third Edition, Revised and Expanded, *edited by Robert L. Bronaugh and Howard I. Maibach*
98. Bioadhesive Drug Delivery Systems: Fundamentals, Novel Approaches, and Development, *edited by Edith Mathiowitz, Donald E. Chickering III, and Claus-Michael Lehr*
99. Protein Formulation and Delivery, *edited by Eugene J. McNally*
100. New Drug Approval Process: Third Edition: The Global Challenge, *edited by Richard A. Guarino*
101. Peptide and Protein Drug Analysis, *edited by Ronald E. Reid*
102. Transport Processes in Pharmaceutical Systems, *edited by Gordon Amidon, Ping I. Lee, and Elizabeth M. Topp*
103. Excipient Toxicity and Safety, *edited by Myra L. Weiner and Lois A. Kotkoskie*
104. The Clinical Audit in Pharmaceutical Development, *edited by Michael R. Hamrell*
105. Pharmaceutical Emulsions and Suspensions, *edited by Francoise Nielloud and Gilberte Marti-Mestres*
106. Oral Drug Absorption: Prediction and Assessment, *edited by Jennifer B. Dressman and Hans Lennernäs*
107. Drug Stability: Principles and Practices, Third Edition, Revised and Expanded, *edited by Jens T. Carstensen and C. T. Rhodes*
108. Containment in the Pharmaceutical Industry, *edited by James Wood*
109. Good Manufacturing Practices for Pharmaceuticals: Fifth Edition, Revised and Expanded, *Sidney H. Willig*
110. Advanced Pharmaceutical Solids, *Jens T. Carstensen*
111. Endotoxins: Pyrogens, LAL Testing, and Depyrogenation, Second Edition, Revised and Expanded, *Kevin L. Williams*
112. Pharmaceutical Process Engineering, *Anthony J. Hickey and David Ganderton*
113. Pharmacogenics, *edited by Werner Kalow, Urs A. Meyer, and Rachel F. Tyndale*
114. Handbook of Drug Screening, *edited by Ramakrishna Seethala and Prabhavathi B. Fernandes*
115. Drug Targeting Technology: Physical • Chemical • Biological Methods, *edited by Hans Schreier*
116. Drug–Drug Interactions, *edited by A. David Rodrigues*
117. Handbook of Pharmaceutical Analysis, *edited by Lena Ohannesian and Anthony J. Streeter*
118. Pharmaceutical Process Scale-Up, *edited by Michael Levin*
119. Dermatological and Transdermal Formulations, *edited by Kenneth A. Walters*
120. Clinical Drug Trials and Tribulations: Second Edition, Revised and Expanded, *edited by Allen Cato, Lynda Sutton, and Allen Cato III*
121. Modern Pharmaceutics: Fourth Edition, Revised and Expanded, *edited by Gilbert S. Banker and Christopher T. Rhodes*

ADDITIONAL VOLUMES IN PREPARATION

Surfactants and Polymers in Drug Delivery, *Martin Malmsten*

Pharmaceutical Process Validation: An International Third Edition, Revised and Expanded, *edited by Robert A. Nash and Alfred H. Wachter*

Transdermal Drug Delivery: Second Edition, Revised and Expanded, *edited by Jonathan Hadgraft and Robert H. Guy*

Simulation for Designing Clinical Trials, *edited by Hui C. Kimko and Stephen Duffull*

Modified-Release Drug Delivery Technology, *edited by Michael J. Rathbone, Jonathan Hadgraft, and Michael S. Roberts*

Modern Pharmaceutics

Fourth Edition, Revised and Expanded

edited by

Gilbert S. Banker
University of Iowa
Iowa City, Iowa

Christopher T. Rhodes
University of Rhode Island
Kingston, Rhode Island

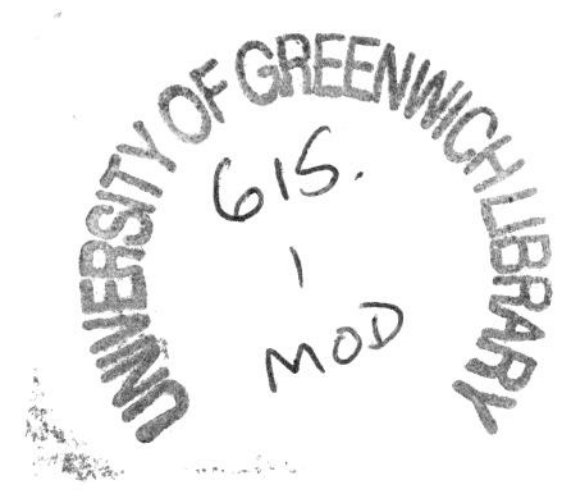

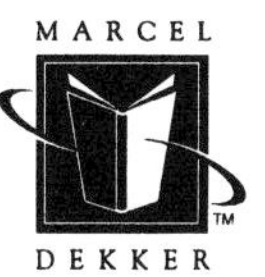

Marcel Dekker, Inc. New York • Basel

ISBN: 0-8247-0674-9

This book is printed on acid-free paper.

Headquarters
Marcel Dekker, Inc.
270 Madison Avenue, New York, NY 10016
tel: 212-696-9000; fax: 212-685-4540

Eastern Hemisphere Distribution
Marcel Dekker AG
Hutgasse 4, Postfach 812, CH-4001 Basel, Switzerland
tel: 41-61-261-8482; fax: 41-61-261-8896

World Wide Web
http://www.dekker.com

The publisher offers discounts on this book when ordered in bulk quantities. For more information, write to Special Sales/Professional Marketing at the headquarters address above.

Current printing (last digit):
10 9 8 7 6 5 4 3 2 1

PRINTED IN THE UNITED STATES OF AMERICA

Preface

The first edition of *Modern Pharmaceutics* was published in 1980, the second in 1989, and the third in 1995. During the more than 20 years since we developed the concept of this text we have been privileged to work with many of the most notable pharmaceutical scientists as chapter authors. Some of our original first edition team are still with us. Others, for a variety of reasons—including change of career focus, retirement, and death—are no longer with us or able to cooperate in this endeavor. We place on record our gratitude to all our colleagues who have so unselfishly assisted us in any or all of our four editions.

We are also grateful to all those readers of our book who have provided comments on their perceptions of the value of *Modern Pharmaceutics* and suggested to us ways in which the book might be improved. We have most carefully considered all such ideas and some of the changes that we have implemented in this edition derive from advice given to us by industrial pharmaceutical scientists, university faculty, and students.

The fourth edition of *Modern Pharmaceutics* follows the same format and has the same goals as previous editions. Chapter 1 sets the stage by reviewing the role of drugs and drug products in treating and preventing disease, while also summarizing their primary quality features. Chapters 2 through 6 provide background that is fundamental to an understanding of drug action and the design of drug products. Chapter 7, on preformulation, is another fundamentals chapter, describing the manner in which drugs are characterized for their physical, chemical, and pharmacokinetic properties to provide a rational and scientific basis for drug product design.

Chapters 8 through 16 describe drug products and dosage forms, together with the routes of administration by which they are given. Chapters 17 through 28 also treat topics critical to drug product quality such as packaging, optimization, and food and drug laws, in addition to examining more specialized product classes and introducing several new chapters. As in previous editions, this book once again ends with a view to the future.

In the planning of this edition, we identified certain areas of recent growth that seemed to merit increased attention in this text, while attempting to further recognize pharmacy's international character. Also, we gave attention to topics that are of relatively more importance than previously. Overall the book has grown in size because there are a number of critical areas that justify significant additional coverage. We have been fortunate in obtaining the services of a number of distinguished individuals to cover topics not allocated whole chapters in previous editions.

The growing importance of botanicals and other natural products has been recognized by devoting one of our new chapters to this topic. Also, we have a new chapter on managed care since this is an area of great importance and impacts all facets of pharmacy. Further, we expect this topic to gain additional recognition in parts of the world where at present the implications of this discipline are not fully recognized. Also, appreciating the growing importance of generic products, especially in North America and the European Union, we have included in this edition a chapter focused on bioequivalence. Finally, recognizing the impact of the information revolution, catalyzed by computers and the Internet, we have included a new chapter on drug information.

With one exception, all the chapters from the third edition of *Modern Pharmaceutics* that appear in the fourth edition have been revised and updated. Many chapters were extensively updated, and some, such as the first and last chapters, were extensively rewritten. Due to the illness of Dr. Robinson, the chapter on sustained and controlled release drug delivery systems was updated with the assistance of Gil Banker, with Dr. Robinson's approval.

Although *Modern Pharmaceutics* continues to evolve, our basic goals remain those which we developed in the 1970s when we first delineated the concept of this comprehensive and integrated treatment of pharmaceutics, with a focus on drug product quality and performance. We are committed to producing an up-to-date, authoritative, multiauthored treatise on pharmaceutics, which can be used by both students and practitioners.

Gilbert S. Banker
Christopher T. Rhodes

Contents

Contributors

Thomas J. Ambrosio, Ph.D. Development Fellow, Package Development, Schering-Plough Research Institute, Kenilworth, New Jersey

Larry L. Augsburger, Ph.D. Shangraw Professor of Industrial Pharmacy and Pharmaceutics, Department of Pharmaceutical Sciences, School of Pharmacy, University of Maryland, Baltimore, Maryland

Narendra B. Barn, Ph.D. Project Management and R&D Strategy, GlaxoSmithKline, Collegeville, Pennsylvania

Gilbert S. Banker, Ph.D. Dean Emeritus and John L. Lach Distinguished Professor of Drug Delivery Emeritus, College of Pharmacy, University of Iowa, Iowa City, Iowa

Lisa Blair Banker, D.V.M. Blair Animal Clinic, West Lafayette, Indiana

Leslie Z. Benet, Ph.D. Professor of Biopharmaceutical Sciences, School of Pharmacy, University of California, San Francisco, California

David W. A. Bourne, Ph.D. Professor of Pharmacy, College of Pharmacy, University of Oklahoma, Oklahoma City, Oklahoma

James C. Boylan, Ph.D. Pharmaceutical Consultant, Gurnee, Illinois

Jens T. Carstensen, Ph.D. Professor Emeritus, School of Pharmacy, University of Wisconsin, Madison, Wisconsin

Masood A. Chowhan, Ph.D. Director of Consumer Products, Alcon Research Ltd., Fort Worth, Texas

Paul R. Dal Monte, Ph.D. Project Management and R&D Strategy, GlaxoSmithKline, Collegeville, Pennsylvania

Michele Danish, Pharm.D. Clinical Manager, Department of Pharmacy, St. Joseph Health Services, Providence, Rhode Island

William R. Doucette, Ph.D. Associate Professor, Division of Clinical and Administrative Pharmacy, University of Iowa, Iowa City, Iowa

Gordon L. Flynn, Ph.D. Professor of Pharmaceutical Science, Department of Pharmaceutical Sciences, College of Pharmacy, The University of Michigan, Ann Arbor, Michigan

Julie M. Ganther, Ph.D. Assistant Professor, Department of Clinical and Administrative Pharmacy, University of Iowa, Iowa City, Iowa

J. Keith Guillory. Ph.D. Professor Emeritus, Division of Pharmaceutics, College of Pharmacy, University of Iowa, Iowa City, Iowa

Anthony J. Hickey, Ph.D. Professor, School of Pharmacy, University of North Carolina, Chapel Hill, North Carolina

Betty-ann Hoener, Ph.D. Professor, Department of Biopharmaceutical Sciences, School of Pharmacy, University of California, San Francisco, California

Wandee Im-Emsap College of Pharmacy, Freie Universität Berlin, Berlin, Germany

Rajni Jani, Ph.D. Senior Director, Department of Pharmaceutics, Alcon Research Ltd., Fort Worth, Texas

Gwen M. Jantzen, Ph.D. School of Pharmacy, University of Wisconsin, Madison, Wisconsin

Teresa Bailey Klepser, Pharm.D. Associate Professor, College of Pharmacy, Ferris State University, Big Rapids, Michigan

Mary Kathryn Kottke, Ph.D. Department of Regulatory Affairs, Cubist Pharmaceuticals, Inc., Lexington, Massachusetts

Vijay Kumar, Ph.D. Assistant Professor, Division of Pharmaceutics, College of Pharmacy, University of Iowa, Iowa City, Iowa

John C. Lang, Ph.D. Director of Emerging Technologies, Consumer Products Research and Development, Alcon Research Ltd., Fort Worth, Texas

Brian R. Matthews, Ph.D. Senior Director of EC Registration, Alcon Laboratories (UK) Ltd., Hemel Hempstead, United Kingdom

Michael Mayersohn, Ph.D. Professor of Pharmaceutical Sciences, College of Pharmacy, University of Arizona, Tucson, Arizona

J. Patrick McDonnell, B.S.Ph. Senior Compliance Auditor, Department of Biologics Quality Assurance, Fort Dodge Animal Health, Charles City, Iowa

Paul J. Missel, Ph.D. Principal Scientist, Department of Drug Delivery, Alcon Research Ltd., Fort Worth, Texas

Steven L. Nail, Ph.D. Associate Professor, Department of Industrial and Physical Pharmacy, Purdue University, West Lafayette, Indiana

Robert E. O'Connor, Ph.D. Pharmaceutical Sourcing Group Americas, a division of Ortho-McNeil Pharmaceutical, Bridgewater, New Jersey

Steven Øie, Ph.D. Professor, Department of Biopharmaceutical Sciences, School of Pharmacy, University of California, San Francisco, California

Ornlaksana Paeratakul, Ph.D. Assistant Professor, Pharmaceutical Technology, Faculty of Pharmacy, Srinakharinwirot University, Nakhonnayok, Thailand

Garnet E. Peck, Ph.D. Professor and Director of the Industrial Pharmacy Laboratory, Department of Industrial and Physical Pharmacy, School of Pharmacy, Purdue University, West Lafayette, Indiana

Rolland Poust, Ph.D. Professor, Pharmaceutical Services Division, College of Pharmacy, University of Iowa, Iowa City, Iowa

Christopher T. Rhodes, Ph.D. Professor, Department of Applied Pharmaceutical Sciences, University of Rhode Island, Kingston, Rhode Island

Joseph R. Robinson, Ph.D. Professor of Pharmacy, School of Pharmacy, University of Wisconsin, Madison, Wisconsin

Denise P. Rodeheaver, Ph.D., D.A.B.T. Assistant Director, Department of Toxicology, Alcon Research Ltd., Fort Worth, Texas

Robert E. Roehrs, Ph.D.* Vice President, Department of Drug Regulatory Affairs, Alcon Research Ltd., Fort Worth, Texas

S. Kathy Edmond Rouan, Ph.D. Vice President, Cardiovascular and Urology Project Team Leadership and Management, Project Management and R&D Strategy, GlaxoSmithKline, Collegeville, Pennsylvania

Edward M. Rudnic, Ph.D. Advancis Pharmaceutical Corp., Gaithersburg, Maryland

Roger L. Schnaare, Ph.D. Philadelphia College of Pharmacy, Philadelphia, Pennsylvania

Joseph B. Schwartz, Ph.D. Philadelphia College of Pharmacy, Philadelphia, Pennsylvania

Hazel H. Seaba, M.S. Professor (Clinical) and Director, Division of Drug Information Service, College of Pharmacy, University of Iowa, Iowa City, Iowa

Juergen Siepmann, Ph.D. Assistant Professor, College of Pharmacy, Freie Universität Berlin, Berlin, Germany

*Retired.

Chapter 1

Drug Products: Their Role in the Treatment of Disease, Their Quality, and Their Status and Future as Drug-Delivery Systems

Gilbert S. Banker

University of Iowa, Iowa City, Iowa

I. ROLE OF DRUGS AND DRUG PRODUCTS IN THE TREATMENT AND PREVENTION OF DISEASE

The methods of treating illness and disease as we enter the twenty-first century include the use of the following forms of therapy: (a) surgery, including organ transplantation; (b) psychotherapy; (c) physical therapy; (d) radiation, and (e) chemo or pharmacotherapy. Of these various methods, pharmacotherapy (treatment with drugs) is the most frequently used technique for treating disease, has the broadest range of application over the greatest variety of disease states, and is usually the most cost-effective and preferred treatment method. Although surgery is the preferred method of treating some ailments or disease states, when alternative methods are available, these methods (usually pharmacotherapy) will be employed first if feasible, in the initial attempt to secure satisfactory relief or control of the condition or a complete cure. As pharmacotherapy continues to improve, it is replacing other forms of treatment as the preferred method of therapy. Pharmacotherapy is, for example, increasingly becoming the treatment of choice in treating various forms of cancer, including breast cancer, replacing the use of radical surgery. Pharmacotherapy is now an effective option to surgery in the treatment of some forms of prostate disease. When cure rates or reliability of disease control by pharmacotherapy can match surgical treatment (e.g., prostate surgery or radical mastectomy), most patients will strongly prefer the chemotherapeutic approach or the use of chemotherapy combined with less radical surgical approaches.

In some surgical procedures, such as organ transplantation, the success of that procedure will be only as great as the course of pharmacotherapy that follows. Organ transplant recipients are required to continue drug therapy for the balance of their lives for control of their immune systems and to prevent organ rejection.

Pharmacotherapy is also very important in the prevention of disease, since vaccines and other immunizing agents are drug products. The impact of vaccines in eliminating or reducing the incidence of six diseases is shown in Fig. 1. Some diseases that previously killed or crippled tens of millions of people worldwide, often reaching epidemic proportions, are now virtually unknown in most of the world. Table 1 shows the average number of deaths in the United States per million people as a result of various diseases in a nonepidemic situation over the last century. The table lists diseases that have been obliterated or nearly obliterated in the United States through drug immunology as shown in Fig. 1, together with diseases that have now been brought largely under control or greatly reduced by the discovery and effective use of anti-infective drugs than can combat bacterial infections. Examples of diseases in this latter category are

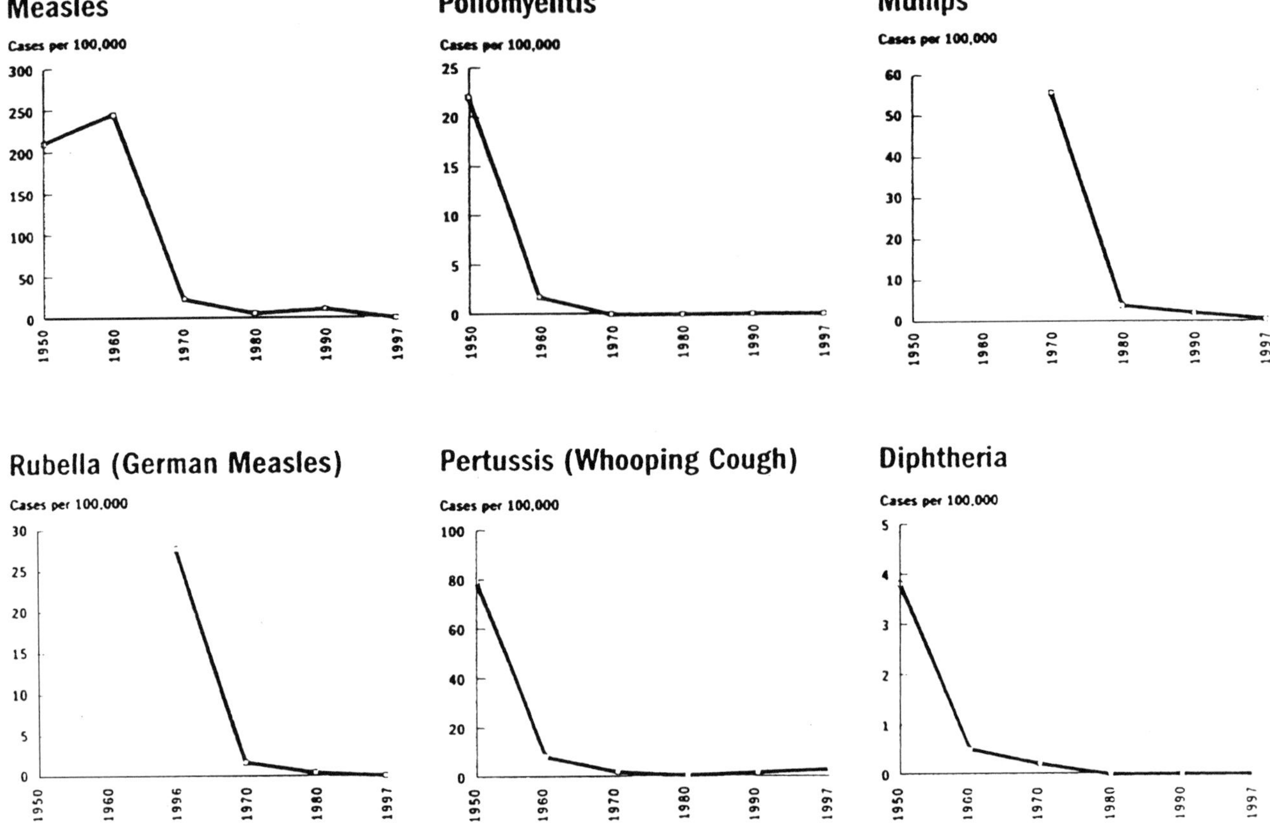

Fig. 1 Impact of vaccines in reducing incidence of diseases.

Table 1 Causes of Death in the United States per Million Population in Nonepidemic Years from Infectious and Other Identifiable Diseases

	Year							
Disease	1900	1920	1940	1960	1975	1985	1990	1999
Influenza and pneumonia	2030	2080	700	310	370	250	3313	311
Tuberculosis (all forms)	2020	1150	460	220	50	8	7	5
Diarrheas and intestinal	1330	540	100	50	40	1	0	0
Kidney diseases	890	890	820	210	110	85	83	95
Bronchitis	460	130	30	20	30	16	1	1
Diphtheria	430	260	10	3	0	0	0	0
Typhoid and paratyphoid	360	80	10	0	0	0	0	0
Syphilis	20	160	140	50	20	0	0	0
Measles	120	90	5	3	0	0	0	0
Whooping cough	120	120	20	7	0	0	0	0
Appendicitis	100	130	100	20	0	2	1	0
Scarlet fever	100	50	5	0	0	0	0	0
Malaria	80	40	10	0	0	0	0	0
Smallpox	20	6	0	0	0	0	0	0

Source: Official Statistics, U.S. Census Bureau.

pneumonia, tuberculosis, certain diarrheal and intestinal disorders, and bronchitis.

Yet other diseases have been largely controlled by improved sanitation and public health procedures, alone or in combination with pharmacotherapy. Bubonic plague (the "Black Death"), malaria, and typhus are in this category. Largely through pharmacotherapy, including the use of immunological agents, epidemics of life-threatening diseases have been greatly reduced and, until recently, were thought to have been eliminated in all but the least developed regions of the world. We now know that this is not the case.

In past centuries epidemics swept entire countries and continents. In one 8-year period in the fourteenth century when bubonic plague was epidemic throughout Europe, two thirds of the population were infected; half of these died, totaling 25 million deaths. In 1918–1919 an influenza epidemic swept most of the world, causing 20 million deaths, with more than a half-million deaths occurring in the United States. Twenty or 30 years ago we thought such pandemics could be prevented. A pandemic occurs when a disease occurs over a wide geographic area and affects an exceptionally high proportion of some populations. As we enter the third millennium we are in the midst of a pandemic that is worse than anything the world has known before, based on numbers of human casualties.

Acquired immunodeficiency syndrome (AIDS) is a virally transmitted disease caused by HIV, a human immunodeficiency retrovirus, whose genetic material is RNA. AIDS is an especially nasty, progressive, and costly disease for which no cure currently exists. When a cure is found it will be a drug cure. The virus uses the enzyme reverse transcriptase to incorporate its genetic material into the infected host cell's genome. The primary host target cells are T_4 (T-helper) cells, which, after a significant level of destruction, compromises the body's immune system. A whole range of opportunistic infections then attack, often in concert, until death inevitably ensues.

Table 2 lists the distribution of HIV/AIDS in various regions of the world. The heavy infection level in sub-Saharan Africa is the result of several factors. First, the disease probably originated there. The oldest HIV sample came from the Republic of the Congo in 1959, but most researchers believe AIDS had been killing people many decades before then. Second, most of the countries in sub-Saharan Africa are underdeveloped and have lacked the resources to fight the disease or implement effective prevention plans. This region of the world now has 70% of the global total of HIV-infected people but only 10% of the world's population. The epidemic in Africa has exploded in the last 20 years. In 1982 only one African country had an HIV prevalence rate in adults above 2%. By 1998 it was estimated that more than 7% of the adults living in 21 African countries were HIV-positive or had AIDS. In two populations 25% of the adults were infected. Life expectancy has fallen to 30 years or less in some of these countries, making HIV an unprecedented catastrophe in the world's history [1]. In addition to the nearly 35 million people estimated to have HIV/AIDS going into the new millennium, to date AIDS has killed 20 million people [2]. It is clearly the most lethal pandemic the world has ever known and represents one of the biggest challenges to public health and pharmacotherapy today.

Table 2 Distribution of HIV/AIDS in Various Regions of the World

Region	Number infected[a]
Sub-Saharan Africa	22,500,000
Southeast Asia	6,700,000
Latin America	1,400,000
North America	890,000
Eastern Europe and Central Asia	560,000
Western Europe	500,000
Caribbean	330,000
Northern Africa and Middle East	210,000
Australia and New Zealand	12,000
Total	34,400,000

[a]As of the end of 1998.
Source: Ref. 1.

Another challenge facing pharmacotherapy as we enter the twenty-first century are diseases known as zoonoses. Zoonoses are animal-borne diseases, which are transmitted to humans. They often develop in a relatively small region of the world initially and then spread. They are often viral in origin and thus produce a far greater challenge to humankind than did many of the bacterial diseases of the past. Although controversy exists, there is compelling evidence that HIV is a variant of viruses that infect nonhuman primates in central Africa and is thus a zoonose disease.

Another recent example of a zoonose infection is the Nipah virus, named after the town in Malaysia where its first known victim lived. The animal vector of this disease has been identified as several species of bats. The Nipah virus has destroyed Malaysia's pig industry and it killed 105 people in 1999. The virus produces a severe form of encephalitis, and about 40% of infected individuals die.

In the United States in recent years several diseases with animal hosts are now infecting humans. The Arena virus has as its host certain desert rodents. Rodent droppings when dry and airborne as dust particles infect humans, often with lethal consequences. The West Nile virus appeared in the United States in 1999. Birds carry this virus, and mosquitoes are the vector to humans. In 1999 the virus was localized in the New York City area. By 2000 it has spread across New York State and into New Jersey and Massachusetts. The West Nile virus is especially lethal when it infects children, the elderly, or those with a compromised immune system.

The subject of zoonoses was extensively discussed at the International Conference on Emerging Infectious Diseases, July 16–19, 2000 in Atlanta, Georgia [3]. A group of researchers from the University of Edinburgh reported that humanity is currently challenged by 1709 known pathogens, including viruses, bacteria, fungi, protozoa, and worms. Of these, 832, or 49%, are zoonotic. Of even greater concern is the fact that of the 156 disease that are considered to be new or "emerging," 114 are zoonoses, a staggering 73%. The diseases produced by these zoonoses often must primarily be challenged by pharmacotherapy. It is clear that much will remain to be done by pharmaceutical scientists in the years ahead, in addition to attacking the leading causes of death and disability.

II. ROLE OF PHARMACOTHERAY IN MORTALITY RATES, LIFE EXPECTANCY, AND QUALITY OF LIFE

Another impact of pharmacotherapy that is not generally recognized has been its effect on life expectancy and on the health of the newborn, infants, and children. Some of the earliest valid historical statistics on the death rates of children are found in parish records of London, England. One parish, St. Botolph's, "which was bordered by the city wall and eastern gate, the Tower of London and the Thames," has detailed records from 1558 to 1626, which have survived the years intact [4]. The population of this region probably enjoyed better medical care than did their rural neighbors. The stillborn death rate in the parish fluctuated between 40.8 and 133.4, averaging 71.6/1000 births. The current overall average stillborn death rate in the United States is about 20/1000 births. Infants dying in the first month in Shakespeare's day in London were known as chrisoms. The average chrisom death rate from 1584 to 1598 was more than 162/1000 (two to four times the average stillborn rate). Thus, about one child out of every three to four was stillborn or failed to survive the first month. By contrast, in the United States today fewer than 10 deaths per 1000 live births occur during the first year of life. Survival rates of infants and older children were equally grim in Shakespeare's England. Of every 100 children born in the late sixteenth century, only about 70 survived to the first birthday, about 48 to their fifth, and only 27–30 survived to their fifteenth birthday.

The death rate statistics of newborns, infants, and older children have greatly improved from the sixteenth, or even the twentieth century, to the opening of the twenty-first century. An interesting exercise when next you visit an old cemetery would be to read tombstones that predate 1900, or even 1940. You will find that one grave marker out of every two or three is for a newborn, infant, or a young child. This was largely related to the inability of the medical and pharmaceutical professions of that day to effectively combat infectious and children's diseases. Many of these diseases affected children almost exclusively among their fatality victims (see Table 1), including measles, scarlet fever, polio, and whooping cough. Added to the infectious "children's diseases" problem was the fact that these diseases often left their young survivors with permanent physiological damage, such as scarred heart valves, brain damage, poorly developed limbs or paralysis, and other defects that remained for the balance of life. The dramatic improvement in the infant mortality rate in the United States over the past 60 years is shown in Fig. 2 [5]. Although great advances have been made, a number of countries in Western Europe have rates that are substantially better than those of the United States.

The increasing life expectancy and the growing number of the elderly in our citizenry over the last century, and in recent decades, is well known (Figs. 3 and 4) [5]. A person born in 1920 could expect to live only 54.1 years. Today we can expect to live over 76 years (about 73 years for men and nearly 80 years for women). The life expectancy for women helps explain the fact that octogenarians (persons over 80) are the fastest-growing segment of any age group in our population. Another interesting way to look at life expectancy is shown in Fig. 5. Here we see the average additional life expectancy a person may have based on their current age. These figures, at all age levels, also show a steady upward progression over the last 27 years.

Figure 3 also shows what many experts predict. Life expectancy is not expected to plateau, but by 2030–2040 the life expectancy for women will be at least 90, and for men will be approaching 85. However, these

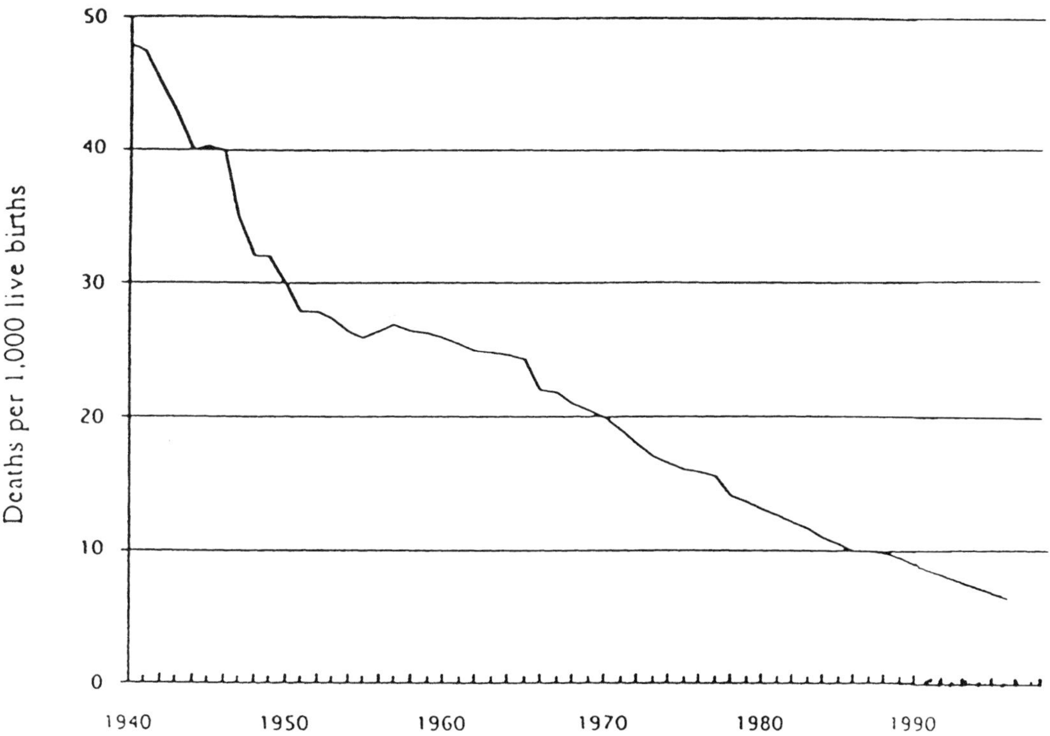

Fig. 2 Infant (under 1 year) mortality rates in the United States, 1940–2000.

numbers could be negatively impacted in the United States by the current AIDS epidemic. Figure 4 shows another result of our increasing life expectancy—the very rapid growth in the over-65 population as a percentage of the U.S. population from 1960 to the year 2000. In a report of the National Institute on Aging [6] it was noted that there are 35 million people in the United States age 65 or older. This number will double by 2030, continuing the dramatic shift to a much larger population of older Americans. Women currently account for about 60% of those over 65, and nearly half of these older women live alone. The percentage of older Americans living in poverty has dropped dramatically in the last 40 years, from 35% to 11%, but there is a disparity between races (8.2% for whites vs. 26.4% for blacks). This dramatic shift in our elderly population will have a large impact on social programs such as Social Security, Medicare, and Medicaid, as well as on the rapidly expanding growth and need for pharmaceutical services and pharmacy care in the years ahead.

The exact contribution of modern pharmaceuticals to our increased longevity can be only estimated and weighed in comparison with improved diet and lifestyles, sanitation, housing, and generally improved public health. However, advances in chemotherapy have certainly been the major factor in extending our life expectancy. Similarly, the contribution of pharmacotherapy to an improved quality of life in recent decades can be only estimated—but it has been a very major factor. It is clearly a leading factor in the well-being of the elderly, allowing them to remain active and essentially healthy through more years and over a greater fraction of their total life span. The role of pharmacotherapy in improving the quality of life of the mentally ill is also clearly evident. Hundreds of thousands of mentally ill patients in the United States alone who are currently being treated as outpatients can live essentially normal lives and can remain with their families through the use of drugs to control their illness. Without the availability of effective psychotherapeutic drug agents, many of these patients would require institutionalization or at least short- to midterm hospitalization.

Other diseases that formerly required long-term hospitalization or complete isolation include tuberculosis and the dreaded leprosy. Only a generation or two ago, for patients to be told that they had such diseases

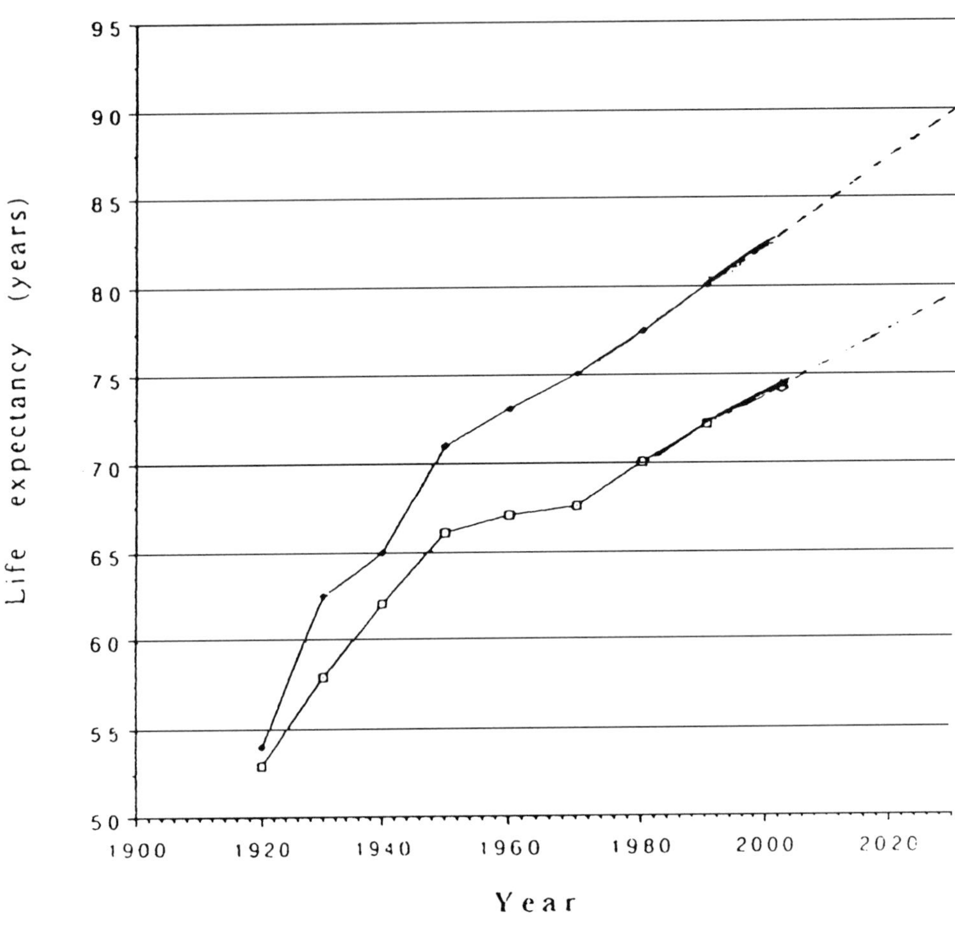

Fig. 3 Expectation of life in years at birth in the United States.

was equivalent to receiving a death sentence, or worse. These diseases are totally curable today by means of chemotherapy, and the patient no longer needs to be isolated in a sanitarium. Other diseases, such as rheumatoid arthritis, frequently drove patients to suicide. Today, even though we still lack cures for some of these diseases, we can contain and control them, permitting patients to lead nearly normal lives.

Great strides have been made in chemotherapy since World War II (1939–1945) and in the decades following the war. Antibiotics and other anti-infective drugs, steroids, psychotherapeutic agents, many new immunizing agents, important cardiovascular agents, antineoplastic agents, and numerous other drug classes and agents have appeared in the last four to five decades. Given the rapid advances in biotechnology, new drug innovation is entering another period of revolutionary growth. Nevertheless pharmaceutical scientists have no cause for complacency. We cannot yet cure the debilitating diseases of cystic fibrosis or muscular dystrophy. Many forms of cancer are treatable with only low to moderate success if detected early; that battle is far from won. Over one-half million Americans are dying each year from cancer, the number 2 cause of death in this country. Although death rates are consistently continuing to decline (Fig. 6), we must continue the battle to effectively combat many degenerative diseases affecting our growing elderly population, notably heart disease, the number 1 killer, which kills three-quarters of a million Americans a year. The growing challenge posed by cardiovascular disease, as Americans continue to age, is shown in Fig. 7. The current third leading cause of death also heavily affecting the elderly, is cerebrovascular disease, which kills about 150,000 Americans a year. This prevalence and estimated annual economic cost of some common diseases as shown in Table 3, further documents some of our remaining challenges in pharmacotherapy and

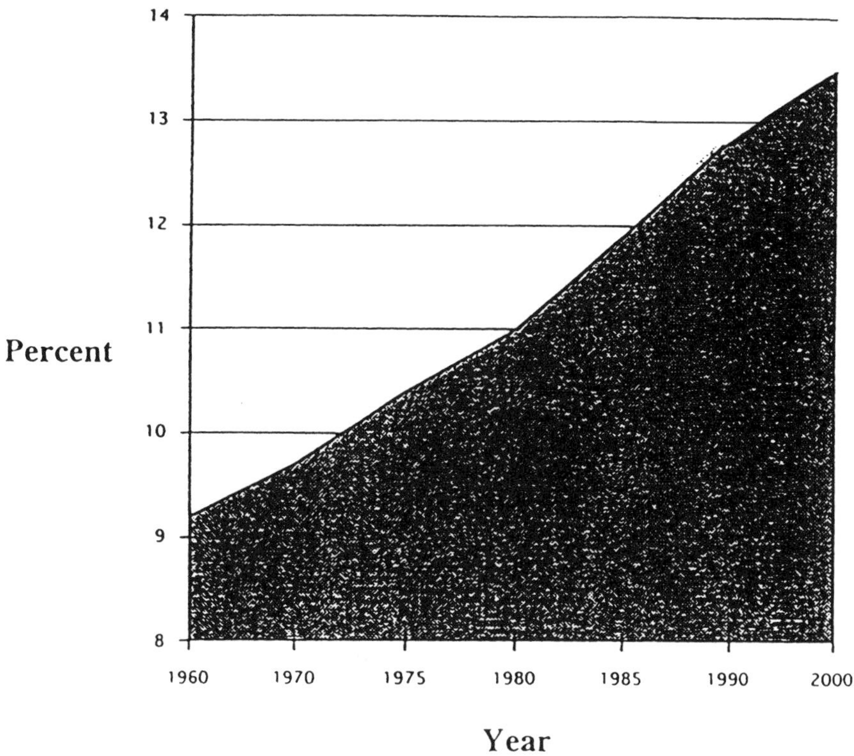

Fig. 4 Percentage of the total U.S. population older than 65 years, 1960–2000. (From Ref. 5.)

health care. The challenge of the AIDS pandemic and other emerging diseases was discussed in the previous section. Accidents are the fourth leading cause of death at 90,000–95,000/year. Pharmacotherapy is expected to provide major answers to most, if not all of these and many other disease challenges in the years to come.

III. DRUG AND DRUG PRODUCT QUALITY AND ITS EVALUATION

A. Reasons for the Drug Product Quality Question

The quality of drugs, which used to be an important discussion topic only for pharmaceutical manufacturers and experts in education, compendial standards, and regulatory enforcement, has now been placed in the spotlight of public attention. The reasons for the broadbased interest in drug product quality are based on the following factors, at least in part: (a) a clear realization that drug products are different from other consumer products; (b) rapidly increasing health care and drug product costs over the last several decades; (c) increasing public advertising of prescription drug products, with identification of price differentials among chemically equivalent generic products; (d) increasing payment of health care costs by third parties; (e) promulgation of the federal "maximum allowable cost" (MAC) regulations; and (f) effects of health care reform and increasing pressure to provide a prescription drug benefit under Medicare.

The greatest difference between drug products and other consumer products is that the principle of *caveat emptor* ("let the buyer beware") cannot operate in the usual way when the layperson acquires prescription drugs. In addition, laypeople lack the skills and sophistication to evaluate the quality and appropriateness of their prescription drug products, whereas they do have some ability to evaluate most other consumer products. Furthermore, consumers do not select prescription products as they do nearly every other product they purchase or use. A consumer is often compelled to buy a specific drug product, whereas he or she has more freedom of choice about when or if they buy other products. In the process, the layperson must usually trust the physician who prescribes the medication and the pharmacist who selects it (if a generic drug) and dispenses it. Other differences are that drug products are

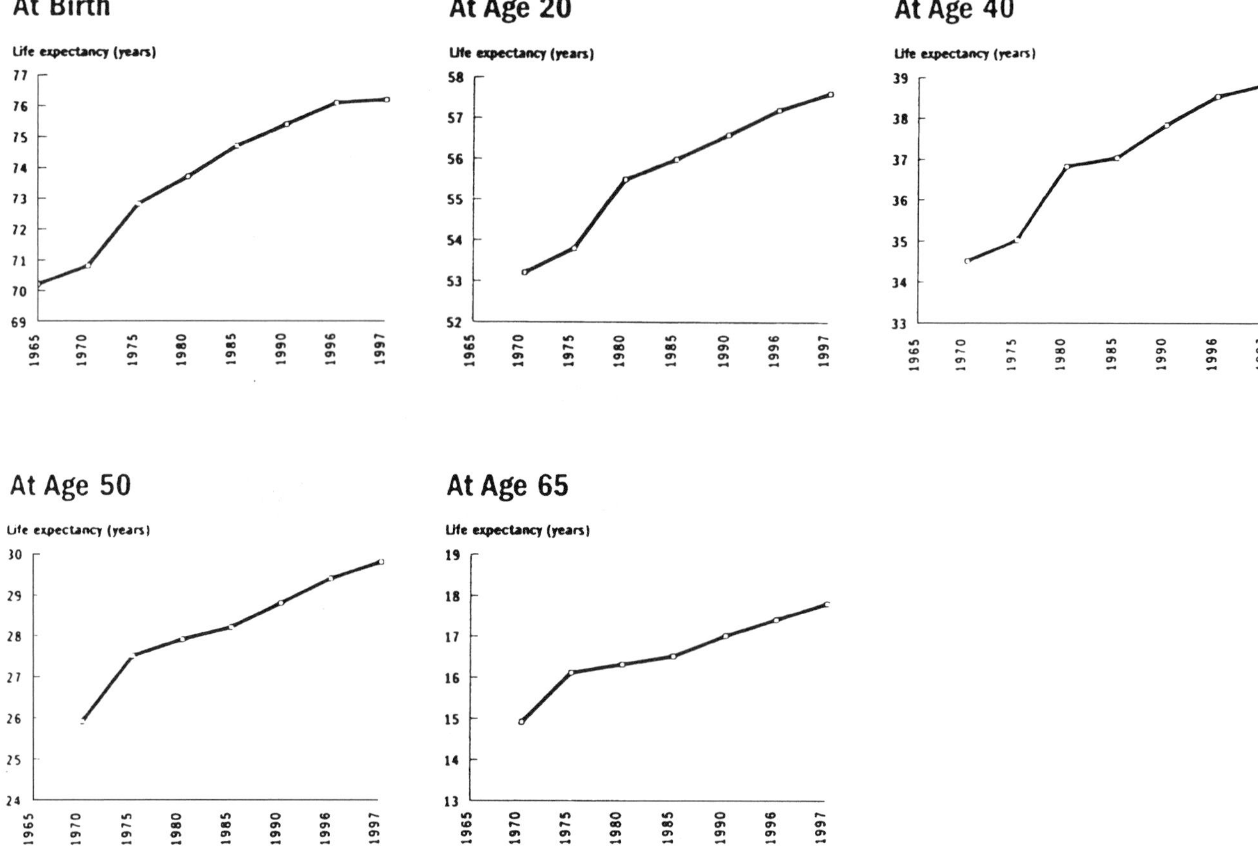

Fig. 5 Additional years of life expectancy at various ages, 1965–1970–1997.

typically more critical to the consumer's well-being than are other products. A poor quality drug product can have more serious consequences than a poor quality consumer product of nearly any other category. Drug products are also more complex than nearly any other class of consumer product. These last two factors are why drug products are subjected to many more tests and controls than are other types of products.

In the last four to five decades national health care expenditures for all types of health-related transactions, including dental, medical, hospital, prescription, and over-the-counter (OTC) drugs, has grown from about 5% of the country's gross domestic product (GDP) (national expenditures on all goods and services) to nearly 14% of the GDP today. Total health expenditures in the United States are now well over $1 trillion annually.

There are many reasons for the cost increases in health care, in addition to inflation, including the following: (a) there are more and more older people, requiring more care; (b) new and additional types of care and treatment are available and they tend to be more expensive, and (c) the quality of treatment has been improving. Aggregate expenditures in the health sector, have been rising at 10% or more a year over the last 15–20 years. While per capita health care expenditures for Americans are the highest in the world, a recent report from the World Health Organization (WHO) ranks the United States as only 37th out of 191 nations in terms of the health services provided to our citizens [7]. In this first ever ranking of United Nations member countries' health systems, some of the factors considered were life expectancy, health quality based on infant/child survival rates, system responsiveness, system cost per population served, fairness of financial contributions, and overall health system performance. The top ranked countries were France, Italy, San Marino, Andorra, Malta, Singapore, Spain, Oman, Austria, and Japan. The bottom ranked countries were all from sub-Saharan Africa plus Burma.

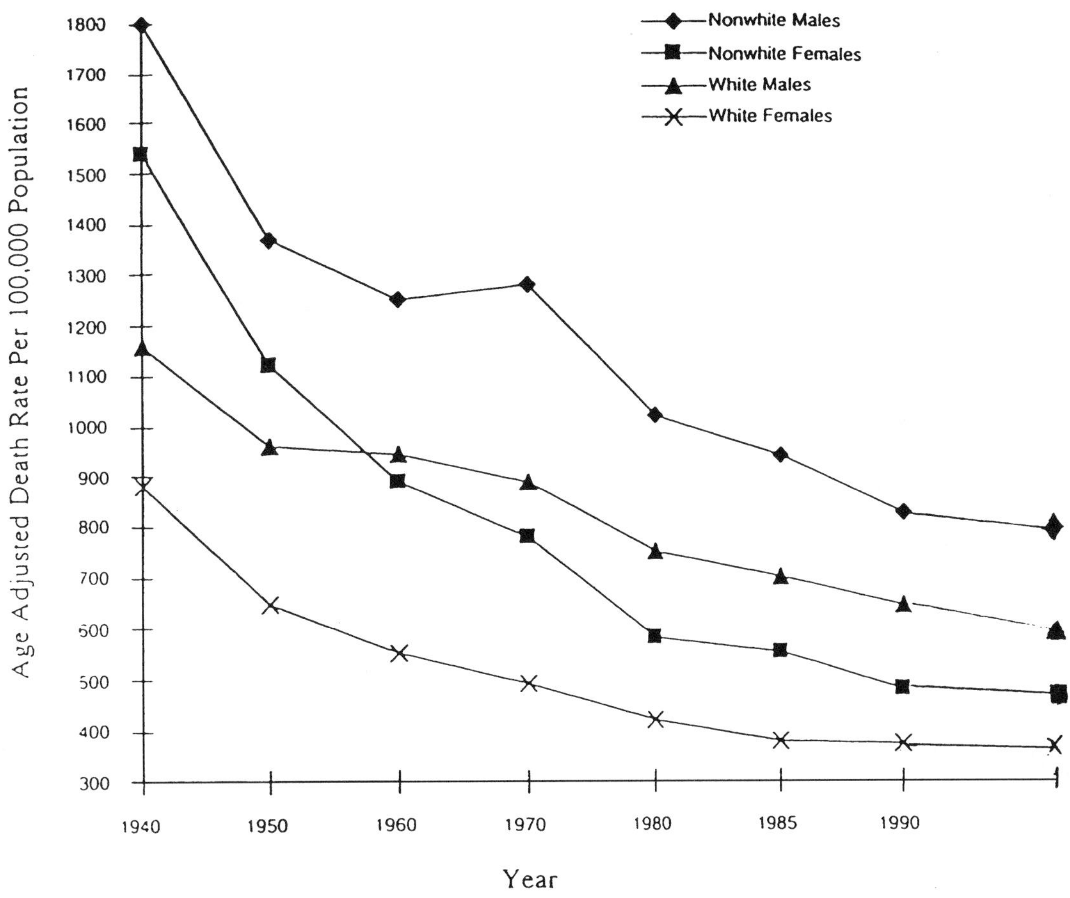

Fig. 6 Age-adjusted death rates in the United States from all causes by sex and by race (white and all others), 1940–1996. (Courtesy of National Center for Health Statistics.)

The WHO report noted that many countries are falling far short of their potential and that expenditures per se do not necessarily produce the best system. This is exemplified by the fact that the United States, which is ranked 37th, spends 13.7% of its gross domestic product on health care, while the United Kingdom, which is ranked 18th, spends only 5.8%.

While rankings are only as meaningful as the criteria on which they are based and the accuracy of their assessments, there is undoubtedly some validity to the WHO study and its rankings. One analysis of the relatively low U.S. ranking noted the large number of Americans who have no health insurance or other coverage and the lower level of healthy life expectancy in the United States compared to other industrialized nations. The WHO analysis also commented on the high rates of heart disease and tobacco-related cancers in the United States, together with the "extremely poor health" of minority groups, notably Native Americans and rural African Americans, as contributing to the relatively low ranking of U.S. health care.

The great majority of health care expenditures are for services—medical services, nursing services, or hospital services. While pharmacy (prescription products and services) constitutes a relatively small percentage of total health care expenditures (9–10% of the total), the pharmacy component has received a great deal of attention in recent years. There are several reasons for this. A product is involved in the pharmacy component, and it is much easier to analyze and attempt to minimize product costs compared to medical or hospital services. Second, a well-defined private industry is involved with the drug component—the pharmaceutical industry. Based in part on the relatively high profits shown by this industry it is a target for criticism by government and politicians. The pharmaceutical industry, its relationships to pharmacy, and the public are discussed in chapter 28. Lastly, the

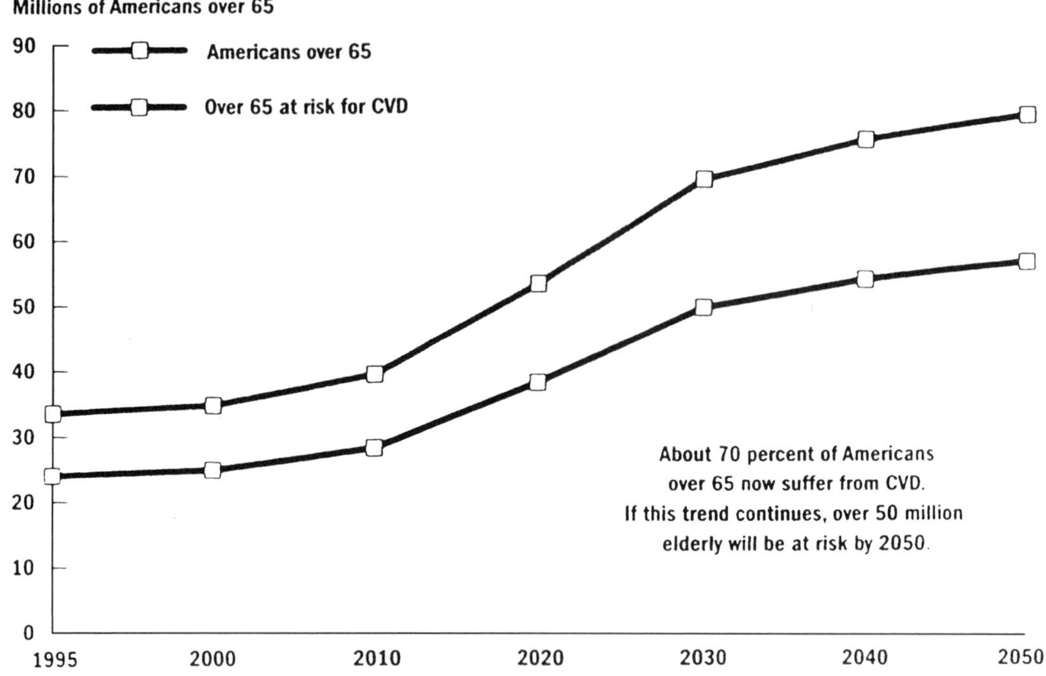

Fig. 7 Aging of baby boomers will dramatically increase population potentially at risk from cardiovascular disease (CVD).

Table 3 Prevalence, Cost, and Medicines in Development for Selected Major Diseases in the United States

Uncured disease	Approximate prevalence	Approximate annual economic cost ($billions)	Number[a] of medicines in development	Source
Alzheimer's disease	4,000,000	100.0	24	National Institute on Aging
Arthritis	43,000,000	54.6	28	Arthritis Foundation
Asthma	14,000,000	6.2	17	National Heart Lung and Blood Institute
Cancer	8,000,000	107.0	354	American Cancer Society
Congestive heart failure	4,900,000	20.2	17	American Heart Association
Coronary heart disease	13,900,000	95.6	38	American Heart Association
Depression	17,600,000	53.0	17	National Institute on Mental Health
Diabetes	15,700,000	98.2	26	National Institute of Diabetes and Digestive and Kidney Diseases
Hypertensive disease	50,000,000	31.7	10[b]	American Heart Association
Osteoporosis	10,000,000	13.8	19	National Osteoporosis Foundation
Schizophrenia	1,500,000	23.0	12	National Institute of Mental Health
Stroke	4,000,000	43.3	19	American Heart Association

Note: HIV/AIDS discussed separately in Chapter 1.
[a]PhRMA data.
[b]Hypertension medicines.
Source: PhRMA, 2000.

pharmaceutical component has been the fastest growing cost component of all health care expenditures, growing since 1993 at a steady 13.3 compound rate.

The U.S. prescription drug market in 1999 increased by 19%, totaling $2.7 billion, representing 2.7 billion prescriptions, a 9% increase over the prior year [8].

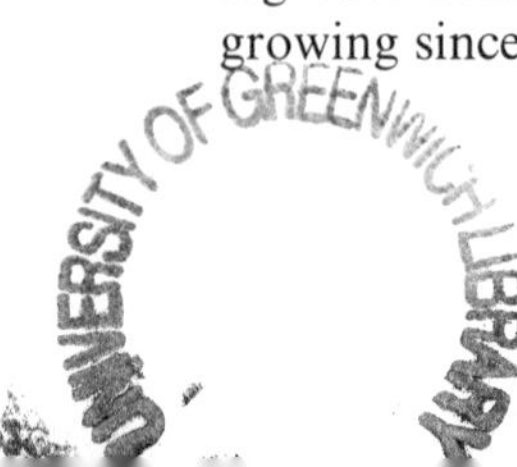

Of this total prescription market the federal government paid about 13% (Medicaid), third parties paid 68%, and the individual paid about 19%[8]. The rapid growth of the prescription market in recent years is the result of numerous factors, but it certainly includes growing managed care utilization which includes some level of drug coverage, the continuing aging of the U.S. population, new product approvals and introductions (which tend to be more expensive), direct to consumer advertising by drug companies, inflation of drug product costs, and a strong economy. The aging-of-America effect is documented by following statistics [9]: the 50-plus age group consume 74% of all prescription drugs, 51% of all over-the-counter (OTC) drug products, and represent 65% of all hospital bed days. By 2005 30% of Americans will be 50 or older. The impact of the rapidly growing drug cost share of total operating expenses for HMOs is discussed in Chapter 27.

B. The Pharmacist's Responsibility and Role in Drug Product Selection

The pharmacist bears a heavy responsibility for the quality and appropriateness of the drug products that she or he dispenses. The Code of Ethics of the American Pharmaceutical Association states (in Section 2): "The pharmacist should never condone the dispensing of drugs and medications which are not of good quality or which do not meet standards required by law." Pharmacists are frequently obliged to make judgments concerning the quality of individual drug products and the various dosage forms and possible presentations available for individual drugs. This occurs as pharmacists serve on formulary committees, therapeutics committees, and in other "official" roles, as well as on a day-to-day basis, in evaluating manufacturers' and other data to select drug products for their patients that are not only cost-competitive, but are also safe and effective. The pharmacist's role in drug and drug product selection has increased dramatically in recent decades with the evolution of clinical pharmacy and pharmaceutical care and with the growth of third-party payments for prescription drugs. Fortunately, the pharmacist is the most knowledgeable expert on available drugs and drug products and criteria affecting drug product quality. Pharmacists are also better qualified and more knowledgeable than other health care professionals when it comes to drug product forms available, relative merits of different dosage forms, even within a given route of administration, and possible or most likely side effects within a given population group such as children or the elderly. Furthermore, pharmacists are well acquainted with the storage requirements for various drugs and drug products and with the physical signs by which deterioration may be detected. The pharmacist is the health care professional in the best position today to know the various drugs a given patient is taking and thus is best able to avert adverse therapeutic effects that can arise from many sources. This is because many patients see more than one physician, and they are increasingly taking a broader range of OTC products, including herbs, natural products, and nutriceuticals.

The questions of drug quality, drug cost, drug selection and effectiveness, and proper drug utilization have become a matter of widespread public interest. It is thus very important for pharmacists to be highly knowledgeable concerning all aspects of drug product quality and optimal drug utilization on an individual patient basis.

C. History and Evolution of Drugs and Drug Products

Every pharmacist and pharmacy student should read one of the many available books on the history of drugs and the drug industry [10–14]. A pictorial history such as *Drugs* [10] in the Life Science Library Series or one of the several illustrated books on the patent remedy era [11,12] is entertaining as well as educational reading. Several U.S. drug companies, on reaching the century mark, have also written interesting histories that also document U.S. pharmacy history [15–17]. Several pharmacy trade associations have written interesting histories directed to pharmacy practice [18,19]. A history of the U.S. Public Health Service also contains important bench marks for pharmacy [20]. These references are only a few of the many interesting historical books on pharmacy that could be cited.

When the history of drugs and drug products is expressed as a time continuum, as shown in Table 4, it is very apparent that most drug and drug product advancements have occurred over the last 50 years. Before the early twentieth century, the only purified organic chemical substances used in chemotherapy were aspirin, quinine, and morphine. For the preceding 4000 years, drugs changed relatively little. Early Egyptian physicians recorded over 70 "drugs" in 800 remedies administered in 14 different forms from pills to ointments and salves and poultices. The drugs were all from natural sources, ranging from spider webs, to animal excretions, to packs of mud, to poppy seeds. Between the eighth and thirteenth centuries, Arabic alchemists greatly advanced pharmaceutical art by

Table 4 Periods and Notable Events in the History of the Development of Drugs and Drug Products

2000 B.C.	First drug records	
Ancient times to Middle Ages	Ancient to medieval pharmacy and medicine	Witch doctors Religious healers
1700		Natural products development
1800		First compendium (U.S.)
1850		First U.S. drug companies
1900	Patent remedy era	Development of analytical standards
1906		Wiley Act—first food and drug law
1938		Second major FDA legislation
1945–1965	Golden age of discovery	Development of sulfa anti-infectives (antibiotics, steroids, etc.)
1962		Kefauver-Harris Amendment
	New regulations	Accelerating development of cancer chemotherapy New drug-delivery systems
1977		Additional drug regulatory legislation—phase IV testing, etc.
1980s	Pharmaceutics advances	Full implementation of bioavailability standards Additional new drug-delivery capabilities
1980s–2000s		Mathematical optimization of drug product safety, effectiveness, and reliability
	Biotechnology era beginning	First recombinant DNA products Human insulin Human growth hormone Interferons, etc. Monoclonal antibodies Nucleotide blockage Growth in use of natural products and neutraceuticals
2000		Pharmaceutical company megamergers continue Sequencing of the human gerome Gene therapy developing Use of human tissues in medicine High throughput screening of potential drugs Combinatorial chemistry, biotechnology, and computers advance rational drug design

introducing extraction and distillation processes to concentrate and purify natural products. However, Arabic drugs did not reach Christian Europe until the late Middle Ages (thirteenth to fifteenth centuries). Pharmaceutical art in colonial America some 200 years ago was little better than that of the Arabic alchemists 1000 years earlier. The patent remedy era that flourished in the second half of the nineteenth century was a colorful period in pharmaceutical history when "cure-alls" were marketed by pitchmen from the backs of horse-drawn wagons, often as a follow-up to some free entertainment used to gather the locals. As depicted in the advertised indications from the label of one popular patent remedy of the day (Fig. 8), the only limit on claims appeared to be the imagination of the label writers [10]. As noted on the advertising copy of Fig. 8, these remedies were expensive in the days when an average wage earner made 15–20 dollars a week. Grandmother Pinkham used pictures of her grandchildren on her advertising and label copy; others, such as the medicinal syrups millionaire G. G. Green, placed on their advertising and labeling illustrations of the mansions that their high-profit "cure-alls" brought them. Most patent remedies contained common plant

MRS. LYDIA E. PINKHAM, OF LYNN, MASS.,
Woman can Sympathize with Woman.
Health of Woman is the Hope of the Race.
Yours for Health
Lydia E. Pinkham
LYDIA E. PINKHAM'S
VEGETABLE COMPOUND.

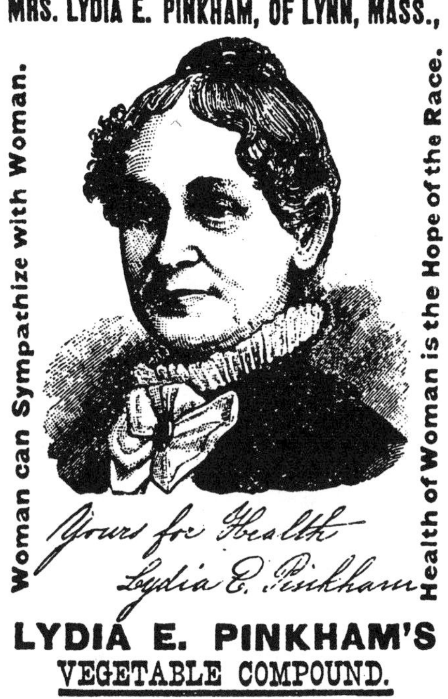

IS A POSITIVE CURE

For all those painful Complaints and Weaknesses so common to our best female population.

It will cure entirely the worst forms of Female Complaints, all Ovarian troubles, Inflammation, Ulceration, Falling and Displacements of the Womb, and the consequent Spinal Weakness, and is particularly adapted to the Change of Life.

It will dissolve and expel Tumors from the Uterus in an early stage of development. The tendency to cancerous humors there is checked very speedily by its use. It removes faintness, flatulency, destroys all craving for stimulants, and relieves weakness of the stomach. It cures Bloating, Headaches, Nervous Prostration, General Debility, Sleeplessness, Depression and Indigestion.

That feeling of bearing down, causing pain, weight and backache, is always permanently cured by its use.

It will at all times and under all circumstances act in harmony with the laws that govern the female system. For the cure of Kidney Complaints of either sex this Compound is unsurpassed.

Lydia E. Pinkham's Vegetable Compound is prepared at Lynn, Mass. Price, $1.00; six bottles for $5.00. Sent by mail in the form of Pills, also in the form of Lozenges, on receipt of price, $1.00 per box, for either. Send for pamphlet. All letters of inquiry promptly answered. Address as above.

No family should be without LYDIA E. PINKHAM'S LIVER PILLS. They cure Constipation, Biliousness, and Torpidity of the Liver. 25 cents per box.

Lydia E. Pinkham's Blood Purifier.

This preparation will eradicate every vestige of Humors from the Blood, and at the same time will give tone and strength to the system.

It is far superior to any other known remedy for the cure of all diseases arising from impurities of the blood, such as Scrofula, Rheumatism, Cancerous Humors, Erysipelas, Canker, Salt Rheum and Skin Diseases.

SOLD BY ALL DRUGGISTS.

Fig. 8 Example of the advertised indication (cures) from the labeling of a widely used patent remedy, before Enactment of the Food, Drug and Cosmetic Act of 1906. (From Ref. 10.)

extracts, such as taraxicum (common dandelion weed), at least 15% alcohol, and occasionally opium or other narcotic or addictive substances to help assure repeat sales. It is interesting to speculate on the number of persons in the temperance era who kept all those around them "dry" and then enjoyed their evening toddy of Lydia Pinkhams or stronger higher proof products before retiring. The Food, Drug, and Cosmetic Act of 1906 was intended to combat the abuses of the patent remedy era, at least in part by requiring labeling of the active ingredients contained in all pharmaceuticals and by broadly limiting fraudulent practices. The 1938 act went further, requiring that at least some principles of rational therapeutics be applied to all products and their claims. The 1962 act required many more proofs of safety and effectiveness. (See Chapter 19 for a more detailed description of the evolution of drug laws.)

One interesting way of examining drug and drug product quality is to analyze the changes in drugs and drug products over the centuries, especially the very rapid changes in the last half-century (see Table 4). Anyone who imagines that current drug products are optimal as to quality features or that we have reached the ultimate in chemotherapeutic capabilities is assuming that the history of drugs is now standing still as well as ignoring the science of pharmaceutics as we currently know it. Although the Middle Ages ended around 1450, historically speaking, drugs and drug products did not progress substantially above the quality and knowledge level of the medieval period until the late nineteenth and early twentieth centuries (Table 4). Drug and drug product advancements during the last 50–60 years have surpassed the total advancement in the field over the entire 4000-year history of drug development (see Chapter 28). As we enter the twenty-first century and the biotechnology scientific era, there is every likelihood that the rate of advancement in pharmacotherapy will overshadow everything we have known in the past.

D. Criteria for Drug and Drug Product Quality

Compendial standards and government regulations require that all drug products, whether ethical prescription or OTC products, meet strict standards of identity, potency, and purity. From about 1900 (see Table 4) until recent decades, standards of identity (the product is what it is actually labeled to be), potency (the active ingredient is present in the labeled amount), and purity [basically limiting nondrug materials as well as describing the amount of active ingredient(s) in natural substances] were thought to define drug quality adequately and were enforced under evolving law and U.S. Food and Drug Administration (FDA) regulation. The addition of a few physical tests, such as weight variation and disintegration time to compendial products such as tablets and capsules, was thought to accurately define the quality of these products. We now know that drug products require very careful evaluation to accurately reflect their quality and performance in clinical roles and that earlier concepts of evaluation required expansion. The designation "quality," applied to a drug product, according to a modern definition, requires that the product:

- Contain the quantity of each active ingredient claimed on its label, within the applicable limits of its specifications
- Contain the same quantity of active ingredient from one dosage unit to the next
- Be free from extraneous substances
- Maintain its potency, therapeutic availability, and appearance until used
- Upon administration, release the active ingredient for full biological availability

In the contemporary definition of quality we see that the concepts of identity, potency, and purity are retained in the first three criteria, but that bioavailability potency maintenance (including maintenance of pharmaceutical elegance and therapeutic availability or full biological availability) are added. The definition recognizes that drug products may undergo changes with time that result in a loss of biological and therapeutic activity, even though the product complies completely with the original potency and purity standards and no significant drug decomposition has occurred. Such losses in therapeutic activity, without any chemical potency change, may occur as a result of a variety of causes, including:

1. Physical changes in the dosage form (moisture loss or gain, crystal changes in excipients, tablet hardening, loss of disintegration/deaggregation properties, etc.)
2. Physical changes in the drug (conversion of a more stable, less readily soluble polymorph, etc.)
3. Chemical changes or interactions involving excipients (such as esterification of coatings, rendering them less polar and less soluble)

As noted in chapters that follow, in vitro tests may not themselves be adequate to assure that a product possesses adequate or full bioavailability and therapeutic activity. Whether or not in vitro tests are adequate quality-control indications depends on their sensitivity to pick-up aging or environmental exposure effects that produce the type of changes noted in the preceding paragraphs or other changes that are of consequence to therapy. The effects on drug potency of environmental stress conditions (e.g., increased temperature, increased humidity, combinations of the two, or temperature cycling) are known for most drug products. The effects of such stress conditions on bioavailability or therapeutic activity are much less well known currently, even for many commercial products.

A drug product can be of no higher quality than the quality of the drug(s) and excipients (nondrug additives) from which the product is made. It is possible, however, for a product to be of much lower quality than its components, since quality and clinical performance are also related to:

1. The rationale of the dosage form design (e.g., if a drug is rapidly destroyed in solution at a pH of 2 or below, the design of an oral product must enable the drug to get through the stomach without substantial dissolution)
2. The method(s) of product manufacture
3. In-process and final quality-control procedures to assure that the quality designed and manufactured into the product is actually there
4. Reasonable convenience and ease of product use to assure patient compliance with prescribed dosages

Some of the factors and considerations in the design of high-quality drug products are shown in Table 5. Various physicochemical and pharmacokinetic properties of drugs that affect dosage form design, and their influence on design of high-quality products, are de-

Table 5 Factors in the Design and Production of High-Quality Drug Products

Input factors	Output factors
A sound development/design manufacturing base	Effectiveness
The preformulation research database	Safety
Physicochemical properties of the drug	
Pharmacokinetic characterization of the drug	Reliability
A rational dosage form design	Stability
Formulation of a stable, reliable system	Physical
	Chemical
Objective preclinical and clinical testing	Microbiological
	Bioavailability
A precise, reproducible manufacturing process	
Well-controlled manufacturing steps	Pharmaceutical
Coordinated manufacturing sequences	Appearance
Efficient, sanitary operation	Organoleptic properties
Modern plant and equipment	
Knowledgeable, well-qualified workers	
	Convenience
A sensitive product control system	Ease of use
Raw material control	Dosing frequency
Processing controls	Consumer acceptance
Final product controls	
Chemical control standards	
Physical properties standards	
Biological and microbiological standards	
Informed, qualified, and responsible personnel	
Management	
Research and development	
Quality control	
Production	
Services	

scribed in Chapter 7 on preformulation. The criteria and properties defining the quality of various dosage forms are discussed in the relevant chapters on dosage forms. The features of an optimized drug are discussed in the relevant chapters on dosage forms. The features of an optimized drug product and the concepts of true drug-delivery systems are described in the next section.

IV. THE DRUG PRODUCT AS A DELIVERY SYSTEM

A. Drug Products, Drug-Delivery Systems, and Therapeutic Systems

Drug substances in their purified state usually exist as crystalline or amorphous powders or as viscous liquids. The majority of drug substances exist as white or light-colored crystalline powders. Although drugs were once commonly dispensed as such in powder papers, this practice is virtually unknown in pharmacy practice today. With the possible exception of the anesthetic gases, all drugs in legitimate commerce are now presented to the patient as drug products. It is now well recognized that the therapeutic efficacy and the therapeutic index [ratio of LD_{50} (lethal dose in 50% of the subjects) to ED_{50} (effective dose in 50% of the subjects)] of a drug product is not totally defined by the chemical constitution of the drug and its inherent pharmacokinetic profile. The actual performance of many drugs in clinical practice is now known to be greatly affected by the method of presentation of the drug to the patient. Factors affecting the presentation include:

- The portal of drug entry
- The physical form of the drug product
- The design and formulation of the product
- The method of manufacture of the drug product
- Various physicochemical properties of the drug and excipients
- Physicochemical properties of the drug product
- Control and maintenance of the location of the drug product at the absorption site(s)
- Control of the release rate of the drug from the drug product

In the late 1940s and early 1950s, sustained-release products appeared as a major new class of pharmaceutical product, in which product design was intended to modify and improve drug performance, by increasing the duration of drug action and reducing the required frequency of dosing. In the mid- to late 1960s, the term "controlled drug delivery" came into being to describe new concepts of dosage form design, which also usually involved controlling and retarding drug dissolution from the dosage form, but with additional or alternative objectives to sustained drug action. These new objectives included improving safety, enhancing bioavailability, improving drug efficiency and effectiveness, enhancing reliability of performance, reducing side effects, facilitating patient use and compliance, or other beneficial effects. In the 1970s, yet another term and concept of drug product design and administration appeared: the therapeutic system. The objective of the therapeutic system is to optimize drug therapy by design of a product that incorporates an advanced engineering systems control approach. Three types of therapeutic systems have been proposed, the first of which is already in use: (a) the "passive preprogrammed" therapeutic system—one containing a controlling "logic element," such as a membrane or series of plastic laminates, which preprograms at the time of fabrication or assembly a predetermined delivery pattern (usually constant zero-order release) that is ideally independent of all in vivo, physical, chemical, and biological processes; (b) the "active, externally programmed or controlled" therapeutic system—wherein the logic element is capable of receiving and converting a signal (such as an electromagnetic signal) sent from a source external to the body to control and properly modulate drug release from the device within the body; and (c) the "active, self-programmed" therapeutic system—containing a sensing element that responds to the biological environment (such as blood glucose concentration in diabetes) to modulate drug delivery in response to that information. Before the sustained-release concepts of the 1940s and 1950s, which also included depot forms of parenteral products, no significant new oral drug-delivery concepts had occurred in the preceding 75 years (since the enteric-coating concept).

B. The Concept of the Optimized Drug Product

The optimized drug product may be viewed as a drug-delivery system for the one or more drugs that it contains. The goal of this drug-delivery system is to release the drug(s) to produce the maximum simultaneous safety, effectiveness, and reliability, as depicted in Fig. 9. Various physicochemical product properties that influence the quality features of safety, effectiveness, and reliability are shown in Table 6. Some physicochemical properties can affect two or all three quality features of Fig. 9. For example, consider chemical stability. As a drug decomposes, if the

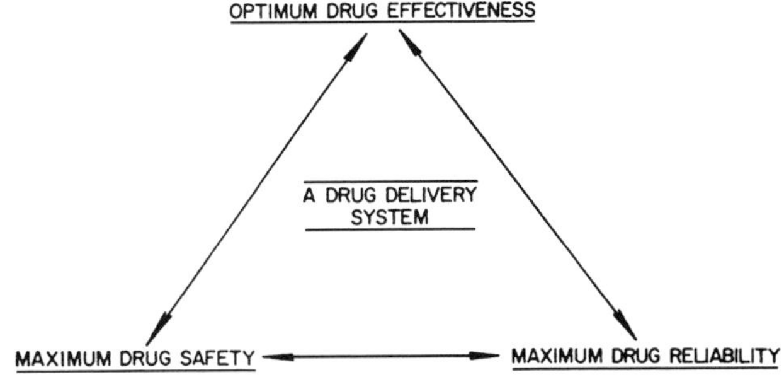

Fig. 9 Features of the optimized drug product.

decomposition product(s) are inactive, this is equivalent to a reduction of the drug dose remaining in the product— in other words, a reduction in product reliability and eventually effectiveness. If the decomposition products are toxic or irritating to the body, product safety is also reduced as the product degrades.

In examining Table 6, the manner in which each physicochemical, physiological, or therapeutic property affects the various quality features will generally be apparent. You will think of and read about many other physicochemical properties that influence the quality features of drugs and drug products as you read various chapters of this book. It should also be noted that the three basic quality features of Fig. 9 are connected by double-headed arrows. Thus, as the pharmaceutical formulator modifies the design of a drug product or its method of manufacture to improve one quality feature or one physicochemical property related primarily to one quality feature, the other properties or quality features may be, and usually are, altered. As an example, it may be our goal to increase the hardness of a tablet by formulation (adding more binder) and/or processing (compressing the tablets harder) to improve tablet gloss and appearance or to reduce tablet friability (powdering and chipping in the bottle). This is a

Table 6 Factors Affecting Drug Product Safety, Effectiveness, and Reliability

Safety	Effectiveness	Reliability
Acute safety quantification	Clinical effectiveness	Chemical stability
Therapeutic index $= LD_{50}/ED_{50}$		
	Generic effectiveness	Physical stability
Long-range safety considerations	Blood levels	
Onset of side effects	Urinary elimination	Microbiological stability
Accumulation	Pharmacological response(s)	Unit-dose precision
Nature of side effects	Bioavailability	Patient acceptance
Severity		Convenience
Reversibility		Pharmaceutical elegance
Frequency of side effects		Bioavailability
		High percentage
Untoward and other reactions		Uniformity
Idiosyncratic responses		Stability
Anaphylaxis		
Tolerance		
Addiction		
Drug interactions		
Number of drugs involved		
Probability of interaction in therapy		
Severity of the interactions		
Frequency of interactions		
Stability considerations		
Chemical stability		
Physical stability		
Microbiological stability		
Bioavailability stability		

worthy objective, but it may also reduce the rate and extent of drug dissolution from the tablet. This, in turn, could reduce the reliability of drug absorption and drug performance from patient to patient, influence transit rate and drug dissolution along the gastrointestinal tract within a given patient, or even reduce effectiveness if the dissolution rate now limits or reduces bioavailability. In the example just cited, maximizing tablet hardness and appearance is a "competing objective" to maximizing drug dissolution and bioavailability.

In Fig. 9 we see the definition of the optimized drug product as the drug-delivery system that balances all these factors against each other to produce the maximum possible effectiveness as the primary objective, while producing the best possible simultaneous safety and reliability as secondary objectives, with mathematical certainty. An alternative optimization approach would be to produce the maximum possible (optimized) product safety as the primary objective, while producing the best effectiveness and reliability as the secondary objectives. Yet a third approach would be to optimize safety and effectiveness as equally weighted primary objectives, while maximizing reliability as the secondary objective. Chapter 18 is devoted to the topic of optimization and treats the manner in which experiments may be designed to establish the necessary factors and relationships between factors (independent and controllable processing, formulation, and other variables) as these influence one another and the product quality features (dependent or response variables). Optimization methods then treat this database to design and manufacture the best possible product from an overall standpoint, considering quality features, which may be competing (i.e., as you improve one feature, another degrades), taking into account primary versus secondary features and numerous possible trade-off decisions. Although it is true that the vast majority of drug products on the market today are reasonably safe and effective, it is also true that relatively few products have been designed as optimized systems. Indeed, until about 25 years ago, formal optimization methods were unknown in the pharmaceutical and most other industries. The significance of drug products not being optimum systems varies with drug product class. For drugs and drug product classes with a high therapeutic index (ratio of LD_{50} to ED_{50}) and minimal dose-related side effects, maximizing safety is of less concern, and if the drug is well absorbed, a good, stable, pure, and potent drug product that is reasonably reliable may be nearly optimum. For drugs that have less of a safety margin, it may be argued that the conventional, rapidly releasing, effective, stable, and typical reliable product that is currently marketed is not optimum.

Figure 10 illustrates the types of blood level concentration profiles that are produced with different doses of a rapidly releasing product versus a controlled-release product. This figure is representative of the oral route of administration but may be extrapolated to other routes of administration, with the blood-level time frame simply being shifted to reflect changes in absorption (and possibly distribution) patterns. For the rapidly releasing product, whether given in a single 100-unit dose (curve A) or three divided doses of 33 units (curve B), the inherent ability of the individual to absorb the drug determines the rate of absorption and the peak blood level obtained. (At the peak, the rate of absorption and elimination are equal.) The conventional rapidly releasing drug product is not controlling the blood level versus time profiles; such a product is simply an uncontrolled "dump system," dumping the drug in the stomach for rapid dissolution and uncontrolled absorption. The body's inherent ability to absorb the drug under the patient's physiological state at a particular time point and the drug's pharmacokinetics dictate the shape of the blood level versus time profile at any particular dosing level or dosing frequency. For the optimized controlled-release form (curve C in Fig. 10), the drug product, which is now a drug-delivery system, is controlling the rate of release of drug in solution for absorption, and the release rate has been optimized to match drug inactivation and elimination, so that nearly constant levels may be maintained while the drug is in an absorption region in the gut. It has been clearly demonstrated that controlled drug delivery can also substantially increase the therapeutic index and safety margins of certain drugs, while retaining full therapeutic effectiveness. This is because many controlled-release systems produce more rounded blood level versus time profiles, without sharp peaks (compare curves A and C in Fig. 10), so that much larger doses of the controlled-release product are required to reach toxic levels. In one study [21], the effectiveness and duration of action of an antihistamine was followed in animals using a histamine vapor challenge test. The drug as a rapidly soluble dispersion or solution had a duration of action of 3.8 hours, whereas the controlled-release form provided protection to histamine vapor of 8.7 hours. Many antihistamines are depressant drugs and are dangerous on overdosage or in combination with other depressant drugs. In the same study, the drug in conventional form was lethal to 85% of the rats dosed within 30

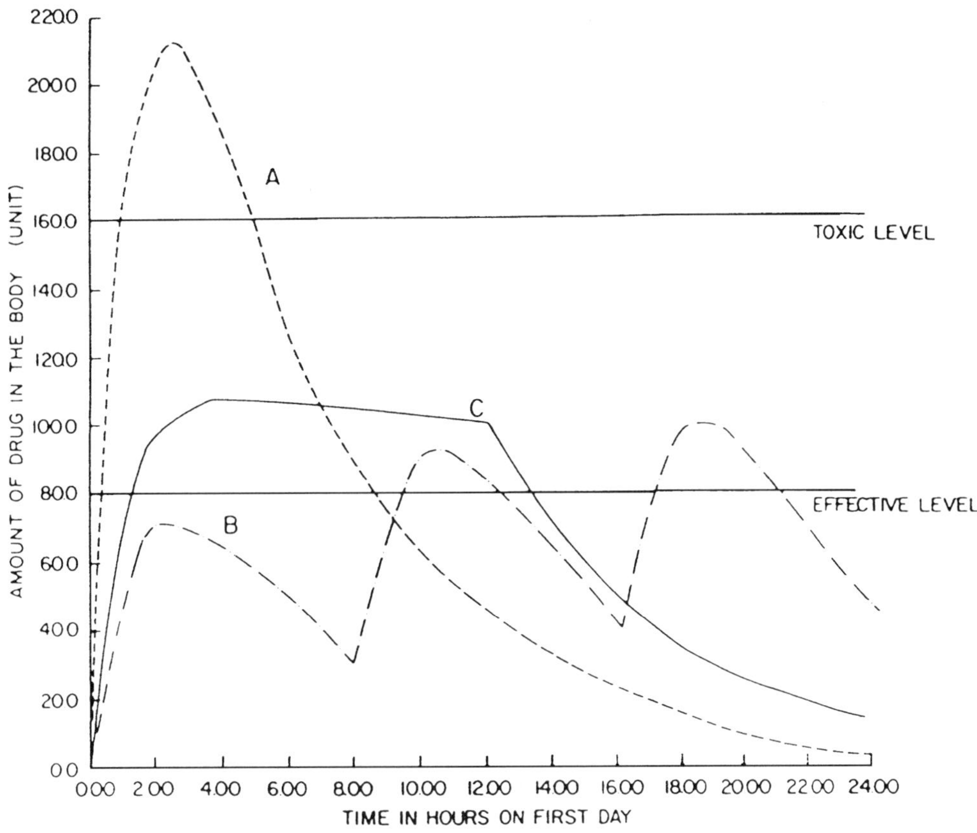

Fig. 10 Blood level versus time profile simulations following: (A) a single dose representing 100 units of a drug from a rapidly releasing dosage; (B) Three divided ddoses of 33 units each from the same rapidly releasing product; and (C) a single 100 unit dose from an optimized controlled-release dosage form. A hypothetical effective level (80 units) and toxic level (160 units) are depicted. The dosing units are typically in mg and the blood level concentration units in μg or ng.

minutes at a dose of 200 mg/kg. The same dose of drug when administered as the active controlled-release form killed none of the rats dosed (LD_0 at 24 h) [21]. Similar studies have demonstrated the ability to improve the safety of a barbiturate drug. In one such study, conventional phenobarbital had an LD_{50} in rats at a dose of 200 mg/kg. Twice the dose from an active controlled-release form had only an LD_{40} [22]. The cost of developing, testing, and gaining approval through the FDA of depressant or hazardous drugs as new products, optimized from a safety as well as effectiveness standpoint, is apparently currently too high to warrant much activity in this area. Nevertheless, we predict that such products will be the rule, rather than the exception, at some point in the future. Not only would such products save lives as a result of the consequences of purposeful or accidental overdosing of potent, depressant, and low therapeutic index drugs, but they might also reduce the severity of some drug interaction effects (especially when alcohol is one of the drugs). By eliminating the spikes in the blood profiles of immediate release dosage forms, sustained release dosage forms have the ability to reduce the frequency and severity of the side effects of some drugs. A number of cardiovascular and other drugs are designed as sustained release products for this reason. Other controlled-delivery forms have the potential of reducing some drug abuse problems, since the formulations and slow drug dissolution from the forms makes it more difficult to produce extemporaneous illegal and hazardous injectable solution forms.

Drug-delivery systems have been designed that are held in the stomach or are bioadhesive at other absorption sites for prolonged and controlled time periods (6–10 h) while releasing drug at controlled rates. Such concepts are bringing us closer to being able to achieve the ideal attributes of drug-delivery systems (Table 7), including control of such factors as variable

Table 7 Ideal Attributes of a Drug-Delivery System

1. Capable of controlled delivery rates to accommodate the pharmacokinetics of various drugs (flexible programming)
2. Capable of precise control of a constant delivery rate (precise programming)
3. Not highly sensitive to physiological variables, such as:
   - Gastric motility and emptying, pH, fluid volume, and contents of the gut
   - Presence/absence or concentration of enzymes
   - State of fasting and type of food present
   - Physical position and activity of subject
   - Individual variability
   - Disease state
4. Predicated on physicochemical principles (not pharmaceutical art)
5. Capable of a high order of drug dispersion (the ultimate is molecular in scale)
6. Drug stability is maintained or enhanced
7. The controlling mechanism adds little mass to the dosage form
8. Applicable to a wide range and variety of drugs

and uncontrolled gastric emptying and transit along the gut, which currently cause the oral route of administration to be the least reliable route of drug administration, even though it is the most popular method of achieving systemic drug effects. Future drug-delivery systems that have controlled, prolonged retention in the stomach (or accessible body cavities) with simultaneously controlled delivery rates will no doubt improve drug effectiveness for some agents by enhancing absorption, reliability, and efficiency. They also offer new possibilities of truly optimizing drug safety by prolonging the time over which the drug can be recovered or neutralized, not only on overdosing, but in acute drug interaction episodes. Bioadhesive systems that can retain drugs on mucosal surfaces for prolonged periods, while promoting drug absorption and delivery, will play a growing role in developing future delivery systems and drug products for some proteins, peptides, and other biotechnology-generated drugs. Such systems will also render the oral mucosal, nasal, vaginal, and rectal routes more useful and reliable for drug delivery. During their working lifetimes pharmacy students of today are certain to see many new drug-delivery concepts reach the marketplace that permit true optimization of drug action and the attainment of the ideal attributes of drug delivery.

REFERENCES

1. HIV and Africa's future. Science 288: 2149–2178, 23 June 2000.
2. XIII International AIDS Conference, Durban, South Africa, reported in Newsweek, July 24, 2000, and other public press.
3. Emerging diseases. Science 289: 518–519, 28 July 2000.
4. R. Forbes. Life and Death in Shakespere's London. Am Sci 58: 511–520 1970.
5. Statistical Abstract. U.S. Dept. of Commerce, Washington, DC, 1999.
6. Report of the National Institute on Aging. Older Americans 2000: Key Indicators of Well Being, Washington, DC, Aug. 10, 2000.
7. World Health Report 2000. World Health Organization, Geneva, Switzerland.
8. F. Deardorff. Changes and Trends in the R_x Market. IMS Health, 1999.
9. K. Dychtwald. Age Power, How the 21st Century Will be Ruled by the New Old. Putnam, New York, 1999.
10. W. Model and A. Lansing. Drugs. Time-Life Books, New York, 1969.
11. A. Hechtlinger. The Great Patent Medicine Era. Galahad Books, New York, 1970.
12. G. Carson. One for a Man, Two for a Horse. Bramhall House, New York, 1971.
13. W. Screiber and F. K. Mathys. Infectious Diseases in the History of Medicine. Kreis and Co., Basel, 1987.
14. P. Boussel, H. Bonnemain, and F. Bove. History of Pharmacy and the Pharmaceutical Industry. Asklepious Press, Paris, 1983.
15. R. Carlisle. A Century of Caring—The Upjohn Story. Benjamin Co., Elmsford, NY, 1987.
16. W. D. Pratt. The Abbott Almanac. Benjamin Co., Elmsford, NY, 1987.
17. L. Galambos et al. Values and Visions. A Merck Century. Merck and Co., 1992.
18. C. F. Williams. A Century of Service and Beyond, 1898 NARD-NCPA 1998. National Community Pharmacy Association, Alexandria, VA 1998.
19. J. Mobley. Prescription for Success, The Chain Drug Story. The Lowell Press, Kansas City, MO, 1990.

20. F. Mullan. Plagues and Politics, A Story of the United States Public Health Service. Basic Books Inc., New York, 1989.
21. H. Goodman and G. Banker. Molecular-scale drug entrapment as a precise method of controlled drug release I: Entrapment of cationic drugs by Polymeric flocculation, J. Pharm. Sci. 59: 1131–1137, 1970.
22. J. Boylan and G. Banker. Molecular-scale drug entrapment as a precise method of controlled drug release II: Entrapment of anionic drugs by polymeric gelation. J. Pharm. Sci. 62: 1177–1184, 1973.

Chapter 2

Principles of Drug Absorption

Michael Mayersohn

University of Arizona, Tucson, Arizona

I. INTRODUCTION

Drugs are most often introduced into the body by the oral route of administration. In fact, the vast majority of drug dosage forms are designed for oral ingestion, primarily for ease of administration. It should be recognized, however, that this route may result in inefficient and erratic drug therapy. Whenever a drug is ingested orally (or by any nonvascular route), one would like to have rapid and complete absorption into the bloodstream for the following reasons:

1. Assuming that there is some relationship between drug concentration in the body and the magnitude of the therapeutic response (which is often the case), the greater the concentration achieved, the greater the magnitude of response.
2. In addition to desiring therapeutic concentrations, one would like to obtain these concentrations rapidly. The more rapidly the drug is absorbed, in general, the sooner the pharmacological response is achieved.
3. In general, one finds that the more rapid and complete the absorption, the more uniform and reproducible the pharmacological response becomes.
4. The more rapidly the drug is absorbed, the less chance there is of drug degradation or interactions with other materials present in the gastrointestinal tract.

In a broad sense, one can divide the primary factors that influence oral drug absorption and thus govern the efficacy of drug therapy into the following categories: physicochemical variables, physiological variables, and dosage form variables. For the most part, these variables will determine the clinical response to any drug administered by an extravascular route. Although often the total response to a drug given orally is a complex function of the aforementioned variables interacting together, the present discussion is limited primarily to the first two categories involving physicochemical and physiological factors. Dosage form variables influencing the response to a drug and the effect of route of administration are discussed in Chapters 4 and 5.

The vast majority of drugs in current use and those under development are relatively simple organic molecules obtained from either natural sources or by synthetic methods. It is important to note, however, the virtual revolution in development of new therapeutic entities—those based upon the incredible advances being made in the application of molecular biology and biotechnology. These new drugs, especially peptides and proteins, are not the traditional small organic molecules stressed in this chapter. Indeed, those compounds have unique physicochemical properties, which are quite different from those of small organic molecules, and they offer remarkable challenges for drug delivery. As a result, new and more complex physical delivery systems are being designed in conjunction with an examination of other, less traditional routes of administration (e.g., nasal, pulmonary, transdermal, etc.). Because of issues of instability in the gastrointestinal tract and poor intrinsic membrane permeability, it appears unlikely that these new biotechnology-derived drugs will employ the oral route for administration. Numerous strategies, however, are being explored and there is evidence that some measure of gastrointestinal absorption can be achieved for certain peptides [1]. One recently reported approach that shows promise involves conjugating the poorly absorbed compound to a so-called molecular transporter. The latter are oligomers of arginine that undergo active cellular uptake [2,3].

II. ANATOMICAL AND PHYSIOLOGICAL CONSIDERATIONS OF THE GASTROINTESTINAL TRACT

The gastrointestinal tract (GIT) is a highly specialized region of the body whose primary functions involve the processes of secretion, digestion, and absorption. Since all nutrients needed by the body, with the exception of oxygen, must first be ingested orally, processed by the GIT, and then made available for absorption into the bloodstream, the GIT represents a significant barrier and interface with the environment. The primary defense mechanisms employed by the gut to rid it of noxious or irritating materials are vomiting and diarrhea. In fact, emesis is often a first approach to the treatment of oral poisoning. Diarrhea conditions, initiated by either a pathological state or a physiological mechanism, will result in the flushing away of toxins or bacteria or will represent the response to a stressful condition. Indeed, the GIT is often the first site of the body's response to stress, a fact readily appreciated by students taking a final exam! The nearly instinctive gut response to stress may be particularly pertinent to patients needing oral drug therapy. Since stress is a fact of our daily lives, and since any illness requiring drug therapy may to some degree be considered stressful, the implications of the body's response to stress and the resulting influence on drug absorption from the gut may be extremely important.

Figure 1 illustrates the gross functional regions of the GIT. The liver, gallbladder, and pancreas secrete materials vital to the digestive and certain absorptive functions of the gut. The lengths of various regions of the GIT are presented in Table 1. The small intestine, comprising the duodenum, jejunum, and ileum, represents greater than 60% of the length of the GIT, which is consistent with its primary digestive and absorptive functions. In addition to daily food and fluid

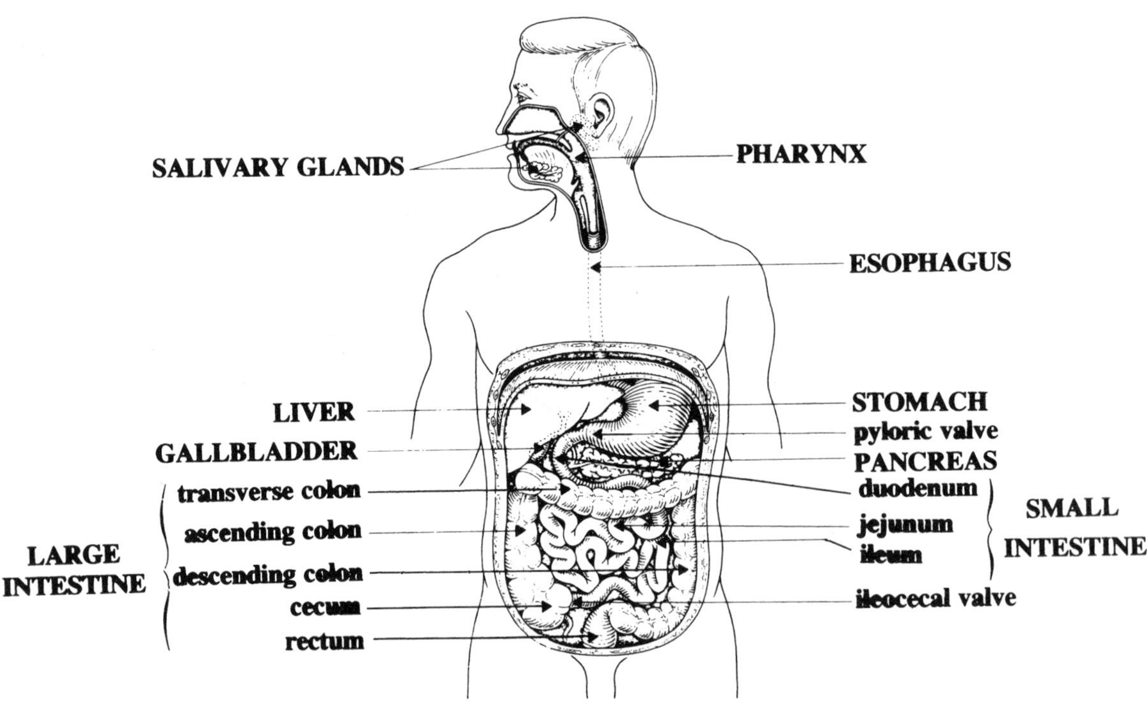

Fig. 1 Diagrammatic sketch of the gastrointestinal tract (and subdivisions of the small and large intestines) along with associated organs. (Modified from Ref. 4.)

Table 1 Approximate Lengths of Various Regions of the Human Gastrointestinal Tract

Region	Length (m)
Duodenum	0.3
Jejunum	2.4
Ileum	3.6
Large Intestine	0.9–1.5

intake (about 1–2 L), the GIT and associated organs secrete about 8 L of fluid per day. Of this total, only 100–200 mL of stool water is lost per day, indicating efficient absorption of water throughout the tract.

A. Stomach

After oral ingestion, materials are presented to the stomach whose primary functions are storage, mixing, and reducing all components to a slurry with the aid of gastric secretions and then emptying these contents in a controlled manner into the upper small intestine (duodenum). All of these functions are accomplished by complex neural, muscular, and hormonal processes. Anatomically, the stomach has classically been divided into three parts: fundus, body, and antrum (or pyloric part), as illustrated in Fig. 2. Although there are no sharp distinctions among these regions, the proximal stomach, made up of the fundus and body, serves as a reservoir for ingested material, and the distal region (antrum) is the major site of mixing motions and acts as a pump to accomplish gastric emptying. The fundus and body regions of the stomach have relatively little tone in their muscular wall, and, as a result, these regions can distend outward to accommodate a meal of up to one liter.

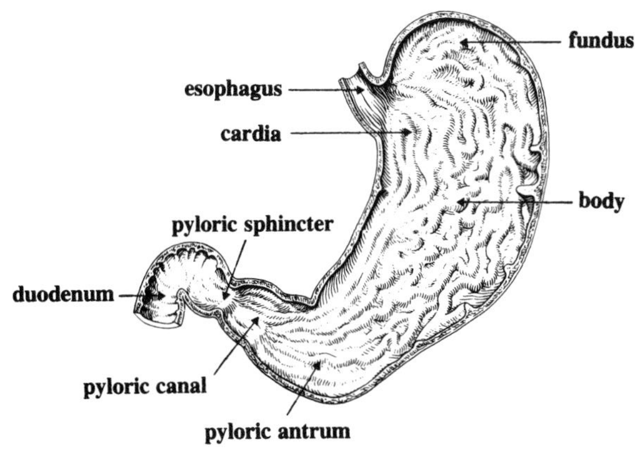

Fig. 2 Diagrammatic sketch of the stomach and anatomical regions. (Modified from Ref. 5.)

A common anatomical feature of the entire GIT is its four concentric layers. Beginning with the luminal (i.e., inner or absorbing) surface these are the mucosa, submucosa, muscularis mucosa, and serosa. The three outer layers are similar throughout most of the tract; however, the mucosa has distinctive structural and functional characteristics. The mucosal surface of the stomach is lined by an epithelial layer of columnar cells, the surface mucous cells. Along this surface are many tubular invaginations, referred to as gastric pits, at the bottom of which are found specialized secretory cells. These secretory cells form part of an extensive network of gastric glands, which produce and secrete about 2 L of gastric fluid daily. The epithelial cells of the gastric mucosa represent one of the most rapidly proliferating epithelial tissues, being shed by the normal stomach at the rate of about a half-million cells per minute. As a result, the surface epithelial layer is renewed every 1 to 3 days. Covering the epithelial cell surface is a layer of mucus 1.0–1.5 mm thick. This material, made up primarily of mucopolysaccharides, provides a protective lubricating coat for the cell lining.

The next region, the muscularis mucosa, consists of an inner circular and an outer longitudinal layer of smooth muscle. This area is responsible for the muscular contractions of the stomach wall needed to accommodate a meal by stretching and for the mixing and propulsive movements of gastric contents. An area known as the lamina propria lies below the muscularis mucosa and contains a variety of tissue types, including connective and smooth muscles, nerve fibers, and the blood and lymph vessels. It is the blood flow to this region and to the muscularis mucosa that delivers nutrients to the gastric mucosa. The major vessels providing a vascular supply to the GIT are the celiac and the inferior and superior mesenteric arteries. Venous return from the GIT is through the splenic and the inferior and superior mesenteric veins. The outermost region of the stomach wall provides structural support for the organ.

B. Small Intestine

The small intestine has the shape of a convoluted tube and represents the major length of the GIT. The small intestine, comprising the duodenum, jejunum, and ileum, has a unique surface structure, making it ideally suited for its primary role of digestion and absorption. The most important structural aspect of the small intestine is the means by which it greatly increases its

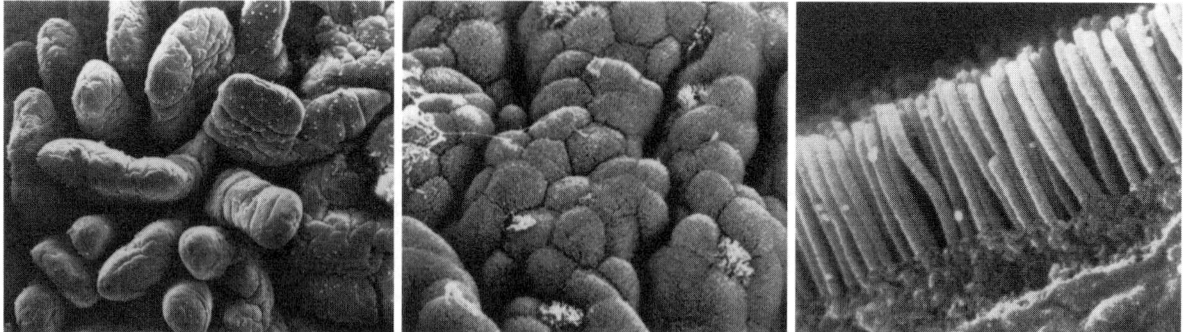

Fig. 3 (A) Photomicrograph of the human duodenal surface illustrating the projection of villi into the lumen (magnification ×75). The goblet cells appear as white dots on the villus surface. (B) Photomicrograph of a single human duodenal villus illustrating surface coverage by microvilli and the presence of goblet cells (white areas) (magnification ×2400). (C) Photomicrograph illustrating the microvilli of the small intestine of the dog (magnification ×33,000). (From Ref. 6.)

effective luminal surface area. The initial increase in surface area, compared to the area of a smooth cylinder, is due to the projection within the lumen of folds of mucosa, referred to as the folds of Kerckring. Lining the entire epithelial surface are finger-like projections, the villi, extending into the lumen. These villi range in length from 0.5 to 1.5 mm, and it has been estimated that there are about 10–40 villi per square millimeter of mucosal surface. Projecting from the villi surface are fine structures, the microvilli (average length, 1 mm), which represent the final large increase in the surface area of the small intestine. There are approximately 600 microvilli protruding from each absorptive cell lining the villi. Relative to the surface of a smooth cylinder, the folds, villi, and microvilli increase the effective surface area by factors of 3, 30, and 600, respectively. The resulting area represents a surface about equal to two thirds of a regulation tennis court! These structural features are clearly indicated in the photomicrographs shown in Fig. 3. A diagrammatic sketch of the villus is shown in Fig. 4.

The mucosa of the small intestine can be divided into three distinct layers. The muscularis mucosa, the deepest layer, consists of a thin sheet of smooth muscle

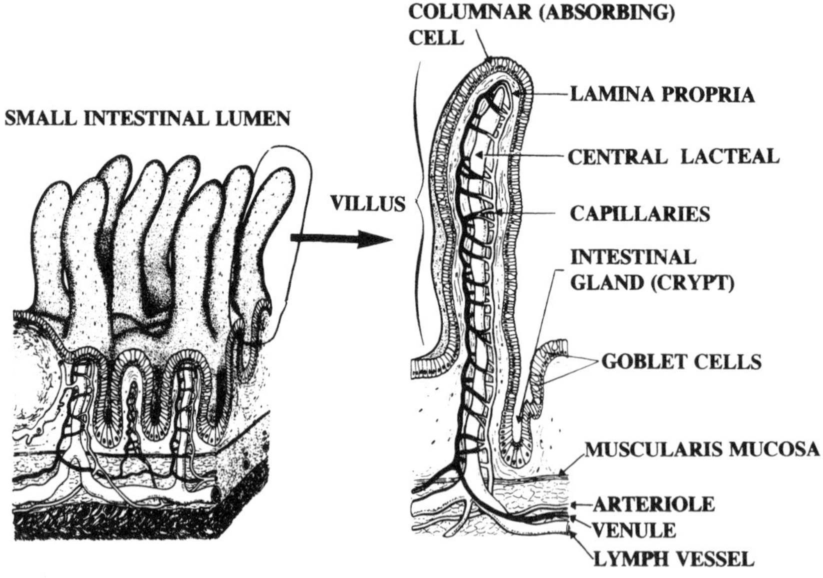

Fig. 4 Diagrammatic sketch of the small intestine illustrating the projection of the villi into the lumen (left) and the anatomic features of a single villus (right). (Modified from Ref. 7.)

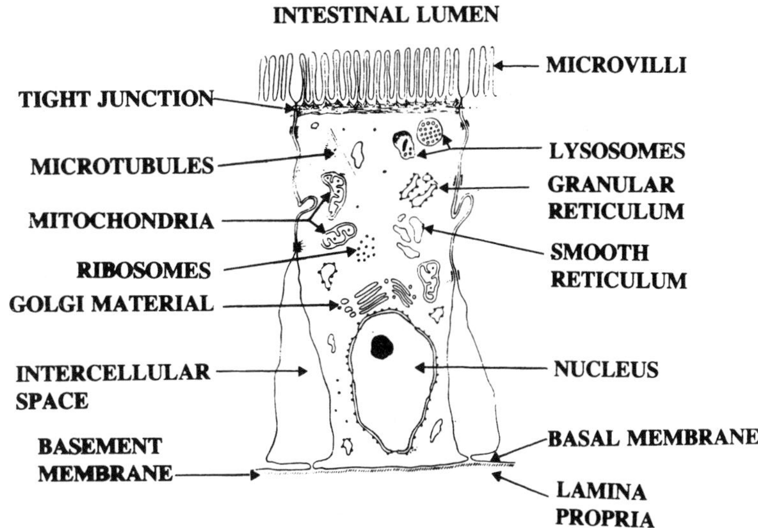

Fig. 5 Diagrammatic sketch of the intestinal absorptive cell. (Modified from Ref. 8.)

3–10 cells thick and separates the mucosa from the submucosa. The lamina propria, the section between the muscularis mucosa and the intestinal epithelia, represents the subepithelial connective tissue space and, together with the surface epithelium, forms the villi structure. The lamina propria contains a variety of cell types, including blood and lymph vessels and nerve fibers. Molecules to be absorbed must penetrate into this region to gain access to the bloodstream.

The third mucosal layer is that lining the entire length of the small intestine and which represents a continuous sheet of epithelial cells. These epithelial cells (or enterocytes) are columnar in shape, and the luminal cell membrane, upon which the microvilli reside, is called the apical cell membrane. Opposite this membrane is the basal (or basolateral) plasma membrane, which is separated from the lamina propria by a basement membrane. A sketch of this cell is shown in Fig. 5. The primary function of the villi is absorption.

The microvilli region has also been referred to as the striated or "brush" border. It is in this region where the process of absorption is initiated. In close contact with the microvilli is a coating of fine filaments composed of weakly acidic sulfated mucopolysaccharides. It has been suggested that this region may serve as a relatively impermeable barrier to substances within the gut such as bacteria and other foreign materials. In addition to increasing the effective luminal surface area, the microvilli region appears to be an area of important biochemical activity.

The surface epithelial cells of the small intestine are renewed rapidly and regularly. It takes about two days for the cells of the duodenum to be renewed completely. As a result of its rapid renewal rate, the intestinal epithelium is susceptible to various factors that may influence proliferation. Exposure of the intestine to ionizing radiation and cytotoxic drugs (such as folic acid antagonists and colchicine) reduces the cell renewal rate.

C. Large Intestine

The large intestine, often referred to as the colon, has two primary functions: the absorption of water and electrolytes and the storage and elimination of fecal material. The large intestine, which has a greater diameter than the small intestine (~ 6 cm), is connected to the latter at the ileocecal junction. The wall of the ileum at this point has a thickened muscular coat called the ileocecal sphincter, which forms the ileocecal valve, whose principal function is to prevent backflow of fecal material from the colon into the small intestine. From a functional point of view the large intestine may be divided into two parts. The proximal half, concerned primarily with absorption, includes the cecum, ascending colon, and portions of the transverse colon. The distal half, concerned with storage and mass movement of fecal matter, includes part of the transverse and descending colon, the rectum, and anal regions, terminating at the internal anal sphincter (see Fig. 1).

In humans, the large intestine usually receives about 500 mL of fluid-like food material (chyme) per day. As

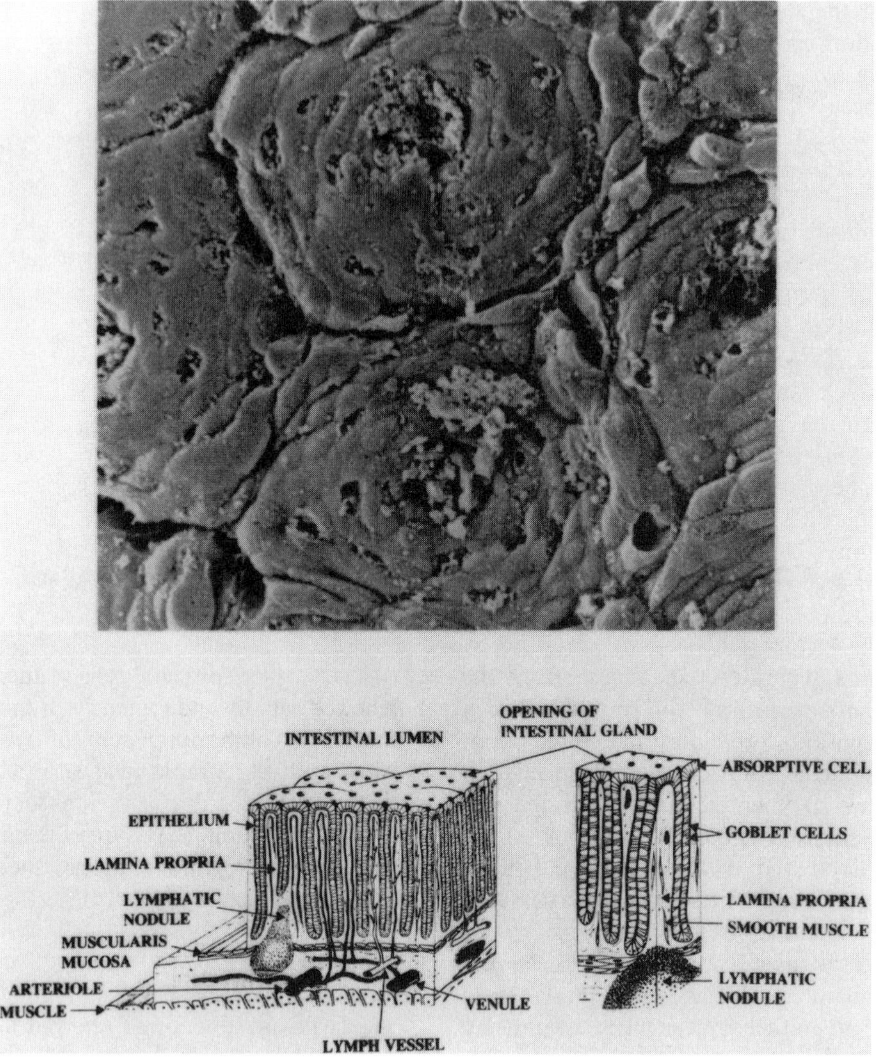

Fig. 6 (A) Scanning electron micrograph of the luminal surface of the large intestine (transverse colon; magnification ×60). (From Ref. 9.) (B) Schematic diagram showing a longitudinal cross section of the large intestine. (C) Enlargement of cross section shown in B. (A and B modified from Ref. 10.)

this material moves distally through the large intestine, water is absorbed, producing a viscous and finally a solid mass of matter. Due to efficient water absorption, of the 500 mL normally reaching the large intestine, approximately 80 mL are eliminated from the gut as fecal material.

Structurally, the large intestine is similar to the small intestine, although the luminal surface epithelium of the former lacks villi. The muscularis mucosa, as in the small intestine, consists of inner circular and outer longitudinal layers. Figure 6 illustrates a photomicrograph and diagrammatic sketches of this region.

D. Pathways of Drug Absorption

Once a drug molecule is in solution, it has the potential to be absorbed. Whether or not it is in a form available for absorption depends on the physicochemical characteristics of the drug (i.e., its inherent absorbability) and the characteristics of its immediate environment (e.g., pH, the presence of interacting materials, and the local properties of the absorbing membrane). Assuming that there are no interfering substances present to impede absorption, the drug molecule must come in contact with the absorbing membrane. To accomplish this, the drug molecule must diffuse from the gastrointestinal fluids to the membrane surface. The most appropriate definition of drug absorption is the penetration of the drug across the intestinal "membrane" and the appearance of the unchanged form in the blood draining the GIT. The latter blood flow will drain into the portal circulation on the way to the liver. A clear distinction must be made between *absorbed* drug and *bioavailable* drug. The former was defined above; the latter refers to the appearance of unaltered drug in the systemic circulation (i.e., beyond the liver). There are two important points to this definition. First, it is often assumed that drug disappearance from the GI fluids represents absorption. This is true only if disappearance from the gut represents appearance in the bloodstream. This may not be the case, for example, if the drug degrades in GI fluids or if it is metabolized within the intestinal cells. Second, the term intestinal "membrane" is rather misleading, since this membrane is not a unicellular structure but a number of unicellular membranes parallel to one another. In fact, relative to the molecular size of most drug molecules, the compound must diffuse a considerable distance. Thus, for a drug molecule to reach the blood, it must penetrate the mucous layer and brush border covering the GI lumen, the apical cell surface, the fluids within this cell, the basal membrane, the basement membrane, the tissue region of the lamina propria, the external capillary membrane, the cytoplasma of the capillary cell, and finally, the inner capillary membrane. Therefore, when the expression intestinal "membrane" is used, we are discussing a barrier to absorption consisting of several distinct unicellular membranes and fluid regions bounded by these membranes. Throughout this chapter the term "intestinal membrane" will be used in that sense.

For a drug molecule to be absorbed from the GIT and gain access to the portal circulation (on its way to the liver), it must effectively penetrate all the regions of the intestine just cited. There are primarily three factors governing this absorption process once a drug is in solution: the physicochemical characteristics of the molecule, the properties and components of the GI fluids, and the nature of the absorbing membrane. Although penetration of the intestinal membrane is obviously the first part of absorption, we discuss the factors controlling penetration extensively in the following section. At this point, assume that the drug molecule has penetrated most of the barriers in the intestine and has reached the lamina propria region. Once in this region the drug may either diffuse through the blood capillary membrane and be carried away in the bloodstream or penetrate the central lacteal and reach the lymph. These functional units of the villi are illustrated in Fig. 4. Most drugs, if not all, reach the systemic circulation via the bloodstream of the capillary network in the villi. The primary reason for this route being dominant over lymphatic penetration is the fact that the villi are highly and rapidly perfused by the bloodstream. Blood flow to the GIT in humans is approximately 500–1000 times greater than lymph flow. Thus, although the lymphatic system is a potential route for drug absorption from the intestine, under normal circumstances it will account for only a small fraction of the total amount absorbed. The major exception to this rule will be drugs (and environmental toxicants, such as insecticides, etc.) that have extremely large oil/water partition coefficients (greater than about 10^5 or log partition of 5). By increasing lymph flow or, alternatively, reducing blood flow, drug absorption via the lymphatic system may become more important. The capillary and lymphatic vessels are rather permeable to most low molecular weight and lipid-soluble compounds. The capillary membrane, however, represents a more substantial barrier than the central lacteal to the penetration of very large molecules or combinations of molecules as a result of frequent separations of cells along the lacteal surface. The lymphatic route of movement is important, for example, for the absorption of triglycerides or emulsified fats in the form of chylomicrons, which are rather large (about 0.5 μm in diameter).

III. PHYSICOCHEMICAL FACTORS GOVERNING DRUG ABSORPTION

A. Oil/Water Partition Coefficient and Chemical Structure

As a result of extensive experimentation it has been found that the primary physicochemical properties of a drug influencing its passive absorption into and across biological membranes are its oil/water partition coefficient ($K_{o/w}$), extent of ionization in biological fluids determined by its pK_a value and pH of the fluid in which it is dissolved, and its molecular weight or volume. The fact that these variables govern drug absorption is a direct reflection of the nature of biological membranes. The cell surface of biological membranes (including those lining the entire GIT) is lipid in nature; as a result, one may view penetration into the intestinal cells as a competition for drug molecules between the aqueous environment, on one hand, and the lipid-like materials of the membrane, on the other. To a large extent, then, the principles of solution chemistry and the molecular attractive forces to which the drug molecules are exposed will govern movement from an aqueous phase to the lipid-like phase of the membrane.

At the turn of this century, Overton examined the osmotic behavior of frog sartorius muscle soaked in a buffer solution containing various dissolved organic compounds. He reasoned that if the solute entered the tissue, the weight of the muscle would remain essentially unchanged, whereas loss of weight would indicate an osmotic withdrawal of fluid and hence impermeability to the solute. He noted that, in general, the tissue was most readily penetrated by lipid-soluble compounds and poorly penetrated by lipid-insoluble substances. Overton was one of the first investigators to illustrate that compounds penetrate cells in the same relative order as their oil/water partition coefficients, suggesting the lipid nature of cell membranes. Using animal or plant cells, other workers provided data in support of Overton's observations. The only exception to this general rule was the observation that very small molecules penetrate cell membranes faster than would be expected based on their $K_{o/w}$ values. To explain the rapid penetration of these small molecules (e.g., urea, methanol, formamide), it was suggested that cell membranes, although lipid in nature, were not continuous but interrupted by small water-filled channels or "pores"; such membranes are best described as being lipid-sieve membranes. As a result, one could imagine lipid-soluble molecules readily penetrating the lipid regions of the membrane while small water-soluble molecules pass through the aqueous "pores". Fordtran et al. [11] estimated the effective pore radius to be 7–8.5 and 3–3.8 Å in human jejunum and ileum, respectively. There may be a continuous distribution of pore sizes—a smaller fraction of larger ones and a greater fraction of smaller pores.

Our knowledge of biological membrane ultrastructure has increased considerably over the years as a result of rapid advances in instrumentation. Although there is still controversy over the most correct biological membrane model, the concept of membrane structure presented by Davson and Danielli of a lipid bilayer is perhaps the one best accepted [12,13]. The most current version of that basic model, illustrated in Fig. 7, is referred to as the "fluid mosaic" model of membrane structure. This model is consistent with what we have learned about the existence of specific ion channels and receptors within and along surface membranes.

Table 2 summarizes some literature data supporting the general dependence of the rate of absorption on

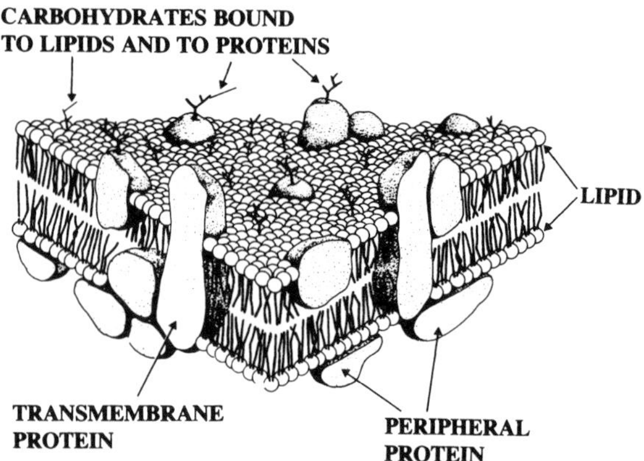

Fig. 7 Diagrammatic representation of the fluid mosaic model of the cell membrane. The basic structure of the membrane is that of a lipid bilayer in which the lipid portion (long tails) points inward and the polar portion (round "head") points outward. The membrane is penenetrated by transmembrane (or integral) proteins. Attached to the surface of the membrane are peripheral proteins (inner surface) and carbohydrates that bind to lipid and protein molecules (outer surface). (Modified from Ref. 14.)

$K_{o/w}$ as measured in the rat intestine [15,16]. As with other examples that are available, as $K_{o/w}$ increases, the rate of absorption increases. One very extensive study [17–19] has examined in depth the physicochemical factors governing nonelectrolyte permeability for several hundred compounds. This study employed an in vitro preparation of rabbit gallbladder, an organ whose mucosal surface is lined by epithelial cells. The

Table 2 Influence of Oil/Water Partition Coefficient ($K_{o/w}$) on Absorption from the Rat Intestine

Compound	$K_{o/w}$	Percentage absorbed
	Olive Oil/Water	
Valeramide	0.023	85
Lactamide	0.00058	67
Malonamide	0.00008	27
	Chloroform/Water	
Hexethal	>100	44
Secobarbital	50.7	40
Pentobarbital	28.0	30
Cyclobarbital	13.9	24
Butethal	11.7	24
Allybarbituric acid	10.5	23
Phenobarbital	4.8	20
Aprobarbital	4.9	17
Barbital	0.7	12

method used to assess solute permeability is based upon measurement of differences in electrical potential (streaming potentials) across the membrane. The more permeable the compound, the smaller the osmotic pressure it exerts and the smaller the osmotic fluid flow it produces in the opposite direction; this results in a small potential difference. If the compound is impermeable, it produces a large osmotic pressure and osmotic fluid flow, resulting in a large potential difference. Experimentally, one exposes the mucosal membrane surface to a buffer solution containing a reference compound to which the membrane is completely impermeable and measures the resulting potential difference. This is followed by exposing the same membrane to a solution of a test compound and again measuring the resulting potential difference. The ratio of the potential difference of the test compound to that of the reference compound is referred to as the reflection coefficient (σ). The reflection coefficient is a measure of the permeability of the test compound relative to a reference solute with the particular membrane being used. The less permeable the test compound, the closer the reflection coefficient approaches one; the more permeable the test compound, the closer the coefficient approaches zero.

Using this method, Wright and Diamond [17–19] were able to reach a number of important conclusions concerning patterns of nonelectrolyte permeability. In general, membrane permeability of a solute increases with $K_{o/w}$, supporting previous findings mentioned earlier. The two classes of exceptions to this pattern are highly branched compounds, which penetrate the membrane more slowly than would be expected based on their $K_{o/w}$, and smaller polar molecules, which penetrate the membrane more readily than would be expected based on their $K_{o/w}$. The latter observation has been noted by other workers, and, as noted earlier, it has resulted in the development of the lipid-sieve membrane concept whereby one envisions aqueous "pores" in the membrane surface. The authors postulate that these small, polar, relatively lipid-insoluble compounds penetrate the membrane by following a route lined by the polar groupings of membrane constituents (i.e., localized polar regions). This concept is an attractive structural explanation of what have been referred to as "pores." The accessibility of this route would be limited primarily by the molecular size of the compound as a result of steric hindrance. In fact, it is the first one or two members of a homologous series of compounds that are readily permeable, but beyond these members it is primarily $K_{o/w}$ that dictates permeability. Table 3 illustrates this effect for several members of various homologous series. Recall that the smaller the σ, the more permeable the compound. In each instance, permeability decreases after the first member, reaches a minimum, and then increases again.

Table 3 Influence of Chain Length on Membrane Permeability within Several Homologous Series[a]

Compound	Reflection coefficient, σ
Urea	0.29 ↑
Methyl urea	0.54 |
Ethyl urea	0.92 |
Propyl urea	0.93 -
Butyl urea	0.70 ↓
Malononitrile	0.09 ↑
Succinonitrile	0.30 -
Glutaronitrile	0.21 ↓
Methylformamide	0.28 ↑
Methylacetamide	0.51 -
Methylproprionamide	0.22 ↓

[a] The reflection coefficient σ is defined in the text. The direction of the arrows indicates an increase in permeability from the least permeable member of the series.

The other anomalous behavior was the smaller-than-expected permeability of highly branched compounds. This deviation has been explained on the basis that membrane lipids are subject to a more highly constrained orientation (probably a parallel configuration of hydrocarbon chains of fatty acids) than are those in a bulk lipid solvent. As a result, branched compounds must disrupt this local lipid structure of the membrane and will encounter greater steric hindrance than will a straight-chain molecule. This effect with branched compounds is not adequately reflected in simple aqueous-lipid partitioning studies (i.e., in the $K_{o/w}$ value).

With the exception of rather small polar molecules, the majority of compounds, including drugs, appear to penetrate biological membranes via a lipid route. As a result, the membrane permeability of most compounds is dependent on $K_{o/w}$. The physicochemical interpretation of this general relationship is based on the atomic and molecular forces to which the solute molecules are exposed in the aqueous and lipid phases. Thus, the ability of a compound to partition from an aqueous to a lipid phase of a membrane involves the balance between solute-water and solute-membrane intermolecular forces. If the attractive forces of the solute-water interaction are greater than those of the solute-membrane interaction, membrane permeability will be relatively poor and vice versa. In examining the permeability of a homologous series of compounds and, therefore, the influence of substitution or chain length on permeability, one must recognize the influence of the substituted group on the intermolecular forces in aqueous and membrane phases (e.g., dipole-dipole, dipole-induced dipole, or van der Waals forces). The membrane permeabilities of the nonelectrolytes studied appear to be largely determined by the number and strength of hydrogen bonds the solute can form with water. Thus, nonelectrolyte permeation is largely a question of physical organic chemistry in aqueous solution. Table 4 summarizes some of the interesting findings of Diamond and Wright with respect to the influence of substituent groups on membrane permeation. These data have been interpreted based on the solutes' ability to form hydrogen bonds with water.

Within a homologous series of compounds the first few small members are readily permeable, due to the polar route of membrane penetration. Permeability decreases for the next several members (i.e., σ increases) and then increases as the carbon chain length increases. The regular influence of chain length on permeability is a result not of increased solubility in the lipid phase of the membrane but of the unique interaction of hydrocarbon chains with water. The nonpolar hydrocarbon molecules are surrounded by a local region of water that has a more highly ordered structure than bulk water. This "iceberg" structure of water results in increased $K_{o/w}$ and membrane permeability as the carbon chain length is increased due to the compound being "pushed out" of the aqueous phase by the resulting gain in entropy.

Based upon a review of the physical chemical properties of marketed drugs, Lipinski and coworkers have proposed an empirical "rule of 5" (20). This rule may help pharmaceutical scientists in reaching an early decision about the potential candidacy for further development of a new chemical entity. The rule states that a chemical candidate is likely to display poor absorption or poor membrane permeability if

1. There are more than 5 hydrogen bond donors
2. There are more than 10 hydrogen bond acceptors
3. The molecular weight is greater than 500
4. Log $K_{o/w}$ is greater than 5
5. The above rules only apply to compounds that undergo passive membrane transport

There have been several, albeit limited, attempts to develop quantitative, structure-activity relationships in drug absorption (e.g., Ref. 21). Such relationships could prove extremely useful in the early stages of drug design in order to produce optimum absorption characteristics. Another very practical approach involves "data mining," whereby large data bases are examined to characterize the properties of those compounds exhibiting good absorption.

B. pK_a and pH

Most drug molecules are either weak acids or bases that will be ionized to an extent determined by the compound's pK_a and the pH of the biological fluid in which it is dissolved. The importance of ionization in drug absorption is based on the observation that the nonionized form of the drug has a greater $K_{o/w}$ than the ionized form and, since $K_{o/w}$ is a prime determinant of membrane penetration, ionization would be expected to influence absorption. The observation that pH influences the membrane penetration of ionizable drugs is not a recent finding. At the turn of the previous century Overton was able to relate pH to the rate of penetration of various alkaloids into cells, and he noted the resulting influence in toxicity. Other investigators have made similar observations with respect to the influence of pH on the penetration of alkaloids through the conjunctival and mammalian skin [22,23]. The rate of penetration of these weak bases is enhanced by alkalinization due to a greater fraction of the nonionized species being present. Travell [24] examined the influence of pH on the absorption of several alkaloids from the stomach and intestine of the cat. After ligation of the proximal and distal ends of the stomach of an anesthetized cat, a 5.0 mg/kg solution of strychnine at pH 8.5 produced death within 24 minutes; however, the same dose at pH 1.2 produced no toxic response. Identical results were found with nicotine, atropine, and cocaine. The same trend was also seen when the drug solution was instilled into ligated intestinal segments and after oral administration (via stomach tube) to ambulatory animals. These results indicate that alkaloids, which are weak bases, will be more rapidly absorbed in the nonionized form (i.e., at high fluid pH) compared to the ionized form (low pH). This fundamental observation has sometimes been overlooked in oral acute drug toxicity studies.

In 1940 Jacobs [25] made use of the Henderson-Hasselbalch equation to relate pH and pK_a to membrane transport of ionizable compounds. Extensive experimentation by a group of investigators in the early 1950s [16,26–30] quantitated many of the aforementioned observations concerning the influence of pH and pK_a on drug absorption from the GIT. These studies have resulted in the so-called "pH partition hypothesis." In essence, this hypothesis states that ionizable compounds penetrate biological membranes primarily in the nonionized form (i.e., nonionic diffusion). As a result, acidic drugs should best be absorbed from acidic solutions where $pH < pK_a$, while basic compounds would best be absorbed from alkaline solutions where $pH > pK_a$. The data in Table 5 illustrate this principle [31].

The investigators noted some inconsistencies in their data, however, as some compounds (e.g., salicylic acid) that were essentially completely ionized in the buffer solution were nevertheless rapidly absorbed. To explain these exceptions it was suggested that there was a "virtual membrane pH" (~5.3), different from the bulk pH of the buffer solution, which was the actual pH determining the fraction of drug nonionized and hence dictating the absorption pattern. Although there may indeed be an effective pH at the immediate surface of the intestinal membrane different from the pH of solutions bathing the lumen, there is overwhelming experimental evidence indicating that many drugs in the ionic form may be well absorbed. Over the years there has been an unqualified acceptance of the pH partition hypothesis, and, as a result, many texts and considerable literature on drug absorption indicate that acidic drugs are best absorbed from the acidic gastric fluids of the stomach and basic drugs best absorbed from the relatively more alkaline intestinal fluids. If all other conditions were the same, the nonionized form of the solution would be more rapidly absorbed than the ionized form. However, conditions along the GIT are not uniform, and hence most drugs, whether ionized or nonionized (i.e., regardless of pH), are best absorbed from the small intestine as a result of the large absorbing surface area of this region. A good example to illustrate this point is presented in Table 6. There are three important comparisons that should be made in examining these data:

1. By comparing gastric absorption at pH 3 and pH 6 where surface area and factors other than pH are constant, one sees that the general principle is supported; acid drugs are more rapidly absorbed from acidic solution, whereas basic drugs are more rapidly absorbed from relatively alkaline solution.
2. At the same pH (i.e., pH 6) acidic and basic drugs are more rapidly absorbed from the intestine compared to the stomach, by virtue of the larger intestinal surface area.
3. Acidic drugs are more rapidly absorbed from the intestine (pH 6), although there is substantial ionization, compared to the rate of gastric absorption, even at a pH where the drug is in a far more acidic solution (pH 3). Again, this is primarily a result of surface area differences.

Interestingly, in an analysis of the original data used in developing the pH partition hypothesis, Benet [32] has shown that these data support the findings in point 3 above. The pH partition hypothesis provides a useful guide in predicting general trends in drug absorption, and it remains an extremely useful concept. There are numerous examples illustrating the general relationship among pH, pK_a, and drug absorption developed in that hypothesis. The primary limitation of this concept is the assumption that only nonionized drug is absorbed, when in fact the ionized species of some compounds can be absorbed, albeit at a slower rate. There is also the presence of unstirred water layers at the epithelial membrane surface, which can alter the rate of drug diffusion. Furthermore, the hypothesis is based on data obtained from drug in solution. In a practical sense, there are other considerations that may also govern the pattern of drug absorption and these include dissolution rate from solid dosage forms, the large intestinal surface area, and the relative residence times of the drug in different parts of the GIT. These factors are discussed below. In general then, drug absorption in humans takes place primarily from the small intestine regardless of whether the drug is a weak acid or base.

C. Mechanisms of Drug Absorption

A thorough discussion of the mechanisms of absorption is provided in Chapter 4. Water-soluble vitamins (B_2, B_{12}, and C) and other nutrients (e.g., monosaccharides, amino acids) are absorbed by specialized mechanisms. With the exception of a number of antimetabolites used in cancer chemotherapy, L-dopa, and certain antibiotics (e.g., aminopenicillins, aminocephalosporins), virtually all drugs are absorbed in humans by a passive diffusion mechanism. Passive diffusion indicates that the transfer of a compound from an aqueous phase through a membrane may be described by physicochemical laws and by the properties of the membrane. The membrane itself is passive in that it does not partake in the transfer process but acts as a simple barrier to diffusion. The driving force for diffusion across the membrane is the concentration gradient (more correctly, the activity gradient) of the compound across that membrane. This mechanism of

Table 4 Influence of Chemical Substitution on the Membrane Permeability of Several Series of Nonelectrolytes

Substituent group	Influence on membrane permeability	Compound	Example	σ[a]
Oxygen and nitrogen functional groups				
Alcoholic hydroxyl group (-OH)	(a) At any given chain length, permeability decreases as the number of -OH groups increases	*n*-Propanol	$CH_3CH_2CH_2OH$	0.02
		1,2-Propanediol	$CH_3CHOHCH_2OH$	0.84
		Glycerol	$CH_2OHCHOHCH_2OH$	0.95
	(b) Intramolecular H-bonds formed between adjacent -OH groups result in greater permeability compared to the same compound with nonadjacent -OH groups due to decreased H-bond formation with water	2,3-Butanediol	$CH_3CHOHHCHOHCH_3$	0.74
		1,3-Butanediol	$CH_3CHOHCH_2CH_2OH$	0.77
		1,4-Butanediol	$CH_2OHCH_2CH_2CH_2OH$	0.86
Ether group (-O-)	Has less of an influence than an -OH group in decreasing permeability	*n*-Propanol	$CH_3CH_2CH_2OH$	0.02
		Ethyleneglycol-methyl ether	$CH_3\text{–}O\text{–}CH_2CH_2OH$	0.15
		1,2-Propanediol	$CH_3CHOHCH_2OH$	0.84
Carbonyl group Ketone (–C=O) Aldehyde (–HC=O)	Has less of an influence than an -OH gourp in decreasing permeability; difficulty in measuring permeability of these compounds per se as many are unstable in solution forming diols and enolic tautomers	Acetone	$CH_3\overset{O}{\overset{\|}{C}}CH_3$	0.01
		2-Propanol	$CH_3CHOHCH_3$	0.10
		2-5-Hexanedione	$CH_3\overset{O}{\overset{\|}{C}}CH_2CH_2\overset{O}{\overset{\|}{C}}CH_3$	0.00
		2,5-Hexanediol	$CH_3CHOHCH_2CH_2CHOHCH_3$	0.59
Ester group $(\text{-}\overset{O}{\overset{\|}{C}}\text{-O-})$	Has less of an influence than an -OH group in decreasing permeability	1,2-Propanediol-1-acetate	$CH_3\overset{O}{\overset{\|}{C}}\text{—}O\text{—}CH_2CHOHCH_3$	0.31
		1,5-Pentanediol	$CH_2OH(CH_2)_3CH_2OH$	0.71
Amide group $\text{-}\overset{O}{\overset{\|}{C}}\text{-}NH_2$	Causes a greater decrease in permeability than any of the above groups	*n*-Propanol	$CH_3CH_2CH_2OH$	0.02
		Acetone	$CH_3\overset{O}{\overset{\|}{C}}CH_3$	0.08
		Ethyleneglycol-methyl ether	$CH_3\text{—}O\text{—}CH_2CH_2OH$	0.15
		Proprionamide	$CH_3CH_2\overset{O}{\overset{\|}{C}}NH_2$	0.66

Urea derivatives $R-NH-C(=O)-NH_2$	These compounds have lower permeability than amides with the same numer of carbons and are about as impermeable as the corresponding dihydroxyl alcohols	*n*-Butanol	$CH_3CH_2CH_2CH_2OH$	0.01 ↑
		n-Butryamide	$CH_3CH_2CH_2C(=O)-NH_2$	0.42
		1,4-Butanediol	$CH_2OHCH_2CH_2CH_2OH$	0.86
		n-Propyl urea	$CH_3CH_2CH_2NHC(=O)NH_2$	0.89
α-Amino acids $R-CH(NH_2)COOH$	These compounds have the lowest $K_{o/w}$ values of all orgainc molecules and are essentially impermeable due to large dipole-dipole interactions with water	Proprionamide	$CH_3CH_2C(=O)NH_2$	0.66 ↑
		1-Amino-2-propanol	$CH_3CHOHCH_2NH_2$	0.89
		1,3-Propanediol	$CH_2OHCH_2CH_2OH$	0.92
		Alanine	$CH_3CH(H_2N)C(=O)-OH$	1.06
Sulfur functional groups Sulfur replacement of oxygen	(a) Sulfur compounds have greater $K_{o/w}$ values and permeate membranes more readily than the corresponding oxygen compound; this is a result of poor H-bond formation between sulfur and water compared to the oxygen analog	1-Thioglycerol	$CH_2OHCHOHCH_2SH$	0.69 ↑
		Glycerol	$CH_2OHCHOHCH_2OH$	0.95
		Thiodiglycol	$(OHCH_2CH_2)_2S$	0.71
		Diethylene glycol	$(OHCH_2CH_2)_2O$	0.92
	(b) Sulfoxides ($R_2S{=}O$) are less permeable than the corresponding ketone ($R_2C{=}O$), due to stronger H-bond formation with water	Acetone	$CH_3C(=O)CH_3$	0.01 ↑
		Dimethyl sulfoxide	$CH_3S(=O)CH_3$	0.92

[a] The reflection coefficient σ is defined in the text. The direction of the arrows indicates an increase in permeability.
Source: Refs. 17–19.

Table 5 Influence of pH on Drug Absorption from the Small Intestine of the Rat[a]

Drug	pK_a	Percentage absorbed			
		pH 4	pH 5	pH 7	pH 8
Acids					
5-Nitrosalicylic acid	2.3	40	27	<2	<2
Salicylic acid	3.0	64	35	30	10
Acetylsalicylic acid	3.5	41	27	—	—
Benzoic acid	4.2	62	36	35	5
Bases					
Aniline	4.6	40	48	58	61
Aminopyrine	5.0	21	35	48	52
p-Toluidine	5.3	30	42	65	64
Quinine	8.4	9	11	41	54

[a] Drug buffer solutions were perfused through the in situ rat intestine for 30 min and percentage of drug absorbed was determined from four subsequent 10 min samples of the buffer solution.

Table 6 Influence of pH on Drug Absorption from the Stomach and Intestine of the Rat[a]

Drug	Apparent first-order absorption rate constant (min^{-1})		
	pH 3	Stomach pH 6	Intestine pH 6
Acids			
Salicylic acid	0.015	0.0053	0.085
Barbital	0.0029	0.0026	0.037
Sulfaethidole	0.004	0.0023	0.022
Bases			
Prochlorperazine	<0.002	0.0062	0.030
Haloperidol	0.0028	0.0041	0.028
Aminopyrine	<0.002	0.0046	0.022

[a] Drug buffer solutions were placed into the GIT of an in situ rat preparation. The apparent first-order absorption rate constants are based upon drug disappearance from the buffer solution.

membrane penetration may be described mathematically by Fick's first law of diffusion, which has been simplified by Riggs [33] and discussed by Benet [32].

$$\left(\frac{dQ_b}{dt}\right)_{g\to b} = D_m \cdot A_m \cdot R_{m/aq}\left(\frac{C_g - C_b}{\Delta X_m}\right) \qquad (1)$$

The derivative on the left side of the equation represents the rate of appearance of drug in the blood (amount/time) when the drug diffuses from the gut fluids (g) to the blood (b). The expression reads, the rate of change of the quantity (Q) entering the blood stream. The other symbols have the following meanings (and units): D_m, the diffusion coefficient of the drug through the membrane (area/time); A_m, the surface area of the absorbing membrane available for drug diffusion (area); $R_{m/aq}$, the partition coefficient of the drug between the membrane and aqueous gut fluids (unitless); $C_g - C_b$, the concentration gradient across the membrane, representing the difference in the effective drug concentration (i.e., activity) in the gut fluids (C_g) at the site of absorption and the drug concentration in the blood (C_b) at the site of absorption (amount/volume); and ΔX_m, the thickness of the membrane (length). This equation nicely explains several of the observations discussed previously. Thus, rate of drug absorption is directly dependent on the membrane surface area available for diffusion, indicating that one would expect more rapid absorption from the small intestine compared to the stomach. Furthermore, the greater the membrane aqueous fluid partition coefficient ($R_{m/aq}$), the more rapid the rate of absorption, supporting the previous discussion indicating the dependence of absorption rate on $K_{o/w}$. We know that pH will produce a net effect on absorption rate by altering several of the parameters in Eq. (1). As the pH for a given drug will determine the fraction nonionized, the value of $R_{m/aq}$ will change with pH, generally increasing as the fraction nonionized increases. Depending on the relative ability of the membrane to permit the diffusion of the nonionized and ionized forms, C_g will be altered appropriately. Finally, the value of D_m may be different for the ionized and nonionized forms of the compound. For a given drug and membrane and under specified conditions, Eq. (1) is made up of a number of constants that may be incorporated into a large constant (P), referred to as the permeability coefficient:

$$\left(\frac{dQ_b}{dt}\right)_{g\to b} = P \cdot (C_g - C_b) \qquad (2)$$

where P incorporates D_m, A_m, $R_{m/aq}$, and ΔX_m and has units of volume/time, which is analogous to a flow or clearance term. Since the volume into which the drug may distribute from the blood is large compared to the gut fluid volume and since the rapid circulation of blood through the GIT continually moves absorbed drug away from the site of absorption, $C_g \gg C_b$. This is often referred to as a "sink condition," indicating a relatively small drug concentration in the bloodstream at the absorption site. As a result, Eq. (2) may be simplified:

$$\left(\frac{dQ_b}{dt}\right)_{g\to b} \cong P \cdot C_g \qquad (3)$$

Equation (3) is in the form of a differential equation describing a first-order kinetic process, and, as a result, drug absorption generally adheres to first-order kinetics. The rate of absorption should increase directly with an increase in drug concentration in the GI fluids.

Figure 8 illustrates the linear dependence of absorption rate on concentration for several compounds placed into the in situ rat intestine. The slopes of these lines represent the constant (P) for absorption in Eq. (3). Alternatively, one may express these data as the percentage absorbed per unit of time as a function of concentration or amount. Several examples illustrating such an analysis are listed in Table 7. As can be seen, the percentage absorbed in any given period is independent of concentration, indicating that these compounds are absorbed by a passive diffusion or first-order kinetic process over the concentration ranges studied. Similar studies by other investigators employing an in situ rat intestine preparation indicate that several other drugs (those listed in Table 6) are absorbed in a first-order kinetic fashion.

It is far more difficult to establish the mechanism(s) of drug absorption in humans. Most investigators analyze drug absorption data in humans (from blood or urine data) by assuming first-order absorption kinetics. For the most part this assumption seems quite

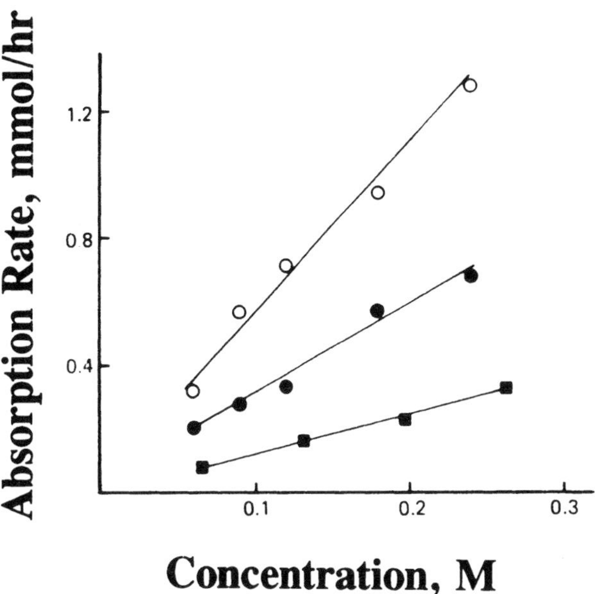

Fig. 8 Influence of concentration on the rate of absorption from the in situ rat intestine. The linear dependence of absorption rate on concentration suggests an apparent first-order absorption process over the range studied. Absorption rates have been calculated from the data in Ref. 15 and the straight lines are from linear regression of the data. Key: (○) erythritol; (●) urea; (■) malonamide.

Table 7 Influence of Concentration on the Absorption of Various Solutes from the In Situ Rat Intestine

Compound	Concentration (mM)	Percentage absorbed	Compound	Concentration (mM)	Percentage absorbed
Urea[a]	60	20.9	Salicylic acid[b]	1	12
	90	19.0		2	12
	120	17.0		10	13
	180	20.0			
	240	17.8	Aniline[b]	1	44
				10	43
Erythritol[a]	60	54.1			
	90	65.0	Benzoic acid[b]	1	12
	120	62.2		2	12
	180	54.4		10	13
	240	55.5			
			Quinine[b]	1	20
Malonamide[a]	66	16.9		10	20
	132	16.8		0.1	58
	198	16.5	Aniline[c]		
	264	18.4		1	54
				10	59
				20	54

[a] Based on data in Ref. 15.
[b] Based on data in Ref. 16.
[c] Based on data in Ref. 29.

valid, and the results of such analyses are consistent with that assumption. As discussed in Chapter 3, one method used to assess the mechanism of drug absorption in humans is based on a pharmacokinetic treatment of blood or urine data and the preparation of log percentage unabsorbed versus time plots. If a straight-line relationship is found, this is indicative of an apparent first-order absorption process, where the slope of that line represents the apparent first-order absorption rate constant. Some cautions must be taken in the application of this method. Although the overall absorption process in humans for many drugs appears consistent with the characteristics of a first-order kinetic process, there are some questions as to which of the sequential steps in the absorption process is rate-limiting. As discussed in a thorough review of mass transport phenomena [34], the oil/water partition coefficient of a solute ($K_{o/w}$) will govern its movement across a lipid-like membrane as long as the membrane is the predominant barrier to diffusion. However, for such membranes, when the $K_{o/w}$ becomes very large, the barrier controlling diffusion may no longer be the membrane but rather an aqueous diffusion layer surrounding the membrane. Thus, for some molecules, depending on their physicochemical characteristics, the rate-limiting step in membrane transport will be movement through or out of the membrane, while for other compounds the rate-limiting step will be diffusion through an aqueous layer. Our incomplete understanding of drug transport across biological membranes is not that surprising given the complexity of the system and the experimental requirements needed to make unequivocal statements about this process on a molecular level.

The analysis of absorption data in humans has moved away from the more traditional modeling and data fitting techniques [35]. Absorption processes are now more often characterized by a mean absorption (or input) time (i.e., the average amount of time that the drug molecules spend at the absorption site) or by a process called deconvolution. The former analysis results in a single value (similar to absorption half-life) and the latter results in a profile of the absorption process as a function of time (e.g., absorption rate or cumulative amount absorbed vs. time). These approaches offer additional ways of interpreting the absorption process.

Most drugs appear to be absorbed in humans by passive diffusion (linear or first-order kinetics). The predominant pathway taken by most drugs is through the epithelial cell, the *transcellular* route. It is this route that requires the compound to have a reasonable $K_{o/w}$

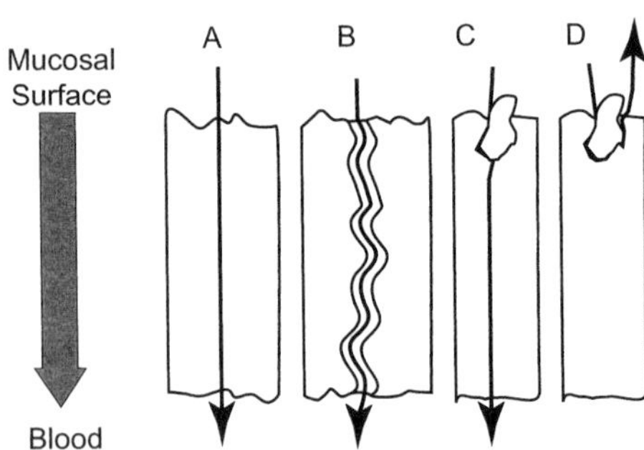

Fig. 9 Schematic representation depicting the movement of molecules from the absorbing (mucosal or apical) surface of the GIT to the basolateral membrane and from there to blood. (A) transcellular movement through the epithelial cell. (B) Paracellular transport via movement between epithelial cells. (C) Specialized carrier-mediated transport into the epithelial cell. (D) Carrier-mediated efflux transport of drug out of the epithelial cell. (Copyright © 2000 Saguaro Technical Press, Inc., used with permission.)

(>1 and $<10^5$). This route is indicated in Fig. 9A as the arrow moving through the cell from the mucosal (or apical) absorbing surface to the basolateral membrane. In contrast, small polar molecules ($K_{o/w} < 1$) may have access to a convoluted route that exists between adjacent epithelial cells but which has a tight junction along the absorbing surface. This route is referred to as being *paracellular* (Fig. 9B). The molecular size cut-off for this route is about 500 Da [36].

Since many essential nutrients (e.g., monosaccharides, amino acids, and vitamins) are water-soluble, they have low oil/water partition coefficients, which would suggest poor absorption from the GIT. However, to ensure adequate uptake of these materials from food, the intestine has developed specialized absorption mechanisms that depend on membrane participation and require the compound to have a specific chemical structure. Since these processes are discussed in Chapter 4, we will not dwell on them here. This carrier transport mechanism is illustrated in Fig. 9C. Absorption by a specialized carrier mechanism (from the rat intestine) has been shown to exist for several agents used in cancer chemotherapy (5-fluorouracil and 5-bromouracil) [37,38], which may be considered "false" nutrients in that their chemical structures are very similar to essential nutrients for which the intestine has a specialized transport mechanism. It would be instructive to examine some studies concerned with riboflavin and ascorbic acid absorption in humans, as these illustrate how one may treat urine data to explore the mechanism of absorption. If a compound is absorbed by a passive mechanism, a plot of amount absorbed (or amount recovered in the urine) versus dose ingested will provide a straight-line relationship. In contrast, a plot of percentage of dose absorbed (or percentage of dose recovered in the urine) versus dose ingested will provide a line of slope zero (i.e., a constant fraction of the dose is absorbed at all doses). If the absorption process requires membrane involvement, the absorption process may be saturated as the oral dose increases, making the process less efficient at larger doses (i.e., there are more drug molecules than sites on the transporter). As a result, a plot of amount absorbed versus dose ingested will be linear at low doses, curvilinear at larger doses, and approach an asymptotic value at even larger doses. One sees this type of relationship for riboflavin and ascorbic acid in Figs. 10A and C, suggesting nonpassive absorption mechanisms in humans [39,40]. This nonlinear relationship is reminiscent of Michaelis-Menten saturable enzyme kinetics, from which one may estimate the kinetic parameters (K_m and V_{max}) associated with the absorption of these vitamins. Figures 10B and D illustrate an alternative plot—percentage absorbed versus dose ingested. For a nonpassive absorption process, the percentage dose absorbed will decrease as the dose increases as a result of saturation of the

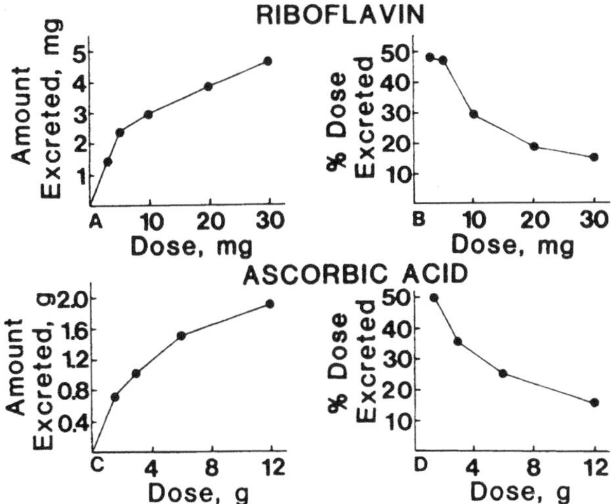

Fig. 10 Urinary excretion of riboflavin (A, B) and ascorbic acid (C, D) in humans as a function of oral dose. Graphs A and C illustrate the nonlinear dependence of absorption on dose, which is suggestive of a saturable specialized absorption process. Graphs B and D represent an alternative graph of the same data and illustrate the reduced absorption efficiency as the dose increases. (Graphs A and C based on data in Ref. 39 and graphs B and D based on data in Ref. 40.)

transport mechanism and of there being a reduction in absorption efficiency. It has been suggested [40] that one means of overcoming the decrease in absorption efficiency is to administer small divided doses rather than large single doses, as illustrated later for ascorbic acid.

Several investigators suggest that L-dopa (L-dihydroxyphenylalanine) absorption may be impaired if the drug is ingested with meals containing proteins [41]. Amino acids formed from the digestion of protein meals, which are absorbed by a specialized mechanism, may competitively inhibit L-dopa absorption if the drug is also transported by the same mechanism. There is evidence (in animals) indicating a specialized absorption mechanism for phenylalanine and L-dopa, and there are data illustrating L-dopa inhibition of phenylalanine and tyrosine absorption in humans [42,43]. L-Dopa appears to be absorbed by the same specialized transport mechanism responsible for the absorption of other amino acids [44]. In a later section several of the complicating factors in L-dopa absorption that influence therapy are discussed.

In addition to some anticancer agents being absorbed by a specialized process in humans (e.g., methotrexate) [45], there is recent evidence to suggest that a similar mechanism exists for the absorption of aminopenicillins (e.g., amoxicillin) [46] and aminocephalosporins (e.g., cefixime) [47]. Absorption of these compounds appears to be linked to cellular amino acid or peptide transporters. Other compounds that have the requisite structural properties may also benefit from those transporting systems (e.g., gabapentin) [48]. This behavior may represent an important observation for the new generation of drugs being developed through the application of biotechnology (e.g., peptides), assuming such compounds are sufficiently stable in the GIT. Calcium channel blockers, such as nifedipine, have been shown to increase the absorption of amoxicillin and cefixime [46,47]. This may result from the role of calcium in the transport process, the inhibition of which (i.e., calcium channel blockers) enhances absorption.

In direct contrast with specialized transport of a drug into the epithelial cell is a process referred to as "efflux transport"; the facilitated movement of a drug out of the cell. This phenomenon explains the resistance of cancerous cells to some chemotherapeutic agents [49]. It is now apparent that this mechanism exists in epithelial cells of numerous organ systems, including the GIT, liver, lung, kidney and brain [50]. There is a cell surface glycoprotein (P-glycoprotein; P-gp), a multidrug-resistance protein (MDR), that is responsible for the efflux mechanism. This protein belongs to a large family of glycosylated membrane proteins referred to as ATP-binding cassette (ABC) transporters. As depicted in Fig. 9D, the cell surface glycoprotein will attach to the drug molecule and escort it out of the cell and back into the gut lumen, hence the term "efflux transporter." The presence of this protein in the GIT has significant implications for drug absorption and bioavailability (e.g., Refs. 51,52). Substrates for this transporter have a diverse range of structures and include compounds such as [51]: anticancer agents (e.g., anthracyclines, taxol, and vinblastine); cardioactive drugs (e.g., digoxin, phenytoin, quinidine, and verapamil); immunosuppressants (e.g., cyclosporine and tacrolimus); erythromycin, quinine, etc. The P-gp protein may be inhibited or induced and the efflux transport process may be saturated. The former is the basis for many potential drug-drug and nutrient-drug interactions, and the latter limits the efficacy of the transporter.

It is difficult to unequivocally implicate P-gp as the mechanism of an interaction resulting in altered absorption. The reason for this is that the absorbing intestinal cells are rich in metabolizing enzymes, especially those responsible for phase I oxidative metabolism, the cytochrome P450 family (CYP450). Within that family the most significant isozyme is CYP3A4, since it is less selective of substrates (a "promiscuous" enzyme), and, as a result, it accounts for about 50% of all drug-drug and nutrient-drug interactions. P-gp and CYP3A4 are present in the same locations, and they both appear to share the same substrates. As a consequence, it is almost impossible to ascribe alterations in absorption to be the exclusive result of either the efflux transporter or the enzyme. This is the case, for example, for cyclosporine, whose absorption is enhanced in the presence of several drugs (e.g., ketoconazole), which may be due to inhibition of P-gp efflux or inhibition of CYP3A4 metabolic activity or both [52,53]. A further complication is the need to consider the systemic effect of altered P-gp activity on drug clearance, an effect that is independent of the absorption process.

The significance of P-gp, however, in affecting absorption and bioavailability of P-gp substrate drugs can be seen in studies in knockout mice that do not have intestinal P-gp. The gene responsible for producing that protein has been knocked out of the genetic repertoire. Those animals evidenced a sixfold increase in plasma concentrations (and AUC, area under the plasma concentration-time curve) of the anticancer drug paclitaxel (Taxol) compared to the control animals [54]. Another line of evidence is the recent report of an interaction between the β-adrenergic blocking agent talinolol and digoxin [55]. Talinolol co-administration resulted in a significant increase in digoxin plasma concentrations (and AUC), and, since talinolol does not appear to be a substrate for CYP3A3, the effect on absorption may be attributed to inhibition of P-gp, which normally modulates digoxin absorption.

IV. PHYSIOLOGICAL FACTORS GOVERNING DRUG ABSORPTION

A. Components and Properties of Gastrointestinal Fluids

The characteristics of aqueous GI fluids to which a drug product is exposed will exert an important influence on what happens to that dosage form in the tract and on the pattern of drug absorption. To appreciate clearly how physiological factors influence drug absorption, one must consider the influence of these variables on the dosage form per se, that is, how these variables influence drug dissolution in the aqueous GI fluids, and finally what influence these variables exert on absorption once the drug is in solution.

One important property of GI fluids is pH, which varies considerably along the length of the tract. The gastric fluids are highly acidic, usually ranging from pH 1 to 3.5. There appears to be a diurnal cycle of gastric acidity, the fluids being more acidic at night and fluctuating during the day, primarily in response to food ingestion. Gastric fluid pH generally increases when food is ingested and then slowly decreases over the next several hours, fluctuating from pH 1 to about 5 [56]. There is considerable intersubject variation, however, in GI fluid pH, depending on the general health of the subject, the presence of local disease conditions along the tract, types of food ingested, and drug therapy. Upper GI fluid pH appears to be independent of gender.

An abrupt change in pH is encountered when moving from the stomach to the small intestine. Pancreatic secretions (200–800 mL/day) have a high concentration of bicarbonate, which neutralizes gastric fluid entering the duodenum and thus helps regulate the pH of fluids in the upper intestinal region. Neutralization of acidic gastric fluids in the duodenum is important to avoid damage to the intestinal epithelium, prevent inactivation of pancreatic enzymes, and prevent precipitation of bile acids, which are poorly soluble at acid pH. The pH of intestinal fluids gradually increases when moving in the distal direction, ranging from approximately 5.7 in the pylorus to 7.7

in the proximal jejunum. The fluids in the large intestine are generally considered to have a pH of between 7 and 8.

Gastrointestinal fluid pH may influence drug absorption in a variety of ways. Since most drugs are weak acids or bases, and since the aqueous solubility of such compounds is influenced by pH, the rate of dissolution from a dosage form, particularly tablets and capsules, is dependent on pH. This is a result of the direct dependence of dissolution rate on solubility, as discussed in Chapter 6. Acidic drugs dissolve most readily in alkaline media and, therefore, will have a greater rate of dissolution in intestinal fluids compared to gastric fluids. Basic drugs will dissolve most readily in acidic solutions, and, thus, the dissolution rate will be greater in gastric fluids compared to intestinal fluids. Since dissolution is a prerequisite step to absorption and is often the slowest process, especially for poorly water-soluble drugs, pH will exert a major influence on the overall absorption process. Furthermore, since the major site of drug absorption is the small intestine, it would seem that poorly soluble basic drugs (e.g., dipyridamole, ketaconazole, and diazepam) must first dissolve in the acidic gastric fluids in order to be well absorbed from the intestine, as the dissolution rate in intestinal fluids will be low. In addition, the disintegration of some dosage forms, depending on their formulation, will be influenced by pH if they contain certain components (e.g., binding agents or disintegrants) whose solubility is pH sensitive. Several studies (e.g., Ref. 57) have indicated that if the specific products being examined were not first exposed to an acidic solution, the dosage form would not disintegrate and thus dissolution could not proceed.

A complication here, however, is noted with those drugs that exhibit a limited chemical stability in either acidic or alkaline fluids. Since the rate and extent of degradation is directly dependent on the concentration of drug in solution, an attempt is often made to retard dissolution in the fluid where degradation is seen. There are preparations of various salts or esters of drugs (e.g., erythromycin) that do not dissolve in gastric fluid and thus are not degraded there but which dissolve in intestinal fluid prior to absorption. A wide variety of chemical derivatives are used for such purposes.

As mentioned previously, pH will also influence the absorption of an ionizable drug once it is in solution, as outlined in the pH partition hypothesis. Most drugs, however, are best absorbed from the small intestine regardless of pK_a and pH. In some instances, especially lower down the GIT, there is the possibility of insoluble hydroxide formation of a drug or insoluble film formation with components of a dosage form, which reduces the extent of absorption of, for example, aluminum aspirin (in chewable tablets) [58,59], and iron [60]. The coadministration of acidic or alkaline fluids with certain drugs may exert an effect on the overall drug absorption process for any of the foregoing reasons.

Moreover, in addition to pH considerations, the GI fluids contain various materials that have been shown to influence absorption, particularly bile salts, enzymes, and mucin. Bile salts, which are highly surface active, may enhance the rate and/or extent of absorption of poorly water-soluble drugs by increasing the rate of dissolution in the GI fluids. This effect has been noted in in vitro experiments and has been seen as well with other natural surface-active agents (e.g., lysolecithin). Increased absorption of the poorly water-soluble drug griseofulvin after a fatty meal [61,62] may reflect the fact that bile is secreted into the gut in response to the presence of fats and the bile salts which are secreted increase the dissolution rate and absorption of the drug. The contrast agent, iopanoic acid, used in visualizing the gallbladder dissolves more rapidly and is better absorbed from the dog intestine in the presence of bile salts. Studies in rats have indicated enhanced intestinal drug absorption from bile salt solutions; however, the implication of these findings for humans are uncertain. Bile salts may also reduce drug absorption (e.g., neomycin and kanamycin) through the formation of water-insoluble, nonabsorbable complexes.

Since intestinal fluids contain large concentrations of various enzymes needed for digestion of food, it is reasonable to expect certain of these enzymes to act on a number of drugs. Pancreatic enzymes hydrolyze chloramphenicol palmitate. Pancreatin and trypsin are able to deacetylate *N*-acetylated drugs, and mucosal esterases appear to attack various esters of penicillin. Oral cocaine ingestion is generally ineffective in producing a pharmacological response because of efficient hydrolysis by esterase enzymes in the gut. This is not true at very large doses, however, such as those resulting from the rupture of bags containing the drug which are ingested to avoid detection at international borders.

Mucin, a viscous mucopolysaccharide that lines and protects the intestinal epithelium, has been thought to bind certain drugs nonspecifically (e.g., quarternary ammonium compounds) and thereby prevent or reduce absorption. This behavior may partially account for the erratic and incomplete absorption of such charged compounds. Mucin may also represent a barrier to drug diffusion prior to reaching the intestinal membrane.

B. Gastric Emptying

Physiologists have for many years been interested in factors that influence gastric emptying and the regulatory mechanisms controlling this process. Our interest in gastric emptying is based on the fact that, since most drugs are best absorbed from the small intestine, any factor that delays movement of drug from the stomach to the small intestine will influence the rate (and possibly the extent) of absorption and therefore the time needed to achieve maximal plasma concentrations and pharmacological response. As a result, and in addition to rate of dissolution or inherent absorbability, gastric emptying may represent a limiting factor in drug absorption. Only in those rare instances where a drug is absorbed by a specialized process in the intestine will the amount of drug leaving the stomach exceed the capacity of the gut to absorb it.

Gastric emptying is determined with a variety of techniques using liquid or solid meals or other markers. Gastric emptying is quantitated by one of several mesurements including emptying time, emptying half-time ($t_{50\%}$), and emptying rate. Emptying time is the time needed for the stomach to empty the total initial stomach contents. Emptying half-time is the time it takes for the stomach to empty one half of its initial contents. Emptying rate is a measure of the speed of emptying. Note that the last two measures are inversely related (i.e., the greater the rate, the smaller the value for emptying half-time).

Gastric emptying and factors that affect that process need to be understood because of the implications for drug absorption and with regard to optimal dosage form design [63]. Gastric-emptying patterns are distinctly different depending upon the absence or presence of food. In the absence of food, the empty stomach and the intestinal tract undergo a sequence of repetitious events referred to as the interdigestive migrating motor (or myoelectric) complex (MMC) [64]. This complex results in the generation of contractions beginning with the proximal stomach and ending with the ileum. The first of four stages is one of minimal activity that lasts for about 1 hour. Stage 2, which lasts 30–45 minutes, is characterized by irregular contractions that gradually increase in strength leading to the next phase. The third phase, while only lasting 5–15 minutes, consists of intense peristaltic waves, which results in the emptying of all remaining gastric contents into the pylorus. The latter phase is sometimes referred to as the "housekeeper" wave. The fourth stage represents a transition of decreasing activity leading to the beginning of the next cycle (i.e., phase 1). The entire cycle lasts about 2 hours. Thus, a solid dosage form ingested on an empty stomach will remain in the stomach for a period of time dependent upon time of dosing relative to the occurrence of the housekeeper. The gastric residence time of a solid dosage form will vary from perhaps 5–15 minutes (if ingested at the beginning of the housekeeper) to about 2 hours or longer (if ingested at the end of the housekeeper wave). It would not be surprising, however, for gastric residence time to be substantially longer. This variability in gastric residence time may explain some of the intersubject variation in rate of absorption, and it raises some question concerning the term "ingested on an empty stomach." While it is quite common in clinical research studies for a panel of subjects to ingest a solid test dosage form following an overnight fast and, therefore, on an empty stomach, it is unlikely that all subjects will be in the same phase of the migrating motor complex. It is the latter point rather than an empty stomach per se, that will determine when emptying occurs and, consequently, when drug absorption is initiated. The above considerations will not apply to liquid dosage forms, however, which are generally able to empty during all phases of the migrating motor complex.

Various techniques have been used to visualize the gastric emptying of dosage forms. Radiopaque tablets were found to undergo relatively mild agitation in the stomach—a point that needs to be considered in the design and interpretation of disintegration and dissolution tests. While single large solid dosage forms (e.g., tablets and capsules) rely upon the housekeeper wave for entry into the small intestine, some controversy remains about the influence of particle (or pellet) size (diameter and volume), shape, and density on gastric emptying. There has been a great deal of recent interest in this issue, which has been investigated primarily with use of gamma scintigraphy (a gamma-emitting material is ingested and externally monitored with a gamma camera). These studies are generally performed with the use of nondisintegrating pellets so that movement throughout the tract may be estimated. Particles as large as 5–7 mm may leave the stomach. It is likely that there is a range of particle sizes that will empty from the stomach, rather than there being an abrupt cut-off value. The range of values among individuals will be affected by the size of the pylorus diameter and the relative force of propulsive contractions generated by the stomach. The interest in this issue stems from the desire to develop sustained-release dosage forms that would have sufficient residence time in the GIT to provide constant drug release over an extended time. Experimental dosage forms that have been investigated include floating tablets, bioadhesives (that attach to the gastric mucosa), dense pellets, and large dimension forms.

Eating interrupts the interdigestive migrating motor complex. Gastric emptying in the presence of solid or liquid food is controlled by a complex variety of mechanical, hormonal, and neural mechanisms. Receptors lining the stomach, duodenum, and jejunum that assist in controlling gastric emptying include mechanical receptors in the stomach which respond to distension; acid receptors in the stomach and duodenum; osmotic receptors in the duodenum, which respond to electrolytes, carbohydrates and amino acids; fat receptors in the jejunum; and L-tryptophan receptors. Neural control appears to be through the inhibitory vagal system (the exact neurotransmitter is not known but may be dopamine and enkephalin). Hormones involved in controlling emptying include cholecystokinin and gastrin, among others.

As food enters the stomach the fundus and body regions relax to accommodate the meal. Upon reaching the stomach, food tends to form layers that are stratified in the order in which the food was swallowed, and this material is mixed with gastric secretions in the antrum. Nonviscous fluid moves into the antrum, passing around any solid mass. Gastric emptying will begin once a considerable portion of the gastric contents become liquid enough to pass the pylorus. Peristaltic waves begin in the fundus region, travel to the prepyloric area, and become more intense in the pylorus. The antrum and pyloric sphincter contract and the proximal duodenum relaxes. A moment later the antrum relaxes and the duodenum regains its tone. The pyloric sphincter will remain contracted momentarily to prevent regurgitation, and the contents in the duodenum are then propelled forward. Emptying is accomplished by the antral and pyloric waves, and the rate of emptying is regulated by factors controlling the strength of antral contraction. Gastric emptying is influenced primarily by meal volume, the presence of acids, certain nutrients, and osmotic pressure. Distension of the stomach is the only natural stimulus known to increase the emptying rate. Fat in any form in the presence of bile and pancreatic juice produces the greatest inhibition of gastric emptying. This strong inhibitory influence of fats permits time for their digestion, as they are the slowest of all foods to be digested. Meals containing substantial amounts of fat can delay gastric emptying for 3–6 hours or more. These various factors appear to alter gastric emptying by interacting with the receptors noted above.

Other than meal volume per se all of the other factors noted above result in a slowing of gastric emptying (e.g., nutrients, osmotic pressure, and acidity). It is important to recognize that a host of other factors are known to influence emptying rate. Thus, a variety of drugs can alter absorption of other drugs via their effect on emptying. For example, anticholinergics and narcotic analgesics reduce gastric-emptying rate, while metoclopramide increases that rate. A reduced rate of drug absorption is expected in the former instance and an increased rate in the latter. The following factors should be recognized: body position (reduced rate lying on left side), viscosity (rate decreases with increased viscosity), and emotional state (reduced rate during depression, increased rate during stress). As an illustration, one recent report indicates that absorption rate (and potentially completeness of absorption) may be altered when comparing posture—lying on the left or right side [65]. Acetaminophen and nifedipine absorption rates were faster when the subjects were lying on the right compared to the left side, suggesting more rapid gastric emptying. In the case of nifedipine, the extent of absorption was greater when the subjects were lying on the right side, which may be due to transient saturation of a presystemic metabolic process (this is discussed in a later section). Miscellaneous factors whose exact effect on emptying may vary, include gut disease, exercise, obesity, gastric surgery, and bulimia.

Many investigators have suggested that gastric emptying takes place by an exponential (i.e., first-order kinetic) process. As a result, plots of log volume remaining in the stomach versus time will provide a straight-line relationship. The slope of this line will represent a rate constant associated with emptying. This relationship is not strictly linear, however, especially at early and later times, but the approximation is useful in that one can express a half-time for emptying ($t_{50\%}$). Hopkins [66] has suggested a linear relationship between the square root of the volume remaining in the stomach versus time. There may be a physical basis for this relationship, since the radius of a cylinder varies with the square root of the volume and the circumferential tension is proportional to the radius. Methods for analyzing gastric emptying data have been reviewed [67].

Gastric-emptying rate is influenced by a large number of factors, as noted above. Many of these factors account for the large variation in emptying among different individuals and variation within an individual on different occasions. Undoubtedly, much of this variation in emptying is reflected in variable drug absorption. Although gastric emptying probably has little major influence on drug absorption from solution, emptying of solid dosage forms does exert an important influence on drug dissolution and absorption. A prime example is enteric-coated tablets, which are designed to prevent drug release in the stomach. Any delay in the gastric emptying of these forms will delay dissolution, absorption, and the onset time for producing a response. Since these dosage forms must empty as discrete units, the drug is either in the stomach or the intestine. The performance of this dosage form can be seriously hampered if it is taken with or after a meal, as emptying is considerably delayed. Furthermore, if the drug is to be taken in a multiple-dosing fashion, there is a possibility that the first dose will not leave the stomach until the next dose is taken, resulting in twice the desired dose getting into the intestine at one time. Blythe et al. [68] administered several enteric-coated aspirin tablets containing $BaSO_4$ and radiologically examined emptying of these tablets. The tablets emptied in these subjects anywhere from 0.5 to 7 hours after ingestion. Tablets will empty more rapidly when given prior to a meal compared to administration after a meal. One potential way of improving the emptying and release pattern of enteric-coated products is to use capsules containing enteric-coated microgranules. The median time for 50% and 90% emptying of such a dosage form has been shown to be 1 and 3–3.5 hours, respectively [69].

Several recent publications have reviewed the effects of food on drug absorption in humans [70–72]. The effect of food on the gastrointestinal absorption of drugs is complex and multidimensional. We are only now beginning to understand this complexity. The physical presence of food in the GIT may play a significant role in affecting the efficient absorption of a drug from an oral dosage form. The ultimate effect of food on the rate and/or extent of gastrointestinal absorption is a function of numerous interacting variables. While some general rules may be postulated, the effect of food on a given drug and its dosage form will require, in general, individual investigation. The U.S. Food and Drug Administration (FDA) has recognized this complexity and requires that all dosage forms that do not immediately release drug (e.g., controlled release formulations) undergo a food-effects study in humans, for which a "Guidance" has been written (these are available on the FDA webpage—fda.gov). The precedence for this requirement is the observation that a sustained release formulation may "dose-dump" its entire contents of drug in the presence of food, and, since the dose is several times the usual single dose, this may lead to toxicity [73,74].

The extent to which food will alter absorption depends upon factors such as physical chemical characteristics of the drug (e.g., aqeuous solubility, oil/water partition coefficient, and stability in gut fluids), the dose of drug, the characteristics of the dosage form, time of drug administration relative to food ingestion, amount of food, and type of food. The schematic in Fig. 11 summarizes the variables that food is able to affect, which in turn are associated with the sequential steps of drug release, dissolution, absorption, systemic availability, and elimination. Notice the two heavy arrows for the dissolution and absorption steps. One of those two processes is generally associated with the rate-limiting step in the overall absorption of a drug. Therefore, when food affects drug absorption, it most often does so by affecting the factors influencing dissolution or transport. Most of the factors noted in Fig. 11 are self-explanatory, but many will be discussed with examples in the following sections.

It is useful to consider the schematic in Fig. 11 and the most important rate-limiting steps in drug absorption in conjunction with what has become known as the Biopharmaceutical Classification System (BCS). The latter system attempts to classify drugs in terms of their aqueous solubility and membrane permeability and, from that classification, predict the most likely behavior of the drug with regard to absorption following oral administration. FDA is proposing to use this approach in establishing regulatory standards for new drug entities and for generic versions of marketed drugs. The BCS can be easily understood from the simple two-by-two matrix illustrated in Fig. 12. Drug behavior with respect to aqueous solubility and membrane permeability may be described by one of four possible conditions noted as I to IV. The effects of food on the absorption behavior of compounds classified according to the BCS has been discussed thoroughly elsewhere [71], and they will be highlighted here.

Class I compounds have both good solubility and permeability and generally offer no problems with regard to having a good absorption profile (e.g., acetaminophen, disopyramide, ketoprofen, metoprolol, nonsteroidal anti-inflammatory agents, valproic acid, verapamil). In general, one would not expect the presence of food to influence the absorption of this class

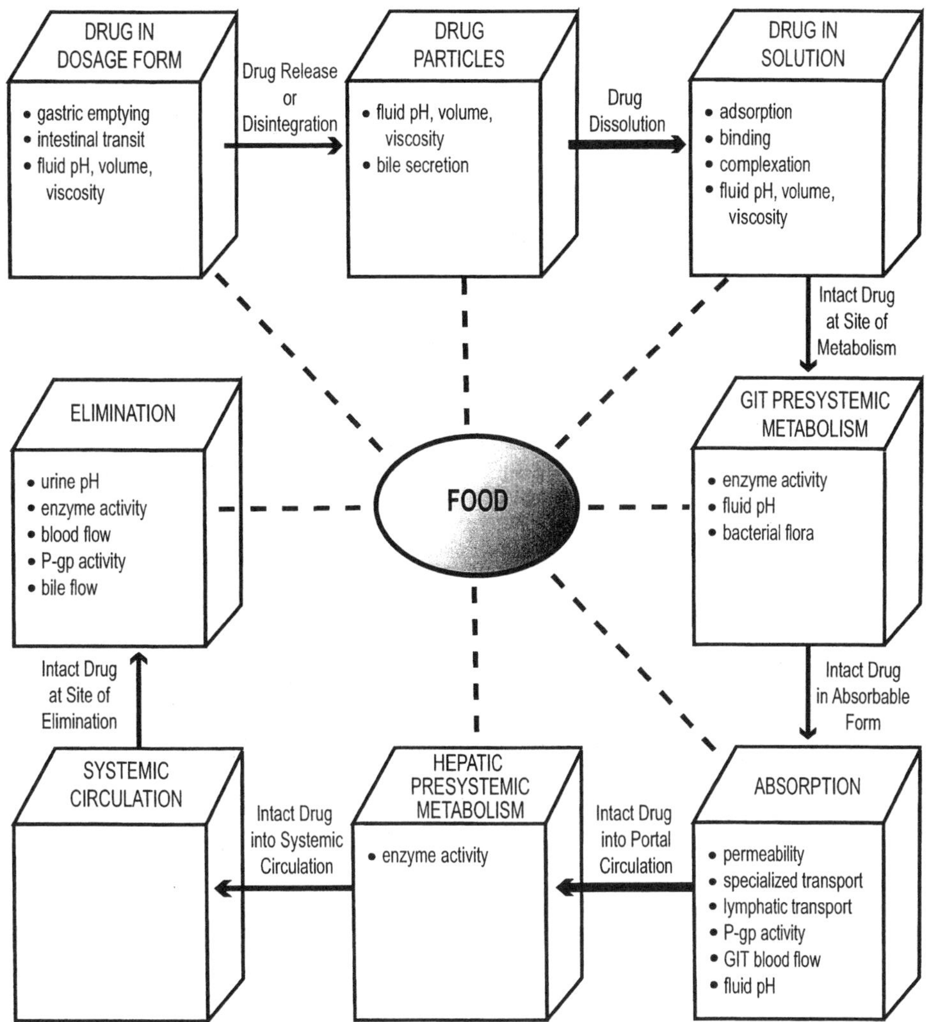

Fig. 11 The influence of food on factors that affect the sequential steps leading to GIT drug absorption, systemic availability, and elimination. (Copyright © 2000 Saguaro Technical Press, Inc., used with permission.)

of drug. The onset or rate of absorption may be delayed by the presence of food as a consequence of reduced gastric-emptying rate, but the completeness of absorption should not be compromised.

Drugs in Class II have low aqueous solubility (but high membrane permeability), and any factor affecting dissolution rate would be expected to have an impact on the absorption of such compounds. Factors that are noted in Fig. 11, such as fluid pH, volume and viscosity, and bile secretion (especially in response to fatty foods), might be expected to play a role in dissolution rate and thereby affect absorption. Compounds that fall into this class include carbamazepine, cyclosporin, digoxin, griseofulvin, and spironolactone. Food would be expected to exert a potentially significant affect on the absorption of the drugs in this class. The absorption of many compounds in this class is improved in the presence of a fatty meal. Improved absorption occurs because of the secretion of bile in response to fat and the surfactant and solubilizing properties that bile salts exert on poorly water-soluble compounds (griseofulvin is a classic example). The presence of food, especially fatty foods, will delay gastric emptying and intestinal transit, which in turn allow for more time for drug dissolution and absorption.

Drugs in Class III have good aqueous solubility but poor membrane permeability (e.g., bidisomide, bisphosphonates, captopril, and furosemide). Food and food components would only be expected to influence absorption of drugs in this class if they affected some aspect

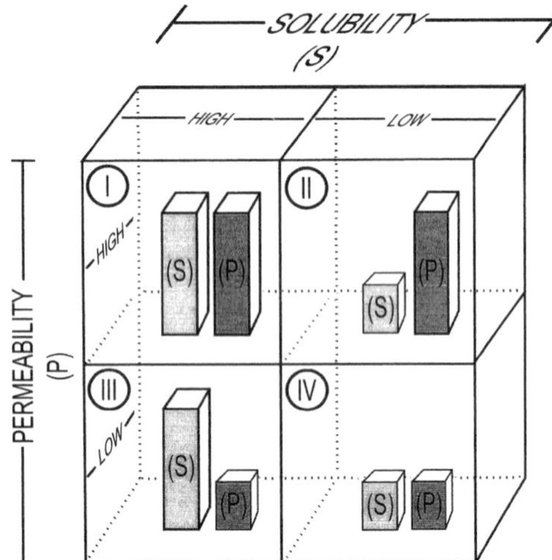

Fig. 12 Illustration of the Biopharmaceutical Classification System (BCS), which classifies drug absorption potential on the basis of aqueous solubility or membrane permeability. (Copyright © 2000 Saguaro Technical Press, Inc., used with permission.)

of membrane permeability or function or if the permeable form of the molecule was altered (e.g., through ionization). Many of these compounds tend to be absorbed in relatively well defined and limited areas of the upper small intestine. As a consequence, the physical presence of food may affect the time during which the drug resides at sites of maximal absorption. Food and the viscous milieu that it creates in gut fluids may also create a significant physical barrier to the diffusion of the drug to sites of absorption along the GIT membrane. Several compounds that fall into this class illustrate reduced absorption in the presence of food.

Class IV drugs have low aqueous solubility and poor membrane permeability and as such are often considered as poor drug candidates for oral administration. Other routes of administration may need to be considered. For example, neomycin falls into this category, and its oral use is to achieve sterilization of the gut. There is too little information about these compounds and the effect of food to offer general observations.

A drug should always be ingested with a cup of water (~ 8 oz) to insure easy transit down the esophagus and to provide fluid for disintegration and dissolution. Whether or not the drug should be taken on an empty stomach (e.g., enteric-coated tablets) or with food will depend upon the specific drug as noted above.

Drugs that should be taken with food include those compounds that are irritating to the tract (e.g., phenylbutazone or nitrofurantoin), those compounds absorbed high in the tract by a specialized mechanism (e.g., riboflavin and ascorbic acid), and those compounds for which the presence of certain food constituents are known to enhance absorption (e.g., griseofluvin). For those compounds that irritate the tract, perhaps the best recommendation is to ingest the drug with or after a light meal that does not contain fatty foods or constituents known to interact with the drug. Nitrofurantoin absorption is improved in the presence of food [75,76]. Riboflavin and ascorbic acid, which are absorbed by a specialized process high in the small intestine, are best absorbed when gastric emptying is delayed by the presence of food [39,77]. As the residence time of the vitamins in the upper portion of the intestine is prolonged, contact with absorption sites is increased and absorption becomes more efficient (i.e., saturation of transporters is avoided). The influence of food on the absorption of those vitamins is illustrated in Fig. 13 along with improved efficacy of ascorbic acid absorption achieved by administering divided doses.

The absorption of griseofulvin, which is a very poorly water-soluble drug, is enhanced when it is coadministered with a fatty meal as discussed previously [61,62]. The importance of gastric emptying can probably be most readily appreciated by those investigators who have examined drug absorption in patients after a partial or total gastrectomy. Muehlberger [78] notes that,

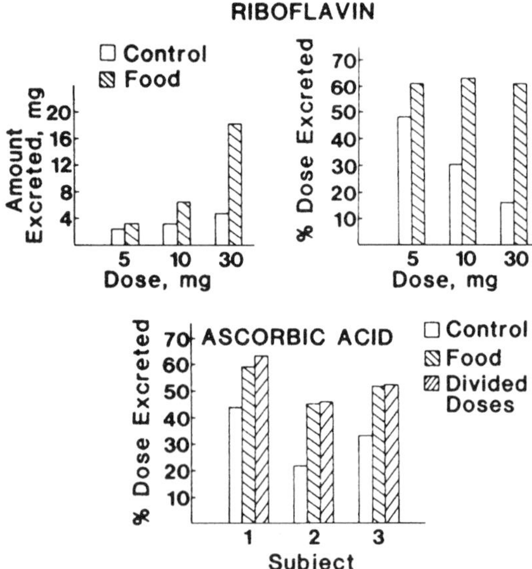

Fig. 13 (Top) Influence of food on the absorption of different doses of riboflavin. (Bottom) Influence of food and divided doses on ascorbic acid absorption in three subjects. (Based on data from Refs. 39 and 77.)

following a near-total gastrectomy, patients often complain of a "sensitivity" to alcohol. This is probably best explained by ethanol moving rapidly from the poorly absorbing surface of the stomach to the small intestine, where absorption will be rapid. Gastric emptying has been shown to be important in oral L-dopa therapy, and it has been noted [79] that patients with a partial gastrectomy or gastrojejunostomy exhibit a prompt response with less than average doses of the drug. This observation is consistent with rapid absorption from the small intestine in such patients and is essentially equivalent to introduction of the drug into the duodenum. Similar conclusions have been reached for aspirin and warfarin absorption [80,81].

For many drugs, as has been shown for acetaminophen, there will be a direct relationship between gastric-emptying rate and maximal plasma concentration and an inverse relationship between gastric-emptying rate and the time required to attain maximal plasma concentrations. Those relationships are illustrated in Figs. 14A and B. Also shown is the influence of a narcotic (heroin) on the gastric emptying and absorption of acetaminophen (Figs. 14C and D). In attempting to predict such relationships, however, it is essential that one consider the physicochemical characteristics of the drug. While increased gastric-emptying rate will probably increase the rate (and possibly the extent) of absorption for drugs best absorbed from the small intestine from rapidly dissolving dosage forms, the converse may be true in other circumstances. For example, if the dosage form must first be exposed to the acidic gastric fluids to initiate disintegration or dissolution, rapid emptying may reduce the rate and extent of absorption. Similarly, if the drug dissolves slowly from the dosage form, a shortened residence time in the gut may reduce the extent of dissolution and absorption. One needs a good deal of fundamental understanding of the chemistry of the drug, its dosage form, and the absorption mechanism before being able to anticipate or rationalize the influence of these various factors on the efficacy of absorption.

A final point that should be mentioned here, although it has received relatively little attention, is that of esophageal transit. Delay in movement down the esophagus will delay absorption and, in addition, for certain drugs, may also cause local mucosal damage. Capsule disintegration has been observed to occur in the esophagus within 3–5 minutes. Esophageal transit is delayed when solid dosage forms are swallowed with little fluid or when the subject is supine [84,85]. Antipyrine absorption from capsules [86] has been shown to be delayed when esophageal transit was prolonged. To avoid this delay the dosage form should be swallowed with water or other fluids, and the subject should be in a standing or sitting position.

C. Intestinal Transit

Once a dosage form empties from the stomach and enters the small intestine, it will be exposed to an

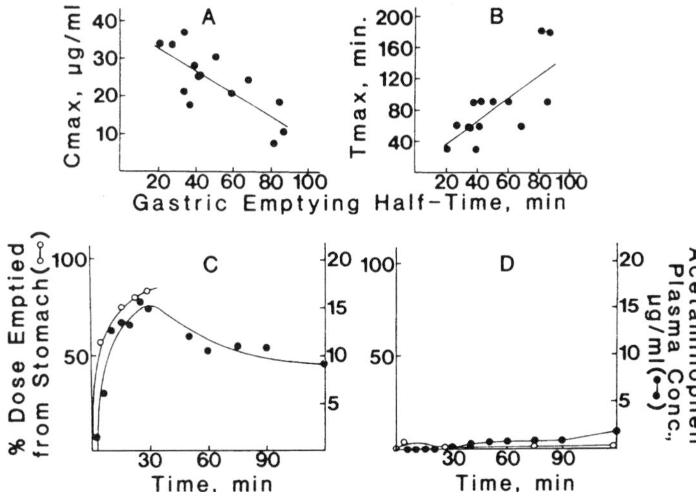

Fig. 14 (A, B) Maximum acetaminophen plasma concentration ($C_{\max}$) and time to achieve that concentration ($T_{\max}$) as a function of gastric emptying half-time. (From Ref. 82.) (C) Percent of an acetaminophen dose emptied from the stomach (O) and acetaminophen plasma concentrations (●) as a function of time in one subject. (D) The same plot and for the same subject as in (C) after a 10 mg intramuscular dose of heroin. (C and D from Ref. 83.)

environment totally different from that in the stomach, as discussed previously. Since the small intestine is the primary site of drug absorption, the longer the residence time in this region, the greater the potential for complete absorption, assuming that the drug is stable in the intestinal fluids and will not form water-insoluble derivatives.

There are primarily two types of intestinal movements: propulsive and mixing. Propulsive movements, generally synonymous with peristalsis, will determine intestinal transit rate and therefore the residence time of a drug in the intestine. This time of residence is important since it will dictate the amount of time the dosage form has in which to release the drug, permit dissolution, and allow for absorption. Obviously, the greater the intestinal motility, the shorter the residence time and the less time there is for those processes to proceed. Intestinal motility will be most important for those dosage forms that release drug slowly (e.g., sustained-release products) or require time to initiate release (e.g., enteric-coated products), as well as those drugs that dissolve slowly or where absorption is maximal only in certain regions of the intestine. Peristaltic waves propel intestinal contents down the tract at about 1–2 cm/s. Peristaltic activity is increased after a meal as a result of the gastroenteric reflex initiated by distension of the stomach and results in increased motility and secretion.

Mixing movements of the small intestine are a result of contractions dividing a given region of the intestine into segments producing an appearance similar to a chain of sausages. These contractions result in the mixing of the intestinal contents with secretions several times a minute. These movements bring the gut contents into optimal contact with the surface epithelium and thereby provide a larger effective area for absorption. In addition, the muscularis mucosa produces folds in the surface epithelium, resulting in an increased surface area and rate of absorption. The villi contract during this process, which results in a "milking" action so that lymph flows from the central lacteal into the lymphatic system.

These mixing motions will tend to improve drug absorption for two reasons. Any factor that increases rate of dissolution will increase the rate (and possibly the extent) of absorption, especially for poorly water-soluble drugs (BCS Classes II and IV). Since rate of dissolution depends on agitation intensity, mixing movements will tend to increase dissolution rate and thereby influence absorption. As rate of absorption depends directly on membrane surface area, and since mixing increases the contact area between drug and membrane, these motions will tend to increase rate of absorption.

Metoclopramide will increase the rate of gastric emptying, which will often, but not always, increase the rate of drug absorption. However, metoclopramide will also increase the rate of intestinal transit and thus reduce the residence time in the intestine. These two effects may have an opposing influence on absorption. The net effect on absorption depends on the characteristics of the drug and its dosage form as well as the mechanism of absorption. Metoclopramide or similar-acting drugs will probably have little if any effect on absorption of a drug given orally in solution, unless the compound (e.g., riboflavin) is absorbed by a specialized process high in the small intestine, in which case there is likely to be a reduction in the amount absorbed. Metoclopramide will probably increase the rate of absorption of a drug from a solid dosage form because of its effect on gastric emptying if the drug is rapidly released and readily dissolved. On the other hand, if the drug dissolves slowly from the dosage form, the extent of absorption may be reduced as a result of shortened residence time in the intestine, even though gastric-emptying rate is increased. Similar reasoning may be applied to the influence on drug absorption of various anticholinergics (e.g., atropine and propantheline) and narcotic analgesics that reduce gastric emptying and intestinal transit rates. While there will be a reduction in gastric-emptying rate and thus a delay in absorption, these compounds will increase intestinal transit time and possibly increase the extent of absorption, particularly for slowly dissolving drugs or dosage forms that release drug slowly.

Transit through the small intestine appears to be quite different in a variety of ways from movement through the stomach. Once emptied from the stomach, material (such as pellets and tablets) will move along the small intestine and reach the ileocecal valve in about 3 hours. While this value may range from about 1 to 6 hours, intestinal residence time appears to be relatively consistent among normal subjects [87]. Values similar to this have been found for food and water movement along the small intestine. Transit appears to be less dependent upon the physical nature of the material (liquid vs. solid and size of solids) compared to the response of the stomach. Furthermore, food appears not to influence intestinal transit as it does gastric emptying.

Three to four hours in the small intestine is a relatively short time for a dosage form to completely dissolve or release drug and then be absorbed. This time would be even more critical to the performance of poorly water-soluble drugs, slowly dissolving coated dosage forms (enteric or polymer coated), and sustained-release forms. Assuming minimal absorption from the colon (discussed below), gastric residence time may prove a critical issue to the performance of certain drugs and drug dosage forms (especially those in the latter categories) as a result of the relatively short intestinal residence time.

There is less information available concerning the factors that may influence intestinal transit time compared to what we know about gastric residence time. Although based upon small populations, there appear to be no gender-related differences in intestinal transit time [88], while vegetarians appear to have longer intestinal transit times compared to nonvegetarians [89]. The latter point may have implications for drug therapy in the third world where the diet is primarily vegetarian. Other factors that result in an increased transit time include reduced digestive fluid secretion, reduced thyroxin secretion, and pregnancy [90–92].

The distal portion of the GIT, the colon (see Fig. 1), has as its primary function water and electrolyte absorption and the storage of fecal matter prior to its being expelled. The proximal half of the colon is concerned with absorption and the distal half with storage. Although there are mixing and propulsive movements in the colon, they tend to be rather sluggish. Large circular constrictions occur in the colon that are similar to the segmenting contractions seen in the small intestine. The longitudinal muscles lining the colon also contract, producing a bulging similar in appearance to sacs and referred to as haustrations. These movements increase the surface area of the colon and result in efficient water absorption.

Contents within the colon are propelled down the tract not by peristaltic waves but by a "mass movement," which occurs only several times a day, being most abundant the first hour after breakfast as a result of a duodenocolonic reflex. The greatest proportion of time moving down the GIT is spent by a meal moving through the colon. In the presence of a diarrheal condition, fluid absorption is incomplete, which results in a watery stool.

Colonic residence time is considerably longer than in other parts of the GIT, and it is also more variable. The transit time can be as short as several hours to as long as 50–60 hours. Transit along the colon is characterized by abrupt movement and long periods of stasis. In one study of 49 healthy subjects the average colonic residence time was 35 hours with the following times associated with different regions: 11 hours in the right (ascending) colon, 11 hours in the left (descending) colon, and 12 hours in the rectosigmoid colon [93]. The latter values do not appear to be influenced by particle size (i.e., pellets vs. tablet), but these times are highly variable and are shortened in response to ingestion of a laxative (average time for a 5 mm tablet in the ascending colon of 8.7 vs. 13.7 hours) [94,95]. Furthermore, the ingestion of food, which is known to increase colonic activity, does not appear to have a dramatic effect on the movement of dosage forms from the ileum into the colon or on the movement within the colon [96]. Any differences in colonic transit times as a function of age and gender are not clear at this time due to conflicting reports and investigation in small populations of subjects.

The colonic mucosal pH varies along the length of the colon: right colon, pH 7.1; transverse colon, pH 7.4; left colon, pH 7.5; sigmoid colon, pH, 7.4; rectum, pH 7.2. These values were determined in a group of 21 subjects (mean age 54 years), and they are somewhat higher than previous estimates (pH $\sim$ 6.7 in the right colon) [97]. Those values contrast with the proximal small intestine with a pH of about 6.6 and the terminal ileum with a pH of about 7.4. This near-neutral pH in conjunction with low enzymatic activity has made the colon an interesting potential site for drug absorption. Indeed, there is active interest in delivery of drug dosage forms to the colon for site-specific absorption, especially for peptides (e.g., Refs. 63,98). Characteristics of the colon that are thought to provide a good environment for drug absorption include mild pH, little enzyme activity, and long residence time. The disadvantages of the colon, however, include several considerations that substantially limit this area for providing good absorption: small surface area, relatively viscous fluid-like environment (which varies along the length of the colon), and the large colonies of bacteria. The latter factors would limit dissolution and contact with the absorbing surface membrane and could result in presystemic drug metabolism.

The intention of colon-specific drug delivery is to prevent the drug from being released from the dosage form (by coating or other release-controlling mechanism) until it reaches the distal end of the large intestine (i.e., the ileocecal valve). Drug release needs to be delayed for about 5 hours, but clearly this delay time will vary from patient to patient and will depend upon a host of factors that may affect gastric emptying and intestinal transit (e.g., food, drugs, etc.). The dosage form should then release drug over the next 10–15 hours while in the colon. The results of studies that have examined colonic absorption are not that encouraging, although they do indicate that absorption does occur but to a variable extent (depending on the drug). The hormone calcitonin provided an absolute bioavailability from the colon of <1%; however, no comparison to oral dosing was made [99]. The relative bioavailability of ranitidine solution from the cecum was about 15% of that following gastric or jejunal administration [100]. Benazepril relative bioavailability following a colonic infusion was about 23% that of an oral solution [101]. Figure 15 illustrates the plasma concentration–time profiles for those two drugs. The long-lasting analog of vasopressin, dDAVP, a nonapeptide, had a relative bioavailability of about 17 and 21% compared to duodenal and gastric (and jejunal) solution administration, respectively. Rectal administration provided absorption comparable to that from the colon [102]. Sumatriptan solution was absorbed from the cecum to an extent of about 23% compared to an oral (and jejunal) dose [103]. In all cases rate of absorption is substantially slower than from the upper regions of the GIT. Furthermore, in some instances the metabolite to parent drug concentration ratios change depending upon the site of administration, which may reflect a number of causes (e.g., different extent of presystemic metabolism, differences in metabolite absorption, etc.). The latter needs to be a consideration for those compounds whose metabolites are either pharmacologically active or toxic.

A relevant consideration of absorption from the colonic area is with regard to rectal drug administration. While this is not a frequently used route, it is employed to some extent, especially in infants, children, and those unable to swallow medication. Absorption from the rectum is generally considered to be relatively poor, at least in comparison to absorption from regions of the upper GIT. The reasons for this are essentially those outlined above for the colon: small absorbing surface area, little fluid content, and poor mixing movements. There are, in addition, two other considerations. First, the presence of fecal material may provide a site for adsorption, which can effectively compete for absorption. Second, the extent of absorption will be dependent upon the retention time of the dosage form in the rectum. This may be a critical issue for infants, who often have irregular bowel movements. The readers are referred to a review of this topic [104].

D. Blood Flow

The entire GIT is highly vascularized and therefore well perfused by the bloodstream. The splanchnic

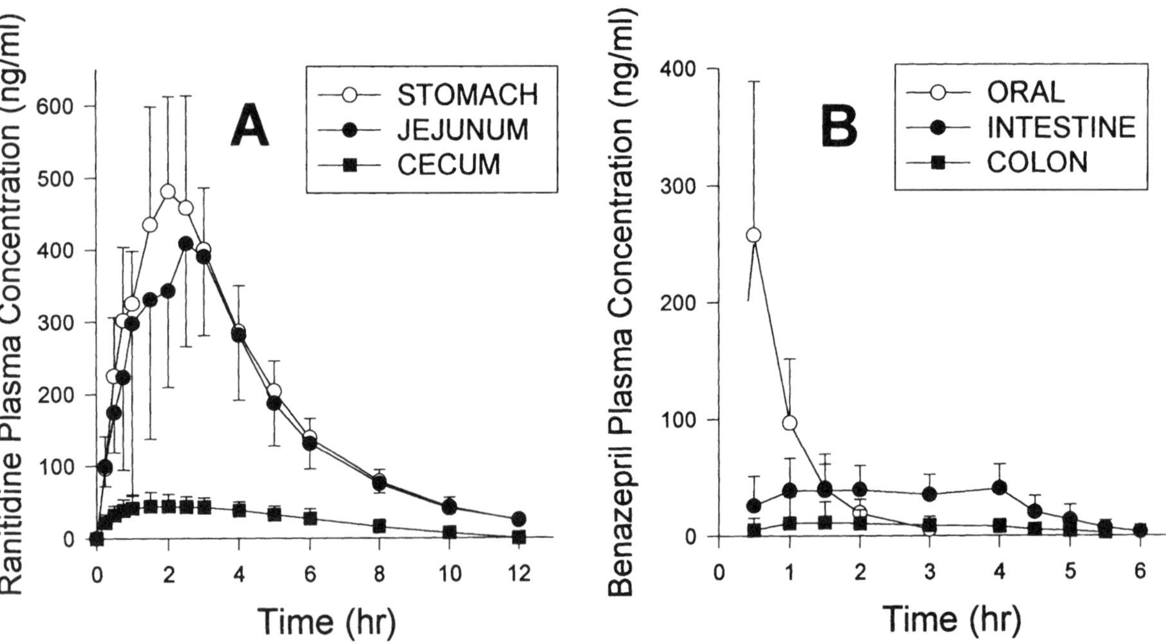

Fig. 15 (A) Ranitidine plasma concentrations as a function of time following administration of a solution into the stomach, jejunum, or cecum. Each value is the mean of eight subjects (the cross-hatched vertical bars are standard deviations). (Based on data in Ref. 100.) (B) Benazepril plasma concentrations as a function of time following a solution dose taken orally or administered as a 4-hour intestinal or 4-hour colonic infusion. Each value is the mean of 7–13 subjects. (Based on data in Ref. 101.)

circulation, which perfuses the GIT, receives about 28% of cardiac output, and this flow drains into the portal vein and then goes to the liver prior to reaching the systemic circulation. An absorbed drug will first go to the liver, which is the primary site of drug metabolism in the body; the drug may be metabolized extensively prior to systemic distribution. This has been referred to as the hepatic "first-pass" effect or presystemic hepatic elimination, and it has important implications in bioavailability and drug therapy.

The fact that the GIT is so well perfused by the bloodstream permits efficient delivery of absorbed materials to the body. As a result of this rapid blood perfusion, the blood at the site of absorption represents a virtual "sink" for absorbed material. Under normal conditions, then, there is never a buildup in drug concentration in the blood at the site of absorption. Therefore, the concentration gradient will favor further unidirectional transfer of drug from the gut to the blood. Usually, then, blood flow is not an important consideration in drug absorption. Generally, the properties of the dosage form (especially dissolution rate) or the compound's inherent absorbability will be the limiting factors in absorption.

There are circumstances, however, where blood flow to the GIT may influence drug absorption. Those compounds absorbed by active or specialized mechanisms require membrane participation in transport, which in turn depends on the expenditure of metabolic energy by intestinal cells. If blood flow and therefore oxygen delivery is reduced, there may be a reduction in absorption of those compounds. This has been shown to be the case in rats for the active absorption of phenylalanine [105].

The rate-limiting step in the absorption of those compounds that readily penetrate the intestinal membrane (i.e., have a large permeability coefficient) may be the rate at which blood perfuses the intestine. However, absorption will be independent of blood flow for those compounds that are poorly permeable. Extensive studies have illustrated this concept in rats [106,107]. The absorption rate of tritiated water, which is rapidly absorbed from the intestine, is dependent on intestinal blood flow, but a poorly absorbed compound, such as ribitol, penetrates the intestine at a rate independent of blood flow. In between these two extremes are a variety of intermediate compounds whose absorption rate is dependent on blood flow at low flow rates but independent of blood flow at higher flow rates. By altering blood flow to the intestine of the dog, as blood flow decreased the rate of sulfaethidole absorption also decreased [108]. These relationships are illustrated in Fig. 16.

An interesting clinical example of the influence of blood flow on drug absorption is that provided by Rowland et al. [109]. After oral ingestion of aspirin, one subject fainted while blood samples were being taken. Absorption ceased at the time of fainting but continued when the subject recovered. Interestingly, there was no reduction in the total amount of aspirin absorbed compared to another occasion when the subject did not faint. Another investigator observed a

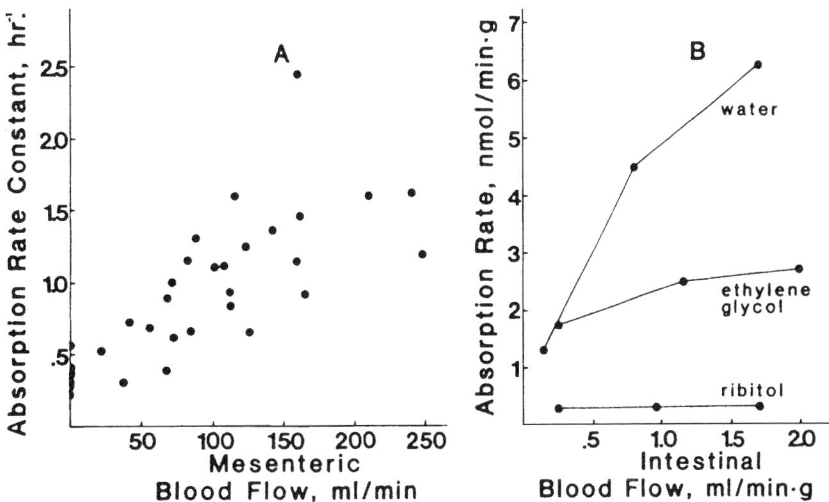

Fig. 16 (A) Absorption rate constant of sulfaethidole in dogs as a function of mesenteric blood flow. (Based on data from Ref. 108.) (B) Absorption rate of several compounds in rats as a function of intestinal blood flow. (Based on data from Ref. 107.)

3-hour delay in the absorption of sulfamethoxy-pyridazine in a patient who fainted [110]. The most reasonable explanation of these observations is the fact that in a fainting episode blood is preferentially shunted away from the extremities and other body organs, including the GIT, thereby reducing blood perfusion of the tract and resulting in a decreased rate of absorption. It is possible that generalized hypotensive conditions may be associated with altered drug absorption. In that regard, consideration needs to be given to the influence of congestive heart failure and other disease conditions that will alter gut blood flow as well as the presence of other drugs that may alter flow. For example, it has been suggested that digoxin absorption is impaired in congestive heart failure but improves after compensation [111]. The influence of such conditions on absorption has been reviewed elsewhere [112], but there is relatively little information available.

Blood flow to the GIT increases shortly after a meal and may last for several hours. Digestive processes in general seem to enhance blood flow to the tract. For the reasons discussed previously, however, coadministration of a drug with a meal would normally not be expected to improve drug absorption. Strenuous physical exercise appears to reduce blood flow to the tract and may reduce absorption rate.

V. COMPLICATING FACTORS IN DRUG ABSORPTION

A. Drug-Food and Drug-Drug Interactions

There are a variety of factors that may affect the rate or extent of absorption. Interactions in absorption are mediated by physical chemical, physiological, or biochemical factors. Physical chemical considerations include the characteristics of the dosage form and altered solubility, dissolution, and chemical stability within the GIT. Physiological factors include residence time in the tract (i.e., gastric emptying and intestinal transit rates) and blood flow to and the characteristics of the absorbing membrane. Biochemical factors would include enzymatic activity in the GIT. Drug-food and drug-drug interactions will alter absorption by one or more of the foregoing mechanisms.

As discussed previously, drug absorption may be impaired or improved when food is present in the GIT. Food may reduce the rate or extent of absorption by virtue of reduced gastric-emptying rate, which is particularly important for compounds unstable in gastric fluids and for dosage forms designed to release drug slowly. Food provides a rather viscous environment that will reduce the rate of drug dissolution and drug diffusion to the absorbing membrane. Drugs may also bind to food particles or react with gastrointestinal fluids secreted in response to the presence of food. An interesting example of the influence of food and gastric emptying on the fate of a drug in the body is that of *para*-aminobenzoic acid. This compound is metabolized in the body (acetylation) by a saturable process. The rate of presentation (i.e., the rate of absorption) of the drug to its site of metabolism will influence the extent of acetylation. The more rapid the absorption, the less the extent of acetylation since the capacity to metabolize is exceeded by the rate of presentation to the enzyme system. When absorption rate is reduced by slowing gastric emptying (e.g., with fat or glucose), a greater fraction of the dose is metabolized [113]. Similar observations have been made with respect to salicylamide absorption rate and metabolism [114].

There are problems as well in the absorption of certain drugs in the presence of specific food components. L-Dopa absorption may be inhibited in the presence of certain amino acids formed from the digestion of proteins [43]. The absorption of tetracycline is reduced by calcium salts present in dairy foods and by several other cations, including magnesium and aluminum [115–117], which are often present in antacid preparations. In addition, iron and zinc have been shown to reduce tetracycline absorption [118]. Figure 17 illustrates several of these interactions. These cations react with tetracycline to form a water-insoluble and nonabsorbable complex. Obviously, these offending materials should not be co-administered with tetracycline antibiotics.

The tetracycline example cited above is one type of physical-chemical interaction that may alter absorption. The relative influence of complexation on drug absorption will depend on the water-solubility of the drug, the water-solubility of the complex, and the magnitude of the interaction (i.e., the complexation stability constant). If the drug itself is poorly water-soluble, the absorption pattern will be governed by rate of dissolution. Often such compounds are incompletely and erratically absorbed. As a result, complexation will probably exert more of an influence on the absorption of such a compound than on one that is normally well absorbed, although this will depend on the nature of the complex. If the complex is water-insoluble, as in the case of tetracycline interactions with various metal cations, the fraction complexed will be unavailable for absorption. Although most complexation interactions are reversible, the greater the stability constant of the

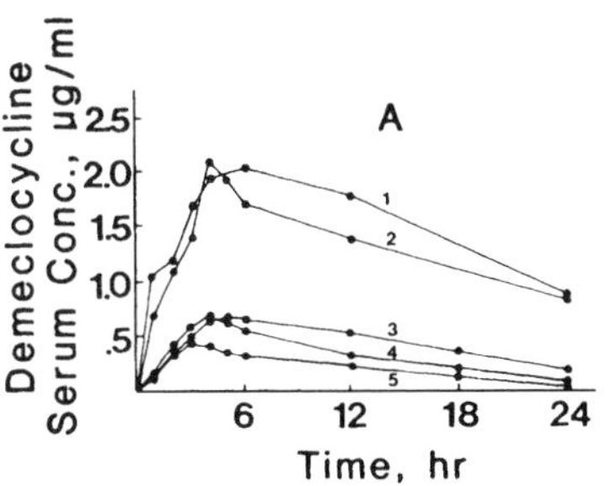

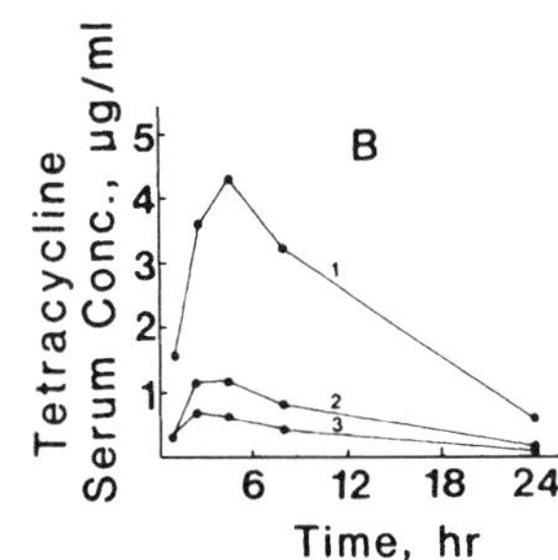

Fig. 17 (A) Demeclocycline serum concentrations as a function of time in four to six subjects after oral ingestion of demeclocycline in the absence or presence of dairy meals. Key: 1, meal (no dairy products); 2, water; 3, 110 g cottage cheese; 4, 240 mL buttermilk; 5, 240 mL whole milk. (Based on data from Ref. 117.) (B) Tetracycline serum concentrations as a function of time in six subjects after oral ingestion of tetracycline in the absence or presence of iron salts (equivalent to 40 mg elemental iron). Key: 1, control; 2, ferrous gluconate; 3, ferrous sulfate. (Based on data from Ref. 118.)

complex, the greater the relative influence on absorption. Generally, however, because the interaction is reversible, complexation is more likely to influence the rate than the extent of absorption.

Drug complexation is sometimes used in preparing pharmaceutical dosage forms to improve stability or solubility or to prolong drug release. There are several examples, however, where a drug complex results in reduced absorption. Amphetamine interacts with sodium carboxymethyl cellulose to form a poorly water-soluble derivative, and a decrease in absorption is seen [119]. Phenobarbital absorption is reduced as a result of interaction with polyethylene glycol 4000 [120]. These large macromolecules have the potential to bind many drugs.

Surface-active agents, because they are able to form micelles above the critical micelle concentration, may bind drugs either by inclusion within the micelle (solubilization) or by attachment to its surface. Below the critical micelle concentration, surfactant monomers have a membrane-disrupting effect, which can enhance drug penetration across a membrane. The latter influence has been seen in drug absorption studies in animals. The influence of surface-active agents on drug absorption will depend on the surfactant concentration and the physicochemical characteristics of the drug. If the drug is capable of partitioning from the aqueous to the micellar phase, and if the micelle is not absorbed, which is usually the case, there may be a reduction in rate of absorption. Micellar concentrations of sodium lauryl sulfate or polysorbate 80 (Tween 80) increase the rectal absorption rate of potassium iodide in the rat but reduce the absorption rate of iodoform and triiodophenol [121,122]. Since potassium iodide is not solubilized by the micelle, the enhanced rate of absorption is attributed to the influence of the surfactant on the mucosal membrane. The other compounds, which partition into the micelle, exhibit a reduced rate of absorption since there is a decrease in their effective concentration. Similar observations, using pharmacological response data in goldfish, have been made for several barbiturates in the presence of varying surfactant concentrations.

In addition to the aforementioned effects of surfactants, one must consider their influence on drug dissolution from pharmaceutical dosage forms. If the drug is poorly water-soluble, enhanced dissolution rate in the presence of a surface-active agent, even if part of the drug is solubilized, will result in increased drug absorption. The absorption rate of sulfisoxazole suspensions given rectally to rats increased with increasing polysorbate 80 concentration. At surfactant concentrations in excess of that needed to solubilize the drug completely, there was a reduced rate of absorption; however, the rate was greater than that from the control suspension (i.e., without surfactant) [123].

Another important type of physical chemical interaction that may alter absorption is that of drug binding or adsorption onto the surface of another material. As with complexation and micellarization, adsorption will reduce the effective concentration gradient between gut fluids and the bloodstream, which is the driving force for passive absorption. While adsorption frequently reduces the rate of absorption, the interaction is often readily reversible and will not affect the extent of absorption. A major exception is adsorption onto charcoal, which in many cases appears to be irreversible, at least during the time of residence within the GIT. As a result, charcoal often reduces the extent of drug absorption. Indeed, this fact along with the innocuous nature of charcoal is what make it an ideal antidote for oral drug overdose. The effectiveness of that form of therapy will depend on the amount of charcoal administered and the time delay between overdose and charcoal dosing. Another interesting aspect of charcoal dosing is its influence on shortening the elimination half-life of several drugs. This is a particularly attractive noninvasive means of enhancing drug elimination from the body (phenobarbital is a good example).

In addition to charcoal, adsorption is often seen with pharmaceutical preparations that contain large quantities of relatively water-insoluble components. A good example is antidiarrheal products and perhaps antacids. The importance of the strength of binding as it influences absorption has been illustrated by Sorby [124], who showed that both attapulgite and charcoal reduce the rate of drug absorption but only charcoal reduced the extent of absorption. Lincomycin is an example of a drug whose absorption in impaired by an antidiarrheal preparation [125]. Another type of compound that has been shown to alter drug absorption due to binding are the anion-exchange resins cholestyramine and colestipol. The foregoing physical chemical interactions, which may alter drug therapy, may be minimized by not coadministering the interacting compounds at the same time but separating their ingestion by several hours.

We noted previously, when discussing mechanisms of drug absorption, that certain calcium channel blockers have been shown to enhance the gastrointestinal absorption of several aminopenicillin and aminocephalosporin derivatives [46,47]. This type of interaction, while perhaps not of practical clinical importance, is very intriguing in terms of promoting absorption efficiency, and it illustrates the useful (rather than deleterious) aspect of a drug-drug interaction. Another interesting and recently observed drug-food (or drug-nutrient) interaction is that between grapefruit juice and certain drugs, especially those with a high hepatic clearance that undergo substantial presystemic (first-pass) metabolism (discussed later). The discovery of this interaction is an excellent example of serendipity and an illustration of Pasteur's famous statement, "In the field of experimentation, chance favors only the prepared mind." In their original study [126], the experimenters were attempting to examine the influence of ethanol on the pharmacokinetics of co-administered drugs. The ethanol was mixed (serendipitously) with grapefruit juice to mask the taste of the ethanol. A substantial interaction was noted with felodipine—an approximate three fold increase in bioavailability. Since that initial observation, numerous studies have indicated that many other drugs with diverse chemical structures having a high metabolic clearance participate in this interaction with grapefruit juice (not ethanol!). Many studies have been devoted to determining the mechanism(s) of this interaction, and the readers are referred to a recent symposium and book chapter that cover this topic [127,128]. While we have a better understanding of the nature of the interaction, it now appears that there may be several processes going on.

The drugs that undergo this interaction are substrates for one of the major drug-metabolizing isozymes in the body, cytochrome P450 3A4 (CYP3A4). This enzyme has been referred to as being "promiscuous" (in a biochemical sense), in that it will accommodate and metabolize a very wide range of drug molecules. Since this isozyme is responsible for the metabolism of many drugs, it is also involved in many drug-drug and, in this case, nutrient-drug interactions. This enzyme and many other isozymes are present in the mucosal surface cells (enterocytes) of the GIT. Therefore, the gut surface represents a potential site for drug metabolism. Some component(s) of grapefruit juice is able to inhibit the CYP3A4 enzyme, resulting in less than usual presystemic gastrointestinal metabolism of the drug. This, in turn, results in greater oral bioavailability of the drug. While it was initially thought that bioflavanoids present in the grapefruit juice were the critical chemical components, it has since been determined that furanocoumarin derivatives are the most likely enzyme inhibitors [129]. Enzyme inhibition could also be expressed in liver enzyme activity (also resulting in increased bioavailability); however, liver enzymes appear to play a less significant role in this interaction than those in the GIT. The latter, however, may be more or less true depending upon the drug whose interaction is under investigation.

A complicating factor, however, in this interaction is that many compounds that are substrates for CYP3A4 are also substrates for P-glycoprotein (P-gp), the efflux transporter protein that resides in the membrane surface of the GIT enterocyte. This transporter was noted in a previous section that discussed the transport process. There is evidence to suggest that the drug interaction with grapefruit juice also involves inhibition of this efflux transporter [127]. Both CYP3A4 metabolic inhibition and P-gp efflux transport inhibition will result in increased drug bioavailability. It is possible that these two mechanisms are acting in tandem in an attempt to limit foreign compounds (such as drugs) from entering the systemic circulation.

Table 8 Drugs Known to Interact with Grapefruit Juice

Anti-infective: artemether, saguinavir
Antilipemic: atorrastatin, lovastatin, simvastatin
Cardiovascular: carvedilol, cilostazole, felodipine, nicardipine, nifedipine, nimodipine, nisoldipine, nitrendipine, verapamil
CNS: buspirone, carbamazepine, diazepam, midazolam, trizolam
Other:
Antihistamine: astemizole, terfenadine
Estrogen: ethinyl estradiol
GI: cisapride
Immunosuppressant: cyclosporine, tacrolimus

Source: Ref. 130.

A recent paper [130] has also indicated that this interaction occurs in elderly patients. This is especially important since most interaction studies are typically performed in young subjects, yet the elderly are more likely to be taking the drugs that undergo this interaction. Table 8 lists drugs in different therapeutic categories that are known to participate in this grapefruit juice interaction [130]. It should also be recognized that these compounds will also interact with any other drug (e.g., ketoconazole) capable of inhibiting CYP3A4 and/or P-gp.

The above illustration should be a clear caution that components of food may interact with drugs, resulting in substantial positive or negative therapeutic effects. As will be noted later, this principle also applies to so-called dietary supplements, including botanicals, used for the treatment of numerous medical conditions.

B. Metabolism

Drug molecules may be chemically or metabolically altered at various sites along the GIT including within gut fluids, within the gut wall, and by microorganisms present in the low end of the tract. These sites are noted in Fig. 18. Several examples of enzymatic

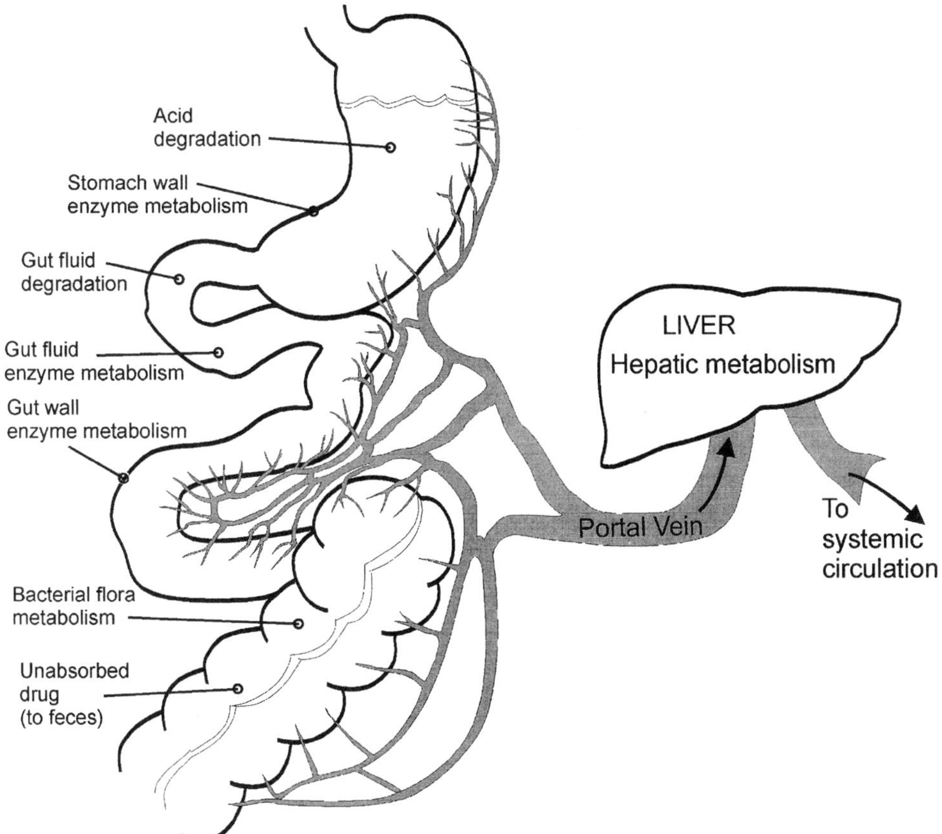

Fig. 18 Diagrammatic sketch indicating sites along the GIT where drug may be chemically altered or enzymatically metabolized. (Copyright © 2000 Saguaro Technical Press, Inc., used with permission.)

alteration of certain drugs in gut fluids have been noted previously. Gut fluids contain appreciable quantities of a variety of enzymes, which are needed to accomplish digestion of food. An additional consideration in that regard is that of acid- or base-mediated drug breakdown. Numerous drugs are unstable in acidic media (e.g., erythromycin, penicillin) and will therefore degrade and provide lower effective doses depending on the pH of the gastric fluid, solubility of the drug, and the residence time of the dosage form in the stomach. Chemical modification of the drug by, for example, salt or ester formation may provide a more stable derivative whose absorption will be influenced to a smaller degree by the factors noted above. An interesting example of a prodrug that must first be acid-hydrolyzed to produce the active chemical form is clorazepate. Upon hydrolysis in the gut fluids the active form, *N*-desmethyldiazepam, is produced. In this instance, unlike the examples cited above, acid hydrolysis is a prerequisite for absorption of the pharmacologically active form. As a result, pH of gastric fluids and gastric-emptying time and variables that influence those factors are expected to affect the absorption profile of clorazapate. Greater concentrations of *N*-desmethyldiazepam are achieved at the lower gastric pH, which is consistent with the more rapid acid hydrolysis at acidic pH [131].

As noted in the preceding section, mucosal cells lining the gut wall represent a significant potential site for drug metabolism. The metabolic activity of this region has been studied by a variety of techniques, ranging from subcellular fractions to tissue homogenates to methods involving the whole living animal. Metabolic reactions include both phase I and II processes. It appears that the entire small intestine, especially the jejunum and ileum, have the greatest enzymatic activity, although most regions of the GIT can partake in metabolism. It is not a simple matter, especially in the whole animal, to distinguish among the several sites of metabolism responsible for presystemic elimination. The latter refers to all processes of chemical or metabolic alteration prior to the drug reaching the systemic circulation and which take place primarily in the gut and liver. It is this presystemic elimination that contributes to differences in drug effects as a function of route of administration and which may seriously compromise the clinical efficiency of certain drugs given orally. Many drugs have been shown to undergo metabolism in the gut wall, including those listed in Table 8 and, among others, aspirin, acetaminophen, salicylamide, *p*-aminobenzoic acid, morphine, ethanol, pentazocine, isoproterenol, L-dopa,

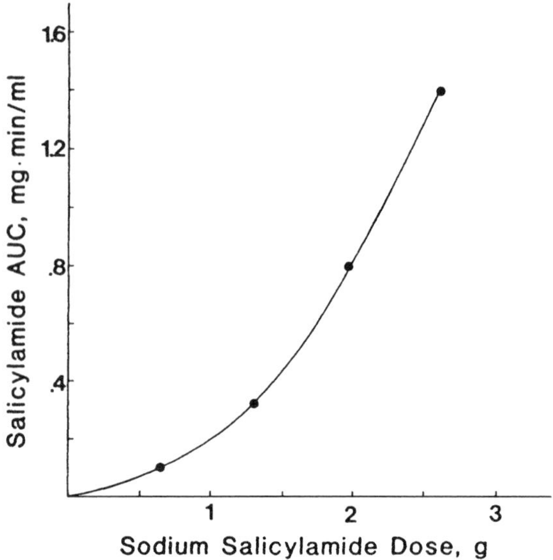

Fig. 19 Area under the salicylamide plasma concentration-time curve (AUC) as a function of the oral dose of sodium salicylamide. Each point is the average of five subjects. (Based on data from Ref. 133.)

lidocaine, and certain steroids. L-Dopa appears to be metabolized by decarboxylase enzymes present in the gastric mucosa, which, as discussed previously, suggests the importance of rapid gastric emptying to achieve maximal absorption of the unchanged compound [132].

Salicylamide and *p*-aminobenzoic acid are interesting examples because they illustrate another aspect of gut metabolism, that of saturation. In addition, factors affecting absorption rate will influence the fraction of the dose that reaches the systemic circulation in the form of intact drug. Figure 19 illustrates the relationship between the area under the salicylamide plasma concentration–time curve (AUC) as a function of the oral dose of sodium salicylamide [133]. Normally, that relationship is expected to be linear and the line should go through the origin. The curvilinearity, especially at low doses, suggests some form of presystemic elimination, which becomes saturated above a certain dose. The drug is metabolized in the gut wall to sulfate and glucuronide conjugates, although metabolism in the liver also occurs on the first pass. Extrapolation of the straight-line segment to the x-axis in Fig. 19 gives an intercept that has been referred to as the "break through" dose, which approximates the dose needed to saturate the enzyme system (about 1–1.5 g for salicylamide). Doses less than that value produce only small plasma concentrations of the unchanged drug.

Another interesting aspect of this phenomenon is that the rate of drug presentation to the enzyme system will influence the fraction of the dose reaching the systemic circulation unchanged and will alter the metabolic pattern. The latter factors, therefore, will be influenced by the dosage form characteristics and the rate of gastric emptying. The more rapid the rate of absorption, the more likely the enzyme system will become saturated. The latter will result in greater plasma concentrations of unchanged drug and a metabolic pattern with a lower percentage of the drug recovered as the saturable metabolite. At any given dose, the more rapidly soluble sodium salicylamide produces greater plasma concentrations of unchanged drug compared to salicylamide. The more rapidly soluble dosage forms of saticylamide (solution and suspension) produce smaller fractions of the dose in the form of the saturable metabolite (sulfate conjugate) compared to a slowly dissolving tablet [134]. Observations similar to the latter have been made for *p*-aminobenzoic acid. In that instance, however, it was shown that a delay in gastric emptying produced a greater percentage of the dose in the form of the saturable metabolite (acetyl derivative), which is consistent with a reduced rate of absorption [135].

An interesting example of gut metabolism and gender-dependent differences is that of ethanol. Females appear to have greater blood ethanol concentrations following an oral dose compared to males given the same dose. The latter is true even if the data are corrected for weight and lean body mass differences. Ethanol is metabolized by alcohol dehydrogenase present in the gastric mucosa, and it appears that this enzyme is present in smaller quantities in females. The lower enzyme concentration results in a greater fraction of the dose not being metabolized compared to males and a subsequent higher blood ethanol concentration. Estimates of absorption suggest that females absorb about 91% of the dose as ethanol compared to about 61% in males [136]. Evidence suggests that alcohol deydrogenase activity is lower in young women (less than about 50 years of age), elderly males, and alcoholics [137]. One review has examined first-pass metabolism in oral absorption and factors that affect that process [138].

The gastrointestinal microflora provide another potential site for drug metabolism within the GIT, and it has received some attention. In normal subjects the stomach and proximal small intestine contain small numbers of microorganisms. Concentrations of these organisms increase toward the distal end of the intestine. A wide variety of aerobic and anaerobic organisms are present in the gut. The microflora, derived primarily from the environment, tend to adhere to the luminal surface of the intestine. Within an individual, the microflora tend to remain rather stable over long periods of time. The primary factors governing the numbers and kinds of microorganisms present in the tract include the activity of gastric and bile secretions, which tend to limit the growth of these organisms in the stomach and upper part of the GIT, and the propulsive motility of the intestine, which is responsible for continually cleansing the tract, thereby limiting the proliferation of microorganisms. Gastric atrophy permits increased numbers of microorganisms to pass into the small intestine, and reduced intestinal motility results in overgrowth.

Studies conducted mostly in animals indicate a wide range of primarily phase I metabolic pathways. Various drugs that are glucuronidated in the body are secreted into the intestine via the bile, and these are subject to cleavage by bacterial glucuronidase enzymes. The cleavage product may then be in a form available for absorption. Various drug conjugates may be similarly deconjugated by other bacterial enzymes (e.g., the glycine conjugate of isonicotinic acid). Although some drugs may be rendered inactive, bacterial metabolism of other drugs may give rise to more active or toxic products. The formation of the toxic compound cyclohexylamine from cyclamate is an example [139].

Salicylazosulfapyridine (sulfasalazine), which is used in treating ulcerative colitis, provides an interesting example of a drug whose metabolites represent the active pharmacological species. The parent drug is metabolized to 5-aminosalicylate and sulfapyridine. In conventional rats, both metabolites and their conjugates appear in urine and feces. In germ-free rats, however, the metabolites are not excreted. This suggests that the intestinal flora play a role in reducing the parent compound and formation of the two metabolites. If this is the case, factors influencing the population and types of intestinal microorganisms may in turn influence the absorption and effectiveness of the drug. For example, concomitant antibiotic therapy, by reducing the population of microorganisms, may prevent the parent drug from being metabolized.

The impact of presystemic elimination may be clearly understood by considering the following relationships among the several steps involved in making the drug available to the systemic circulation. The significance of this relationship is its multiplicative nature, since most of the processes are sequential. These relationships assume linear or first-order kinetics (i.e., there is no nonlinearity or saturation effects).

$$F_{\text{systemic}} = f_{\text{released}} \times f_{\text{absorbed}} \times f_{\text{hepatic}} \quad (4)$$

The fraction of the orally administered dose that is bioavailable to the systemic circulation ($F_{systemic}$) is dependent upon the fraction of the dose that is released from the dosage form ($f_{released}$), multiplied by the fraction that is absorbed into the portal circulation on its way to the liver ($f_{absorbed}$; this is the fraction that escapes gut metabolism), multiplied by the fraction of the dose that escapes the hepatic first-pass effect ($f_{hepatic}$). Since this is a multiplicative process if, for example, $f_{released}$ is 1.0 and $f_{absorbed}$ is 0.5 and $f_{hepatic}$ is 0.5, then the overall $F_{systemic}$ is 0.25 (i.e., 25% of the dose reaches the systemic circulation). The absorption process can be broken down further into its component parts

$$F_{systemic} = f_{released}(f_{gut\ fluid} \times f_{gut\ wall} \times f_{gut\ flora}) f_{hepatic} \quad (5)$$

where $f_{gut\ fluid}$, $f_{gut\ wall}$ and $f_{gut\ flora}$ are the fractions of the dose of drug that escape metabolism in the gut fluid, gut wall, and gut flora, respectively. In the above example, an $f_{absorbed}$ of 0.5 represents the product of the three processes noted that affect absorption. It is often common to express the fraction surviving a specific process as one minus the extraction ratio (ER) for that process. Thus, the above relationship may be written as,

$$F_{systemic} = f_{released}(1 - ER_{gut\ fluid}) \times (1 - ER_{gut\ wall}) \times (1 - ER_{gut\ flora}) \times (1 - ER_{hepatic}) \quad (6)$$

A change in the ER value for any of the above processes will have an effect on the systemically available dose of the orally administered drug. For example, in the previous section it was noted that grapefruit juice inhibits CYP3A4 metabolism of many drugs. The factor most affected by this interaction is the intrinsic metabolic clearance of the drug by enzymes present in the gut wall. The latter would be expressed by a decrease in the value of $ER_{gut\ wall}$, and a consequent increase in $F_{systemic}$.

In addition to food- or nutrient-based interactions in the metabolism of drugs, it has become quite clear in recent years that so-called dietary supplements including botanicals have the potential to participate in such interactions. The latter observation has special relevance because of the extensive use of such products worldwide (~ $12 billion per year in the United States alone), their easy commercial availability (no prescription required), and their common use with prescribed drugs. Furthermore, many people consider such "natural" products to be safe and free of any bad effects (it should be pretty easy to recall many poisons that occur in nature and are, therefore, "natural"). Several recent examples of botanical-drug interactions should serve as a warning that we have just begun to see the tip of the iceberg. This should not be at all surprising when one considers the large number and variety of chemicals (phytochemicals) present in botanicals that are ingested for medicinal value.

St. John's wort, which has become very popular for the treatment of depression, has been shown to induce intestinal P-gp and intestinal and hepatic CYP3A4 in humans [140]. That mechanism explains the significant reduction in cyclosporin and anti-aids (e.g., indinavir) plasma concentrations. It is likely that similar effects will be noted with the compounds listed in Table 8 (although the effects noted in Table 8 are in the opposite direction of those seen in the presence of St. John's wort).

C. Disease States

Gastrointestinal disorders and disease states have the potential to influence drug absorption. Although this important area has not been explored thoroughly, numerous studies have addressed this issue. Unfortunately, many of these studies have not been correctly designed, and this has resulted in conflicting reports and our inability to reach generally valid conclusions. The majority of these studies are conducted by administration of an oral dose and measurement of the area under the plasma concentration–time curve (AUC). The latter parameter is frequently used in assessing bioavailability. The resulting AUC is compared to that from a control group of different subjects or within the same subject during the time the disorder is present and compared to the value prior to or after the disorder is resolved. The problem here is that a value for AUC depends as much on the body's ability to clear or eliminate the drug as it does on absorption (i.e., AUC = dose absorbed/clearance). Differences in the former parameter are likely to be present between subjects as well as within a subject from time to time (especially in the presence of a disease). Therefore, values of AUCs after oral dosing may lead to incorrect conclusions. To use such a value properly, one must be certain that drug clearance is not different between or within a subject. In the ideal situation an intravenous dose would be given to establish the correctness of that assumption. This is an approach, unfortunately, that is not generally used. The influence of gastrointestinal disease on drug absorption has been reviewed [141].

Elevated gastric pH is seen in subjects with achlorhydria as a result of reduced acid secretion. The absorption of tetracycline, which is most soluble at acidic pH, appears to be unaffected by achlorhydria and after surgery where the acid-secreting portion of the stomach was removed [142,143]. The absorption of clorazepate would be expected to be reduced in achlorhydria (for the reasons discussed above), but as yet the data are not conclusive. The clinical significance of altered gut pH with regard to drug absorption is not clearly established. Alterations in drug absorption due to changes in gut pH will most likely be mediated by its influence on dissolution rate.

Changes in gastric emptying are expected to influence the rate and possibly the extent of absorption for the reasons discussed previously. Emptying may be severely hampered and absorption altered soon after gastric surgery as a result of pyloric stenosis and in the presence of various disease states. Riboflavin absorption is increased in hypothyroidism and reduced in hyperthyroidism, conditions that alter gastric emptying and intestinal transit rates [144].

Diarrheal conditions may decrease drug absorption as a result of reduced intestinal residence time. The absorption of several drugs was decreased in response to lactose- and saline-induced diarrhea [145]. Digoxin absorption from tablets was impaired in one subject who developed chronic diarrhea as a result of x-ray treatment [146]. Abdominal radiation or the underlying disease has been shown to reduce digoxin and clorazepate absorption [147]. A dosage form that provides rapid drug dissolution (e.g., solution) may partially resolve this problem.

Various malabsorption syndromes are known to influence the absorption of certain nutrients. Although not thoroughly investigated, such syndromes may exert an influence on the efficacy of drug absorption. Heizer et al. [148] noted reduced absorption of digoxin in patients with sprue, malabsorption syndrome, and pancreatic insufficiency. The dosage form of digoxin, especially dissolution rate from tablets, will partially determine the influence of malabsorption states on absorption, the problem being compounded by poorly dissolving tablets. Phenoxymethyl penicillin absorption is reduced in patients with steatorrhea [149], and ampicillin and nalidixic acid absorption appears to be impaired in children with shigellosis [150].

There are a variety of other disease states whose influence on drug absorption has been reported, including cystic fibrosis, villous atrophy, celiac disease, diverticulosis, and Crohn's disease. The results of these studies are frequently divergent, and therefore general statements cannot be made. A thorough discussion of these findings is beyond the scope of this chapter, and the interested reader is referred to a recent review [141].

As most drugs are best absorbed from the small intestine, any surgical procedure that removes a substantial portion of the small intestine is likely to influence absorption; however, and as discussed previously, the characteristics of the dosage form may affect the findings. Although the procedure has fallen out of favor, intestinal bypass surgery has been used in treatment of the morbidly obese. A number of studies have been conducted to examine absorption prior to and after surgery. As noted in the introduction to this section, care must be exercised in study design and evaluation of data, as large weight loss may alter drug elimination from the body compared to the presurgery condition. Further complications include the time that the study is conducted relative to the time of surgery and the length and sections of the intestine removed.

One excellent study [151] employed intravenous and oral dosing at each of several times postsurgery (1–2 weeks, 6 and 12 months). This design permits valid conclusions about the absorption process. There was a significant reduction after surgery in ampicillin absorption but no change in propylthiouracil absorption.

In those instances where a patient's response to a drug is less than expected, and there is reason to believe that this is a result of impaired absorption due to any of the pathological conditions or disease states cited earlier, a first attempt in seeking to improve drug therapy is to optimize absorption from the GIT. To do this, a practical approach might well be to administer the drug in a form readily available for absorption. In most cases, if such a form is marketed or easily prepared, administration of a drug in solution will represent the best way to achieve maximal absorption, as this will eliminate the time for drug dissolution in the gut needed by solid oral dosage forms. When absorption cannot be sufficiently improved by use of a drug solution, alternative routes of administration must be considered (e.g., intramuscular).

D. Age

The majority of the information discussed to this point and most of the literature concerned with drug absorption involve studies performed in young, healthy (usually male) adults. In contrast, there is considerably less information concerning absorption in subjects at either end of the age spectrum (i.e., pediatric and geriatric populations). For a variety of reasons, one would expect the absorption process in the latter groups to be different from that in young adults; unfortunately, at this time there is little information to present valid general statements.

The pediatric population (neonates, infants, and children) presents a particularly difficult group in which to conduct clinical experimentation because of ethical considerations. A further complication is the rapid development of organ function, which is likely to influence results even over a relatively short experimental period (e.g., 2–4 weeks), especially in neonates and infants. An additional consideration in the latter groups is whether the neonate is premature or full-term. Most often, plasma concentration–time data are obtained after an oral dose for the purpose of estimating elimination half-life or to provide a basis for the development of a multiple dosing regimen. Such data provide very limited information about the rate or extent of absorption. Indeed, most reviews of drug disposition in the pediatric population indicate the lack of rigorous information about absorption. There have been recent initiatives to encourage the study of drugs in the pediatric population, and this will undoubtedly result in useful new information.

Gastric fluid is less acidic in the newborn than in adults since acid secretion is related to the development of the gastric mucosa. This condition appears to last for some time, as pH values similar to the adult are not reached until after about 2 years. The higher gastric fluid pH along with smaller gut fluid volume may influence dissolution rate and the stability of acid-unstable drugs. The gastric-emptying rate appears to be slow, approaching adult values after about 6 months. An interesting example in support of that suggestion is a study that examined riboflavin absorption in a 5-day-old and a 10-month-old infant [152]. The maximum urinary excretion rate was considerably greater in the infant, while excretion rate in the neonate was constant and prolonged. These data suggest more rapid absorption in the infant, while absorption in the neonate proceeds for a longer time. For the reasons discussed previously, these data suggest slower emptying and/or intestinal transit rates in the neonate (recall that riboflavin is absorbed by a specialized process high in the small intestine). Intestinal transit tends to be irregular and may be modified by the type of food ingested and the feeding pattern.

Intestinal surface area and total blood flow to the GIT are smaller than in adults and may influence the efficiency of absorption. With regard to the use of rectal suppositories, one must keep in mind that the completeness of absorption will be a function of retention time in the rectum. Since bowel movements in the neonate and infant are likely to be irregular, the retention time may limit the efficiency of absorption by that route. In light of the little information available about absorption in the young, it would seem reasonable to attempt to optimize absorption by using solution or suspensions rather than solid dosage forms.

Only in recent years has there been any substantial progress made in better understanding drug disposition in the elderly. Active research programs in gerontology have begun to provide more information about rational drug dosing in the elderly. There are a number of important and unique characteristics of the elderly that make a compelling argument for the need for such information (e.g., they ingest more drugs per capita, their percentage of the population is increasing, they suffer from more disease and physical impairments, etc.). As noted for the pediatric population, a variety of complex issues are associated with the conduct of research in the elderly. Careful consideration must be given to experimental design and data analysis. Some considerations include the appropriate definition of age, cross-sectional versus longitudinal study design, and health status of the subject [153,154].

There have been numerous statements in the literature to the effect that GI absorption in the elderly is impaired and less efficient than in young adults. Although there have been few data to support the suggestion, one basis for that statement has been the results obtained from the application of the so-called xylose tolerance test, which is often used in assessing malabsorption. This conclusion of impaired absorption in the elderly presents a good example of the need for careful study design and appropriate pharmacokinetic analysis of data. Figure 20 illustrates the results of several studies that have examined xylose absorption [155]. Most studies indicate an inverse relationship between urinary xylose recovery and age after an oral dose (lines B and C). It is this observation that has suggested reduced absorption with age. However, the same inverse relationship is found after an intravenous dose (line A), an observation that is not explained by impaired absorption but, rather, by reduced renal clearance of xylose. Line D shows the ratio of urinary recovery (oral to intravenous), which suggests that absorption is not altered with age. A more complete study in which each subject (age range, 32–85 years) received both an oral and an intravenous dose indicates no relationship between xylose bioavailability and age [156].

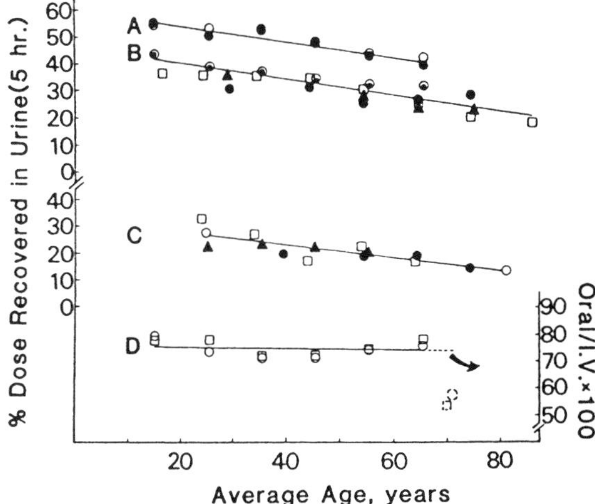

Fig. 20 Percentage xylose dose recovered in urine as a function of age after a 5 g intravenous dose (A), 5 g oral dose (B), and 25 g oral dose (C). Line D is the ratio of urinary recoveries (oral to intravenous) after 5 g doses (*y*-axis on right). Symbols represent data obtained from different studies. (From Ref. 155.)

There are substantial changes in a variety of physiological functions in the elderly, which may influence drug absorption [153], including a greater incidence of achlorhydria, altered gastric emptying, reduced gut blood flow, and smaller intestinal surface area. One recent example indicates that gastric pH may be an important determinant of drug absorption in the elderly [157]. Dipyridamole is a poorly water-soluble weak base whose dissolution would be optimal in an acidic environment. Elevated gastric pH due to achlorhydria (a condition more prevalent in the elderly than the young) results in impaired absorption of dipyridamole. The ingestion of glutamic acid by achlorhydric subjects improves absorption. Other factors that may influence absorption include a greater incidence of GI disease, altered nutritional intake and eating habits, and ingestion of drugs, which may affect the absorption of other drugs. Although data are still somewhat limited, the general impression is that the rate of absorption is frequently reduced, while there is little if any change in the extent of absorption [153]. This is a tentative statement that needs to be qualified for the specific drug and for the health status of the subject. For example, the absorption of drugs that undergo hepatic first-pass metabolism (e.g., propranolol) may be improved in the elderly as a consequence of reduced hepatic clearance with age.

REFERENCES

1. JD Verhoff, HE Bodde, AG deBoer, JA Bouwstra, HE Junginger, FWHM Merkus DD Breimer. Transport of peptide and protein drugs across biological membranes. Eur J Drug Metab Pharmacokin 15:83–93, 1990.
2. PA Wender, DJ Mitchell, K Pattabiraman, ET Pelkey, L Steinman, JB Rothbard. The design, synthesis, and evaluation of molecules that enable or enhance cellular uptake: Peptoid molecular transporters. Proc Natl Acad Sci USA 97:13003–13008, 2000.
3. JB Rothbard, S Garlington, Q Lin, T Kirschberg, E Kreider, PL McGrane, PA Wender, PA Khavari. Conjugation of arginine digomers to cyclosporin: A facilitates topical delivery and inhibition of inflammation. Nat Med 6:1253–1257, 2000.
4. JW Hole. Human Anatomy and Physiology. 2nd ed. Dubuque, IA: Wm. C. Brown Company, 1981, p. 414.
5. H Leonhardt. Color Atlas/Text of Human Anatomy. Vol. 2. 4th ed. New York: Thieme Medical Publishers, 1993, p. 213.
6. T Fujita, K Tanaka, J Tokunaga. SEM Atlas of Cells and Tissues. New York: Igaku-Shoin, 1981, pp. 122, 123, 129.
7. JW Hole. In: SEM Atlas of Cells and Tissues. New York: Igaku-Shoin, 1981, p. 439.
8. JS Trier. Morphology of the epithelium of the small intestine. In: CF Code, ed. Handbook of Physiology. Vol. III, Intestinal Absorption. Washington, DC: American Physiological Society,1968, p. 1133.
9. T Fujita, K Tanaka, J Tokunaga. In: CF Code, ed. Handbook of Physiology. Washington DC: American Physiological Society, 1968, p. 135.
10. GJ Tortora, NP Anagnostakos. Principles of Anatomy and Physiology. 6th ed. New York: Harper and Row, 1990, p. 770.
11. JS Fordtran, FC Rector, Jr., MF Ewton, N Soter, J Kinney. Permeability characteristics of the human small intestine. J Clin Invest 44:1935–1944, 1965.
12. JF Danielli, H Davson. A contribution to the theory of permeability of thin films. J Cell Comp Physiol 5:495–508, 1935.
13. H Davson, JF Danielli. The Permeability of Natural Membranes. 2nd ed. New York: Cambridge University Press, 1952.
14. LC Junqueira, J Carneiro, RO Kelley. Basic Histology. 6th ed. East Norwalk, CT: Appleton and Lange, 1989, p. 32.
15. R Hober, J Hober. Experiments on the absorption of organic solutes in the small intestine of rats. J Cell Comp Physiol 10:401–422, 1937.
16. LS Schanker. Absorption of drugs from the rat colon. J Pharmacol Exp Ther 126:283–290, 1959.
17. EM Wright, JM Diamond. Patterns of non-electrolyte permeability. Proc Royal Soc B 172:203–225, 1969.

18. EM Wright, JM Diamond. Patterns of non-electrolyte permeability. Proc Royal Soc B 172:227–271, 1969.
19. JM Diamond, EM Wright. Molecular forces governing nonelectrolyte permeation through cell membranes. Proc Royal Soc B 172:273–316, 1969.
20. CA Lipinski, F Lombardo, BW Dominy, PF Feeney. Experimental and computational approaches to estimate solubility and permeability in drug discovery and development settings. Adv Drug Deliv Rev 23:3–25, 1997.
21. Y Yoshimura, N Kakeya. Structure-gastrointestinal absorption relationship of penicillins. Int J Pharm 17:47–57, 1983.
22. T Sollmann. The comparative efficiency of local anesthetics. J Am Med Assoc 70:216–219, 1918.
23. JM Faulkner. Nicotine poisoning by absorption through the skin. J Am Med Assoc 100:1664–1665, 1933.
24. J Travell. The influence of the hydrogen ion concentration on the absorption of alkaloids from the stomach. J Pharmacol Exp Ther 69:21–33, 1940.
25. MH Jacobs. Some aspects of cell permeability to weak electrolytes. Cold Spring Harbor Symp Quant Biol 8:30–399, 1940.
26. PA Shore, BB Brodie, CAM Hogben. The gastric secretion of drugs: a pH partition hypothesis. J Pharmacol Exp Ther 119:361–369, 1957.
27. LS Schanker, PA Shore, BB Brodie, CAM Hogben. Absorption of drugs from the stomach. I. The rat. J Pharmacol Exp Ther 120:528–539, 1957.
28. CAM Hogben, LA Schanker, DJ Tocco, BB Brodie. Absorption of drugs from the stomach. II. The human. J Pharmacol Exp Ther 120:540–545, 1957.
29. LS Schanker, DJ Tocco, BB Brodie, CAM Hogben. Absorption of drugs from the rat small intestine. J Pharmacol Exp Ther 123:81–87, 1958.
30. CAM Hogben, DJ Tocco, BB Brodie, LS Schanker. On the mechanism of intestinal absorption of drugs. J Pharmacol Exp Ther 125:275–282, 1959.
31. JT. Doluisio, NF Billups, LW Dittert, ET Sugita, JV Swintosky. Drug absorption. I. An in situ rat gut technique yielding realistic absorption rates. J Pharm Sci 58:1196–1200, 1969.
32. LZ Benet. Biopharmaceutics as a basis for the design of drug products. In: EJ Ariens, ed. Drug Design, Vol. 4. New York: Academic Press, 1973, pp. 26–28.
33. DS Riggs. The Mathematical Approach to Physiological Problems. Baltimore: Williams & Wilkins, 1963, pp. 181–185.
34. GL Flynn, SK Yalkowsky, TJ Roseman. Mass transport phenomena and models: theoretical concepts. J Pharm Sci 63:479– 510, 1974.
35. M Mayersohn. Drug absorption. J Clin Pharmacol 27:634–638, 1987.
36. Y-L He, S Murby, G Warhurst, L Gifford, D Walker, J Ayrton, R Eastmond, M Rowland. Species differences in size discrimination in the paracellular pathway reflected by oral bioavailability of poly (ethylene glycol) and D-peptides. J Pharm Sci 87: 626–633, 1998.
37. LS Schanker, JJ Jeffrey. Active transport of foreign pyrimidines across the intestinal epithelium. Nature 190:727–728, 1961.
38. DF Evered, HG Randall. The absorption of amino acid derivatives of nitrogen mustard from rat intestine in vitro. Biochem Pharmacol 11:371–376, 1962.
39. G Levy, WJ Jusko. Factors affecting the absorption of riboflavin in man. J Pharm Sci 55:285–289, 1966.
40. M Mayersohn. Ascorbic acid absorption in man-pharmacokinetic implications. Eur J Pharmacol 19:140–142, 1972.
41. NG Gillespie, I Mena, GC Cotzias, MA Bell. Diets affecting treatment of parkinsonism with levodopa. J Am Diet Assoc 62:525–528, 1973.
42. DN Wade, PT Mearrick, JL Morris. Active transport of L-Dopa in the intestine. Nature 242:463–465, 1973.
43. MH van Woert. Phenylalanine and tyrosine metabolism in Parkinson's disease treated with levodopa. Clin Pharmacol Ther 12:368–375, 1971.
44. H Lennernas, D Nilsson, S-M Aquilonius, D Ahrenstedt, L Knutson, LK Paalzow. The effect of L-leucine on the absorption of levodopa, studied by regional jejunal perfusion in man. Br J Clin Pharmacol 35:343–250, 1993.
45. J Zimmerman. Methotrexate transport in the human intestine. Biochem Pharmacol 43:2377–2383, 1992.
46. J-F Westphal, J-H Trouvin, A Deslandes, C Carbon. Nifedipine enhances amoxicillin absorption kinetics and bioavailability in human. J Pharmacol Exp Ther 255:312–317, 1990.
47. C Duverne, A Bouten, A Deslandes, J-F Westphal, J-H Trouvin, R Farinotti, C Carbon. Modification of cifixime bioavailability by nifedipine in humans: involvement of the dipeptide carrier system. Antimicrob Agents Chemother 36:2462–2467, 1992.
48. BH Stewart, AR Kugler, PR Thompson, NN Bockbrader. A saturable transport mechanism in the intestinal absorption of gabapentin is the underlying cause of the lack of proportionality between increasing dose and drug levels in plasma. Pharmaceut Res 10:276–281, 1993.
49. II Gottesman, I Pastan. Biochemistry of multidrug resistance mediated by the multidrug transporter. Ann Rev Biochem 62:385–427, 1993.
50. Y Tanigawara. Role of p-glycoprotein in drug disposition. Ther Drug Monitor 22:137–140, 2000.
51. JV Asperen, OV Tellingen, JH Beijnen. The pharmacological role of *p*-glycoprotein in the intestinal epithelium. Pharmacol Res 37:429–435, 1998.

52. V Wacher, JA Silverman, Y Zhang, LZ Benet. Role of *p*-glycoprotein and cytochrome P4503A in limiting oral absorption of peptides and peptidomimetics. J Pharm Sci 87:1322–1330, 1998.
53. J Wacher, L Salphati, LZ Benet. Active secretion and enterocyte drug metabolism barriers to drug absorption. Adv Drug Del Rev 20:99–112, 1996.
54. A Sparreboom, J van Asperen, U Mayer, AH Schinkel, JW Smit, DKF Meijer, P Borst, WJ Nooijen, JH Beijnen, O van Tillingen. Limited oral bioavailability of taxol and active epithelial secretion of paclitaxel (Taxol) caused by *p*-glycoprotein in the intestine. Proc Nat Acad Sci USA 94:2031–2035, 1997.
55. K Westphal, A Weinbrenner, T Giessmann, M Stuhr, G Franke, M Zschiesche, R Oertel, B Terhaag, HK Kroemer, W Siegmund. Oral bioavailability of digoxin is enhanced by talinolol: evidence for involvement of intestinal p-glycoprotein. Clin Pharmacol Ther 68:6–12, 2000.
56. JB Dressman, GL Amidon, C Reppas, VP Shah. Dissolution testing as a prognostic tool for oral drug absorption: immediate release dosage forms. Pharm Res 15:11–22, 1998.
57. TR Bates, JM Young, CM Wu, HA Rosenberg. pH-dependent dissolution rate of nitrofurantoin from commercial suspensions, tablets and capsules. J Pharm Sci 63:643–645, 1974.
58. G Levy, BA Sahli. Comparison of the gastrointestinal absorption of aluminum acetylsalicylate and acetylsalicylic acid in man. J Pharm Sci 51:58–62, 1962.
59. G Levy, JA Procknal. Unusual dissolution behavior due to film formation. J Pharm Sci 51:294, 1962.
60. CE Blezek, JL Lach, JK Guillory. Some dissolution aspects of ferrous sulfate tablets. Am J Hosp Pharm 27:533–539, 1970.
61. RG Crounse. Human pharmacology of griseofulvin. The effect of fat intake on gastrointestinal absorption. J Invest Dermatol 37:529–533, 1961.
62. M Kraml, J Dubuc, D Beall. Gastrointestinal absorption of griseofulvin. I. Effect of particle size, addition of surfactants and corn oil on the level of griseofulvin in the serum of rats. Can J Biochem Physiol 40:1449–1451, 1962.
63. AJ Moes. Gastroretentive dosage forms. Crit Rev Therap Drug Carrier Sys 10:143–195, 1993.
64. H Minami, RW McCallum. The physiology and pathophysiology of gastric emptying in humans. Gastroenterol 86:1592–1610, 1984.
65. AG Renwick, CH Ahsan, VF Challenor, R Daniels, BS MacKlin, DG Waller, CF George. The influence of posture on the pharmacokinetics of orally administered nifedipine. Br J Clin Pharmacol 34:332–336, 1992.
66. A Hopkins. The pattern of gastric emptying: a new view of old results J Physiol 182:144–149, 1966.
67. JD Elashoff, TJ Reedy, JH Meyer. Analysis of gastric emptying data. Gastroenterology 83:1306–1312, 1982.
68. RH Blythe, GM Grass, DR MacDonnell. The formulation and evaluation of enteric coated aspirin tablets. Am J Pharm 131:206–216, 1959.
69. M Alpsten, C Bogentoft, G Ekenved, L Solveil. Gastric emptying and absorption of acetylsalicylic acid administered as enteric-coated micro-granules. Eur J Clin Pharmacol 22:57–61, 1982.
70. P Welling. Effects of food on drug absorption. Ann Rev Nutr 16:383–415, 1996.
71. D Fleisher, C Li, Y Zhou, L-H Pao, A Karim. Drug, meal and formulation interactions influencing drug absorption after oral administration. Clin Pharmacokin 36:233–254, 1999.
72. WN Charman, CJH Porter, S Mithani, JB Dressman. Physicochemical and physiological mechanisms for the effects of food on drug absorption: the role of lipids and pH. J Pharm Sci 86:269–282, 1997.
73. L Hendeles, M Weinberger, G Milavetz, M Hill III, L Vaughan. Food-induced ‘dose-dumping’ from a once-a-day theophylline product as a cause of theophylline toxicity. Chest 87:758–765, 1985.
74. MN Gai, A Isla, MT Andonaegui, AM Thielemann, C Seitz. Evaluation of the effect of 3 different diets on the bioavailability of 2 sustained release theophylline matrix tablets. Int J Clin Pharmacol Ther 35:565–571, 1997.
75. TR Bates, JA Sequeira, AV Tembo. Effect of food on nitrofurantoin absorption. Clin Pharmacol Ther 16:63–68, 1974.
76. HA Rosenberg, TR Bates. The influence of food on nitrofurantoin bioavailability. Clin Pharmacol Ther 20:227–232, 1976.
77. S Yung, M Mayersohn, JB Robinson. Ascorbic acid absorption in man: influence of divided dose and food. Life Sci 28:2505–2511, 1981.
78. CW Meuhlberger. The physiological action of alcohol. J Am Med Assoc 167:1842–1845, 1958.
79. J Fermaglich, S O’Doherty. Effect of gastric motility on levodopa. Dis Nerv Syst 33:624–625, 1972.
80. M Siurala, O Mustala, J Jussila. Absorption of acetylsalicylic acid by a normal and strophic gastric mucosa. Scand J Gastroenterol 4:269–273, 1969.
81. M Kekki, K Pyorola, O Justala, H Salmi, J Jussila, M Siurala. Multicompartment analysis of the absorption kinetics of warfarin from the stomach and small intestine. Int J Clin Pharmacol 5:209–214, 1971.
82. RC Heading, J Nimmo, LF Prescott, P Tothill. The dependence of paracetamol absorption on the rate of gastric emptying. Br J Pharmacol 47:415–421, 1973.
83. LF Prescott, WS Nimmo, RC Heading. Drug absorption interactions. In: DG Grahame-Smith, ed. Drug Interactions. Baltimore: Macmillan, 1977, p. 45.
84. KS Channer, J Virjee. Effect of posture and drink volume on the swallowing of capsules. Br Med J 285:1702, 1982.

85. H Hey, F Jorgenson, K Sorensen, H Hasselbalch, T Wamberg. Oesophageal transit of six commonly used tablets and capsules. Br Med J 285:171–179, 1982.
86. KS Channer, CJC Roberts. Effect of delayed esophageal transit on acetaminophen absorption. Clin Pharmacol Ther 37:72–76, 1985.
87. SS Davis, JG Hardy, JW Fara. Transit of pharmaceutical dosage forms through the small intestine. Gut 27:886–892, 1986.
88. JL Madsen. Effects of gender, age, and body mass index on gastrointestinal transit times. Digest Dis Sci 37:1548–1553, 1992.
89. JMC Price, SS Davis, IR Wilding. The effect of fibre on gastrointestinal transit times in vegetarians and omnivores. Int J Pharmaceut 76:123–141, 1991.
90. F Pirk. Changes in the motility of the small intestine in digestive disorders. Gut 8:486–490, 1967.
91. AC Guyton. Basic Human Physiology: Normal Functions and Mechanisms of Disease. Philadelphia: WB Saunders, 1971, p. 428.
92. E Parry, R Shields, AC Turnbull. Transit time in the small intestine in pregnancy. J Obstet Gynaecol 77:900–901, 1970.
93. AM Metcalf, SF Phillips, AR Zinsmeister, RL MacCarty, RW Beart, BG Wolff. Simplified assessment of segmental colonic transit. Gastroenterology 92:40–47, 1987.
94. PJ Watts, L Barrow, KP Steed, CG Wilson, RC Spiller, CD Melia, MC Davis. The transit rate of different sized model dosage forms through the human colon and the effects of a lactulose-induced catharsis. Int J Pharmaceut 87:215–221, 1992.
95. DA Akin, SS Davis, RA Sparrow, IR Wilding. Colonic transit of different sized tablets in healthy subjects. J Controlled Release 23:147–156, 1993.
96. JMC Price, SS Davis, RA Sparrow, IR Wilding. The effect of meal composition on the gastrocolonic response: implications for drug delivery to the colon. Pharmaceut Res 10:722–726, 1993.
97. CJ McDougall, R Wong, P Scudera, M Lesser, JJ De Cosse. Colonic mucosal pH in humans. Digest Dis Sci 38:542–545, 1993.
98. DR Friend. Colon-specific drug delivery. Adv Drug Del Rev 7:149–199, 1991.
99. KH Antonin, V Saano, P Bleck, J Hastewell, R Fox, P Low, M MacKay. Colonic absorption of human calcitonin in man. Clin Sci 83:627–631, 1992.
100. MF Williams, GF Dukes, W Heizer, Y-H Han, DJ Hermann, T Lampkin, LJ Hak. Influence of gastrointestinal site of drug delivery on the absorption characteristics of ranitidine. Pharmaceut Res 9:1190–1194, 1992.
101. KKH Chan, A Buch, RD Glazer, VA John, WH Barr. Site-differential gastrointestinal absorption of benazepril hydrochloride in health volunteers. Pharmaceut Res 11:432–437, 1994.
102. L d'Agay-Abensour, A Fjellestad-Paulsen, P Hoglund, Y Ngo, O Paulsen, JC Rambaud. Absolute bioavailability of an aqueous solution of 1-deamino-8-D-arginine vasopressin from different regions of the gastrointestinal tract in man. Eur J Clin Pharmacol 44:473–476, 1993.
103. PE Warner, KLR Brouwer, EK Hussey, GE Dukes, WD Heizer, KH Donn, IM Davis, JR Powell. Sumatriptan absorption from different regions of the human gastrointestinal tract. Pharmaceut Res 12:138–143, 1995.
104. AG De Boer, F Moolenaar, LGJ de Leede, DD Breimer. Rectal drug administration: clinical pharmacokinetic considerations. Clin Pharmacokinet 7:285–311, 1982.
105. D Winne. The influence of blood flow on the absorption of L- and D-phenylalanine from the jejunum of the rat. Arch Pharmacol 277:113–138, 1973.
106. D Winne. Formal kinetics of water and solute absorption with regard to intestinal blood flow. J Theoret Biol 2:1–18, 1970.
107. D Winne, J Remischovsky. Intestinal blood flow and absorption of nondissociable substances. J Pharm Pharmacol 22:640–641, 1970.
108. WG Crouthamel, L Diamond, LW Dittert, JT Doluisio. Drug absorption.VII. Influence of mesenteric blood flow on intestinal drug absorption in dogs. J Pharm Sci 64:664–671, 1975.
109. M Rowland, S Riegelman, PA Harris, SD Sholkoff. Absorption kinetics of aspirin in man following oral administration of an aqueous solution. J Pharm Sci 61:379–385, 1972.
110. E Kruger-Thiemer. Pharmacokinetics and dose-concentration relationships. In: EJ Ariens, ed. Physico-Chemical Aspects of Drug Action. Elmsford, NY: Pergamon Press, 1968, pp. 63–113.
111. GC Oliver, R Tazman, R Frederickson. Influence of congestive heart failure on digoxin level. In: O Storstein, ed. Symposium on Digitalis. Oslo: Gyldendal Norsk Forlag, 1973, pp. 336–347.
112. NL Benowitz. Effects of cardiac disease on pharmacokinetics: pathophysiologic considerations. In: LZ Benet, N Massoud, JG Gainbertoglio, eds. Pharmacokinetics Basis for Drug Treatment. New York: Raven Press, 1984, pp. 89–103.
113. MM Drucker, SJ Blondheim, L Wislicki. Factors affecting acetylation in vivo of *para*-aminobenzoic acid by human subjects. Clin Sci 27:133–141, 1964.
114. G Levy, T. Matsuzawa. Pharmacokinetics of salicylamide elimination in man. J Pharmacol Exp Ther 156:285–293, 1967.
115. KE Price, Z Zolli, Jr, JC Atkinson, HG Luther. Antibiotic inhibitors. I. The effect of certain milk constituents. Antibiot Chemother 7:672–688, 1957.
116. KE Price, Z Zolli, Jr, JC Atkinson, HG Luther. Antibiotic inhibitors. II. Studies on the inhibitory action

of selected divalent cations for oxytetracyctine. Antibiot Chemother 7:689–701, 1957.

117. J Scheiner, WA Altemeier. Experimental study of factors inhibiting absorption and effective therapeutic levels of declomycin. Surg Gynecol Obstet 114:9–14, 1962.

118. PJ Neuvonen, H Turakka. Inhibitory effect of various iron salts on the absorption of tetracycline in man. Eur J Clin Pharmacol 7:357–360, 1974.

119. JG Wagner. Biopharmaceutics: absorption aspects. J Pharm Sci 50:359–387, 1961.

120. P Singh, JK Guillory, TD Sokoloski, LZ Benet, VN Bhatia. Effect of inert tablet ingredients on drug absorption. I. Effect of polyethylene glycol 4000 on the intestinal absorption of four barbiturates. J Pharm Sci 55:63–68, 1966.

121. S Riegelman, WJ Crowell. The kinetics of rectal absorption. II. The absorption of anions. J Am Pharm Assoc Sci Ed 47:123–127, 1958.

122. S Riegelman, WJ Crowell. The kinetics of rectal absorption. III. The absorption of undissociated molecules. J Am Pharm Assoc Sci Ed 47:127–133, 1958.

123. K Kakemi, T Arita, S Muranishi. Absorption and excretion of drugs. XXVII. Effect of nonionic surface-active agents on rectal absorption of sulfonamides. Chem Pllarm Bull 13:976–985, 1965.

124. DL Sorby. Effect of adsorbents on drug absorption. I. Modification of promazine absorption by activated attapulgite and activated charcoal. J Pharm Sci 54:677–683, 1965.

125. JG Wagner. Design and data analysis of biopharmaceutical studies in man. Canad J Pharm Sci 1:55–68, 1966.

126. DG Bailey, JD Spence, C Munoz, JMO Arnold. Interaction of citrus juices with felodipine and nifedipine. Lancet 337:268–269, 1991.

127. SD Hall, KE Thummel, PB Watkins, KS Lown, LZ Benet, MF Paine, RR Mayo, DK Turgeon, DG Bailey, RJ Fontana, SA Wrighton. Molecular and physical mecahnisms of first-pass extraction. Drug Metab Dispos 27:161–166, 1999.

128. DG Bailey, JMO Arnold, JD Spence. Inhibitors in the diet: grapefruit juice-drug interactions. In: RH Levy, KE Thummel, WE Trager, PD Hansten, M Eichelbaum, eds. Metabolic Drug Interactions: New York: Lippincott Williams & Wilkins, 2000, pp. 661–667.

129. P Schmeidlin-Ren, DJ Edwards, ME Fitzsimmons, K He, KS Lown, PM Woster, A Rahman, KE Thummel, JM Fisher, PF Hollenberg, PB Watkins. Mechanisms of enhanced oral availability of CYP3A4 substrates by grapefruit constituents: decreased enterocyte CYP3A4 concentration and mechanism-based inactivation by furanocoumarins. Drug Metab Dispos 25:1228–1233, 1997.

130. GK Dresser, DG Bailey, SG Carruthers. Grapefruit juice-felodipine interaction in the elderly. Clin Pharmacol Ther 68:28–34, 2000.

131. CW Abruzzo, T Macasieb, R Weinfeld, JA Rider, SA Kaplan. Changes in the oral absorption characteristics in man of dipotassium clorasepate at normal and elevated gastric pH. J Pharmacokinet Biopharm 5:377–390, 1977.

132. L Rivera-Calimlim, CA Dujovne, JP Morgan, L Lasagna, JR Bianchine. Absorption and metabolism of L-dopa by the human stomach. Eur J Clin Invest 1:313–320, 1971.

133. L Fleckenstein, GR Mundy, RA Horovitz, JM Mazzullo. Sodium salicylamide: relative bioavailability and sujective effects. Clin.Pharmacol Ther 19:451–458, 1976.

134. G Levy, T Matsuzawa. Pharmacokinetics of salicylamide in man. J Pharmacol Ther 156:285–293, 1967.

135. MM Drucker, SJ Blondheim, L Wislicki, Factors affecting acetylation in vivo of *para*-aminobenzoic acid by human subjects. Clin Sci 27:133–141, 1964.

136. M Frezza, C Di Padova, G Pozzato, M Terpin, E Baraona, CS Lieber. High blood alcohol levels in women: the rold of decreased gastric alcohol dehydrogenase and first-pass metabolism. N Engl J Med 322:95–99, 1990.

137. HK Seitz, G Egerer, UA Simanowski, R Waldherr, R Eckey, DP Agarwal, HW Goedde, J-P von Wartourg. Human gastric alcohol dehydrogenase activity: effect of age, sex and alcoholism. Gut 34:1433–1437, 1993.

138. YK Tam. Individual variation in first-pass metabolism. Clin Pharmacokin 25:300–332, 1993.

139. RL Smith. The role of the gut flora in the conversion of inactive compounds to active metabolites. In: A Symposium on Mechanisms of Toxicity. WN Aldridge, ed. New York: Macmillan, 1971, pp. 228–244.

140. D Durr, B Stieger, GA Kullak-Ublick, KM Rentsch, HC Steinert, PJ Meier, K Fattinger. St. John's wort induces intestinal *p*-glycoprotein/MDR1 and intestinal and hepatic CYP3A45. Clin Pharmacol Ther 68:598–604, 2000.

141. WA Ritschel, DD Denson. Influence of disease on bioavailability. In: PG Welling, FLS Tse, SV Dighe, eds. Pharmaceutical Bioequivalence. New York: Marcel Dekker, 1991, pp. 67–115.

142. PA Kramer, DJ Chapron, J Benson, SA Merik. Tetracycline absorption in elderly patients with achlorhydria. Clin Pharmacol Ther 23:467–472, 1978.

143. HR Ochs, DJ Greenblatt, HJ Dengler. Absorption of oral tetracycline in patients with Billroth-II gastrectomy. J Pharmacokinet Biopharm 6:295–303, 1978.

144. G Levy, MH MacGillivray, JA Procknal. Riboflavin absorption in children with thyroid disorders. Pediatrics 50:896–900, 1972.

145. LF Prescott. Gastrointestinal absorption of drugs. Med Clin North Am 58:907–916, 1974.
146. WJ Jusko, DR Conti, A Molson, P Kuritzky, J Giller, R Schultz. Digoxin absorption from tablets and elixir: the effect of radiation-induced malabsorption. J Am Med Assoc 230:1554–1555, 1974.
147. GH Sokol, DJ Greenblatt, BL Lloyd, A Gecrgotas, MD Allen, JS Harmatz, TW Smith, RI Shader. Effect of abdominal radiation therapy on drug absorption in humans. J Clin Pharmacol 18:388–396, 1978.
148. WD Heizer, TW Smith, SE Goldfinger. Absorption of digoxin in patients with malabsorption syndromes. N Engl J Med 285:257–259, 1971.
149. AE Davis, RC Pirola. Absorption of phenoxymethyl penicillin in patients with steatorrhea. Aust Ann Med 17:63–65, 1968.
150. JD Nelson, S Shelton, HT Kusmiesz, KC Haltalin. Absorption of ampicillin and nalidixic acid in infants and children with acute shigellosis. Clin Pharmacol Ther 13:879–886, 1972.
151. JP Kampmann, H Klein, B Lumholtz, JEM Hansen. Ampicillin and propylthiouracil pharmacokinetics in intestinal bypass patients followed up to a year after operation. Clin Pharmacokinet 9:168–176, 1984.
152. WJ Jusko, N Khanna, G Levy, L Stern, SJ Yaffe. Riboflavin absorption and excretion in the neonate. Pediatrics 45:945–949, 1970.
153. M Mayersohn. Special pharmacokinetic considerations in the elderly. In: WE Evans, JJ Schentag, WJ Jusko, eds. Applied Pharmacokinetics: Principles of Therapeutic Drug Monitoring. 3rd ed. Vancouver, WA: Applied Therapeutics, 1992, pp. 9-1–9-43.
154. M Mayersohn. Pharmacokinetics in the elderly. Environ Health Perspect 102 (suppl 11):119–124, 1994.
155. M Mayersohn, The ‘‘xylose test’’ to assess gastrointestinal absorption in the elderly: a pharmacokinetic evaluation of the literature. J Gerontol 37:300–305, 1982.
156. SL Johnson, M Mayersohn, KA Conrad. Gastrointestinal absorption as a function of age: xylose absorption in healthy adult subjects. Clin Pharmacol Ther 38:331–335, 1985.
157. TL Russell, RR Berardi, JL Barnett, TL O'Sullivan, JG Wagner, JB Dressman. pH-related changes in the absorption of dipyridamole in the elderly. Pharmaceut Res 11:136–143, 1994.

Chapter 3

Pharmacokinetics

David W. A. Bourne

University of Oklahoma, Oklahoma City, Oklahoma

I. INTRODUCTION

Drug therapy is a dynamic process. When a drug product is administered, absorption usually proceeds over a finite time interval, and distribution, metabolism, and excretion (ADME) of the drug and its metabolites proceed continuously at various rates. The relative rates of these "ADME processes" determine the time course of the drug in the body, most importantly at the receptor sites that are responsible for the pharmacological action of the drug.

The usual aim of drug therapy is to achieve and maintain effective concentrations of drug at the receptor site. However, the body is constantly trying to eliminate the drug, and, therefore, it is necessary to balance absorption against elimination so as to maintain the desired concentration. Often the receptor sites are tucked away in a specific organ or tissue of the body, such as the central nervous system, and it is necessary to depend upon the blood supply to distribute the drug from the site of administration, such as the gastrointestinal tract, to the site of action.

Since the body may be viewed as a very complex system of compartments, at first it might appear to be hopeless to try to describe the time course of the drug at the receptor sites in any mathematically rigorous way. The picture is further complicated by the fact that, for many drugs, the locations of the receptor sites are unknown. Fortunately, body compartments are connected by the blood system, and distribution of drugs among the compartments usually occurs much more rapidly than absorption or elimination of the drug. The net result is that the body behaves as a single homogeneous compartment with respect to many drugs, and the concentration of the drug in the blood directly reflects or is proportional to the concentration of the drug in all organs and tissues. Thus, it may never be possible to isolate a receptor site and determine the concentration of drug around it, but the concentration at the receptor site usually can be controlled if the blood concentration can be controlled.

The objective of pharmacokinetics is to describe the time course of drug concentrations in blood in mathematical terms so that (a) the performance of pharmaceutical dosage forms can be evaluated in terms of the rate and amount of drug they deliver to the blood, and (b) the dosage regimen of a drug can be adjusted to produce and maintain therapeutically effective blood concentrations with little or no toxicity. The primary objective of this chapter will be to describe the graph paper and calculator-level mathematical tools needed to accomplish these aims when the body behaves as a single homogeneous compartment and when all pharmacokinetic processes obey first-order kinetics.

On some occasions, the body does not behave as a single homogeneous compartment, and multicompartment pharmacokinetics are required to describe the time course of drug concentrations. In other instances certain pharmacokinetic processes may not obey first-order kinetics and saturable or nonlinear models may be required. Additionally, advanced pharmacokinetic analyses require the use of various computer programs, such as those listed on the website http://www.boomer.org/pkin/soft.html.

Readers interested in such advanced topics are referred to a number of texts that describe these more complex pharmacokinetic models in detail [1–5] and to the website http://www.boomer.org/pkin/.

II. PRINCIPLES OF FIRST-ORDER KINETICS

A. Definition and Characteristics of First-Order Processes

The science of kinetics deals with the mathematical description of the rate of the appearance or disappearance of a substance. One of the most common types of rate processes observed in nature is the first-order process in which the rate is dependent upon the concentration or amount of only one component. An example of such a process is radioactive decay in which the rate of decay (i.e., the number of radioactive decompositions per minute) is directly proportional to the amount of undecayed substance remaining. This may be written mathematically as follows:

$$\text{Rate of radioactivity decay} \propto [\text{undecayed substance}] \tag{1}$$

or

$$\text{Rate of radioactive decay} = k\,(\text{undecayed substance}) \tag{2}$$

where k is a proportionality constant called the first-order rate constant.

Chemical reactions usually occur through collision of at least two molecules, very often in a solution, and the rate of the chemical reaction is proportional to the concentrations of all reacting molecules. For example, the rate of hydrolysis of an ester in an alkaline buffered solution depends upon the concentration of both the ester and hydroxide ion:

$$\text{Ester} + \text{OH}^- \rightarrow \text{Acid}^- + \text{Alcohol} \tag{3}$$

The rate of hydrolysis may be expressed as follows:

$$\text{Rate of hydrolysis} \propto [\text{Ester}] \bullet [\text{OH}^-] \tag{4}$$

or

$$\text{Rate of hydrolysis} = k[\text{Ester}] \bullet [\text{OH}^-] \tag{5}$$

where k is the proportionality constant called the second-order rate constant.

But in a buffered system, $[\text{OH}^-]$ is constant. Therefore, at given pH, the rate of hydrolysis is dependent only on the concentration of the ester and may be written:

$$\text{Rate of hydrolysis}_{(\text{pH})} = k^* \bullet [\text{Ester}] \tag{6}$$

where k^* is the pseudo-first-order rate constant at the pH in question. (The pseudo-first-order rate constant, k^*, is the product of the second-order rate constant and the hydroxide ion concentration: $k^* = k \bullet [\text{OH}^-]$).

Fortunately, most ADME processes behave as pseudo-first-order processes—not because they are so simple, but because everything except the drug concentration is constant. For example, the elimination of a drug from the body may be written as follows:

$$\begin{bmatrix}\text{Drug}\\ \text{in}\\ \text{body}\end{bmatrix} + \begin{bmatrix}\text{Enzymes;}\\ \text{membranes;}\\ \text{pH; protein}\\ \text{binding; etc.}\end{bmatrix} \longrightarrow \begin{matrix}\text{Metabolized or}\\ \text{excreted drug}\end{matrix} \tag{7}$$

If everything except the concentration of drug in the body is constant, the elimination of the drug will be a pseudo-first-order process. This may seem to be a drastic oversimplification, but most in vivo drug processes, in fact, behave as pseudo-first-order processes.

B. Differential Rate Expressions

In the previous discussion of radioactive decay, it was noted that the rate of decay is directly proportional to the amount of undecayed substance remaining. In a solution of a radioactive substance, a similar relationship would hold for the concentration of undecayed substance remaining. If a solution of a radioactive substance were allowed to decay and a plot were constructed of the concentration remaining versus time, the plot would be a curve such as that shown in Fig. 1.

In this system, the rate of decay might be expressed as a change in concentration per unit time, $\Delta C/\Delta t$, which corresponds to the slope of the line. But the line in Fig. 1 is curved, which means that the rate is constantly changing and therefore cannot be expressed in terms of a finite time interval. By resorting to differential calculus, it is possible to express the rate of decay in terms of an infinitesimally small change in concentration (dC) over an infinitesimally small time interval (dt). The resulting function, dC/dt, is the slope of the line, and it is this function that is proportional to concentration in a first-order process. Thus,

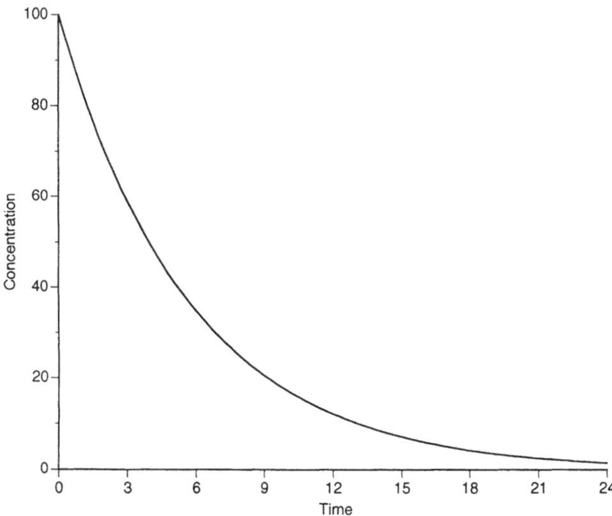

Fig. 1 Plot of concentration remaining versus time for a first-order process (e.g., radioactive decay).

$$\text{Rate} = \frac{dC}{dt} = -kC \tag{8}$$

The negative sign is introduced because the concentration is falling as time progresses.

Equation (8) is the differential rate expression for a first-order reaction. The value of the rate constant, k, could be calculated by determining the slope of the concentration versus time curve at any point and dividing by the concentration at that point. However, the slope of a curved line is difficult to measure accurately, and k can be determined much more easily using integrated rate expressions.

C. Integrated Rate Expressions and Working Equations

Equation (8) can be rearranged and integrated as follows:

$$\frac{dC}{C} = -k\,dt \tag{9}$$

$$\int \frac{dC}{C} = -k \int dt$$

$$\ln C = -kt + \text{constant} \tag{10}$$

where ln C is the natural logarithm (base e) of the concentration.

The constant in Eq. (10) can be evaluated at zero time when $kt = 0$ and $C = C_0$, the initial concentration. Thus,

$$\ln C_0 = \text{constant}$$

and

$$\log C = -kt + \ln C_0 \tag{11}$$

Equation (11) is the integrated rate expression for a first-order process and can serve as a working equation for solving problems. It is also in the form of the equation of a straight line:

$$y = mx + b$$

Therefore, if ln C is plotted against t, as shown in Fig. 2, the plot will be a straight line with an intercept (at $t = 0$) of ln C_0, and the slope of the line (m) will be $-k$. Such plots are commonly used to determine the order of a reaction; that is, if a plot of ln C versus time is a straight line, the reaction is assumed to be a first-order or pseudo-first-order process.

The slope of the line and the corresponding value of k for a plot such as that shown in Fig. 2 may be calculated using the following equation:

$$\text{slope}(m) = \frac{\ln C_1 - \ln C_2}{t_1 - t_2} = -k \tag{12}$$

Example. A solution of ethyl acetate in pH 10.0 buffer (25°C) 1 hour after preparation was found to contain 3 mg/mL. Two hours after preparation, the solution contained 2 mg/mL. Calculate the

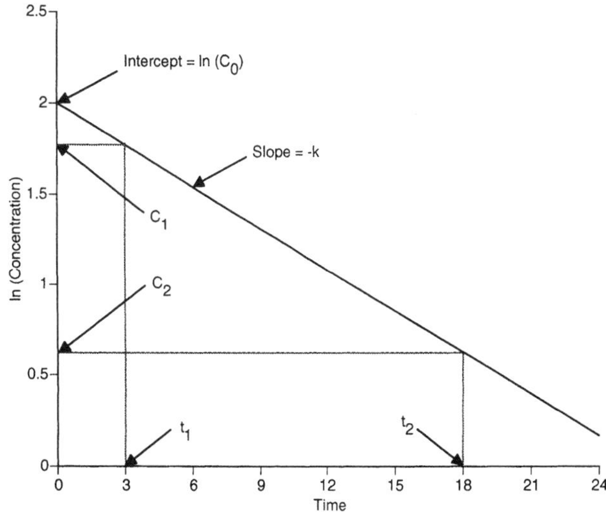

Fig. 2 Plot of ln (Concentration remaining) versus time for a first-order process.

pseudo-first-order rate constant for hydrolysis of ethyl acetate at pH 10.0 (25°C).

$$\text{slope}(m) = \frac{\ln 3 - \ln 2}{(1-2)\,\text{h}} = -k$$
$$= \frac{1.099 - 0.693}{-1}$$
$$= -0.406\,\text{h}^{-1} = -k$$

$$k = 0.406\,\text{h}^{-1}$$

Note that since ln C is dimensionless, the rate constant, k, has the dimensions of reciprocal time (i.e., day^{-1}, h^{-1}, min^{-1}, s^{-1}, etc.).

Another useful working equation can be obtained by rearranging Eq. (11) as follows:

$$\ln C - \ln C_0 = -kt$$
$$\ln C_0 - \ln C = kt \tag{13}$$
$$\ln \frac{C_0}{C} = kt$$

Equation (13) shows that since k is a constant for a given process, the value of t is determined solely by the ratio C_0/C. For example, when C_0/C is equal to 2, the value t will be the same, no matter what was the value of the initial concentration (C_0).

Example. For the ethyl acetate hydrolysis above ($k = 0.406\,\text{h}^{-1}$), if $C_0 = 3\,\text{mg/mL}$, when would $C = 1.5\,\text{mg/mL}$?

$$\ln \frac{C_0}{C} = kt$$

$$\ln \frac{3}{1.5} = 0.406 \times t$$

$$\ln 2 = 0.406 \times t$$

$$0.693 = 0.406 \times t$$

$$t = 1.71\,\text{h}$$

If $C_0 = 1.5\,\text{mg/mL}$, when would $C = 0.75\,\text{mg/mL}$?

$$\ln \frac{C_0}{C} = kt$$

$$\ln \frac{1.5}{0.75} = 0.406 \times t$$

$$\log 2 = 0.406 \times t$$

$$t = 1.71\,\text{h}$$

The time required for the concentration to fall to $C_0/2$ is called the half-life, and the foregoing example shows that the half-life for a first-order or pseudo-first-order process is a constant throughout the process; it also demonstrates that a first-order process theoretically never reaches completion, since even the lowest concentration would only fall to half its value in one half-life.

Table 1 Approach to Completeness with Increasing Half-Lives

Number of half-lives elapsed	Initial concentration remaining (%)	"Completeness" of process (%)
0	100.0	0.0
1	50.0	50.0
2	25.0	75.0
3	12.5	87.5
4	6.25	93.75
5	3.13	96.87
6	1.56	98.44
7	0.78	99.22

For most practical purposes, a first-order process may be deemed complete if it is 95% or more complete. Table 1 shows that five half-lives must elapse to reach this point. Thus the elimination of a drug from the body may be considered to be complete after five half-lives have elapsed (i.e., 97% completion). This principle becomes important, for example, in crossover bioavailability studies in which the subjects must be rested for sufficient time between each drug administration to ensure that "washout" is complete.

The half-life of a first-order process is very important. Since it is often desirable to convert a half-life to a rate constant, and vice versa, a simple relationship between the two is very useful. The relationship may be derived as follows:

$$\ln \frac{C_0}{C} = kt$$

When $C_0/C = 2$ and $t = t_{1/2}$. Thus,

$$\ln 2 = kt_{1/2}$$

$$0.693 = kt_{1/2}$$

$$k = \frac{0.693}{t_{1/2}} \tag{14}$$

$$t_{1/2} = \frac{0.693}{k} \tag{15}$$

D. Examples of Calculations

Equations (13), (14), and (15) can be used to solve three types of problems involving first-order processes.

These types of problems are illustrated in the following examples:

Type 1

Given the rate constant or half-life and the initial concentration, calculate the concentration at some time in the future.

Example. A penicillin solution containing 500 units/mL has a half-life of 10 days. What will the concentration be in 7 days?

$$k = \frac{0.693}{t_{1/2}} = \frac{0.693}{10\,\text{day}} = 0.069\,\text{day}^{-1}$$

$$\ln\frac{C_0}{C} = kt$$

$$\ln\frac{500\ \text{units/mL}}{C} = 0.069\,\text{day}^{-1} \times 7\,\text{days} = 0.483$$

$$\frac{500}{C} = \text{anti}\ \ln(0.483) = e^{0.483} = 1.62$$

$$C = 308\,\text{units/mL}$$

Type 2

Given the half-life or rate constant and the initial concentration, calculate the time required to reach a specified lower concentration.

Example. A penicillin solution has a half-life of 21 days. How long will it take for the potency to drop to 90% of the initial potency?

$$k = \frac{0.693}{21\ \text{days}} = 0.033\,\text{day}^{-1}$$

$$\ln\frac{C_0}{C} = kt$$

$$\ln\frac{100\%}{90\%} = 0.033 \times t$$

$$t = 3.2\,\text{days}$$

Type 3

Given an initial concentration and the concentration after a specified elapsed time, calculate the rate constant or half-life.

Example. A penicillin solution has an initial potency of 125 mg/5 mL. After 1 month in a refrigerator, the potency is found to be 100 mg/5 mL. What is the half-life of the penicillin solution under these storage conditions?

$$\ln\frac{C_0}{C} = kt$$

$$\ln\frac{125\,\text{mg/5\,mL}}{100\,\text{mg/5\,mL}} = k \times 30\,\text{day}$$

$$k = 0.0074\,\text{day}^{-1}$$

$$t_{1/2} = \frac{0.693}{0.0074\,\text{day}^{-1}} = 94\,\text{days}$$

For each type of problem the following assumptions are made: (a) the process follows first-order kinetics, at least over the time interval and concentration range involved in the calculations, and (b) all time and concentration values are accurate.

The latter assumption is particularly critical in solving problems such as type 3, where a rate constant is being calculated. It would be unwise to rely on only two time points to calculate such an important value. Normally, duplicate or triplicate assays would be performed at six or more time points throughout as much of the reaction as possible. The resulting mean assay values and standard deviation values would be plotted on semilogarithmic graph paper and a straight line carefully fitted to the data points. The half-life could then the determined using Eq. (14).

Example. A solution of ethyl acetate in pH 9.5 buffer (25°C) was assayed in triplicate several times over a 20-hour period. The data obtained are presented in Table 2. The results were plotted on semilogarthmic graph paper as shown in Fig. 3. Calculate the psuedo-first-order rate constant for the hydrolysis of ethyl acetate at pH 9.5 (25°C).

By fitting a straight line ("best-fit" line) through the data points in Fig. 3 (this can be done by eye using a transparent straight edge) and extrapolating to $t = 0$,

Table 2 Assay of Ethyl Acetate

Time (h)	Concentration (mg/mL) ± SD
2	1.83 ± 0.15
4	1.01 ± 0.09
6	0.58 ± 0.07
8	0.33 ± 0.06
10	0.18 ± 0.04
12	0.10 ± 0.02
16	0.031 ± 0.006
20	0.012 ± 0.002

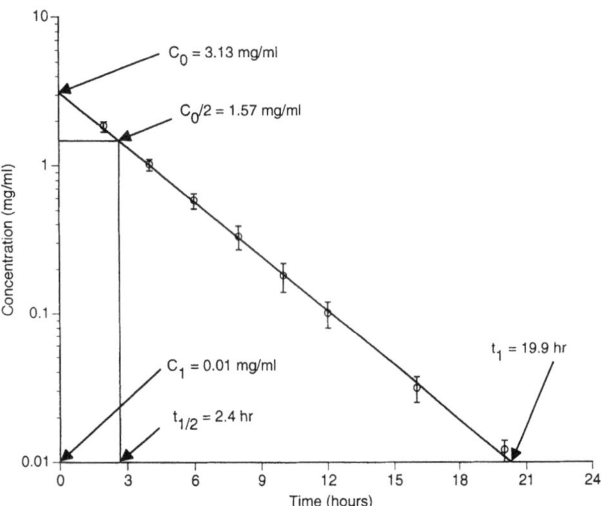

Fig. 3 Semilogarithmic plot of concentration versus time for the hydrolysis of ethyl acetate. (Data shown in Table 2. One standard deviation is indicated by error bars.)

the intercept C_0 is found to be 3.13 mg/mL. The half-life is the time at which the concentration equals 1.57 mg/mL, and this is found by interpolation to be 2.4 hours. The value of k can be given by

$$k = \frac{0.693}{t_{1/2}} = \frac{0.693}{2.4\,\text{h}} = 0.289\,\text{h}^{-1}$$

A value for k can also be determined directly from points on the line using Eq. (12). In Fig. 3, values for C_0, C_1, t_0, and t_1 can read from the "best-fit" line as 3.13 mg/mL, 0.01 mg/mL, 0 hour, and 19.9 hours. Thus:

$$k = -\text{slope} = \frac{\ln C_0 - \ln C_1}{t_1 - t_0}$$

$$k = \frac{\ln 3.13 - \ln 0.01}{19.9 - 0.0} = 0.289\,\text{h}^{-1}$$

Semilogarithmic graph paper is readily available from many graph paper manufactures. It consists of a logarithmic scale on the y-axis and a cartesian scale on the x-axis (see Fig. 3). On the logarithmic scale, the spatial distribution of lines is such that the position of each line is proportional to the logarithm of the value represented by the mark. For example, plotting a concentration of 1.83 mg/mL on semilog paper is equivalent to looking up the logarithm of 1.83 and plotting it on a Cartesian scale. This type of graph paper is extremely useful for kinetic calculations because raw concentration data can be plotted directly without converting to logarithms, and concentration values can be extrapolated and interpolated from the plot without converting logs to numbers.

For example, to determine the half-life in the preceding example, the C_0 value and the time at which $C = C_0/2$ were both read directly from the graph. If Fig. 3 had been a plot of ln C (on a Cartesian scale) versus time, it would have been necessary to read ln C_0 from the graph, convert it to C_0, divide by 2, convert back to ln $(C_0/2)$, then read the half-life off the graph. If the rate constant is determined for this example using Eq. (12), the slope must be calculated. To calculate the slope of the line it is necessary first to read two concentrations from the graph and then take the logarithm of each concentration as described in Eq. (12).

III. FIRST-ORDER PHARMACOKINETICS: DRUG ELIMINATION FOLLOWING RAPID INTRAVENOUS INJECTION

It was mentioned previously that drug elimination from the body most often displays the characteristics of a first-order process. Thus, if a drug is administered by rapid intravenous (IV) injection, after mixing with the body fluids its rate of elimination from the body is proportional to the amount remaining in the body.

Normally, the plasma concentration is used as a measure of the amount of drug in the body, and a plot of plasma concentration versus time has the same characteristics as the plot in Fig. 1. A semilogarithmic

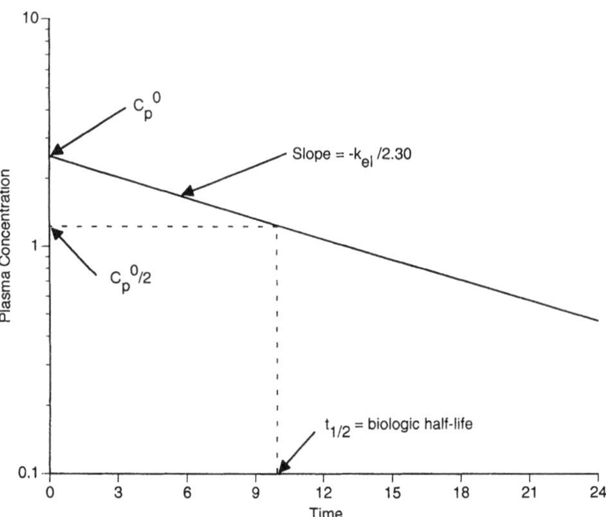

Fig. 4 Semilogarithmic plot of plasma concentration versus time for a drug administered by rapid intravenous injection.

plot of plasma concentration versus time is a straight line and allows the calculation of k_{el} from the slope, where k_{el} is the overall elimination rate constant. The intercept at $t = 0$ is C_p^0, the hypothetical plasma concentration after the drug is completely mixed with body fluids but before any elimination has occurred.

A typical semi-log plasma concentration versus time plot is shown in Fig. 4. This figure shows that pharmacokinetic data can also be expressed in terms of a half-life, called the biological half-life, which bears the same relationship to k_{el} as that shown in Eqs. (14) and (15).

Since all the kinetic characteristics of the disappearance of a drug from plasma are the same as those for the pseudo-first-order disappearance of a substance from a solution by hydrolysis, the same working equations [Eqs. (11) and (13)] and the same approach to solving problems can be used.

Example. A 250 mg dose of tetracycline was administered to a patient by rapid IV injection. The initial plasma concentration (C_p^0) was 2.50 μg/mL. After 4 hours the plasma concentration was 1.89 μg/mL. What is the biological half-life ($t_{1/2}$) of tetracycline in this patient?

$$\ln \frac{C_p^0}{C_p} = k_{el}t$$

$$\ln \frac{2.50}{1.89} = k_{el} \times 4$$

$$k_{el} = \frac{0.280}{4} = 0.0699\,\text{h}^{-1}$$

$$t_{1/2} = \frac{0.693}{0.0699\,\text{h}^{-1}} = 9.91\,\text{h}$$

Note that this approach involves the following assumptions: (a) the drug was eliminated by a psuedo-first-order process, and (b) the drug was rapidly distributed so that an "initial plasma concentration" could be measured before any drug began to leave the body. The latter assumption implies that the body behaves as a single homogeneous compartment throughout which the drug distributes instantaneously following IV injection. In pharmacokinetic terms, this is referred to as the one-compartment model. Although most drugs do not, in fact, distribute instantaneously, they do distribute very rapidly, and the one-compartment model can be used for may clinically important pharmacokinetic calculations.

An important parameter of the one-compartment model is the apparent volume of the body compartment, because it directly determines the relationship between the plasma concentration and the amount of drug in the body. This volume is called the apparent volume of distribution, V_d, and it may be calculated using the relationship:

$$\text{Volume} = \frac{\text{amount}}{\text{concentration}}$$

The easiest way to calculate V_d is to use C_p^0, the plasma concentration when distribution is complete (assumed to be instantaneous for a one-compartment model) and the entire dose is still in the body. Thus,

$$V_d = \frac{\text{dose}}{C_p^0} \tag{16}$$

Example. Calculate V_d for the patient in the previous example;

$$V_d = \frac{250\,\text{mg}}{2.50\,\mu\text{g/mL}}$$

$$V_d = 100\,\text{L}$$

Note: Since 1 μg/mL = 1 mg/L, dividing the dose in milligrams by the plasma concentration in micrograms per milliliter will give V_d in liters.

The apparent volume of distribution of a drug very rarely corresponds to any physiological volume, and even in cases where it does, it must never be construed as showing that the drug enters or does not enter various body spaces. For example, the 100 L volume calculated in the foregoing example is much greater than either plasma volume (about 3 L) or whole blood volume (about 6 L) in a standard (70 kg) man; it is even greater than the extracellular fluid volume (19 L) and total body water (42 L) in the same average man. Based on the calculated value of V, it cannot be said that tetracycline is restricted to the plasma or that it enters or does not enter red blood cells, or that it enters or does not enter any or all extracellular fluids.

A discussion of all the reasons for this phenomenon is beyond the scope of this chapter, but a simple example will illustrate the concept. Highly lipid-soluble drugs, such as pentobarbital, are preferentially distributed into adipose tissue. The result is that plasma concentrations are extremely low after distribution is complete. When the apparent volumes of distribution are calculated, they are frequently found to exceed total body volume, occasionally by a factor of 2 or more. This would be impossible if the concentration in the entire body compartment were equal to the plasma concentration. Thus, V_d is an empirically fabricated number relating the concentration of drug in plasma (or blood) with the amount of drug in the body. For drugs such as pentobarbital the ratio of the concentration in adipose tissue to the concentration in plasma is much greater than unity, resulting in a large value for V_d.

IV. PHARMACOKINETIC ANALYSIS OF URINE DATA

Occasionally, it is inconvenient or impossible to assay the drug in plasma, but it may be possible to follow the appearance of the drug in urine. If the drug is not metabolized to any appreciable degree, the pharmacokinetic model may be written as shown in Scheme 1.

$$D_B \xrightarrow{k_{el}} D_U$$

Scheme 1

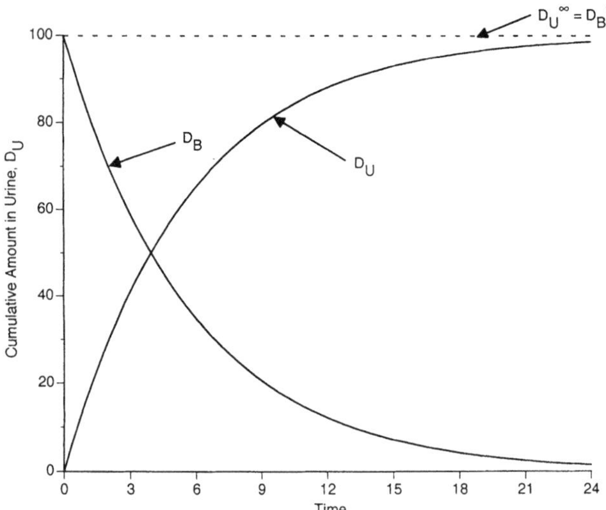

Fig. 5 Plot of cumulative amount of drug in urine, D_U (solid line), and the amount of drug in body, D_B (dashed line), versus time according to Scheme 1.

A plot of cumulative amount of drug appearing in urine (D_U) versus time will be the mirror image of a plot of amount of drug remaining in the body (D_B) versus time. This is illustrated in Fig. 5, which shows that the total amount of drug recovered in urine throughout the entire study (D_U^∞) is equal to the dose (D_B^0) and, at any time, the sum of drug in the body (D_B) plus drug in urine (D_U) equals the dose (D_B^0).

A kinetic equation describing urine data can be developed as follows. If

$$\frac{dD_B}{dt} = -k_{el}D_B$$

then,

$$\frac{dD_U}{dt} = +k_{el}D_B$$

But if

$$D_B + D_U = D_U^\infty$$
$$= \text{amount recovered in urine}$$

Then,

$$D_B = D_U^\infty - D_U$$

Therefore,

$$\frac{dD_U}{dt} = k_{el}(D_U^\infty - D_U)$$

or

$$\frac{dD_U}{D_U^\infty - D_U} = k_{el}\,dt$$

Integration gives

$$\int \frac{dD_U}{D_U^\infty - D_U} = k_{el} \int dt$$

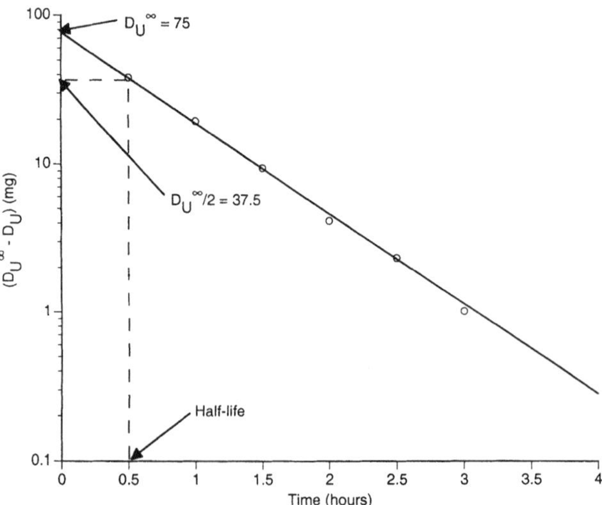

Fig. 6 Semilogarithmic plot of amount of drug remaining to be excreted (ARE) into urine, $D_U^\infty - D_U$, versus time.

Table 3 Drug Excreted into the Urine Versus Time

Time interval (h)	Amount excreted (mg)	Cumulative amount excreted, D_U^a (mg)	$D_U^\infty - D_U$ (mg)
0.0–0.5	37.5	37.5	37.8
0.5–1.0	18.5	56.0	19.3
1.0–1.5	10.0	66.0	9.3
1.5–2.0	5.2	71.2	4.1
2.0–2.5	1.8	73.0	2.3
2.5–3.0	1.3	74.3	1.0
3.0–6.0	1.0	75.3	0.0
6.0–12.0	0.0	75.3	0.0

[a] $D_U^\infty = 75.3$ mg.

$$-\ln(D_U^\infty - D_U) + \ln(D_U^\infty - D_U^0) = k_{el}t$$

Since $D_U^0 = 0$ (there is no drug in urine when $t = 0$),

$$\ln(D_U^\infty - D_U) - \ln D_U^\infty = -k_{el}t$$

$$\ln(D_U^\infty - D_U) = -k_{el}t + \ln D_U^\infty \tag{17}$$

Equation (17) is in the form of the equation for a straight line ($y = mx + b$), where t is one variable (x), $-k_{el}$ is determined from the slope (m), ln D_U^∞ is the constant (b), and ln $(D_U^\infty - D_U)$ the other variable (y). Thus a plot of ln $(D_U^\infty - D_U)$ versus time is a straight line with a slope providing a value of k_{el} and an intercept of ln D_U^∞. Since D_U^∞ is the total amount excreted and D_U is the amount excreted up to time t, $D_U^\infty - D_U$ is the amount remaining to be excreted (ARE). A typical ARE plot is shown in Fig. 6.

Example. The plot in Fig. 6 was constructed using the data shown in Table 3. Note that the concentration of the drug in each urine specimen is not the information analyzed. The total amount excreted over each time interval and throughout the entire study must be determined. As a result, the experimental details of a urinary excretion study must be very carefully chosen, and strict adherence to the protocol is required. Loss of a single urine specimen, or even an unknown part of a urine specimen, makes construction of an ARE plot impossible.

V. CLEARANCE RATE AS AN EXPRESSION OF DRUG-ELIMINATION RATE

A clearance rate is defined as the volume of blood or plasma completely cleared of drug per unit time. It is a useful way to describe drug elimination because it is related to blood or plasma perfusion of various organs of elimination, and it can be directly related to the physiological function of these organs. For example, the renal clearance rate (RCR) of a drug can be calculated using the following equation:

$$\text{RCR} = \frac{\text{amount excreted in urine per unit time}}{\text{plasma concentration}} \tag{18}$$

Example. In the example plotted in Fig. 6, the amount of drug excreted over the 0- to 0.5-hour interval was 37.5 mg. If the plasma concentration at 0.25 hour (the middle of the interval) was 10 µg/mL, what was the renal clearance rate? From Eq. (18),

$$\begin{aligned}\text{RCR} &= \frac{37.5\,\text{mg}/0.5\,\text{h}}{10\,\mu\text{g/mL}}\\ &= 7.5\,\text{L/h}\\ &= 125\,\text{mL/min}\end{aligned}$$

The glomerular filtration rate (GFR) in normal males is estimated to be 125 mL/min, and the results of the example calculation suggest that the drug is cleared by GFR. If the RCR had been less than 125 mL/min, tubular reabsorption of the drug would have been suspected. If it had been greater than 125 mL/min, tubular secretion would have been involved in the drug elimination.

Drugs can be cleared from the body by metabolism as well as renal excretion, and when this occurs it is not possible to measure directly the amount cleared by metabolism. However, the total clearance rate (TCR), or total body clearance, of the drug can be calculated from its pharmacokinetic parameters using the following equation:

$$\text{TCR} = k_{el}V_d \tag{19}$$

Example. The biological half-life of procaine in a patient was 35 minutes, and its volume of distribution was estimated to be 58 L. Calculate the TCR of procaine.

$$k_{el} = \frac{0.693}{35\text{ min}} = 0.0198\text{ min}^{-1}$$

$$\begin{aligned}\text{TCR} &= k_{el}V_d\\ &= 0.0198\,\text{min}^{-1} \times 58\,\text{L}\\ &= 1.15\,\text{L/min}\end{aligned}$$

When a drug is eliminated by both metabolism and urinary excretion, it is possible to calculate the metabolic clearance rate (MCR) by the difference between TCR and RCR:

$$\text{MCR} = \text{TCR} - \text{RCR} \tag{20}$$

The RCR can be determined from urine and plasma data using Eq. (18), and the TCR can be determined from the pharmacokinetic parameters using Eq. (19). Alternately, the RCR can be calculated by multiplying the TCR by the fraction of the dose excreted unchanged into urine, f_e:

$$\text{RCR} = f_e\text{TCR} \tag{21}$$

If it is assumed that the fraction of the dose not appearing as unchanged drug in urine has been metabolized, the MCR can be calculated as follows:

$$\text{MCR} = (1 - f_e)\text{TCR} \tag{22}$$

Example. Sulfadiazine in a normal volunteer had a biological half-life of 16 hours and a volume of distribution of 20 L. Sixty percent of the dose was recovered as unchanged drug in urine. Calculate TCR, RCR, and MCR for sulfadiazine in this person.

$$k_{el} = \frac{0.693}{16\,\text{h}} = 0.0433\,\text{h}^{-1}$$

$$\begin{aligned} \text{TCR} &= k_{el}V_d \\ &= 0.0433\,\text{h}^{-1} \times 20\,\text{L} \\ &= 0.866\,\text{L/h} \\ &= 14.4\,\text{mL/min} \end{aligned}$$

$$\begin{aligned} \text{RCR} &= f_e\text{TCR} \\ &= 0.6 \times 14.4\,\text{mL/min} \\ &= 8.64\,\text{mL/min} \end{aligned}$$

$$\begin{aligned} \text{MCR} &= (1 - f_e)\text{TCR} \\ &= (1 - 0.6) \times 14.4\,\text{mL/min} \\ &= 5.76\,\text{mL/min} \end{aligned}$$

It should be emphasized that the assumption that any drug not appearing as unchanged drug in urine has been metabolized may introduce a great amount of error into the values of the clearance rates estimated using Eqs. (21) and (22). By this assumption unchanged drug eliminated in the feces would be included with metabolized drug, as would any orally administered drug that was unabsorbed.

VI. PHARMACOKINETICS OF DRUG ELIMINATED BY SIMULTANEOUS METABOLISM AND EXCRETION

Although some drugs are excreted unchanged in urine, most are partially eliminated by metabolism. Usually

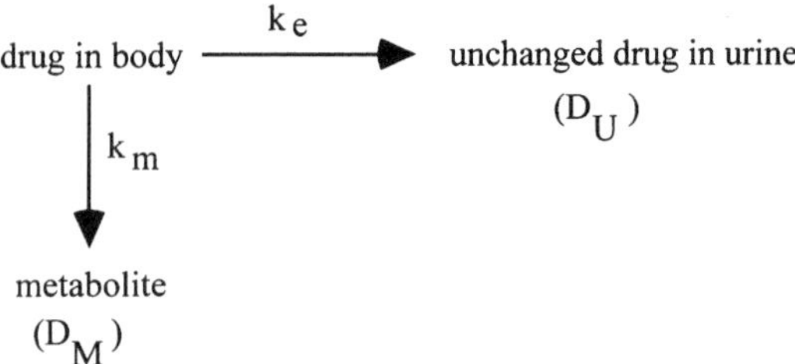

Scheme 2

both the urinary excretion of unchanged drug and the metabolism are first-order processes, with the rate of excretion and metabolism dependent upon the amount of unchanged drug in the body. This results in a "branch" in the kinetic chain representing exit of drug in the body as depicted in the accompanying pharmacokinetic model (Scheme 2).

In this scheme, the rate of loss of drug from the body is determined by both k_e and k_m, and this can be written in differential form as follows:

$$\begin{aligned} \frac{dD_B}{dt} &= -k_eD_B - k_mD_B \\ &= -(k_e + k_m)D_B \end{aligned} \tag{23}$$

Thus, the overall elimination rate constant (k_{el}) here is the sum of the urinary excretion rate constant (k_e) and the metabolism rate constant (k_m):

$$k_{el} = k_e + k_m \tag{24}$$

For drugs that are both metabolized and excreted unchanged, semilogarithmic plots of plasma concentrations versus time will provide values of k_{el}.

Urine data are required to determine the individual values of k_e and k_m. The required equations are derived next.

Derivation. From Scheme 2, the differential equation describing overall rate of disappearance of drug from the body may be written:

$$\frac{dD_B}{dt} = -k_{el}D_B$$

and the following integrated equation can be written [see also Eq. (10)]:

$$\ln D_B = \ln D_B^0 - k_{el}t$$

Taking antilogs yields

$$D_B = D_B^0 \exp(-k_{el}t) \tag{25}$$

It should be noted that Eq. (25) is another form of an integrated rate equation. This form makes use of an exp $(-x)$ term and may be referred to as an exponential rate expression. These expressions are useful for visualizing the characteristics of a first-order process. For example, when $t = 0$, $\exp(-k_{el}t) = 1$, and $D_B = D_B^0$. When $t = t_{1/2}$, $\exp(-k_{el}t_{1/2}) = 0.5$, and $D_B = 0.5 \times D_B^0$. When $t = \infty$, $\exp(-k_{el}t) = 0$, and $D_B = 0$. Thus, the value of exp $(-k_{el}t)$ varies from 1 to 0 as time varies from 0 to ∞. At any time between 0 and ∞, the fraction of the dose remaining in the body is equal to exp $(-k_{el}t)$.

Exponential rate expressions are also useful in deriving kinetic equations because they can be substituted into differential equations, which can then be integrated. For example, from Scheme 2 the differential equation describing the rate of appearance of unchanged drug in urine may be written:

$$\frac{dD_U}{dt} = +k_e D_B \tag{25a}$$

substituting Eq. (25) into Eq. (25a) gives:

$$\frac{dD_U}{dt} = +k_e[D_B^0 \exp(-k_{el}t)]$$

$$dD_U = +k_e[D_B^0 \exp(-k_{el}t)]dt$$

Integration yields:

$$D_U = -\frac{k_e}{k_{el}} D_B^0 \exp(-k_{el}t) + \text{constant}$$

at $t = 0$, $D_U = 0$, and $\exp(-k_{el}t) = 1$; therefore, the constant equals $(k_e/k_{el})D_B^0$, and

$$D_U = \frac{k_e}{k_{el}} D_B^0[1 - \exp(-k_{el}t)] \tag{26}$$

At $t = \infty$ after elimination is complete, the total amount of drug excreted unchanged in urine (D_U^∞) can be calculated using Eq. (26) as follows:

$$D_U^\infty = \frac{k_e}{k_{el}} D_B^0(1 - 0)$$

$$\frac{D_U^\infty}{D_B^0} = \frac{k_e}{k_{el}} = f_e \tag{27}$$

Equation (27) shows that the fraction of the dose appearing as unchanged drug in urine (f_e) is equal to the fraction of k_{el} attributable to k_e. [An equation analogous to Eq. (27) for D_M^∞ and k_m could be derived in much the same way.]

Substituting Eq. (27) into Eq. (26) and rearranging gives:

$$D_U^\infty - D_U = D_U^\infty \exp(-k_{el}t)$$

Taking logarithms yeilds

$$\ln(D_U^\infty - D_U) = -k_{el}t + \ln D_U^\infty \tag{28}$$

Equation (28) is identical to Eq. (17), for the case in which all eliminated drug was excreted unchanged in urine. $(D_U^\infty - D_U)$ is the amount remaining to be excreted (ARE), and Eq. (28) shows that an ARE plot of unchanged drug in urine versus time will be a straight line with a slope providing a value of k_{el} even when the drug is partially eliminated by metabolism (see Figs. 6 and 7). Using Eq. (27) and the total amount of unchanged drug excreted in urine (D_U^∞), it is possible to calculate k_e. Also, k_m can be calculated from Eq. (24). Thus, all the rate constants in Scheme 2 can be calculated solely on the basis of urinary excretion of unchanged drug.

Example. Five hundred milligrams of a drug was administered IV to a normal healthy volunteer, and various amounts of unchanged drug were recovered from the urine over the 24-hour postdrug period (Table 4). Calculate k_{el}, k_e, and k_m for this drug. A plot of $(D_U^\infty - D_U)$ on a log scale versus time is shown in Fig. 7. A half-life of 1.2 hours can be estimated from the line in Fig. 7.

$$k_{el} = \frac{0.693}{1.2\,\text{h}} = 0.578\,\text{h}^{-1}$$

From Eq. (27):

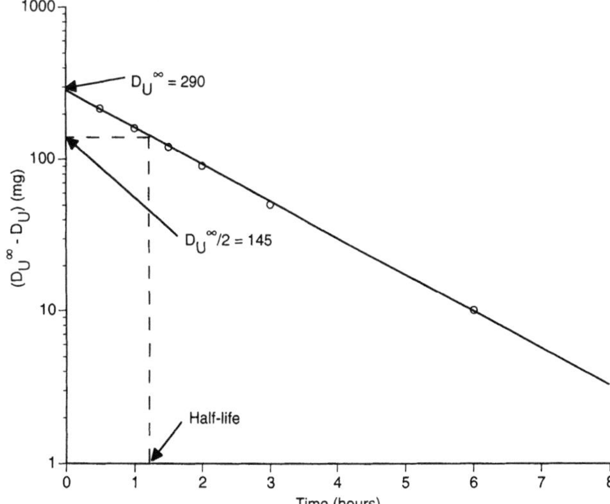

Fig. 7 Semilogarithmic plot of amount of unchanged drug remaining to be excreted into urine, $D_U^\infty - D_U$, versus time according to Scheme 2.

Table 4 Drug Recovered in Urine

Time interval (h)	Amount excreted unchanged (mg)	Cumulative amount excreted unchanged, D_U^a (mg)	$D_U^\infty - D_U$ (mg)
0.0–0.5	75	75	215
0.5–1.0	55	130	160
1.0–1.5	40	170	120
1.5–2.0	30	200	90
2.0–3.0	40	240	50
3.0–6.0	40	280	10
6.0–12.0	10	290	0
12.0–24.0	0	290	0

[a] $D_U^\infty = 290\,\text{mg}$.

$$\frac{D_U^\infty}{D_B^0} = \frac{k_e}{k_{el}}$$

$$\frac{290\,\text{mg}}{500\,\text{mg}} = \frac{k_e}{0.578\,\text{h}^{-1}}$$

$$k_e = 0.335\,\text{h}^{-1}$$

From Eq. (24),

$$k_{el} = k_e + k_m$$

$$k_m = 0.578 - 0.335 = 0.243\,\text{h}^{-1}$$

It is important to reemphasize the following assumptions inherent in this type of calculation:

1. It must be assumed that urine collections were accurately timed and that complete urine specimens were obtained at each collection time. It is also assumed that the assay procedure is accurate and reproducible.
2. It is assumed that all processes of elimination obey first-order kinetics.
3. It is assumed that any drug not appearing unchanged in urine has been metabolized. Furthermore, if the drug is not administered by IV injection, it must also be assumed that the dose is completely absorbed. (The IV route was chosen for the preceding example specifically to avoid the need to introduce this assumption.)

A. Significance of k_e and k_m in Patients with Kidney or Liver Disease

In the foregoing example, the drug was administered to a healthy subject who had normal kidney and liver function. The estimated biological half-life in this person was 1.2 hours. If the same drug were administered to a person with no kidney function but with a normal liver, it would be impossible for this individual to excrete unchanged drug. They would, however, be able to metabolize the drug at the same rate as a normal individual. The net result would be that the overall k_{el} would be reduced to the value of k_m, and the biological half-life would increase to

$$\frac{0.693}{k_m} = \frac{0.693}{0.243\,\text{h}^{-1}} = 2.85\,\text{h}$$

Thus, the biological half-life of a drug can increase dramatically when the organs of elimination are diseased or nonfunctional; it may increase to varying degrees if these organs are partially impaired.

At the present time no simple relationship exists between clinical measurements of liver function and the value of k_m. Fortunately, kidney function can be measured quantitatively using standard clinical tests, and it is directly related to k_e for a number of drugs. Great success has been achieved in using kidney clearance measurements to predict the biological half-lives of a number of drugs. This is best illustrated with a drug that is eliminated exclusively by urinary excretion.

Example. Kanamycin is a member of the aminoglycoside class of antibiotics, all of which are eliminated exclusively by glomerular filtration. Creatinine is a natural body substance that is cleared almost exclusively by glomerular filtration, and creatinine clearance rate is frequently used as a diagnostic tool to determine glomerular filtration rate. The relationship

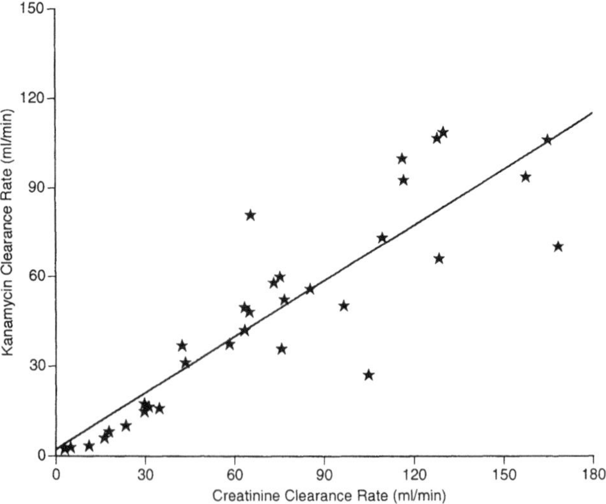

Fig. 8 Plot of kanamycin clearance rate versus creatinine clearance rate.

between creatinine clearance rate and kanamycin clearance rate is shown in Fig. 8. Creatinine clearance rate can be determined as a standard clinical procedure, and the corresponding kanamycin clearance rate can be determined by interpolation on the plot in Fig. 8. Since clearance rate $= k_{el}V_d$ [see Eq. (19)], the kanamycin clearance rate can be converted to kanamycin elimination rate constant by dividing by the V_d value for kanamycin, estimated to be about 27% of the patient's body weight.

Although determination of creatinine clearance rate is a standard clinical procedure, it is difficult to carry out mainly because accurate collection of total urine output over a 24-hour period is required. It can never be certain that this requirement has been met. Since creatinine is produced continuously in muscle and is cleared by the kidney, renal failure is characterized by elevated serum creatinine levels. The degree of elevation is directly related to the degree of renal failure—if it is assumed that the production of creatinine in the muscle mass is constant and that renal function is stable. When these assumptions are valid, there is a direct relationship between serum creatinine level and kanamycin half-life, as shown in Fig. 9. The equation of the line in Fig. 9 is

Kanamycin half-life (h)
$= 3 \times$ serum creatinine concentration (mg/100 mL)

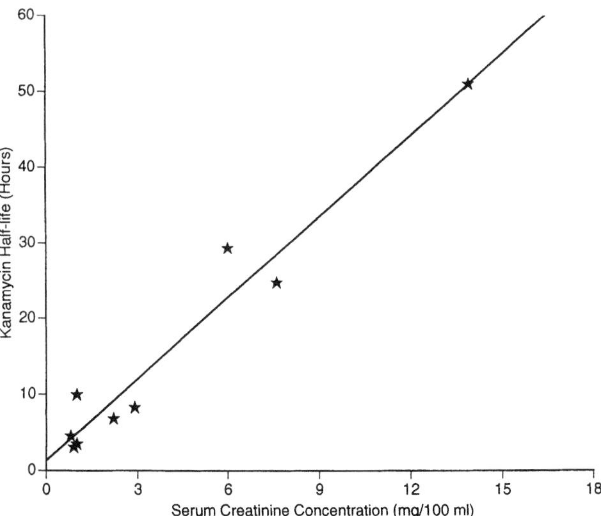

Fig. 9 Plot of kanamycin elimination half-life versus serum creatinine concentration in patients with varying degrees of (stable) renal failure.

Thus, kanamycin half-lives (h) can be predicted in patients with varying degrees of (stable) renal failure by multiplying the serum creatinine level (in mg/100 mL) by 3.

VII. KINETICS OF DRUG ABSORPTION

For all commonly used routes of administration except intravenous, the drug must dissolve in body fluids and diffuse through one or more membranes to enter the plasma. Thus, all routes except intravenous are classed as extravascular routes, and absorption is defined as appearance of the drug in plasma.

The most common extravascular route is oral. When a solution or a rapidly dissolving solid dosage form is given orally, the absorption process often obeys first-order kinetics. In these cases, absorption can be characterized by evaluating the absorption rate constant, k_a, using plasma concentration versus time data.

A. The Method of "Residuals" ("Feathering" the Curve)

When absorption is first-order, the kinetic model may be written as shown in Scheme 3:

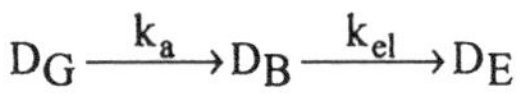

$$D_G \xrightarrow{k_a} D_B \xrightarrow{k_{el}} D_E$$

Scheme 3

where D_G = drug at the absorption site (gut)
D_B = drug in the body
D_E = eliminated drug
k_a = first-order absorption rate constant
k_{el} = overall elimination rate constant

The differential equations describing the rates of change of the three components of Scheme 3 are:

$$\frac{dD_G}{dt} = -k_a D_G \tag{29}$$

$$\frac{dD_B}{dt} = k_a D_G - k_{el} D_B \tag{30}$$

$$\frac{dD_E}{dt} = +k_{el} D_B \tag{31}$$

To determine k_a from plasma concentration versus time data, it is necessary to integrate Eq. (30). This is best achieved through exponential expressions. First, integration of Eq. (29) gives

$$D_G = D_G^0 \exp(-k_a t) \tag{32}$$

where D_G^0 is the initial amount of drug presented to the absorbing region of the gut. (D_G^0 = dose, if absorption is complete.)

Substituting Eq. (32) into Eq. (30) gives

$$\frac{dD_B}{dt} = +k_a D_G^0 \exp(-k_a t) - k_{el} D_B \tag{33}$$

Integration of Eq. (33) may be accomplished with Laplace transforms.* The result is

$$D_B = \frac{D_G^0 k_a}{k_a - k_{el}} [\exp(-k_{el} t) - \exp(-k_a t)] \tag{34}$$

Thus, amount of drug in the body following administration of an extravascular dose is a constant $[(D_G^0 k_a)/(k_a - k_{el})]$ multiplied by the difference between two exponential terms—one representing elimination $[\exp(-k_{el} t)]$ and the other representing absorption $[\exp(-k_a t)]$.

Dividing both sides of Eq. (34) by V_d yields an equation for plasma concentration versus time:

$$C_p = \frac{D_G^0 k_a}{V_d(k_a - k_{el})} [\exp(-k_{el} t - \exp(-k_a t)] \tag{35}$$

Equation (35) describes the line in Fig. 10, which is a semilog plot of C_p versus time for an orally administered drug absorbed by a first-order process. The plot begins as a rising curve and becomes a straight line with a negative slope after 6 hours. This behavior is the result of the biexponential nature of Eq. (35). Up to 6 hours, both the absorption process $[\exp(-k_a t)]$ and the elimination process $[\exp(-k_{el} t)]$ influence the plasma concentration. After 6 hours, only the elimination process influences the plasma concentration.

This separation of the processes of absorption and elimination is the result of the difference in the values of k_a and k_{el}. If k_a is much larger than k_{el} (a good rule is that it must be at least five times larger), the second exponential term in Eq. (35) will approach zero much more rapidly than the first exponential term. And at large values of t, Eq. (35) will reduce to

$$C_p = \frac{D_G^0 k_a}{V_d(k_a - k_{el})} [\exp(-k_{el} t)] \tag{36}$$

* Full details of this integration may be found in M. Mayersohn, M. Gibaldi, Am J Pharm Ed 34: 608, 1970, Eq. (27).

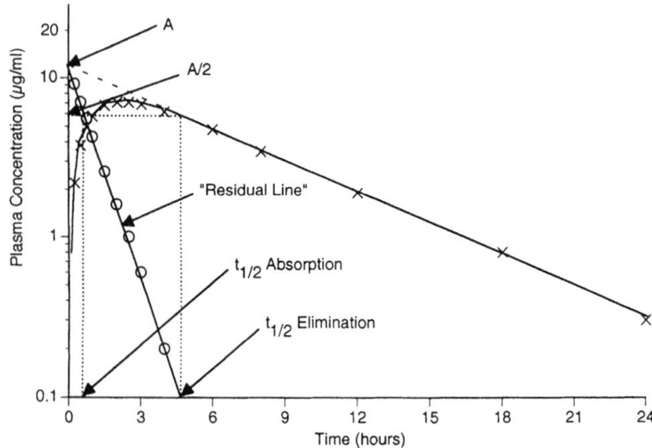

Fig. 10 Semilogarithmic plot of observed plasma concentrations (crosses) and "residuals" (circles) versus time for an orally administered drug absorbed by a first-order process.

or

$$C_p = A \cdot \exp(-k_{el} t)$$

where A is a constant term.

Converting to logarithms, we obtain

$$\ln C_p = -k_{el} t + \ln A \tag{37}$$

Thus after 6 hours the semilog plot of C_p versus time shown in Fig. 10 becomes a straight line and k_{el} can be determined from the slope. Therefore, the overall elimination rate constant for a drug may be accurately determined from the "tail" of a semilog plot of plasma concentration versus time following extravascular administration if k_a is at least five times larger than k_{el}.

The value of k_a can also be determined from plots like Fig. 10 using the following logic: In Fig. 10 the curved line up to 6 hours is given by

$$C_{p1} = A \cdot \exp(-k_{el} t) - A \cdot \exp(-k_a t)$$

The straight line after 6 hours and the extrapolated (dashed) line before 6 hours is given by

$$C_{p2} = A \cdot \exp(-k_{el} t)$$

The difference ("residual") between the curved line and the extrapolated (dashed) line up to 6 hours is given by

$$\text{Residual} = C_{p2} - C_{p1}$$
$$= A \cdot \exp(-k_a t)$$

Converting to logs:

$$\ln(\text{residual}) = -k_a t + \ln A \tag{38}$$

Table 5 Plasma Concentrations and "Residuals" Versus Time

Time (h)	Observed C_p (μg/mL)	Extrapolated C_p (μg/mL)	Residuals (μg/mL)
0.0	0.0	11.8	11.8
0.25	2.2	11.4	9.2
0.5	3.8	10.9	7.1
0.75	5.0	10.6	5.6
1.0	5.8	10.1	4.3
1.5	6.8	9.4	2.6
2.0	7.1	8.7	1.6
2.5	7.1	8.1	1.0
3.0	6.9	7.5	0.6
4.0	6.2	6.4	0.2
6.0	4.8	4.8	—
8.0	3.5	3.5	—
12.0	1.9	1.9	—
18.0	0.8	0.8	—
24.0	0.3	0.3	—

As shown in Fig. 10, a semilog plot of residuals versus time is a straight line with a slope of $-k_a$.

It should be noted that the intercepts (A) for both the extrapolated (dashed) line [Eq. (37)] and the residuals line [Eq. (38)] are the same and are equal to the constant in Eq. (35):

$$A = \frac{D_G^0 k_a}{V_d(k_a - k_{el})} \tag{39}$$

A is a function of the two rate constants (k_a and k_{el}), the apparent volume of distribution (V_d), and the amount of drug absorbed (D_G^0). After k_a and k_{el} have been evaluated and A has been determined by extrapolation, a value for V_d can be calculated if it is assumed that D_G^0 is equal to the dose administered, i.e., absorption is 100% complete.

Example. Fig. 10 is a plot of the data shown in Table 5. The extrapolated value of A is 11.8 μg/mL.

The $t_{1/2}$ (elimination) is the time at which the elimination line crosses $A/2 = 4.5$ hour:

$$k_{el} = \frac{0.693}{t_{1/2}(\text{elimination})} = 0.154\ \text{h}^{-1}$$

The $t_{1/2}$ (absorption) is the time at which the residuals line crosses $A/2 = 0.7$ hour:

$$k_a = \frac{0.693}{t_{1/2}(\text{absorption})} = 0.990\ \text{h}^{-1}$$

Assuming that the 100-mg dose of drug was completely absorbed, the V_d can be calculated from Eq. (39):

$$A = 11.8\ \mu\text{g/mL} = \frac{100\ \text{mg} \times 0.990\ \text{h}^{-1}}{V_d(0.990 - 0.154)\ \text{h}^{-1}}$$

$$V_d = 10.0\ \text{L}$$

This method of calculation is often referred to as the "method of residuals" or "feathering the curve." It is important to remember that the following assumptions were made:

1. It is assumed that k_a is at least five times larger than k_{el}; if not, neither constant can be determined accurately.
2. It is assumed that the absorption and elimination processes are both strictly first order; if not, the residuals line and, perhaps, the elimination line will not be straight.
3. It is assumed that absorption is complete; if not, the estimate of V_d will be erroneously high.

B. The Wagner-Nelson Method*

A major shortcoming of the method of residuals for determining the absorption rate constant from plasma concentration versus time data following administration of oral solid dosage forms is the necessity to assume that the absorption process obeys first-order kinetics. Although this assumption is often valid for solutions and rapidly dissolving dosage forms for which the absorption process itself is rate determining, if release of drug from the dosage form is rate determining, the kinetics are often zero-order, mixed zero- and first-order, or even more complex processes.

The Wagner-Nelson method of calculation does not require a model assumption concerning the absorption process. It does require the assumption that (a) the body behaves as a single homogeneous compartment and (b) drug elimination obeys first-order kinetics. The working equations for this calculation are developed next.

Derivation. For any extravascular drug administration, the mass balance equation can be written as amount absorbed (A) equals amount in body (W) plus amount eliminated (E), or

$$A = W + E$$

Taking the derivative with respect to time yields

$$\frac{dA}{dt} = \frac{dW}{dt} + \frac{dE}{dt}$$

* See J.G. Wagner, E. Nelson, J Pharm Sci 53:1392, 1964.

But

$$W = V_d C_p$$

or

$$\frac{dW}{dt} = V_d \frac{dC_p}{dt}$$

and

$$\frac{dE}{dt} = k_{el} W$$
$$= k_{el} V_d C_p$$

Therefore,

$$\frac{dA}{dt} = V_d \frac{dC_p}{dt} + k_{el} V_d C_p$$

$$dA = V_d dC_p + k_{el} V_d C_p \, dt$$

Integrating from $t = 0$ to $t = t$

$$\int_0^t dA = V_d \int_0^t dC_p + k_{el} V_d \int_0^t C_p \, dt$$

$$A_t = V_d C_p^t + k_{el} V_d \int_0^t C_p \, dt$$

Rearranging, we have

$$\frac{A_t}{V_d} = C_p^t + k_{el} \int_0^t C_p \, dt \tag{40}$$

where A_t/V_d is the amount of drug absorbed up to time t divided by the volume of distribution, C_p^t is plasma (serum or blood) concentration at time t, and $\int_0^t C_p \, dt$ is the area under the plasma (serum or blood) concentration versus time curve up to time t (see Sec. VIII.A). An equation similar to Eq. (40) can be derived by integration from $t = 0$ to $t = \infty$. Since $C_p = 0$ at $t = \infty$, the equation becomes

$$\frac{A_{\max}}{V_d} = k_{el} \int_0^\infty C_p \, dt \tag{41}$$

where $A_{\max}$ is the total amount of drug absorbed from the dosage form divided by the volume of distribution and $\int_0^\infty C_p \, dt$ is the area under the entire plasma (serum or blood) concentration versus time curve (see Sec. VIII.A).

Equation (41) is useful for comparing the bioavailabilities of two dosage forms of the same drug administered to the same group of subjects. If it is assumed that k_{el} and V_d are the same for both administrations, it can be seen that the relative availabilities of the dosage forms is given by the ratio of the areas under the plasma concentration versus time curves:

$$\frac{A_{\max_1}}{A_{\max_2}} = \frac{\int_0^\infty (C_p \, dt)_1}{\int_0^\infty (C_p \, dt)_2} \tag{42}$$

Other methods of comparing bioavailabilities will be discussed in a later section.

A great deal can be learned about the absorption process by applying Eqs. (40) and (41) to plasma concentration versus time data. Since there is no model assumption with regard to the absorption process, the calculated values of A_t/V_d can often be manipulated to determine the kinetic mechanism that controls absorption. This is best illustrated by an example.

Example. A tablet containing 100 mg of a drug was administered to a healthy volunteer and the plasma concentration (C_p) versus time data shown in Table 6 were obtained. Figure 11 shows a semi-log plot of these C_p versus time data. The half-life for elimination of the drug can be estimated from the straight line "tail" of the plot to be 4.7 hours. The overall elimination rate constant is then

$$k_{el} = \frac{0.693}{4.7\,\text{h}} = 0.147\,\text{h}^{-1}$$

Table 6 illustrates the steps involved in carrying out the Wagner-Nelson calculation. The third column ($\int_0^t C_p \, dt$) shows the area under the C_p versus time curve calculated sequentially from $t = 0$ to each of the time points using the trapezoidal rule (see Sec. VIII.A). The fourth column ($k_{el} \int_0^t C_p \, dt$) shows each of the preceding areas multiplied by k_{el} (as estimated from the "tail")

Table 6 Data Illustrating the Wagner-Nelson Calculation

Time (h)	C_p (μg/ml)	$\int_0^t C_p \, dt$	$k_{el} \int_0^t C_p \, dt$	$\frac{A_t}{V_d}$	$\frac{A_{\max}}{V_d} - \frac{A_t}{V_d}$
0.25	0.6	0.1	0.0	0.6	9.4
0.50	1.2	0.3	0.1	1.3	8.7
0.75	1.8	0.7	0.1	1.9	8.1
1.0	2.3	1.2	0.2	2.5	7.5
1.5	3.4	2.6	0.4	3.8	6.2
2.0	4.3	4.5	0.7	5.0	5.0
3.0	6.0	9.7	1.5	7.5	2.5
6.0	5.6	27.1	4.1	9.7	0.3
12.0	2.3	50.8	7.6	9.9	0.1
18.0	0.9	60.4	9.1	10.0	—
24.0	0.4	64.3	9.6	10.0	—

[a] $A_{\max}/V_d = 10.0$.

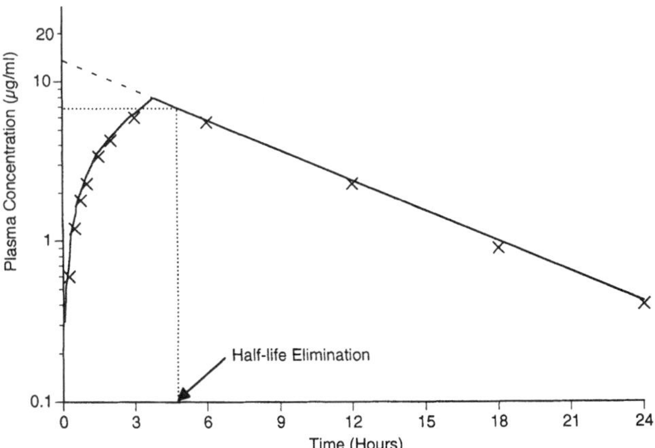

Fig. 11 Semilogarithmic plot of observed plasma concentrations (crosses) versus time for an orally administered drug absorbed by a zero-order process. (Data shown in Table 6.)

constituting the second term of the Wagner-Nelson equation [see Eq. (40)]. The fifth column (A_t/V_d) shows the sums of the values indicated in the second and fourth columns according to Eq. (40). $A_{\max}/V_d$ is the maximum value in the fifth column (i.e., 10.0), and the sixth column shows the residual between $A_{\max}/V_d$ and each sequential value of A_t/V_d in the fifth column.

If the absorption process obeyed first-order kinetics, a semilog plot of the residuals in the sixth column would be a straight line and k_a can be determined from the slope. However, the regular Cartesian plot of the residuals shown in Fig. 12 is a straight line showing the absorption process obeys zero-order kinetics; that is, the process proceeds at a constant rate (25 mg/h), stopping abruptly when the dose has been completely absorbed.

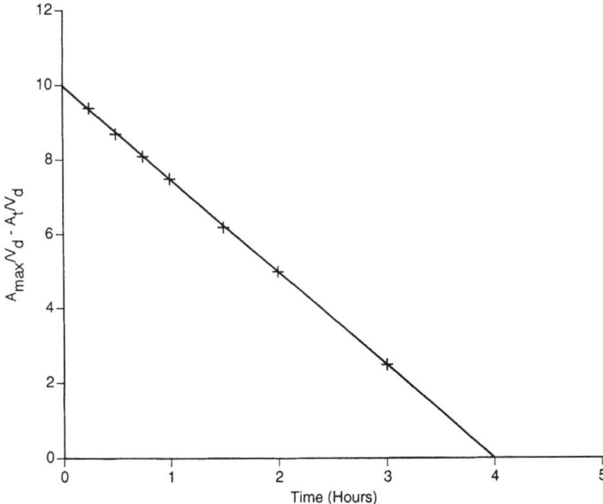

Fig. 12 Plot of the residuals (crosses) between $A_{\max}/V_d$ and A_t/V_d versus time (last column of Table 6).

This example illustrates the usefulness of the Wagner-Nelson calculation for studying the mechanism of release of drugs from dosage forms in vivo. Whereas the absorption process itself usually obeys first-order kinetics, dissolution of capsules, tablets, and especially sustained-release dosage forms often must be described by more complex kinetic mechanisms. Although pure zero-order absorption, such as that just illustrated, is almost never observed in practice, many sustained-release dosage forms are designed to produce as close to zero-order release as possible since constant absorption produces constant plasma levels.

C. The Method of "Inspection"

Often it is unnecessary to calculate an exact value for an absorption rate constant. For example, when several oral tablets containing the same drug substance are all found to be completely absorbed, it may be sufficient to merely determine if the absorption rates are similar to conclude that the products would be therapeutically equivalent. In another instance, it would be possible to choose between an elixir and a sustained-release tablet for a specific therapeutic need without assigning accurate numbers to the absorption rate constant for the two dosage forms.

In these instances, the "*time of the peak*" in the plasma concentration versus time curve provides a convenient measure of the absorption rate. For example, if three tablets of the same drug are found to be completely absorbed and all give plasma peaks at 1 hour, it can be safely concluded that all three tablets are absorbed at essentially the same rate. (In fact, if all tablets are completely absorbed and all peak at the same time, it would be expected that all three plasma concentration versus time curves would be identical, within experimental error.)

The time of the peak can also be used to roughly estimate the absorption rate constant. If it is assumed that k_a is at least $5 \times k_{el}$, then it can be assumed that absorption is at least 95% complete at the peak time; that is, the peak time represents approximately five absorption half-lives (see Table 1). The absorption half-life can then be calculated by dividing the time of the peak by 5, and the absorption rate constant can be calculated by dividing the absorption half-life into 0.693.

Example. Inspection of Fig. 10 gives a peak time of about 2.5 hours. The absorption half-life can be estimated to be 0.5 h and the absorption rate constant, to be $1.4\,h^{-1}$.

VIII. BIOAVAILABILITY (EXTENT OF ABSORPTION)

If a drug is administered by an extravascular route and acts systemically, its potency will be directly related to the amount of drug the dosage form delivers to the blood. Also, if the pharmacological effects of the drug are related directly and instantaneously to its plasma concentration, the rate of absorption will be important because the rate will influence the height of the plasma concentration peak and the time at which the peak occurs. Thus, the *bioavailability of a drug product is defined in terms of the amount of active drug delivered to the blood and the rate at which it is delivered.*

Whenever a drug is administered by an extravascular route, there is a danger that part of the dose may not reach the blood (i.e., absorption may not be complete). When the intravenous route is used, the drug is placed directly in the blood; therefore an IV injection is, by definition, 100% absorbed. The absolute bioavailability of an extravascular dosage form is defined relative to an IV injection. If IV data are not available, the relative bioavailability may be defined relative to a standard dosage form. For example, the bioavailability of a tablet may be defined relative to an oral solution of the drug.

In Sec. VII we dealt with methods of determining the rate (and mechanism) of absorption. In this section we will deal with methods of determining the extent of absorption. In every example, the calculation will involve a comparison between two studies carried out in the same group of volunteers on different occasions. Usually it will be necessary to assume that the volunteers behaved identically on both occasions, especially with regard to their pharmacokinetic parameters.

A. Area Under the Plasma Concentration Versus Time Curve

In the development of equations for the Wagner-Nelson method of calculation, the following equation was derived [see Eq. (42)]:

$$\frac{A_{\max_1}}{A_{\max_2}} = \frac{\int_0^\infty (C_p\,dt)_1}{\int_0^\infty (C_p\,dt)_2}$$

This equation shows that the amounts of drug absorbed from two drug products (i.e., the relative bioavailability of product 1 compared with product 2) can be calculated as the ratio of the areas under the plasma concentration versus time curves (AUCs), assuming k_{el} and V_d were the same in both studies. This assumption is probably valid when the studies are run with the same group of volunteers and within a few weeks of one another.

If dosage form 2 [Eq. (42)] is an intravenous dosage form, the *absolute bioavailability* of the extravascular dosage form (dosage form 1) is given by:

$$\begin{array}{c}\text{Absolute bioavailability}\\ \text{(extravascular dosage form)}\end{array} = \frac{\mathrm{AUC}_{\text{extravascular}}}{\mathrm{AUC}_{\text{IV}}} \tag{43}$$

The AUC for a plasma concentration versus time curve can be determined using the trapezoidal rule. For this calculation, the curve is divided into vertical segments, as shown in Fig. 13. The top line of each segment is assumed to be straight rather than slightly curved, and the area of the segment is calculated as though it were a trapezoid; for example, the area of segment 10 is

$$\text{area}_{10} = \frac{C_{p9} + C_{p10}}{2} \times (t_{10} - t_9) \tag{44}$$

The total AUC is then obtained by summing the areas of the individual segments. [Equation (44) can be programmed into a microcomputer that will calculate the areas and sum them as rapidly as the C_p values can be entered.]

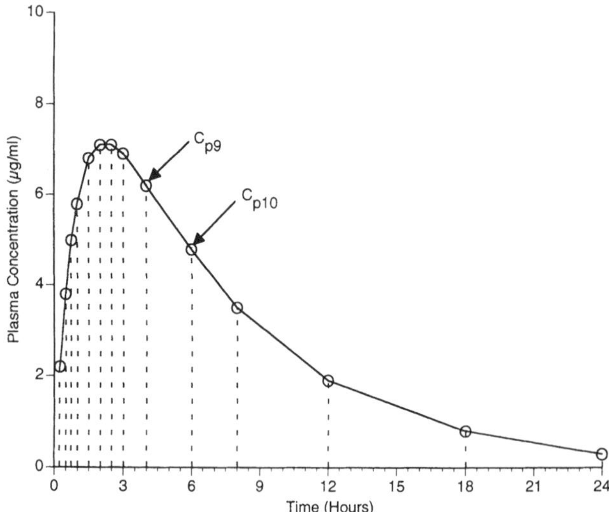

Fig. 13 Plot of plasma concentrations (circles) versus time with the curve divided into vertical segments. (Data shown in Table 7.)

It should be readily apparent that the trapezoidal rule does not measure AUC exactly. However, it is accurate enough for most bioavailability calculations, and the segments are chosen on the basis of the time intervals at which plasma was collected.

Example. The AUC for Fig. 10 can be calculated from the data given in Table 7.

Assuming that the AUC for a 100 mg IV dose given to the same group of volunteers was 86.7 h.μg/mL, the absolute bioavailability of the extravascular dosage form is

Table 7 Calculation of Area Under the Plasma Concentration Versus Time Curve (AUC) Using the Trapezoidal Rule

Time (h)	C_p (μg/mL)	Area of segment (h·μg/mL)	Cumulative area up to time t (h·μg/mL)
0.0	0.0		
		0.275	0.275
0.25	2.2		
		0.75	1.025
0.5	3.8		
		1.1	2.125
0.75	5.0		
		1.35	3.475
1.0	5.8		
		3.15	6.625
1.5	6.8		
		3.475	10.10
2.0	7.1		
		3.55	13.65
2.5	7.1		
		3.50	17.15
3.0	6.9		
		6.55	23.70
4.0	6.2		
		11.0	34.70
6.0	4.8		
		8.3	43.0
8.0	3.5		
		10.8	53.8
12.0	1.9		
		8.1	61.9
18.0	0.8		
		3.3	65.2
24.0	0.3		
		2.0	67.2[a]
∞	—		

[a]$AUC_\infty = 67.2$ h.μg/m.

$$\text{Absolute bioavailability} = \frac{\text{AUC}_\infty}{\text{AUC}_{\text{IV}}} \times 100$$
$$= \frac{67.2}{86.7} \times 100 = 77.5\%$$

It is not necessary to apply the trapezoidal rule to the entire plasma concentration versus time curve in order to calculate the total AUC. After the semilog plot becomes a straight line, the remaining area out to $t =$ can be calculated using the following equation:

$$\text{AUC}_{(t \text{ to } \infty)} = \frac{C_p^t}{k_{el}} \tag{45}$$

Once a semilog plasma concentration versus time plot begins to follow simple first-order elimination kinetics, the remaining AUC can be calculated in one step using Eq. (45).

Example. In the previous problem, the AUC from 24 hours to infinity is given by

$$\text{AUC}_{(24\,\text{h to }\infty)} = \frac{0.3\,\mu\text{g/mL}}{0.15\,\text{h}^{-1}} = 2.0\,\text{h}\cdot\mu\text{g/mL}$$

It follows that if the entire semilog plot were straight, as would be the case for a one-compartment drug following IV administration, the total AUC would be given by

$$\text{AUC}_{\text{IV}} = \frac{C_p^0}{k_{el}} \tag{45a}$$

Example. For IV administration in the foregoing problem, the AUC was calculated as follows:

$$\text{AUC}_{\text{IV}} = \frac{13.0\,\mu\text{g/mL}}{0.15\,\text{h}^{-1}} = 86.7\,\text{h}.\mu\text{g/mL}$$

B. Cumulative Urinary Excretion

In the development of equations for calculating urine data when the drug is partially metabolized and partially excreted unchanged in urine, the following equation was derived [see Eq. (27)]:

$$\frac{D_U^\infty}{D_B^0} = f_e$$

where $D_U^\infty$is the amount of drug recovered from urine, D_B^0 is the amount of drug absorbed, and f_e is the fraction of the absorbed amount recovered as unchanged drug in urine. Equation (27) may be rearranged and written for two dosage forms as follows:

$$D_{U_1}^\infty = D_{B_1}^0 \times f_{e_1}$$

and

$$D_{U_2}^{\infty} = D_{B_2}^{0} \times f_{e_2}$$

Dividing the first equation by the second gives:

$$\frac{D_{U_1}^{\infty}}{D_{U_2}^{\infty}} = \frac{D_{B_2}^{0} \times f_{e_2}}{D_{B_2}^{0} \times f_{e_2}}$$

Assuming that $f_{e_1} = f_{e_2}$, we have

$$\frac{D_{U_1}^{\infty}}{D_{U_2}^{\infty}} = \frac{D_{B_2}^{0}}{D_{B_2}^{0}} = \text{relative bioavailability} \qquad (46)$$

Similarly,

$$\frac{D_{U(\text{extravascular})}^{\infty}}{D_{U(\text{IV})}^{\infty}} = \text{absolute bioavailability} \qquad (47)$$

Thus, if it is assumed that the same fraction of absorbed drug always reaches the urine unchanged, the bioavailability can be calculated as the ratio of total amounts of unchanged drug recovered in urine.

Example. When potassium penicillin G was administered IV to a group of volunteers, 80% of the 500 mg dose was recovered unchanged in urine. When the same drug was administered orally to the same volunteers, 280 mg was recovered unchanged in urine. What is the absolute bioavailability of potassium penicillin G following oral administration? From Eq. (47),

$$\text{Absolute bioavailability} = \frac{280}{400} \times 100$$
$$= 70\%$$

For this calculation, it is unnecessary to assume that V_d and/or k_{el} are the same for the two studies. It is only necessary that f_e be the same in both studies. This is usually a valid assumption unless the drug undergoes a significant amount of "first-pass" metabolism in the gut wall or liver following oral administration or a significant amount of decomposition at an intra muscular (IM) injection site. When this occurs, the availability of the extravascular dosage form may appear to be low, but the fault will not lie with the formulation. The bioavailability will be a true reflection of the therapeutic efficacy of the drug product, and reformulation may not increase bioavailability.

C. The Method of "Inspection"

Bioavailability studies are frequently carried out for the sole purpose of comparing one drug product with another with the full expectation that the two products will have identical bioavailabilities; that is, their rates and extents of absorption will be identical. Such studies are called *bioequivalence studies* and are often employed when a manufacturer wishes to market a "generic equivalent" of a product already on the market. To take advantage of the safety and efficacy data the product's originator has filed with the FDA, the second manufacturer must show that their product gives an *identical plasma concentration versus time curve*.

In these cases it is not necessary to determine the absolute bioavailability or the absorption rate constant for the product under study. It is only necessary to prove that the plasma concentration versus time curve is not significantly different from the reference product's curve. This is done by comparing the means and standard deviations of the plasma concentrations for the two products at each sampling time using an appropriate statistical test.

A discussion of the statistical methods used in analyzing the data from bioequivalence studies is beyond the scope of this chapter. For a discussion of these considerations, the reader is referred to a description by Westlake [6].

IX. MULTIPLE DOSING REGIMENS (REPETITIVE DOSING)

Drugs are infrequently used in single doses to produce an acute effect, the way aspirin is used to relieve a headache. More often, drugs are administered in successive doses to produce a repeated or prolonged effect, the way aspirin is used to relieve the pain and inflammation of arthritis. A properly designed multiple dosing regimen will maintain therapeutically effective plasma concentrations of the drug while avoiding toxic concentrations. Such regimens are easily designed if the pharmacokinetic parameters of the drug are known.

When drugs are administered on a multiple dosing regimen, each dose (after the first) is administered before the preceding doses are completely eliminated. This results in a phenomenon known as *accumulation*, during which the amount of drug in the body (represented by plasma concentration) builds up as successive doses are administered. The phenomenon of accumulation for a drug administered IV is shown in Fig. 14.

Figure 14 shows that the plasma concentrations do not continue to build forever but reach a plateau where the same maximum ($C_{\max}$) and minimum ($C_{\min}$) con-

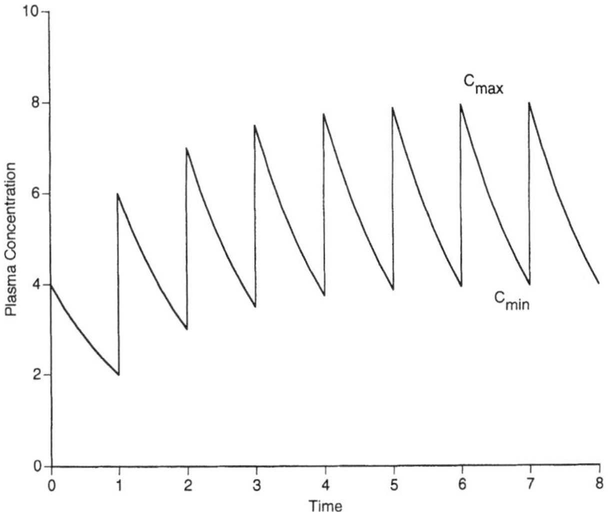

Fig. 14 Plot of plasma concentration versus time showing accumulation following multiple intravenous injections.

centrations are reproduced over and over. The objectives of designing a dosing regimen are to keep $C_{\min}$ above the *minimum effective concentration* (MEC) and to keep $C_{\max}$ below the *minimum toxic concentration* (MTC).

A. Repetitive Intravenous Dosing

The plasma concentrations in Fig. 14 can be calculated as follows: from Eq. (25) the plasma concentration at the end of the first dosing interval, T, is given by:

$$C_{p_1}^T = C_{p_1}^0 \exp(-k_{el}T) \tag{48}$$

Immediately after the second dose is given, the plasma concentration will be,

$$C_{p_2}^0 = C_{p_1}^T + C_{p_1}^0 = C_{p_1}^0 \exp(-k_{el}T) + C_{p_1}^0 \tag{49}$$

and so on.

It is now helpful to define the parameter R as the fraction of the initial plasma concentration that remains at the end of any dosing interval; R is given by the following equation:

$$R = \exp(-k_{el}T) \tag{50}$$

As was pointed out in Sec. VI, when $T = t_{1/2}$, $R = 0.5$. The plot in Fig. 14 was constructed using these conditions; therefore, the plasma concentration at the end of each dosing interval is half the concentration at the beginning of the dosing interval.

Equations (48) and (49) can be simplified to

$$C_{p_1}^T = C_{p_1}^0 R$$

for the plasma concentration at the end of the first dosing interval, and

$$C_{p_2}^0 = C_{p_1}^0 R + C_{p_1}^0$$

for the plasma concentration at the beginning of the second dosing interval.

The series can be carried further for more doses:

$$C_{p_2}^T = (C_{p_1}^0 R + C_{p_1}^0)R$$

$$C_{p_3}^0 = (C_{p_1}^0 R + C_{p_1}^0)R + C_{p_1}^0$$

$$C_{p_3}^T = [(C_{p_1}^0 R + C_{p_1}^0)R + C_{p_1}^0]R$$

etc.

The plasma concentrations at the beginning and end of the nth dosing interval are given by the following power series:

$$\text{Beginning} = C_{p_1}^0 + C_{p_1}^0 R + C_{p_1}^0 R^2 + \cdots + C_{p_1}^0 R^{n-1} \tag{51}$$

$$\text{End} = C_{p_1}^0 R + C_{p_1}^0 R^2 + C_{p_1}^0 R^3 + \cdots + C_{p_1}^0 R^n \tag{52}$$

Since R is always smaller than 1, R^n becomes smaller as n increases. For example, if $R = 0.5$, $R^{10} = 0.001$. Therefore, the high power terms in Eqs. (51) and (52) become negligible as n increases, and additional doses do not change the value of $C_{p_n}^0$ or $C_{p_n}^T$ significantly. This explains why the plasma concentrations reach a plateau instead of continuing to rise as more doses are given.

Hence, $C_{\max}$ and $C_{\min}$ (see Fig. 14) are defined as the plasma concentrations at the beginning and end, respectively, of the nth dosing interval after the plateau has been reached (i.e., $n = \infty$). When $n = \infty$, Eqs. (51) and (52) become

$$C_{\max} = \frac{C_{p_1}^0}{1 - R} \tag{53}$$

$$C_{\min} = C_{\max} R = \frac{C_{p_1}^0 R}{1 - R} \tag{54}$$

Thus, the maximum and minimum plasma concentrations on the plateau of a repetitive IV dosing regimen can be calculated if the dosing interval (T), the overall elimination rate constant (k_{el}), and the initial plasma concentration (C_p^0) are known.

Example. A drug has a biologic half-life of 4 hours. Following an IV injection of 100 mg, C_p^0 is found to be 10 μg/mL. Calculate C_{max} and C_{min} if the 100-mg IV dose is repeated every 6 hour until a plasma concentration plateau is reached.

$$k_{el} = \frac{0.693}{4\ \text{h}} = 0.173\ \text{h}^{-1}$$
$$\begin{aligned} R &= \exp(-k_{el}T) \\ &= \exp(-0.173 \times 6) \\ &= \exp(-0.451) \\ &= 0.354 \end{aligned}$$
$$C_{max} = \frac{10\ \mu\text{g/mL}}{1 - 0.354} = 15.5\ \mu\text{g/mL}$$
$$C_{min} = 15.5\ \mu\text{g/mL} \times 0.354 = 5.49\ \mu\text{g/mL}$$

Example. As indicated earlier, when $T = t_{1/2}$, $R = 0.5$. As a result, on the plateau in Fig. 14,

$$C_{max} = \frac{C_p^0}{1 - 0.5} = 2 \times C_p^0$$

$$C_{min} = \frac{C_p^0 \times 0.5}{1 - 0.5} = C_p^0$$

Thus, when a dose is administered every half-life, C_{max} will be twice C_p^0 and C_{min} will be half C_{max} or equal to C_p^0.

The second example illustrates a very simple and often-used dosage regimen; i.e., administration of a maintenance dose every half-life. The calculations indicate that on this regimen, C_{min} will be $C_{max}/2$ and C_{max} will be $2 \times C_p^0$. Figure 14 indicates that approximately five half-lives will be required to reach the plasma concentration plateau. If the drug has a relatively long half-life, many hours, perhaps days, may be required for the plasma concentrations to reach the ideal range. If the patient's condition is serious, the physician may not want to wait for this to happen. It is under these circumstances that a loading dose is indicated. The loading dose immediately puts the plasma concentrations in the plateau range, and the maintenance dose maintains that condition.

For IV administration, the easiest way to determine the loading dose is in terms of C_p^0 and C_{max}. For example, if the desired C_{max} is 20 μg/mL and a dose of 100 mg gives a C_p^0 of 10 μg/mL, a loading dose of 200 mg should give a C_p^0 of 20 μg/mL, which is the desired C_{max}. If this loading dose is followed by maintenance doses of 100 mg every half-life, the plasma concentrations can be maintained at the plateau from the very beginning and throughout the entire dosing regimen. Thus, for the maintenance dose every half-life regimen, the ideal loading dose is twice the maintenance dose.

Example. Kanamycin is an aminoglycoside antibiotic that exerts a toxic effect on the hearing. If the plasma concentrations are allowed to remain above 35 μg/mL (MTC) for very long, permanent hearing loss may result. The minimum effective concentration (MEC) of kanamycin in plasma is estimated to be about 10 μg/mL for most organisms against which it is used. Thus, kanamycin is a classic example of a drug with a narrow therapeutic index for which a very precise dosing regimen is an absolute necessity. (In fact, this is true of all aminoglycosides.) When kanamycin is administered IV in a dose of 7.5 mg/kg to adults, it yields a C_p^0 of about 25 μg/mL and a half-life of about of 3 hours. What would be a good dosing regimen for kanamycin?

Since 25 μg/mL is well above the MEC but below the MTC, a loading dose of 7.5 mg/kg might be given initially. After one half-life (3 h), the plasma concentration should be 12.5 μg/mL. Since this is just above the MEC and corresponds to half the initial 25 μg/mL, a maintenance dose of 3.75 mg/kg could be administered. With repeated 3.75 mg/kg maintenance doses every 3 hours, C_{max} should be 25 μg/mL and C_{min} should be 12.5 μg/mL, which would allow some margin for error on either side.

Example.The kanamycin problem could be solved more aggressively as follows: let C_{max} = 35 μg/mL and C_{min} = 10 μg/mL. From Eqs. (53) and (54), the value of R on the plateau may be calculated as follows:

$$C_{p_1}^0 = C_{max}(1 - R) = (35\ \mu\text{g/mL})(1 - R)$$

$$C_{p_1}^0 = \frac{C_{min}(1 - R)}{R} = \frac{(10\ \mu\text{g/mL})(1 - R)}{R}$$

$$35\ \mu\text{g/mL}(1 - R) = \frac{(10\ \mu\text{g/mL})(1 - R)}{R}$$

$$\begin{aligned} R &= \frac{10}{35} = 0.286 \\ &= 10 \exp(-k_{el}T) \qquad \left(k_{el} = \frac{0.693}{3\ \text{h}} = 0.231\ \text{h}^{-1}\right) \end{aligned}$$

$$0.268 = \exp(-0.231 \times T)$$

$$-1.25 = -0.231 \times T$$

$$T = 5.41\ \text{h (dosing interval)}$$

A loading dose that produces a $C^0_{p_1}$ of 35 μg/mL is desired, and this can be calculated as follows [from Eq. (16)]:

$$\frac{\text{dose}_1}{C^0_{p_1}} = \frac{\text{dose}_2}{C^0_{p_2}}$$

$$\frac{7.5\,\text{mg/kg}}{25\,\mu\text{g/mL}} = \frac{x\,\text{mg/kg}}{35\,\mu\text{g/mL}}$$

$$\text{Loading dose} = 10.5\,\text{mg/kg}$$

The amount of drug remaining in the body at the end of the first dosing interval can be calculated in a similar way from the known $C_{\min}$:

$$\frac{7.5\,\text{mg/kg}}{25\,\mu\text{g/mL}} = \frac{x\,\text{mg/kg}}{10\,\mu\text{g/mL}}$$

$$\text{Amount remaining} = 3\,\text{mg/kg}$$

The maintenance dose needed to replace the amount lost over the dosing interval is the difference between the loading dose and the amount remaining at the end of the interval:

$$\text{Maintenance dose} = (10.5 - 3)\,\text{mg/kg} = 7.5\,\text{mg/kg}$$

Thus, the regimen would be a loading dose of 10.5 mg/kg, followed by maintenance doses of 7.5 mg/kg every 5.41 hours. This regimen is not only impractical but, were it carried out, it would produce $C_{\max}$ and $C_{\min}$ concentrations too close to the limiting values to allow for any errors. A better approach would be to define clinicially relevant $C_{\max}$ and $C_{\min}$ values and use the approach in the previous section to develope a useful dosing regimen.

B. Repetitive Extravascular Dosing

Although the equations become considerably more complex than for the IV case, $C_{\max}$ and $C_{\min}$ can be calculated when the drug is administered by an extravascular route. The required equations may be developed as follows: The equation describing the plasma concentration versus time curve following one extravascular administration was discussed previously. Equation (35) may be written as follows:

$$C_p = \frac{FD}{V_d} \times \frac{k_a}{k_a - k_{el}}[\exp(-k_{el}t) - \exp(-k_a t)] \quad (55)$$

where D is the dose administered and F is the fraction of the administered dose absorbed [$FD = D^0_G$ in Eq. (35)].

If n doses of the drug are administered at fixed time intervals (T), the plasma concentrations following the nth dose are given by

$$C_p = \frac{FD}{V_d} \times \frac{k_a}{k_a - k_{el}}\left[\frac{1-\exp(-nk_{el}T)}{1-\exp(-k_{el}T)}\exp(-k_{el}t') - \frac{1-\exp(-nk_aT)}{1-\exp(-k_aT)}\exp(-k_at')\right] \quad (56)$$

where t' is the time elapsed after the nth dose. When n is large (i.e., when the plasma concentrations reach a plateau), the terms $\exp(-nk_{el}T)$ and $\exp(-nk_aT)$ become negligibly small, and Eq. (56) simplifies to

$$C_p = \frac{FD}{V_d} \times \frac{k_a}{k_a - k_{el}} \times \left[\frac{\exp(-k_{el}t')}{1-\exp(-k_{el}T)} - \frac{\exp(-k_at')}{1-\exp(-k_aT)}\right] \quad (57)$$

Equation (57) can be used to calculate the $C_{\max}$ and $C_{\min}$ values on the plasma concentration plateau by substituting values for t' that correspond to the "peaks" and "valleys" in the C_p versus t curve. Thus, if $t' = t_{\max}$ (the time of the peak), Eq. (57) gives $C_{\max}$:

$$C_{\max} = \frac{FD}{V_d} \times \frac{k_a}{k_a - k_{el}} \times \left[\frac{\exp(-k_{el}t_{\max})}{1-\exp(-k_{el}T)} - \frac{\exp(-k_at_{\max})}{1-\exp(-k_aT)}\right] \quad (58)$$

If $t' = 0$ (the time at which another dose is to be given), Eq. (57) gives $C_{\min}$:

$$C_{\min} = \frac{FD}{V_d} \times \frac{k_a}{k_a - k_{el}} \times \left[\frac{1}{1-\exp(-k_{el}T)} - \frac{1}{1-\exp(-k_aT)}\right] \quad (59)$$

Example. The results of a single IM dose of kanamycin show that the dose is completely absorbed (F = 1.0), $V_d = 20\,\text{L}$, $k_{el} = 0.3\,\text{h}^{-1}$, and the time of the peak is about 1 hr ($k_a = 3.47\,\text{h}^{-1}$). If 800 mg doses of kanamycin are administered IM every 6 h, what will $C_{\max}$ and $C_{\min}$ be when the plasma concentration plateau is reached?

$$C_{\max} = \frac{1.0 \times 800\,\text{mg}}{20\,\text{L}} \times \frac{3.47\,\text{h}^{-1}}{(3.47-0.3)\,\text{h}^{-1}} \times \left[\frac{\exp(-0.3\times 1)}{1-\exp(-0.3\times 6)} - \frac{\exp(-3.47\times 1)}{1-\exp(-3.47\times 6)}\right] = 37.5\,\mu\text{g/mL}$$

From Eq. (59),

$$C_{\min} = \frac{1.0 \times 800\,\text{mg}}{20\,\text{L}} \times \frac{3.47\,\text{h}^{-1}}{(3.47 - 0.3)\,\text{h}^{-1}} \times \left[\frac{1}{1 - \exp(-0.3 \times 6)^{-1}} \frac{1}{1 - \exp(-3.47 \times 6)}\right]$$
$$= 8.67\,\mu\text{g/mL}$$

Note: The value of exp($-x$) can be calculated directly with a scientific calculator or as the inverse or antilog(base e).

The foregoing example shows the calculation of the two most important features of a repetitive dosing regimen, the maximum and minimum plasma concentrations on the plateau. But if Eq. (56) had been used, it would have been possible to calculate the plasma concentration at any time throughout an entire dosing regimen. Although these calculations are complex and laborious when done by hand, relatively inexpensive programmable calculators and now personal computers can solve Eq. (56) in seconds. As a result, a plasma concentration versus time plot can be generated for an entire dosing regimen in a very short time. The next example illustrates such a calculation.

Example. The following personal computer spreadsheet will solve Eq. (56) with an added loading dose for any time during a repetitive dosing regimen (see Fig. 15).

Comments: This spreadsheet has been written to be as flexible as possible for use in clinical situations; therefore many parameters are entered in a form different from their form in Eq. (56). The following comments should clarify the relationships:

1. The spreadsheet accepts half-lives for the elimination and absorption processes and converts them into rate constants, but both half-lives must be in the same time units! (If the half-life for absorption is unknown, the time of the peak divided by 5 gives a reasonable estimate; see Sec. VII.C.)
2. The fraction of the dose absorbed must be estimated in a separate study or from past experience.
3. The volume of distribution is expressed as a fraction of the body weight, and the spreadsheet calculates V_d in liters using the subject weight in kilograms.
4. Since loading doses are often used clinically, the spreadsheet accepts both a loading dose and a

B14 =($B$7*$B$8*$E$4/($E$6*($E$4-$E$3)))*(EXP(-$E$3*($B$11*$B$10+A14))-EXP(-$E$4*($B$11*$B$10+A14)))+($B$7*$B$9*$E$4/($E$6*($E$4-$E$3)))*(((1-EXP(-$B$11*$E$3*$B$10))/(1-EXP(-$E$3*$B$10)))*EXP(-$E$3*A14)-((1-EXP(-$B$11*$E$4*$B$10))/(1-EXP(-$E$4*$B$10)))*EXP(-$E$4*A14))

	A	B	C	D	E	F
1	Figure 15					
2						
3	Elimination Half-life	2.3	hr	kel	0.30	hr(-1)
4	Absorption Half-life	0.2	hr	ka	3.47	hr(-1)
5	Volume of Distribution	0.27	L/kg			
6	Body Weight	74	kg	Vd	19.98	L
7	Fraction Absorbed (F)	1				
8	Loading Dose	800	mg			
9	Maintenance Dose	800	mg			
10	Dosing Interval (T)	6	hr			
11	Number of Doses (n)	2				
12						
13	Time Since Last Dose (t')	Cp (mg/L)				
14	0	8.3684				
15	0.25	29.9937				
16	0.5	37.1647				
17	0.75	38.3977				
18	1	37.2635				
19	1.25	35.2539				

Fig. 15 Spreadsheet illustrating the calculation of plasma concentrations after multiple extravascular doses, calculated using Eq. (56).

maintenance dose. If no loading dose is given, these two entries are the same value.

5. The time units for the dosing interval (T) and the step interval (int) must be the same as those for the half-lives of elimination and absorption.
6. Once the number of maintenance doses (n) is entered the spreadsheet calculates C_p for the nth dosing interval.
7. This spreadsheet can be used in the following ways:

   (a) The entire plasma concentration versus time profile for a repetitive dosing regimen can be calculated by starting with $n = 0$ and calculating C_p for the first dosing interval. Then $n = 1$ is entered, and the second interval C_p values calculated. The process can be repeated for as many dosing intervals as desired.

   (b) The plasma concentration versus time profile for a dosing interval on the plateau can be calculated by entering $n = 50$. The values of C_{min} and C_{max} can then be determined by noting the maximum and minimum values calculated. [Note: When $n = 50$ or some other large number, Eq. (56) becomes Eq. (57). Thus, calculations involving Eqs. (57), (58), and (59) can also be performed with this spreadsheet if a large number is entered for n.]

   (c) The entire plasma concentration versus time profile for a single dose administration can be calculated if the dose is entered as the loading dose (D_0), 50 (or any large number) is entered for T, and 0 is entered for d_0 and n. [Equation (56) becomes Eq. (55).]

Example. Calculate C_p at quarter-hourly intervals for the first 24 hours of the kanamycin dosing regimen described in the first example in this subsection. The entry data are as follows:

Half-life for elimination = 2.3 h
Half-life for absorption = 0.2 h
Fraction of body weight equal to volume of distribution = 0.27
Subject weight = 74 kg
Fraction of the dose absorbed = 1.0
Loading dose (D_0) = 800 mg
Maintenance dose (d_0) = 800 mg
Dosing interval (T) = 6 h
Time interval = 0.25 h
Number of maintenance doses (n) = 0 to 4

The results of the calculation are shown in Fig. 16. Note that C_{max} and C_{min} are identical to the values calculated in the aforementioned example.

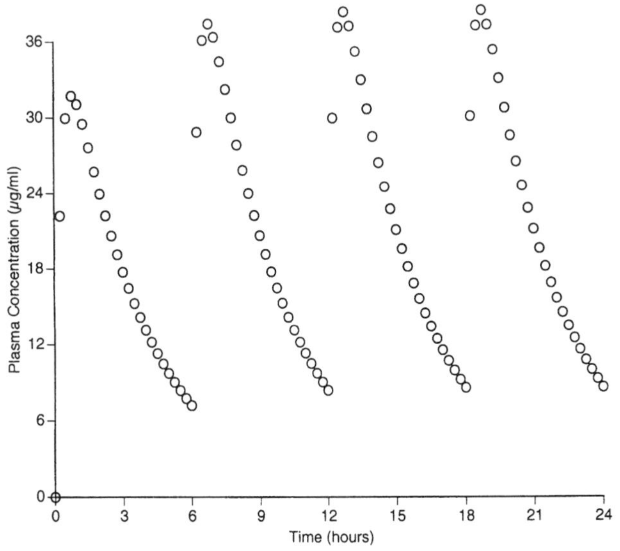

Fig. 16 Plot of kanamycin plasma concentrations (circles) versus time following multiple IM injections, calculated using Eq. (56).

REFERENCES

1. DWA Bourne. Mathematical Modeling of Pharmacokinetic Data. Lancaster, PA: Technomic Publishing Company, 1995.
2. RE Notari. Biopharmaceutics and Clinical Pharmacokinetics. 4th ed. New York, Marcel Dekker, 1987.
3. M Rowland, TN Tozer. Clinical Pharmacokinetics. 2nd ed. Philadelphia, PA: Lea & Febiger, 1989.
4. L. Shargel, ABC Yu. Applied Biopharmaceutics and Pharmacokinetics. 4th Ed, Stamford, CT: Appleton & Lange, 1999.
5. ME Winter. Basic Clinical Pharmacokinetics. 3rd ed. Vancouver, WA: Applied Therapeutics, 1994.
6. WJ Westlake. The design and analysis of comparative blood-level trails In: J Swarbrick, ed. Current Concepts in the Pharmaceutical Sciences: Dosage Form Design and Bioavailability. Philadelphia, PA: Lea & Febiger, 1973.

Chapter 4

Factors Influencing Drug Absorption and Drug Availability

Betty-ann Hoener and Leslie Z. Benet

University of California, San Francisco, California

I. INTRODUCTION

In this chapter we examine dosage forms as drug-delivery systems. The scope of the examination will, however, be limited to those oral dosage forms in which the drug is not in solution when taken by the patient. Usually the absorption of drugs from aqueous solutions can be defined by the principles discussed in Chapter 2. However, occasionally drugs in solution may precipitate in the gastrointestinal (GI) fluids and effectively be considered as suspensions. Nevertheless, the dosage forms considered in this chapter are tablets, capsules, and suspensions. In addition, the discussion is limited to drugs absorbed by passive diffusion that thus appear to obey first-order linear absorption kinetics.

The successful transposition of a drug from an oral dosage form into the general circulation can be described as a four-step process: first, delivery of the drug to its absorption site; second, getting the drug into solution; third, movement of the dissolved drug through the membranes of the gastrointestinal tract (GIT); and, finally, movement of the drug away from the site of absorption into the general circulation. Each of these four steps is considered in turn. However, the order of the first two steps is not absolute; that is, the drug may dissolve either before or after reaching its absorption site. It is imperative, however, as discussed in Chapter 2, that the drug be in solution before it can be absorbed. The slowest of the four steps will determine the rate of availability of the drug from an oral dosage form. The rate and extent of availability of a drug from its dosage form will be influenced by many factors in all four of these steps. Those factors related to the physicochemical properties of the drug and the design and production of the dosage form will be called pharmaceutical variables. Those variables resulting from the anatomical, physiological, and pathological characteristics of the patient are called patient variables. The pharmacist, who is the one member of the health care team knowledgeable about both the patient and the dosage form, is uniquely qualified to evaluate the influence of both the pharmaceutical and patient variables on rational drug therapy.

II. GETTING THE DRUG TO ITS SITE OF ABSORPTION

When an oral dosage form is swallowed by a patient, it will travel through the gastrointestinal tract (Fig. 1). During this passage the dosage form will encounter great anatomical and physiological variations. These patient variables have been discussed in Chapter 2. Two of these variables are most important in effecting the delivery of the drug from its dosage form. The first variable, hydrogen ion concentration, exhibits a 10^7-fold difference between the mucosal fluids of the stomach and the intestine. The second variable, available surface area of the absorbing membranes, changes dramatically between different regions of the GIT (see Chapter 2).

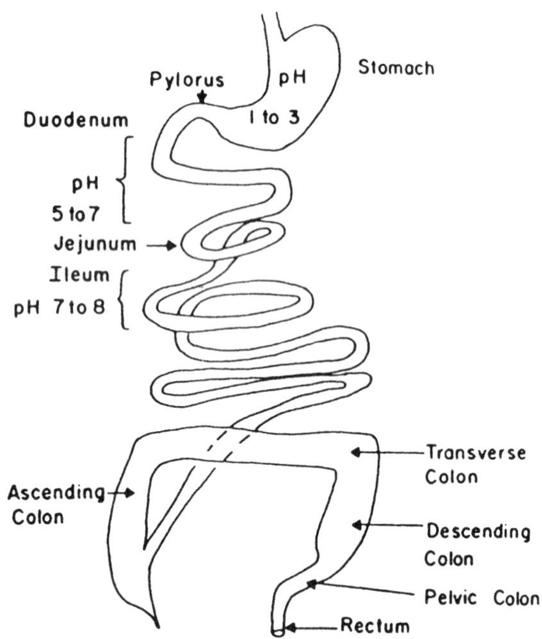

Fig. 1 Diagram of the gastrointestinal tract showing the variations of pH. (From Ref. 1.).

A. Gastric Emptying

Since various factors, principally increased membrane surface area and decreased thickness of the membrane, favor the small intestine versus the stomach as the primary site for drug absorption, the rate at which the drug gets to the small intestine can significantly affect its rate of absorption. Hence, gastric-emptying rate may well be the rate-determining step in the absorption of a drug. As has been discussed in Chapter 2, light physical activity will stimulate stomach emptying, but strenuous exercise will delay emptying [2,3]. If a patient is lying on the left side, the stomach contents will have to move uphill to get into the intestine [2,3]. The emotional state of the patient can either reduce or speed up the stomach-emptying rate [2,3]. In addition, numerous pathological conditions may alter gastric-emptying rate [4]. Other drugs may affect the stomach-emptying rate by influencing GI motility. It should be noted that any substance in the stomach delays emptying and, therefore, can delay the absorption of a drug. The stomach serves to protect the intestine from extreme conditions. Thus, if the stomach contents differ appreciably in pH, temperature, osmolarity, or viscosity from those conditions normally expected in the intestine, the stomach will delay emptying until those conditions approach normal [2,3]. Food, by altering the foregoing factors, can affect the rate of stomach emptying. Moreover, the volume, composition, and caloric content of a meal can alter the stomach-emptying rate [2,3].

Thus, the timing of meals relative to the timing of the oral dosing of a drug can influence the rate, and possibly the extent, of drug availability. It can be anticipated that taking a drug shortly before, after, or with a meal may delay the rate of drug availability as a function of decreased-emptying rate. However, the effect of food on the extent of availability cannot be so readily predicted. Figure 2 illustrates the mean serum concentration versus time curves obtained following administration of three 2.5-mg tablets of methotrexate to normal healthy volunteers [5]. The tablets were taken on an empty stomach or with a standard, high-fat content breakfast. Food significantly decreased the rate of availability of methotrexate from these tablets, as indicated by the shift to the right of the peak time. However, there was no significant change in the area under the curve and, therefore, no change in the extent of availability of methotrexate from these tablets.

In contrast with these results, Fig. 3 illustrates the decreased extent of availability of erythromycin when two 250-mg tablets of erythromycin were taken on a fasting stomach with 20 or 250 mL of water or with 250 mL of water immediately after high-fat, high-protein, and high-carbohydrate meals [6]. The rate of availability of this poorly absorbed water-soluble, acid-labile antibiotic was not affected by food (i.e., peak time was approximately the same for all dosings), indicating that stomach emptying is not the rate-determining step in the absorption of erythromycin from this drug-delivery system. The extent of availability was, however, markedly decreased. This decrease might be due to complexation between drug and food or, more likely, to degradation of the antibiotic when it is retained in the acid environment of the stomach for longer periods. (The effect of the volume of water is considered later in the chapter.)

A third possibility, an increase in the extent of availability of a drug taken with food, is illustrated in Fig. 4. Here the cumulative amount of unmetabolized nitrofurantoin excreted in the urine is plotted against time. Healthy male volunteers took nitrofurantoin as a capsule containing 100 mg of the drug in a *macro*crystalline form (circles) or as a tablet containing 100 mg of the drug in the *micro*crystalline form (squares). (The significance of the macro- and microcrystalline forms are discussed later in this chapter.) The dosage forms were taken with 240 mL of

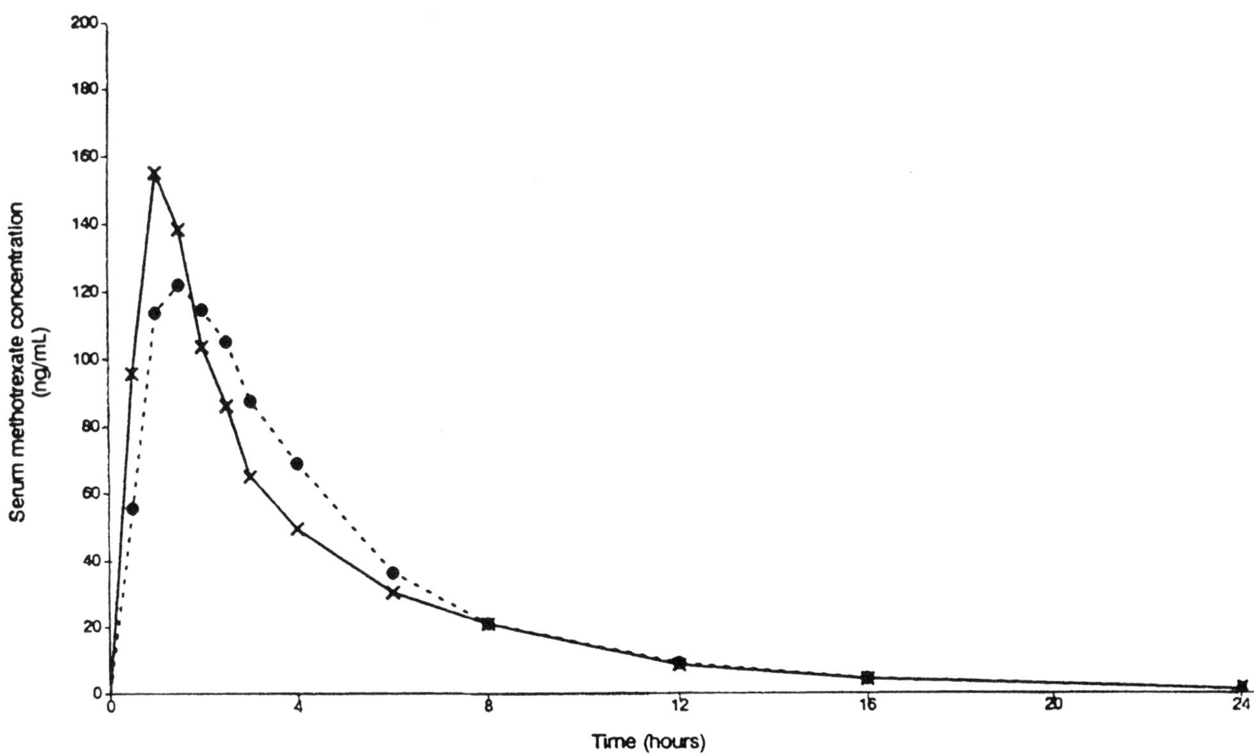

Fig. 2 Mean serum concentration of methotrexate in healthy volunteers who took three 2.5-mg tablets: ×, on a fasting stomach; ●, with breakfast. (From Ref. 5.).

water either on an empty stomach (open symbols) or immediately after a standard breakfast (solid symbols). It can be seen that food delays the absorption of nitrofurantoin from both the tablet and the capsule dosage forms, as indicated by the initial phase of each plot. However, food enhanced the extent of availability of the drug from both dosage forms, as indicated by the cumulative amount of drug excreted at 24 hours. It appears that delaying the rate of transit of nitrofurantoin through the GIT gives this poorly soluble drug more time to dissolve in the GI fluids. Thus, more nitrofurantoin gets into solution, and, therefore, more is absorbed.

In summary, food will delay stomach emptying and, as a result, may decrease the rate of availability of a drug from its oral dosage form. The extent of availability of that drug, however, may be increased, decreased, or unaffected by meals. Thus, it is important for the pharmacist to counsel patients on the importance of timing the taking of their medications relative to their mealtimes.

Large objects, such as nondisintegrating dosage forms, are handled by the stomach quite differently from liquids and particles smaller than about 2 mm in diameter [8]. These larger particles will remain in the stomach pouch until they are swept out by a series of contractions called a migrating motor complex (MMC). This MMC occurs about every 3 hours in the fasted stomach [9]. However, when a patient has eaten a meal, the MMC does not occur until after most of the food has left the stomach [8]. Thus, there could be a considerable delay in the absorption of drugs from solid dosage forms that do not disintegrate or release their contents by some other mechanism while in the stomach. This effect of size on the rate of delivery of the drug from its dosage form may or may not also affect the extent of availability.

B. Gastrointestinal Motility

Other patient variables may affect GI motility and, thereby, the extent or rate of availability of a drug from a delivery system. As illustrated in Chapter 2, the degree of physical activity, age, disease state, and emotional condition of a patient may increase or de-

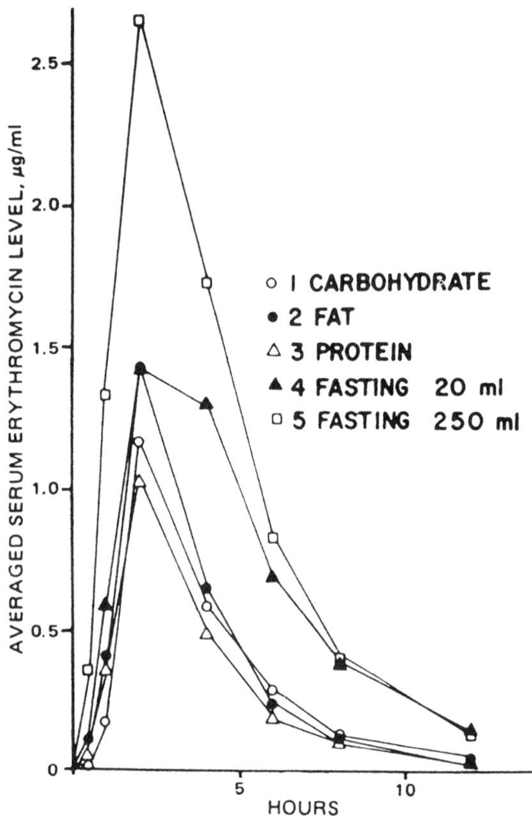

Fig. 3 Mean serum erythromycin levels in healthy volunteers given 500 mg of erythromycin stearate with 20 mL of water (▲), 250 ml of water (□), or 250 mL of water immediately after a high-carbohydrate meal (○), 250 mL of water immediately after a high-fat meal (●), and 250 mL of water immediately after a high-protein meal (△). (From Ref. 6.).

crease GI motility. Other drugs taken concurrently may affect GI motility and, thus, indirectly affect the rate and extent of availability of a particular drug. This concurrent therapy may increase or decrease GI motility, thereby increasing or decreasing the rate at which a drug reaches its absorption site. Such changes in GI motility may increase, decrease, or have no effect on the extent of availability of a drug from an oral dosage form.

Average serum digoxin levels for an elderly female patient taking 0.375 mg of digoxin daily in a tablet dosage form are shown in Fig. 5A. When the patient was also given three daily 10-mg oral doses of metoclopramide, a drug that increases GI motility, the serum digoxin levels dropped (see Fig. 5B), probably indicating a decrease in the extent of digoxin availability. It is possible that this decreased extent of availability occurred because there was insufficient time for the digoxin to be released from its dosage form, or to dissolve in the fluids of the stomach or small intestine, before it was moved completely through the GI tract.

An increase in GI motility will not, however, always decrease the extent of availability of a drug. Figure 6 illustrates the plasma level versus time curves obtained after oral administration of a 100-mg tablet of atenolol to six healthy male volunteers. When the atenolol was given 1 hour after a 25-mg dose of metoclopramide, a slight increase in the rate of availability was observed (i.e., shorter peak time), but the extent of availability of the atenolol was not significantly different from when atenolol was administered alone. Therefore it appears that, under these study conditions, stomach emptying is not the rate-determining step in absorption, nor does an increase in gastrointestinal motility significantly affect the amount of drug available to the general circulation.

Concurrent drug therapy may also decrease the motility of the GIT. Figure 5C shows again average digoxin serum levels in an elderly female patient receiving 0.375 mg of digoxin daily in tablet form. After receiving three daily doses of a 15-mg tablet of propantheline, a drug that slows GI motility, the patient's serum digoxin level increased significantly. Since the digoxin tablet was moving more slowly through its principal site of absorption, the small intestine, it is probable that there was more time for the tablet to disintegrate or for the digoxin to dissolve, thereby increasing the extent of availability.

Returning to Fig. 6, it can be seen that the oral administration of two 15-mg tablets of propantheline 1.5 hours before atenolol delayed the rate of availability of this β-blocker, while increasing its extent of availability [11]. This increased extent might be due to more complete dissolution of the drug, resulting from its increased time in the gastrointestinal tract.

Blood levels versus the time curves obtained after oral administration of two 0.5-g tablets of sulfamethoxazole to male patients are pictured in Fig. 7. (Each subject took the drug with 300 mL of lightly sugared tea.) When a 15-mg tablet of propantheline was taken 30 minutes before the sulfamethoxazole was given and a second propantheline tablet taken with it, both the rate and extent of availability of the sulfa drug from the tablet dosage form decreased (see dotted line in Fig. 7). Here, it is possible that slowing the passage of a drug through the GIT increased the opportunity for drug degradation to take place.

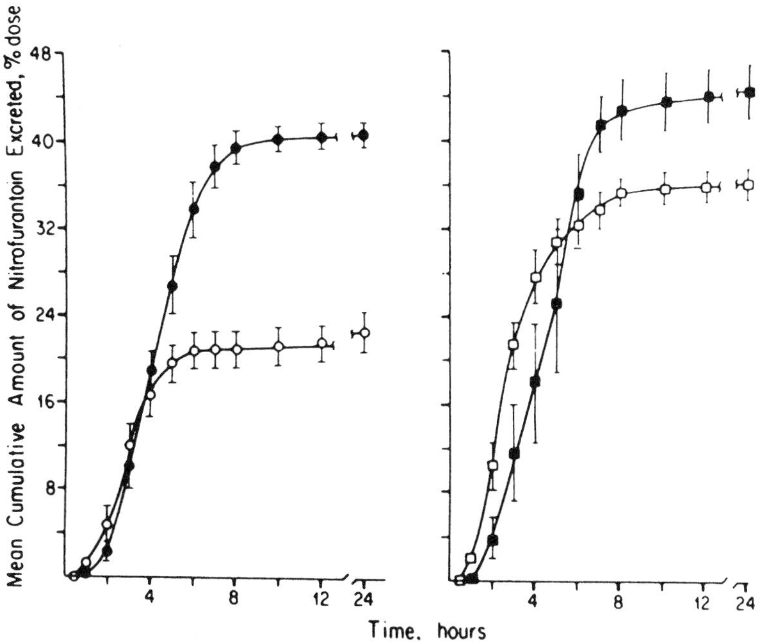

Fig. 4 Mean cumulative urinary excretion of nitrofurantoin after oral administration of a 100-mg macrocrystalline capsule of fasting (○) and nonfasting (●) subjects and a 100-mg microcrystalline tablet to fasting (■) and nonfasting (□) subjects. Vertical bars represent standard errors of the mean. (From Ref. 7.).

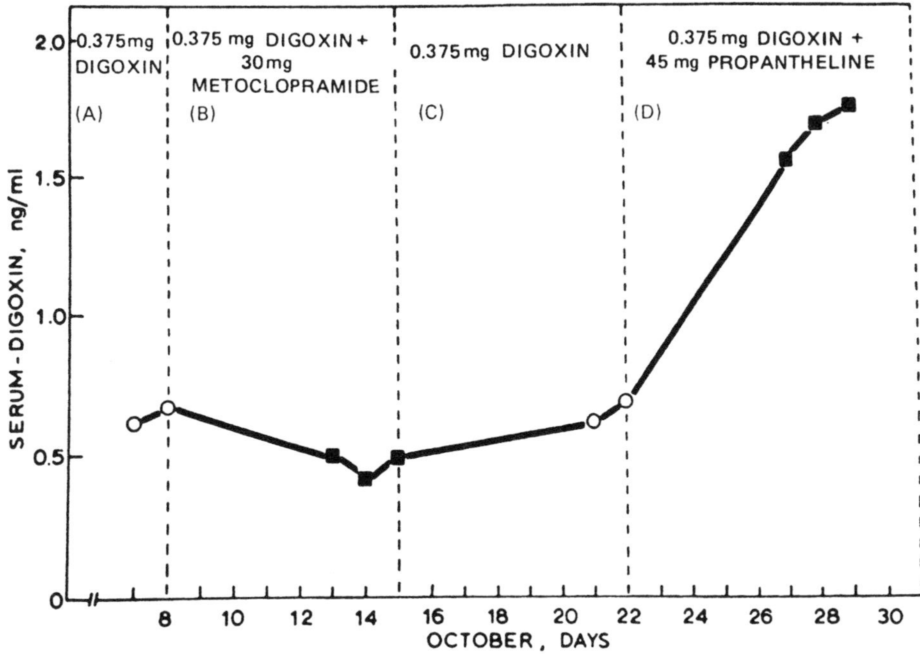

Fig. 5 Variations in serum digoxin concentration in an elderly female patient during treatment with digoxin and metoclopramide or propantheline. (From Ref. 10.).

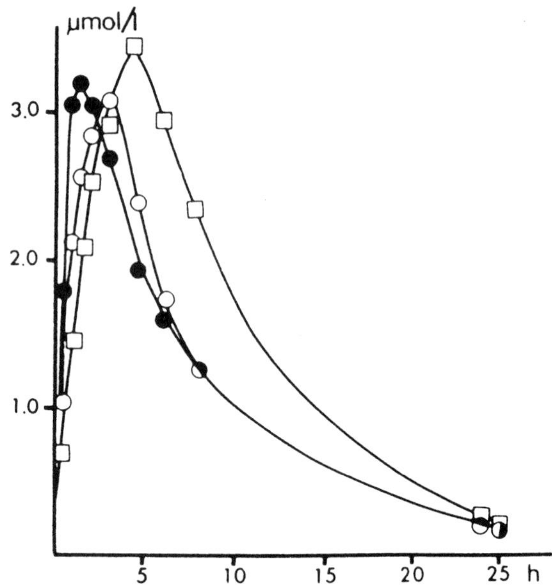

Fig. 6 Mean plasma levels of atenolol in six male volunteers after a 100-mg tablet alone (○), with 25 mg of metoclopramide (●), or with 30 mg of propantheline (□). (From Ref. 11.).

Thus, drugs that alter GI motility may increase or decrease the rate of availability of another drug. In addition, concurrent therapy may increase, decrease, or not affect the extent of availability of a drug. It should be noted that knowledge of the effect of a drug on GI motility usually can lead to an accurate prediction of its potential effect on the rate of availability of a second drug, if, and only if, this is the rate-determining step in absorption, but this knowledge usually does not allow the pharmacist to predict how changes in motility may affect the extent of availability for the second drug. To make such a prediction, additional information, such as degradation and binding mechanisms along the GI tract, must be known.

Since gastric emptying can significantly affect the availability of a drug, it might be suspected that patients who have undergone partial or total gastrectomies will exhibit abnormal rates or extents of availability. Figure 7 illustrates the increased rate of availability of sulfamethoxazole in a patient who had previously undergone a partial gastrectomy. Since the patient had most of his stomach removed, the drug could reach its principal site of absorption, the small intestine, without delay. Some pathological conditions are also accompanied by altered gastrointestinal motility, which may affect availability [4].

The pharmacist, as a drug therapist, should advise both the physician and the patient of the potential problems involved in either initiating or discontinuing concurrent therapy of drugs known to alter GI motility. The pharmacist can also advise the physician

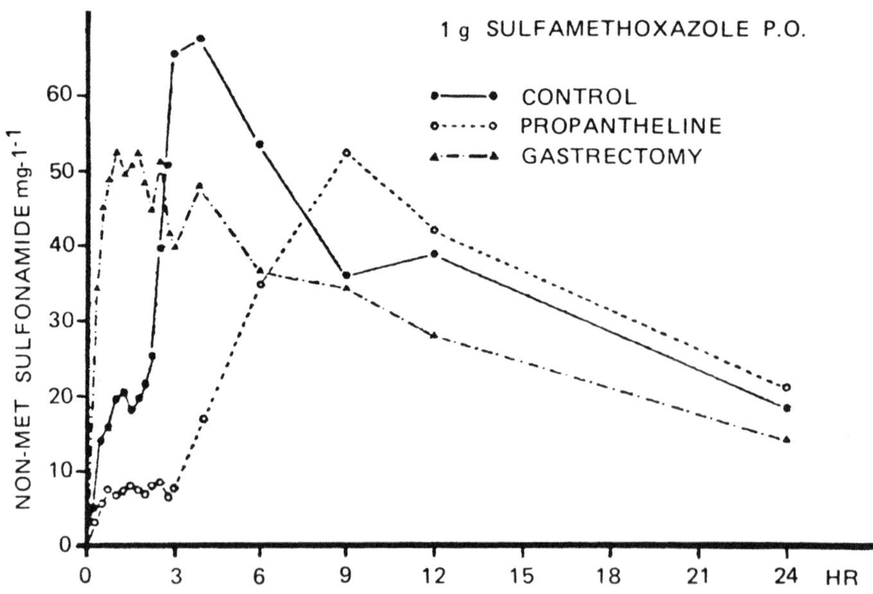

Fig. 7 Blood levels of nonmetabolized sulfamethoxazole following oral administration of 1.0 g, as two 0.5-g tablets, under three different conditions. (From Ref. 12.).

on rational drug therapy in patients in whom the gastrointestinal tract has been altered surgically or by disease.

C. Degradation in the Gastrointestinal Tract

Absorption is not the only process that can occur along the GIT. A drug may be degraded or metabolized before it can be absorbed. Chemical degradation, especially pH-dependent reactions, can occur in the solubilizing fluids of the GIT. Drugs that structurally resemble nutrients, such as polypeptides, nucleotides, or fatty acids, may be especially susceptible to enzymatic degradation [2,3]. Digestion of these molecules would result as a consequence of the normal functions of the GIT. Moreover, the GIT is rich in microflora. These microorganisms could metabolize drug molecules before absorption. The variety of degradations attributable to bacteria has been reviewed [14]. In addition, both the fluids and the microflora of the GIT may be altered in disease states. As a result, drug therapy may need to be modified if the rate and extent of availability are affected by these changes [4].

It would seem that metabolism and degradation of a drug within the GIT would serve primarily to reduce its extent of availability. In some instances, however, these processes may enhance availability. For example, clindamycin palmitate is less soluble than clindamycin HCl. A suspension of the palmitate ester is a more stable, better-tasting dosage form than a solution of clindamycin HCl. The palmitate ester is rapidly hydrolyzed in the GIT to free the more soluble active parent antibiotic drug, which becomes rapidly available to the systemic circulation [13]. Molecules such as clindamycin palmitate are chemical derivatives of drugs. These derivatives, called prodrugs, are made to enhance the pharmaceutical properties of the parent molecule. These prodrugs may depend on degradation in the GIT to release the active parent molecule. Consequently, although metabolism or degradation in the GIT decreases the extent of availability for most drugs, with some prodrugs the degradative processes may be essential for complete bioavailability.

The pharmacist should certainly know which drug dosage forms have been designed as delivery systems for prodrugs and also understand the mechanism whereby the active form is made available within the body. Only then can the pharmacist counsel the physician about why a certain product may be inappropriate for such individuals as an achlorhydric patient, a patient with a gastrectomy, or even possibly a patient with a hepatoportal bypass, if liver metabolism is responsible for conversion of the prodrug into the active form.

III. GETTING THE DRUG INTO SOLUTION: FACTORS AFFECTING THE RATE OF DISSOLUTION

Once the dosage form reaches the absorption site, it must break down and release its therapeutic agent. Figure 8 depicts the disintegration and dissolution processes involved in the gastrointestinal absorption of a drug administered in a tablet dosage form. Figure 9 indicates more comprehensively the various solubility problems that may be encountered after the administration of a drug in an oral dosage form. Arrows drawn with heavy dark lines indicate primary pathways that most drugs administered in a particular dosage form undergo. Arrows drawn with dashed lines indicate that the drug is administered in this state in the dosage form. Arrows drawn as thin, continuous lines and labeled "precipitation" indicate situations in which a drug is already in solution, but then precipitates out as fine particles, usually owing to a change in pH of the aqueous environment that causes a change in drug solubility. Other thin arrows indicate secondary pathways that are usually inconsequential in achieving therapeutic efficacy. The dissolution process is primarily dependent on pharmaceutical variables, with the possible exception of a pH dependency, which may be a patient variable. The relative importance of the various processes in Fig. 9 may be explained in terms of the equation developed by Nernst and Brunner [16] whereby dissolution is described by a diffusion layer model:

$$\frac{dQ}{dt} = \frac{D}{h} S(C_s - C_g) \qquad (1)$$

where

Q = amount of drug involved
t = time
D = diffusion coefficient of the drug in the solubilizing fluids of the GIT
S = effective surface area of the drug particles
h = thickness of a stationary layer of solvent around the drug particle
C_s = saturation solubility of the drug in the stationary layer, h
C_g = concentration of drug in the bulk fluids of the GIT

In deriving this equation, it was assumed that the drug dissolved uniformly from all surfaces of the

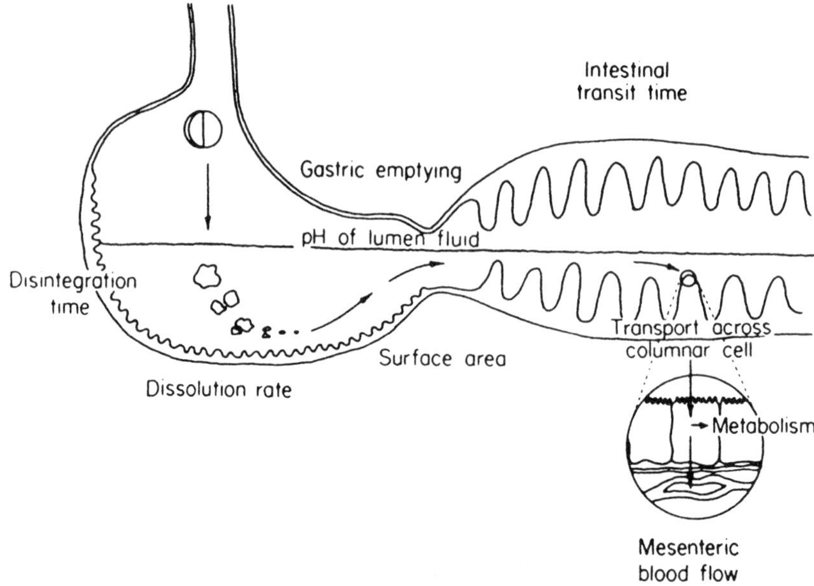

Fig. 8 Factors affecting the rate of absorption of drug from the gastrointestinal tract. (From Ref. 15.).

particles. The particles were assumed to be spherical and all of the same size. In addition, h was assumed to be constant, and both h and C_s were assumed to be independent of particle size. Figure 10 schematically illustrates the relationship of the terms in Eq. (1) to the dissolution process. It should be emphasized that this crude model does not completely describe the dissolution process. The model has, however, helped to explain many experimental results. The following subsections will consider the pharmaceutical implications of the terms given in Eq. (1).

A. Effective Surface Area of the Drug, *S*

Particle Size

The smaller the drug particles, the greater the surface area for a given amount of drug (e.g., 1 g). Thus Eq. (1) predicts that dissolution rate will increase as particle size decreases. Figure 11 confirms this expectation. The smaller granules of phenacetin dissolve more quickly than the larger granules, and there is a graded response; that is, for the five size ranges an increasing amount of drug dissolves over a specified time as the particle size decreases and surface area increases. However, in this example the hydrophobic drug phenacetin has been manipulated by a pharmaceutical manufacturing process called granulation (see Chapter 9 for further discussion) whereby the hydrophilic diluent gelatin has been incorporated into the particle. An opposite effect is seen when phenacetin particles themselves are dissolved in 0.1 *N* HCl (see the solid lines in the lower portion of Fig. 12). In this dissolution study of the hydrophobic drug, the dissolution rate increases with increasing particle size and decreasing particle surface area, in direct contradiction of Eq. (1). However, when a suface-active agent, Tween 80, is added to the 0.1 *N* HCl medium, the dissolution rate of phenacetin particles increases as the particle size decreases (see the dashed lines in the upper portion of Fig. 12). It is probable that decreasing the particle size of a hydrophobic drug actually decreases its *effective* surface area (i.e., the portion of the surface actually in contact with the dissolving fluids). In fact, the smaller phenacetin particles had more air adsorbed on their surfaces and actually floated on the dissolution medium. When a surface-active agent was added to the dissolution medium, the smaller particles were more readily wetted. Thus, their absolute surface area became their effective surface area. In Fig. 11 the granulation process has incorporated the hydrophobic phenacetin particles into the hydrophilic granules where the surface area of the granule approximated the effective surface area.

Figure 13 compares the dissolution rate of pure phenacetin particles with the granulated particles of the same size and with tablets prepared from these granules. These comparisons were made by using

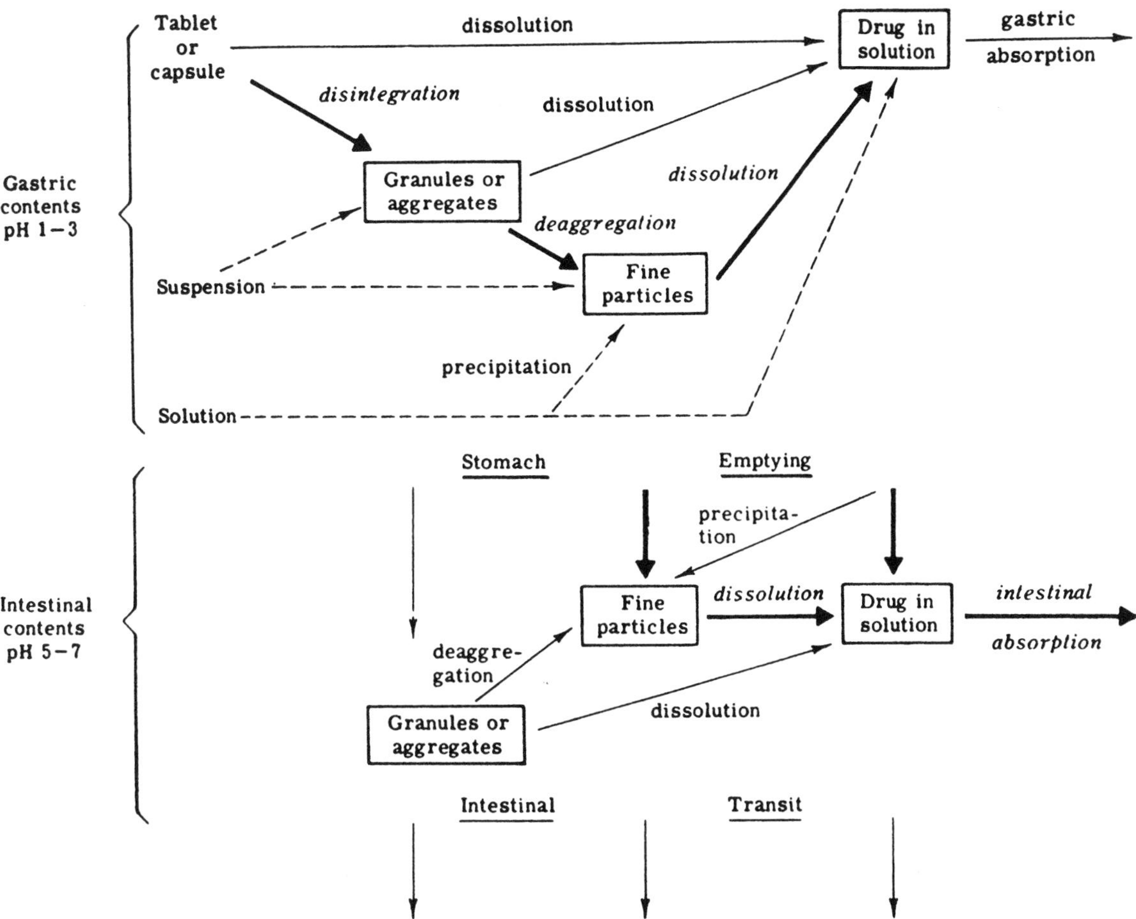

Fig. 9 Processes involved in getting a drug into solution in the GIT so that absorption may take place. Heavy arrows indicate primary pathways that the majority of drugs administered in a particular dosage form undergo. Dashed arrows indicate that the drug is administered in this state in the dosage form. Thin continuous arrows indicate secondary pathways, which are usually inconsequential in achieving therapeutic efficacy. (From Ref. 15.).

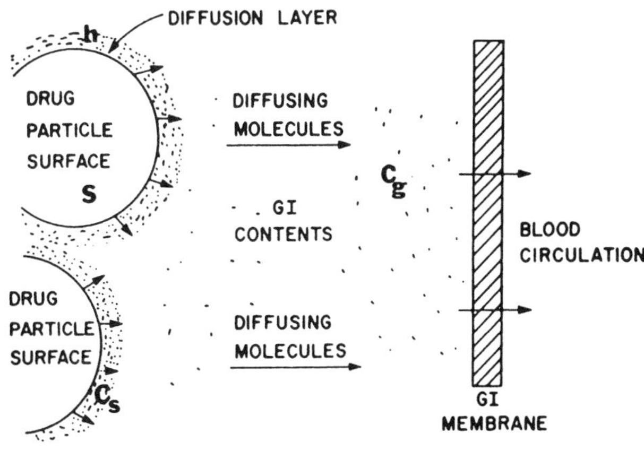

Fig. 10 Schematic diagram of the dissolution process. (From Ref. 1.).

dilute gastric juice as the dissolution medium. Gastric juice has a relatively low surface tension, 42.7 dyn/cm, compared with water, which has a surface tension of approximately 70 dyn/cm. The low surface tension of the gastric juice aids in the wetting of both the hydrophobic particles and the hydrophilic granules. When these hydrophilic granules were compressed into tablets, the dissolution rate of phenacetin decreased but remained greater than the rate of dissolution for the hydrophobic powder. It is possible that the large tablets do not rapidly disintegrate into the smaller granules, as indicated by the apparent lag time before dissolution begins. However, when the tablets do disintegrate, the hydrophilicity of the granules enables them to be more readily wetted than the powdered form.

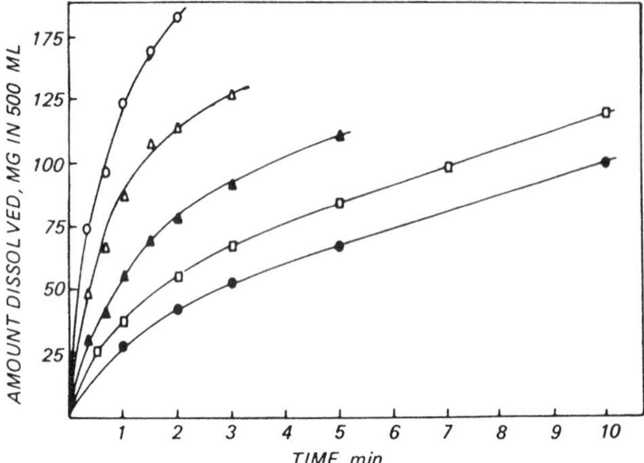

Fig. 11 Effect of particle size of phenacetin on dissolution of drug from granules containing starch and gelatin. ○, particle size 0.11–0.15 mm; △, particle size 0.15–0.21 mm; ▲, particle size 0.21–0.30 mm; □, particle size 0.30–0.50 mm; ●, particle size 0.50–0.71 mm. (From Ref. 17.).

In addition to these in vitro demonstrations of the importance of the effective surface area of drug particles on dissolution rate, many in vivo studies are available. Phenacetin plasma levels versus time are plotted for three different particle sizes of phenacetin in Fig. 14. Healthy adult volunteers received 1.5-g doses of phenacetin as an aqueous suspension on an empty stomach. The results show that both the rate and extent of availability of the phenacetin increase as particle size decreases. Since the large particles dissolve very slowly, the dosage form may pass through the GIT before dissolution is complete. When Tween 80 is added to the dosage form, the rate and extent of availability of the phenacetin increases even more, perhaps as a result of increasing the wettability of the particles, as shown in Fig. 12 for an in vitro study.

The effect of particle size reduction on the bioavailability of nitrofurantoin was shown in Fig. 4. The microcrystalline form (<10 μm) is more rapidly and completely absorbed from the tablet dosage form than is the macrocrystalline form (74–177 μm) from the capsule dosage form. This is not a completely satisfactory illustration of the effect of particle size on the rate and extent of availability, since other manufacturing variables have not been held constant. Nevertheless, it does suggest some correlation between particle size, dissolution rate, and rate of availability.

In summary, it is the effective surface area of a drug particle that determines its dissolution rate. The effective surface area may be increased by physically reducing the particle size, by adding hydrophilic diluents to the final dosage form, or by adding surface-active agents to the dissolution medium or to the dosage form.

Disintegration and Deaggregation

The rate of disintegration of the dosage form and the size of the resulting aggregates can be the rate-limiting

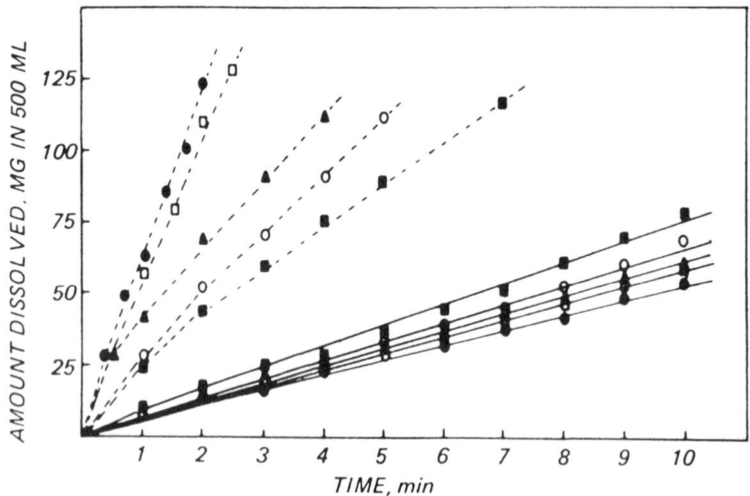

Fig. 12 Effect of particle size on dissolution of phenacetin. ●, particle size 0.11–0.15 mm; □, particle size 0.15–0.21 mm; ▲, particle size 0.21–0.30 mm; ○, particle size 0.30–0.50 mm; ■, particle size 0.50–0.71 mm; —, dissolution medium, 0.1 *N* HCl; - - -, dissolution medium, 0.1 *N* HCl containing 0.2% tween 80. (From Ref. 17.).

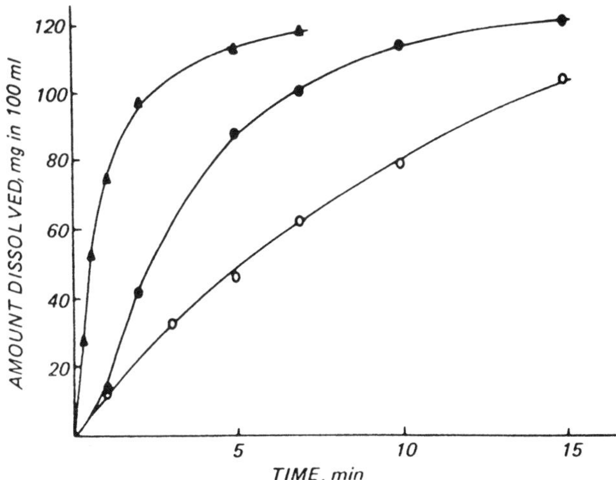

Fig. 13 Rate of dissolution of phenacetin from powder, granules, and tablets in diluted gastric juice (Surface Tension, 42.7 dyn/cm; pH 1.85). ○, Phenacetin Powder; ▲, Phenacetin Granules; ●, Phenacetin Tablets. (From Ref. 17.).

step in the dissolution process. Disintegration is a particularly important step in the dissolution of drugs from coated dosage forms. Tablets or pellets of drugs contained within tablets or capsules are coated for several reasons, as will be discussed in Chapter 10. Rationales for the use of coating include the need to protect a drug during storage or from the very low pH of the stomach. Dosage forms may be coated so that they release their active ingredients slowly for prolonged action. Some drugs are coated to protect the patient's GIT from local irritation. Whatever the reason, these coats are made from materials having various degrees of hydrophilicity that may or may not break down and allow their active ingredients to dissolve. Some poorly formulated coated tablets do not break down at all, and these dosage forms can be recovered intact in the feces. Pharmacists must be aware of such pharmaceutical failures. They must assure themselves that the particular dosage forms they are dispensing to their patients meet all bioavailability standards, as discussed in Chapter 3.

As illustrated in Fig. 9, after a dosage form disintegrates into large particles, these large particles must deaggregate to yield fine particles. Hence, deaggregation may be a rate-limiting step in the dissolution process. Chloramphenicol plasma level versus time curves obtained after the oral administration to healthy volunteers of two 250 mg capsules of each of four different brands of chloramphenicol are plotted in Fig. 15. The in vitro deaggregation rate of the same four brands of chloramphenicol increased in the order $D < B \simeq C < A$. Thus, the in vivo rate and extent of availability of chloramphenicol from these capsule dosage forms correlates well with their in vivo deaggregation rate.

Table 1 summarizes in vitro studies on the effect of pH, a potential patient variable, on the dissolution rate of phenytoin from two different brands of capsules containing 100 mg of sodium phenytoin. Preparation

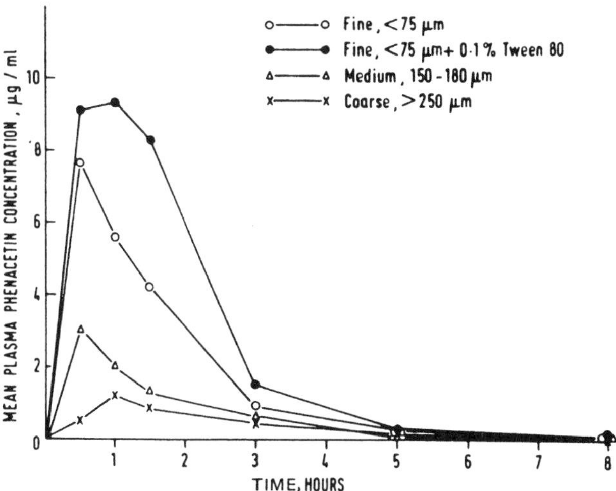

Fig. 14 Mean plasma phenacetin concentrations in six adult volunteers following administration of 1.5-g doses (in aqueous suspensions containing 200 mg of phenacetin per milliliter). (From Ref. 18.).

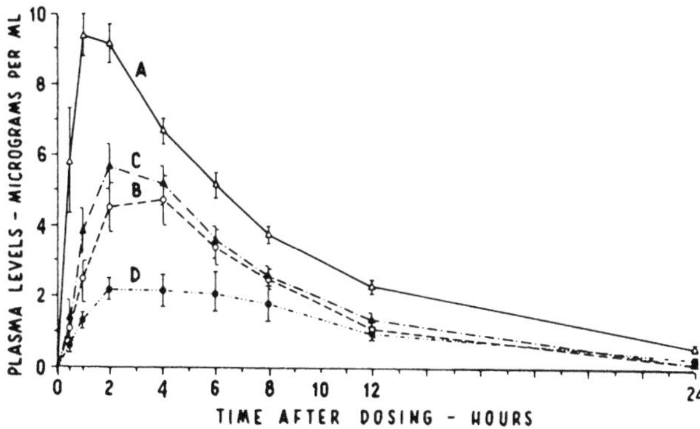

Fig. 15 Mean plasma levels for groups of ten human subjects receiving single 0.5-g doses (as two 250-mg capsules) of chloramphenicol: preparations A, B, C, or D. Vertical lines represent one standard error on either side of the mean. (From Ref. 19.).

Table 1 In Vitro Dissolution Characteristics[a] of Two Commercial Phenytoin Sodium Capsule

Solvent system	Initial pH	Time for 50% dissolution (min); average of five capsules (SD)	
		Preparation A	Preparation B
175 mL 0.1 *N* HCl and 175 mL 0.1 *N* NaOH	~7	42.4 (5.6)	12.3 (3.2)
175 mL 0.1 *N* HCl for 30 min, then addition of 175 mL 0.1 *N* NaOH	~1	34.9[b] (5.6)	80.0[b] (26.2)
175 mL 0.01 *N* HCl for 30 min, then addition of 175 mL 0.01 *N* NaOH	~2	32.6[b] (10.4)	25.2[b] (8.6)

[a]Modified Levy-Hayes method, 55 rpm, 17°C.
[b]Time after addition of NaOH; less than 5% dissolved in HCl solution.
Source: Ref. 20.

A retained its compact capsule shape no matter what the initial pH of the dissolution medium. Moreover, the dissolution rate of phenytoin from preparation A was pH-independent. Preparation B, however, broke down into fine particles. When the initial pH was neutral, these particles rapidly dissolved. As the initial pH was lowered, these fine particles precipitated. Since these precipitated particles then dissolved very slowly, it would appear that the precipitate was not the freely soluble sodium phenytoin, but the poorly soluble acid form of phenytoin. Since capsule A did not disintegrate or deaggregate, most of the sodium phenytoin was not exposed to the lower pH media and, as a result, was not converted to its very slowly dissolving acid form.

Effect of Manufacturing Processes

Various manufacturing processes can affect dissolution by altering the effective surface area of drug particles. Each of the individual processes mentioned here is discussed in more detail in Chapter 9. The effect of adding hydrophilic granulating agents to a dosage form has been discussed earlier (see Sec. III.A).

Lubricating agents are often added to capsule or tablet dosage forms so that the powder mass or the finished dosage forms will not stick to the processing machinery. When the hydrophilic lubricating agent sodium lauryl sulfate was added, 325-mg salicylic acid tablets dissolved in 0.1 *N* HCl more rapidly than did control tablets containing no lubricant, as shown in Fig. 16. If, however, the hydrophobic lubricant magnesium stearate was added, the dissolution rate decreased. Most lubricants, and all the effective lubricants, are very hydrophobic, and they act by particle coating. Thus they must be properly formulated to avoid reducing dissolution rate and bioavailability. Once again, increasing hydrophilicity of a dosage form enhanced its dissolution rate in an aqueous medium, but increasing its hydrophobicity decreased its dissolution rate.

Disintegrating agents, such as starch, tend to swell with wetting. In swelling the starch can break apart the dosage form. As seen in Fig. 17, again for 325-mg salicylic acid tablets, as more starch was added to the tablets the drug dissolved more quickly because the dosage form disintegrated more quickly.

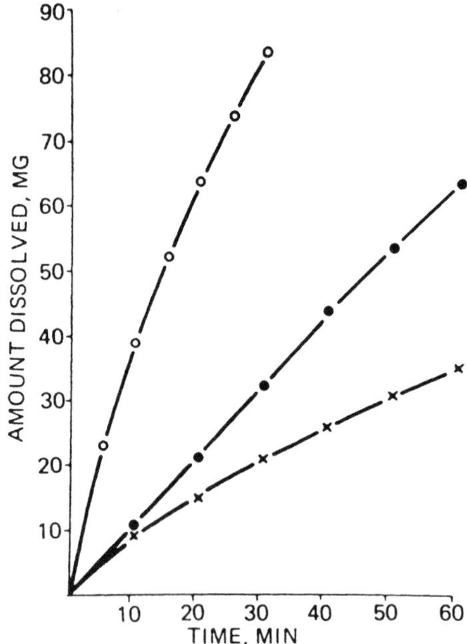

Fig. 16 Effect of lubricant on dissolution of rate of salicylic acid contained in compressed tablets. ×, 3% magnesium stearate; ●, no lubricant; ○, 3% sodium lauryl sulfate. (From Ref. 21.).

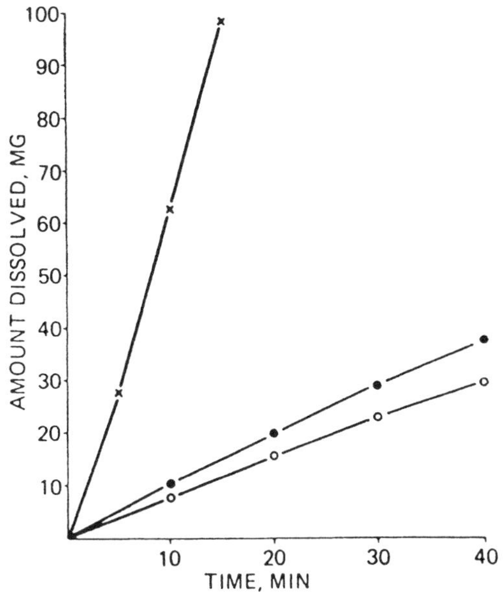

Fig. 17 Effect of starch content of granules on dissolution rate of salicylic acid contained in compressed tablets. ○, 5%; ●, 10%; ×, 20% starch in granules. (From Ref. 22.).

The possible effects on dissolution rate of the force used in compressing the drug-diluent mixture into a tablet dosage form have been summarized in Fig. 18. As compression force is increased, the particles may be more tightly bound to one another. (Part I of Fig. 18 best represents this possibility.) On the other hand, it is also possible that higher pressures may fracture the particles so that they break into yet smaller particles (see part III of Fig. 18). Depending on which of these two extremes is dominant for a given formulation, any of the combinations illustrated in Fig. 18 is possible. Furthermore, a sum of any of them may result. Thus, the effect of the compression force on the dissolution rate of a tablet dosage form would appear to be unpredictable.

The packing density, as illustrated in Fig. 19, may affect the rate of release of a drug (not identified in these studies) from a capsule dosage form [23]. For the rapidly dissolving formulation (see Fig. 19a), packing density had no effect on release rate. For the slowly dissolving formulation (see Fig. 19b), however, increasing packing density decreased dissolution rate. It is probable that further studies of the effect of packing density on dissolution rate for different drugs from different formulations would results in both increasing and decreasing dissolution rates.

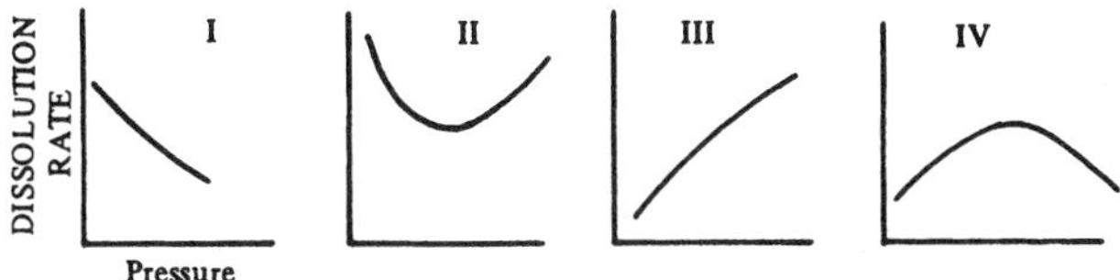

Fig. 18 Effect of compression pressure on dissolution rate. See the text for an explanation. (From Ref. 17.).

From the very few studies discussed here of the many that have been published, it would appear that manufacturing processes can determine the dissolution rate of a drug from its final dosage form. Whether changes in these manufacturing variables are beneficial or detrimental to the ultimate bioavailability of a drug depends on the physicochemical properties of the drug and its dosage form. Pharmacists should be aware of the possible effects that "inert" ingredients and manufacturing methods, which are usually carefully guarded trade secrets, may have on the bioavailability of the drug products they select to dispense to their patients.

B. Saturation Solubility of the Drug, C_s

The next term in Eq. (1) that can be manipulated is C_s, the saturation solubility of the drug. This variable can be influenced by both patient and pharmaceutical variables. The patient variables include the changes in pH as well as the amounts and types of secretions along the GIT. Additionally, both the physical and chemical properties of a drug molecule can be modified to increase or decrease its saturation solubility.

Salt Form of the Drug

Since the salt form of a drug is more soluble in an aqueous medium, the dissolution rate for the salt form of a drug should be greater than the dissolution rate of the nonionized form of the drug. However, the solubility of the salt depends on the counterion; generally, the smaller the counterion, the more soluble the salt. If dissolution is the rate-determining step in absorption, then, for a series of salts and the nonionized form of a drug, it can be anticipated that the rate of availability of the drug will increase as solubility increases. The weakly acidic drug *p*-aminosalicylic acid (PAS) is available as the potassium, calcium, or sodium salt. The solubility of nonionized PAS is 1 g/600 mL of water; of KPAS, 1 g/10 mL; of CaPAS, 1 g/7 mL; and of NaPAS, 1 g/2 mL. Healthy adult volunteers took, on a fasting stomach with 250 mL of water, tablets containing either 4 g of PAS or tablets containing 4 g of

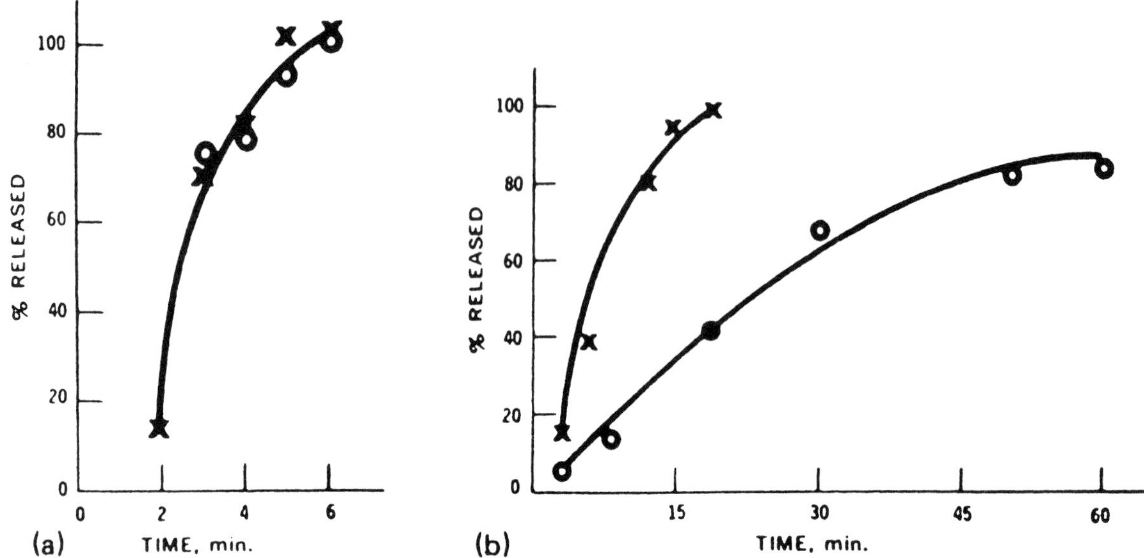

Fig. 19 Influence of packing density on dissolution of drug from capsules in simulated gastric fluid. ×, regular packing: 355 mg/No. 2 capsule; ○, dense packing: 400 mg/No. 2 capsule. (a) Drug, $CaHPO_4$; (b) Drug, $CaHPO_4$, 5% magnesium stearate. (From Ref. 23.).

one of the salts (containing 2.6–2.8 g of PAS) [24]. Mean plasma concentrations (corrected to a 4-g dose of PAS) versus time curves are shown in Fig. 20. Although the rates of availability of the salts are not significantly different, their rank order does correlate with solubility. All the salt forms were more rapidly available than the nonionized PAS to a significant extent. Furthermore, the extent of availability of the acid form is only about 77% of that of the salt forms, indicating that the drug may not have completely dissolved before the dosage form moved through the GIT. Since commercial tablets were used, it is probable that other dosage form variables (as discussed in Sec. III.A) were not held constant. Thus, the decrease in rate and extent of availability of the PAS may not be exclusively due to differences in solubility.

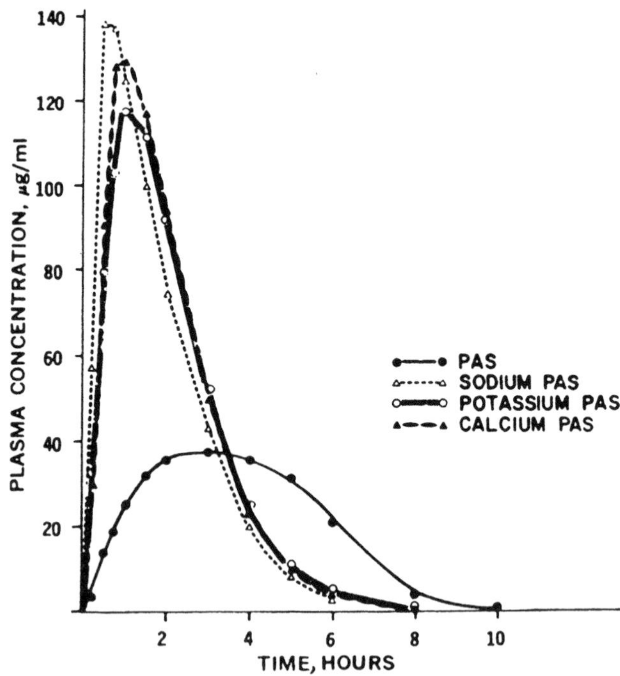

Fig. 20 Mean plasma concentrations of unchanged drug from 12 subjects following administration of four different preparations of *p*-aminosalicylic acid (PAS). Data were corrected to 70 kg of body weight and to a dose equivalent of 4 g of free acid. (From Ref. 24.).

pH Effect

As indicated, the ionized form of a drug will be more soluble than the nonionized form in the aqueous fluids of the GIT. The classic studies on the beneficial effects of changing nonionized drugs into salt forms were reported by Nelson for tetracycline [25], and Nelson et al. for tolbutamide [26]. Table 2 combines portions of the data from each study. Urinary excretion of the drug or its metabolite was taken as the in vivo measure of the relative absorption rate for the salt and the nonionized

Table 2 Correlation of Dissolution Rates with Biological Measurements for Tolbutamide and Tetracycline Absorption in Humans

Drug as nondisintegrating pellet	In vitro dissolution rate[a] ($mg\,cm^{-2}h^{-1}$): 0.1 *N*HCl[b] or simulated gastric fluid[a]	pH 7.2 buffer[b] or simulated neutral intestinal fluid[c]	Average amount excreted (mg) to time indicated[d]: 1 h	2 h	3 h	Lowering of blood sugar level (mg/100 mL) after 1 h
Tolbutamide	0.21 (N → N)	3.1 (N → I)	5	7	12	5.2
Sodium tolbutamide	1069 (I → N)	868 (I → I)	21	65	117	9.1
Tetracycline	2.6 (N → I)	0.001 (N → N)	0.2	1.5	3.3	
Tetracycline HCl	4.1 (I → I)	7.8 (I → N)	3.0	12.0	20.4	

[a]The N → N, etc. designations for the dissolution data are explained in the text.
[b]Tolbutamide study.
[c]Tetracycline study.
[d]Tolbutamide excretion measured as the carboxytolbutamine metabolite.
Source: Refs. 25 and 26.

form of each drug. No comparison can be made between the two drugs, and they are combined here only to illustrate that the same principles hold for both positively and negatively charged drug ions. Note that the salt forms of the drug dissolve much faster than the nonionized forms (or zwitterion for tetracycline) in all media and that more of the salt forms of the drug are absorbed and subsequently excreted in each period. For a dissociable drug, either an acid or a base, such as tolbutamide or tetracycline, the pH of the GI fluids will determine whether the drug is ionized or nonionized. The dependence of the dissolution rate of a drug on pH is not evident in the Nernst-Brunner as written in Eq. (1). That equation may be rewritten as

$$\frac{dQ}{dt} = \frac{DS}{h}(C_h - C_g) \tag{2}$$

where Q, t, D, S, h, and C_g are defined as before, and C_h = saturation solubility of the drug in the boundary layer, h, at any particular pH; $C_h = C_s$ when the drug is dissolving in an aqueous solution in which it is totally nonionized. Then, for a weakly acidic drug:

$$\mathrm{AH} \overset{K_a}{\rightleftharpoons} \mathrm{A^-} + \mathrm{H^+}; \quad K_a = \frac{[\mathrm{A^-}][\mathrm{H^+}]}{[\mathrm{AH}]}$$

$$C_h = [\mathrm{AH}] + [\mathrm{A^-}]$$

$$C_h = [\mathrm{AH}]\left(1 + \frac{K_a}{[\mathrm{H^+}]}\right) \quad \text{but,} \quad C_s = [\mathrm{AH}]$$

and, therefore,

$$C_h = C_s\left(1 + \frac{K_a}{[\mathrm{H^+}]}\right)$$

so

$$\frac{dQ}{dt} = \frac{DS}{h}\left\{C_s\left(1 + \frac{K_a}{[\mathrm{H^+}]}\right) - C_g\right\} \tag{3}$$

Therefore, as pH increases, the dissolution rate of a week *acid* increases. Similarly, for a weak base:

$$\mathrm{BH^+} \overset{K_a}{\rightleftharpoons} \mathrm{B} + \mathrm{H^-}; \quad K_a = \frac{[\mathrm{B}][\mathrm{H^+}]}{[\mathrm{BH^+}]}$$

$$C_h = [\mathrm{BH^+}] + [\mathrm{B}]$$

$$C_h = [\mathrm{B}]\left(1 + \frac{[\mathrm{H^+}]}{K_a}\right) \quad \text{but,} \quad C_s = [\mathrm{B}]$$

and, therefore

$$C_h = C_s\left(1 + \frac{[\mathrm{H^+}]}{K_a}\right)$$

so

$$\frac{dQ}{dt} = \frac{DS}{h}\left\{C_s\left(1 + \frac{[\mathrm{H^+}]}{K_a}\right) - C_g\right\} \tag{4}$$

Thus, as the pH increases, the dissolution rate of a weak *base* decreases. Referring to Table 2, we can see that, for the weak acid tolbutamide, the dissolution rate increases as pH is increased, as predicted by Eq. (3). Additionally, for the weak base tetracycline, as predicted by Eq. (4), the dissolution rate decreases as pH is increased. Thus far, the more rapid dissolution of the salt forms of these drugs and the direction of change of the dissolution rate with pH have been accounted for with Eqs. (1) to (4). However, there are six possible dissolution rate comparisons that can be made for each set of nonionized drug and its salt in the two buffers, as discussed by Benet [15]. The letters in Table 2 indicate similar measurements in the two studies. Thus N → N indicates a nonionized solid drug dissolving in a medium in which the dissolved solute in the bulk solution will be nonionized; N → I indicates a nonionized solid drug dissolving in a medium in which the dissolved solute in the bulk solution will be ionized; I → I indicates an ionized solid drug dissolving in a medium in which the dissolved solute will be ionized; and I → N indicates an ionized solid drug becoming nonionized solute after dissolution.

Process I → I should be faster than process N → N, since the solubility of the dissolving substance will be much greater for the salt than for the nonionized molecule. A similar explanation can be used for (I → N)>(N → N) and (I → I)>(N → N) and (I → I)>(N → I), but it must be remembered that according to Eqs. (1), (3), and (4), C_s is the saturation solubility of the drug in the diffusion layer, not in the bulk solution. It is believed that the dissolving solid acts as its own buffer and changes the pH of the liquid environment immediately surrounding the solid particle; thus, the dissolution rate should be governed by the solubility of the drug in the buffered diffusion layer. The I → N and N → N comparison is especially significant in the oral administration of weakly acidic drugs and their salts, since the acidic region of the stomach is the first solvent medium encountered following normal oral dosing. Frequently, administering the sodium or potassium salt of an acidic drug actually speeds up absorption by increasing the effective surface area of the solid drug according to the following hypothesized process. The salt acts as its own buffer in the diffusion layer and goes into solution in this layer. However, when the salt molecules diffuse out of the layer and encounter the bulk solution, they precipitate out as very fine nonionized prewetted particles. The large surface area thus precipitated favors rapid dissolution when additional fluid becomes available for one of the following reasons: (a) dissolved particles are absorbed; (b) more fluid accumulates in the stomach; or (c) the fine particles are emptied into the intestine. The classic study of Lee et al. [27] comparing serum levels of penicillin V following administration of the salt and free acid to dogs is explained by this phenomenon also. However, in at least three cases—aluminum acetylsalicylate [28], sodium warfarin [29], and the pamoate salt of benzphetamine [30]—administration of the salt slowed dissolution of the drug and subsequent absorption as compared with the nonionized form. This decrease appears to be due to precipitation of an insoluble particle or film on the surface of the tablet, rather than in the bulk solution. Precipitation of an insoluble particle or film onto the surface of the tablet decreases the effective surface area by preventing deaggregation of the particles.

The comparison of I → N and N → I may also be explained by the buffered pH in the diffusion layer and leads to an interesting comparison between a process under kinetic control versus one under thermodynamic control. Because the bulk solution in process N → I favors formation of the ionized species, a much larger quantity of drug could be dissolved in the N → I solvent if the dissolution process were allowed to reach equilibrium. However, the dissolution rate will be controlled by the solubility in the diffusion layer; accordingly, faster dissolution of the salt in the buffered diffusion layer (process I → N) would be expected. In comparing N → I and N → N, or I → N and I → I, the pH of the diffusion layer is identical in each set, and the differences in dissolution rate must be explained either by the size of the diffusion layer or by the concentration gradient of drug between the diffusion and the bulk solution. It is probably safe to assume that a diffusion layer at a different pH than that of the bulk solution is thinner than a diffusion layer at the same pH because of the acid-base interaction at the interface. In addition, when the bulk solution is at a different pH than that of the diffusion layer, the bulk solution will act as a sink and C_g can be eliminated from Eqs. (1), (3), and (4). Both a decrease in the h and C_g terms in Eqs. (1), (3), and (4) favor faster dissolution in processes N → I and I → N as opposed to N → N and I → I, respectively.

Although the explanation for (N → I)>(N → N) and (I → N)>(I → I) is self-consistent for a nonionized drug and its salt form and reflects the experimentally observed values in Table 2, Nelson [31] studied a series of weak organic acids and found (I → I)>(I → N) for the sodium salt of four of these compounds. For example, the dissolution rate of sodium benzoate in pH 6.83 buffer was 1770 mg/100 min cm^2 versus 980 mg/100 mm cm^2 in a pH 1.5 solution. Corresponding values of I → I and I → N were 820 versus 200 for sodium phenobarbital, 2500 versus 1870 for sodium salicylate, and 810 versus 550 for sodium sulfathiazole. The acid forms of these drugs all showed the expected (N → I)>(N → N) relationship, and we cannot yet explain the salt data [33]. As stated earlier, the preceding explanation of the data in Table 2 is presented with reference to a specific theory of dissolution. Although this theory may not be acceptable to some, it does provide a basis for understanding the general principles that dictate the (I → N) ≈ (I → I) >(N → I)>(N → N) relationship observed in dissolution rate measurements for a nonionized drug and its salt form.

The pH of a solution affects not only the active ingredients of a dosage form, but also the inert ingredients. Returning to Table 1, the pH dependence of two different commercial capsules of sodium phenytoin were studied [20]. For one capsule, dissolution rate was independent of the initial pH of the dissolution media. For the second capsule, dissolution rate was very much dependent, as has been discussed, on the initial pH. Similar studies have been made using three commercial dosage forms of nitrofurantoin (Table 3). Nitrofurantoin is a weak acid with $pK_a = 7.2$. Equation (3) predicts that as the pH of the dissolution medium increases, the dissolution half-life of nitrofurantoin should decrease. For the suspension of microcrystalline nitrofurantoin and for the capsule, containing 100 mg of nitrofurantoin in the macrocrystalline form, the experimental results follow this prediction. For the tablet, containing 100 mg of nitrofurantoin in the microcrystalline form, the dissolution half-life increases with increasing pH. However, the tablet did not disintegrate at pH 7.20. Thus, for the tablet, it would appear that the physicochemical properties of the dosage form, rather than physicochemical properties of the drug, determined the rate of release of the drug from its dosage form. Interestingly, both the capsule and tablet, which must both disintegrate, are less rapidly available than the suspension. (See the dissolution scheme shown in Fig. 9.)

It has been mentioned that the pH of the bulk fluids may not reflect the pH of the stationary diffusion layer. As the active or inert ingredients of a dosage form dissolve, they may alter the pH of the microenvironment of the stagnant diffusion layer, without significantly changing the pH of the bulk fluids. Moreover, it is possible to intentionally add buffering agents to a capsule of tablet dosage forms. The small amount of buffer may not alter the pH of the bulk fluids of the GIT but can buffer the pH in the diffusion layer to a pH favoring rapid dissolution of the active ingredient. Such an effect was hypothesized when dissolution rates were compared for buffered versus plain (no alkaline additives) tablets of aspirin [33]. Later, more extensive studies on the effects of a variety of buffers on the dissolution of aspirin tablets were carried out [34]. Hydrophilic buffers and buffers that released carbon dioxide increased the dissolution rate; however, hydrophobic buffers decreased the dissolution rate, possibly by effectively waterproofing the tablets.

Table 3 Effect of pH on the Dissolution Half-Life of Nitrofurantoin from Commercial Dosage Forms at 37°C

	Mean dissolution half-life[a] (min)	
Commercial dosage form	pH 1.12	pH 7.20
Aqueous suspension[b]	12.5 (1.2)	2.64 (0.34)
Compressed tablet[c]	77.9 (19.0)	167.0 (35)
Gelatin capsule[d]	212.0 (44)	160.0 (24)

[a]Determined from log-normal probability plots of individual rate data. Mean of five determinations (SD).
[b]Furadantin suspension containing microcrystalline (< 10 μm) drug.
[c]Furadantin tablets containing microcrystalline (< 10 μm) drug.
[d]Macrodantin capsules containing microcrystalline (74–177 μm) drug.
Source: Ref. 32.

In summary, the effect of pH on the dissolution rate of a drug from an oral dosage form depends on (a) the pH of the GI fluids, a patient variable; (b) the acid or base strength of the drug, a pharmaceutical variable; as well as (c) the physicochemical properties of the dosage form, another pharmaceutical variable. Furthermore, by intentionally designing the dosage form such that it buffers the diffusion layer, we can control a patient variable by a pharmaceutical variable.

Pharmacists are probably the only health professionals who, by training, understand pH effects on drug solubility and transport. They must be aware of why different drugs are prepared as different salt forms and how changes in the acid-base environment of the GIT will influence availability. Usually, drugs in a salt form will be more quickly available and, often, available to a greater extent. However, there are instances when the drug may not be formulated in the salt form, even when a proper, stable formulation of the salt may be produced. Such an example was shown in Table 2. Sodium tolbutamide dissolves faster than tolbutamide when both in vitro dissolution data and in vivo urinary excretion measurements are compared. As would be expected, the pharmacological effect (i.e., lowering of the blood sugar level) is also more pronounced after 1 hour for the salt form. However, the product is actually formulated containing the acidic nonionized tolbutamide, because the manufacturer does not want to induce such a rapid decrease in blood sugar, which might lead to diabetic coma.

Solvate Formation

Another variable that influences the saturation solubility of a drug molecule is its degree of solvation. Since the anhydrous, hydrated, and alcoholated forms of a drug have slightly different solubilities, they may well have different dissolution rates and, therefore, different rates of absorption. However, these differences may not be clinically significant [35].

Polymorphism

Yet another property of a drug that may affect its saturation solubility and, hence, its dissolution rate is its crystalline state. Many drugs exhibit polymorphism [36]; that is, they are available in an amorphous or several different crystalline states. Chloramphenicol palmitate is available in at least two different forms, A and B. The B form is the more soluble. Figure 21 shows the mean serum level of chloramphenicol versus time curves obtained after oral administration to male volunteers of chloramphenicol palmitate suspensions containing the equivalent of 1.5 g of chloramphenicol [37]. The fraction of the B form of chloramphenicol palmitate ranges from 0% in suspension M to 100% in suspension L. Since the suspensions were identical except for the crystalline form, it would appear that the increase in rate and extent of availability with an increasing percentage of the B form is due to the increasing rate of dissolution. A warning, however, is necessary. In general, the more soluble polymorph is the least stable thermodynamically. Thus, older dosage forms may contain more of the more stable, but less soluble, polymorph. Aging may significantly affect the bioavailability of drugs exhibiting polymorphism. Pharmacists must, for this and many other reasons, be aware of the storage requirements of all drugs dispensed. They must also counsel their patients on the proper storage of their medicines and the importance of discarding out-of-date drugs.

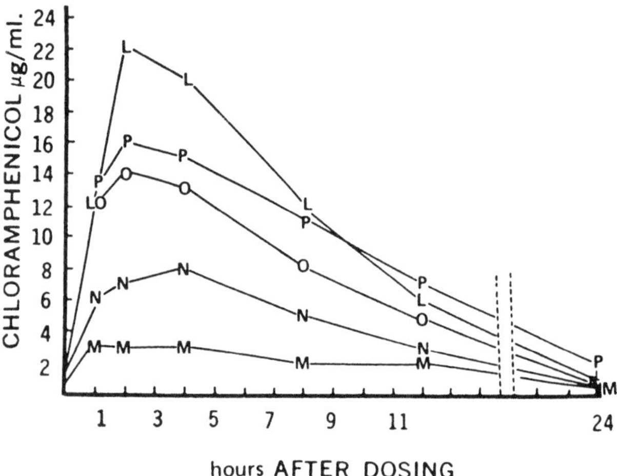

Fig. 21 Comparison of mean blood serum levels obtained with chloramphenicol palmitate suspensions containing varying ratios of A and B polymorphs, following a single oral dose equivalent to 1.5 g of chloramphenicol. Percentage of polymorph B in the suspension: M, 0%; N, 25%; O, 50%; P, 75%;L, 100%. (From Ref. 37.).

Complexation

Several studies have examined the effects of complex formation on the rate and extent of drug availability. A drug may complex with both absorbable and nonabsorbable excipients in a dosage form. This complexation may occur within the dosage form or in the solubilizing fluids, and the resulting complex may be more or less soluble than the drug itself. The rate and extent of availability of promazine from a suspension of the drug adsorbed on either activated charcoal or the clay attapulgite were compared with the availability of the drug from an aqueous solution [38]. Healthy adults took, on an empty stomach, 45 mL of either the solution or one of the suspensions with 4 oz (0.12 L) of water. The rate of availability of promazine from the attapulgite suspension was less than from the solution, but the extent of absorption was the same. When compared with the solution, the promazine-activated charcoal suspension showed both a decreased rate and a decreased extent of availability. However, the association constant for the promazine-attapulgite complex was greater than for the promazine-activated charcoal complex. Thus, it appears that it is not the magnitude of the association constant of the complex, but the rate at which the complex dissociates, that determines whether absorption of the drug is as rapid or as complete as in the absence of complex formation.

In addition to possible complexation with other ingredients in the dosage form, a drug may complex with the natural components of the GIT. The mucin, enzymes, bile, and physiological surfactants found in the mucosal fluids may interact with a given drug. The influence of these interactions on the availability of the drug will depend on the physicochemical properties of the drug and those of the endogenous compound, as discussed in Chapter 2. It seems probable that both increased and decreased drug solubilities will be encountered. Thus, for drugs for which the rate of availability is dissolution rate-limited, such interactions may be beneficial or detrimental. Once again, patient variables may control the availability of the drug from its dosage form.

Solid-Solid Interactions

Preparing a solid solution of a drug is one additional way of controlling its dissolution rate. For this chapter, the term *solid solution* will be used to describe any solid system in which one component is dispersed at the molecular level within another [39]. In deriving Eq. (1) it was assumed that C_s is independent of particle size. However, for extremely small particles, such as those found in solid solutions, the saturation solubility (C_s) of the drug may increase as particle size decreases. This increase in solubility can be described by the Kelvin equation [40]:

$$C_s^{\text{micro}} = C_s \exp\left(\frac{2\gamma M}{r\rho RT}\right) \tag{5}$$

where

C_s^{micro} = saturation solubility of the microscopic particle
C_s = saturation solubility of drug (macroparticles)
γ = interfacial tension between drug particles and the solubilizing fluids
M = Molecular weight of the drug
r = radius of the microscopic drug particle
R = ideal gas constant
ρ = density of the microscopic drug particle
T = absolute temperature

Figure 22 depicts the dissolution rates of griseofulvin, an insoluble antifungal agent, and griseofulvin–succinic acid samples as described by Goldberg et al. [41]. Several conclusions can be drawn from these experiments. The first is that physically reducing the particle size of the griseofulvin by micronization increased the rate of dissolution in accordance with Eq. (1) but did not increase the concentration of drug above its equilibrium solubility. Second, physical mixtures of griseofulvin and succinic acid, at ratios corresponding to those in the solid solution and eutectic mixture, had dissolution rates similar to griseofulvin alone. Therefore, succinic acid does not itself increase the solubility of griseofulvin (by a complexation mechanism, for example). Finally, the solid solution and the eutectic mixture were very rapidly soluble. Both gave supersaturated solutions, as predicted by Eq. (5), because of the extremely small—approaching molecular—size of the griseofulvin particles in these states. Solid solutions and eutectic mixtures have been used, at least in research laboratories, to increase the rate of dissolution of drugs, presumably by decreasing the particle size of the drug molecules [42]. However, since the drug is in an unstable thermodynamic state, it is critical that the stability of the formulation be maintained. Otherwise, the preparation may revert to a state of having even less favorable dissolution properties than those of a micronized formulation, as shown by the dissolution characteristics of the physical mixtures in Fig. 22. Pharmacists should be aware of the potential problems of such formulations and may, once again, take an active role in advising patients of proper storage conditions.

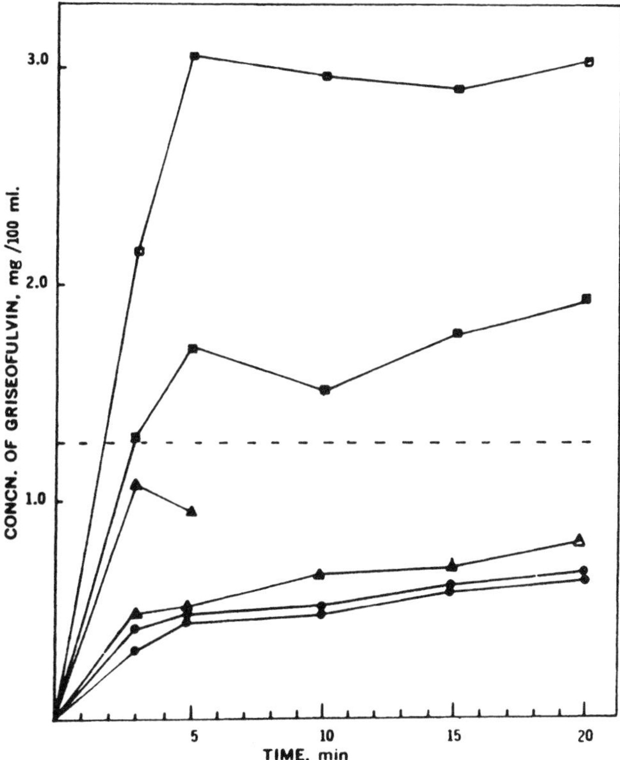

Fig. 22 Dissolution fates of various griseofulvin and griseofulvin-succinic acid samples as determined by the oscillating bottle method. ●, griseofulvin, crystalline; ▲, griseofulvin, micronized; ■, eutectic mixture; ○, physical mixture at eutectic composition; □, solid solution; △, physical mixture at solid solution composition. The dashed line indicates the equilibrium solubility of griseofulvin in water. (From Ref. 41.).

C. Concentration of the Dissolved Drug in Bulk Solution, C_g

In Eq. (1), the saturation solubility of the drug in the diffusion layer does not of itself determine dissolution rate. The determinant is, rather, the difference between C_s and C_g, the concentration of dissolved drug in the bulk fluids of the GIT. Thus, the driving force for dissolution is the concentration gradient, $C_s - C_g$. It is usually assumed that C_g is much smaller than C_s, meaning that dissolution occurs under sink conditions. If a drug is absorbed through the GI membrane very slowly, drug concentration in the GIT fluids may build up. This buildup would, by decreasing the gradient, decrease the dissolution rate. Additionally, the bulk fluids may not be identical with the solubilizing fluids of the diffusion layer. A drug may be more soluble in the boundary layer and then precipitate in the bulk fluids, especially if the pH differs between these two sites. However, these precipitated particles should be quite small, and thus may rapidly redissolve (see the dissolution scheme presented in Fig. 9). On the other hand, the drug may be more soluble in the bulk fluids than in the boundary layer because of a difference in pH or by complexation with other components. Here, the gradient may decrease and dissolution may slow down or even stop. However, the volume of the bulk fluids is much larger than the volume of the boundary layer. Thus, a large absolute amount of drug in the bulk fluids may still give a small value of C_g.

Figure 3 illustrates a situation in which this may not be true. When 250 mL of water was taken with erythromycin tablets, the extent of absorption was much greater than when the tablets were taken with only 20 mL of water. In the latter case, dissolution probably did not occur under sink conditions. Hence, the dissolution rate decreased, and it appears that not all of the erythromycin had a chance to dissolve in the GIT. Note than the dissolution was not, however, the rate-determining step in absorption, since the time to reach the peak concentration was the same in all situations.

Usually, an increase in C_g that would affect the dissolution rate would occur only when another process, such as membrane transport or stomach emptying, becomes the rate-limiting step in drug absorption. As a general rule pharmacists should advise patients to take their oral medications with a full glass of water to ensure that dissolution occurs under optimal conditions.

D. Diffusion Coefficient Divided by the Thickness of the Stationary Diffusion Layer, D/h

Although it is possible to control the dissolution rate of a drug by controlling its particle size and solubility, the pharmaceutical manufacturer has very little, if any, control over the D/h term in the Nernst-Brunner equation, Eq. (1). In deriving the equation it was assumed that h, the thickness of the stationary diffusion layer, was independent of particle size. In fact, this is not necessarily true. The diffusion layer probably increases as particle size increases. Furthermore, h decreases as the "stirring rate" increases. In vivo, as GI motility increases or decreases, h would be expected to decrease or increase. In deriving the Nernst-Brunner equation, it was also assumed that all the particles were spherical and of the same size. In fact, particles in pharmaceutical systems are neither spherical nor uniform. Furthermore, pharmaceutical systems are usually mixtures of different compounds, the particle sizes of which are not identical. Thus pharmaceutical systems are polydisperse and multiparticulate [43]. Their size distribution in terms of number of particles tends to be skewed toward the smaller particles. Furthermore, as dissolution proceeds, the particles become smaller. Hence h can vary considerably initially and throughout the dissolution process.

The other virtually uncontrollable term in Eq. (1) is D, the diffusion coefficient of the drug. For a spherical, ideal drug molecule in solution,

$$D = \frac{kt}{6\pi\eta r}$$

where

k = Boltzmann's constant
T = absolute temperature
r = radius of molecule in solution
η = viscosity of the solution

Both k and 6π are constants. The radius r is a property of the drug molecule not subject to manipulation. The viscosity η of the GI fluids can vary. Increasing the viscosity will decrease dissolution. In addition, increasing the viscosity of the stomach contents will slow gastric emptying, thereby delaying delivery of the drug to the absorption site. Increasing the temperature of the GI fluids tends to increase diffusion. Patients might be advised to take oral dosage forms with warm liquids. However, extremely hot liquids will delay stomach emptying. In summary, D and h are largely uncontrollable factors, although they may influence drug availability.

IV. GASTROINTESTINAL MEMBRANE TRANSPORT

Once a drug is in solution at the absorption site, it must move through the GIT membrane and then into the general circulation. In Chapter 2 Fick's law was used to describe this transport:

$$\left(\frac{dQ_b}{dt}\right)_{g\to b} = D_m A_m R_{m/\text{aq}} \left[\frac{(C_g - C_b)}{X_m}\right] \tag{6}$$

Paradoxically, the larger the value of C_g, the more quickly the drug will more through the membrane. This C_g is the same concentration of drug in the bulk fluids that was minimized in Eq. (1) to increase the rate of dissolution. A second paradox is the relation between $R_{m/aq}$ and C_g. The bulk fluids of the GIT are aqueous. Thus, C_g will increase as the water solubility of the drug increases; $R_{m/aq}$ will, however, decrease. Thus, to be absorbed, a drug cannot be so lipid-soluble that it will not dissolve in the aqueous fluids of the GIT, nor so water-soluble that it will not penetrate the lipid GI membrane. Recently, Lipinski and colleagues presented the empirically derived Rule of 5 (Table 4) [44]. These guidelines allow drug developers to select as drug candidates molecules with acceptable hydrophilicity and acceptable lipophilicity, that is, molecules likely to have good oral availability. Although diffusion across the GI membrane is one of the major rate-limiting steps in oral absorption, it has been extensively covered in Chapter 2 and will not receive further treatment here.

The GI wall is not, however, an inert barrier. Some drugs may be actively transported into the enterocytes, as discussed in Chapter 2. Additionally, it is now known that there are efflux transporters in these cells. The most studied is P-glycoprotein (Pgp), which is a relatively nonselective carrier for a wide variety of drugs [45]. In addition, the enterocytes also contain drug-metabolizing enzymes, particularly cytochrome P4503A4 (CYP3A4), which metabolizes a significant number of marketed drugs [46]. To further complicate the picture, some drugs are substrates of both Pgp and CYP 3A4 [45]. Thus, drug molecules that are absorbed from the lumen of the GI tract may be pumped back out and/or metabolized before they reach the blood. This will limit the overall availability of these drugs. As if this were not enough of a challenge, both Pgp and/or CYP3A4 can be both upregulated and/or downregulated by other drugs, herbal products, and food [45–48]. Pharmacists can be invaluable resources for other clinicians and patients in integrating the multitude of potential interactions and advising them about how to maximize drug effectiveness.

Table 4 The Rule of 5: Drugs That Have More Than 2 Strikes Are Likely to Be Poorly Absorbed

1. There are more than 5 H-bond donors (expressed as sum of OHs and NHs)
2. There are more than 10 H-bond acceptors (expressed as the sum of Ns and Os)
3. Molecular weight is > 500
4. log P is > 5
5. Compounds that are substrates for biological transporters are exceptions to the rule

Source: Ref. 44.

V. MOVING THE DRUG AWAY FROM THE SITE OF ABSORPTION

The fourth basic process that may influence drug absorption is moving the drug away from the site of absorption. Drugs that have crossed the GI membrane are primarily removed as a function of blood flow [50]. It can be seen in Eq. (6) that if there were no blood flow, the concentration of drug in the blood, C_b, would quickly approach C_g, and net transfer of drug across the GIT would cease. Thus, a decreased blood flow might decrease the rate or removal of passively absorbed drugs [51,52]. Decreased flow could possibly also interfere with active transport systems owing to the reduction of the supply of oxygen to the tissues. Winne and Ochsenfahrt [52] and Winne [53] have developed models and derived equations for GI absorption considering blood flow and countercurrent exchanges, respectively. For the following theoretical discussion, a simplified equation is presented as a modification of Eq. (6) [50]:

$$\left(\frac{dQ_b}{dt}\right)_{g\to b} = \frac{C_g - C_b}{1/P_m A_m + 1/\alpha\ \mathrm{BF}} \tag{7}$$

where

$P_m = D_m R_{m/aq}/X_m$
α = fraction of blood flowing through the capillaries near the GI membrane
BF = GI blood flow

The other terms are defined in Chapter 2. The denominator of Eq. (7) can be interpreted as the resistance of the region between the GI lumen and the blood pool. Winne and Remischovsky [54] divided this resistance into two parts (first and second terms of the denominator): (a) the resistance to transport of the region between the gastrointestinal lumen and the capillary blood (mainly resistance of the membrane), and (b) the resistance to drainage by blood. Figure 23 indicates the influence of blood flow on the rate of intestinal absorption for eight substances from the jejunum of the rat. The absorption of highly permeable materials [those with a small first term in the denominator of Eq. (7)], such as very lipid-soluble or pore-diffusable substances, should be blood flow–limited. Conversely, the absorption rate of drugs characterized by low membrane permeability [those with a large first term in the denominator of Eq. (7)] may be independent of blood flow. From Fig. 23 it may be seen that the absorption of freely permeable tritiated water is very sensitive to blood flow, but that ribitol, a sugar that penetrates the GI

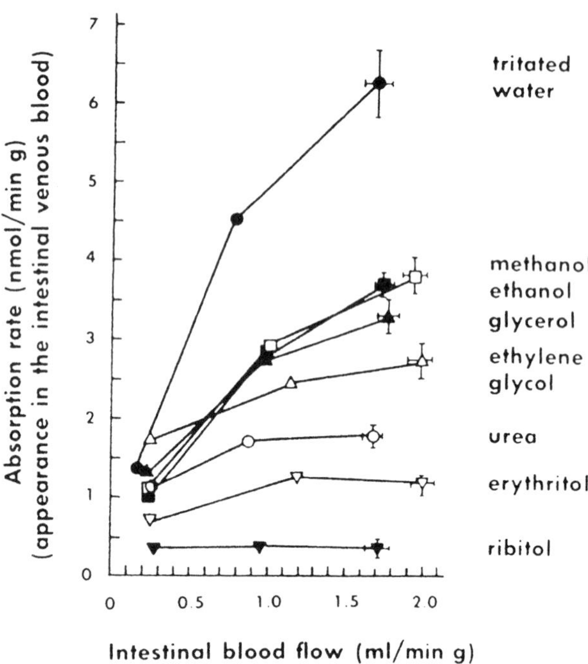

Fig. 23 Dependence of intestinal absorption on blood flow as reported by Winne and Remischovsky. All data are corrected to a concentration of 50 nmol/mL in the solution perfusing jejunal loops of rat intestine. Bracketed points indicate the 50% confidence intervals. (From Ref. 54.).

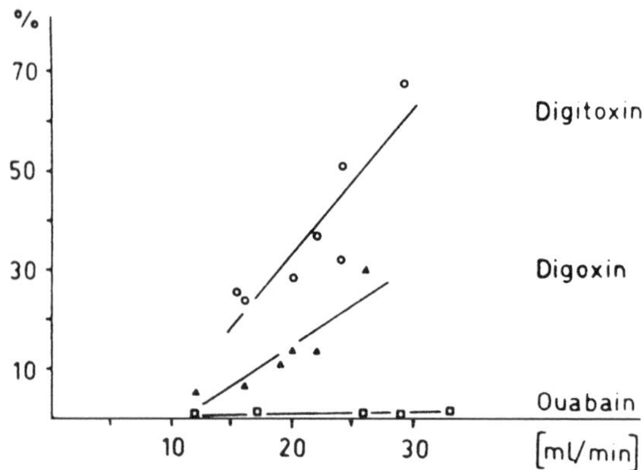

Fig. 24 Total amount of radioactivity absorbed during 1 hr, plotted versus portal blood flow. Ordinate: absorption as a percentage of the amount infused into the duodenum. Abscissa: mean portal blood flow in milliliters per minute. Each point represents one guinea pig. (From Ref. 56).

membrane with great difficulty, is essentially unaffected by changes in the intestinal blood flow in the range studied. As would be expected from Eq. (7), the absorption rate of intermediate substances, such as urea, appear to be flow-limited at low blood flow rates, but then become insensitive to blood flow at higher rates. Winne and coworkers [51–54] have reported a blood flow dependence for several relatively small drug molecules. Crouthamel et al. [55] also noted a decrease in the absorption rate of sulfaethidole and haloperidol as a function of decreased mesenteric blood flow rates, using an in situ canine intestinal preparation. Haas and coworkers [56], using a guinea pig model, found a strong correlation between spontaneously varying portal blood flow and the amount of digitoxin and digoxin absorbed following intraduodenal infusion of the drug. As can be seen in Fig. 24, digitoxin, the most lipophilic of the three cardiac glycosides, showed the most pronounced effects as a function of the blood flow. Digoxin also showed increasing absorption rates as a function of blood flow. However, ouabain, the most hydrophilic of the three, showed no dependence on blood flow. These results are consistent with the predictions of Eq. (7) for the effects of blood flow on the absorption rate of drugs.

These animal studies should indicate to the pharmacist that blood flow can, under certain circumstances, be an important patient variable that may affect the absorption of drugs. Patients in heart failure would generally be expected to have a decreased cardiac output and, therefore, a decreased splanchnic blood flow. This could lead to a decreased rate of absorption for drugs when the blood flow rates in Eq. (7) become rate-limiting. In addition, redistribution of cardiac output during cardiac failure may lead to splanchnic vasoconstriction in patients [57]. Other disease states and physical activity can also decrease blood flow to the GIT [2–4]. Thus, the pharmacist must be aware of the possible effect of blood flow rate, especially alterations in the rate, on the availability of drugs.

VI. PHYSICOCHEMICAL VERSUS BIOCHEMICAL FACTORS INFLUENCING DRUG ABSORPTION AND DRUG AVAILABILITY

As described in Chapter 2, the extent of oral drug availability (F_{oral}) may be described as the product of absorption availability (F_{abs}), the extent of availability through the gastrointestinal membranes (F_G), and the availability through the liver (F_H):

$$F_{oral} = F_{abs} F_G F_H \quad (8)$$

First-pass loss in the gut will be due to metabolic processes within the intestinal membrane (due primarily to CYP3A and phase 2 enzymes present in the intestine such as glucuronosyltransferases, sulfotransferases, and glutathione S-transferases). First-pass hepatic loss will be due to liver metabolism as well as biliary excretion. Although transporters present in the intestinal epithelium can effect F_G, their consequences are probably reflected as a result of changes in intestinal metabolism. Absorption transporters should decrease intestinal metabolism by speeding the drug through the intestinal membrane and allowing less access of drug to intestinal enzymes, while efflux transporters would increase intestinal metabolism since the drug molecule may be repeatedly absorbed by passive processes increasing access to intestinal enzymes [49].

The physicochemical processes described in detail in this chapter (disintegration, dissolution, saturation solubility, and diffusion) will primarily affect the F_{abs} term in Eq. (8). However, the physicochemical processes, together with gastric emptying and gastrointestinal motility, can also affect the rate of absorption, as described earlier in this chapter. For a drug susceptible to GI metabolism, F_G could be expected to increase if absorption rate could increase to the point that intestinal metabolsm could be saturated, leading to further increases in F_G. In a similar manner a fast absorption rate could also possibly lead to saturation of hepatic enzymes during first pass resulting in an increase in F_H.

VII. SUMMARY

Drug availability following oral dosing may be thought of as the result of four basic steps: (a) getting the drug to its absorption site, (b) getting the drug into solution, (c) moving the dissolved drug through the membranes of the GIT, and (d) moving the drug away from the site of absorption into the general circulation. Although steps a, c, and d were discussed briefly, these topics are also found in Chapter 2 and 5. Step b, the combination of factors influencing the dissolution rate of a drug from its dosage form, served as the major topic of this chapter. Dissolution rate was discussed in terms of the parameters found in the Nernst-Brunner equation. Although this equation [Eq. (1)] is derived in terms of a specific model for dissolution, which, in fact, may not accurately describe the physical process, we believe that the treatment gives pharmacists a point of reference from which they can predict and interpret availability date that are rate-limited by the dissolution step. Two terms in the Nernst-Brunner equation are of major importance and are susceptible to manipulation by the pharmaceutical manufacturer in preparing the dosage form, by the patient in the manner in which he or she takes the drug and stores it between drug dosing, and by the biological system, specifically the GIT of the patient, through interactions with the dosage form and the drug. These two variables are the surface area of the drug particles and the saturation solubility of the particular chemical form of the drug. We believe that pharmacists must be aware of these variables and how they can change in each of the three situations listed previously before they can make rational judgments about which of many pharmaceutical alternatives should be dispensed under a specific set of conditions. Knowledge of these variables and their potential for change also allows pharmacists to make a rational guess about possible drug-related factors that may be responsible for inefficacious drug treatment. Under these conditions, pharmacists may be able to recommend an alternative formulation that will prove to be efficacious.

REFERENCES

1. D. E. Cadwallader, *Biopharmaceutics and Drug Interactions*, 3rd Ed., Raven Press, New York, 1983.
2. W. H. Bachrach, Physiology and pathologic physiology of the stomach, Ciba Clin. Symp., 11, 1–28 (1959).
3. H. W. Davenport, Gastric digestion and emptying: Absorption, in *Physiology of the Digestive Tract*, 3rd Ed., Year Book Medical Publishers, Chicago, 1971, pp. 163–171.
4. L. Z. Benet and B. Hoener, Pathological limitations in the application of rate control systems, in *Proceeding of the 2nd International Conference of Drug Absorption Rate Control in Drug Therapy*, (L. Prescott, ed.), Edinburgh, 1983, pp. 155–165.
5. G. D. Kozloski, J. M. De Vito, J. C. Kisicki, and J. B. Johnson, The effect of food on the absorption of methotrexate sodium tablets in healthy volunteers, Arthritis Rheum., 35, 761–764 (1992).
6. P. G. Welling, H. Huang, P. F. Hewitt, and L. L. Lyons, Bioavailability of erythromycin stearate: Influence of food and fluid volume, J. Pharm. Sci., 67, 764–766 (1978).
7. T. R. Bates, J. A. Sequeria, and A. V. Tembo, Effect of food on nitrofurantoin absorption, Clin. Pharmacol. Ther., 16, 63–68 (1974).
8. J. W. Fara, Physiological limitations: Gastric emptying and transit of dosage forms, in *Proceedings of the 2nd International Conference on Drug Absorption, Rate Control in Drug Therapy* (L. Prescott, ed.), Edinburgh, 1983, pp. 144–150.

9. C. P. Dooley, C. Di Lorenzo, and J. E. Valenzuela, Variability of migrating motor complex in humans, Dig. Dis. Sci., 37, 723–728 (1992).
10. V. Manninen, J. Melin, A. Apajalahti, and M. Karesoja, Altered absorption of digoxin in patients given propantheline and metoclopramide, Lancet, 1, 398–400 (1973).
11. C. G. Regardh, P. Lundborg, and B. A. Persson, The effect of antacid, metoclopramide and propantheline on the bioavailability of metoprolol and atenolol. Biopharm. Drug Dispos., 2, 79–87 (1981).
12. J. A. Antonioli, J. L. Schelling, E. Steininger, and G. A. Borel, Effect of gastrectomy and of an anticholinergic drug on the gastrointestinal absorption of a sulfonamide in man, Int. J. Clin. Pharmacol., 5, 212–215 (1971).
13. W. H. Barr and S. Riegelman, Intestinal drug absorption and metabolism. I. Comparison of methods and models to study physiological factors in vitro and in vivo intestinal absorption, J. Pharm. Sci., 59, 154–163 (1970).
14. R. R. Scheline, Metabolism of foreign compounds by gastrointestinal microorganisms, Pharmacol, Rev., 25, 451–523 (1973).
15. L. Z. Benet, Biopharmaceutics as a basis for the design of drug products, in *Drug Design*, Vol. 4 (E. J. Ariens, ed.), Academic Press, New York, 1973, pp. 1–35.
16. W. Nernst and E. Brunner, Z. Phys. Chem., 47, 52–102 (1904).
17. P. Finholt, Influence of formulation on dissolution rate, in *Dissolution Technology* (L. J. Leeson and J. T. Carstensen, eds.), Academy of Pharmaceutical Sciences, American Pharmaceutical Association, Washington, DC, 1974, pp. 106–146.
18. L. F. Prescott, R. F. Steel, and W. R. Ferrier, The effects of particle size on the absorption of phenacetin in man, Pharmacol. Ther., 11, 496–504 (1970).
19. A. J. Glazko, A. W. Kinkel, W. C. Alegnani, and E. L. Holmes, An evaluation of the absorption characteristics of different chloramphenicol preparations in normal human subject, Clin. Pharmacol. Ther., 9, 472–483 (1968).
20. K. Arnold, N. Gerber, and G. Levy, Absorption and dissolution studies on sodium diphenlyhydantoin capsules, Can. J. Pharm. Sci., 5, 89–92 (1970).
21. G. Levy and R. H. Gumtow, Effect of certain tablet formulation factors on dissolution rate of the active ingradient. III. Tablet lubricants, J. Pharm. Sci., 52,1139–1141 (1963).
22. G. Levy, J. M. Antkowiak, J. A. Procknal, and D. C. White, Effect of certain tablet formulation factors on dissolution rate of the active ingredients. II. Granule size, starch concentration, and compression pressure, J. Pharm. Sci., 52, 1047–1051 (1963).
23. J. C. Samyn and W. Y. Jung, In vitro dissolution from several experimental capsule formulations, J. Pharm. Sci., 59, 169–175 (1970).
24. S. H. Wan, P. J. Pentikainen, and D. L. Azarnoff, Bioavailability of aminosalicylic acid and its various salts in humans. III. Absorption from tablets, J. Pharm. Sci., 63, 708–711 (1974).
25. E. Nelson, Influence of dissolution rate and surface on tetracycline absorption, J. Am. Pharm. Assoc. Sci. Ed., 48, 96–103 (1959).
26. E. Nelson, E. L. Knoechel, W. E. Hamlin, and J. G. Wagner, Influence of the absorption rate of tolbutamide on the rate of decline of blood sugar levels in normal humans, J. Pharm. Sci., 51, 509–514 (1962).
27. C. C. Lee, R. O. Froman, R. C. Anderson, and K. C. Chen, Gastric and intestinal absorption of potassium penicillin V and the free acid, Antibiot. Chemother., 8, 354–360 (1958).
28. G. Levy and B. A. Sanai, Comparison of the gastrointestinal absorption of aluminum acetylsalicylic and acetylsalicylic acid in man, J. Pharm. Sci., 51, 58–62 (1962).
29. R. A. O'Reilly, E. Nelson, and G. Levy, Physicochemical and physiologic factors affecting the absorption of warfarin in man, J. Pharm. Sci., 55, 435–437 (1966).
30. W. I. Higuchi and W. E. Hamlin, Release of drug from a self-coating surface: Benzphetamine pamoate pellet, J. Pharm. Sci., 52, 575–579 (1963).
31. E. Nelson, Comparative dissolution rates of weak acids and their sodium salts, J. Am. Pharm. Assoc. Sci. Ed., 47, 297–299 (1958).
32. T. R. Bates, J. M. Young, C. M. Wu, and H. A. Rosenberg, pH-dependent dissolution rate of nitrofurantoin from commercial suspensions, tablets and capsules, J. Pharm. Sci., 63, 643–645 (1974).
33. G. Levy, J. R. Leonards, and J. A. Procknal, Development of in vitro dissolution tests which correlate quantitatively with dissolution rate-limited drug absorption in man, J. Pharm. Sci., 54, 1719–1722 (1966).
34. K. A. Javaid and D. E. Cadwallader, Dissolution of aspirin from tablets containing various buffering agents, J. Pharm. Sci., 61, 1370–1373 (1972).
35. J. W. Poole, G. Owen, J. Silverio, J. N. Freyhot, and S. B. Roseman, Physicochemical factors influencing the absorption of the anhydrous and trihydrate forms of ampicillin, Curr. Ther. Res., 10, 292–303 (1968).
36. J. Hableblian and W. McCone, Pharmaceutical application of polymorphism, J. Pharm. Sci., 58, 911–929 (1969).
37. A. J. Aguiar, J. Krc. A. W. Kinkel, and J. C. Samyn, Effect of polymorphism on the absorption of chloramphenicol palmitate, J. Pharm. Sci., 56, 847–853 (1967).
38. D. L. Sorby, Effect of adsorbents on drug absorption. I. Modification of promazine absorption by activated attapulgite and activated charcoal, J. Pharm. Sci., 54, 677–683 (1965).
39. K. C. Kwan and D. J. Allen, Determination of the degree of crystallinity in solid-solid equilibria, J. Pharm. Sci., 58, 1190–1193 (1969).

40. E. N. Hiestand, W. I. Higuchi, and N. F. H. Ho, Theories of dispersion techniques, in *Theory and Practice of Industrial Pharmacy*, 2nd Ed. (L. Lachman, H. A. Lieberman, and J. L. Kanig, eds.), Lea & Febiger, Philadelphia, 1976, p. 159.
41. A. H. Goldberg, M. Gibaldi, and J. L. Kanig, Increasing dissolution rates and gastrointestinal absorption of drugs via solid solutions and eutectic mixtures. III. Experimental evaluation of griseo-fulvin-succinic acid solid solution, J. Pharm. Sci., 55, 487–492 (1966).
42. A. Goldberg, Methods of increasing dissolution rates, in *Dissolution Technology* (I. J. Leeson and J. T. Carstensen, eds.), Academy of Pharmaceutical Sciences, American Pharmaceutical Association, Washington, DC, 1974, pp. 147–162.
43. L. Z. Benet, Theories of dissolution: Multi-particulate systems, in *Dissolution Technology* (I. J. Leeson and J. T. Carstensen, eds.), Academy of Pharmaceutical Sciences, American Pharmaceutical Association, Washington, DC, 1974, pp. 29–57.
44. C. A. Lipinski, F. Lombardo, B. W. Dominy, and P. J. Feeney, Experimental and computational approaches to estimate solubility and permeability in drug discovery and development settings, Adv. Drug Del. Rev., 23, 3–25 (1997).
45. V. J. Wacher, L. Salphati, and L. Z. Benet, Active secretion and enterocytic drug metabolism barriers to drug absorption, Adv. Drug Del. Rev., 20, 99–122 (1996).
46. W. E. Evans and M. V. Relling, Pharmacogenomics: translating functional genomics into rational therapeutics, Science, 286, 487–491 (1999).
47. A. Johne, J. Brockmoller, S. Bauer, A. Maurer, M. Langheinrich, and I. Root, Pharmacokinetic interaction of digoxin with an herbal extract from St. John's wort (*Hypericum perforatum*). Clin. Pharmacol. Ther., 66, 338–345 (1999).
48. S. C. Piscitelli, A. H. Burstein, D. Chaitt, R. M. Alfaro, and J. Falloon, Indinavir concentrations and St. John's wort, Lancet, 355, 547–548 (2000).
49. V. J. Wacher, J. A. Silverman, Y. Zhang, and L. Z. Benet, Role of P-glycoprotein and cytochrome P450 3A in limiting oral absorption of peptides and peptidomimetics, J. Pharm. Sci., 11, 1322–1330 (1998).
50. L. Z. Benet, A. Greither, and W. Meister, Gastrointestinal absorption of drugs in patients with cardiac failure, in *The Effect of Disease States on Drug Pharmacokinetics* (L. Z. Benet, ed.), Academy of Pharmaceutical Association, Washington, D.C., 1976, pp. 33–50.
51. L. Ther and D. Winne, Drug absorption, Annu. Rev. Pharmacol., 11, 57–70 (1971).
52. D. Winne and H. Ochsenfahrt, Die formale Kinetic der Resorption unter Berücksichtigung der Darmdurchblutung, J. Theor. Biol., 14, 293–315 (1967).
53. D. Winne, The influence of villous countercurrent exchange on intestinal absorption, J. Theor. Biol., 53, 145–176 (1976).
54. D. Winne and J. Remischovsky, Intestinal blood flow and absorption of nondissociable substances, J. Pharm. Pharmacol., 22, 640–641 (1970).
55. W. G. Crouthamel, L. Diamond, L. W. Dittert, and J. T. Doluisio, Drug absorption. VII. Influence of mesenteric blood flow on intestinal drug absorption in dogs, J. Pharm, Sci., 64, 661–671 (1975).
56. A. Haas, H. Lullman, and T. Peters, Absorption rates of some cardiac glycosides and portal blood flow, Eur. J. Pharmacol., 19, 366–370 (1972).
57. J. Ferrer, S. E. Bradley, H. O. Wheeler, Y. Enson, R. Presig, and R. M. Harvey, The effect of digoxin on the splanchnic circulation in ventricular failure, Circulation, 32, 524–537 (1965).

Chapter 5

The Effect of Route of Administration and Distribution on Drug Action

Svein Øie and Leslie Z. Benet

University of California, San Francisco, California

I. THE DOSE-EFFICACY SCHEME

When a health practitioner administers (or "inputs") a dose of drug to a patient, usually the ultimate goal is solely directed to the usefulness of the drug under abnormal conditions. That is, the drug must be efficacious and must be delivered to its site of action in an individual experiencing a particular physiological anomaly or pathological state. Pharmaceutical scientists, on the other hand, concent\ate their attention to solving problems inherent in drug delivery to deliver the optimal dose to the site(s) of action.

The general pathway a drug takes from residence in a dosage form until its clinical utility is depicted in Fig. 1. Ideally, the drug should be placed directly at the site of action, as illustrated by the stippled arrow in Fig. 1, to maximize the effect and minimize side effects relating to unwanted responses at sites other than the target tissue. However, delivery directly to the site of action is, more often than not, impractical or not possible. Instead, we have to settle for the most convenient routes of delivery. This is illustrated by the solid arrows in Fig. 1. That is, the drug is placed directly in the vascular systems or in close proximity to some biological membrane through which the drug can traverse to reach body fluids or the vascular system. The delivery system is generally designed to release the drug in a manner that is conducive to this passage through the membrane. Previous chapters have discussed how drug-delivery systems may be optimized in terms of dissolution in the fluids surrounding the membrane to allow the desired rate of passage through the membrane. Subsequent chapters will deal with specific drug-delivery systems and their optimization. Once the drug has passed through the membrane and into the blood stream adjacent to the site of absorption, a general distribution of the drug will take place throughout the biological system. As pointed out in Chapter 3, the degree of dilution (referred to as the apparent volume of distribution) will dictate the initial concentration of drug in the general circulation, as sampled from a peripheral vein. Usually, the dose of the drug administered to the patient was chosen to give sufficiently high blood levels so that an adequate quantity of the drug would reach the site of action. The rate of input needed to achieve adequate levels of the drug at the site of action is not only influenced by the distribution and general elimination in the body, but may also be modified by the loss processes that are unique to a specific route of administration. This chapter will deal primarily with the distribution and loss processes that result uniquely from the physiological parameters inherent in the use of a particular route of administration.

Unfortunately, no drug is yet so specific that it interacts with only the target site in the target tissue and will not give rise to hyperclinical activity. Too much drug at the wrong place or too high a concentration at the right place may result in unwanted or toxic effects. Thus the practitioner must determine the usefulness of any dose of a drug from a particular drug-delivery

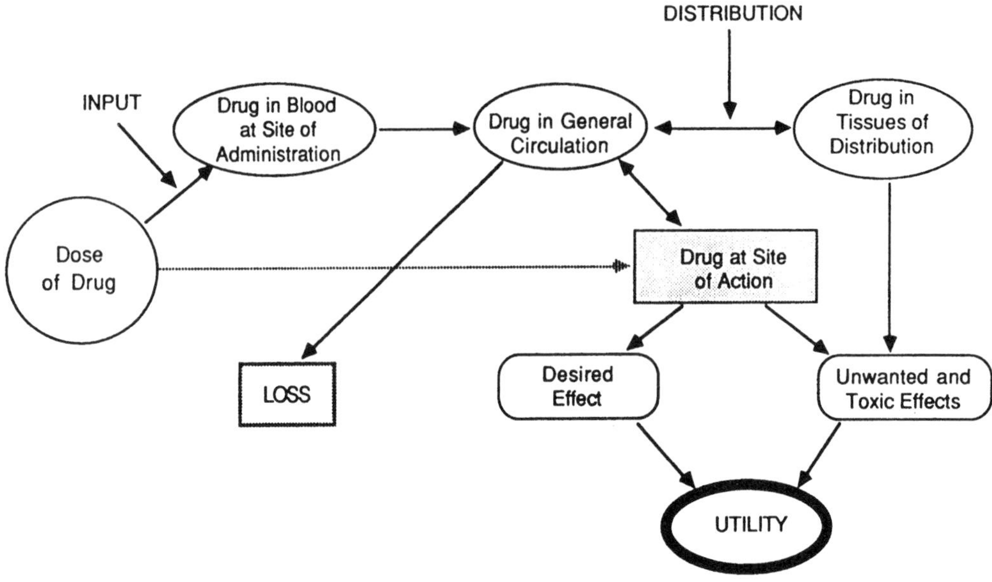

Fig. 1 A schematic representation of the dose-efficacy relationship for a drug.

system by balancing the efficacy achieved from the clinical effect against the toxic reactions observed.

Most drug-delivery systems achieve the required drug levels at the site of action as a result of attaining adequate blood levels in the general circulation (see Fig. 1, solid arrows). This process is followed because of the ease with which present drug-delivery systems can "input" drugs into the general circulation and the inherent difficulties in delivering the drug selectively to a relatively inaccessible site (e.g., pituitary gland). In addition, for many compounds the exact site of action is still unknown. However, when the site of drug action is sufficiently defined, Fig. 1 illustrates the advantage of delivering the drug directly to the site of action. By direct administration to the active site, a lower dose could be used to achieve the clinical effect because the drug no longer is diluted or eliminated en route. As a result, drug concentrations at unwanted sites of action could be kept to a minimum; in addition, clinically effective levels at the site of action might be attained much more rapidly, since the process of distribution throughout the entire body could be avoided. One should not forget that, in addition to the obvious clinical advantage of direct administration, there is also an economical one. By delivering the drug to the site of action, the amount of drug needed is much smaller than by more traditional delivery methods. This is particularly important for many of the newer recombinant compounds that can be very expensive. Much work is currently being carried out in an attempt to achieve selectiveness such as that described in Fig. 1.

II. PHYSIOLOGICAL CONSIDERATIONS FOR THE VARIOUS ROUTES AND PATHWAYS OF DRUG INPUT

A. Drug Input at or Close to the Site of Action

Figure 2 illustrates a number of sites where drug-delivery systems have historically been used to input drug directly to its site of action [1,2]. Various classic dosage forms were developed to take advantage of these input sites: eye, ear, and nose drops; inhalation, oral, topical, and vaginal aerosols; topical solutions, creams, and ointments; and rectal solutions, enemas, and suppositoires. Each of the sites for local drug administration requires specific formulation to allow the drug to remain at the site of application for a sufficient length of time to allow the drug to penetrate through the particular membrane(s) so that it can reach the actual site of action adjacent to the site of application. For example, some opthalmic preparations may be given to elicit a superficial anti-infective effect, such as treatment of an inflammation of the conjuctiva. Thus, only topical effects are desired, and there is no need for the drug to penetrate into the eyeball. Formulation of such products would be quite different than formulation of a drug-delivery system for which the drug must be absorbed into the in-

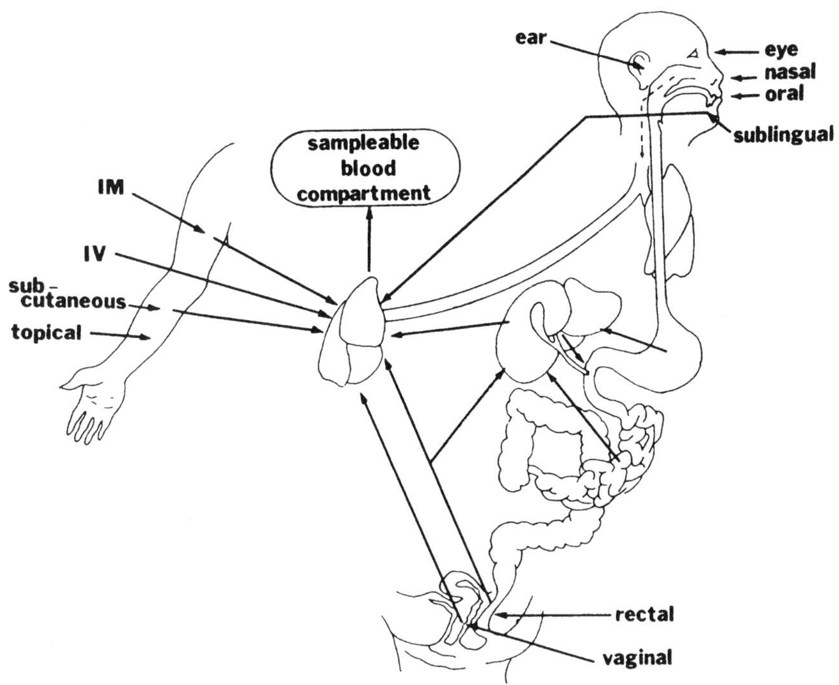

Fig. 2 Various routes and pathways by which a drug may be "input" into the body. The position of one lung is distorted to emphasize that the lungs are in an excellent position for cleansing the blood. The diagram is especially useful in explaining the first-pass effect following oral dosing, for which drug absorbed from the small intestine or stomach must first pass through the liver and, therefore, is subject to metabolism or biliary excretion before reaching the sampleable blood. (From Ref. 2.)

terior of the eye to produce a response, such as miotics, mydriatics, anti-inflammatory drugs that act in the anterior segment of the eye, and, occasionally, drugs for treatment of infections. A detailed description of the factors involved in the development of such opthalmic preparations, as well as the particular physiological characteristics of the eye, will be presented in Chapter 13. Similar types of design problems arise for many of the other sites that are traditionally treated by direct local application. One of the most difficult problems facing the formulator is that the behavior of the diseased tissue may be different from that for healthy individuals, and it may also change over the course of treatment. For example, diseased skin is often more permeable than healthy skin; therefore, the drug may disappear faster from the site of administration that desired, and the effect will be less than expected. Should the formulation be designed to accommodate this phenomenon, one must be mindful of the fact that as the pathological condition improves, the absorption may also change.

Although the classic dosage forms mentioned earlier can be used to put drug directly into the site of action, many of them have a degree of "messiness" that prevents good patient acceptance and adherence. Not only is there an initial psychological barrier that must be overcome, but the general public has an aversion to taking drugs by routes other than oral. There is, in addition, a general dislike for sticky creams, drippy drops, greasy ointments, and the like. Over the last two decades much work has been directed toward developing more acceptable delivery systems than the traditional ones. Emphasis has been placed on long-acting drug-delivery systems that may be more convenient, since they would only require self-administration once a week or possibly at even longer intervals.

A large number of new devices have been developed, and new ones are constantly being investigated. Plastic disks for placement in the eye (similar to a contact lens) that slowly release drug into the humoral fluid; drug-impregnated plastic rings or loops that when placed in the uterus will release controlled amounts of contraceptive agents; bioadhesive tablets or disks that can be placed buccally, nasally, or vaginally for local release; hydrogels for slow release in the eye are examples of such new delivery systems that input drug directly to the site of action.

In a more ambitious move, many groups have also embarked on site-specific delivery to less accessible sites than those given in Fig. 2. Although numerous experimental systems have been designed, few have reached the clinical stage. The simplest and most direct method when a specific target organ can be located is cannulation (direct access port). A catheter is placed in an appropriate artery or vein. If a vein is used, the catheter has to reach the organ, otherwise the drug will be flowing away from the target tissue, be diluted with blood from the rest of the body, and not be different than a systematic intravenous administration. Catheters can also be placed in the peritoneum, the bladder, and the cerebrospinal fluid. A drug can now be administered directly into the desired tissues at a rate that can be well controlled. Although catheter delivery is a direct method, it is limited in that it is essentially restricted to inpatient use. Use of implants in the desired tissue, or a drug carrier (e.g., liposomes, nano-particles, and such) that will either home in on the desired tissue by specific receptors or release their content at the desired site by an external stimulus (e.g., magnetic fields, light, current), are drug systems currently being explored for target-specific delivery.

Although the method of direct delivery is a very attractive one, it also has its regulatory problems. Benet [1] has noted that assessing the bioavailability of this system can create difficulties because the manufacturer may not be able to devise a control procedure that can measure drug concentration at the site of action. For example, the extent and rate of availability of an orally administered drug can easily be assessed by measuring blood levels, whereas for a drug input into a site of action, significant blood levels would indicate distribution away from that site. Frequently, significant blood levels of a drug that is administered at a site of action (such as a topical preparation, an eye drop, a nasal insufflation, or an antiobiotic that acts on intestinal flora) indicate either a poor drug-delivery system or substantial overdosing. For this class of drug-delivery system, clinical efficacy necessarily has to serve as the best measurement of drug availability and dosage form efficacy.

B. Drug Input into the Systemic Circulation

The overwhelming majority of existing drugs are, however, given by general routes; that is, by routes that do not deliver the drug directly to the site of action. These modes of drug input rely on a passive delivery of drug through distribution by the vascular system. The most commonly accepted method is oral administration. As will be discussed later, oral administration is not ideal, as one needs to be concerned about whether the drug can be destroyed in the stomach, in the gastrointestinal fluid, in its passage through the gut wall, through the liver, or simply not be absorbed in time before it is expelled from the gastrointestinal tract. Several alternative routes of delivery are being used or are being developed to diminish these potential losses. The advantages and problems inherent in the individual routes of administration will now be discussed.

Parenteral Administration: Intravascular

Of the routes of input depicted in Fig. 2, intravenous (IV) administration yields one of the fastest and most complete drug availabilities. However, intra-arterial injections might be employed when an even faster and more complete input of drug to a particular organ is desired. By administering the drug through an artery, the total drug delivered will enter the organ or tissue to which the artery flows. Intravenously administered drug will first be diluted in the venous system as the venous blood is pooled in the superior and inferior vena cava. It then enters the heart and is subsequently pumped to the lung before it can enter the arterial system and reach the target organ(s). In addition, the fraction of the drug reaching a desired site is dependent on the fraction of the arterial blood flow reaching that site. Additional drug can reach the target tissue only by being recirculated from the other organs. In comparison with intra-arterial administration, IV administration reaches the target slower, and initially at a lower concentration. Although intra-arterial injections appear superior, they are infrequently used because they are considered much more dangerous than IV administration. Intra-arterial administration has been associated with patient discomfort, bleeding, and thrombosis.

In addition to the dilution factor resulting from mixing with larger volumes of blood after intravenous administration, one also needs to consider the possibility of temporary or permanent loss of drug during its passage through the lung. The position of the lungs in Fig. 2 has been distorted to emphasize the point that the lungs are in an excellent strategic position for cleansing the blood, since all of the blood passes through the lungs several times a minute. Apart from their respiratory function and the removal of carbon dioxide from the pulmonary circulation, the lungs serve other important cleansing mechanisms, such as filtering emboli and circulating leukocytes, as well as excretion of volatile substances. The lungs also have metabolic capacity [3] and may serve as a metabolic site for certain drugs [4] or as an excretory route for compounds with a high vapor pressure. The lungs can also act as good temporary storage site for a number of drugs, especially basic compounds, by partitioning of the drug into lipid tissues, as well as serving a filtering function for particulate matter that may be given by IV injection. Accumulation of lipophilic compounds and filtering of any compounds in solid form can be viewed as a temporary clearing or dilution of the drug, as it will eventually leach back into the vascular system. Thus the lung serves as a dampening or clearing device, which is not present following intra-arterial injection. Drugs given by the IV route may, therefore, not necessarily be completely available to the site of action,

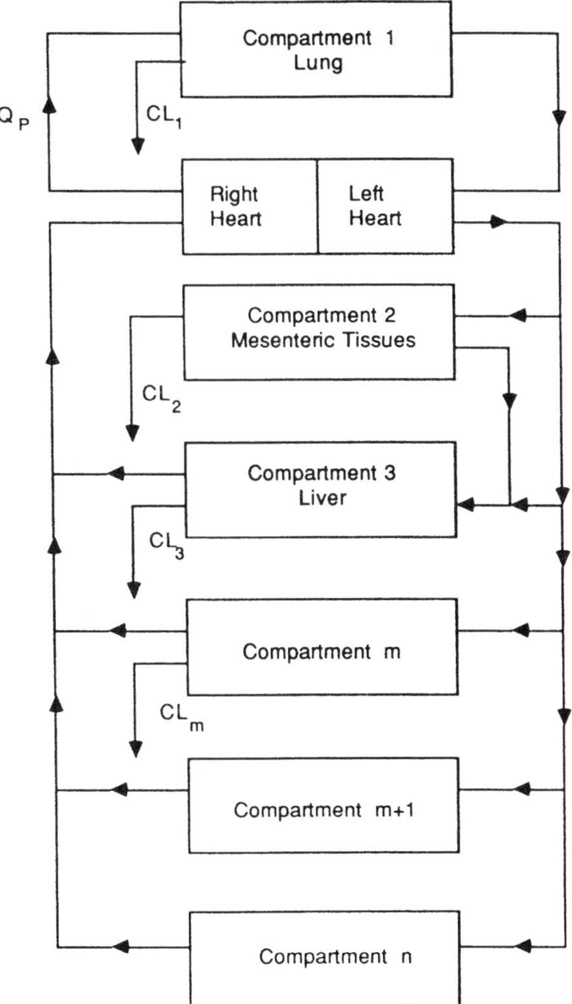

Fig. 3 The body depicted as a physiological perfusion model. Compartment m must be considered as a summation of the individual tissues that metabolize the drug and compartment m + 1 through n as noneliminating tissues.

since a certain fraction of the drug could be eliminated by the lung before entering into the general circulation [5]. This might be called a "lung first-pass effect."

The foregoing concepts may be visualized by referring to Fig. 3. In this figure one can readily see the difference between intra-arterial and intravenous administration of drugs. Let us assume that compartment n is the target tissue. Administration into any vein (i.e., into any of the efferent arrows on the left-hand side of the figure) would lead the drug to the heart and, from there, to the lung. Drug that enters the lung can leave by only one of two routes, as illustrated in Fig. 4: by the blood that leaves the lung, or by being eliminated. The result is that there is a competition between the two routes for the drug, and the greater the ability of the lung to eliminate the drug in comparison with the pulmonary blood flow, the more drug will be extracted. If we assume that the pulmonary blood flow in Q_P and that the intrinsic elimination clearance of the organ is CL_{Int}, and no plasma protein binding occurs ($Cu = C_{\text{out}}$), then the extraction ratio can be expressed as

$$E = \frac{C_{\text{out}} CL_{\text{Int}}}{(C_{\text{out}} CL_{\text{Int}}) + (C_{\text{out}}\, Q_P)} = \frac{CL_{\text{Int}}}{CL_{\text{Int}} + Q_P} \tag{1}$$

In perfusion models, as depicted in Fig. 3, it is assumed that distribution into and out of the organ is perfusion rate–limited such that drug in the organ is in equilibrium with drug concentration in the emergent blood [6]. The intrinsic clearance of an organ is different from the value we normally think of as the clearance of the organ. The *clearance of the organ* is defined as the rate of loss in relation to the incoming concentration, whereas the *intrinsic clearance* is defined as the rate of loss in relation to the organ concentration (or exiting concentration). In addition, it is also clear that, of the

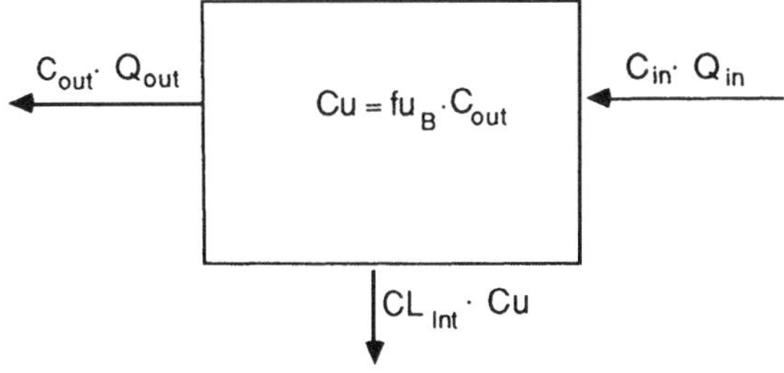

Fig. 4 Flow model of an eliminating organ. The drug enters the body by the organ blood flow, CL_{in} and is immediately mixed in the organ. The drug leaves the organ by either being eliminated ($CL_{\text{int}}Cu$) or by the exiting blood flow.

drug that escapes elimination in the lung, only a small fraction goes to compartment n, while the rest is distributed to other organs. Drugs that enter these organs will be exposed to elimination in these organs and must necessarily recirculate through the heart and lungs before they again have the opportunity to reach compartment n.

Parenteral Administration: Depot

The other parenteral routes depicted in Fig. 2, intramuscular (IM) and subcutaneous (SC) injections, may also be considered in terms of Fig. 3. Drug absorbed from the IM and SC sites into the venous blood will return to the heart and pass through the lungs before being distributed to the rest of the body. However, there will be an initial lag between the time when the drug is injected and when it enters the circulation. Thus, the kinetics for drugs administered by these parenteral routes would be expected to show a decreased *rate* of availability and may also show a decreased *extent* of availability in comparison with intravenous administration, if loss processes take place at the site of injection. For example, we could consider that drug is now injected directly into compartment m in Fig. 3 and that this compartment is the muscle. The rate at which the drug leaves the muscle will depend primarily on blood flow in relation to the size (apparent volume of distribution) of the organ.

Evans and coworkers [7] measured resting human muscle blood flow through the gluteus maximus, vastus lateralis, and deltoid muscles. Deltoid muscle blood flow was significantly greater than gluteus muscle blood flow, with vastus being intermediate. Because the two sites most commonly used for IM injections are the deltoid and the gluteus muscles, we might expect to see differences in rates of drug absorption following injection to these sites. Lidocaine is one drug that has been investigated for its effect in response to the site of injection [8,9]. Deltoid injection gave higher peak levels than lateral thigh injection, which, in turn, gave higher levels than gluteal injection. Schwartz et al. [9] demonstrated that therapeutic plasma levels for a particular lidocaine dose were reached only when the deltoid injection site was used. Evans et al. [7] concluded, "This demonstrates that the site of injection can influence the plasma level achieved and that the deltoid muscle should be used to achieve therapeutic blood levels as rapidly as possible." Likewise, if a sustained or a prolonged release is desired, this would more readily be achieved by injection into a lower blood flow muscle, such as the gluteus.

Loss processes may also account for a decrease in the extent of availability following an IM injection. This can be visualized by assuming that the dose is injected into compartment m, which, as depicted in Fig. 3, is capable of eliminating the drug. As shown in Fig. 4, the drug can leave the tissue only by one of two routes: either by the blood leaving the organ, or by being eliminated by metabolism in the muscle. In addition, the drug that leaves the site of administration will also be subject to the additional distribution and elimination in the lung, similar to intravenous administration. In other words, drug given by intramuscular administration may not only be further delayed in its distribution to the target organ, but may also show a decreased extent of distribution to the organ, in comparison with the intravenous dose. For example, degradation can take place in the muscle, as shown by Doluisio et al. [10] for ampicillin. These workers found that only 77–78% of an IM does of ampicillin sodium solution was absorbed, as compared with the IV solution. The most likely explanation is that the drug may have been decomposed chemically or enzymatically at the injection site. In addition, temporary losses may also occur. For example, intramuscular doses of phenytoin result in a marked decreased rate and extent of absorption in comparison with IV or oral doses. Wilensky and Lowden [11] demonstrated that this could be due to precipitation of the drug as crystals in the muscle. Although these crystals eventually dissolve, the drug is essentially lost during a normal dosing interval.

Oral Administration

First-Pass Effect. Metabolism in the Gastrointestinal Fluids and Membranes. When a dosage form is administered by the oral route, drug particles come in contact with varying pH solutions, different enzymes, mucus, gut flora, and bile all of which may contribute to decreasing the extent of availability of degradation, binding, or sequestering mechanisms. These factors, as well as the possibility of drug metabolism in the intestinal membrane itself, have been well covered in Chapter 2 and will not be discussed here

Hepatic Metabolism: Linear Systems. As depicted in both Figs. 2 and 3, drug that is absorbed from the gastrointestinal tract must pass through the liver before reaching the sampleable circulation and the rest of the body. Thus, if a drug is metabolized in the liver or excreted into the bile, some of the active drug absorbed from the gastrointestinal tract will be inactivated by hepatic processes before the drug can reach the general circulation and be distributed to its site(s) of action. An exception would be if the liver itself were the target organ, as we then would have to contend with only losses in the gastrointestinal tract and in the gut wall before reaching the site of action.

For many drugs, the fraction of the dose eliminated on the first pass through the liver is substantial. The fraction eliminated is often referred to as the hepatic extraction ratio, designated herein as E_H. Many drugs are known or suspected to have a high hepatic extraction ratio. A short list of some of the better-known compounds is given in Table 1. The hepatic first-pass phenomenon is not restricted to any particular pharmacological or chemical group of drug substances, and the foregoing list includes acids, bases, and neutral compounds.

The available fraction (F) of an oral dose appearing in the sampleable blood circulation will, therefore, be governed by not only the extent of drug absorbed from the gastrointestinal tract, as discused in Chapter 4, but also by the fraction metabolized in the gut membranes (E_G) and the fraction metabolized or excreted into the bile following passage through the liver (E_H), where E_G and E_H are the extraction ratios for the gut and liver, respectively. If it is assumed that a drug is completely absorbed from the gastrointestinal tract and not degraded during passage through the gut membranes, this would be equivalent to an injection of the drug into the hepatic portal vein. Under these conditions the unmetabolized fraction (F_H) of an oral dose appearing in the sampleable blood circulation would equal $1 - E_H$. If the drug elimination in the liver follows first-order kinetics, Rowland [12] has shown that F_H, the fraction of the oral dose that is available following the liver first pass, may be related to liver blood flow (Q_H) and the hepatic clearance for an IV does of the drug ($CL_{H,\mathrm{iv}}$).

$$F_H = 1 - E_H = 1 - \frac{CL_{H,\mathrm{iv}}}{Q_H} \tag{2}$$

Table 1 Drugs Suspected to Have High Hepatic Extraction Ratios

Acetylsalicylic acid	Alprenolol	Aldosterone
Cocaine	Desipramine	Doxorubicin
Fluorouracil	Isoproteranol	Imipramine
Lidocaine	Lorcainide	Morphine
Nitroglycerin	Prazepam	Propranolol

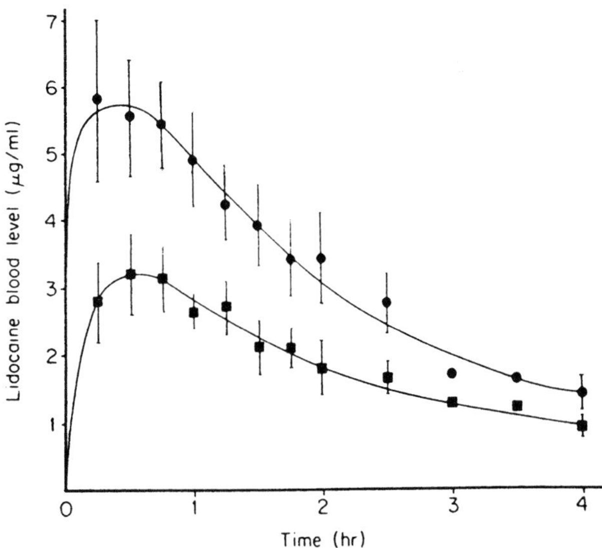

Fig. 5 Mean blood levels of lidocaine hydrochloride in five beagles after exponential IV infusion through a peripheral vein (●) and in the portal vein (■). Vertical bars represent standard errors of the mean. (From Ref. 13.)

This hepatic first-pass effect, as discussed by Boyes et al. [13], is well illustrated in Fig. 5. Identical doses of lidocaine hydrochloride were injected into dogs (beagles) by an exponential infusion process. The upper curve describes the mean levels found when the drug was infused into a peripheral vein, whereas the lower curve describes the lidocaine levels following hepatic portal vein infusion (thereby eliminating any effects caused by gastrointestinal degradation either in the fluids of the tract or in the intestinal membrane). The area under the curve (AUC) measurements for the two curves show that the extent of bioavailability following portal vein infusion is only 60% of that found following infusion into a peripheral vein (i.e., $F_H = 0.6$). This "oral" availability could be predicted for a drug such as lidocaine for which drug elimination occurs predominantly in the liver when the hepatic clearance—calculated by dividing the dose by the area under the peripheral vein infusion curve—and the hepatic blood flow are substituted into Eq. (2). An even greater first-pass effect is found for oral administration of lidocaine to humans, $F_H = 0.25$–0.48 [14].

Thus, if the hepatic clearance for a drug is largely relative to the hepatic blood flow, the extent of availability for this drug will be low when it is given by a route that yields first-pass effects. The decrease in availability is a function of only the anatomical site form which absorption takes place, and no amount of dosage form redesign can improve the availability. Of course, therapeutic blood levels can be reached by this route of administration if larger doses are given, but the health practitioner and pharmacist must be aware that levels of the drug metabolite may increase significantly over that seen following IV administration.

Lidocaine is not normally administered by the oral route, but many of the drugs listed earlier are routinely given orally. For these drugs, analysis of Eq. (2) leads to the conclusion that small variations in plasma or blood clearance of a drug throughout a population may yield significant differences in availability when the drug is given by a route subject to significant first-pass effects. For example, data from a study of Shand et al. [15] for oral and IV administration of propranolol in five men are shown in Table 2. Although the clearance following an IV dose of the drug (column 6) varies by only 67% from the smallest to the largest, the oral availability (column 5) varies by 275%. As would be expected from Eq. (2), the oral availability decreases as the IV clearance increases.

Hepatic Metabolism: Nonlinear Systems. The discussion of the first-pass effect has thus far assumed linear first-order kinetics. Under this condition, the hepatic extraction will be independent of the rate of drug availability. That is, no matter when a drug molecule is absorbed form the gastrointestinal tract and at whatever dose administered, the hepatic extraction and the extent of availability [see Eq. (2)] for that drug will remain constant. This would not be true for a drug for which saturation of the hepatic enzymes is a possibility. Under such a condition, the extraction ratio would vary depending on the concentration of drug in the hepatic portal vein. If the concentration were high, the hepatic enzymes would become partially saturated, and a large amount of drug would pass through the liver without being metabolized (i.e., E_H would be low). Saturable metabolism during the first passage through the liver is not an unusual occurrence even for a drug that, after intravenous administration, fails to show saturable metabolism. The main reason is that drug absorbed from the gastrointestinal tract is diluted to only a small degree before it enters the liver (in the portal blood only), and the concentrations can be relatively high. On the other hand, intravenously administered drug is generally quickly distributed to individual tissues, and the concentration reaching the liver during the elimination process is sufficiently low that no saturation of the metabolism is achieved. However, if the concentration in the hepatic portal vein were low, either because of administration of a low dose or because of very slow absorption of the drug, then the enzymes would not be saturated, and most of the drug could be metabolized on passage through the liver (i.e., E_H would approach 1). In a similar manner, metabolism in the gastrointestinal membranes could also be saturated or not, depending on the dose and the rate of absorption (i.e., E_G would vary from 0 to 1).

Salicylamide appears to be a drug for which the first-pass extraction may be dose-dependent. When a 300-mg oral dose of salicylamide is administered as a solution, the area under the plasma concentration time curve is less than 1% of the area seen following a similar IV dose [16]. Even following a 1-g oral dose, most of the drug is found in the systemic circulation as the inactive glucuronide and sulfate conjugates. However, when a 2-g dose was given to a particular subject (Fig. 6), the area under the plasma concentration time curve for unmetabolized salicylamide increased dramatically (>200 times increase over that seen for a 1-g dose). This very large increase is probably related to saturation of enzymes in the gastrointestinal mucosa as well as in the liver. Saturation of the hepatic enzymes not only increases the extent of oral availability, but a

Table 2 Peak Plasma Levels and Areas Under Plasma Concentration Time Curves Following Oral and Intravenous Administration to Men

	Propranolol, 80 mg fasting orally		Propranolol, 10 mg IV		
Subject	Peak (ng/ml)	Area (ng/ml · hr)	Area (ng/ml · hr)	$\frac{AUC_{Oral}}{AUC_{IV}} \cdot \frac{10}{80} \cdot 100$	Clearance, IV (ml/min)
OF	212	1400	292	60	570
DS	100	480	220	30	756
GY	94	510	200	32	833
JC	45	290	183	20	909
JF	36	220	175	16	950

Source: After Ref. 15.

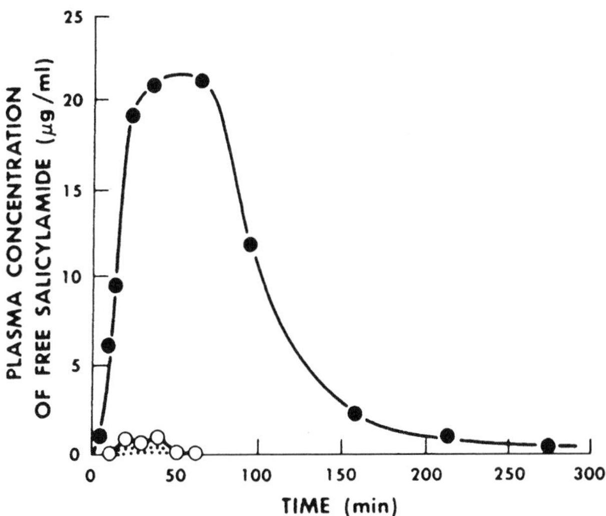

Fig. 6 Comparison of plasma concentrations of intact salicylamide when given as 1-g (○) and a 2-g (●) dose in solution to the same subject. Dotted lines show the plasma concentrations of a 0.5-g dose and 0.3-g dose. (From Ref. 16.)

sufficient amount of unchanged drug is allowed to enter the systemic circulation, thereby decreasing the rate of drug metabolism during the postabsorptive phase as well. This phenomenon is due to enzyme saturation. Thus, the extraction ratio [see Eq. (1)] and, thereby, the drug clearance, change continuously during both the absorption and elimination processes. Under these conditions AUC measurements can no longer be used to determine the extent of drug availability (as described in Chapter 3 for linear systems.)

The effects of stomach emptying on drug availability are discussed in Chapters 2 and 4, relative to processes within the gastrointestinal system. In addition, Benet [1] has interpreted data for *p*-aminobenzoic acid (PABA) as reflecting an example for which the rate of drug absorption modified by changes in stomach emptying causes changes in the extent of drug availability owing to saturation of first-pass metabolism. Table 3 represents a situation in which the drug PABA is completely absorbed from the gastrointestinal tract, yet there is a decrease in the extent of drug available to the systemic circulation as a function of food [17].

The data for the oral solution, single-dose studies suggest that all of the drug is being absorbed, since the total amount of PABA found in the urine (both as unchanged drug and acetyl metabolite) equals the dose administered. It appears that the decreasing fraction of the acetyl metabolite found in the urine with increasing doses would indicate that a saturable metabolic process was operable. For the second series of studies listed in Table 3, the oral solution dose remains constant at 1 g, while increasing amounts of sweet cream are added to the solution. With increasing amounts of fat, there is a concomitant increase in the percentage of dose excreted as the acetyl metabolite. This may be explained by assuming that the fat decreases the rate of stomach emptying, causing the drug to be emptied from the stomach more slowly and to be absorbed over a longer time period. If plasma concentration were maintained at lower levels by slowing absorption, the metabolic site would not reach the same degree of saturation and a greater fraction of the metabolite should appear in the urine. Even if gastric absorption of PABA did occur, owing to retention of the drug in the stomach, the absorption rate should be significantly lower than that seen for the oral solutions without fat, thereby maintaining plasma concentrations of PABA at lower levels. The prolonged administration of the smaller oral and IV doses in the third part of Table 3 yields high levels of metabolite in the urine, which is consistent with the saturable enzyme hypothesis (i.e., when plasma concentrations are maintained at a low level, extensive metabolism will occur).

Biliary Excretion. The effects of significant hepatic extraction as a result of biliary secretion, with or without metabolism, would be expected to follow the same principles just outlined for hepatic metabolism. In fact, a whole class of compounds that serve as biliary contrast agents for radiological examination depend on significant first-pass biliary secretion to be effective.

Several studies in rats have shown that certain acidic and basic compounds can be actively secreted into the bile. Thus, one might expect to see saturation of the biliary excretion process, although data in humans describing this phenomenon have not, as yet, been reported for orally dosed drugs.

Oral Dosing Without a First-Pass Effect. If a drug is not metabolized in the gut wall or the liver and if the drug is not subject to biliary excretion, there will be no first-pass effect following oral dosing. In addition, with drugs for which the hepatic clearance is significantly less than hepatic blood flow [see Eq. (2)], the hepatic extraction will be negligible (i.e., $F_H \approx 1$). Most orally administered drugs used today fall into this latter category. Examination of Fig. 2 indicates that another form of oral administration, sublingual dosing, may avoid first-pass metabolism as well as the degradation

Table 3 Extent of Urinary Excretion of *p*-Aminobenzoic Acid (PABA) and Its Acetyl Metabolite as a Function of Route of Administration and Ingestion of Fat

Route	Dose Na-PABA to 61-kg man (g)	Total PABA in urine as percentage of dose in 24 hr	Acetyl-PABA in urine as percentage of total PABA excreted in 24 hr
Oral solution			
Single dose	1	103	51
	2	103	47
	4	102	36
	8	102	30
Fat added to oral dose			
60 g sweet cream	1	95	76
90 g sweet cream	1	104	83
120 g sweet cream	1	99	90
Prolonged administration			
10 oral doses given every 30 min	0.365	95	97
Intravenous infusion, 270 min	0.365	90	95
Intravenous bolus	1	102	51

Source: Ref. 17.

process that may occur in the gastrointestinal fluids. This route of administration has been used predominantly in dosing organic nitrates in patients experiencing angina.

Rectal Administration

As can be seen in Fig. 2, the first-pass effect can be partially avoided by rectal administration. The capillaries in the lower and middle sections of the rectum drain into the inferior vena cava, thus bypassing the liver. However, suppositories tend to move upward in the rectum into a region where veins (such as the superior hemorrhoidal vein) drain predominantly into the portal circulation [18]. In addition, there are extensive anastomoses between the middle and superior hemorrhoidal veins. Thus, Schwarz [19] has suggested that only about 50% of a rectal dose can be assumed to bypass the liver and its first-pass extraction. Again referring to Fig. 2, we can see that absorption of drugs from the vagina would bypass the first-pass effect, although almost no drugs where systemic levels are desired have been formulated using this route of administration.

Other Routes of Administration

It is clear from the foregoing discussion that none of the methods traditionally used for systemic administration are ideal. Intravenous administration requires hospital staff and, therefore, is rarely used in an outpatient setting. Intramuscular and subcutaneous doses may be metabolized at the site of administration, may be significantly delayed, and may run the risk of infections and meet with public reluctance for self-administration, although subcutaneous administration has been met with great success in insulin-dependent diabetics. Oral administration must run through a series of elimination sites before the drug can enter the general circulation. Rectal administration can also be exposed to hepatic first-pass and must also contend with a public reluctance in its usage. Because of these factors, several other routes for systemic administration of drugs have been explored over the years. Significant acceleration in these areas has occurred as a response to the increased interest in the use of peptide and protein drugs made by recombinant techniques. Peptides and proteins are notoriously prone to degradation in the gastrointestinal tract, and the only modes of administration have been parenteral administrations. This limits the use by outpatients, and great efforts are being made to develop alternative routes of delivery.

Nasal Administration. The nasal mucosa is relative permeable to small molecular weight compounds. The most notorious example is cocaine. Cocaine that is snorted is both rapidly and extensively absorbed. Small peptides have also been successfully administered nasally, although the bioavailability is low. However, where the availability is not critical, nasal administration of peptides has been successful. The best example is calcitonin, which shows an activity after nasal administration similar to that seen after intravenous administration, although the plasma concentrations achieved after nasal delivery were lower [20]. This is a compound that has a relatively large therapeutic index for which a variable bioavailability is not critical.

During the absorption process through the nasal lining, the drug has to cross not only lipophilic barriers, but it must also pass through the nasal epithelia, which have a significant capability to metabolize drugs. Nasally administered drug can, in addition to this loss by metabolism, also be removed by mucous flow and ciliary movement and be swallowed. Nasal administration can, under circumstances during which significant amounts are swallowed, be thought of as being similar to administering the drug in part as an oral dose. To increase the absorption by the nasal epithelia, the use of bioadhesive drug-delivery forms and many exciting absorption enhancer techniques are being explored. Chemicals that disrupt the lipophilic membranes as well as opening the tight junction between the cells have resulted in a dramatic increase in the availability. The opening of the tight junctions is particularly interesting, as the compounds pass between the cells, thereby avoiding exposure to the metabolizing enzymes in the nasal epithelia. Whether these absorption enhancement techniques are the ways of the future as a means to reduce first-pass elimination, or if, in the end, they will be judged to invoke too much tissue damage for continuous use, still needs to be evaluated.

Transdermal Absorption. If transdermal delivery of drugs to the systemic circulation is to be successful, it must mimic subcutaneous injection in terms of yielding minimal first-pass skin elimination. The main barrier to absorption is the thick lipophilic keratin layer of the skin. Few nonlipophilic compounds penetrate the skin to a sufficient degree that this mode of delivery can be used for systematic absorption without modification. Highly lipophilic drugs, on the other hand, penetrate the skin with relative ease, although the absorption usually takes a long time. Several drugs are successfully given by dermal administration (e.g., nitroglycerin, scopolamine, nicotine, progesterone). To increase the absorption of hydrophilic compounds, including peptides and proteins, strategies similar to those described previously for nasal absorption have been studied (i.e., use of hydration and chemical enhancers). In addition, use of nonchemical enhancement methods (i.e., iontophoresis) is also being explored. This technique uses a low electric charge to force fluid and solutes to cross the skin. Although it was introduced more than 200 years ago [21], it is only recently that the method appears to have reached a practical stage [22]. These methods not only allow the drug to bypass the gastrointestinal tract and the liver, they also may be employed to achieve very attractive long-term sustained delivery.

Pulmonary Inhalation. Although aerosol preparations now serve primarily as a convenient drug-delivery system that can input drug directly to its site of action, new interest has recently been generated in this delivery system as a potential route for systemic administration of drug. The lung has a relatively large surface area and is relatively permeable to lipophilic compounds and, to some degree, even to protein [23]. Several barriers to absorption by the lungs do exist. The barrier to absorption is greatest in the upper bronchi and decreases in the alveoli. In the upper bronchi the mucus is relatively thick, the surface area small, and ciliar movement tends to move impacted particles up the bronchi and into the esophagus. The particle size of therapeutic inhalation aerosols determines the site of deposition in the lungs and, thus, the clinical effectiveness of a particular formulation. Particles that are too large will impact in the upper bronchi, and those too small will not readily impact on the wall of the lung and, therefore, will simply be exhaled. Particle sizes in the order of 0.3–1 μm are usually considered to be most effective. Sciarra [24] has suggested that almost all drugs given by IV injection can be reformulated into a suitable aerosol, provided that the drug is capable of being deposited in the respiratory tract and is nonirritating. However, the total availability of the pulmonary route will, to a large degree, depend on how much drug is deposited in the lung and, again, how much metabolized during first pass. It is expected that the first-pass bioavailability will be lower than that seen after intravenous administration because the drug has to pass the epithelial cell layer before it can reach the general circulation. From intravenous administration, only the amount of drug that is actually taken up by the lung tissue will be exposed to metabolism and exhalation.

III. DRUG DISTRIBUTION

Figure 1 indicates that distribution will take place as the drug reaches the general circulation. This will dilute the drug and influence the levels at the site of action. Thus, an understanding of drug distribution is critical in designing appropriate drug dosage regimens. This has led to the determination of "apparent" volumes of distribution (as discussed in Chapter 3), which can be used to related the amount of drug in the body (or in a hypothetical compartment) to a measured plasma or blood concentration. The volume of distribution is a function of four major factors: (a) the size of the organs into which the drug distributes; (b) the partition coefficient of drug between the organ and the circulating blood; (c) the blood flow to the distributing organs; and (d) the extent of protein binding of the drug both in the plasma and in various tissues.

A. Organ Size, Blood Flow, and Partition Coefficient

A particular organ in the body may act as a site of distribution or as a site of both distribution and elimination. The relative importance of the various organs as storage or elimination sites depends on how fast the drug gets to each organ and how much space or volume is available to hold the drug. Table 4 presents a compilation of the volumes and blood flows of the different regions of the human body for a standard man, as compiled as Dedrick and Bischoff [25] using the mean estimates of Mapleson [26].

The various regions of the body are listed in decreasing order relative to blood flow per unit volume of tissue (adrenals highest and bone cortex lowest). This value essentially describes how fast a drug can be delivered to a body region per unit volume of tissue and reflects the relative rates at which tissues may be expected to come to equilibrium with the blood. How much drug can be stored or distributed into a tissue will depend on the size of the tissue (volume) and the ability of the drug to concentrate in the tissue (i.e., the partition coefficient between the organ and blood, $K_{O/B}$). For

Table 4 Volumes and Blood Supplies of Different Body Regions for a Standard Man[a]

Tissue	Reference letters	Volume (liters)	Blood flow (ml/min)	Blood flow (ml/100 ml)	Volume of blood in equilibrium with tissue (ml)
Adrenals	A	0.02	100	500	62
Kidneys	B	0.3	1240	410	765
Thyroid	C	0.02	80	400	49
Gray matter	D	0.75	600	80	371
Heart	E	0.3	240	80	148
Other small glands and organs	F	0.16	80	50	50
Liver plus portal system	G	3.9	1580	41	979
White matter	H	0.75	160	21	100
Red marrow	I	1.4	120	9	74
Muscle	J	30	300/600/1500	1/2/5	185/370/925
Skin				1/2/5	18/37/92
Nutritive	K	3	30/60/150		
Shunt	L		1620/1290/300	54/43/10	
Nonfat subcutaneous	M	4.8	70	1.5	43
Fatty marrow	N	2.2	60	2.7	37
Fat	O	10.0	200	2.0	123
Bone cortex	P	6.4	≈0	≈0	≈0
Arterial blood	Q	1.4			
Venous blood	R	4.0			
Lung parenchymal tissue	S	0.6			
Air in lungs	T	2.5 + half			1400[b]
		Tidal volume			999/795/185[c]
Total		70.0[d]	6480		5400

[a]Standard man = 70-kg body weight, 1.83-m^2 surface area, 30–39 years old.
[b]Arterial blood.
[c]Skin-shunt venous blood.
[d]Excluding the air in the lung.

example, the blood flow per unit volume of thyroid gland (see Table 4) is one of the highest in the body, whereas the gland itself is quite small. Thus, if partition of the drug between the thyroid and blood were approximately 1, we would expect to see that the drug in the tissue would rapidly come into equilibrium with that in the blood but that relatively little drug would be found in the thyroid. However, for certain drugs containing iodine moieties, $K_{O/B}$ is enormous, and a significant amount of drug will distribute into this small gland relatively rapidly. In addition, Table 4 lists the volume of blood contained within each tissue and believed to be in equilibrium with the tissue. Thus, the volume of the thyroid in Table 4 is considered to be 20 mL of tissue and 49 mL of blood. Note that total volume of all tissues in column 3 is 70 L, including the 5.4 L of blood volume. This blood volume is broken down into 1.4 L of arterial blood (listed in the last column as being in equilibrium with the air in the lungs) and 4 L of venous blood (in equilibrium with tissues A through O). Since different muscle masses throughout the body receive different blood flows (discussed in Sec. II.B, with reference to drug input following IM injection), Mapleson [26] lists only a range for this tissue as well as for the skin. Dedrick and Bischoff [25] suggest an average blood flow value of 3.25 mL/(100 mL tissue × min) for tissues J and K, corresponding to average total flows of 980 and 98 mL/min for muscle and skin, respectively. Note that total blood flow in column 4 corresponds to the cardiac output, 6.48 L/min.

When discussing drug distribution, if it often convenient to lump various tissue regions into general categories. For example, following an IV bolus injection, the heart, brain, liver, and kidneys achieve the highest and earliest drug concentrations, with equilibrium between these tissues and blood being rapidly achieved. Thus, Dedrick and Bischoff [25] have combined these tissues and other well-perfused regions (see A through H in Table 4) into a well-perfused compartment that they designate as viscera. Similarly, regions I, J, K, and M are lumped into a less well-perfused compartment, the lean tissues, whereas poorly perfused regions N and O are designated as the adipose compartment. Blood flows, volumes, and such, for these lumped compartments can be calculated by summing the appropriate terms in Table 4. By using a perfusion model containing these three lumped compartments and a blood compartment, Bischoff and Dedrick [27] were able to describe thiopental concentrations in various tissues as shown in Fig. 7.

Levels in the dog liver, representative of the visceral tissues, are already at a maximum by the time the first sample is taken, since very rapid equilibrium is achieved between these tissues and the blood. Drug uptake into the less well-perfused skeletal muscle, representative of the lean tissue, is slower—peaking at about 20 minutes, but still achieving apparent distribution equilibrium between 1 and 2 hours. Uptake into the poorly perfused adipose tissue in even slower. In fact, peak levels in this tissue have not even been reached by the time the last samples are taken.

Since the site of action for the barbiturates is the brain, we might expect the pharmacological action to correspond to the time course of thiopental concentrations in the viscera, which, in turn, would be reflected by blood levels, since a rapid equilibrium is attained between viscera and blood. Although the pharmacological action may terminate quickly (within an hour) owing to decreased blood levels, traces of the drug may be found in the urine for prolonged periods (days) owing to accumulation in the fatty tissues. Note

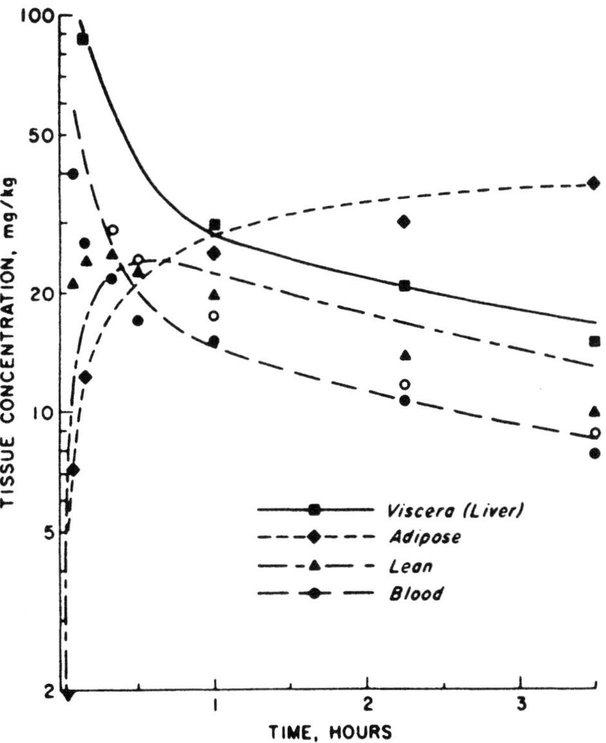

Fig. 7 Thiopental concentrations in various tissues following 25-mg/kg IV bolus doses. Solid symbols indicate data in dogs; the open circles are from data in humans. Lines correspond to predicted values in various tissues using a perfusion model containing compartments corresponding to the blood, viscera, lean, and adipose tissues. (From Ref. 26.)

that the partition coefficient for the drug between tissues and blood is greater than 1 for all three tissue groups (i.e., at distribution equilibrium tissue concentrations greater than blood concentrations) but that the $K_{O/B}$ for adipose tissue is very large. This can be deducted from the fact that drug continues to distribute into adipose tissue, even when the concentration in the fat is significantly greater than the blood concentration. At 3½ hours, most of the lipid-soluble thiopental left in the body is in the fat, and at later times this percentage may even increase before distribution equilibrium is reached. At these later times the removal rate of the barbiturate from the body will be controlled by the slow movement of drug out of the fatty tissue as a result of the high partition into the fat and the low blood flow to this region.

B. Protein Binding

One of the major determinants of drug distribution is the extent of protein binding. Many drugs bind to plasma proteins, mainly to albumin and α_1-acid glycoprotein (orosomucoid), but sometimes to lipoproteins, various globulins, and specific binding proteins as well. Up to the present time, most studies of drug protein binding have examined the interaction between drugs in the plasma and plasma albumin and plasma α_1-acid glycoprotein. Total plasma albumin for a 70-kg man is about 120 g. Total interstitial albumin is approximately 156 g [28]. Thus almost 60% of total albumin in the body is found outside the plasma. The total extracellular α_1-acid glycoprotein is approximately 3 g, of which approximately 45% is located extravascularly [29]. α_1-Acid glycoprotein has also been found intracellularly and exists as a membrane-bound form [30], but its total cellular amount is unknown. The extracellular amount of α_1-acid glycoprotein can increase significantly in many diseases (inflammation, infections, cancers) as well as during trauma. The increase is variable and usually averages a twofold change, although increases up to fivefold have been reported. Binding to tissue components is also assumed to be important for the overall distribution, although direct evidence is difficult to obtain. However, albumin and α_1-acid glycoprotein represent only approximately 1% of the "dry tissue" in the body, of which a large fraction is proteins. One might, therefore, expect that the binding of drugs to tissue would affect drug distribution significantly and frequently much more than the binding of drugs to plasma proteins. The binding of drugs to plasma proteins has been studied extensively, primarily because the experiments can be easily carried out. Tissue-binding studies do not have this advantage, and thus knowledge of the qualitative and quantitative aspects of the binding of drugs to tissue components is poorly understood. The partition coefficients between body organs and blood, $K_{O/B}$, discussed in the previous section will be considerably influenced by binding. It is probably for this reason that attempts to correlate drug distribution, drug action, and membrane transport with oil/water partition coefficients have succeeded only infrequently, necessitating the use of different organic solvents in different correlations to obtain at least an approximate rank order correlation.

Effect on Distribution

The extent of distribution to an organ is usually expressed as the apparent volume of distribution of the organ, V_i. Because the blood concentration is used as a reference, the apparent volume of an organ, V_i, can usually be expressed in the following way:

$$V_i = V_T K_{O/B} = V_T \left(\frac{fu}{fu_T} \right) \tag{3}$$

where V_T is the physical volume of the tissue, fu is the unbound fraction of drug in the blood and fu_T is the unbound fraction of drug in the tissue. This relationship indicates that the partition coefficient $K_{O/B}$ essentially reflects the strength of binding to the tissues in comparison with the binding to blood proteins, which will be particularly true for hydrophilic compounds. Decreased binding to proteins in a tissue will increase the value of fu_T, as the fraction of drug in the tissue that is not bound is now increased and the apparent volume of the tissue decreases. Similarly, if the binding to blood proteins is decreased, the relative affinity for the tissue increases and the apparent volume of distribution is increased. Often, volumes of distribution and protein binding are defined in terms of plasma measurements, rather than in blood, as used here. Such an approach is correct as long as one defines explicitly the reference fluid of measurement. We prefer to use blood measurements throughout, because, as described in the next section, the relationship of clearance to organ elimination capacity must be defined in terms of the total flow to each organ.

Effect on Clearance

The *clearance* of an organ can be viewed as the volume of blood completely cleared of drug per unit time. Given this definition, the blood clearance of an organ will be equal to the blood flow through the organ multiplied by the extraction ratio (equal to the fraction of the blood completely cleared of drug). From Eq. (1) we, therefore, obtain

$$CL = QE = Q\left(\frac{CL_{\text{Int}}}{Q + CL_{\text{Int}}}\right) = \frac{Q\,CL_{\text{Int}}}{Q + CL_{\text{Int}}} \tag{4}$$

Equation (1) was derived assuming no protein binding, whereas, in fact, CL_{Int} should be defined in terms of the maximum ability of the organ to remove *unbound* drug because only unbound drug can bind to enzymes and excretory molecules. By including the unbound fraction of drug in Eq. (4) one obtains

$$CL_{\text{organ}} = \frac{Q\,fu\,CL_{\text{Int}}}{Q + fu \cdot CL_{\text{Int}}} \tag{5}$$

where *fu* is the fraction of drug unbound in the blood. [Note that all the discussions in this chapter have related clearances and flows to blood concentrations (i.e., drug concentrations in the actual transporting fluid). Blood concentrations must be used when any physiological interpretation is placed on the clearance process. However, it is easier to carry out studies measuring plasma concentrations and plasma protein binding. These measured parameters may be converted to blood values if one knows the blood/plasma concentration ratio.]

When the intrinisic clearance of an organ is very high compared with blood flow, such that $fu\ CL_{\text{Int}} \gg Q$, the extraction ratio approaches 1 and $CL_{\text{organ}} \to Q$. Thus, according to Eq. (5), if a drug is cleared exclusively in the liver with an extraction ratio approaching unity, organ clearance will be very sensitive to changes in liver blood flow and essentially independent of blood binding [31]. Likewise, for drugs eliminated in the kidney by active-transport processes, elimination appears to be independent of the extent of blood binding. Under these conditions, kidney blood flow becomes the rate-limiting step.

However, for many drugs, blood flow is significantly greater than the intrinsic organ clearance ($Q \gg fu\,CL_{\text{Int}}$) and then Eq. (5) reduces to

$$CL_{\text{organ}} = fu\,CL_{\text{Int}} \tag{6}$$

indicating that organ clearance is dependent on binding in blood and is proportional to the unbound fraction of drug in blood. This phenomenon is valid for both hepatic and renal elimination. For example, the glomerulus in the kidneys will filter approximately 120 mL of plasma per minute. High molecular weight compounds (i.e., most of the plasma proteins) will not be filtered. Likewise, drugs bound to these proteins will be retained. In other words, one could view the filtration process as being filtration of plasma water and of the small molecular weight compounds dissolved therein. Plasma water contains only unbound drug. Increases in binding will lower the fraction of the drug in plasma in unbound form and, therefore, decrease the filtration clearance. For hepatic elimination, data for several compounds have been published over the years that show a correlation between the clearance and the unbound fraction in plasma [32]. We expect similar relationships between the organ clearance and the unbound fraction to be also valid for other organs.

Effect on Availability

Should changes in protein binding have a significant effect on first-pass availability? Combining Eqs. (2) and (5), we obtain:

$$F = 1 - E = 1 - \frac{CL}{Q} = 1 - \left[\frac{fu\,CL_{\text{Int}}}{Q + fu \cdot CL_{\text{Int}}}\right]$$
$$= \frac{Q}{Q + fu \cdot CL_{\text{Int}}} \tag{7}$$

This indicates that the first-pass availability is a function of organ flow, protein binding, and intrinisic clearance of the organ. When $fu\ CL_{\text{Int}} \gg Q$ (i.e., when we have relatively large extraction ratios), the first-pass bioavailability is equal to

$$F = \frac{Q}{fu\,CL_{\text{Int}}} \tag{8}$$

Under this circumstance, the first-pass bioavailability is inversely proportional to the unbound fraction, and changes in the binding are expected to have a significant effect. It is also clear that changes in both the blood flow and the intrinsic clearance of the first-pass organ may have a significant effect when the extraction ratio is high ($fu\ CL_{\text{Int}} \gg Q$). On the other hand, if $Q \gg fu\,CL_{\text{Int}}$, then Eq. (7) simply says that the first-pass bioavailability is approximately 1 (i.e., little or no drug is eliminated in a first pass), and changes in binding, blood flow, and intrinsic clearance are not expected to have any effect on *F*.

Combined Kinetic Effect of Binding Alterations

Changes in binding can occur in many situations. In some diseases, the concentrations of binding proteins may be altered, and accumulation of endogenous inhibitors of binding may occur. For example, in renal failure the albumin level may decrease, resulting in decreased binding. In renal failure, accumulation of waste products also occurs, and this, in turn, may further suppress the binding. In other diseases (e.g., inflammations), the level of α_1-acid glycoprotein increases, which may lead to increased drug binding. Concomitant administration of compounds that compete for the same binding sites may also decrease the binding and increase the unbound fraction. These changes will lead to changes in the apparent volume of distribution, in clearance, and in the first-pass availability, as discussed earlier, but will they lead to changes in the time required for the drug to reach the target organ and in the activity of the drug? The answer is not simple, as it depends on the actual values of clearance and volume of distribution, as well as on whether the target tissue is among the highly or poorly perfused tissues.

To begin answering this question we must realize that the effect of drugs in the body is related to the unbound and not the total concentration in the body [33]. Only non–protein-bound drug can interact with receptors and, therefore, elicit an effect. Therefore, it is important to look at how the *unbound* concentration changes. Let us assume that a situation of decreased binding exists in blood and that no changes in the tissue binding have occurred. If a dose is given, we expect no changes in the first-pass bioavailability if the extraction ratio in the first-pass tissue is low. If the extraction ratio is high, on the other hand, we expect a significant decrease in the first-pass bioavailability if the extraction [see Eq. (8)] of either an IV administration (if first-pass in the lung is significant) or an oral administration (first-pass effect both in the liver and lung). When it comes to other routes of administration, we need to be more cautious. For example, let us look at dermal administration. If the major first-pass elimination occurs before the drug reaches the blood (i.e., in its passage through the epithelial cells), we do not expect the blood-binding changes to be important. On the other hand, if the major first-pass elimination relates to cell downstream from where the drug enters the blood, changes in the binding will cause changes predictable from Eq. (8).

Will the drug be delayed on its way to the target tissue in the foregoing example? A decreased blood binding is equivalent to increasing the $K_{O/B}$ value. Distribution into various tissues, including the target tissue, therefore, is expected to be more extensive and swifter. However, because the drug usually has to pass the lungs before it can reach the target tissue, high $K_{O/B}$ values in the lung will significantly reduce the amount available to other tissues when the $K_{O/B}$ value increases for the lung. Consequently, a delay of distribution here can occur. On the other hand, if the $K_{O/B}$ value in the lung is low, the amount sequestered by the lung will be too small to delay the distribution. In this situation, no delay is expected in distribution of drug to the target tissue, if the target tissue is highly perfused. However, if the target tissue is a poorly perfused tissue, a delay may still occur. In this situation, a higher $K_{O/B}$ value will mean that the highly perfused tissues can take up more of the initial drug presented to them. In turn, the diffusion out of the hihgly perfused tissues will be slower, and may take longer before the redistribution to poorly perfused tissues is completed. Therefore, if the effect is in the poorly perfused tissues, the effect will lag.

On the continuous administration, the drug's effect is dependent on the average unbound steady-state concentration. The unbound concentration is dependent on the average rate of dosing, bioavailability, clearance, and degree of binding in plasma. Let us, for the moment, assume that the bioavailability and dosing rate remain constant. The change in the steady-state unbound concentration now depends on whether the extraction ratio is low or high (or whether $Q \gg fu\,CL_{\text{Int}}$ or $fu\,CL_{\text{Int}} \gg Q$ in addition to the alteration of the binding. For a low-extraction ratio compond, the average unbound concentration, Cu_{ss} is

$$Cu_{ss} = \frac{F(\text{rate of dosing})}{CL_{\text{Int}}} \tag{9}$$

For a high-extraction ratio, the value is

$$Cu_{ss} = \frac{F(\text{rate of dosing})}{Q/fu} \tag{10}$$

Under the assumptions of constant bioavailability and dosing rate, a high-extraction ratio compound is expected to have an increased unbound steady-state concentration when the plasma binding is decreased, and a low-extraction ratio compound is not affected by binding changes. Now, however, we also need to evaluate whether the first-pass availability is affected by a change in the binding and adjust our expectation accordingly. Under special circumstances for which the first-pass organ is the major metabolizing organ, some simplified concepts can be established. For a low-extraction ratio compound in this situation, neither the first-pass bioavailability nor the clearance relative to unbound drug will be affected, and the result is that there is no overall effect on the average unbound steady-state concentration and the activity of the drug. For a high-extraction ratio compound both the clearance realative to unbound drug [Eq. (5)] and the first-pass bioavailability [see Eq. (7)] will increase proportional to the increase in the unbound fraction in plasma, and the result is again that the average unbound concentration is not affected by a change in the plasma binding. If the first-pass organ is different from the major eliminating organ, the extraction ratio in these organs may be different, and their dependence on binding may differ (i.e., the unbound clearance and bioavailability may be affected to a different extent). If saturation of the first-pass takes place, there is also likely to be different effect of binding on the first-pass bioavailability and unbound clearance, even if the first-pass organ is the major eliminating organ.

Changes in tissue binding have effects only on the tissue distribution and not on clearance. Tissue-binding changes, therefore, are not expected to affect the first-pass bioavailability, but are expected to alter the distribution [See Eq. (3)] and $K_{O/B}$ value. If the value of $K_{O/B}$ is reduced, we expect a smallar sequestering of drug in its passage through the body, higher initial concentrations will reach the target tissue, and the effect will occur more swiftly and, initially, more potently. But because the apparent volume of distribution is smaller, the half-life will also be smaller:

$$t_{1/2} = \frac{0.693V}{CL} \tag{11}$$

and the concentration and the effect will fall off faster. Documentation for such changes is difficult to obtain, because we cannot measure the tissue binding directly, and we can make only inferences from overall changes in the kinetic parameters and changes in plasma-binding values [34].

A third possibility—that the binding in plasma and tissue changes to the same degree—is not expected to affect the apparent volume of distribution to the individual organs [see Eq. (3)], and the value of $K_{O/B}$ will not be changed. The clearance, on the other hand, is affected only by changes in binding in blood and will change as described in Sec. III.B, the section describing the effect of protein-binding changes on clearance. Assuming that the first-pass bioavailability is not affected, this will mean that sequestering of drug will not increase, and the total concentration reaching the target tissue should not be significantly affected. However, because the unbound fraction in plasma is increased (decreased), the unbound concentration will be increased (decreased), the unbound concentration initially reaching the target tissue will be higher (lower), and the initial pharmacological activity will be higher (lower). The duration of this change will depend on the half-life of the drug, which will be altered according to Eq. (11).

IV. SUMMARY

The extent and time course of drug action can be markedly affected by the route of drug administration into the patient as well as the pattern of drug distribution within the patient. Drug efficacy can be improved, and drug toxicity probably decreased, if the drug can be administered directly to its site of action. However, several factors prevent direct application of drugs to the site of action, including incomplete knowledge about the action site and also poor patient adherence owing to the inconvenience of using direct application formulations. Because of these factors, most drug products have been formulated as oral, solid dosage forms.

Drugs that are rapidly cleared by hepatic processes will show a decreased extent of availability following oral administration owing to metabolism of the drug on its first pass through the liver. The magnitude of this first-pass effect will depend on the blood flow to the liver and the intrinsic clearing ability of the liver (i.e., the ability of the organ to eliminate the drug independently of the rate at which drug is brought to the organ). This first-pass elimination by metabolic or biliary excretion processes can be excluded if the drug is absorbed from a sublingual site. The rectal administration of drugs eliminates approximately one-half the first-pass metabolism. Absorption through nasal, dermal, and other sites may also give rise to lower first-pass elimination and higher bioavailability than oral administration if the metabolic capacity of these sites for the drug in question is small.

Drug distribution in the patient will depend on the blood blow to various sites in the body as well as on the partition coefficient of the drug between the blood and distributive organs. Protein binding, both in the blood and in the tissues, will markedly affect this distribution. However, free drug concentrations are generally believed to be the effective determinant in drug therapy. Often a redistribution owing to changes in protein binding will have little effect on the therapeutic efficacy, since, although total drug distribution changes, the average unbound concentrations at steady state in blood remain essentially similar. An understanding of the effects of the route of administration as well as the distribution of the drug within the body is critical to the pharmacist in planning appropriate drug dosage regimens.

REFERENCES

1. L. Z. Benet, Biopharmaceutics as a basis for the design of drug products, in *Drug Design*, Vol. 4, (E. Ariens, Ed.), Academic Press, New York, 1973, pp. 1–35.
2. L. Z. Benet, Input factors as determinants of drug activity: route, dose, dosage regimen, and the drug delivery system, in *Principles and Techniques of Human Research and Therapeutics*, Vol. 3, (F. G. McMahon, Ed.), Futura, New York, 1974, pp. 9–23.
3. T. E. Gram, The metabolism of xenobiotics by the mammalian lung, in *Extrahepatic Metabolism of Drugs and Other Foreign Compounds* (T. E. Gram, Ed.), S.P. Medical and Scientific Books, New York, 1980, pp. 159–209.
4. J. R. Vane, The role of the lungs in the metabolism of vasoactive substances, in *Pharmacology and Pharmacokinetics* (T. Teorell, R. L. Dedrick, and P. G. Condliffe, Eds.), Plenum Press, New York, 1974, pp. 195–207.
5. W. L. Chiou, Potential pitfalls in the conventional pharmacokinetic studies: Effects of the initial mixing of drug in blood and the pulmonary first-pass elimination, J. Pharmacokinet. Biopharm., 7, 527–536 (1979).
6. M. Rowland, L. Z. Benet, and G. G. Graham, Clearance concepts in pharmacokinetics, J. Pharmacokinet. Biopharm., 1, 123–136 (1973).
7. E. F. Evans, J. D. Proctor, M. J. Fraktin, J. Velandia, and A. J. Wasserman, Blood flow in muscle groups and drug absorption, Clin. Pharmacol. Ther., 17, 44–47 (1975).
8. L. S. Cohen, J. E. Rosenthal, D. W. Horner, Jr., J. M. Atkins, O. A. Matthews, and S. F. Sarnoff, Plasma levels of lidocaine after intramuscular administration, Am. J. Cardiol., 29, 520–523 (1972).
9. M. L. Schwartz, M. B. Meyer, B. G. Covino, R. M. Narange, W. Sethi, A. J. Schwartz, and P. Kemp, Antiarrhythmic effectiveness of intramuscular lidocaine: Influence of different injection sites, J. Clin. Pharmacol., 14, 77–83 (1974).
10. J. T. Doluisio, J. C. LaPiana, and L. W. Dittert, Pharmacokinetics of ampicillin trihydrate, sodium ampicillin, and sodium dicloxacillin following intramuscular injection, J. Pharm. Sci., 60, 715–719 (1971).
11. A. J. Wilensky and J. A. Lowden, Inadequate serum levels after intramuscular administration of diphenylhydantoin, Neurology, 23, 318–324 (1973).
12. M. Rowland, Influence of route of administration on drug availability, J. Pharm. Sci., 61, 70–74 (1972).
13. R. N. Boyes, J. H. Adams, and B. R. Duce, Oral absorption and disposition kinetics of lidocaine hydrochloride in dogs, J. Pharmacol. Exp. Ther. 174, 1–8 (1970).
14. M. Rowland, Effect of some physiologic factors on bioavailability of oral dosage forms, in *Dosage Form Design and Bioavailability* (J. Swarbrick, Ed.), Lea & Febiger, Philadelphia, 1973, pp. 181–222.
15. D. G. Shand, E. M. Nuckolls, and J. A. Oates, Plasma propranolol levels in adults with observations in four children, Clin. Pharmacol. Ther., 11, 112–120 (1970).
16. W. H. Barr, Factors involved in the assessment of systemic or biologic availability of drug products, Drug Inf. Bull., 3, 27–45 (1969).
17. M. Drucker, S. H. Blondheim, and L. Wislicki, Factors affecting acetylation in vivo of *para*-aminobenzoic acid by human subjects, Clin. Sci., 27, 133–141 (1964).
18. A. G. De Boer, D. D. Breimer, H. Mattie, J. Pronk, and J. M. Gubbens-Stibbe, Rectal bioavailability of lidocaine in man: Partial avoidance of "first-pass" metabolism, Clin. Pharmacol. Ther., 26, 701–709 (1979).
19. T. W. Schwarz, in *American Pharmacy*, 6th ed., (J. B. Sprowls, Jr. and H. M. Beal, Eds.), J. B. Lippincott, Philadelphia, 1966, pp. 311–331.
20. A. E. Pontiroli, M. Alberetto, and G. Pozza, Intranasal calcitonin and plasma calcium concentrations in normal subjects, Br. Med. J., 290, 1390–1391 (1985).
21. Y. W. Chien and K. Banga, Iontophoretic (transdermal) delivery of drugs: Overview of historic development, J. Pharm. Sci., 78, 353–354 (1989).
22. D. Parasrampuria and J. Parasrampuria, Percutaneous delivery of proteins and peptides using iontophoretic techniques, J. Clin. Pharm. Ther., 16, 7–17 (1991).
23. D. T. O'Hagan and L. Illum, Absorption of peptides and proteins from the respiratory tract and the potential for development of locally administered vaccine, Crit. Rev. Ther. Drug Carrier Syst., 7, 35–97 (1990).
24. J. J. Sciarra, Aerosols, in *Prescription Pharmacy*, 2nd ed. (J. B. Sprowls, Jr., Ed.), J. B. Lippincott, Philadelphia, 1970, pp. 280–328.
25. R. L. Dedrick and K. B. Bischoff, Pharmacokinetics in applications of the artifical kidney, Chem. Eng. Progr. Symp. Ser., 64, 32–44 (1968).
26. W. W. Mapleson, An electric analogue for uptake and exchange of inert gases and other agents, J. Appl. Physiol., 18, 197–204 (1963).
27. K. B. Bischoff and R. L. Dedrick, Thiopental pharmacokinetics, J. Pharm. Sci., 57, 1347–1357 (1968).
28. J. G. Wagner, *Fundamentals of Clinical Pharmacokinetics*. Drug Intelligence Publishers, Hamilton, IL, 1975, pp. 24–26.
29. F. Bree, G. Houin, J. Barre, J. L. Moretti, V. Wirquin, and J.-P. Tillement, Pharmacokinetics of intravenously administered ^{125}I-labelled human alpha-1-acid glycoprotein, Clin. Pharmacokinet, 11, 336–342 (1986).
30. C. G. Gahmberg and L. C. Anderson, Leucocyte surface origin of human alpha-1-acid glycoprotein (orosomucoid), J. Exp. Med., 148, 507–521 (1978).
31. T. W. Guenthert and S. Øie, Effect of plasma protein binding on quinidine kinetics in the rabbit, J. Pharmacol. Exp. Ther., 215, 165–171 (1980).

32. T. F. Blaschke, Protein binding and kinetics of drugs in liver disease, Clin. Pharmacokinet, 2, 32–44 (1977).
33. S. Øie and J.-D. Huang, Binding, should free drug levels be measured? in *Topics in Pharmaceutical Sciences 1983* (D. D. Breimer and P. Speiser, Eds.), Elsevier, Amsterdam, 1983, pp. 51–62.
34. B. Fichtl, Tissue binding of drugs: Methods of determination and pharmacokinetic consequences, in *Plasma Binding of Drugs and Its Consequences* (F. Belpaire, M. Bogaert, J. P. Tillement, and R. Verbeeck, Eds.), Academia Press, Ghent, 1991, pp. 149–158.

Chapter 6

Chemical Kinetics and Drug Stability

J. Keith Guillory and Rolland I. Poust

University of Iowa, Iowa City, Iowa

I. INTRODUCTION

In the rational design and evaluation of dosage forms for drugs, the stability of the active components must be a major criterion in determining their suitability. Several forms of instability can lead to the rejection of a drug product. First, there may be chemical degradation of the active drug, leading to a substantial lowering of the quantity of the therapeutic agent in the dosage form. Many drugs (e.g., 5-fluorouracil, carbamazepine, digoxin, and theophylline) have narrow therapeutic indices, and they need to be carefully titrated in individual patients so that serum levels are neither too high as to be potentially toxic nor too low as to be ineffective. In these cases it is of paramount importance that the dosage form reproducibly deliver the same amount of drug.

Second, although chemical degradation of the active drug may not be extensive, a toxic product may be formed in the decomposition process [1]. Dearborn [2] described several examples in which the products of degradation are significantly more toxic than the original therapeutic agent. Thus, the conversions of tetracycline to epianhydrotetracycline, arsphenamine to oxophenarsine, and *p*-aminosalicylic acid to *m*-aminophenol in dosage forms give rise to potentially toxic agents that, when ingested, can cause undesirable effects. Nord et al. [3] have reported that the antimalarial chloroquine can produce toxic reactions that are attributable to the photochemical degradation of the substance. Phototoxicity has also been observed to occur following administration of chlordiazepoxide and nitrazepam [4]. Another example of an adverse reaction due to a degradation product was provided by Neftel et al. [5], who showed that infusion of degraded penicillin G led to sensitization of lymphocytes and formation of antipenicilloyl antibodies.

Third, instability of a drug product can lead to a decrease in its bioavailability rather than loss of drug or formation of toxic degradation products. This reduction in bioavailability can result in a substantial lowering in the therapeutic efficacy of the dosage form. This phenomenon can be caused by physical and/or chemical changes in the excipients in the dosage form, independent of whatever changes the active drug may have undergone. A more detailed discussion of this subject is given in Sec. II.B.

Fourth, there may be substantial changes in the physical appearance of the dosage form. Examples of these physical changes include mottling of tablets, creaming of emulsions, and caking of suspensions. Although the therapeutic efficacy of the dosage form may be unaffected by these changes, the patient will most likely lose confidence in the drug product, which then has to be rejected.

Fifth, while the drug substance itself may retain its potency, excipients such as antimicrobial preservatives, solubilizers, emulsifying or suspending agents may degrade, compromising the integrity of the drug product.

A drug product, therefore, must satisfy stability criteria chemically, toxicologically, therapeutically, and physically. Basic principles in pharmaceutical kinetics can often be applied to anticipate and quantify the undesirable changes so that they can be circumvented by stabilization techniques. Some chemical compounds, called prodrugs [6,7], are designed to undergo chemical or enzymatic conversion in vivo to pharmacologically active drugs. Prodrugs are employed to solve one or several problems presented by active drugs (e.g., short biological half-life, poor dissolution, bitter taste, inability to penetrate through the blood-brain barrier, etc.). They are pharmacologically inactive as such but are converted back in vivo to their parent (active) compounds. Naturally, the rate and extent of this conversion (governed by the same laws of kinetics described in this chapter) are the primary determinants of the therapeutic efficacy of these agents.

In the present chapter, stability problems and chemical kinetics are introduced and surveyed. The sequence employed is as follows: first, an overview of the potential routes of degradation that drug molecules can undergo; then, a discussion of the mathematics used to quantify drug degradation; a delineation of the factors that can affect degradation rates, with an emphasis on stabilization techniques; and finally a description of stability-testing protocols employed in the pharmaceutical industry. It is not the intent of this chapter to document stability data of various individual drugs. Readers are referred to the compilations of stability data [8] and to literature on specific drugs (e.g., Ref. 9 and earlier volumes) for this kind of information.

II. ROUTES BY WHICH PHARMACEUTICALS DEGRADE

Since most drugs are organic molecules, many pharmaceutical degradation pathways are, in principle, similar to reactions described for organic compounds in standard organic chemistry textbooks. On the other hand, different emphases are placed on the types of reactions that are commonly encountered in the drug product stability area as opposed to those seen in classical organic chemistry. In the latter case, reactions generally are described as tools for use by the synthetic chemist; thus, the conditions under which they are carried out are likely to be somewhat drastic. Reactive agents (e.g., thionyl chloride or lithium aluminum hydride) are employed in relatively high concentrations (often >10%), and exaggerated conditions, such as refluxing or heating in a pressure bomb are common. Reactions are effected in relatively short periods of time (hours or days). In contrast, the active drug components in pharmaceuticals are usually present in relatively low concentrations. For example, dexamethasone sodium phosphate, a synthetic adrenocorticoid steroid salt, is present only to the extent of about 0.4% in its injection, 0.1% in its topical cream or opthalmic solution, and 0.05% in its opthalmic ointment. The decomposition of a drug is likely to be mediated not by reaction with another active ingredient but by reaction with water, oxygen, or light. Reaction conditions of interest usually are ambient or subambient. Reactions in pharmaceuticals ordinarily occur over months or years as opposed to the hours or days required for completion of reactions in synthetic organic chemistry.

Reactions such as the Diels-Alder reaction and aldol condensations, which are important in synthetic and mechanistic organic chemistry, are of only minor importance when drug degradation is being considered. Pharmaceutical scientists need to refocus their attention on reactions such as hydrolysis, oxidation, photolysis, racemization, and decarboxylation, the routes by which most pharmaceuticals degrade.

A familiarity with reactions of particular functional groups is important if one is to gain a broad view of drug degradation. It is a difficult task to recall degradative pathways of all commonly used drugs. Yet, through the application of functional group chemistry it is possible to anticipate the potential mode(s) of degradation that drug molecules will likely undergo. In the following discussion, therefore, degradative routes are demonstrated by calling attention to the reactive functional groups present in drug molecules. The degradative routes are described, through the use of selected examples, as *chemical* when new chemical entities are formed as a result of drug decomposition and as *physical* when drug loss does not produce distinctly different chemical products. For further information about chemical functional group reactivity, the interested reader should consult a recent review ([10] and the comprehensive text by K. A. Connors [11]).

A. Chemical Degradative Routes

Solvolysis

In this type of reaction the active drug undergoes decomposition following reaction with the solvent present. Usually the solvent is water, but sometimes the reaction may involve pharmaceutical cosolvents such as ethyl alcohol or polyethylene glycol. These solvents can act as nucleophiles, attacking the electropositive centers in drug molecules. The most common solvolysis reactions encountered in pharmaceuticals are those involving "labile" carbonyl compounds such as esters, lactones, and lactams (Table 1).

Table 1 Some Functional Groups Subject to Hydrolysis

Drug type		Examples
Esters	RCOOR'	Aspirin, alkaloids
	$ROPO_3M_x$	Dexamethasone sodium phosphate
	$ROSO_3M_x$	Estrone sulfate
	$RONO_2$	Nitroglycerin
Lactones	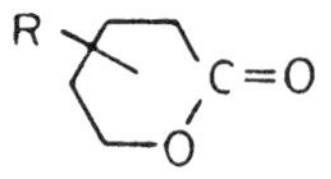 R–(ring)–C=O, –O–	Pilocarpine Spironolactone
Amides	$RCONR'_2$	Thiacinamide Chloramphenicol
Lactams	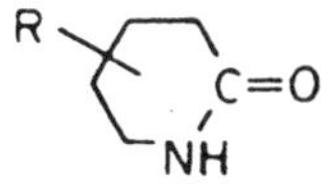 R–(ring)–C=O, –NH–	Penicillins Cephalosporins
Oximes	$R_2C = NOR$	Steroid oximes
Imides	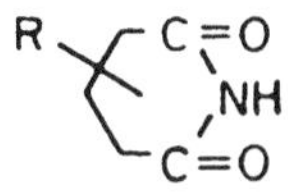 R–(ring)–C=O, NH, C=O	Glutethimide Ethosuximide
Malonic ureas	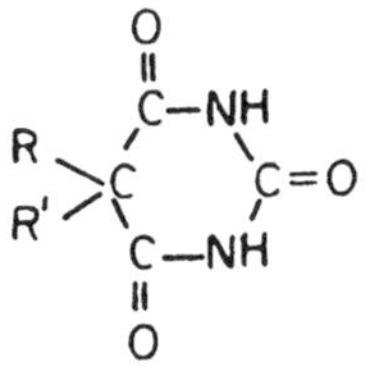 R, R'>C(C(=O)–NH)₂C=O	Barbiturates
Nitrogen mustards	$R\text{-}N(CH_2CH_2Cl)_2$	Melphalan

Although all the functional groups cited are, in principle, subject to solvolysis, the rates at which they undergo this reaction may be vastly different. For example, the rate of hydrolysis of a β-lactam ring (a cyclized amine) is much greater than that of its linear analog. The half-life (the time needed for half of the drug to decompose) of the β-lactam in potassium phenethicillin at 35°C and pH 1.5 is about 1 hour. The corresponding half-life for penicillin G is about 4 minutes [12]. In contrast, the half-life for hydrolysis of the simple amide propionamide in 0.18 molal H_2SO_4 at 25°C is about 58 hours [13]. It has been suggested that the antibacterial activity of β-lactam antibiotics arises from a combination of their chemical reactivity and their molecular recognition by target enzymes. One aspect of their chemical reactivity is their acylating power, and while penicillins are not very good acylating agents, they are more reactive than simple, unsubstituted amides [14]. Unactivated or "normal" amides undergo nonenzymatic hydrolysis slowly except under the most extreme conditions of pH and temperature because the N-C(O) linkage is inherently stable, yet when the amine function is a good leaving group (and particularly if it has a pK_a greater than 4.5), amides can be susceptible to hydrolysis at ordinary temperatures. (For a review on this subject see Ref. 15.) Acyl-transfer reactions in peptides, including the transfer to water (hydrolysis), are of fundamental importance in biological systems where the reactions proceed at normal temperatures and enzymes serve as catalysts.

The most frequently encountered hydrolysis reaction in drug instability is that of the ester, but curtain esters can be stable for many years when properly formulated. Substituents can have a dramatic effect on reaction rates. For example, the *tert*-butyl ester of acetic acid is about 120 times more stable than the methyl ester, which, in turn, is approximately 60 times more stable than the vinyl analog [16]. Structure-reactivity relationships are dealt with in the discipline of physical organic chemistry. Substituent groups may exert electronic (inductive and resonance), steric, and/or hydrogen-bonding effects that can drastically affect the stability of compounds. A detailed treatment of substituent effects can be found in a review by Hansch et al. [17] and in the classical reference text by Hammett [18].

A dramatic decrease in ester stability can be brought about by intramolecular catalysis. This type of facilitation is effected mostly by neighboring groups capable of exhibiting acid-base properties (e.g., $-NH_2$, -OH, -COOH, COO^-, etc.). If neighboring-group participation leads to an enhanced reaction rate, the group is said to provide anchimeric assistance [19]. For example, the ethyl salicylate anion undergoes hydrolysis in alkaline solution at a rate 10^6 times greater than the experimental value for the uncatalyzed cleavage of ethyl *p*-hydroxybenzoate. The rate advantage is attributed to intramolecular general base catalysis by the phenolate anion [20]. Self-associated insulin degrades at a rate approximately 2.5 times greater than the monomer at pH 2 and 3 due to intramolecular catalysis by the unionized carboxyl terminus of the A chain [21].

Oxidation

Oxidation reactions are important pathways of drug decomposition. In pharmaceutical dosage forms, oxidation is usually mediated through reaction with atmospheric oxygen under ambient conditions, a process commonly referred to as autoxidation. Oxygen is, itself, a diradical, and most autoxidations are free radical reactions. A free radical is a molecule or atom with one or more unpaired electrons. Of considerable importance to pharmaceutical scientists is a reliable method for determining and controlling oxygen concentration in aqueous solutions [22]. Sensitivity to oxidation of a drug can be ascertained by investigating its stability in an atmosphere of high oxygen tension. Usually a 40% oxygen atmosphere allows for a rapid evaluation. Results are compared against those obtained under inert (nitrogen or argon) or ambient atmospheres. A thorough review of autoxidation and of antioxidants has been published [23].

The mechanisms of oxidation reactions are usually complex, involving multiple pathways for the initiation, propagation, branching, and termination. Many oxidation reactions are catalyzed by acids and bases [23]. Often autoxidation reactions are initiated by trace amounts of impurities such as metal ions or hydroperoxides. Thus, ferric ion catalyzes the degradation reaction and decreases the induction period for the oxidation of the compound procaterol [24]. As little as 0.0002 M copper ion has been shown to increase the rate of vitamin C oxidation by a factor of 10^5 [25]. Hydroperoxides contained in polyethylene glycol suppository bases have been implicated in the oxidation of codeine to codeine-*N*-oxide [26]. Peroxides apparently are responsible for the accelerated degradation of benzocaine hydrochloride in aqueous cetomacrogol solution [27] and of a corticosteriod in polyethylene glycol 300 [28,29]. Butyl *p*-hydroxybenzoate, formulated in a suspension containing poly(ethylene glycol) and polysorbate 80, was found to turn yellow under ambient conditions if not adequately protected from oxygen. The degradation product, oxalamidine, may be formed by the reaction of butamben with an oxidation product of poly(-ethylene glycol) [30].

The formation of peroxides and formaldehyde in the high-purity polyoxyethylene surfactants in toiletries has been shown to lead to contact dermatitis [31]. Peroxides in hydrogenated castor oil can cause autoxidation of miconazole [32]. Oxidative decomposition of the polyoxyethylene chains occurs at elevated temperature, leading to the formation of ethylene glycol, which may then be oxidized to formaldehyde. When polyethylene glycol and poloxamer were used to prepare solid dispersions of bendroflumethiazide, a potent, lipophilic diuretic drug, the drug reacted with the formaldehyde to produce hydroflumethiazide [33].

In the case of nucleotides, oxidation mainly involves the reactions of reactive oxygen species such as the hydroxyl radical (·OH), hydrogen peroxide (H_2O_2), superoxide ($\cdot O_2^-$), and/or singlet oxygen ($^1O_2$). They are generated by ionizing irradiation, photolysis, and/or the metal-catalyzed reduction of oxygen or decomposition of peroxides [34].

A list of some functional groups that are subject to autoxidation is shown in Table 2. The products of oxidation are usually electronically more conjugated; thus, the appearance of, or a change in,

Table 2 Some Functional Groups Subject to Autoxidation

Functional group		Examples
Phenols	HO–C_6H_4–R	Phenols in steroids
Catechols	$(HO)_2C_6H_3$–R	Catecholamines (dopamine, isoproterenol)
Ethers	R–O–R'	Diethylether
Thiols	RCH_2SH	Dimercaprol (BAL)
Thioethers	R–S–R'	Phenothiazines (chlorpromazine)
Carboxylic acids	RCOOH	Fatty acids
Nitrites	RNO_2	Amyl nitrite
Aldehydes	RCHO	Paraldehyde
Amines	R(R')N-H	Morphine Clozapine (to N-oxides)

color in a dosage form is suggestive of the occurrence of oxidative degradation.

Photolysis

Normal sunlight or room light may cause substantial degradation of drug molecules. The energy from light radiation must be absorbed by the molecules to cause a photolytic reaction. If that energy is sufficient to achieve activation, degradation of the molecule is possible. Saturated molecules do not interact with visible or near-ultraviolet light, but molecules that contain π-electrons usually do absorb light throughout this wavelength range. Consequently, compounds such as aromatic hydrocarbons, their heterocyclic analogs, aldehydes, ketones, etc., are most susceptible to photolysis. In general, drugs that absorb light at wavelengths below 280 nm have the potential to undergo decomposition in sunlight, and drugs with absorption maxima greater than 400 nm have the potential for degradation in both sunlight and room light. Fortunately, most pharmaceuticals can be protected adequately from photodegradation by the use of appropriate packaging.

A dramatic example of photolysis is the photodegradation of sodium nitroprusside in aqueous solution. Sodium nitroprusside, $Na_2Fe(CN)_5NO{\cdot}2\ H_2O$, is administered by intravenous infusion for the management of acute hypertension. If the solution is protected from light it is stable for at least one year; if exposed to normal room light, it has a shelf life of only 4 hours [35].

Photolysis reactions often are associated with oxidation because the latter category of reactions frequently can be initiated by light. The photooxidation of phenothiazines with the formation of N- and S-oxides is typical. But photolysis reactions are not restricted to oxidation. In the case of sodium nitroprusside, it is believed that degradation results from loss of the nitroligand from the molecule, followed by electronic rearrangement and hydration. Photo-induced reactions are common in steroids [36]; an example is the formation of 2-benzoylcholestan-3-one following irradiation of cholest-2-en-3-ol benzoate. Photoadditions of water and of alcohols to the electronically excited state of steroids have also been observed [37].

Phototoxicity caused by drugs is a problem that is being observed with greater frequency. The primary reactions responsible for initiating phototoxicity can usually be described in terms of basic photochemical reaction patterns. These often involve generation of singlet state excited oxygen. Phototoxic drugs include furosemide, acetazolamide, triamterine, thiocolchicoside, and chlorthalidone [38].

A guideline for evaluation of the photostability of new drug substances and dosage forms was published in 1997 [39]. Subsequently, a joint study was undertaken by the U.S. Food and Drug Administration (FDA) and Pharmaceutical Research and Manufacturers of America to evaluate the ICH guideline. A draft chapter for the United States Pharmacopeia, based on the guideline and the joint study, has been published in Pharmacopeial Forum [40].

Dehydration

The preferred route of degradation for prostaglandin E_2 and tetracycline is the elimination of a water molecule from their structures. The driving force for this type of covalent dehydration is the formation of a double bond that can then participate in electronic resonance with neighboring functional groups. In physical dehydration processes, such as those occurring in theophylline hydrate and ampicillin trihydrate [41], water removal does not create new bonds but often changes the crystalline structure of the drug. Since it is possible that anhydrous compounds may have different dissolution rates compared to their hydrates [42,43], dehydration reactions involving water of crystallization may potentially affect the absorption rate of the dosage form.

Racemization

The racemization of pharmacologically active agents is of interest because enantiomers often have significantly different absorption, distribution, metabolism, and excretion, in addition to differing pharmacological actions [44]. The best known racemization reactions of drugs are those that involve epinephrine, pilocarpine, ergotamine, and tetracycline. In these cases, the reaction mechanism appears to involve an intermediate carbonium ion or carbanion, which is stabilized electronically by the neighboring substituent group. For example, in the racemization of pilocarpine [45], a carbanion is produced and stabilized by delocalization to the enolate. In addition to the racemization reaction, pilocarpine is also degraded through hydrolysis of the lactone ring.

Most racemization reactions are catalyzed by acid and/or by base. A notable exception is the "spontaneous" racemization of the diuretic and antihypertensive agent, chlorthalidone, which undergoes facile S_N1 solvolysis of its tertiary hydroxyl group to form a planar carbonium ion. Chiral configuration is then restored by nucleophilic attack (S_N2) of a molecule of water on the carbonium ion with subsequent elimination of a proton [46].

When configurational stability is truly low and results in half-lives of racemization or epimerization, which are on the order of minutes or hours, the phenomenon has pharmacological significance. On the other hand, when the half-lives are on the order of months or years, the phenomenon has pharmaceutical significance and may shorten the shelf life of drugs [47].

Incompatibilities

Chemical interactions between two or more drug components in the same dosage form, or between active ingredient and a pharmaceutical adjuvant, occur frequently. An example of drug-drug incompatibility is the inactivation of cationic aminoglycoside antibiotics, such as kanamycin and gentamycin, by anionic penicillins in IV admixtures. The formation of an inactive complex between these two classes of antibiotics occurs not only in vitro but apparently also in vivo in patients with severe renal failure [48]. Thus, when gentamycin sulfate was given alone to patients on long-term hemodialysis, the biological half-life of gentamycin was greater than 60 hours. But, when carbenicillin disodium (CD) was given with gentamycin sulfate (GS) in the dose ratio CD/GS = 80:1, the gentamycin half-life was reduced to about 24 hours.

Incompatibilities have also been observed in solid dosage forms. A typical tablet contain binders, disintegrants, lubricants and fillers. Compatibility screening for a new drug should consider two or more excipients from each class. Serajuddin et al. have developed a drug-excipient compatibility screening model to predict interactions of drug substances with excipients [49].

Many pharmaceutical incompatibilities are the result of reactions involving the amine functional group. A summary of the potential interactions that can occur between various functional groups is given in Table 3. The Maillard reaction between simple amines or amino acids, peptides or proteins, and carbonyl compounds, such as the "glycosidic" hydroxyl group of reducing sugars, is typical and often results in mottling of tablets. It is a variant of the Schiff's base reaction. One would think that pharmaceutical scientists would realize by now that combinations of lactose and primary or secondary amines will lead to Amadori rearrangement products, which are responsible for browning reactions; however, this topic remains the subject of many reports [50,51].

Table 3 Some Potential Drug Incompatibilities

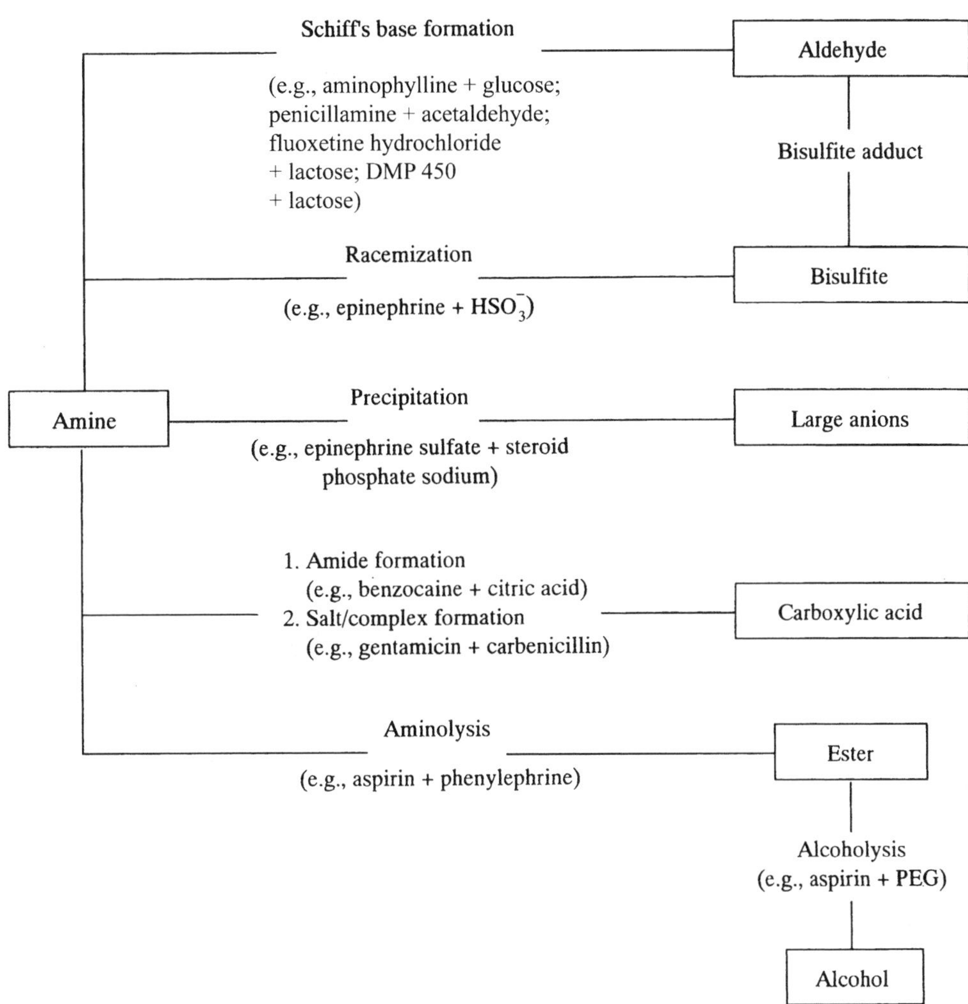

The Maillard reaction is likely to take on additional significance with the introduction of many new protein and peptide pharmaceuticals. For example, Tarelli et al. have demonstrated that lysine vasopressin undergoes rapid glycation in the presence of reducing sugars in both aqueous and solid formulations and that the N-terminal adduct can form rapidly even at $-20°C$ [52]. A textbook that deals with the consequences for the chemical and life sciences of the Maillard reaction has been published [53].

Other Chemical Degradation Reactions

Other chemical reactions, such as hydration, decarboxylation, or pyrolysis, are also potential routes for drug degradation. For example, cyanocobalamin may absorb about 12% of water when exposed to air, and *p*-aminosalicyclic acid decomposes with evolution of carbon dioxide to form *m*-aminophenol when subjected to temperatures above 40°C. The temperature at which pyrolytic decomposition of terfenadine occurs has been used as a criterion for determining which of several tablet excipients will be preferable with respect to long-term stability of the drug substance [54].

B. Physical Degradative Routes

Polymorphs are different crystal forms of the same compound [55]. They are usually prepared by crystallization of the drug from different solvents under diverse conditions. However, exposure to changes in temperature, pressure, relative humidity, and comminution which are encountered in processes such as drying, granulation, milling, and compression may also lead to polymorphic transformations.

Steroids, sulfonamides, and barbiturates are notorious for their propensity to form polymorphs [56]. Yang and Guillory [57] attempted to correlate the frequency of occurrence of polymorphism in sulfonamides with certain aspects of chemical structure. They found that sulfonamides that did not exhibit polymorphism have somewhat higher melting points and heats of fusion than those that were polymorphic. The absence of polymorphism in sulfacetamide was attributed to the stronger hydrogen bonds formed by the amide hydrogen in this molecule. These stronger hydrogen bonds were not readily stretched or broken to form alternate crystalline structures.

Since polymorphs differ from one another in their crystal energies, the more energetic ones will seek to revert to the most stable (and the least energetic) crystal form. When several polymorphs and solvates (substances that incorporate solvent in a stoichiometric fashion into the crystal lattice) are present, the conditions under which they may interconvert can become quite complex, as is true of fluprednisolone [58].

Polymorphs may exhibit significant differences in important physicochemical parameters such as solubility, dissolution rate, and melting point [59]. Thus the conversion from one polymorph to another in a pharmaceutical dosage form may lead to a drastic change in the physical characteristics of the drug. A well-known example of this phenomenon is the conversion of a more soluble crystal form (form II) of cortisone acetate to a less soluble form (form V) when the drug is formulated into an aqueous suspension [60]. This phase change leads to caking of the cortisone acetate suspension.

The phenomenon of pseudopolymorphism is also observed, i.e., compounds can crystallize with one or more molecules of solvent in the crystal lattice. Conversion from solvated to nonsolvated, or hydrate to anhydrous, and vice versa, can lead to changes in solid-state properties. For example, a moisture-mediated phase transformation of carbamazepine to the dihydrate has been reported to be responsible for whisker growth on the surface of tablets. The effect can be retarded by the inclusion of Polyoxamer 184 in the tablet formulation [61].

Another physical property that can affect the appearance, bioavailability, and chemical stability of pharmaceuticals is degree of crystallinity. Amorphous materials tend to be more hygroscopic than their crystalline counterparts. Also, there is a substantial body of evidence that indicates that the amorphous forms of drugs are less stable than their crystalline counterparts [62]. It has been reported, for example, that crystalline cyclophosphamide [63] is much more stable than the amorphous form. Paradoxically, M. J. Pikal and D. R. Rigsbee have reported that in the case of biosynthetic human insulin, the amorphous form is more stable [64].

Vaporization

Some drugs and pharmaceutical adjuvants possess sufficiently high vapor pressures at room temperature that their volatilization constitutes a major route of drug loss. Flavors, whose constituents are mainly ketones, aldehydes, and esters, and cosolvents (low molecular weight alcohols) may be lost from the formulation in this manner. The most frequently cited example of a pharmaceutical that "degrades" by this route is nitroglycerin, which has a vapor pressure of 0.00026 mm at 20°C and 0.31 mm at 93°C [65]. Significant drug loss to the environment can occur during patient storage and use. In 1972, FDA issued special regulations governing the types of containers that may be used for dispensing sublingual nitroglycerin tablets [66].

Reduction of vapor pressure and, hence, of volatility of drugs such as nitroglycerin can be achieved through dispersion of the volatile drug in macromolecules that can provide physicochemical interactions. The addition of macromolecules such as polyethylene glycol, polyvinylpyrrolidone, and microcrystalline cellulose allows for preparation of "stabilized" nitroglycerin sublingual tablets [67,68]. A β-cyclodextrin-nitroglycerin tablet is currently being marketed in Japan to achieve the same purpose.

Another aspect of nitroglycerin instability has been observed by Fusari [68]. When conventional (unstabilized) nitroglycerin sublingual tablets are stored in enclosed glass containers, the high volatility of the drug gives rise to redistribution of nitroglycerin among the stored tablets. Interestingly, this redistribution leads to an increase in the standard deviation of the drug contents of the tablets, rather than the reverse. This migration phenomenon results in a deterioration in the uniformity of the tablets upon storage.

"Aging"

The most interesting and perhaps the least-reported area of concern regarding the physical instability of pharmaceutical dosage forms is generally termed "aging." This is a process through which changes in the disintegration and/or dissolution characteristics of the dosage form are caused by subtle, and sometimes unexplained, alterations in the physicochemical properties of the inert ingredients or the active drug in the dosage form [69]. Since the disintegration and dissolution steps may be the rate-determining steps in the absorption of a drug, changes in these processes as a function of the "age" of the dosage form may result in corresponding changes in the bioavailability of the drug product.

An example of this phenomenon was provided by deBlaey and Rutten-Kingma [70], who showed that the melting time of aminophylline suppositories, prepared from various bases, increased from about 20 minutes to over an hour after 24 weeks of storage at 22°C. Like the dissolution time for solid dosage forms, the melting time for suppositories can be viewed as an in vitro index of drug release. Thus, an increase in melting time can perceivably lead to a decrease in bioavailability. The mechanism responsible for this change appeared to involve an interaction between the ethylenediamine in aminophylline and the free fatty acids present in the suppository bases. Interestingly, no increase in melting time was detected when the suppositories were stored at 4°C, even up to 15 months.

"Aging" of solid dosage forms can cause a decrease in their in vitro rate of dissolution [71], but a corresponding decrease in in vivo absorption cannot be assumed automatically. For example, Chemburkar et al. [72] showed that when a methaqualone tablet was stored at 80% relative humidity for 7–8 months, the dissolution rate as measured by in vivo absorption was not affected. This lack of in vitro dissolution–in vivo absorption correlation for the aged product was observed even though the particular dissolution method (that of the resin flask) was shown by the same workers to be capable of discriminating between the absorption of several trial dosage forms of the same drug.

Adsorption

Drug-plastic interaction is increasingly being recognized as a major potential problem when intravenous solutions are stored in bags or infused via administration sets that are made from polyvinyl chloride (PVC). For example, up to 50% drug loss can occur after nitroglycerin is stored in PVC infusion bags for 7 days at room temperature [73]. This loss can be attributed to adsorption rather than chemical degradation because the drug can be recovered from the inner surface of the container by rinsing with a less polar solvent (methanol in this case). Similarly, more than 40% of a dose of quinidine gluconate was lost when the drug was administered with a conventional PVC intravenous administration set. Drug loss was reduced by using a winged intravenous catheter and shorter tubing [74]. A diverse array of drugs, including diazepam [75], insulin [76], isosorbide dinitrate [77], and others [78], has shown substantial adsorption to PVC. The propensity for significant adsorption is related to the oil/water partition coefficient of the drug since this process depends on the relative affinity of the drug for the hydrophobic PVC (dielectric constant of about 3) and the hydrophilic aqueous infusion medium.

Physical Instability in Heterogeneous Systems

The stability of suspensions, emulsions, creams, and ointments is dealt with in other chapters. The unique characteristics of solid-state decomposition processes have been described in reviews by D. C. Monkhouse [79,80] and in the monograph on drug stability by J. T. Carstensen [81]. Baitalow et al. have applied an unconventional approach to the kinetic analysis of solid-state reactions [82]. The recently published monograph on solid-state chemistry of drugs also treats this topic in great detail [83].

III. QUANTITATION OF RATE OF DEGRADATION

Before undertaking a discussion of the mathematics involved in the determination of reaction rates is undertaken, it is necessary to point out the importance of proper data acquisition in stability testing. Applications of rate equations and predictions are meaningful only if the data utilized in such processes are collected using valid statistical and analytical procedures. It is beyond the scope of this chapter to discuss the proper statistical treatments and analytical techniques that should be used in a stability study. Some perspectives in these areas can be obtained by reading the comprehensive review by Meites [84], the paper by P. Wessels et al. [85], and the section on statistical considerations in the stability guidelines published by FDA in 1987 [86] and in the more recent *Guidance for Industry* published in June 1998 [87].

A. Kinetic Equations

Consider the reaction

$$aA + bB \rightarrow mM + nN \tag{1}$$

where A and B are the reactants, M and N the products, and $a, b, m,$ and n the stoichiometric coefficients describing the reaction. The rate of change of the concentration C of any of the species can be expressed by the differential notations $-dC_A/dt$, $-dC_B/dt$, dC_M/dt, and dC_N/dt. Note that the rates of change for the reactants are preceded by a negative sign, denoting a decrease in concentration relative to time (rate of disappearance). In contrast, the differential terms for the products are positive in sign, indicating an increase in concentration of these species as time increases (rate of appearance). The rates of disappearance of A and B and the rates of appearance of M and N are interrelated by equations that take into account the stoichiometry of the reaction:

$$-\frac{1}{a}\frac{dC_A}{dt} = -\frac{1}{b}\frac{dC_B}{dt} = \frac{1}{m}\frac{dC_M}{dt} = \frac{1}{n}\frac{dC_N}{dt} \tag{2}$$

The Rate Expression

The rate expression is a mathematical description of the rate of the reaction at any time t in terms of the concentration(s) of the molecular species present at that time. By using the hypothetical reaction $aA + bB \rightarrow$ products, the rate expression can be written as

$$-\frac{dC_A}{dt} = -\frac{dC_B}{dt} \propto C^a_{A(t)} C^b_{B(t)} \tag{3}$$

Equation (3) in essence states that the rate of change of the concentration of A at time t is equal to that of B and that each of these changes at time t is proportional to the product of the concentrations of the reactants raised to the respective prowers. Note that $C_{A(t)}$ and $C_{B(t)}$ are time-dependent variables. As the reaction proceeds, both $C_{A(t)}$ and $C_{B(t)}$ will decrease in magnitude. For simplicity, these concentrations can be denoted simply by C_A and C_B, respectively.

$$-\frac{dC_A}{dt} = -\frac{dC_B}{dt} = kC^a_A C^b_B \tag{4}$$

where k is a proportionality constant, commonly referred to as the reaction rate constant or the specific rate constant. The format for rate expressions generally involves concentration terms of only the reactants and very rarely those of the products. The latter occurs only when the products participate in the reaction once it has been initiated.

The order of the reaction, n, can be defined as $n = a + b$. Extended to the general case, the order of a reaction is the numerical sum of the exponents of the concentration terms in the rate expression. Thus if $a = b = 1$, the reaction just described is said to be second-order overall, first-order relative to A, and first-order relative to B. In principle, the numerical value of a or b can be integral or fractional.

Special attention is directed to those instances in which the rate of reaction is apparently independent of the concentration of one of the reactants, even though this reactant is consumed during the reaction. For example, in the reaction between an ester and water (hydrolysis) in a predominantly aqueous environment, the theoretical rate expression for the ester can be written in terms of the concentrations of the ester (C_E) and water (C_W):

$$-\frac{dC_E}{dt} = kC_E C_W \tag{5}$$

If the initial concentration of the ester is 0.5 M or less, complete hydrolysis of the ester will bring about a corresponding decrease in the concentration of water of 0.5 M or less. Since the initial water concentration is 1000/18, which is about 55 M for an aqueous solution, the loss of water through reaction is insignificantly small and C_W can be considered a constant throughout the entire course of the reaction. Thus, in practice,

$$-\frac{dC_E}{dt} = k_\pi C_E \tag{6}$$

where $k_\pi = kC_W$. The reaction is thus apparently first-order relative to ester and zero-order relative to water; the overall reaction is known as a pseudo-first-order reaction and k_π the pseudo-first-order constant.

This type of kinetics is observed whenever the concentration of one of the reactants is maintained constant, either by a vast excess initial concentration or by rapid replenishment of one of the reactants. Thus, if one of the reactants is the hydrogen ion or the hydroxide ion, its concentration, though probably small when compared with that of the drug, can be kept constant throughout the reaction by using buffers in the solution. Similarly, the concentration of an unstable drug in solution can be maintained invariant by preparing a drug suspension, thus providing excess solid in equilibrium with the drug in solution.

Simple Reactions

It is obvious that to quantify the rate expression, the magnitude of the rate constant k needs to be determined. Proper assignment of the reaction order and accurate determination of the rate constant is important when reaction mechanisms are to be deduced from the kinetic data. The integrated form of the reaction equation is easier to use in handling kinetic data. The integrated kinetic relationships commonly used for zero-, first-, and second-order reactions are summarized in Table 4. [The reader is advised that basic kinetic

Table 4 Rate Expressions for Zero-, First-, and Second-Order Reactions

	Zero-order	First-order	Second-order: $a = b = c_0$	Second-order: $a \neq b$
Differential rate expression	$-\frac{dc}{dt} = k$	$-\frac{dc}{dt} = kc$	$-\frac{dc}{dt} = kc^2$	$-\frac{dc}{dt} = kc_a c_b$
Integrated rate expression	$k = \frac{c_0 - c}{t}$	$k = \frac{1}{t}\ln\frac{c_0}{c}$	$\frac{1}{c} - \frac{1}{c_0} = kt$	$k = \frac{1}{t(a-b)}\ln\frac{b(a-x)}{a(b-x)}$
$t_{1/2}$	$\frac{c_0}{2k}$	$\frac{0.693}{k}$	$\frac{1}{c_0 k}$	(i) When $x = 0.5a$ $\frac{1}{k(a-b)}\ln\frac{0.5ab}{a(b-0.5a)}$ (ii) When $x = 0.5b$ $\frac{1}{k(a-b)}\ln\frac{b(a-0.5b)}{0.5ab}$
$t_{90\%}$	$\frac{c_0}{10k}$	$\frac{0.105}{k}$	$\frac{0.11}{c_0 k}$	(i) When $x = 0.1a$ $\frac{1}{k(a-b)}\ln\frac{0.9ab}{a(b-0.1a)}$ (ii) When $x = 0.1b$ $\frac{1}{k(a-b)}\ln\frac{b(a-0.1b)}{0.9ab}$

theory is also extensively exploited in pharmacokinetics; for further information on this subject, see Chapter 3.] The concentration symbols in Table 4 are defined as follows: c is the concentration of the drug at any time t and c_0 is the initial concentration. In the last column describing a second-order reaction in which the reactants A and B do not have the same initial concentrations, these are designated as a and b, respectively; x is the concentration reacted at time t.

In a reaction of either zero-order or second-order, the time to reach a certain fraction of the initial concentration, for example, $t_{1/2}$ or $t_{90\%}$ [the time required for the drug concentration to decrease to 90% of its original value (i.e., 10% degradation)] is dependent on c_0. This is illustrated in Fig. 1, in which a zero-order reaction (Fig. 1a) and a second-order reaction (Fig. 1b) are plotted with two initial concentrations. It is readily seen that for a zero-order reaction, the $t_{1/2}$ increases

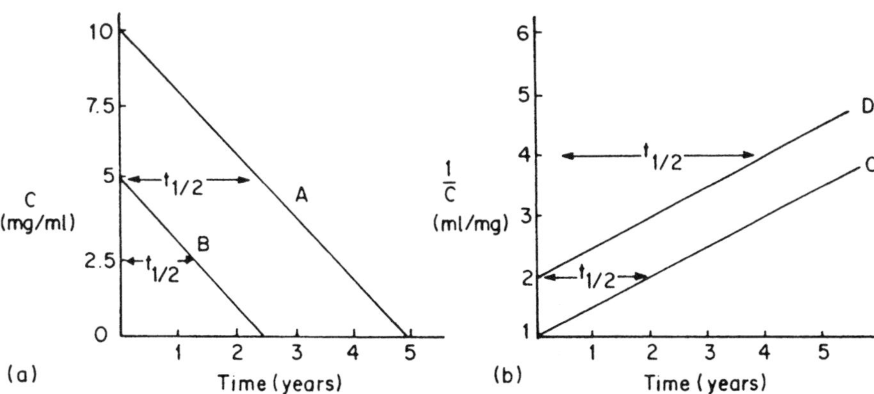

Fig. 1 Effect of initial concentration on the half-life of (a) a zero-order and (b) a second-order reaction. In (a), $k = 2$ mg/year-mL; curve A, initial concentration $c_0 = 10$ mg/mL, $t_{1/2} = 2.5$ years; curve B, $c_0 = 5$ mg/mL, $t_{1/2} = 1.25$ years. In (b), $k = 0.5$ mL/mg-year; curve C, $c_0 = 1$ mg/mL, $t_{1/2} = 2$ years; curve D, $c_0 = 0.5$ mg/mL, $t_{1/2} = 4$ years.

with a higher initial concentration. Conversely, for a second-order reaction, $t_{1/2}$ decreases with increasing initial concentration. For a reaction obeying first-order kinetics, the $t_{1/2}$ or $t_{90\%}$ is independent of c_0.

Complex Reactions

Parallel First-Order Reactions. In many instances, the active drug may degrade through more than one pathway:

$$A \xrightarrow{k_1} B, \quad A \xrightarrow{k_2} C, \quad A \xrightarrow{k_3} D \tag{7}$$

If the concentration of the active drug, A, can be monitored, the composite rate constant, $k' = k_1 + k_2 + k_3$, can easily be determined from the relationship $[A] = [A]_0 e^{-k't}$, where $[A]_0$ is the initial concentration and [A] is the concentration at time t. If the concentrations of A cannot be determined because of assay difficulties, it is still possible to determine k' by monitoring one of the degradation products. For example, if the concentrations of B can be assayed as a function of time, and the concentration of B at time infinity, $[B]_\infty$, is also determined, the following relationships can be derived:

$$[B] = \frac{k_1}{k'}[A]_0(1 - e^{-k't}) \tag{8}$$

$$[B]_\infty = \frac{k_1}{k'}[A]_0 \tag{9}$$

$$\ln\left(1 - \frac{[B]}{[B]_\infty}\right) = -k't \tag{10}$$

Approach to Equilibrium Through First-Order Reactions. This type of reaction can be represented by Eq. (11):

$$A \underset{k_2}{\overset{k_1}{\rightleftharpoons}} B \tag{11}$$

The concentrations of A and B as a function of time can be derived:

$$[A] = \frac{k_2}{k_1 + k_2}[A]_0 + \frac{k_1}{k_1 + k_2}[A]_0(e^{-(k_1+k_2)t}) \tag{12}$$

$$[B] = \frac{k_1}{k_1 + k_2}[A]_0(1 - e^{-(k_1+k_2)t}) \tag{13}$$

The combined constants $(k_1 + k_2)$ can be obtained through Eq. (14), and the individual rate constants k_1 and k_2 can now be calculated through Eq. (15):

$$\ln([A] - [A]_\infty) = \ln [B]_\infty - (k_1 + k_2)t \tag{14}$$

$$k_1[A]_\infty = k_2[B]_\infty \tag{15}$$

Fractional Order. In the decomposition of pure solids, the kinetics of reactions can often be more complex than simple zero- or first-order processes. Carstensen [88] has reviewed the stability of solids and solid dosage forms as well as the equations that can be used in these cases. In addition to zero- and first-order kinetics, solid-state degradations are often described by fractional-order equations.

More complicated reactions schemes, including first-order reversible consecutive processes and competitive consecutive reactions, are considered in a textbook by Irwin [89]. Professor Irwin's textbook also includes computer programs written in the BASIC language. These programs can be used to fit data to the models described.

B. Energetics of Reactions

According to the transition state theory, the reaction between two molecules, A and B, to form products C and D proceeds through a transition state, X:

$$A + B \overset{K^\ddagger}{\rightleftharpoons} X \rightarrow C + D \tag{16}$$

Here $K^\ddagger$ is a thermodynamic equilibrium constant that can be expressed as a function of the activities [Eq. (17)] or of the activity coefficients γ_X, γ_A, and γ_B [Eq. (18)]:

$$K^\ddagger = \frac{a_X}{a_A a_B} \tag{17}$$

$$K^\ddagger = \frac{[X]}{[A][B]}\frac{\gamma_X}{\gamma_A \gamma_B} \tag{18}$$

The rate of the reaction $-d[A]/dt$ is proportional to the concentration of the transition state

$$-\frac{d[A]}{dt} = k'[X] \tag{19}$$

where k' is a proportionality constant. Combining Eqs. (18) and (19) yields

$$-\frac{d[A]}{dt} = k'K^\ddagger[A][B]\frac{\gamma_A \gamma_B}{\gamma_X} \tag{20}$$

If the activity coefficients are assumed to be unity, the specific rate constant k is then identical to $k'K^{\ddagger}$. It can be shown that

$$k' = \frac{k_B T}{h} \tag{21}$$

where k_B is Boltzmann's constant, h is Planck's constant, and T is the absolute temperature. Thus,

$$k = \frac{k_B T}{h} K^{\ddagger} \tag{22}$$

and

$$\ln k = \ln \frac{k_B}{h} + \ln T + \ln K^{\ddagger} \tag{23}$$

Differentiating relative to T, we obtain

$$\frac{d \ln K^{\ddagger}}{dT} = \frac{d \ln k}{dt} - \frac{1}{T} \tag{24}$$

Since

$$\frac{d \ln K^{\ddagger}}{dT} = \frac{\Delta H^{\ddagger}}{RT^2} \tag{25}$$

where $\Delta H^{\ddagger}$ is the enthalpy of activation, Eq. (26) can be obtained by combining Eqs. (24) and (25):

$$\frac{d \ln k}{dT} = \frac{\Delta H^{\ddagger} + RT}{RT^2} \tag{26}$$

The classic Arrhenius equation is given by Eq. (27), where E_a is the energy of activation:

$$\frac{d \ln k}{dT} = \frac{E_a}{RT^2} \tag{27}$$

On comparing Eqs. (26) and (27), it follows that

$$\Delta H^{\ddagger} = E_a - RT \tag{28}$$

The other thermodynamic parameters, $\Delta G^{\ddagger}$ and $\Delta S^{\ddagger}$, the free energy and entropy of activation, respectively, can also be obtained from the foregoing relationships:

$$\Delta G^{\ddagger} = -RT \ln K^{\ddagger} = -RT \ln \frac{kh}{k_B T} \tag{29}$$

and

$$\Delta S^{\ddagger} = -\frac{\Delta G^{\ddagger} + \Delta H^{\ddagger}}{T} = R \ln \frac{kh}{k_B T} + \frac{E_a - RT}{T} \tag{30}$$

The magnitudes of the thermodynamic parameters, $\Delta H^{\ddagger}$ and $\Delta S^{\ddagger}$, sometimes provide evidence supporting proposed mechanisms of drug decomposition. The enthalpy of activation is a measure of the energy barrier that must be overcome by the reacting molecules before a reaction can occur. As can be seen from Eq. (28), its numerical value is less than the Arrhenius energy of activation by the factor RT. At room temperature, RT is only about 0.6 kcal/mol. The entropy of activation can be related to the Arrhenius frequency factor (i.e., the fraction of molecules possessing the requisite energy that actually reacts). This parameter includes steric and orientation requirements of the reactants, the transition state, and the solvent molecules surrounding them. For unimolecular reactions, $\Delta S^{\ddagger}$ has a value of near zero or slightly positive. For bimolecular reactions, $\Delta S^{\ddagger}$ is more negative. For example, in the hydrolysis of esters and anhydrides, the entropy of activation is on the order of -20 to -50 entropy units, reflecting a transition state in which several solvent molecules are immobilized for solvation of the developing charges [90].

IV. THE ARRHENIUS EQUATION AND ACCELERATED STABILITY TESTING

The purpose of stability testing is to assess the effects of temperature, humidity, light, and other environmental factors on the quality of a drug substance or product. The data produced are used to establish storage conditions, retest periods, shelf loss, and to justify overages included in products for stability reasons. The most useful equation relating temperature and reaction rate is the Arrhenius equation. This equation (27) may be integrated and rewritten as Eqs. (31) and (32).

$$k = Ae^{-E_a/RT} \tag{31}$$

$$\ln \frac{k_1}{k_2} = \frac{E_a}{R}\left(\frac{1}{T_2} - \frac{1}{T_1}\right) \tag{32}$$

where E_a is a constant and the subscripts 1 and 2 denote the two different temperature conditions. A plot of $\ln k$ as a function of $1/T$, referred to as the *Arrhenius plot*, is linear according to Eq. (31) if E_a is independent of temperature. It is thus possible to conduct kinetic experiments at elevated temperatures and obtain estimates of rate constants at lower temperatures by extrapolation of the Arrhenius plot. This procedure, commonly referred to as accelerated stability testing, is most useful when the reaction at ambient temperatures is too slow to be monitored conveniently and when E_a is relatively high. For example, for a reaction with an E_a of 25 kcal/mol, an increase from 25 to 45°C brings about a 14-fold increase in the reaction rate constant. In comparison, a rate increase of just threefold is obtained for the same elevation in temperature when E_a is 10 kcal/mol. The magnitude of E_a for a reaction can be obtained from the slope of its Arrhenius plot.

Hydrolysis reactions typically have an E_a of 10–30 kcal/mol, while oxidation and photolysis reactions have smaller energies of activation [91].

The elevated temperatures most commonly used are 40, 50, and 60°C in conjunction with ambient humidity. Occasionally, higher temperatures are used. The samples stored at the highest temperatures are examined weekly for physical and chemical changes. If a substantial change is seen, samples stored at lower temperatures are examined. If there is no change after 30 days at 60°C, the stability prognosis is excellent. Corroborative evidence must be obtained by monitoring the samples stored at lower temperatures for longer durations.

An underlying assumption of the Arrhenius equation is that the reaction mechanism does not change as a function of temperature (i.e., E_a is independent of temperature). Since accelerated stability testing of pharmaceutical products normally employs a narrow range of temperature (typically, 35°C to at most 70°C), it is often difficult to detect nonlinearity in the Arrhenius plot from experimental data, even though such nonlinearity is expected from the reaction mechanism [92]. Thus, even complex biological processes may show Arrhenius behavior within certain temperature ranges; Laidler [93] cited such phenomena as the frequency of flashing of fireflies and the rate of the terrapin's heartbeat as examples.

Non-Arrhenius behavior has been observed in pharmaceutical systems [94]. This may be attributed to the possible evaporation of solvent, multiple reaction pathways, change in physical form of the formulation, and so on [95] when the temperature of the reaction is changed. An interesting case of non-Arrhenius behavior is the increased rate of decomposition of ampicillin upon freezing. Savello and Shangraw [96] showed that for a 1% sodium ampicillin solution in 5% dextrose, the percentage of degradation at 4 hours is approximately 14% at −20°C, compared to 6% at 0°C and 10% at 5°C. This decrease in stability in frozen solutions is observed most frequently when the reaction obeys second- or higher-order kinetics. For example, the formation of nitrosomorpholine from morpholine and nitrite obeys third-order kinetics [97], and the rate of nitrosation is drastically enhanced in frozen solutions (Fig. 2). A marked acceleration in the hydrolytic degradation of methyl, ethyl, and *n*-propyl 4-hydroxybenzoates in the frozen state has also been reported by Shiva et al. [98]. These authors found that although pseudo-first-order conditions found in the liquid state are also observed in the frozen state, the rate of reaction under frozen state conditions showed very much less dependency on the initial hydroxide ion concentration.

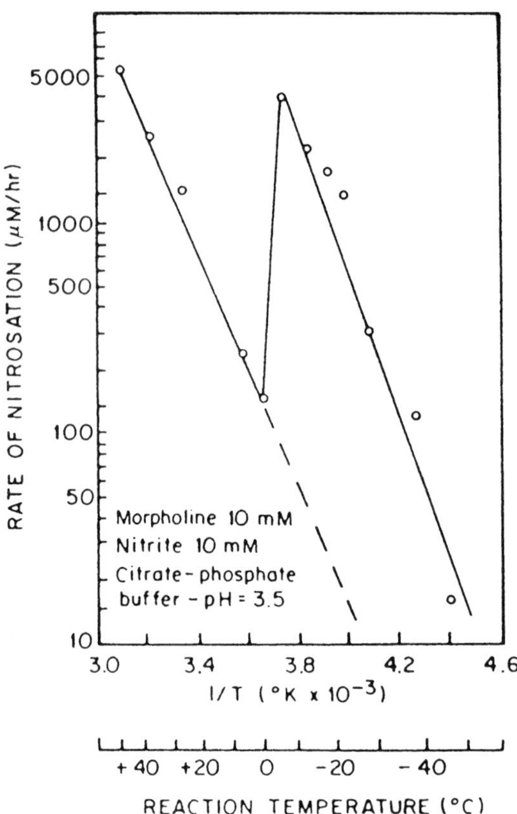

Fig. 2 Effect of temperature on the rate of nitrosation of morpholine with nitrite in citrate-sodium phosphate buffer for temperatures above and below the freezing temperature. (From Ref. 97.). Reproduced with the permission of the Copyright holder, the American Chemical Society, © 1975.

The mechanism for rate enhancement in frozen solutions has been reviewed by Pincock [99]. In reactions following second- or higher-order kinetics, an increase in rate may be brought about by concentration of the reactants in the liquid phase, the solute molecules being excluded from the ice lattice when the solution freezes. In some cases an increase in rate may be due to a change in pH upon freezing. Fan and Tannenbaum [97] reported that citrate–sodium hydroxide and citrate–potassium phosphate buffers do not change pH upon freezing, but citrate–sodium phosphate buffer at pH 8 decreases to pH 3.5 and sodium hydrogen phosphate at pH 9 decreases to pH 5.5 upon freezing. A possible explanation for this phenomenon is now available [100]. Monosodium phosphate forms supersaturated solutions on cooling that become amorphous, with no precipitation of the salt. The disodium and monopotassium salts, on the other hand, readily precipitated when the initial solution concentration was >0.2 M. The possibility of a pH change and rate acceleration should be considered when evaluating the stability of freeze-dried products. Proteins are particularly sensitive to changes in pH, folding or unfolding to varying degrees in response to changes in pH. Proteins tend to be most stable at their isoelectric point due to electrostatic interactions [101], but when a solution is adjusted to the optimum pH for stability at room temperature using buffers, that pH may not be maintained throughout the lyophilization cycle, and the protein may aggregate or undergo denaturation.

Nonlinearity in Arrhenius plots frequently is observed in following the temperature dependence of protein degradation. Degradation mechanisms in proteins often change with temperature [102]. At 60°C, the aggregation of interleukin 1β (1L-1β) in aqueous solution follows apparent first-order behaviour to 30% drug remaining, but at or below 55°C the aggregation deviates from apparent first-order and becomes biphasic (slow and fast) [103].

Considerable interest has been generated in the use of accelerated stability testing based on a single condition of elevated temperature and humidity. For Abbreviated New Drug Applications (ANDAs) the FDA stability guidelines [86,87] suggest that a tentative expiration date of 24 months may be granted for a drug product if satisfactory stability results can be documented under a stressed condition of 40°C *and* 75% relative humidity. The simplicity of such a guideline is naturally attractive because a substantial saving in time can be obtained in advancing a drug product to the marketplace [104].

V. ENVIRONMENTAL FACTORS THAT AFFECT REACTION RATE

A rational way to develop approaches that will increase the stability of fast-degrading drugs in pharmaceutical dosage forms is thorough study of the factors that can affect such stability. In this section, the factors that can affect decomposition rates are discussed; it will be seen that under certain conditions of pH, solvent, presence of additives, and so on, the stability of a drug may be drastically affected. Equations that may allow prediction of these effects on reaction rates are discussed.

A. pH

The pH of a drug solution may have a very dramatic effect on its stability. Depending on the reaction mechanism, a change of more than 10-fold in rate constant may result from a shift of just one pH unit. When drugs are formulated in solution, it is essential to construct a pH versus rate profile so that the optimum pH for stability can be located. Many pH versus rate profiles are documented in the literature, and they have a variety of shapes. The majority of these pH versus rate profiles can be rationalized using an approach in which the reaction of each molecular species of the drug with hydrogen ion, water, and with hydroxide ion is analyzed as a function of pH. The discussion that follows is divided according to the ionization capability of the drug.

1. When the drug is nonionizable in water, three hydrolytic pathways are available [Eq. (33)]: it can degrade by specific acid catalysis represented by the first kinetic term in Eq. (33), water hydrolysis (second term), and specific base catalysis (third term):

$$-\frac{dc}{dt} = k_1[\mathrm{H}^+]c + k_2c + k_3[\mathrm{OH}^-]c \tag{33}$$

Equation (33) can be rearranged to give

$$-\frac{dc}{c\,dt} = k_{\mathrm{obs}} = k_1[\mathrm{H}^+] + k_2 + k_3[\mathrm{OH}^-] \tag{34}$$

Note that k_1 and k_3 are second-order constants, whereas k_2 is a pseudo-first-order constant. The pH versus rate profile can be constructed by considering, in turn, that one of the three kinetic terms is predominating, thus:

(a) When $k_1[\mathrm{H}^+] >> k_2 + k_3[\mathrm{OH}^-]$,

$$k_{\mathrm{obs}} = k_1[\mathrm{H}^+] \text{ and } \log k_{\mathrm{obs}} = \log k_1 - \mathrm{pH} \tag{35}$$

(b) When $k_2 >> k_1[\mathrm{H}^+] + k_3[\mathrm{OH}^-]$,

$$k_{\mathrm{obs}} = k_2 \text{ and } \log k_{\mathrm{obs}} = \log k_2 \tag{36}$$

(c) When $k_3[\mathrm{OH}^-] >> k_1[\mathrm{H}^+] + k_2$,

$$k_{\mathrm{obs}} = k_3[\mathrm{OH}^-] \text{ and}$$

$$\log k_{\mathrm{obs}} = \log k_3 + \mathrm{pH} \tag{37}$$

Equations (35) through (37) are plotted and shown in Fig. 3a. The lines are stippled to indicate that the relative positions of the lines are not fixed, but are dependent on the relative magnitudes of the rate constants. For example, when $k_3[\mathrm{OH}^-] > k_2 >> k_1[\mathrm{H}^+]$, a $\log k_{\mathrm{obs}}$ versus pH profile such as the one depicted in Fig. 3b may result. On the other hand, if $k_1[\mathrm{H}^+]$ and $k_3[\mathrm{OH}^-]$ are both much greater than k_2, a $\log k_{\mathrm{obs}}$ versus pH profile may resemble the curve shown in Fig. 3c. When $k_1[\mathrm{H}^+] > k_2 >> k_3[\mathrm{OH}^-]$, the $\log k_{\mathrm{obs}}$ versus pH profile

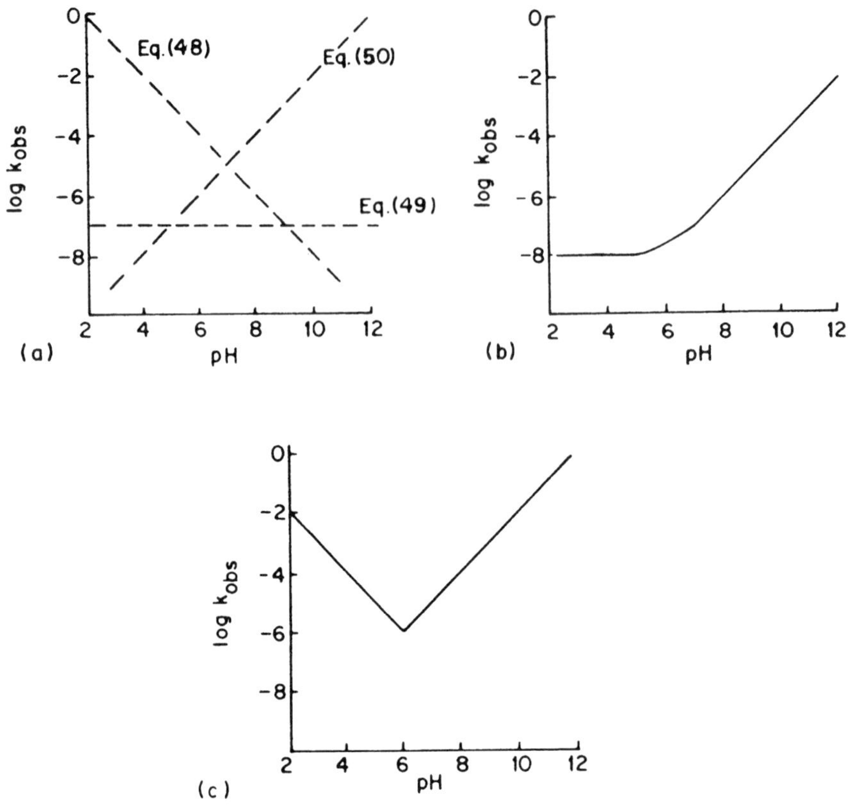

Fig. 3 The log k_{obs} versus pH profiles of nonionizable drugs.

will be a mirror image of Fig. 3b; and when $k_2 >> k_1[H^+] + k_3[OH^-]$, the rate constant will be pH-independent.

2. When the drug is either monoacidic or monobasic, an equation similar to Eq. (34) can be written. Here, however, three kinetic terms are written for the acidic form of the drug, HA, and three terms for the basic form, A (electronic charges on HA and A are not designated here because either HA or A can be charged):

$$k_{obs} = k_1[H^+]f_{HA} + k_2 f_{HA} + k_3[OH^-]f_{HA} + k_4[H^+]f_A + k_5 f_A + k_6[OH^-]f_A$$

where

$$f_{HA} = \frac{[HA]}{[HA] + [A]} = \frac{[H^+]}{[H^+] + K_a} \quad (39)$$

and

$$f_A = \frac{[A]}{[HA] + [A]} = \frac{K_a}{[H^+] + K_a} \quad (40)$$

Again, Eq. (38) can be analyzed by considering each individual term as a function of pH. Since the magnitudes of both f_{HA} and f_A are dependent on the relative magnitudes of K_a and H^+, the kinetic terms can be evaluated under three conditions: (a) when $[H^+] >> K_a$, (b) when $[H^+] = K_a$, and (c) when $[H^+] << K_a$ (Table 5). The log k_{obs} versus pH profile for each kinetic term is shown in Fig. 4, using a hypothetical pK_a of 6 and the condition that $k_1 = 10^7 k_2 = k_3 = K_4 = 10^7 k_5 = k_6 = 1$. Compared with the curves shown in Fig. 3a, the profiles in Fig. 4 show one break each in the lines, with a change of slope of 1 unit at the breaks. It is also seen that term (b) is equivalent to term (d) and that term (c) is equivalent to term (e), as far as their dependency on pH is concerned (see Table 5 and Fig. 4). These terms, therefore, are kinetically equivalent and are indistinguishable from each other in a rate expression. Equation (38), then, can be reduced to a combination of only four terms. The shape of the overall log k_{obs}/pH profile of any drug is determined by the relative magnitudes of the four kinetic terms over the pH range considered. Each log k_{obs} versus pH profile of a

Table 5 Kinetic Expressions for Each Term in Eq. (38)

Logarithm of kinetic term	$\log k_{obs}$ When $[H^+] \gg K_a$	When $[H^+] = K_a$	When $K_a \gg [H^+]$
$\log k_1[H^+]f_{HA}$	$\log k_1 - pH$	$\log \frac{k_1 K_a}{2}$	$\log \frac{k_1}{K_a} - 2\ pH$
$\log k_2 f_{HA}$	$\log k_2$	$\log \frac{k_2}{2}$	$\log \frac{k_2}{K_a} - pH$
$\log k_3[OH^-]f_{HA}$	$\log k_3 K_w + pH$	$\log \frac{k_3 K_w}{2K_a}$	$\log \frac{k_3 K_w}{K_a}$
$\log k_4[H^+]f_A$	$\log k_4 K_a$	$\log \frac{k_4 K_a}{2}$	$\log k_4 - pH$
$\log k_5 f_A$	$\log k_5 K_a + pH$	$\log \frac{k_5}{2}$	$\log k_5$
$\log k_6[OH^-]f_A$	$\log k_6 K_w K_a + 2\ pH$	$\log \frac{k_6 K_w}{2K_a}$	$\log k_6 K_w + pH$

monoacidic or monobasic drug can be adequately described by a combination of no more than four terms. Figure 5 illustrates this principle by showing the log k_{obs} versus pH profiles of idoxuridine [105] and acetylsalicylic acid [106]. The hydrolysis of idoxuridine (see Fig. 5a) as a function of pH can be rationalized by the equation $k_{obs} = k_2 f_{HA} + k_5 f_A^- + k_6[OH^-]f_A^-$ (three kinetic terms), whereas the hydrolysis of acetylsalicylic

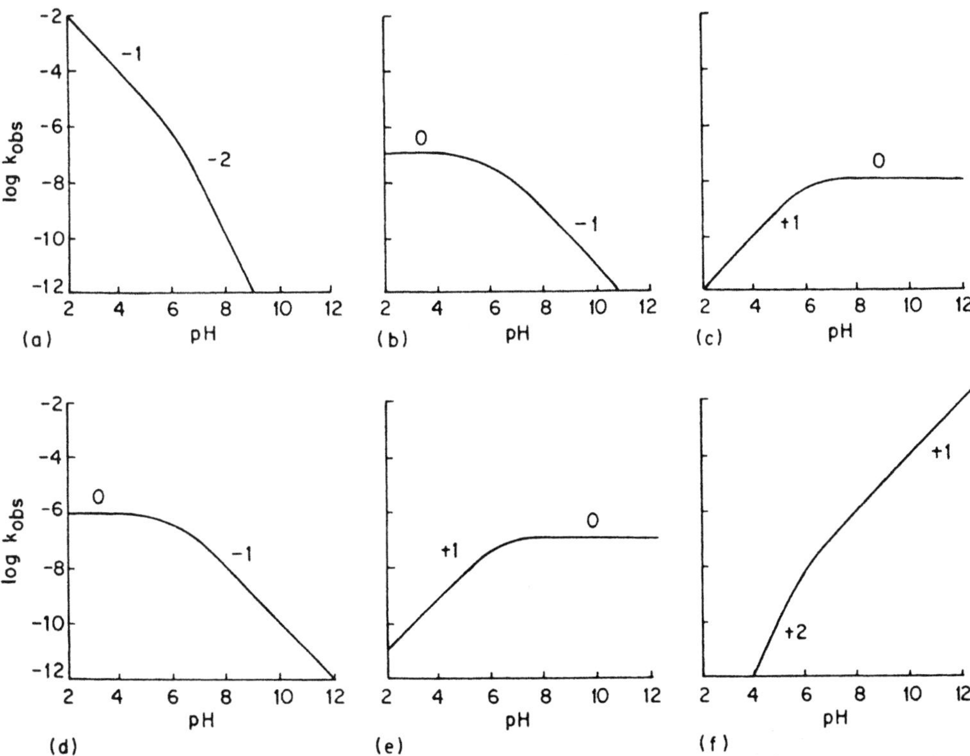

Fig. 4 The $\log k_{obs}$ versus pH profile for each kinetic term in Eq. (38): $k_1 = 10^7$, $k_2 = k_3 = k_4 = 10^7$, $k_5 = k_6 = 1$; $K_a = 10^{-6}$. Each number next to the curve indicates the slope of that portion of the curve.

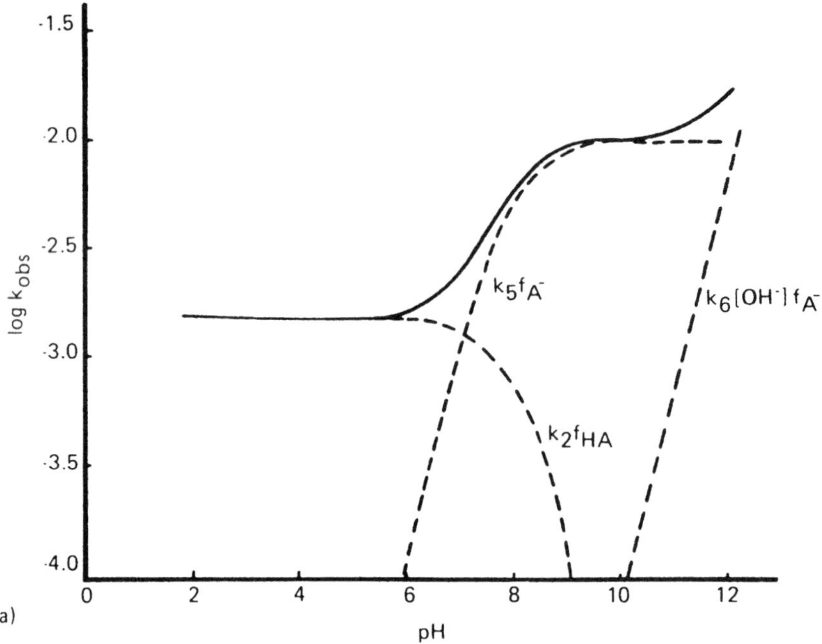

Fig. 5 (a) The pH versus log hydrolysis rate constant profile of idoxuridine at 60°C (solid line). The dashed lines indicate the individual contributions of each kinetic term. (b) pH versus log hydrolysis rate constant profile of acetylsalicylic acid (solid line). The dashed lines indicate the individual contribution of each kinetic term. Adapted from Refs. 105 and 106.

acid (see Fig. 5b) can be decided only by using all four kinetic terms ($k_{obs} = k_1[H^+]f_{HA} + k_4[H^+]f_A^- + k_5 f_A^- + k_6[OH^-]f_A^-$).

Some compounds exhibit pH behavior in which a bell-shaped curve is obtained with maximum instability at the peak [107]. The peak corresponds to the intersection of two sigmoidal curves that are mirror images. The two inflection points imply two acid and base dissociations responsible for the reaction. For a dibasic acid (H_2A) for which the monobasic species (HA^-) is most reactive, the rate will rise with pH as [HA^-] increases. The maximum rate occurs at $pH = (pK_1 + pK_2)/2$ (the mean of the two acid dissociation constants). Where an acid and base react, the two inflections arise from the two different molecules. The hydrolysis of penicillin G catalyzed by 3,6-bis(dimethylaminomethyl)catechol [108], is a typical example. For a systematic interpretation of pH-degradation profiles, see the review papers by van der Houwen et al. [109] and Connors [110].

B. Solvent

In many pharmaceutical dosage forms, it may be necessary to incorporate water-miscible solvents to solubilize the drug. These solvents are generally low molecular weight alcohols such as ethanol, propylene glycol, and glycerin or polymeric alcohols such as the polyethylene glycols. Solvent effects can be quite complicated and difficult to predict. In addition to altering the activity coefficients of the reactant molecules and the transition state, changes of the solvent system may bring about concomitant changes in such physicochemical parameters as pK_a, surface tension, and viscosity, thus indirectly affecting the reaction rate. In some cases, an additional reaction pathway may be generated, or there may be a change in the product mix.

The angiotensin-converting enzyme inhibitor, moexipril, undergoes hydrolysis as well as a cyclization reaction leading to the formation of diketopiperazines. In mixed solvent (75–90% ethanol) systems the hydrolysis reaction is suppressed, but the rate of the cyclization reaction increases by 5.5 to 29-fold [111]. In the presence of increasing concentrations of ethanol in the solvent, aspirin degrades *via* an extra route forming the ethyl ester of acetylsalicylic acid [112]. On the other hand, a solvent change may bring about stabilization of a compound. The hydrolysis of barbiturates occurs 6.7-fold faster in water than in 50% ethanol and 2.6-fold faster in water than in 50% glycerol [113].

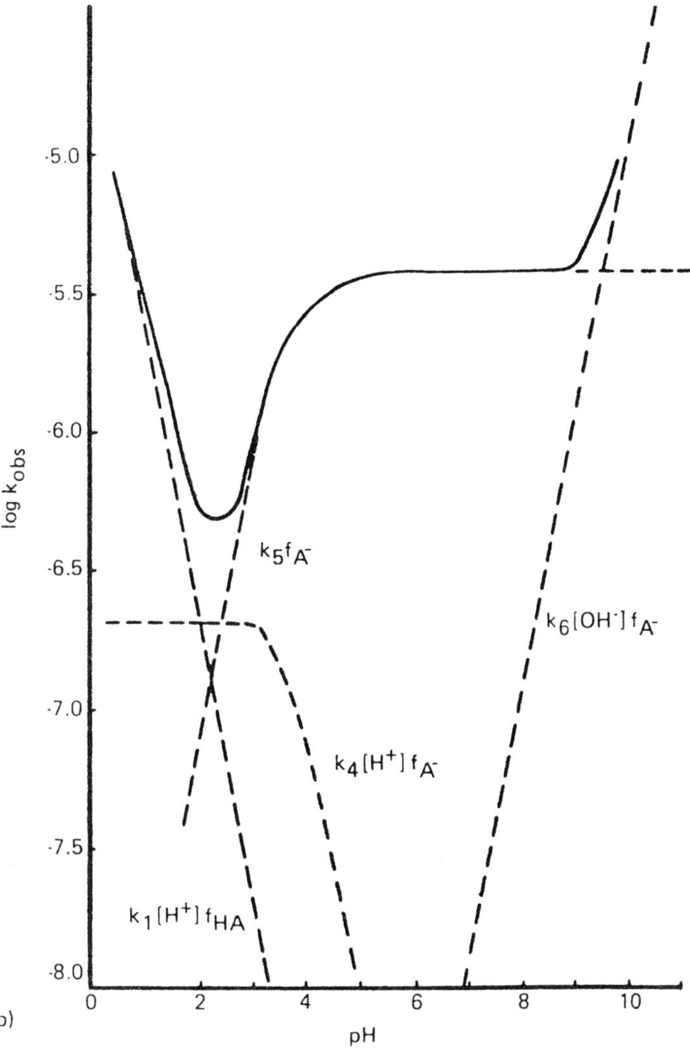

Fig. 5 (b)

Many approaches have been used to correlate solvent effects. The approach used most often is based on the electrostatic theory, the theoretical development of which has been described in detail by Amis [114]. The reaction rate is correlated with some bulk parameter of the solvent, such as the dielectric constant or its various algebraic functions. The search for empirical parameters of solvent polarity and their applications in multiparameter equations has recently been intensified, and this approach is described in the book by Reichardt [115] and more recently in the chapter on medium effects in Connor's text on chemical kinetics [110].

Although the solvent effect on reaction rate could, in principle, be large, the limited availability of nontoxic solvents suitable for pharmaceutical products has rendered this stabilization approach somewhat impractical in most circumstances.

C. Solubility

As mentioned earlier in this chapter, penicillins are very unstable in aqueous solution by virtue of hydrolysis of the β-lactam ring. A successful method of stabilizing penicillins in liquid dosage forms is to prepare their insoluble salts and formulate them in suspensions. The reduced solubility of the drug in a suspension decreases the amount of drug available for hydrolysis. An example of improved stability of a

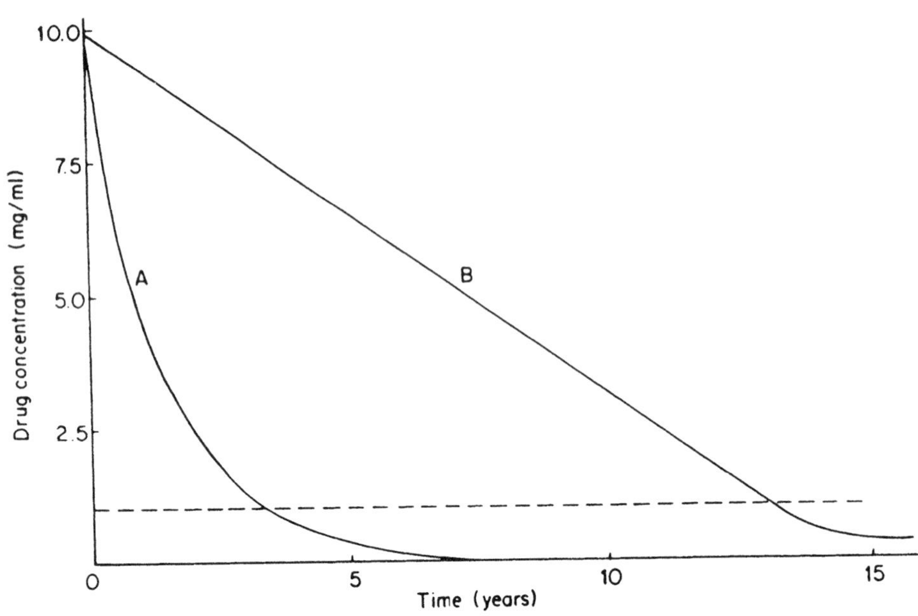

Fig. 6 Solubility effects on drug stability: curve A, drug formulated as 10 mg/mL solution ($t_{1/2} = 1$ year); curve B, drug formulated as a suspension with a saturated solubility of 1 mg/mL ($t_{1/2} = 7.3$ years).

suspension over that of a solution is illustrated in Fig. 6, in which a hypothetical drug is formulated as a 10 mg/mL solution (curve A) and as a suspension containing the same total amount of drug but with a saturated solubility of 1 mg/mL (curve B). It is seen that the drug in solution undergoes first-order degradation with a half-life of 1 month. In the suspension, the drug degrades through zero-order kinetics until there is no more excess solid present, after which point first order kinetics is operative.

D. Additives

Buffer Salts

In many drug solutions, it is necessary to use buffer salts in order to maintain the formulation at the optimum pH. These buffer salts can affect the rate of drug degradation in a number of ways. First, a primary salt effect results because of the effect salts have on the activity coefficient of the reactants. At relatively low ionic strengths, the rate constant, k_μ, is related to the ionic strength, μ, according to

$$\ln k_\mu = \ln k_0 + 1.02\, z_A z_B \sqrt{\mu} \tag{41}$$

where k_0 is rate constant at $\mu = 0$, z_A and z_B are the ionic charges of reactants A and B, respectively, and the constant 1.02 is applicable to aqueous solutions at 25°C. According to Eq. (41), a plot of ln k_μ as a function of $\sqrt{\mu}$ should yield a slope approximately equal to the product $z_A z_B$, which in theory should always be an integer because both z_A and z_B are integral numbers. In practice, however, the slope is often fractional. The sign of the slope is sometimes informative in identifying the reactants that participate in the rate-limiting step in the reaction mechanism. But one must avoid drawing such conclusions in instances where a choice is to be made between kinetically equivalent rate terms [110].

Buffer salts also can exert a secondary salt effect on drug stability. From Table 5 and Fig. 5 it is clear that the rate constant for an ionizable drug is dependent on its pK_a. Increasing salt concentrations, particularly from polyelectrolytes such as citrate and phosphate, can substantially affect the magnitude of the pK_a, causing a change in the rate constant. (For a review of salt effects, containing many examples from the pharmaceutical literature see Ref. 116.)

Lastly, buffer salts can promote drug degradation through general acid or general base catalysis. In these cases, the rate expression will contain additional kinetic terms describing the applicable reactions between different molecular species of the drug and buffer components. The efficiency of general acid or base catalysis by the buffer components is often described by the Brønsted relationship:

$$k_A = G_A K_A^{\alpha}$$

and

$$k_B = G_B K_B^{\beta} \tag{42}$$

where k_A and k_B are the catalytic constants for general acid and base catalysis, respectively, K_A and K_B are the acid and base ionization constants, respectively, and G_A, G_B, α, and β are constants characteristic of the reaction, the solvent, and the temperature [117, 118].

Surfactants

Addition of surface-active agents may accelerate or decelerate drug degradation. Because micellar catalysis may provide a model for enzyme reactions, acceleration of rate due to the presence of surfactants is well documented [119]. Millionfold accelerations of reaction rates have been reported [120]. Stabilization of drugs through the addition of surfactants, is, by comparison, less frequently reported. An example in which both effects are observed is especially rare. The hydrolysis of aspirin in the plateau region (pH 6–8) is inhibited by the presence of micelles of cetyltrimethylammonium bromide and cetylpridinium chloride, while in the region where the normal base-catalyzed reaction occurs (pH > 9), the reaction is catalyzed by micelles of these same surfactants. The mechanism of hydrolysis in the plateau region has been shown to involve intramolecular general base catalysis by the adjacent ionized carboxyl group both in the presence and absence of micelles. This reaction is inhibited in the presence of micelles because the substrate molecules are solubilized into the micelle and water is less available in this environment than in normal aqueous solutions [121].

Complexing Agents

Higuchi and Lachman [122] pioneered the approach of improving drug stability by complexation. They showed that aromatic esters can be stabilized in aqueous solutions in the presence of xanthines such as caffeine. Thus, the half-lives of benzocaine, procaine hydrochloride, and tetracaine are increased by approximately two- to fivefold in the presence of 2.5% caffeine. This increase in stability is attributed to the formation of a less reactive complex between caffeine and the aromatic ester. Professor K. A. Connors has written a comprehensive textbook that describes methods for the measurement of binding constants for complex formation in solution—along with discussions of pertinent thermodynamics, modeling statistics, and regression analysis [123]. The various experimental methods useful for measuring equilibrium constants are also discussed.

A good deal of attention recently has been directed towards the use of derivatives of cyclodextrin for the solubilization and stabilization of pharmaceuticals [124–126]. One cautionary note—complexation may adversely affect the dissolution an/or permeability characteristics of the drug, thereby possibly decreasing drug bioavailability.

Antioxidants and Chelating Agents

Antioxidants and chelating agents are used to protect drugs against autoxidation. Mechanistically, some antioxidants such as ascorbic acid, ascorbyl palmitate, sodium bisulfite, sodium metabisulfite, sodium sulfite, acetone sodium bisulfite, sodium formaldehyde sulfozylate, thioglycerol, and thioglycolic acid act as reducing agents. They are easily oxidized, preferentially undergo autoxidation, thus consuming oxygen and protecting the drug or excipient. They are often called oxygen scavengers because their autoxidation reaction consumes oxygen. They are particularly useful in closed systems where the oxygen cannot be replaced once it is consumed [23]. Primary or true antioxidants act by providing electrons or labile H^+, which will be accepted by any free radical to terminate the chain reaction. In pharmaceuticals, the most commonly used primary antioxidants are butylated hydroxytoluene (BHT), butylated hydroxyanisole (BHA), the tocopherols (vitamin E) and propyl gallate. Chelating agents act by forming complexes with the heavy metal ions that often are required to initiate oxidation reactions. The chelating agents used most often are ethylenediamine tetraacetic acid derivatives and salts, citric acid, and tartaric acid.

E. Light and Humidity

The mathematical relationship between light intensity and drug degradation is much less developed than those describing pH and temperature effects. Part of the reason, perhaps, is that light effects on stability can be substantially avoided by using amber containers, which shield off most of the ultraviolet light. Another deterrent to careful study of the kinetics of these reactions is the fact that multiple products of reaction often are obtained. In the case of nifedipine, for example, six degradation products were isolated from tablets exposed for 30 days under exposure to normal room light [127]. Regulatory authorities usually require a statement on the photostability of products and the means of protection, if required. Often both daylight and artificial light sources are employed for tests on drug substances [128].

Humidity is a major determinant of drug product stability in solid dosage forms. Elevation of relative humidity usually decreases stability, particularly for those drugs highly sensitive to hydrolysis [129]. In addition, increased humidity also can accelerate the "aging" process [49,71,72]. Humidity does not always affect drug stability adversely. Cyclophosphamide in lyophilized cakes containing mannitol or sodium bicarbonate was found to undergo rapid ($t_{90} \approx 15$ days) degradation in the solid state. The cyclophosphamide was found to be in the amorphous state in these formulations. However, on exposure to high humidity the cyclophosphamide was converted to the crystalline monohydrate form, which exhibited greatly improved stability [63]. Reviews dealing with the effects of moisture on the physical and chemical stability of drugs are available [130,131]. As peptides and proteins have become more important as therapeutic agents, the role residual moisture plays in their stabilization has attracted a good deal of attention [132, 133].

VI. STABILITY TESTING IN THE PHARMACEUTICAL INDUSTRY

Stability testing of drug substances and drug products begins as part of the drug discovery/synthesis development/preformulation effort and ends only with the demise of the compound or commercial product. Activities include testing of drug substance, of compatibility with excipients, of preclinical formulations, of phase I formulations and modifications, of the final NDA (commercial) formulation, and of postapproval formulation changes. The regulatory basis for the various aspects of stability testing is established in 21 CFR 211.137, 211.160, 211.170, 211.190, 314.50, 314,70, and 314.81 [134–140]. In addition, FDA guidelines for submitting stability data were published several years ago [86]. More recently, FDA has issued a draft guidance titled "Stability Testing of Drug Substances and Drug Products" [87], which covers all aspects of drug substance and drug product stability testing.

While the Code of Federal Regulations establishes the statutory basis for carrying out stability testing, the FDA and the Expert Working Group of the International Conference on Harmonization (ICH) of Technical Requirements for the Registration of Pharmaceuticals for Human Use have published guidances for conducting the actual studies [86,87, 141,142]. These guidances provide definitions of key terms and principles used in the stability testing of drug substances and drug products. Certain aspects of these guidances will be discussed later in this chapter.

Another valuable source of information on the establishment and maintenance of stability testing programs can be found in Carstensen and Rhodes [81].

A. Resources

Personnel

The number and types of personnel are dictated by the size of the program, the functions contained within the program, and the nature of the program. Some companies maintain separate development and commercial product programs; other integrate the two. It is important, both for operating efficiency and regulatory compliance, that all personnel, regardless of their function, receive adequate and well-documented training in both cGMPs and in the technical aspects of their jobs.

Education and Experience. The program is generally headed by a professional with several years of experience in the company. Experience in some aspect of formulation development or in the stability testing program itself may be as important as the education level of the person heading the program. People with a bachelor's degree in pharmacy, chemistry, or related science as well as people with masters or doctoral level degrees have led successful programs. If the size of the program warrants, intermediate-level scientists, usually at the bachelor's level, may assume responsibility for specific functions within the program, *e.g.*, chemical and physical testing, documentation, etc. Technicians generally have a high-school education or equivalent with clerical and /or scientific experience or interest. Clerical and data entry personnel have traditional training and experience in their respective areas.

Organization. Functions are often divided into testing (chemical, physical and biological), documentation, and clerical/computer operations, if the information system is computerized. Successful manual or paper systems are possible without the aid of computers. However, custom-designed software or commercially available database programs can also be programmed to automate the program. The documentation function usually consists of one or more persons who prepare the stability sections or regulatory documents. Persons specifically trained in technical writing or scientists with an interest and talent in document preparation generally perform well in this capacity.

Facilities

Storage Chambers. Several chambers capable of accurately maintaining different temperatures and combinations of temperature and humidity are needed. For most drug products, these include, as outlined in recent FDA [87] and ICH [142] guidances, −15°C ± 5°C, 5°C ± 3°C/ambient humidity, 25°C± 2°C/60%RH ± 5%, 30°C ± 2°C/60% RH ± 5%, 40°C± °C/75%RH ± 5%. For liquid products stored in semi-permeable containers subject to water loss, exposure to lower humidities, *e.g.*, 25° ± 2°C/ 40%RH ± 5%, 30°C ± 2°C/40%RH ± 5%, 40°C± 2°C/15%RH ± 5%, is needed. Also, a high-intensity light cabinet and a cycling chamber capable of cycling both temperature and humidity are needed. These chambers should be calibrated periodically according to a standard operating procedure, and records of these calibrations should be maintained in a logbook for each chamber.

For drug products normally stored at room temperature, long-term stability testing should be done at 25°C/ 60%RH or 25°C/40%RH. Stress testing should be done at 40°C/75%RH or 40°C/15%RH for 6 months. If "significant change" occurs at these stress conditions, then the product should be tested at an intermediate condition, *i.e.*, 30°C/75%RH or 30°C/40%RH. "Significant change" is defined in the guidelines.

Storage chambers should be validated with respect to their ability to maintain the desired conditions, and, if so equipped, the ability to sound an alarm if a mechanical or electrical failure causes the temperature to deviate from preestabilished limits. They should also be equipped with recording devices, which will provide a continuous and permanent history of their operation. Logbooks should be maintained and frequent readings or mercury-in-glass, National Institute of Science and Technology–traceable thermometers recorded.

Bench Space. Adequate laboratory bench, desk, and file space are needed for physical, chemical, and microbiological testing, for documentation, and for storing records, respectively.

Equipment

Chemical Testing. Adequate instrumentation for a variety of different test methods should be available. Most stability-indicating chemical assays are performed by high-performance liquid chromatography. Occasionally, gas chromatography, infrared spectrophotometry, or spectrofluorimetry are used. Test methods should be validated [143–146] and stability indicating, *i.e.*, able to distinguish the active ingredient from its degradation products so that the active can be accurately measured. Also, methods are needed for identifying and quantitating degradation products present at levels of 0.1% or greater.

Biological Testing. A portion of the laboratory may be reserved for biological testing, or this work can be done by the company's microbiology laboratory. The ability to perform sterility, pyrogen, LAL, preservative challenge, and bioburden tests is needed to support the stability program. As is the case for chemical assays, test methods should be validated and operator familiarity should be documented.

Physical Testing. Equipment and trained personnel should be available for performing such tests as pH, tablet hardness, etc. One important and sometimes overlooked aspect of physical testing is the recording of product appearance. Carefully defined descriptions of appearance and standard descriptions of changes in appearance should be developed, especially when there is a high probability that the person who made the observation at the previous sampling time will not be the person making the observation at the next sampling time. Some companies maintain samples at a lower-than-label storage condition, *e.g.*, refrigeration, to use as standards, assuming that minimal or no appearance change will occur at this condition. The same argument for standard nomenclature applies to other test parameters which are subjective in nature.

Computers. A certain number of personal computers are necessary for report generation and regulatory submission preparation. In addition, these may be useful for record keeping, depending on the type of stability information system that the company chooses to use. Alternatively, if the information system is intended to be accessible (read only) to many users, it may be more efficient to develop a local area network of mini-computers. The size of the database will help determine the nature of the software/hardware configuration used for this function.

B. Program

Scope and Goals

Activities encompassed by the stability program include sample storage of either development or production batches (or both), data collection and storage/retrieval, physical, chemical, and microbiological testing, document preparation of regulatory submissions, and package evaluation. In certain companies, personnel in separate departments may perform some of these functions, *e.g.*, regulatory document preparation. Nonetheless, the function is part of the company's overall stability program.

Protocols

FDA stability guidelines [87] and ICH guidelines [142] are rather detailed regarding sampling times, storage conditions, and specific test parameters for each dosage form. Generally, samples stored at the product label storage condition—controlled room temperature for most products—are tested initially and after 3, 6, 9, 12, 18, and 24 months and annually thereafter. Accelerated testing is generally done more frequently and for a shorter duration, *e.g.*, at 1, 2, 3, and 6 months. Three batches should be tested to demonstrate batch-to-batch uniformity. The number three represents a compromise between a large number desired for statistical precision and the economics of maintaining a manageable program. Generally real-time data obtained at the label storage conditions on the final formulation in the final packaging configuration(s) are needed for an NDA. Supportive data obtained from drug substance stability studies, preformulation studies, and investigational formulations tested during clinical trials and formulation development may be used to supplement primary stability data. Requirements for the IND are less defined, the only requirement being that there should be adequate data to support the clinical batch(es) for the duration of the trials.

There are instances, especially in the case of solid, oral dosage forms, where several package types and configurations are desired by marketing and three or more strengths are needed for flexibility in dosing. In these situations, it may be feasible to apply the principles of bracketing and/or matrixing to reduce the amount of testing. Bracketing refers to reduced testing of either an intermediate dosage strength or package size when the formulation characteristics of all strengths are virtually identical or when the same container/closure materials are used for all package sizes. Matrixing refers to reduced testing regardless of strength or container in situations where there are similarities in formulation or container/closure. Bracketing and matrixing are acceptable only when the product is chemically and physically very stable and does not interact with the container/closure. Demonstration of this chemical and physical stability must be documented by preformulation, drug substance stability, and early formulation stability data. Although not as common, it may be possible to utilize bracketing and matrixing with other types of dosage forms. In all cases, discussions of such strategies with FDA prior to implementation are imperative.

Documentation

The need for adequate documentation of laboratory operations is established not only by good science but also by regulatory requirements [137].

Documentation of all facets of the operation is necessary. This includes validation and periodic calibration of storage chambers, instrumentation, and computer programs. Logbooks for the storage chambers and instruments are also necessary. Standard operating procedures are needed for, among other things, the stability program itself, use of instrumentation, documentation of experiments and their results, determination of expiration dates, investigation of specification failures, and operation of a computerized record-keeping system.

Many companies have developed or purchased computer software for the purpose of storing stability data for a large number of studies. Examples of commercially available systems are "SLIM" [147] and "Stability System" [148]. These systems can perform other functions as well, including work scheduling, preparation of summaries of selected or all studies in the system, tabulation of data for individual studies, label printing, statistical analysis and plotting, and search capabilities. Such systems should be validated to keep pace with current regulatory activity [149].

C. Regulatory Concerns

cGMP Compliance

Current Good Manufacturing Practices [135] establish the requirements for maintaining a stability program and require that most pharmaceutical dosage forms have an established expiration date supported by test data [134]. There are few allowable exceptions.

FDA Stability Guidelines

The guidelines under which stability programs operate and corresponding documentation is prepared were issued in 1987 [86]. A draft revision was issued in 1998 [87]. Although the agency emphasizes that these are guidelines and not regulations, it is generally prudent to follow specific recommendations as indicated in the guidelines. Deviations or omissions should be addressed, and the reasons should be supported with data where applicable.

Regulatory Submissions

An easy-to-read stability summary document will go a long way toward rapid approval of any regulatory submission. Such a document should include a number of items. A clear statement of the objective(s) of the studies included in the submission and the approach that was taken to achieve the objective(s) is critical. This statement of objective(s) should accompany basic information including product and drug substance names, dosage forms and strengths, and type(s) and container/closure systems. Although the objective is usually stated in the summary letter accompanying the submission, a brief reminder to the reviewing chemist is helpful.

A discussion of each of the parameters tested in the course of the evaluation, including test methods and specifications for each, should then follow. These parameters should follow those recommended in the stability guidelines [87] for the specific dosage form. It is especially important to provide a rationale for those parameters not studied. Next should come the study design itself, which should include a list of batch identification number, size, and date of manufacture as well as packaging configuration, storage conditions, and sampling times for each batch. The strategy and rationale for any bracketing or matrixing should also be presented.

The actual data, including replicates, mean, and range, in tabular form should follow, accompanied by a brief discussion of the data. It is important to explain any out-of-specification data. Statistical analyses for all parameters, which lend themselves to such analyses along with conclusions, should be incorporated into the document at this point. These statistical analyses should be accompanied by the results of experiments conducted to determine the "poolability" of batches, or commonality of slopes and intercepts of individual batches. Graphs of these data should be included as part of the documentation.

Protocols for these batches and a commitment to continue them along with a "tentative" expiry date should also be included. Approval of these protocols will allow extension of the expiry date without a special supplement as long as the data remain within specifications. These data will ultimately be reported to FDA as part of periodic reports following NDA approval. Protocols intended for use on commercial batches should also be submitted.

Finally, the three-part commitment to mount studies for the first three production batches and a statistically determined number (at least one) each year, to update current studies in annual reports, and to withdraw any lots not meeting specifications should appear in the submission. Statistical sampling of production batches is usually based on $\log N$, $\sqrt{N}$, etc., where N is the number of batches produced per year. These batches are generally spread over various package types and manufacturing campaigns. There should be a standard operating procedure to handle specification deviations including confirmation of the result, cause-and-effect investigation, impact analysis, final report to management, and field alert or batch recall notice to FDA.

Annual Product Review

Once a product gains FDA approval for marketing, the sponsor should maintain a readily retrievable profile of commercial batches. This includes individual batch release data and stability data. These data should be compiled throughout the year and tabulated prior to the anniversary of NDA approval for submission in the annual product report to FDA. By maintaining an ongoing database, which is reviewed as new information is added, changing trends in the data can be observed and management notified if any of these trends are unfavorable.

REFERENCES

1. T. L. Paal and E. Liptak-Csekey, Acta Pharm. Jugosl. 40, 199 (1990).
2. E. H. Dearborn, in *The Dating of Pharamaceuticals* (J. J. Windheuser and W. L. Blockstein, Eds.), University Extension, University of Wisconsin, Madison, WI, 1970, p. 29.
3. K. Nord, J. Karlsen, and H. H. Tønnesen, Int. J. Pharm., 72, 11 (1991).
4. P. J. G. Cornelissen, G. M. J. Beijersbergen van Henegouwen and K. W. Gerritsma, Int. J. Pharm, 1, 173 (1978).
5. K. A. Neftel, M. Walti, H. Spengler, and A. L. deWeck, Lancet, 986 (1982).
6. V. J. Stella, T. J. Mikkelson, and J. D. Pipkin, in *Drug Delivery Systems* (R. L. Juliano, Ed.), Oxford University Press, New York, 1980.
7. M. D. Taylor, Adv. Drug Delivery Rev., 19, 131 (1996).
8. K. A. Connors, G. L. Amidon, and V. J. Stella, *Chemical Stability of Pharmaceuticals: A Handbook for Pharmacists*, 2nd ed., Wiley, New York, 1986.
9. H. G. Brittain, Ed., *Analytical Profiles of Drug Substances and Excipients*, Vol. 27, Academic Press, Inc., San Diego, 2000.
10. F. Pellerin, D. Baylocq and N. Chanon, Rev. Anal. Chem. 11, 171 (1992).

11. K. A. Connors, *Reaction Mechanisms in Organic Analytical Chemistry*, Wiley Interscience, New York, 1970.
12. M. A. Schwartz, A. P. Granatek, and F. H. Buckwalter, J. Pharm. Sci., 51, 523 (1962).
13. V. K. Krieble and K. A. Holst, J. Am. Chem. Soc., 60, 2976 (1938).
14. L. A. Casey, R. Galt, and M. I. Page, J. Chem. Soc. Perkin Trans. 2, 23 (1993).
15. R. S. Brown, A. J. Bennet, and H. Slebocka-Tilk, Acc. Chem. Res., 25, 481 (1992).
16. H. B. Mark, Jr., and G. A. Rechnitz, in *Chemical Analysis*, Vol. 24 (P. J. Elving and I. M. Kolthoff, Eds.), Wiley-Interscience, New York, 1970.
17. C. Hansch, A. Leo, and R. W. Taft, Chem. Rev., 91, 165 (1991).
18. L. P. Hammett, *Physical Organic Chemistry*, 2nd ed., McGraw-Hill, New York, 1970.
19. B. Capon and S. P. McManus, *Neighboring Group Participation*, Plenum, New York, 1976.
20. M. N. Khan and S. K. Gambo, Int. J. Chem. Kinetics, 17, 419 (1985).
21. R. T. Darrington and B. D. Anderson, Pharm. Res. 11, 784 (1994).
22. R. E. Lindstrom, S. N. Patel, and P. K. Wilkerson, J. Parenter. Drug Assoc., 34, 5 (1980).
23. D. M. Johnson and L. C. Gu, Autooxidation and antioxidants, in *Encyclopedia of Pharmaceutical Technology*, J. Swarbrick and J. C. Boylan, Eds., Marcel Dekker, New York, 1988, pp. 415–449.
24. T. M. Chen and L. Chafetz, J. Pharm. Sci., 76, 703 (1987).
25. P. Finholt, H. Kristiansen, L. Kyowezynski, and T. Higuchi, J. Pharm. Sci., 55, 1435 (1966).
26. J. Schulz and K.-H. Bauer, Acta Pharm. Technol., 32, 78 (1986).
27. R. Hamburger, E. Azaz, and M. Donbrow, Pharm. Acta Helv., 50, 10 (1975).
28. J. W. McGinity, J. A. Hill, A. L. La Via, J. Pharm. Sci., 64, 356 (1975).
29. J. W. McGinity, T. R. Patel, A. H. Naqvi, and J. A. Hill, Drug Dev. Comm., 2, 505 (1976).
30. E. J. Ginsburg, D. A. Stephens, P. R. West, A. M. Buko, D. H. Robinson, L. C. Li, and A. R. Bommireddi, J. Pharm. Sci., 89, 776 (2000).
31. M. Bergh, K. Magnusson, J. L. G. Nilsson, and A. T. Karlberg, Contact Dermatitis, 39, 14 (1998).
32. M. Nishikawa and K. Fuji, Chem. Pharm. Bull., 39, 2408 (1991).
33. R. Frontini and J. B. Mielck, Int. J. Pharm., 114, 121 (1995).
34. D. Pogocki and C. Schöneich, J. Pharm. Sci., 89, 443 (2000).
35. M. J. Frank, J. B. Johnson, and S. H. Rubin, J. Pharm. Sci., 65, 44 (1976).
36. K. Thoma and R. Kerker, Pharm. Ind., 54, 551 (1992).
37. J. A. Waters, Y. Kondo, and B. Witkop, J. Pharm. Sci., 61, 321 (1972).
38. F. Vargas, H. Mendez, J. Sequera, J. Rojas, G. Fraile, and M. Velasquez, Tox. Subst. Mech., 18, 53 (1999).
39. Fed. Reg. 62(95), 27115–27122 (1997).
40. Pharmacopeial Forum, 26, 384 (2000).
41. E. Shefter, H.-L. Fung, O. Mok, J. Pharm. Sci., 62, 791 (1973).
42. E. Shefter and T, Higuchi, J. Pharm. Sci., 52, 781 (1963).
43. K. R. Morris, Structural aspects of hydrates and solvates, in *Polymorphism in Pharmaceutical Solids* (H. G. Brittain, Ed.), Marcel Dekker, New York, 1999, p. 132.
44. F. Jamali, R. Mehon, F. M. Pasutto, J. Pharm. Sci., 78, 695 (1989).
45. M. A. Nunes and E. Brochmann-Hanssen, J. Pharm. Sci., 63, 716 (1974).
46. G. Severin, Chirality, 4, 111 (1992).
47. M. Reist, B. Testa, and P.-A. Carrupt, Enantiomer, 2, 147 (1997).
48. L. J. Riff and G. G. Jackson, Arch. Intern. Med., 130, 887 (1972).
49. A. T. M. Serajuddin, A. B. Thakur, R. N. Ghoshal, M. G. Fakes, S. A. Ranadive, K. R. Morris, and S. A. Varia, J. Pharm. Sci., 88, 696 (1999).
50. R. D. Vickery and M. B. Maurin, J. Pharm. Biomed. Anal., 20, 385 (1999).
51. D. D. Wirth, S. W. Baertschi, R. A. Johnson, S. R. Maple, M. S. Miller, D. K. Hallenbeck and S. M. Gregg, J. Pharm. Sci., 87, 31 (1998).
52. E. Tarelli, P. H. Corran, B. R. Bingham, H. Mollison, and R. Wait, J. Pharm. Biomed. Anal. 12, 1355 (1994).
53. R. Ikan, Ed., *The Maillard Reaction: Consequences for the Chemical and Life Sciences*, John Wiley & Sons, New York, 1996.
54. M. D. Santos-Buelga, M. J. Sanchez-Martin, and M. Sanches-Camazano, Thermochim. Acta, 210, 255 (1992).
55. J. Haleblian and W. McCrone, J. Pharm. Sci., 58, 911 (1969).
56. M. Kuhnert-Brandstätter, *Thermomicroscopy in the Analysis of Pharmaceuticals*, Pergamon Press, Oxford, 1971, pp. 37–42.
57. S. S. Yang and J. K. Guillory, J. Pharm. Sci., 61, 26 (1972).
58. J. Haleblian, R. T. Koda, and J. A. Biles, J. Pharm. Sci., 60, 1485 (1971).
59. H. G. Brittain, Ed., *Polymorphism in Pharmaceutical Solids*, Marcel Dekker, Inc., New York, 1999.
60. T. J. Macek, U.S. Patent, 2,671,750, March 9, 1954.
61. S. Luthala, Acta Pharm. Nordica, 4, 271 (1992).
62. S. R. Byrn, R. R. Pfeiffer and J. G. Stowell, *Solid-State Chemistry of Drugs*, 2nd ed., SSCI, Inc., West Lafayette, IN, 1999, p. 256.
63. T. R. Kovalcik and J. K. Guillory, J. Parenter. Sci. Tech., 42, 29 (1998).

64. M. J. Pikal and D. R. Rigsbee, Pharm. Res., 14, 1379 (1997).
65. S. Budavari, Ed., *The Merck Index*, 11th ed., Merck & Co., Rahway, NJ, 1989.
66. Fed. Reg., 37, 15959 (1972).
67. H.-L. Fung, S. K. Yap, and C. T. Rhodes, J. Pharm. Sci., 63, 1810 (1974).
68. S. A. Fusari, J. Pharm. Sci., 62, 2021 (1973).
69. Z. Chowhan, Pharm. Tech., 6 (9) 47 (1982).
70. C. J. deBlaey and J. J. Rutten-Kingma, Pharm. Acta Helv., 51, 186 (1976).
71. S. T. Horhota, J. Burgio, L. Lonski, and C. T. Rhodes, J. Pharm. Sci., 65, 1746 (1976).
72. P. B. Chemburkar, R. D. Smyth, J. D. Buehler, P. B. Shah, R. S. Joslin, A. Polk, and N. H. Reavey-Cantwell, J. Pharm. Sci., 65, 529 (1976).
73. B. L. McNiff, E. F. McNiff, and H.-L. Fung, Am. J. Hosp. Pharm., 36, 173 (1979).
74. D. Darbar, S. DellOrto, G. R. Wilkinson, and D. M. Roden, Am. J. Health-Syst. Pharm., 53, 655 (1996).
75. W. A. Parker, M. E. Morris, and C. A. Shearer, Am. J. Hosp. Pharm., 36, 505 (1979).
76. J. I. Hirsch, J. H. Wood, and R. B. Thomas, Am. J. Hosp. Pharm., 38, 995 (1981).
77. P. A. Cossum and M. S. Roberts, Eur. J. Clin. Pharmacol., 19, 181 (1981).
78. E. A. Kowaluk, M. S. Roberts, H. D. Blackburn, and A. E. Pollack, Am. J. Hosp. Phar., 38, 1308 (1981).
79. D. C. Monkhouse and L. Van Campen, Drug Dev. Ind. Pharm., 10, 1175 (1984).
80. D. C. Monkhouse, Drug Dev. Ind. Pharm., 10, 1373 (1984).
81. J. T. Carstensen and C. T. Rhodes, *Drug Stability, Principles and Practices*, 3rd ed., Marcel Dekker, Inc., New York, 2000.
82. F. Baitalow, H.-G. Schmidt, and G. Wolf, Thermochim. Acta 337, 111 (1999).
83. S. R. Byrn, R. R. Pfeiffer, and J. G. Stowell, *Solid-State Chemistry of Drugs*, 2nd ed., SSCI, Inc., West Lafayette, IN, 1999.
84. L. Meites, CRC Crit. Rev. Anal. Chem., 8, 55 (1979).
85. P. Wessels, M. Holz, F. Erni, K. Krummen, and J. Ogorka, Drug Dev. Ind. Pharm., 23, 427 (1997).
86. Guideline for Submitting Documentation for the Stability of Human Drugs and Biologics, February, 1987, Center for Drugs and Biologics, Food and Drug Administration, Rockville, MD.
87. Guidance for Industry: Stability Testing of Drug Substances and Drug Products: Draft Guidance, June, 1998, Center for Drug Evaluation and Research and Center for Biologics Evaluation and Research, U. S. Department of Health and Human Services, Food and Drug Administration, Rockville, MD.
88. J. T. Carstensen, J. Pharm. Sci., 63, 1 (1974).
89. W. J. Irwin, *Kinetics of Drug Decomposition, Basic Computer Solutions*, Elsevier Science, Amsterdam, 1990.
90. W. P. Jencks, *Catalysis in Chemistry and Enzymology*, McGraw-Hill, New York, 1969, p. 513.
91. L. Lachman, P. DeLuca, and M. J. Akers, Kinetic principles and stability testing, in *The Theory and Practice of Industrial Pharmacy*, 3rd ed. (L. Lachman, H. A. Lieberman, and J. L. Kanig, Eds.), Lea & Febiger, Philadelphia, 1986, p. 766.
92. H.-L. Fung and S.-Y. P. King, in *Pharm Tech Conference '83 Proceedings*, Aster Publishing, Springfield, OR, 1983.
93. K. J. Laidler, J. Chem. Educ., 49, 343 (1972).
94. M. J. Pikal, A. L. Lukes, and J. E. Lang, J. Pharm. Sci., 66, 1312 (1977).
95. A. J. Woolfe and H. E. C. Worthington, Drug Dev. Commun., 1, 185 (1974).
96. D. R. Savello and R. F. Shangraw, Am. J. Hosp. Pharm., 28, 754 (1971).
97. T.-Y. Fan and S. R. Tannenbaum, J. Agric. Food Chem., 21, 967 (1973).
98. R. Shija, V. B. Sunderland, and C. McDonald, Int. J. Pharm., 80, 203 (1992).
99. R. E. Pincock, Acc. Chem. Res., 2, 97 (1969).
100. N. Murase, P. Echlin, and F. Franks, Cryobiology, 28, 364 (1991).
101. T. Chen, Drug Dev. Ind. Pharm., 18, 1311 (1992).
102. W. Wang, Int. J. Pharm., 185, 129 (1999).
103. L. C. Gu, E. A. Erdös, and H.-S. Chang, Pharm. Res. 8, 485 (1991).
104. H.-L. Fung and S.-Y. P. King, in *Pharm Tech Conference '83 Proceedings*, Aster Publishing, Springfield, OR, 1983.
105. L. J. Ravin, C. A. Simpson, A. F. Zappala, and J. J. Gulesich, J. Pharm. Sci., 53, 106 (1964).
106. E. R. Garrett, J. Am. Chem. Soc., 79, 3401 (1957).
107. J. I. Wells, *Pharmaceutical Preformulation*, Ellis Horwood Ltd., West Sussex, England, 1988.
108. M. A. Schwartz, J. Pharm. Sci., 53, 1433 (1964).
109. O. A. G. J. van der Houwen, M. R. de Loos, J. H. Beijnen, A. Bult, and W. J. M. Underberg, Int. J. Pharm., 155, 137 (1997).
110. K. A. Connors, *Chemical Kinetics: The Study of Reaction Rates in Solution*, VCH Publishers, Inc., New York, 1990, pp. 273–292.
111. L. Gu and R. G. Strickley, Int. J. Pharm., 60, 99 (1990).
112. E. R. Garrett, J. Org. Chem., 26, 3660 (1961).
113. K. Thoma and M. Struve, Pharm. Ind., 47, 1078 (1985).
114. F. S. Amis, *Solvent Effects on Reaction Rates and Mechanisms*, Academic Press, New York, 1966.
115. C. Reichardt, *Solvents and Solvent Effects in Organic Chemistry*, 2nd ed. VCH Verlagsgesellschaft mbH, Weinheim, 1988.
116. J. T. Carstensen, J. Pharm. Sci., 59, 1140 (1970).
117. B. G. Cox, A. J. Kresge and P. E. Sørensen, Acta Chem. Scand., A24, 202, (1988).

118. A. J. Kresge, Chem. Soc. Rev., 2, 475 (1973).
119. C. A. Bunton and G. Savelli, in *Advances in Physical Organic Chemistry*, Vol. 22 (V. Gold and D. Bethell, Eds.) Academic Press, Orlando, FL, 1986, pp. 213–309.
120. S. Otto, J. B. F. N. Engberts, and J. C. T. Kwak, J. Am. Chem. Soc., 120, 9517 (1998).
121. T. J. Broxton, Aust. J. Chem., 35, 1357 (1982).
122. T. Higuchi and L. Lachman, J. Am. Pharm. Assoc. Sci. Ed., 44, 521 (1955).
123. K. A. Connors, *Binding Constants: The Measurement of Molecular Complex Stability*, John Wiley and Sons, New York, 1987.
124. J. V. Stella and R. A. Rajewski, Pharm. Res., 14, 556 (1997).
125. D. O. J. Thompson, Crit. Revi. Ther. Drug Carrier Syst., 14, 1 (1997).
126. T. Loftsson, Drug Stability, 1, 22 (1995).
127. N. Hayase, Y. Itagaki, S. Ogawa, S. Akutsu, and Y. Abiko, Y., J. Pharm. Sci. 83, 532 (1994).
128. N. H. Anderson, D. Johnson, M. A. McLelland, and P. Munden, J. Pharm. Biomed. Anal., 9, 443 (1991).
129. D. Genton and U. W. Kesselring, J. Pharm. Sci., 66, 676 (1977).
130. J. T. Carstensen, Drug Dev. Ind. Pharm. 14, 1927 (1988).
131. C. Ahlneck and G. Zografi, Int. J. Pharm., 62, 87 (1990).
132. T. Chen, Drug. Dev. Ind. Pharm., 18, 1311 (1992).
133. M. J. Hageman, Drug. Dev. Ind. Pharm., 14, 2047 (1988).
134. Code of Federal Regulations, Title 21, Food and Drugs, Part 211, Current good manufacturing practice for finished pharmaceuticals, Subpart G, §211.137 Expiration Dating.
135. Code of Federal Regulations, Title 21, Food and Drugs, Part 211, Current good manufacturing practice for finished pharmaceuticals, Subpart I, §211.166 Stability Testing.
136. Code of Federal Regulations, Title 21, Food and Drugs, Part 211, Current good manufacturing practice for finished pharmaceuticals, Subpart I, §211.170 Reserve Samples.
137. Code of Federal Regulations, Title 21, Food and Drugs, Part 211, Current good manufacturing practice for finished pharmaceuticals, Subpart J, §211.194 Laboratory Records.
138. Code of Federal Regulations, Title 21, Food and Drugs, Part 314, Applications for FDA approval to market a new drug or antibiotic drug, Subpart B, §314.50 Content and format of an application.
139. Code of Federal Regulations, Title 21, Food and Drugs, Part 314, Applications for FDA approval to market a new drug or antibiotic drug, Subpart B, §314.70 Supplements and other changes to an approved application.
140. Code of Federal Regulations, Title 21, Food and Drugs, Part 314, Applications for FDA approval to market a new drug or antibiotic drug, Subpart B, §314.81 Other postmarketing reports.
141. ICH Expert Working Group, Q1A Stability Testing of New Drug Substances and Products, International Conference on Harmonisation of Technical Requirements for the Registration of Pharmaceuticals for Human Use, 1994.
142. ICH Expert Working Group, Q1A (R) Stability Testing of New Drug Substances and Products (draft), International Conference on Harmonisation of Technical Requirements for the Registration of Pharmaceuticals for Human Use, 2000.
143. Guideline for Submitting Samples and Analytical Data for Methods Validation, February 1987, Center for Drugs and Biologics, Food and Drug Administration, Rockville, MD.
144. ICH Expert Working Group, Q2B Validation of Analytical Procedures: Methodology, International Conference on Harmonisation of Technical Requirements for the Registration of Pharmaceuticals for Human Use, 1996.
145. E. Debesis, J. P. Boehlert, T. E. Givand, and J. C. Sheridan, Pharm. Tech., 6(9), 120–137 (1982).
146. United States Pharmacopeia 24, <1225>, Validation of Compendial Methods, 2000, pp. 2149–2152.
147. Stability Lab Information Manager, Metrics, Inc., P.O. Box 4035, Greenville, NC 27836.
148. Stability System, ScienTek Software, Inc., P.O. Box 323, Tustin, CA 92781.
149. R. F. Tetzlaff, Pharm. Tech., 16(5), 70 (1992).

Chapter 7

Preformulation

Jens T. Carstensen

University of Wisconsin, Madison, Wisconsin

I. INTRODUCTION

Historically, preformulation evolved in the late 1950s and early 1960s as a result of a shift in emphasis in industrial pharmaceutical product development. Up until the mid-1950s, the general emphasis in product development was to develop elegant dosage forms and organoleptic considerations far outweighed such (as yet unheard of) considerations as whether a dye used in the preparation might interfere with stability or with bioavailability. In fact, pharmacokinetics and biopharmaceutics were in their infancy, and although stability was a serious consideration, most analytical methodology was such that even gross decomposition often went undetected.

It was, in fact, improvement in analytical methods that spurred the first programs that might bear the name "preformulation." Stability-indicating methods would reveal instabilities not previously known, and reformulation of a product would be necessary. When faced with the problem of attempting to sort out the component of incompatibility in a 10-component product, one might use many labor hours. In developing new products, therefore, it would be logical to check, ahead of time, which incompatibilities the drug exhibited (testing it against common excipients). This way the disaster could be prevented in advance.

A further cause for the birth of preformulation was the synthetic organic programs started in many companies in the 1950s and 1960s. Pharmacological screens would show compounds to be promising, and pharmacists were faced with the task of rapid formulation. Hence they needed a fast screen (i.e., a preformulation program) to enable them to formulate intelligently. The latter adverb implies that some of the physical chemistry had to be known, and this necessitated determination of physicochemical properties, a fact that is also part of preformulation. The approach was so logical, indeed, that it eventually became part of official requirements for INDs and NDAs [1]:

> New drug substances in Phase I submission. For the drug substance, the requirement includes a description of its physical, chemical, or biological characteristics. We in the reviewing divisions regard stability as one of those characteristics. The requirement for NDA submissions . . . stability information is required for both the drug substance and drug product. A good time to start to accumulate information about the appropriate methodology and storage stations for use in dosage form stations for use in dosage form stability studies, therefore, is with the unformulated drug substance. . . . Stress storage conditions of light, heat and humidity are usually used for these early studies, so that the liable structures in the molecule can be quickly identified. . . . If degradation occurs, the chemical reaction kinetics of the degradation should be determined. . . . Physical changes such as changes from one polymorph to another polymorph should be examined. . . . With the drug substance stability profile thus completed, the information should be submitted in the IND submission.

II. TIMING AND GOALS OF PREFORMULATION

The goals of the program are, therefore, (1) to establish the necessary physicochemical parameters of a new drug substance, (2) to determine its kinetic rate profile,

(3) to establish its physical characteristics, and (4) to establish its compatibility with common excipients. To view these in their correct perspective, it is worthwhile to consider where (i.e., at what time) in an overall industrial program preformulation takes place. The following events take place between the birth of a new drug substance and its eventual marketing (most investigational drug substances never make it to the marketplace for one reason or another):

1. The drug is synthesized and tested in a pharmacological screen.
2. The drug is found sufficiently interesting to warrant further study.
3. Sufficient quantity is synthesized to (a) perform initial toxicity studies, (b) do initial analytical work, and (c) do initial preformulation.
4. Once past initial toxicity, phase I (clinical pharmacology) begins and there is a need for actual formulations (although the dose level may not yet be determined).
5. Phase II and III clinical testing then begins, and during this phase (preferably phase II) an order of magnitude formula is finalized.
6. After completion of the above, an NDA is submitted.
7. After approval of the NDA, production can start (product launch).

III. PHYSICOCHEMICAL PARAMETERS

Physicochemical studies are usually associated with great precision and accuracy and in the case of a new drug substance would include (1) pK (if the drug substance is an acid or base), (2) solubility, (3) melting point and polymorphism, (4) vapor pressure (enthalpy of vaporization), (5) surface characteristics (surface area, particle shape, pore volume), and (6) hygroscopicity. Unlike usual physicochemical studies, an abundance of material is usually not at hand for the first preformulation studies: in fact, at the time the function starts, precious little material is supplied, and, therefore, the formulator will often settle for good estimates rather than attempting to generate results with four significant figures.

There is another good reason not to aim "too high" in the physicochemical studies of the first sample of drug substance. In most cases the synthesis is only a first scheme; in later scale-up it will be refined, and in general the first small samples contain some small amounts of impurities, which may influence the precision of the determined constants. But it is necessary to know, grosso modo, important properties such as solubility, pK, and stability.

A. pK_a and Solubility

One important goal of the preformulation effort is to devise a method for making solutions of the drug. Frequently, the drug is not sufficiently soluble in water itself to allow for the desired concentrations, for example, for injection solutions. Solubilities are determined by exposing an excess of solid to the liquid in question and assaying after equilibrium has been established. This usually is in the range of 60–72 hours, and to establish that equilibrium indeed has been established, sampling at earlier points is necessary. Unstable solutions pose a problem in this respect and are dealt with in more detail later. Solubilities cannot be determined by precipitative methods (e.g., by solubilizing an acid in alkali and then lowering the pH to the desired pH) because of the so-called meta-stable (solubility) zone [2]. In this chapter drug substances are subdivided into two categories: (1) ionizable substances and (2) (virtually) nonionizable substances.

Ionizable Substances

For substances that are carboxylic acids (HA) it is advantageous to determine the pK_a since this property is of importance in a series of considerations. For carboxylic acid the species A^- usually absorbs in the ultraviolet (UV) region, and its concentration can be determined spectrophotometrically [3]; HA, on the other hand, will absorb at a different wavelength.

The molar absorbances of the two species at a given wavelength are denoted ε_0 and ε_- (and it is assumed that at the wavelength chosen $\varepsilon_0 < \varepsilon_-$) and it can be shown that if the solution is m_0 molar in total A, then

$$A^-/HA = (\varepsilon - \varepsilon_0 m_0)/(m_0\varepsilon_- - \varepsilon) \quad (1)$$

so that ratio A^-/HA can be determined in a series of buffers of different pH. Hence the pK can be found as the intercept by plotting pH as a function of $\log[(A^-)/(HA)]$ by Henderson-Hasselbach:

$$\mathrm{pH} = \mathrm{p}K + \log(A^-/HA) \quad (2)$$

If several buffer concentrations are used, extrapolation can be carried out to zero ionic strength, and the pK_a can be determined. For initial studies, however, a pK in

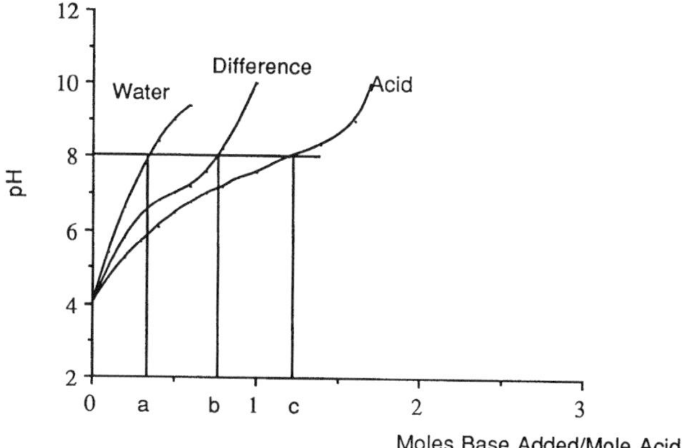

Fig. 1 Typical titration curves. The "water" curve indicates the amount of alkali needed to "titrate" the water, and the "acid" curve is a conventional titration curve. The difference curve is the horizontal difference between the "acid" and the "water" curve, and is the adjusted titration curve, e.g., point b is c−a. The pK is the point of inflection, which is also the point at where half of the acid is neutralized.

the correct range (i.e., ±0.2 unit) will suffice, so that the determination above can be done at one buffer concentration only.

The conventional approach is, of course, to do titrations (Fig. 1) that will yield graphs of fraction neutralized as a function of pH. Usually, the water is titrated as well [4], and what is presented in Fig. 1 is the "difference." The pK is then the pH at half neutralization (which is also the inflection point). The pH-solubility curve can now be constructed simply by determining the solubility of HA (at low pH) and A^- (e.g., of NaA) at high pH (e.g., at pH 10). It is noted that at a given pH the amount in solution in a solubility experiment is:

$$S = S_{HA} + C_{A^-} \tag{3}$$

where S denotes solubility. The last term can be determined from knowledge of the pH and use of Eq. (2).

For drugs that are amines, the free base is frequently poorly soluble, and in this case the pK is often estimated by performing the titration in a solvent containing some organic solvent (e.g., ethanol). By doing this at different organic solvent concentrations (e.g., 5, 10, 15, 20%), extrapolation can be carried out to 0% solvent concentration to estimate the aqueous pK.

Solubility profiles paralleling pH curves have been reported by Granero et al. [5].

Nonionizable Substances

For hydrophobic, (virtually) nonionizable substances [i.e., those that show no ionic species of significance in the pH range 1 to 10 (e.g., diazepam)], solubility can usually be improved by addition of nonpolar solvents. Aside from solubility, stability is also affected by solvents in either a favorable or a nonfavorable direction [6]. Theoretical equations for solubility in water [7] and in binary solvents [8] have been reported in literature, but in general the approach in preformulation is pseudoempirical. Most often the solubility changes as the concentration of nonpolar solvent C_2, increases. For binary systems it may simply be a monotonely changing function [9], as shown in Fig. 2. The solubility is usually tied to the dielectric constant, and in a case such as that shown by the squares, the solubility is often log-linear when plotted as a function of inverse dielectric constant, E, that is,

$$\ln S = -e_1/(\varepsilon + e_2) \tag{4}$$

where ε is the dielectric constant and the e-terms are constants [3].

Frequently, however, the solubility curve has a maximum (as shown by circles in Fig. 2, when plotted as both a function of C_2 and ε [10]. In either case it is possible to optimize solubility by selection of a solvent system with a given value of ε; that is, once the curve has been established, the optimum water/solvent ratio for another solvent can be calculated from known dielectric constant relationships [11].

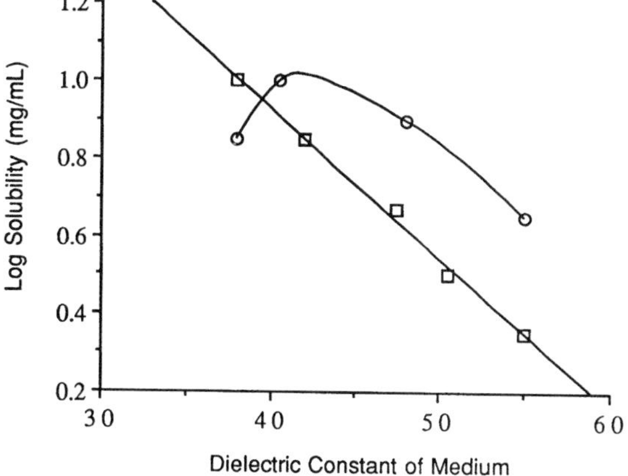

Fig. 2 Squares: Solubility of 7-chloro-1,3-hydro-5-phenyl-2H-1, 4-benzodiazepine-2-one-4-oxide in aqueous propylene glycol. (Data from Ref. 9) Circles: Solubility of another benzodiazepine. (Unpublished data.)

Ternary Systems and Optimization

Frequently, *ternary* solvent systems are resorted to. Examples are water–propylene glycol–benzyl alcohol and water–propylene glycol–ethanol. In such cases the solubility profile is usually presentable by a ternary diagram [12]. This type of diagram usually demands a fair amount of work; that is, solubility of the drug substance in many solvent compositions must be determined. A priori, it would therefore seem that they would be out of place in a situation where only limited quantities of drug are available. However, their principle gives some validity to optimization procedures.

The diagram can be one of two types, as shown in Figs. 3 and 4. In the first type, the solubility may be assumed to be of the type

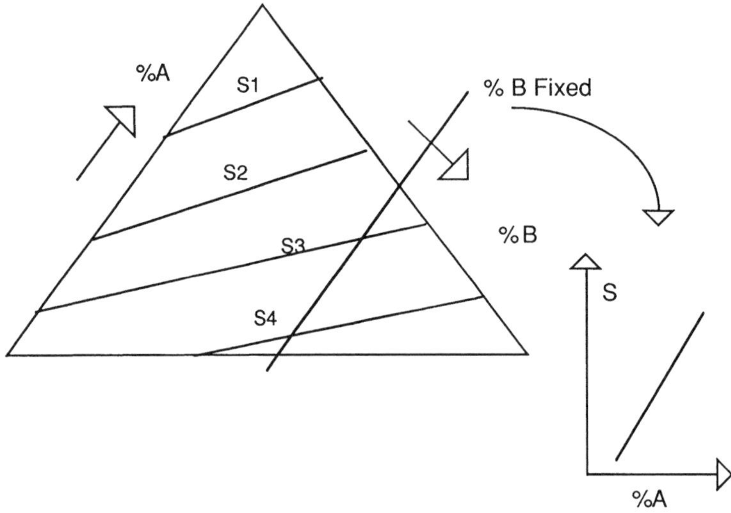

Fig. 3 Ternary diagram of solubility of a compound in a ternary mixture with linear solubility response. (Inset) Concentration of drug in compositions with constant concentration of B. The composition of the solute is the constant concentration of B, the concentration of A in the abscissa, and the complement concentration of the third component. The drug solubility response is linear in the A concentration in this case.

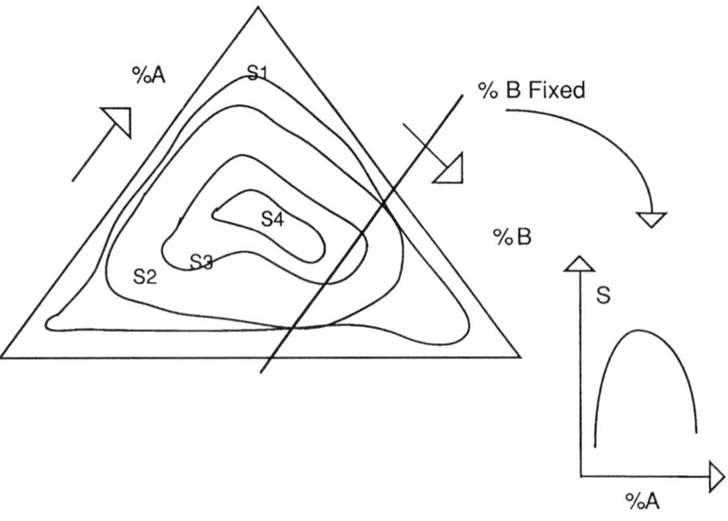

Fig. 4 Ternary diagram and tie line concentration in a nonlinear system.

$$S = a_{10} + a_{11}C_1 + a_{12}C_2 \tag{5}$$

where C denotes concentrations of nonaqueous solvents. An example of this is shown on the right of the figure. In Eq. 5 the subscripts to C denote the two nonaqueous solvents. Hence, three solubility experiments would determine the relationship (with zero degrees of freedom). It is usual to do at least five and determine possible curvature [i.e., inclusion of more terms in Eq. (5)].

In the second case in Fig. 4, each tie line will give a parabolic-type curve as shown on the right of the figure. Hence at a given concentration of C_2 the solubility can be approximated by

$$S = b_{10} + b_{11}C_1 + b_{12}C_1^2 \tag{6}$$

where, in the simplest case,

$$b_{10} = C_{20} + C_{21}C_2 \tag{7}$$

Hence optimization can be achieved by five (or more) experiments, with zero (or in general $n-5$) degrees of freedom.

The effects of pH and of mixed solvent systems have been described by Tongaree et al. [13].

Prediction of Solubility

It is advantageous with a new drug substance to be able to estimate what its solubility will be prior to carrying out dissolution experiments. There are several systems of solubility prediction, most notably those published by Amidon and Yalkowsky [14–16] in the 1970s. Their equation for solubility of *p*-aminobenzoates in polar and mixed solvents is a simplified two-dimensional analog of the Scatchard-Hildebrand equation and is based on the product of the interfacial tension and the molecular surface area of the hydrocarbon portion of a molecule.

More recently Bodor et al. [17] developed a semi-empirical solubility predictor based on 20 variables (S = molecular surface in Å^2, I_a = indicator variable for alkanes, D = calculated dipole moment in Debyes; Q_n = square root of sum of squared charges on oxygen atoms; Q_o = square root of sum of squared charges on oxygen atoms; V = molecular volume in Å^2, S_2 = square of molecular surface; C = constant; MW = molecular weight, $\{O\}$ = ovality of molecule, A_{bh} = sum of absolute values of atomic charges on hydrogen atoms, A_{bc} = sum of absolute values of atomic charges on hydrogen atoms, A_m = indicator variable for aliphatic amines, and N_h = number of N–H single bonds in the molecule.)

The aqueous solubilities, W, of 331 compounds were found to follow the following equation (with tolerances omitted):

$$\begin{aligned}\log W = {} & -56.039 + 0.32235D - 0.59143I_a \\ & + 38.443Q_n^4 - 51.536Q_n^2 + 18.244Q_n \\ & + 34.569Q_o^4 - 31.835Q_o^2 + 15.061Q_o \\ & + 1.9882A_m + 0.15689N_h + 0.00014102S^2 \\ & + 0.40308S - 0.59335A_{bc} + -0.42352V \\ & + 1.3168A_{bh} + 108.80\{O\} - 61.272\{O\}^2\end{aligned} \tag{8}$$

Of the parameters listed, only the ovality and the indicator value for the alkanes I_a are unfamiliar entities that are obtained from literature [17].

Dissolution

The importance of dissolution will be discussed in more detail later. A short note on the topic is, however, necessary at this point. According to Noyes-Whitney [18];

$$dm/dt = VdC/dt = -kA(S - C) \tag{7}$$

where

m = mass not dissolved
V = liquid volume
t = time
k = so-called intrinsic dissolution rate constant (cm/s)
A = surface area of the dissolving solid

Many criticisms have been voiced against Eq. (7), but in general it is correct, and it will be assumed to be so in the following. If an experiment is carried out with constant surface (as, e.g., using a Wood's apparatus [19]) or with smaller amounts, making a small pellet and encasing it in wax and exposing only one face to a dissolution medium, or if an excess of solid prevails throughout the dissolution experiment, then Eq. (7) may be integrated to give

$$\ln[1 - (C/S)] = -(kA/V)t \tag{8}$$

or

$$C = S[1 - \exp(-\{kA/V\}t)] \tag{9}$$

A typical curve following Eq. (9) is shown as "C" in Fig. 5.

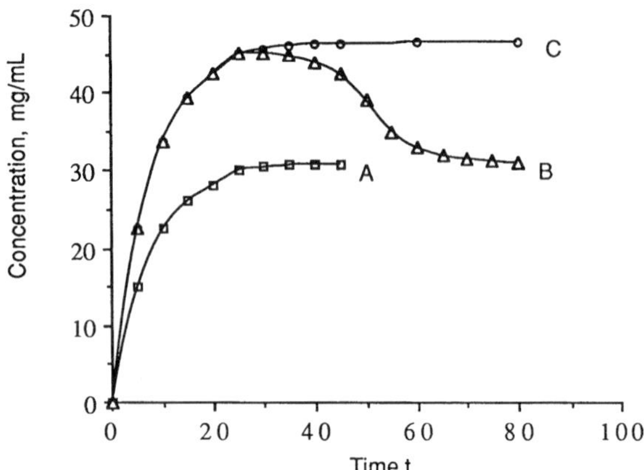

Fig. 5 Dissolution profiles obtained from the solubility determination of two polymorphic forms of the same drug substance. A is the stable form with solubility 31 mg/mL. B is the profile of the metastable form with solubility 46 mg/mL. This solubility (circles) is not achieved in many instances, and precipitation of the stable form occurs at a point beyond the solubility of A, and the trace becomes B. C is the hypothetical profile of the metastable form.

Solubility of Unstable Compounds

Quite often a compound is rather unstable in aqueous solution. Hence the long exposure to liquid required for traditional solubility measurements will cause decomposition, and the resulting solubility results will be unreliable. In this particular case a method known as Nogami's method may be used. If a solution experiment is carried out as a dissolution experiment with samples taken at equal time intervals, δ, it can be shown [20] that when the amount dissolved at time $t+\delta$ is plotted versus the amount dissolved at time t, a straight line will ensue (Fig. 6). When the concentration at time $t+\delta$ is plotted versus the concentration, at t the following relationship holds:

$$C(t+\delta) = S[1 - \exp(-k\delta)] + \exp(-k\delta)C(t) \quad (10)$$

hence such a plot (as shown in Fig. 6) will give k from the slope, and inserting this in the intercept expression will give S. The advantage of the method is that it can be carried out in a short period of time and will reduce the effect of decomposition; the disadvantages is that it is not as precise as ordinary solubility determinations.

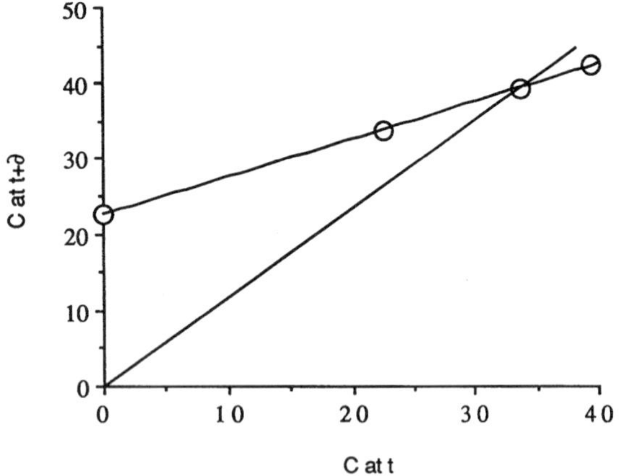

Fig. 6 The Nogami method applied to the data in Fig. 5.

Solubility of Metastable Polymorphs

Polymorphism is an important aspect of the physical properties of a drug substance. One of the characteristics of a metastable polymorph (to be discussed in some detail at a later point) is that it is more soluble than its stable counterpart. The solubility profile of the polymorph will be as shown in Fig. 5; A is the stable form, with solubility of 31 mg/mL. B is the profile of the metastable form, with solubility of 46 mg/mL. This solubility (circles) is usually not achieved, and precipitation of the stable form occurs at a point beyond the solubility of A, and the trace becomes B.

In such cases, the Nogami method can be applied to the early points curve (Fig. 6) and the solubility, S', of the polymorph can be assessed. One of the important aspects of metastable polymorphs in pharmacy is exactly their higher solubility, since the dissolution rate will also be higher [Eq. (7)]. Hence the bioavailability will be increased where this is dissolution rate limited [21].

Polymorphism

Solids exist as either amorphous compounds or crystalline compounds [22]. In the latter, the molecules are positioned in lattice sites. Usually, amorphous substances decompose by first-order kinetics, and as such distinguish themselves from crystalline compounds [23].

A lattice is a three-dimensional array, and there are eight systems known. Inorganic substances are usually defined by one crystal system by the so-called radius-ratio rule [22], but organic compounds often have the capability of existing in more than one crystal form, a phenomenon referred to as polymorphism.

Powder diffraction x-ray analysis and DSC are the methods most often used to distinguish between different polymorphs. Single crystal x-ray analysis [24] will give information about the position of molecular groups within the crystal and thus actually defines the difference between the different forms. Often, however, crystals cannot be grown to an adequate size to allow this to be carried out. Stephenson [25] reported that recent advances in crystallographic computing have made it possible to solve by powder diffraction methods structures that have not been possible to solve by single-crystal methods.

If a compound exhibits polymorphism, one of the forms will be more stable (physically) than the other forms; that is, of n existing forms $n-1$ forms will possess thermodynamic tendency to convert to the nth, stable form (which then has the lowest Gibbs energy; it should be noted that in the preformulation stage it is not known whether the form on hand is the stable polymorph or not).

One manner in which different polymorphs are created is by way of recrystallizing them from different solvents, and at a point in time when sufficient material (and this need not be very much) is available, the preformulation scientist should undertake recrystallization from a series of solvents.

Knowledge of polymorphic forms is of importance in preformulation because suspension systems should never be made with a metastable form (i.e., a form other than the stable crystal form). Conversely, a metastable form is more soluble than a stable modification, and this can be of advantage in dissolution [Eq. (9)]. There are two types of polymorphism, a fact illustrated in the following discussion.

If the vapor pressure or solubility of a compound is plotted as a function of temperature, a plot such as that shown in Fig. 7 will result. Here form I is the form that is stable at temperature of 20°C. If the compound exists in the two forms I and II, the phenomenon is referred to as an entiotropic system, since, on heating to the temperature T_2, form I will transform into form II. Form II may exist below temperature T_2, but perturbations (e.g., presence of moisture) will convert it to form I, and the energy involved in the transformation will be

$$E = \mathrm{RT}\ \ln[S_2/S_1] \tag{11}$$

where S_2 and S_1 are solubilities of II and I.

If the compound is present as form I at room temperature and heated up fast it will melt at T', which is lower than the melting point of form II (T'').

A different situation exists if the compound exists as form I and form III. This is referred to as a monotropic system, and here III is unstable relative to I over the whole solid range. In this case, however, the melting point of the "unstable" polymorph is lower than that of the stable (T''' is lower than T').

If a metastable polymorph is kept dry, it may be stable for eons, and it is therefore not referred to as an unstable but, rather, a metastable polymorph. An even more energetic state is, of course, represented by amorphous forms, which may be considered supercooled liquids. Today, polymorphism is checked for in two fashions. Thermal methods will give information as to whether a polymorph is stable, enantiotropic, or monotropic. If the system possesses a transition point, ΔG is zero at this point. In a fashion like the melting process, where ΔG is also zero, the transition is associated with an enthalpy change, which is endothermic. Hence, if a sample of a compound is heated up and a change in enthalpy occurs below the melting point, it is an enantiotropic transformation if the point is reproducible and if it occurs again after the sample has been cooled back down and shows the same enthalpy change upon heating. Otherwise, it is monotropic, in which case, as shown in Fig. 8, there either will be a (lower) melting point (T''') with a single endotherm or there will be a melting followed by a recrystallization into the more stable forms, which then melt [denoted III(Alternate) in Fig. 8]. An amorphous compound has no melting point, and above glass transition temperatures its vapour pressure curve simply continues into that of the melt.

Second, x-ray diffraction will, directly, give spacings in the crystal and reveal differences between samples. Finally, solubility curves can be carried out, and if a nick in the solubility curve is found (Fig. 9), this is a transition temperature. If no nick is found, there is no transition temperature, but if the dissolution curves are as shown in Fig. 5, there is polymorphism, and it may

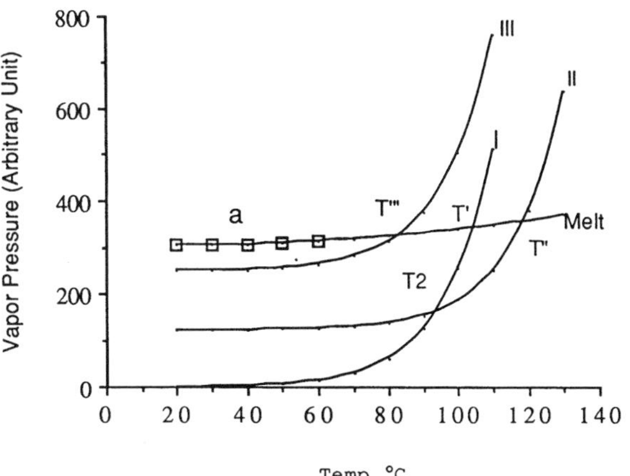

Fig. 7 Dependence of vapor pressure and solubility for an enantiotropic pair (I/II), a monotropic pair (I/III), and an amorphous compound (a).

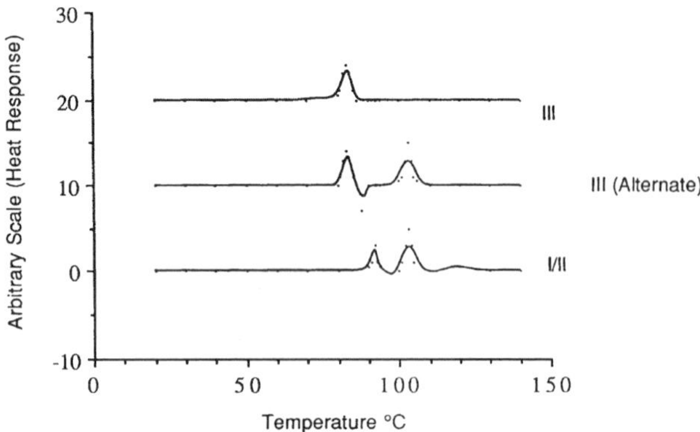

Fig. 8 DSC tracings of the polymorphs shown in Fig. 7.

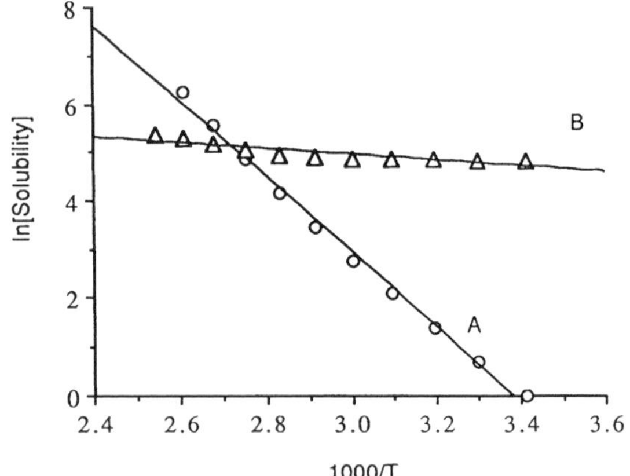

Fig. 9 Solubility curves of an enantiotropic pair.

be concluded that a monotropic system exists, if this is true at all texperatures.

C. Partition Coefficient

Partition coefficients between water and an alkanol (e.g., octanol) should be determined in preformulation programs [26]. The partition coefficient of a compound that exists as a monomer in two solvents is given by

$$K = C_1/C_2 \tag{12}$$

If it exists as an n-mer in one of the phases, the equation becomes

$$K = (C_1)^n/C_2 \tag{13}$$

or

$$\log k = n \log C_1 - \log C_2 \tag{14}$$

The easiest way to determine the partition coefficient is to extract V_1 cm^3 of saturated aqueous solution with V_2 cm^3 of solvent, and determine the concentration C_2 in the latter. The amount left in the aqueous phase is $(C_1V_1 - C_2V_2) = M$, so that the partition coefficient is given by

$$K = M/(V_1C_1) \tag{15}$$

If it is assumed that the species is monomeric in both phases, the partition coefficient becomes the ratio of the solubilities, and it is simply sufficient to determine the solubility of the drug substance in the solvent (since it is assumed that the solubility is already known in water):

$$K = S_1/S_2 \tag{16}$$

D. Vapor Pressure

In general, vapor pressures are not all that important in preformulation, but it should always be kept in mind that a substance may have sufficiently high vapor pressure to (a) become lost to a sufficient extent to cause apparent stability problems and content uniformity problems and (b) exhibit a potential for interaction with other compounds and adsorption onto or sorption into package components [27].

Most drug substances are, substantially, not volatile. As an initial screen, it can be determined whether the drug is sufficiently volatile to cause concern by placing a weighed amount of it in a vacuum desiccator and weighing it daily for a period of time. It is better to have a high-vacuum system for this, and the use of a vacuum electrobalance is best for this purpose. A good estimate of the vapor pressure can be obtained [28] by using a pierced thermal analysis cell, placing it on a vacuum electrobalance, and monitoring the weight loss rate. Using a substance with known vapor pressure can then be used for calibration, the loss rates being proportional to the vapor pressures.

Moisture isotherms were, up until recently, not considered part of preformulation. However, with the advent of microcalorimetry, moisture isotherms and surface areas may be determined with mg quantities of drug substance [29,30].

E. Surface Characteristics

The surface characteristics of a batch of a drug substance may greatly influence its properties in processing (flow, dissolution). Crystals may crystallize in different habits (plate, needle, cube), and these may not be due to morphology; depending on crystallization circumstances, they could all be the same crystal form, but of different habit [31].

It is a good practice, during development of a new drug, all the way through to the NDA, to take photomicrographs of each new batch of drug substance delivered to the product development department. In this manner there will exist a permanent reference record, and when deviations from expected behavior occur during the product development sequence, the photomicrograph will be one record that may throw light on the problem. Aside from this, the specific surface area (A'', cm^2/g) of each batch of drug substance should be measured.

Shape and Fractal Dimension

Shape is of great interest and affects many properties, and it is important to have a record of how a shape changes as the synthesis of the raw material changes during the development process. In the simplest form microscopy of all batches used in product development should be carried out to determine the ratio of longest to shortest dimension (average of 10 measurements). This is a type of shape factor.

Shape Factors

A series of definitions have been developed to describe the shape of a particle [32,33].

A commonly used shape factor converts the volume of a particle, v, to its volumetric mean diameter, a_v:

$$v = \alpha_v a_v^3 \tag{17}$$

Similarly, a shape factor may defined which converts the surface area, s, of a particle to its surface mean diameter, a_s:

$$s = \alpha_s a_s^2 \tag{18}$$

Another, more practical, frequently used shape factor is the overall shape factor Γ, given by:

$$\Gamma = SV^{-2/3} = N^{1/3}\alpha_s a_s^2/\{a_v^2[\alpha_v]^{2/3}\} \tag{19}$$

If a small polydisperse sample of powder is dissolved under sink conditions, then the dimensions, b, of the particle will decrease linearly with respect to time [33–37]:

$$b = b_0 - Kt \tag{20}$$

where b_0 is the initial size of the particle, t is time, and K is a constant. It is noted that the initial distribution function of the powder sample (obtainable from a small sample by electronic counting, for example) can be used to calculate the mass undissolved until the critical time, t^*. At a critical time, t^*, the smallest particle will disappear from the dissolution medium, and up to this point in time (t^*) the total number, N, of particles in the system remains the same [33,34].

If the powder sample is allowed to dissolve at times $t < t^*$, then the mass undissolved will be

$$M = \int_{b_{min}}^{b_{max}} \{\{N\rho f(b_0)\}(\alpha_{v_0})(b_0 - Kt)^3\}db_0 \tag{21}$$

where ρ is density and the subscript zero denotes initial condition. If the cubed term is expanded, then:

$$M = A_1 - B_1 t + C_1 t^2 - D_1 t^3 \tag{22}$$

The coefficients A_1, B_1, C_1, and D_1 are elaborated on below. An example is shown in Fig. 10.

$$A_1 = N\rho\alpha_{v_0} \int_{b_{min}}^{b_{max}} f(b_0)b_0^3\, db_0 = N\rho\alpha_{v_0}\mu_3 \tag{23}$$

This term is obviously the original mass of the powder sample, and μ_3 is the third moment of the probability

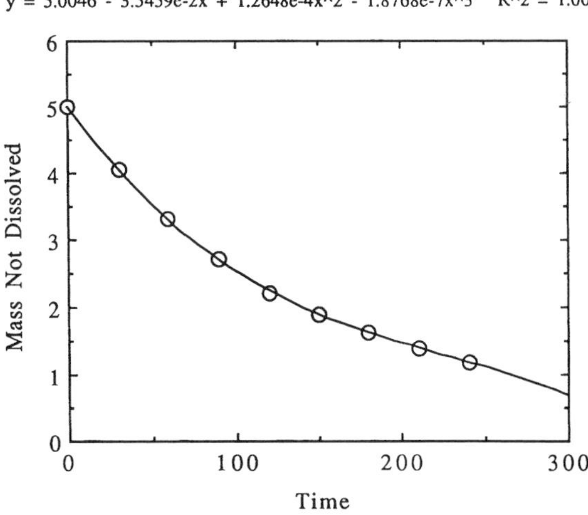

Fig. 10 Dissolution data of an oxalic acid mesh cut, plotted by way of third-order polynomial.

distribution function [38]. The third coefficient in Eq. (22) is

$$C_1 = 3N\rho K^2\alpha_{v_0} \int_{b_{min}}^{b_{max}} f(b_0)b_0\,db_0 = 3K^2N\rho\alpha_{v_0}\mu_1 \quad (24)$$

where μ_1 is the first moment of the probability density function and also the mean of the distribution [38].

The second coefficient in the expansion is

$$B_1 = 3N\rho K\alpha_{v_0} \int_{b_{min}}^{b_{max}} f(b_0)b_0^2\,db_0 = 3KN\rho\alpha_{v_0}\mu_2 \quad (25)$$

where μ_2 is the second moment of the probability density function [38].

The variance of the powder population is given by:

$$s^2 = \mu_2 - \mu_1^2 \quad (26)$$

The coefficient to the last term is given by:

$$D_1 = N\rho K^3\alpha_{v_0} \int_{b_{min}}^{b_{max}} f(b_0)db_0 = K^3N\rho\alpha_{v_0} \quad (27)$$

where use has been made of the fact that the probability density function as used is normalized:

$$D_1 = \int_{b_{min}}^{b_{max}} f(b_0)db_0 = 1 \quad (28)$$

Eq. (22) may be divided through by $A_1 = M_0$, in which case it takes the form:

$$M/M_0 = 1 - B_2t + C_2t^2 - D_2t^3 \quad (29)$$

and the coefficients with subscript 2 are then the coefficients with subscript 1 divided by M_0.

The coefficients of the terms in t, t^2, and t^3 in Eq. (29) are given by the following equations:

$$B_2 = K\mu_2/\mu_3 \quad (30)$$

$$C_2 = K^2\mu_1/\mu_3 \quad (31)$$

$$D_2 = K^3/\mu_3 \quad (32)$$

In a typical research and development setting, in the event that a new drug candidate is recognized by the drug-discovery group, then the dissolution rate constant K for that compound under specified hydrodynamic conditions can be determined from powder dissolution data and practical size analysis by microscopy.

This can be done via Eqs. (29) through (32). From the dissolution data, the coefficient B_2 is obtained and through the results from microscopy the moments μ_2 and μ_3 can be evaluated. By knowing N, the initial number of particles, and the density of the solid, the average initial volume shape factor for a polydisperse powder can be estimated.

The same problem can be considered in the opposite direction [34]. Knowing the K-value for a compound (e.g., oxalic acid dihydrate) under specified hydrodynamic conditions and the fraction undissolved as a function of time, the moments of the distribution function of a "dimension of significance" can be obtained.

At the critical time, there is a change in slope in the cube root law plot [37,39].

The fraction undissolved data until the critical time can be least-square fitted to a third degree polynomial in time as dictated by Eq. (29). The moments of distribution μ_1, μ_2, and μ_3 can be evaluated from Eqs. (30) through (32), with three equations used to solve for three unknowns. These values may be used as first estimates in a nonlinear least-squares fit program, and the curve will, hence, reveal the best values of both shape factor, size distribution, and K-value.

However, more sophisticated methods may be used to attain a good feel for the shape factor, namely its fractal dimension. This is most conveniently carried out by use of imaging techniques.* The general principle of this is shown in Figs. 11 and 12.

As an example (and this is a hypothetical example only), a particle is shown in Fig. 11 such as might appear on a microscope slide. This particle is gridded out in the form shown in the upper lefthand corner of Fig. 11. The number of squares in which parts of the trace of the particle is located is counted. This number is N, and the length of the grid size is g. The grid size is arbitrarily set equal to one in this example. The grid

*An example of an excellent system is that of Universal Imaging Concepts Image 1 Softward 486 66 Computer (Data Store, INc), Hamamatsu C2400-77H BYW Chip Camera (CCD Camera Control), Sony 19″ PVM1943MD Color Monitor, UP5000 (Sony) Color Printer Nikon Model Labophot-2 $40 \times$ ocular $\times$ 10 on screen magnification.

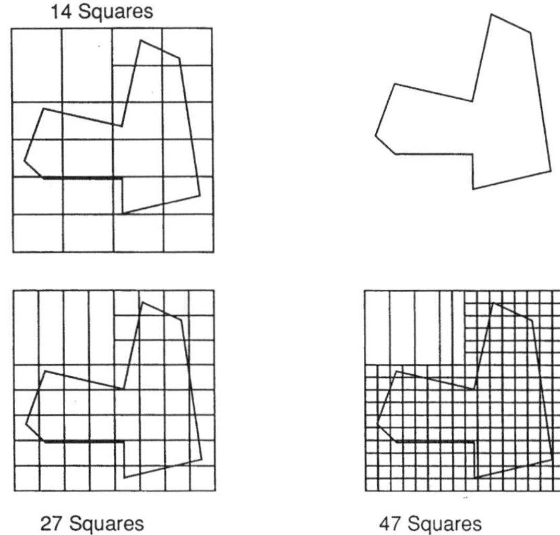

Fig. 11 Dividing the field containing a particle into more and more squares, by dividing the grid length by 2.0 in each step.

length is now halved, and the number of squares counted again, and this is repeated a number of times. The fractal equation is then given by:

$$\ln[N] = -n \ln[g] + q \tag{33}$$

where n and q are constants, and where n, the slope of the line, is the fractal dimension [40]. This dimension is characteristic for shapes, and its determination constitute a record of how shape may change during synthesis.

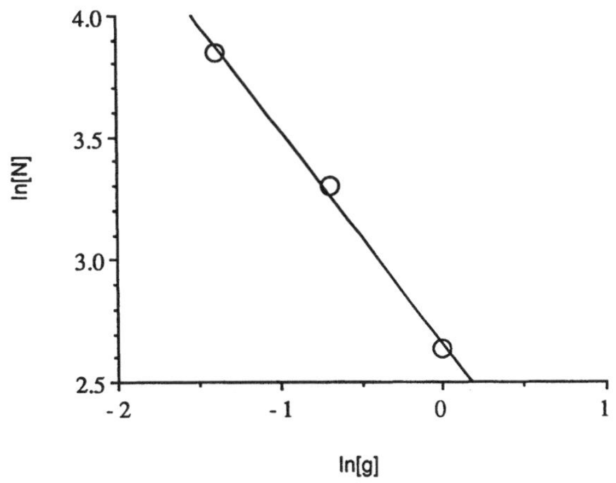

Fig. 12 Fractal graph of the data in Fig. 11. The least-squares fit for the equation is $\ln[N] = 2.6575 - 0.8735 \ln[g]$.

The number of decreases in the so-called "measuring stick" (in this case the grid) is of great importance, and it is the behavior at the smaller end of the measuring stick size that is important. In fact, the small number of iterations leading to Eq. (18) may well be falacious, but at the lower end of the scale the relationship will still be correct (but the true fractal dimension may or will be different from the value found in Fig. 11).

Particle Size and Size Distributions

The size of particles is of great importance, and particle size determinations should be carried out in preformulation as well in formulation functions. For small particle sizes, simple microscopy [41] may be used, but again imaging techniques, particularly with motorized stages, are more representative and much easier to carry out [42].

When characterizing a powder, it is important to know what type of diameter is being described, since various techniques give different types of diameter.

The volume-surface mean diameter, d_{sv}, can be determined by permeamitry (e.g., Fisher Sub-Sieve Sizer) for a fine powder [41]. It is given by

$$d_{sv} = 6V/A'' \tag{34}$$

where V is the solids volume of the sample and A'' is the geometric surface area. A'' can be obtained for a coarse powder by sieve analysis:

$$A'' = \{6/\rho\}\sum w_i/d_i \tag{35}$$

where ρ is the solids density (g/cm^3), d_i the mean diameter of the ith mesh cut, and w_i the weight retained by the ith screen. If the drug substance is not porous,

$$G = A/A'' \tag{36}$$

where G is the rugosity and is a measure of the surface roughness.

Pore Size Distribution

With the advent of mercury intrusion porosimeters, it is advantageous to perform a pore size distribution of investigational batches of a drug [43]. The Washburn equation [44] states that the pressure, P, necessary to intrude a pore is given by

$$\ln P = -q\gamma(1/r)\cos[\theta] \tag{37}$$

where

q = a constant
γ = interfacial tension
θ = contact angle
r = radius of the pore being penetrated

Since mercury has a contact angle with most solids of about 140°, it follows that its cosine is negative (i.e., it takes applied pressure to introduce mercury into a pore). In a mercury porosimeter, a solids sample is evacuated in a cell, mercury is then intruded, and the volume, V, is noted (it actually reads out), and the pressure, P, is then increased stepwise. In this fashion it is possible to deduce the pore volume of a particular radius [corresponding to P by Eq. (21)]. A pore size distribution will give the total internal pore area as well, which can be of importance in dissolution.

Hygroscopicity

Hygroscopicity is, of course, an important characteristic of a powder. It can be shown, roughly, for a fairly soluble compound that the hygroscopicity is related to its solubility [45,46], although it has been shown that the heat of solution plays an important part in what is conceived as "hygroscopicity" [47–49]. A hygroscopicity experiment is carried out most easily by exposing the drug substance to an atmosphere of a known relative humidity (e.g., storing it over saturated salt solutions in desiccators). Each solution will give a certain relative humidity (RH), and the test is simply to weigh the powder from time to time and determine the amount of moisture adsorbed (weight gained). This does not work with drug substances that decompose (e.g., effervescent mixtures will start losing weight due to carbon dioxide evolution) [50].

It can be shown that if the air space is sufficiently agitated to prevent vapor pressure gradients, the initial uptake rate (g H_2O/g solid per hour) is related to relative humidity by

$$L = a_{21}[\mathrm{RH} - \mathrm{RH}_0] \tag{38}$$

where RH_0 is the vapor pressure of a saturated solution of the drug substance in water. The latter can be estimated by an ideality assumption; if the solubility is expressed as a mole fraction X_s, the vapor pressure over a saturated solution will be P' given by

$$P' = (1 - X_s)P^* \tag{39}$$

where P^* is water's vapor pressure at that temperature.

The experiments above are rather easy to carry out and should always be part of a preformulation program, since hygroscopicity can be so important that it will dictate whether or not a particular salt should be used. Dalmane, for instance, is a monosulfate and is used as such since the disulfate, desirable in many other respects, is so hygroscopic that it will remove water from a hard-shell capsule and make it exceedingly brittle.

IV. STABILITY

Stability of a drug substance and product is monitored throughout the development and clinical phases. This monitoring requires stability-indicating assay methodology, and this is a subject that is separate from performulation per se. In most instances, the major, feasible decomposition products are identified early [51], and as such it is known if the pathways are hydrolytic, oxidative, or photochemical.

High-performance liquid chromatography (HPLC) is the usual chemical method employed, although "older" methods, such as thin layer chromatography (TLC) can be of use. Microcalorimetry can also be of use [52].

It should again be emphasized that at the onset of a new drug program, there are only small amounts of drug substance at hand. One of the first tasks for the preformulation scientist is to establish the framework within which the first clinical batches can be formulated. To this end it is important to know with which common excipients the drug is compatible. Below, the distinction will be made between solid and liquid dosage forms.

A. Compatibility Test for Solid Dosage Forms

It is important for the formulator of a new drug substance to know with which excipients he can work and with which he cannot. Some pharmaceutical incompatibilities are known to the formulator, e.g., magnesium stearate/aspirin, and glucose/amines [53].

To assess unknown incompatibilities it is customary to make a small mix of drug substance with an excipient [54,55], place it in a vial, place a rubber stopper in the vial, and dip the stopper in molten carnauba wax (to render it hermetically sealed). The wax will harden and form a moisture barrier up to 70°C. A list of common excipients characteristic of this type of test is shown in Table 1. At times it is possible to obtain quantitative relationships of

Table 1 Categories for Two-Component Systems

	Identical	Worse: 17–27 months at 25°C	Worse: 10 days at 55°C	Total score: 25°C	Total score: 55°C
Drug per se					
Dry	15	4	1	38	31
5% H_2O	9	8	3	49	38
+ Magnesium stearate					
Dry	16	3	1	34	30
5% H_2O	15	4	1	43	35
+ Calcium stearate					
Dry	13	4	3	37	32
5% H_2O	12	5	3	38	35
+ Stearic acid					
Dry	15	5	0	42	31
5% H_2O	7	11	2	60	38
+ Talc					
Dry	14	5	1	38	30
5% H_2O	10	8	2	45	34
+ Acid-washed talc					
Dry	12	8	0	44	31
5% H_2O	10	9	1	49	35
+ Lactose					
Dry	12	5	3	38	32
5% H_2O	9	7	4	65	56
+ $CaHPO_4$, anhydrous					
Dry	12	6	2	46	36
5% H_2O	9	8	3	66	53
+ Cornstarch					
Dry	12	5	3	39	34
5% H_2O	10	5	5	40	37
+ Mannitol					
Dry	10	7	3	39	31
5% H_2O	8	7	5	47	45
+ Terra alba					
Dry	14	6	0	41	28
5% H_2O	11	6	3	50	45
+ Sugar 4x					
Dry	12	6	2	41	34
5% H_2O	9	7	4	63	61

Source: Ref. 54.

excipient characteristics and interaction rates [55,56]. In addition to the test as described, a similar set of samples are set up where 5% moisture is added. A storage period of 2 weeks at 55°C (except for stearic acid and dicalcium phosphate, where 45°C is used) is employed, after which time the sample is observed physically for (1) caking, (2) liquefaction, (3) discoloration, and (4) odor or gas formation. It is then assayed by TLC or HPLC.

It is noted that one of the samples set up is the drug by itself. This is done for several reasons, one of which is that it is now required by FDA for IND submissions [1]. One more reason is that at the onset of a program, the organic synthesis of the compound may lack the refinement it will later have, and it is not uncommon that there will be several weak spots (impurities) on a TLC chromatogram of a compound obtained by initial laboratory synthesis. Hence, in selecting the excipients with which the drug substance is deemed to be compatible, it is customary to use as criteria that (after accelerated exposure of a drug/excipient mix) no new spots have developed and that the intensity of the spots in the drug stored under similar conditions (2 weeks at 55°C) are the same as in the acceptable excipient. This type of program is used by many companies with good success (i.e., the formulas developed based on the findings from the compatibility program are stable).

It should be noted that liquefaction at times occurs because of eutectic formation (e.g., often with caffeine combinations) and that this may not necessarily be associated with decomposition. On the other hand, discoloration (e.g., amines and sugars) usually is.

Finally, the reason for not forcing dicalcium phosphate (a very valuable formulation aid in direct compression) beyond 50°C is that at higher temperatures (actually [57] above 70°C) it converts to the anhydrate, a conversion that is, curiously enough, catalyzed by water. In other words, the dihydrate will be autocatalytic in this respect at elevated temperatures, and it should not be ruled out based on high-temperature findings.

B. Kinetic pH Profiles

In preformulation one task is to establish the stability of the drug substance in both solid and dissolved state. In the latter case it is important, with small samples of drug substance, to assess (a) the effect of buffer type, (b) the effect of buffer concentration, (c) the effect of pH in a practical range, (d) the effect of temperature, and (e) the kinetic salt effect.

At times the solubility of a drug in water is insufficient at room temperature to allow a meaningful kinetic study, in which case it can, at times, be carried out at elevated temperature [58]. If done at several different temperatures, it may be possible to estimate the stability at room temperature by extrapolation. Frequently, a broad screen of stability is performed on the initial small sample used for initial performulation; this is frequently referred to as "forced decomposition studies" [59], in which the drug is exposed to "acid degradation," "base degradation," "aqueous degradation," "drug powder degradation," and "light degradation." More refined studies are eventually needed.

For any compound marketed by a pharmaceutical concern, at one time during its development there should be a concerted effort to establish a very exact pH profile. To do this correctly is a time-consuming undertaking. However, the information that can be gleaned from it is very important with regard to formulations, and it is therefore customary to carry out an approximate kinetic pH profile [60] early in the development stage. This will allow formulation of solutions for injections and for oral products as well, at a pH and using buffers that will give the best stability. Without it, formulation is essentially guesswork.

Most drug decompositions are hydrolyses, where the drug concentration C decreases with time via

$$dC/dt = -k_2 C_{\mathrm{H_2O}} C \tag{40}$$

Since the water concentration hardly changes, this (bimolecular) reaction scheme is reduced to the pseudo-first-order expression

$$dC/dt - KC \tag{41}$$

where K is the first-order rate constant. This integrates to the well-known form

$$\ln[C/C_0] = -Kt \tag{42}$$

Hence semilog plotting of concentration versus time (Fig. 13) will give a straight line with a slope from which K is calculated. But most reactions are catalyzed by buffers, by hydrogen ions, and by hydroxyl ions, so K will be of the form

$$K = k + k_+(\mathrm{H}) + k_-(\mathrm{OH}) + k_B(B) \tag{43}$$

where B denotes buffer concentration and k is a rate constant. A decomposition experiment is now carried out at, say, five pH values, each using two buffer concentrations. A graph is constructed (Fig. 14) versus (B) at the various pH values. At low pH (where hydroxyl ion concentration can be disregarded), Eq. (43) becomes

$$K = k_+(\mathrm{H}) + k_B(B) \tag{44}$$

so that the plot in Fig. 14 will give

$$K = k_+(\mathrm{H}) \tag{45}$$

as intercept and k_B as slope. The above allows assessment of the effect of the buffer (which is an important point in the buffer selection). Taking the 10 logarithms of Eq. (45) now gives

$$\log K = -\mathrm{pH} + \log(k_+) \tag{46}$$

A similar argument will show that at high pH

$$\log K = \mathrm{pH} - 14 + \log(k_-) \tag{47}$$

This explains why the extremes of a pH profile (Fig.15) often have slopes of plus or minus unity [61,63].

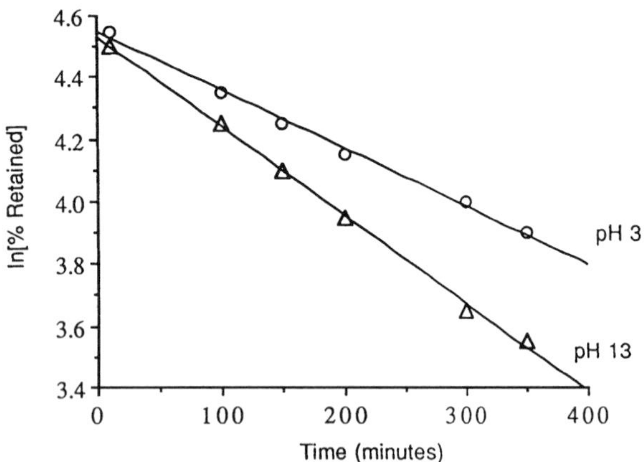

Fig. 13 Pseudo-first-order decompositions of carbuterol at 85°C at an ionic strength of 0.5 (Graphs plotted from data in Refs. 61 and 62.)

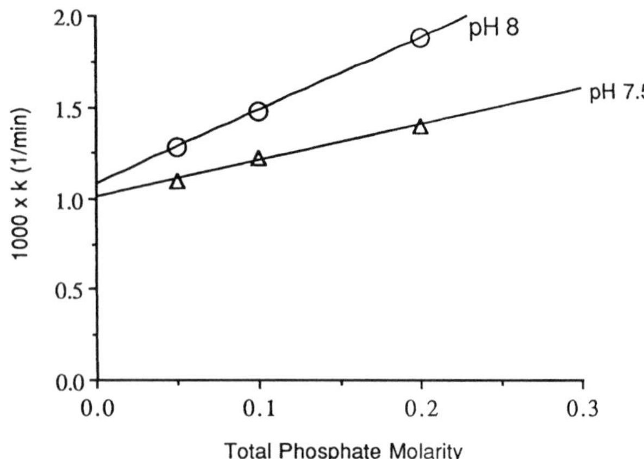

Fig. 14 Buffer concentration dependence of carbuterol at 85°C at an ionic strength of 0.5 (Graphs plotted from data in Refs. 61 and 62.)

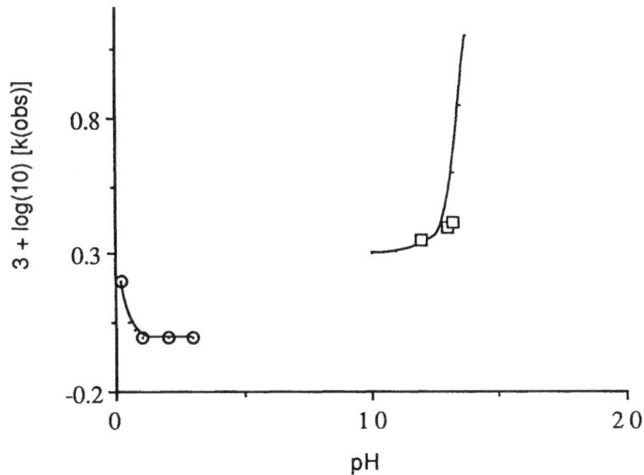

Fig. 15 Kinetic pH profile at low (circles) and high (squares) pH of carbuterol at 85°C. (Graphs plotted from data in Refs. 61 and 62.)

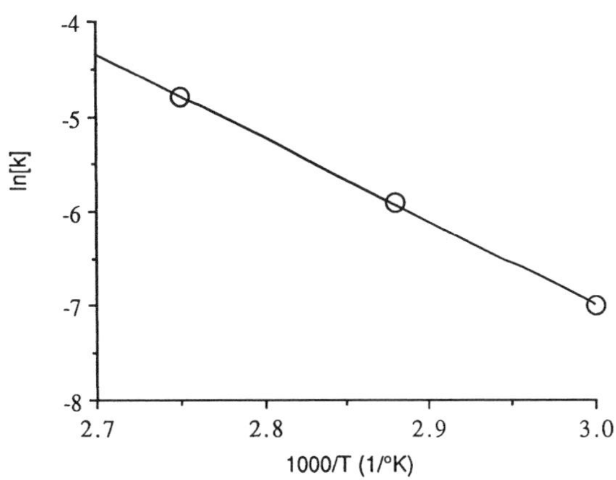

Fig. 16 Arrhenius plotting of carbuterol rate constants at pH 4 of carbuterol. (Graph plotted from data in Refs. 61 and 62.)

The horizontal part is due to the uncatalyzed rate constant, k_+, in Eq. (43). A pH profile can be done at, for example, six pH values, and since there are two kinetic points (times) and two buffer concentrations at each, a total of 24 assays are needed, which is not insurmountable. This number may be minimized and optimized by careful selection of pH and buffer concentrations [60]. Later in the program the pH profile should be repeated but with multiple points and several buffer concentrations, but this is beyond the point of preformulation. An example of a "full" pH profile is one running from pH 1 to pH 11 [61–64].

C. Liquid Compatibilities

The pH profile is the most important part of liquid compatibilities. However, two component systems are set up in aqueous (or other types of) solutions and treated as in Sec. IV.A. This is now required in the stability guidelines [1], which state that "it is suggested that the following conditions . . . be evaluated in studies on solutions or suspensions of bulk drug substances: acidic and alkaline pH, high oxygen and nitrogen atmospheres, and the presence of added substances, such as chelating agents and stabilizers" and it is suggested "that stress testing conditions . . . include variable temperature (e.g., 5, 50, 75°C)."

Aqueous Solution Capability

In general, such studies are carried out by placing the drug in a solution of the additive. These can be (and usually are) a heavy metal (with or without chelating agents present) or an antioxidant (in either oxygen or nitrogen atmosphere). Usually, both flint and amber vials are used, and in many cases an autoclaved condition is included. This will provide answers to questions about susceptibility to oxidation, to light exposure, and to heavy metals. These are important questions as far as injectable compatibilities are concerned. Exposure to various plugs is frequently included at this point so that early injectable preparations can be formulated.

For preparations for oral use, knowledge of the desired dosage form is important, but compatibility with ethanol, glycerin, sucrose, corn syrup, preservatives, and buffers is usually carried out. This type of study also gives an idea of the activation energy, E, of the predominant reaction in solution. The Arrhenius plots (Fig. 16) for compounds in solution are usually quite precise.

Denoting the rate constant by k, absolute temperature by T, the gas constant by R, and a collision factor by Z:

$$k = Z \exp[-E/(RT)] \tag{48}$$

or its more useful logarithmic cousin,

$$\ln k = \ln Z - [E/(R)](1/T) \tag{49}$$

Nonaqueous Liquid

With transdermal dosage forms being of great importance of late, it is advisable to test for compatibilities with "ointment" excipients and with polymers (e.g., ethylvinyl polymer, if that is the desired barrier).

In the case of transdermals, the dosage form is either directly placed in a stirred liquid or it is placed in a

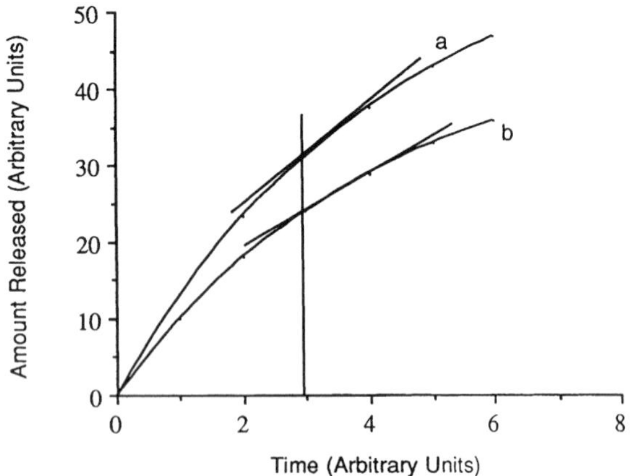

Fig. 17 Slope determination of flux of ointment release and release from ointment + membrane.

cell with an appropriate membrane (e.g., cadaver skin) to estimate the release characteristics of the drug from the ointment [65].

It should be noted here that if the overall flux is J, then

$$1/J = [1/(J_{\text{ointment}})] + [1/(J_{\text{membrane}})] \tag{50}$$

where subscripts refer to the respective phase. J_{membrane} can be obtained from curves such as shown in Fig. 17 where first the overall flux is obtained (with the membrane in place), giving the value of J. Then the release is obtained without the membrane in place, giving J_{ointment}, that is,

$$J = [1/A]\, dm_1/dt \tag{51}$$

and

$$J_{\text{ointment}} = (1/A)\, dm_2/dt \tag{52}$$

J_{membrane} is then obtained as the difference of the reciprocals.

In vivo testing is usually carried out by applying the dosage form to hairless rats followed by subsequent sacrifice. Since the skin consists of a number of layers with differing hydrophilicity, the overall fate of the drug is of importance.

V. DISSOLUTION OF DRUG SUBSTANCE AND DOSAGE FORM

In the time path solid dosage forms (tablets or capsules) must eventually to be manufactured for the clinic (e.g., in phase II). If possible, the drug substance per se is subjected to a dissolution test in a Wood's apparatus [19]. This test is useful, although quite dependent on hydrodynamic conditions. It consists of placing the powder in a type of tablet die, compressing the tablet, and exposing the flat, exposed side of the tablet (with surface area A) to a dissolution liquid (usually water or N/10 HC1) in which it has a solubility S. Under these conditions [66] the intrinsic dissolution rate constant (cm/s) can be obtained by Eq. (8), which under sink conditions* (i.e., where C is 15% of S) becomes

$$C = (SkA/V)t \tag{53}$$

It has been suggested [67] that if k is obtained under sink conditions over a pH range of 1–8 at 37°C in a USP vessel by way of Eq. (53) at 50 rpm, then if the dissolution rate constant (kA/V) is greater than 1 mg $\text{min}^{-1}\ \text{cm}^{-2}$, the drug is prone not to give dissolution-rate–limited absorption problems. On the other hand, if the value is less than 0.1, such problems can definitely be anticipated, and compounds with values of kA/V of 0.1–1 mg $\text{min}^{-1}\ \text{cm}^{-2}$ are in a gray area. For compound selectivity it is frequently useful to express dissolution findings in terms of k (i.e., in cm/s).

For small amounts of powder, dissolution of the particulate material can often be assessed (and compared with that of other compounds) by placing the powder in a calorimeter [68] and measuring the heat evolved as a function of time. The surface area must be assessed microscopically (or by image analyzer), and the data must be plotted by a cube root equation [39]:

$$1 - [M/M_0]^{1/3} = -(2kS/\rho r)t \tag{54}$$

where M is mass not dissolved, M_0 the initial amount subjected to dissolution, is true density, S is solubility, and r is the mean "radius" of the particle. The method is simply comparative, not absolute, due to the hydrodynamics being different in the calorimeter than it would be in a dissolution apparatus.

The stability of the drug substance in the dissolution liquid is of importance and has been reported on by Shishoo et al. [69].

*Strictly speaking, sink conditions are when the amount dissolved plotted versus time yields a line which, within experimental error, is linear. When the surface area, A, is constant, then this corresponds to 15% dissolved. When the surface area changes (e.g., during particulate dissolution), then this number may be smaller.

A. Biopharmaceutical Aspects

One important aspect of drug dosage form development is, of course, to obtain a dosage form that is absorbed in a desired fashion. In most cases this implies a rapidly and completely absorbed dosage form. This means that it is necessary to test the drug substance itself for in vivo release characteristics. A good indication as to whether a drug may give problems in this respect is a comparison of LD_{50} values by parenteral and oral routes. If the former toxicity is much greater than the latter, there is often an absorption problem. In the following, it is assumed that the problems are dissolution dictated.

B. Semi In Vivo Testing

The general goal is, of course, to submit an IND for the drug and to get it into testing in humans in the clinic. Frequently biological absorption characteristics are checked by such procedures as the everted sac technique [70]. Here a segment of the small intestine of a rat is everted. The ends are then tied off, and physiological fluid containing no drug (placebo liquid) is filled into the sac. It is then placed in a vessel containing a solution of the drug in a buffer solution. The setup is kept at 37°C, and all the while oxygen is being supplied to the solution. After a given interval the contents of the sac are assayed for content of the drug. This can then be repeated for other times. Collections of several samples from the same intestine segment is possible [71], and this greatly facilitates the procedure. Other methods, such as that suggested by Dolusio et al. [72], exist and are used in preformulation efforts. Here rats are anesthetized and the ileal and duodenal ends of their intestines are then cannulized, allowing sampling and liquid introduction.

C. In Vivo Testing

For preformulation purposes, some animal testing is usually performed prior to phase I. This could be in rats, dogs, or other species. The animals are tested by being given a specific dose on a specific regimen (e.g., fasting, single dose, or after each meal), and blood is then collected at various intervals. In this fashion a blood-level curve is obtained (Fig. 18). The ultimate value of this is not an absolute. To extrapolate from one species to another is a dubious undertaking, and the ramifications of this are beyond the scope of the chapter. General conclusions can be drawn and methods are briefly described below.

It is customary to do one set of tests by the parenteral route and at this stage (Fig. 18) to assume or define that 100% of the dose is absorbed [73]. Depending on pathways, this may later be modified, but the correctness of the assumption is of lesser importance at this point, as will be seen shortly. Next, a solution (or if solubility is limited, a suspension) is administered, giving a different blood level (curve II in Fig. 18). Finally, the drug is administered dry (e.g., in a capsule), giving rise to curve III in Fig. 18.

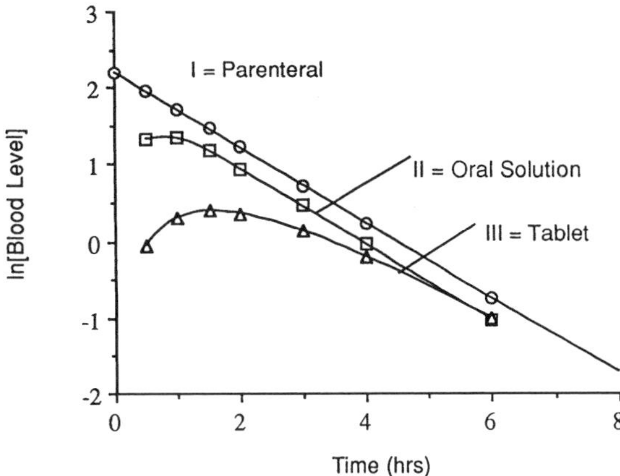

Fig. 18 Blood-level curves of identical doses of a drug by parenteral route (I) and by oral route as a solution (II) and as a tablet (III).

If the areas under the curves are denoted by A, then (based on equal dose) AII/AI is the fraction absorbed by oral route. $AIII/AII$ is the fraction efficiency of the solid dosage form. The reason for this latter is, of course, that the solid dosage form has to dissolve before the drug contained in it is available for absorption. It is the latter ratio that is important to the investigating pharmaceuticist, and therefore the outcome of the parenteral form is actually not a consideration from a formulation point of view. It is critical overall and if it is low, it may, at the point of parenteral data acquisition, be advisable to stop the program and evaluate the possibility of derivatives that would give better availability.

There are large volumes of literature written on this subject, but the simplest manner of evaluating the formula efficiency by way of blood-level data is the following simplified model: It is assumed that upon ingestion the tablets or capsules disintegrate into (N) particles, and that the drug then dissolves from these particles [74,75]. Each particle will release its content in T time units. The number of particles not dislodged from the dosage form at time t is

$$N_t = N_0 \exp(-kt) \tag{55}$$

It can be shown that for this type of situation the blood levels, B, will be a function of time by an equation of the type

$$B = A[\exp(-k_1 t) - \exp(-k_2 t)] \tag{56}$$

where k_1 is an elimination rate constant and k_2 is a function of dissolution and absorption rate constants. Figure 18 shows a case in point, where

$$B\text{II} = 7[\exp(-0 - 494t) - \exp(-2 - 813t)] \tag{57}$$

$$B\text{III} = 4.48[\exp(-0.472t) - \exp(-0.85t)] \tag{58}$$

It is noted that the k_1 values are about the same, as they should be, and that the difference, k'', between the k_2 values,

$$k'' = 2.81 - 0.85 = 2.0 \tag{59}$$

is a parameter indicative of the retardation due to disintegration and dissolution. The areas under the curves, Q, are

$$Q = (1/k_1) - (1/k_2) \tag{60}$$

In the cases in Fig. 18, the areas would be 0.942 μg h/cm^3 for the tablet and 1.67 for the solution. The formulation efficiency is 0.94/1.67 = 56% by this criterion, and the tablet formulation could stand some improvement.

REFERENCES

1. R. C. Schultz, Stability of Dosage Forms, FDA-Industry Interface Meeting, Washington, DC, Oct. 7, 1983; Stability Guidelines, Congressional Record, May 7, 1984.
2. N. Rodriguez-Hornedo, Ph.D. thesis, University of Wisconsin, 1984.
3. W. J. W. Underberg and H. Lingeman, J. Pharm. Sci., 72, 553 (1983).
4. T. Parke and W. Davis, Anal. Chem., 25, 642 (1954).
5. G. Granero, M. M. deBertorello and M. C. Brinon, Int. J. Pharm., 190, 41 (1999).
6. S. K. Bakar and S. Niazi, J. Pharm. Sci., 72, 1024 (1983).
7. S. H. Yalkowsky and S. C. Valvani, J. Pharm. Sci., 72, 912 (1983).
8. W. E. Acree and J. H. Rytting, J. Pharm. Sci., 72, 293 (1983).
9. J. T. Carstensen, K. S. Su, P. Maddrell, and H. Newmark, Bull. Parenter. Drug. Assoc., 25, 193 (1971).
10. A. N. Paruta and S. A. Irani, J. Pharm. Sci., 54, 1334 (1964).
11. G. Cave, F. Puisieux, and J. T. Carstensen, J. Pharm. Sci., 68, 424 (1979).
12. D. Sroby, R. Bitter, and J. Webb, J. Pharm. Sci., 52, 1149 (1963).
13. S. Tongaree, D. R. Flanagan, and R. I. Poust, Pharm. Dev. Tech., 4, 571 (1999).
14. S. H. Yalkowsky, G. L. Flynn, and G. L. Amidon, J. Pharm. Sci., 61, 983 (1972).
15. G. L. Amidon, S. H. Yalkoskky, and S. Leung, J. Pharm. Sci., 63, 1858 (1974).
16. S. H. Yalkowsky, G. L. Amidon, G. Zografi, and G. L. Flynn, J. Pharm. Sci., 64, 48 (1975).
17. N. Bodor, Z. Gabanyi, C. -K. Wong, J. Am. Chem. Soc., 111, 3783 (1989).
18. A. Noyes and W. Whitney, J. Am. Chem. Soc., 23, 689 (1897).
19. J. H. Wood, G. Catacalos, and S. Lieberman, J. Pharm. Sci., 52, 296 (1963).
20. H. Nogami, T. Nagai, and A. Suzuki, Chem. Pharm. Bull., 14, 329 (1966).
21. M. Shibata, H. Kokobu, K. Morimoto, K. Morisaka, T. Ishida, and M. Inoue, J. Pharm. Sci., 72, 1436 (1983).
22. J. T. Carstensen, *Advanced Pharmaceutical Solids*, Marcel Dekker, New York, 2001, p. 117, 118.
23. J. T. Carstensen, *Advanced Pharmaceutical Solids*, Marcel Dekker, New York, 2001, p. 227.
24. P. J. Cox and J. L. Wardell, Int. J. Pharm., 194, 147 (2000).
25. G. A. Stephenson, J. Pharm. Sci., 89, 958 (2000).
26. S. H. Yalkowsky, S. C. Valvani, and T. J. Roseman, J. Pharm. Sci., 72, 866 (1983).
27. M. Pikal and A. L. Lukes, J. Pharm. Sci., 65, 1269 (1976).
28. J. T. Carstensen and R. Kothari, J. Pharm. Sci., 70, 1095 (1981).
29. M. Pudipeddi, T. D. Sokoloski, S. P. Duddu, and J. T. Carstensen, J. Pharm. Sci., 85, 381 (1995).
30. M. Ohta, Y. Tozuka, T. Oguchi, and K. Yamamoto, Drug Dev. Ind. Pharm., 26, 643 (2000).
31. J. T. Carstensen, *Pharmaceutics of Solids and Solid Dosage Forms*, Wiley-Interscience, New York, 1977, pp. 6, 41.
32. J. M. Dallavalle, in *Micromeritics*, 2nd. ed., Pitman Publishing Co., New York, 1948, p. 142.
33. J. T. Carstensen and M. N. Musa, J. Pharm. Sci., 61, 223 (1972).
34. J. T. Carstensen, *Advanced Pharmaceutical Solids*, Marcel Dekker, New York, 2001, pp. 79–80.
35. M. V. Dali and J. T. Carstensen, Pharm. Res., 13, 155 (1996).
36. I. C. Edmundson and K. A. Lees, J. Pharm. Pharmacol., 17, 193, (1945).

37. J. T. Carstensen and M. Patel, J. Pharm. Sci., 64, 1770 (1975).
38. C. A. Bennett and N. L. Franklin, *Statistical Analysis in Chemistry and the Chemical Industry*, Wiley and Sons Inc., New York, 1961.
39. A. Hixson and J. Crowell, Ind. Eng. Chem., 23, 923 (1931).
40. J. T. Carstensen and M. Franchini, Drug Dev. Ind. Pharm., 18, 85 (1992).
41. B. Kaye, in *The Fractal Approach to Heterogeneous Chemistry*, D. Avnir, (Ed.), John Wiley and Sons, Chichester, NY, 1989, p. 62.
42. J. T. Carstensen, *Pharmaceutics of Solids and Solid Dosage Forms*, John Wiley, New York, 1977, pp. 56, 226, 228.
43. J. T. Carstensen and X. P. Hou, J. Pharm. Sci., 74, 466, (1985).
44. E. H. Washburn, Phys. Rev. 17, 273 (1921).
45. J. T. Carstensen, *Pharmaceutics of Solids and Solid Dosage Forms*, Wiley-Interscience, New York, 1977, pp. 11–15.
46. L. Van Campen, G. Zografi, and J. T. Carstensen, Int. J. Pharm. 5, 1 (1980).
47. L. Van Campen, G. L. Amidon, and G. Zografi, J. Pharm. Sci., 72, 1381 (1983).
48. L. Van Campen, G. L. Amidon, and G. Zografi, J. Pharm. Sci., 72, 1388 (1983).
49. L. Van Campen, G. L. Amidon, and G. Zografi, J. Pharm. Sci., 72, 1394 (1983).
50. J. T. Carstensen and F. Usui, J. Pharm. Sci., 74, 1293 (1984).
51. P. J. Jansen, M. J. Akers, R. M. Amos, S. W. Baertschi, G. G. Cooke, D. Dorman, C. A. J. Kemp, S. R. Maple, and K. A. Mccune, J. Pharm. Sci., 89, 885 (2000).
52. L. Ljunggren, N. Vokova and H. Hansson, Int. J. Pharm., 202, 71 (2000).
53. H. Lucida, J. E. Parkin, and V. B. Sunderland, Int. J. Pharm., 202, 47 (2000).
54. J. T. Carstensen, J. B. Johnson, W. Valentine, and J. Vance, J. Pharm. Sci., 53, 1050 (1964).
55. K. J. Hartauer, G. N. Abuthnot, S. W. Baertschi, R. A. Johnson, W. D. Luke, N. G. Pearson, E. C. Rickard, C. A. Tiongle, P. K. S. Tsang, and R. E. Wiens, Pharm. Dev., Tech., 5, 303 (2000).
56. P. R. Perrier and U. W. Kesselring, J. Pharm. Sci., 72, 1072 (1983).
57. A. D. F. Toy, Inorganic phosphorous chemistry, in *Comprehensive Inorganic Chemistry* (J. C. Bailar, Jr., H. J. Emelius, R. Nyholm, and A. F. Trotman-Dickenson, Eds.), A. Wheaton and Co., Exeter, England, pp. 389–543.
58. Z. Zhivkova and I. Stankova, Int. J. Pharm., 200, 181 (2000).
59. J. E. Bodnar, J. R. Chen, W. H. Johns, E. P. Mariani, and E. C. Shinal, J. Pharm. Sci., 72, 535 (1983).
60. J. T. Carstensen, M. Franchini, and K. Ertel, J. Pharm. Sci., 81, 303 (1992).
61. J. T. Carstensen, *Drug Stability*, Marcel Dekker, New York, 1991, p. 60.
62. L. J. Ravin, E. S. Rattie, A. Peterson, and D. E. Guttman, J. Pharm. Sci., 67, 1528 (1978).
63. C. M. Won, T. E. Molnar, V. L. Windisch, and R. E. McKean, Int. J. Pharm., 190, 1 (1999).
64. M. Yanatan, B. Z. Chowdhry, I. C. Ashurst, M. J. Snowden, C. Davies-Cutting, and S. Gray, Int. J. Pharm., 200, 279 (2000).
65. Y. W. Chien, P. R. Keshary, Y. C. Huang, and P. P. Sarpotdar, Drug. Dev. Ind. Pharm., 72, 968 (1983).
66. J. T. Carstensen, in *Dissolution Technology* (L. Leeson and J. T. Carstensen, eds.), The Academy of Pharmaceutical Sciences, American Pharmaceutical Association, Washington, DC, 1974, p. 5.
67. S. Riegelman, Dissolution Testing in Drug Development and Quality Control, The Academy of Pharmaceutical Sciences Task Force Committee, American Pharmaceutical Association, 1979, p. 31.
68. K. Iba, E. Arakawa, T. Morris, and J. T. Carstensen, Drug Dev. Ind. Pharm., 17, 77 (1991).
69. C. J. Shishoo, S. A. Shah, I. S. Rathod, S. S. Savale, J. S. Kotecha, and P. B. Shah, Int. J. Pharm., 190, 109 (1999).
70. T. H. Wilson and G. Wiseman, J. Physiol., 123, 116 (1954).
71. R. K. Crane and T. H. Wilson, J. Appl. Physiol., 12, 145 (1958).
72. J. T. Dolusio, N. F. Billups, L. W. Dittert, E. J. Sugita, and J. V. Swintosky, J. Pharm. Sci., 58, 1196 (1969).
73. J. T. Carstensen, *Pharmaceutics of Solids and Solid Dosage Forms*, Wiley-Interscience, New York, 1977, pp. 99, 101.
74. J. T. Carstensen, J. L. Wright, K. W. Blessel, and J. Sheridan, J. Pharm. Sci., 67, 48 (1978).
75. J. T. Carstensen, J. L. Wright, K. W. Blessel, and J. Sheridan, J. Pharm. Sci., 67, 982 (1978).

Chapter 8

Cutaneous and Transdermal Delivery—Processes and Systems of Delivery

Gordon L. Flynn

The University of Michigan, Ann Arbor, Michigan

I. INTRODUCTION

The skin forms the body's defensive perimeter against what is in reality the biologically hostile environment we humans live in. As such, in the normal course of living, it suffers more physical and chemical insult than any other tissue of the body. It is inadvertently scraped, abraded, scratched, bruised, cut, nicked, and burned. Insects bite it, sting it, and occasionally furrow through it. It is exposed to detergents, solvents, and myriad other chemicals and residues. Bacteria, yeasts, molds, and fungi live on its surface and within its cracks and crevices. It is brushed, smeared, dusted, sprayed, and otherwise anointed with toiletries, cosmetics, and drugs. Any of these exposures can rile the skin and/or provoke allergy. If there is only minor damage associated with such insults, the skin repairs itself in short order without a trace left of the injury. If the insult is severe, its reconstruction takes far longer and may occur with scarring. Such repair is essential in that humans cannot survive for long with an extensively damaged skin because it is the skin that keeps us from losing water and life's other essential chemicals to the external environment. In its intact state the skin is a formidable barrier, resistant to chemicals and tissue-harmful ultraviolet rays and virtually impenetrable to life-threatening microorganisms. To perform these necessary functions, the skin has to be tough and at the same time flexible, for it is stretched and flexed continually as we move around within it. In its healthy state it is thus a remarkable fabric, strong and far more complex than any man-made material [1].

Myriad medicated products are applied to the skin or readily accessible mucous membranes that in some way either augment or restore a fundamental function of the skin or pharmacologically modulate an action in the underlying tissues. Such products are referred to as *topicals* or *dermatologicals*. A *topical delivery* system is one that is applied directly to any external body surface either by inuncting it (spreading and rubbing in a semisolid with the fingers), by spraying or dusting it on, or by instilling it (applying a liquid as drops). Thus, "topical" is frequently used in contexts where the application is to the surface of the eye (cornea and conjunctival membranes), the external ear, the nasal mucosa or the lining of the mouth (buccal mucosa), or even the rectum, the vagina, or the urethral lining. The term "dermatological," on the other hand, describes products that are only to be applied to the skin or the scalp. An "external use only" label is used to denote such restricted use. The distinction between general topical use and external use is not trivial. Mucous membranes allow the rapid absorption of many locally applied substances that do not pass readily through intact, normal skin. This raises the potentials both drugs and excipients have to be locally irritating and/or systemically toxic. Consequently, many drugs can be applied to the external skin with impunity that should not be placed in contact with moist mucosal surfaces. Upon applying an external use only label to a package, the pharmacist warns the patient of such dangers. This chapter mainly deals with dermatological products, but general concepts and drug-delivery rationale are applicable to other modes of topical therapy as well.

The distinctions pharmacists have to make concerning topical dosage forms and their suitability for use obviously go far deeper than merely appreciating the significance of external use only labels. Pharmacological, toxicological, and risk-benefit valuations must be made for every dispensed product. An attending physician usually has such issues in mind when he or she prescribes. But even before the physician or pharmacist sees a product, the manufacturer has to establish its safety and effectiveness to the FDA's satisfaction. As part of the process, the delivery system for the drug is subjected to intense FDA scrutiny. Despite this regulatory oversight, the system isn't failsafe. Consequently, the dispensing pharmacist's lack of input into drug and drug-delivery system development does not abrogate his or her responsibility for assuring that every dispensed pharmaceutical conforms to high standards. The consummate professional thus takes every opportunity evaluate, by literature or by personal observation, how the various products he or she dispenses measure up to established standards. A pharmacist should be continually asking the following questions. Is the drug bioavailable as administered? Are the drug and its dosage form stable? Is the formulation free of contamination? Is the product pharmaceutically elegant? Attribute particulars of course vary by dosage form type and the route of administration. In any case, a "no" to any of the first three questions is reason to remove a product from distribution. Elegance is sometimes sacrificed relative to other function, but only in degree. A goal of this chapter is to elucidate the attributes of dermatological dosage forms that are helpful in evaluating and selecting products.

II. THE STRUCTURE AND FUNCTION OF SKIN

In order to answer questions regarding the therapeutic and cosmetic uses of the myriad dermatological concoctions available, a pharmacist must be knowledgeable about the anatomical structure and physiological functions of the skin and the chemical compositions and physicochemical properties of its constituent tissues. Some understanding of how its properties are affected by disease and damage is a must, as is knowledge of how the skin's physiology and function vary with age, race, environmental conditions, and other factors. Rational approaches to topical therapy rest on having such insights.

A. Skin Functions

General functions of the skin are outlined in Table 1. These functions include containment of tissues and organs, multifaceted protections, environmental sensing, and body temperature regulation. Some skin functions are inextricably entwined. For instance, containment and the barrier functions are to some extent inseparable. Active sweating is accompanied by increased peripheral blood flow, which in turn is tied in with greater nourishment of the cells of the skin as needed to promote their proliferation, differentiation, and specialization.

Let us consider how the skin is structured to better understand how this tissue performs some of its vital functions. Consider the cross section of the skin sketched in Fig. 1. This illustration shows the readily distinguishable layers of the skin, from the outside of the skin inwards: the ~10 μm thin, fully differentiated, devitalized outer epidermal layer called the stratum corneum; the ~100 μm thin live, cellular epidermis; and the ~1000 μm thin (1 mm thin) dermis. Note that all the thicknesses specified here are representative only, for the actual thickness of each stratum varies severalfold from place to place on the body. Dispersed

Table 1 Functions of the Skin

Containment of body fluids and tissues
Protection from harmful external stimuli (barrier functions)
Microbial barrier
Chemical barrier
Radiation barrier
Thermal barrier
Electrical barrier
Reception of external stimuli
Tactile (pressure)
Pain
Thermal
Regulation of body temperature
Synthesis and metabolism
Disposal of biochemical wastes (through secretions)
Intraspecies identification and/or attraction (apocrine secretions)
Blood pressure regulation

Source: Refs. 2 and 3.

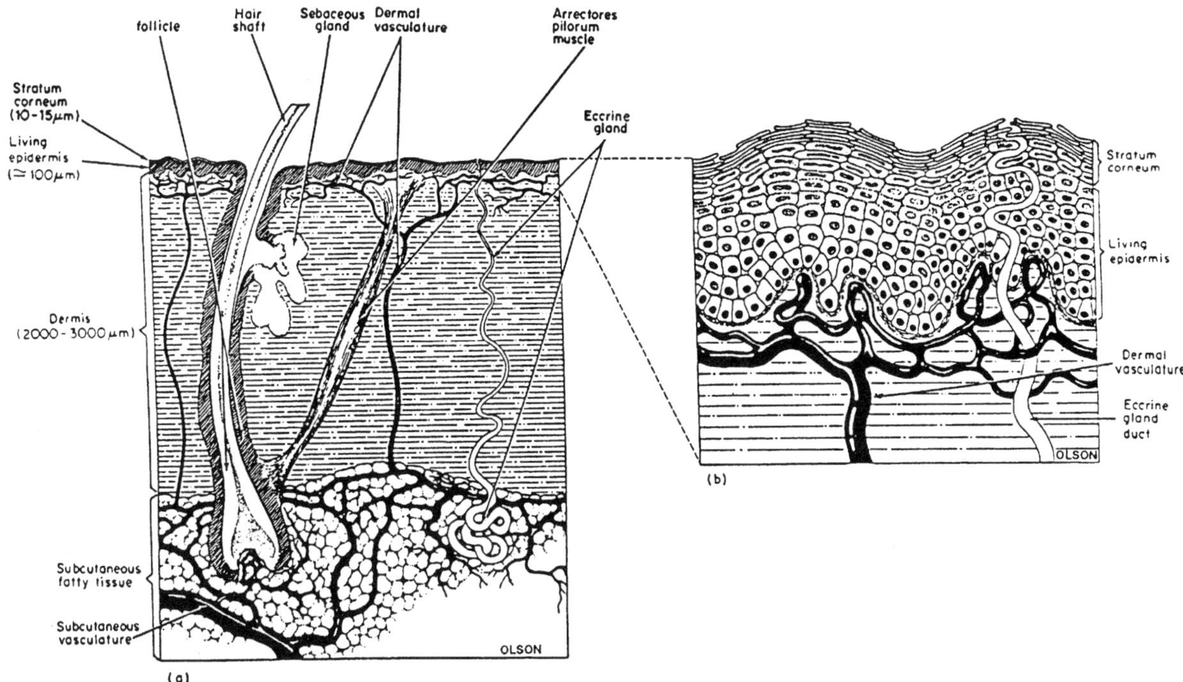

Fig. 1 Sketch of the skin.

throughout the skin, varying in number and size depending on body site, are several glands and appendages. These include (a) hair follicles and their associated sebaceous glands (pilosebaceous glands), (b) eccrine sweat glands, (c) apocrine sweat glands, and (d) nails of the fingers and toes. Each appendage has unique population densities and body distributions. The appendages also exhibit characteristic structural differences from one location to another on the body.

A highly complex network of arteries, arterioles, and capillaries penetrates the dermis from below and extends up to the surface of, but not actually into, the epidermis. A matching venous system siphons the blood and returns it to the central circulation. Blood flow through the vasculature is linked to the production and movement of lymph through a complementary dermal lymphatic system. The dermis is laced with tactile, thermal, and pain sensors.

B. Stratum Corneum

The outermost layer of the skin appearing in the exploded epidermal sketch of Fig. 1(b) represents the stratum corneum (the horny layer). The principal barrier element of the skin, it is an essentially metabolically inactive tissue comprised of acutely flattened, stacked, hexagonal cell–building blocks formed from once-living cells. These cellular building blocks are layered 15–25 cells deep over most of the body [2]. At some sites the cells appear to be stacked in neat columns. At other body locations the cellular arrangement appears random. The stratum corneum exhibits regional differences in thickness, being as thick as several hundred micrometers on the friction surfaces of the body (palms and soles). However, over most of the body, the tissue measures only about 10 μm thick, dimensionally less than a fifth of the thickness of an ordinary piece of paper [2,4]. It is a dense tissue, about 1.4 g/cm^3 in the dry state, a fact that has led it to also be referred to as the stratum compactum.

The stratum corneum is continuously under formation. Microscopic flakes (squamae) dislodged from the surface through wear and tear are replaced with new cells from beneath, with complete turnover of the horny layer occurring roughly every 2 weeks in normal individuals [5]. In humans the cells that give rise to the stratum corneum originate exclusively in the basal layer (also called basement, germinative, or proliferative layer) of the epidermis. Cell division in the basal layer begins an extraordinary process in which daughter cells are pushed outwards, first to form a layer of so-called spinous or prickle cells and then, serially, the granular, lucid, and horny layers. As suggested in Fig. 1, during their transit through the epidermal mass the cells flatten acutely. The protein and lipid components that eventually characterize the fully differentiated horny layer are synthesized in transit, with the initial strands of the structural protein that will eventually fill the cell interior being formed in the basal layer. During their inexorable migration to the stratum corneum, the protein content of the cells expands to the point that massed proteins of several kinds are distinguishable as they merge into the granular layer. Filagrin (*fila*ment ag*gr*egating prote*in*), a basic protein that stains deeply, thereby giving the granular layer some of its characteristic histological appearance, is found here. Released in one of the culminating events of formation of the stratum corneum, filagrin induces individual helical strands of soluble protein to twist together into multistranded, slightly helical fibers. These fibers, in turn, spontaneously bundle into larger helical arrays. In culmination, the intracellular space of the fully differentiated horny cell is literally packed with structural protein, namely semi-crystalline α-keratin intermixed with more amorphous β-keratin. Nothing but keratin is visible inside the fully differentiated horny cell by electron microscope. The intracellular space is dense, offering little freedom of movement to organic molecules that may become dissolved within it. Moreover, because of its remarkable ionic character, the intracellular keratin mass borders on being thermodynamically impenetrable to organic molecules.

Lipid synthesized during a keratinocyte's epidermal transit is collected in small vesicles that become visible within the granular layer. These were designated membrane-coating granules long before their content and function were known. As granular cells undergo transformation, the "coating granules" gravitate to the outermost cell membrane and are passed exocytotically into the intercellular space. A lipid "mortar" is formed that seals the horny structure. Virtually all the lipid of the stratum corneum is in the interstitial space, much of it being present in liquid crystalline, bilayer assemblage [6]. The densely packed keratin platelets caulked with intercellular lipid make the stratum corneum, pound for pound, an incredibly resistive moisture barrier. An exoskeleton (infrastructure) of residual cell membranes bound together by desmosomes and tonofibrils acts to separate the keratin and lipid domains. The lipid content of the horny layer represents about 20% of the stratum corneum's dry weight, while the endoskeleton contributes roughly 5% to the weight (see Table 2) [2,5,7].

In its normal state at ordinary relative humidity, the stratum corneum takes up moisture to the extent of 15–20% of its dry weight [2]. The ionic character of keratin is certainly a factor of consequence here. Should the skin become waterlogged, the water content of horny tissue covering the friction surfaces (callused surfaces) can rise to several multiples of the tissue's dry weight. The water content of ordinary stratum corneum appears to be less affected under the same circumstance for it seems that the stratum corneum covering the greater part of the human body has less capacity to imbibe water. Nevertheless, all horny tissue becomes hydrated to some degree when the natural evaporation of water, so-called insensible perspiration, from the skin's surface is held in check upon applying an occlusive dressing. The horny tissue thus becomes more pliable. Consequently, molecules diffuse through it with greater facility. It is likely that some substances may exhibit greater solubility within the hydrated horny mass, adding further to their ease of permeation. Conversely, the stratum corneum becomes brittle when it dries out. Ultra-dry, inelastic horny tissue splits and fissures when stretched, giving rise to the common conditions we know as chapped lips, windburn, and dishpan hands.

The stratum corneum is thus a dense, polyphasic epidermal sheathing made from dehydrated and

Table 2 Composition of the Stratum Corneum

Tissue component	Gross composition	Percentage of dry weight
Cell membrane	Lipid, protein	~5
Intercellular space	Mostly lipid, some protein and polysaccharide	~20
Intracellular space	Fibrous protein (~65–70%), nonfibrous (soluble) protein (~5–10%)	~75
Overall protein	Water soluble (10%), keratin (~65%), cell wall (~5%)	70–80
Overall lipid		10–20
All other		Up to 10
Water (normal hydration)		15–20
Water (fully hydrated)		Upwards of 300

Source: Data from Refs. 2 and 4.

internally filamented former cells held together by desmosomes, tonofibrils (intercellular anchors), and interstitial lipid. It has been estimated that it contains 10 times the fibrous material of the living epidermis in roughly one-tenth the space [8]. The stratum corneum is in contact with the living epidermal mass at its undersurface. Its external surface interfaces the environment. Cells at the basement of the stratum corneum contain water at the high thermodynamic activity of the physiological milieu, whereas air at the surface of the skin tends to have a far lower water activity. As a result, under ordinary circumstances, water diffuses out through the skin (down the implied activity gradient) and into the environment. This process is known as insensible perspiration. About 5 mL of water is lost this way per square meter of intact body surface per hour (or 0.5 $mg/cm^2/h$) [9]. An adult has upwards of 2 m^2 of body surface area, whereas a 2-year-old has about 0.75 m^2 and an infant roughly 0.25 m^2. Consequently, an adult loses about 250 mL (~8 oz) of water per day by insensible perspiration. A small child loses less than half this amount. Such water loss can increase to alarming proportions, as much or more than 100 $mL/h/m^2$, over skin ravaged by disease or damage. Evaporation rates as the latter over expansive areas of the skin can carry away sufficient body water and heat to gravely dehydrate a patient and lower his or her core body temperature to hypothermic levels.

C. Viable Epidermis

The animate cells of the epidermis make a sharp, upper interface with the lifeless stratum corneum. They also have a well-demarcated, deep interface with the dermis (Fig. 1). When physicochemically considered, the viable epidermis is nothing more than a wedge of tightly massed, live cells. Consequently, the whole of this live, cellular mass is regarded as a singular diffusional field (resistance) in percutaneous absorption models, although, when viewed under microscope, the tissue is clearly multilayered. The identifiable strata, bottom to top, are: (a) the basal layer (s. germinativum), a single layer of cubical or columnar cells that is unremarkable in appearance, (b) the multicellular spinous or prickle layer (s. spinosum) in which the cells exhibit sharp surface protuberances, and (c) the granular layer (s. granulosum), a thin layer that stains to yield a mottled appearance. In some histological displays a fourth, upper transitional and translucent layer is also distinguishable (s. lucidum). These layers reflect the progressive differentiation of the cells that eventuates in their death and placement as "bricks" within the horny structure. As elsewhere in the body, water found in the live epidermis has an activity equivalent to that of a highly dilute, isotonic NaCl solution (0.9% NaCl). The density and consistency of the live epidermal composite are only a little greater than found for water. The interface the viable epidermis makes with the stratum corneum is flat. However, the interface with the dermis is papillose (mounded). Myriad tiny bulges of the epidermis fit with exacting reciprocity over dermal depressions and ridges. It is these ridges that give the friction surfaces of the body their distinctive patterns (e.g., fingerprints). Importantly, since hair follicles and eccrine glands have epidermal origins, cells capable of regenerating the epidermis actually extend well into and through the dermis by way of these tiny glands (Fig. 1). When the skin is superficially injured, surviving cells at the base of these glands regenerate a scar-free surface. Discounting these deep rootages, the epidermis is on the order of 100–250 μm thick [10].

Keratinocytes account for most of the cells of the epidermis. One also finds Langerhans cells of white blood cell progeny here. The latter well-dispersed cells function as antigen-presenting cells (APCs) in the skin's immunological responses. Yet another group of cells, melanocytes, are strategically placed in the epidermis just above the epidermal-dermal junction (Table 3). Acting under the influence of melanocyte-stimulating hormone (MSH), these synthesize and deposit the pigment granules into skin that give the human races their unique skin colorations. Melanocytes are also set into action by ultraviolet radiation. Their activities in this circumstance lead to skin darkening. Migrant macrophages and lymphocytes are occasion-

Table 3 Cells of the Skin

Cell type	Principal function
Cells of the epidermis	
Keratinocytes	Form keratinized structures
Langerhans cells	Antigen presentation
Melanocytes	Pigment synthesis
Macrophages, lymphocytes	Migrant cells, immune responses
Cells of the dermis	
Fibroblasts	Fiber synthesis
Mast cells	Make ground substance, histamine
Blood cells	
Endothelial cells	Form the blood vessels
Nerve cells and endings	Sensors

Source: Data from Refs. 2 and 11.

ally found in skin sections. Such cells can be numerous in traumatized skin.

D. Dermis

The dermis appears in Fig. 1 as a nondescript region lying between the epidermis and a region of subcutaneous fat. In reality it is a complex structure held together by a meshwork of structural fibers, collagen, reticulum, and elastin. Most of the space between fibers is filled with a mucopolysaccharidic gel called the ground substance [2]. Approximate proportions of these phases are indicated in Table 4. The dermis ranges from about 1 mm (1000 μm) to about 5 mm in thickness [11]. The upper one fifth or so of the wedge of tissue, the papillary layer by name, is finely structured and the support for the delicate capillary plexus which nurtures the epidermis. The papillary dermis merges into a far coarser fibrous matrix, the reticular dermis. This deepest layer of the true skin is the main structural element of the skin. Of considerable importance, the microcirculation that subserves the skin is entirely located in the dermis. The dermis is also penetrated by sensory nerve endings (pressure, temperature, and pain) and houses an extensive lymphatic network. Fibroblasts, cells that synthesize the structural fibers, are found here [2], and one also finds mast cells scattered about (Table 3). The latter are thought to synthesize the ground substance. They are known to be a source of histamine that is released when the skin is immunologically provoked.

E. Skin's Circulatory System

Arteries entering the skin arise from more substantial vessels located in the subcutaneous connective tissue. These offshoots form a plexus just beneath the dermis [11]. Branches from this subcutaneous network directly supply blood to the hair follicles, the glandular appendages, and the subcutaneous fat. Branches to the upper skin from this deep plexus divide again within the lower dermis, forming a deep subpapillary network. Arterioles reaching the upper dermis out of this plexus are on the order of 50 μm in diameter. They exhibit arteriovenous anastomoses, shunt-like connections that link the arterioles directly to corresponding venules. The dermal arterioles then further branch to form the shallower subpapillary plexus of capillary loops that bring a blood supply up into the papillae at the dermal/epidermal interface. The epidermis itself is avascular.

The veins of skin are organized along the same lines as the arteries in that there are both subpapillary and subdermal plexuses [11]. The main arteriole communication to these is the capillary bed. Copious blood is passed through capillaries when the core body is either feverish or overheated, far more than needed to sustain the life force of the epidermis, and this rich perfusion lends a red coloration to skin. When there is opposite physiological need, the capillary bed is short-circuited as blood is passed directly into the venous drainage by way of the arteriovenous anastomoses. Fair skin noticeably blanches when this occurs. These mechanisms act in part to regulate body temperature and blood pressure.

The vascular surface available for exchange of substances between the blood and local tissue has been estimated to be of the same magnitude as that of the skin, i.e., 1–2 cm^2 per square centimeter of skin. At room temperature about 0.05 mL of blood flows through the skin per minute per gram of tissue. This perfusion increases considerably when the skin is warmed [4,12]. Sufficient blood courses to within 150 μm of the skin's surface to efficiently draw chemicals into the body that have percutaneously gained access to this depth [7]. Blood circulation at this level is turned off by vasoconstrictors (e.g., glucocorticoids) and turned up by vasodilators (e.g., nicotine), respectively. These vasoactivities are so reliable that vasoconstriction (blanching) has become an FDA-sanctioned measure of the penetration of corticosteroids through the skin [13,14]. The relationships between capillary blood flow and local clearances of percutaneously absorbed drugs, including the influences of vasoconstriction and vasodilation, are not well drawn.

The lymphatic system of the skin extends up and into the papillary layers of the dermis. A dense, flat meshwork of lymphatic capillaries is found here [11]. Lymph passes into a deeper network at the lower boundary of the dermis. Serum, macrophages, and lymphocytes readily negotiate through the skin's lymphatic and vascular networks.

Table 4 Composition of the Dermis

Component	Approximate % composition
Collagen	75.0
Elastin	4.0
Reticulin	0.4
Ground substance	20.0

Source: Data from Refs. 2 and 11.

F. Skin Appendages

Hair follicles and their associated sebaceous glands (pilosebaceous glands), eccrine glands, apocrine glands, and finger and toenails are all considered skin appendages. Hair follicles are found everywhere within the skin except for the soles of the feet, the palms of the hand, the red portion (vermilion border) of the lips, and the external genitalia. All are formed from fetal epidermal cells. Hair differs markedly in its prominence from place to place over the body. Delicate primary hair is found on the fetus; secondary hair or down covers the adult forehead; terminal hair ordinarily blankets the scalp and is found as pubic and axillary (underarm) hair [2]. A hair (hair shaft) emerges from a follicle, as shown in Fig. 1. Each follicle is set within the skin at a slight angle. Each consists of concentric layers of cellular and noncellular components positioned on a slight angle. Each is anchored to the surrounding connective tissue by an individual strand of smooth muscle, the arrector pilorum. Contraction of this muscle causes the hair to stand upright, merely raising goose pimples on human skin. In animals like cats, hair stands on end and makes the animal more imposing as part of the fight-or-flight response.

The hair shaft is formed continuously by cell division, differentiation, and compaction within the bulb (base) of each active hair follicle, a process that is completed deep in the follicle. Hair, like stratum corneum, is thus a compact of fused, keratinized cells. Collectively, hair follicles occupy about one thousandth of the skin's surface [10,15], a factor that sets a limit on the role that follicular orifices can play as a route of penetration. Each hair follicle possesses one or more flask-like sebaceous glands (Fig. 1). These have ducts that vent into the open space surrounding the hair shaft just below the skin's surface. The cells of sebaceous glands, or sebocytes, are programmed to divide, differentiate, and die. Before they die and disintegrate, they pack themselves full of lipid-containing vesicles. The residue left behind at their death is mixed with other follicular debris below the follicular orifice to form an oily substance called sebum. Sebum is then forced upwards around the hair shaft and onto the skin surface. The follicular outlets for sebum exhibit diameters ranging from 200 to 2000 μm (2 mm) depending on body location [11]. Glands with the largest openings are found on the forehead, face, nose, and upper back. These large follicles contain an almost microscopic hair, if they contain one at all, and are therefore referred to as sebaceous follicles. With about 100 follicles per cm^2 of skin, the follicular route takes up roughly a thousandth of the skin surface.

Eccrine glands (salty sweat glands) are found over the entire body except the genitalia and lips. They appear as tubes extending from the skin surface all the way to the footings of the dermis. Here the tube coils into a ball roughly 100 μm in diameter (Fig. 1) [11]. By anatomical count, there are between 150 and 600 glands per cm^2 of body surface depending on body site [16]. They are particularly concentrated in the palms and soles, attaining densities in these locations well in excess of 400 glands/cm^2. However, since many of these glands remain dormant, estimates of their numbers are appreciably lower if based on actual sweating units. Each gland has an approximately 20 μm diameter orifice at surface of the skin from which its secretions are spilled. In total, these glandular openings represent approximately one ten-thousandth of the skin's surface [10]. Eccrine sweat is a dilute (hypotonic), slightly acidic (pH$\sim$5.0 due to traces of lactic acid) aqueous solution of salt. Its secretion is stimulated when the body becomes overheated through warm temperatures or exercise. Evaporation of the water of the sweat cools the body's surface and thus the body. Since the gland is innervated by the autonomic nervous system, eccrine sweating is also stimulated emotionally (the clammy handshake).

Apocrine glands are found only in the axillae (armpits), in the anogenital region, and around the nipples. Along with other secondary sexual characteristics, these glands develop at puberty. We know that they are innervated emotionally and through concupiscence. In the mature female they exhibit cyclical activities in harmony with the menstrual cycle. Like eccrine glands, they are coiled tubular structures, but the coils are roughly 10 times larger. They extend well into the subcutaneous layer beneath the skin [2,11]. Each gland is paired with a hair follicle; its secretion is vented into the sebaceous duct of the follicle beneath the surface of the skin. Because this secretion is minor in amount and combines with sebum before reaching the skin's surface, its exact chemical make-up remains an enigma. What is not a mystery is that bacterial decomposition of the secretion is responsible for human body odor.

III. SKIN FUNCTIONS

The skin's main physiological roles are outlined in Table 1. Of these, the chemical barrier function is central to the use of topical drugs because deposition of a topical drug into the deeper, living strata of skin is a prerequisite for achieving its pharmacological effect. Degeneration in some of the functions can be pathognomonic of disease. Even where specific functions do not relate materially to the skin's state of health, they are tied in with cosmetic practices and thereby are of interest to pharmacists.

A. Containment

The containment function relates specifically to the ability of the skin to confine underlying tissues and restrain their movements. The skin draws the strength it needs to perform this mechanical role from its tough, fibrous dermis [2]. Ordinarily, the skin is taut even when under resting tension, yet it stretches easily and elastically when the body is in motion, quickly returning to normal contours when the stretching ceases. This extensibility of the skin is attributable to an alignment of collagen fibers under tension and in the direction of a load, which are otherwise nonaligned in the ground tension state. Elastin fibers attached to individual collagen strands relax and, in doing so, restore the irregular order of the restive state. As one ages, the resilience of these dermal fibers decreases and the tensile strength of the tissue increases. Eventually, the skin becomes stretched beyond its ability to elastically restore its initial condition and it folds over itself, or wrinkles. Lost elasticity is advanced through extended exposure to ultraviolet (UV) radiation (sunlight), and thus wrinkling is often pronounced on dedicated sunbathers.

The behavior of the epidermis when distended is also of importance. Obviously, this layer should not be torn or broken when placed under mechanical stress, for an intact epidermis is the body's first line of defense against infection. It is the stratum corneum's role to fend against tearing [2]. Pound for pound, this tissue is actually stronger than the dermal fabric, and, as a rule, it is sufficiently elastic to adjust to stretching. Its pliability, however, is conditional, and it fissures and cracks if stretched when excessively dry. Arid atmospheres alone can produce this condition (windburn). Detergents and solvents, which extract essential, water-sequestering lipids from the stratum corneum, and diseases such as psoriasis associated with a malformed horny structure render the stratum corneum brittle and prone to fissuring.

Although much is still to be learned about the factors that contribute to the pliability of the stratum corneum, it is generally accepted that its elasticity is dependent on a proper balance of lipids, hygroscopic, water-soluble substances, and water, all in conjunction with its keratin proteins. Water is its principal plasticizer, or softening agent, and it takes roughly 15% moisture to maintain adequate pliability. The capacity of the stratum corneum to bind and hold onto water is greatly reduced by extracting it with lipid solvents such as ether and chloroform. Moreover, there is a further significant decrease in the water-binding capacity of callus, a thickened stratum corneum found on the palms and soles, when it is extracted with water after having first been treated with a lipid solvent. The latter observation seems to tell us that amino acids, hydroxy acids, urea, and inorganic ions, cosmetically referred to at the skin's natural moistening factor, and the stratum corneum's lipids both assist the stratum corneum in retaining moisture necessary to plasticize its mosaic, filamented matrix. In effect, the water makes the tissue less crystalline through its interposition between polymer strands.

B. Microbial Barrier

Normal stratum corneum, taken in its entirety, is a dense molecular continuum penetrable only by molecular diffusion. It is virtually an absolute barrier to microbes, preventing them from reaching the viable tissues and an environment suitable for their growth. The outermost stratum corneum is continuously being shed in the form of microscopic scales (natural desquamation) and to a limited depth is laced with tiny crevices. Many microorganisms, pathogens and harmless forms alike, are found in these rifts. Surgeons know well that superficial washing is insufficient to remove these surface microbes, and therefore the surgical scrub is an energetic and intense cleansing with a disinfectant soap. The microorganisms residing on and in the skin can and do initiate infections if seeded into living tissues as a result of abrasive or disease-induced stratum corneum damage. Consequently, antiseptics and antibiotics are widely used to chemically sanitize wounds.

Beyond physical barrier protection, several natural processes lead to skin surface conditions unfavorable to microbial growth. Both sebaceous and eccrine secretions are acidic, lowering the surface pH of the skin below that welcomed by most pathogens. This acid mantle (pH$\sim$5) [16] is moderately bacteriostatic. Sebum also contains a number of short-chain fungistatic and bacteriostatic fatty acids, including propanoic, butanoic, hexanoic, and heptanoic acids [17]. That the skin's surface is dry also offers a level of protection. It comes as no surprise that fungal infections and other skin infections are more prevalent in the skin's folds during warm weather as intensified sweating leaves the skin continually moist in these regions.

Glandular orifices provide possible entry points for microbes. The duct of the eccrine sweat gland is tiny and generally evacuated. Experience tells us that this is not an easy portal of entry, although localized infection is seen occasionally in infants suffering prickly heat. Pilosebaceous glands seem more susceptible to infection, particularly those on the forehead, face, and upper back, referred to as sebaceous follicles. Glands at these specific locations have an almost imperceptible hair surrounded by a massive sebaceous apparatus and are especially prone to occlusion and subsequent infection (acneform pimples and blackheads). Such sebaceous gland infections are usually localized. However, if the infected gland ruptures and spews it contents internally, deep infection is possible. The body defends against this by walling off the lesion (forming a sac, or cyst) and then destroying and eliminating the infected tissue. The destruction of cystic acne is deep, so much so that facial scarring is associated with it. In hair follicles containing prominent hairs, the growing hair shaft acts as a sebum conveyer, which unblocks the orifice. It may be strictly coincidental, but such follicles seem less prone to clogging and infection.

C. Chemical Barrier

The intact stratum corneum also acts as a barrier to chemicals brought into contact with it. Its diffusional resistance is orders of magnitude greater than found in other barrier membranes of the body. Externally contacted chemicals can, in principle, bypass the stratum corneum by diffusing through the ducts of the appendages. The ability of each chemical to breach the skin and the diffusional route or routes it takes are dependent on its own physicochemical properties and the interactions it has within the skin's various conduit regimes. Being central to the effectiveness of dermatological products, exposition of the skin's barrier properties is made in following sections.

D. Radiation Barrier

Ultraviolet wavelengths of 290–310 nm from the UV-B band of radiation constitute the principal tissue-damaging rays of the sun, which are not fully atmospherically filtered. An hour's exposure to the summer sun and its damaging rays can produce a painful burn with a characteristic erythema. The skin has natural mechanisms to prevent or minimize such sun-induced trauma, but it takes time to set these into place. Upon stimulation by ultraviolet rays, particularly longer, lower-energy rays above 320 nm, melanocytes at the epidermal-dermal junction produce the pigment melanin. Melanin's synthesis begins in the corpus of the melanocyte, forming pigment granules that migrate outwards to the tips of the long protrusions of these star-like cells. Adjacent epidermal cells endocytotically engulf these projections. Through this cellular cooperation melanin, which absorbs and diffracts harmful UV rays, becomes dispersed throughout the epidermis and a person tans, with his or her capacity to sunburn declining accordingly. It should be realized that tanning takes time, several days in fact, and is incapable of protecting a person on first exposure. Damaging ultraviolet exposure also stimulates epidermal cell division and thickening of the epidermis (acanthosis). Such thickening, too, takes several days. When effected, it also lends protection to the underlying tissues.

Pharmacists should tell their sun-deprived, fair-skinned patrons not to spend more than 15–20 minutes in the mid-day sun (10:00 a.m. to 3:00 p.m.) on first exposure when traveling to vacation spots such as Florida [18]. This is ample, safe exposure to initiate the tanning response in those who are able to tan. Exposures can be increased incrementally by 15 minutes a day until a 45-minute tolerance is developed, which is generally an adequate level of sun protection in conjunction with the use of sunscreens. It should be obvious that dark-skinned people are already heavily pigmented and thus far less susceptible to burning. Other individuals don't tan at all and must apply sunscreens with high protection factors before sun bathing.

E. Electrical Barrier

Dry skin offers high impedance to the flow of an electrical current [3]. Stripping the skin by successively removing layers of the stratum corneum with an adhesive tape reduces the electrical resistance about sixfold, which tells us that the horny layer is the skin's prime electrical insulator. Its high impedance complicates the measurement of body potentials, as is done in electroencephalograms and electrocardiograms. Consequently, electrodes having large contact areas are used to monitor the brain's and the heart's electrical rhythms. Granular salt suspensions or creams and pastes containing high percentages of electrolytes are placed between the electrode surface and the skin to assure that electrical conductance is adequate to make the measurements.

F. Thermal Barrier and Body Temperature Regulation

The body is basically an isothermal system fine-tuned to 37°C (98.6°F). The skin has major responsibility in temperature maintenance. When the body is exposed to chilling temperatures that remove heat faster than the body's metabolic output can replace it, changes take place in the skin to conserve heat. Conversely, when the body becomes overheated, physiological processes come into play that lead to cooling.

The skin's mechanism of heat conservation involves its very complex circulatory system [2,3]. To conserve heat, blood is diverted away from the skin's periphery by way of the arteriovenous anastomoses. The externalmost circulation of the blood is effectively shut down, leading to a characteristic blanching of the skin in fair-skinned individuals. Less heat is irradiated and convectively passed into the atmosphere. Furry mammals have yet another mechanism to conserve body heat. Each tiny arrector pilorum stands its hair up straight, adding appreciable thickness to the insulating air layer entrapped in the fur, reducing heat loss.

When the body is faced with the need to cast out thermal energy, the circulatory processes are reversed and blood is sent coursing through the skin's periphery, maximizing radiative and convective heat losses. This process produces a reddening in light skin, a phenomenon that is particularly noticeable following strenuous exercise. Exercise also leads to profuse eccrine sweating, a process that is even more efficient in heat removal. Watery sweat evaporates, with the heat attending this process (heat of vaporization) cooling the skin's surface. Factors that accelerate the evaporative process, such as the gentle flow of air produced by a fan, accelerate cooling. Low humidity favors evaporation, and one is more comfortable and sweating is less noticeable when the air's moisture content is low. Pharmacists should be aware that eccrine sweating is a vital process not to be tampered with. Coverage of the body with a water-impermeable wrapping, as has occasionally been done in faddish weight control programs, may result in hyperthermia, particularly if there is concurrent exercise. In its extreme, hyperthermia can be fatal.

IV. RATIONALE FOR TOPICALS

One's grasp of topical dosage forms and their functioning can be nicely organized into several broad usage categories. For instance, many products exist to augment the skin barrier (Table 5). Sunscreens and anti-infective drugs obviously do this. The barrier is made pliable and restored in function by emollients. Pastes are sometimes used to directly block out sunlight and at other times to sequester irritating chemicals that would otherwise penetrate into the skin. Even insect repellants add function to the barrier.

Table 5 Barrier Augmentation by Topical Products

Product type	Barrier effect
Sunscreens	Enhance radiation barrier
Topical anti-infectives	Augment microbial barrier
Emollients	Moisturize stratum corneum, restore barrier
Insect repellents	Add a chemical barrier to insects
Poison ivy products	Negate antigens, augment chemical barrier
Diaper rash products	Build up moisture and chemical barrier

A second general purpose of topical application involves the selective access drugs have to epidermal and dermal tissues when administered this way. Penetration of the skin can drench the local tissues with the drug prior to the systemic dissemination and dilution. As a result, the drug's systemic levels are kept low and pharmacologically inconsequential. In contrast, systemic treatment of local conditions bathes highly blood-perfused tissues with the drug first, with the drug's systemic effects or its side effects sometimes overpowering the actions sought for it in the skin.

In a few instances, drugs are applied to the skin to actually elicit their systemic effects. This is called transdermal therapy. Transdermal therapy is set apart from local treatment on several counts. It is only possible with potent drugs that are also highly skin permeable. To be used transdermally, compounds must be free of untoward cutaneous actions as well. When these demanding conditions are met, transdermal therapy offers an excellent means of sustaining the action of a drug. Transdermal delivery also skirts frequently encountered oral delivery problems such as first-pass metabolic inactivation and gastrointestinal (GI) upset. Transdermal therapy is actually an old medical strategy, as compresses and poultices have been used for centuries, although never with certainty of effect. The current effective use of small adhesive patches to treat systemic disease or its symptoms has revolutionized the practice.

A. Therapeutic Stratification of the Skin

How does a person best organize his or her thinking relative to these different rationales? One can start by asking what the topical drug is supposed to do. Is it to be applied to suppress inflammation? Eradicate infectious microorganisms? Provide protection from the sun? Stop glandular secretions? Provide extended relief from visceral pain? Regardless of which feat the drug is to perform, the answer to the question directs us to where and sometimes how the drug must act to be effective or to the target for the drug. Once knowing the locus of action, one can then consider its accessibility. Clearly, if the drug cannot adequately access its target, little or no therapeutic benefit will be realized.

Sundry drug targets exist on, within, or beneath the skin. These include: (1) the skin surface itself (external target), (2) the stratum corneum, (3) any one of several levels of the live epidermis, (4) the avascular, upper dermis, (5) any one of several deeper regions of the dermis, (6) one or another of the anatomically distinct domains of the pilosebaceous glands, (7) eccrine glands, (8) apocrine glands, (9) the local vasculature, and, following systemic absorption, (10) any of numerous internal tissues. As these targets become increasingly remote, delivery to them becomes sparser as the result of dilution via tissue distribution, and, consequently, adequacy of delivery becomes less certain. Moreover, the specific properties of these targets and their negotiability are very much determined by the state of health of the skin. Disease and damage alter the barrier characteristics of the skin and therefore target accessibility itself.

Causes of skin damage and/or eruptions are diverse and may alternatively be traced to damage, irritant or allergic reactions, an underlying pathophysiological condition, or an infection. Depending on the problem, the entire skin or only a small part of it may be involved. Moreover, disease may be manifest in one part of a tissue as a consequence of a biochemical abnormality in another. For instance, the cardinal expression of psoriasis is its thickened, silvery, malformed stratum corneum (psoriatic scale), but the disease actually results from maverick proliferation of keratinocytes in the germinal layer of the epidermis. Humankind suffers many skin problems, each unique in expression to the well-trained eye. The names of some common afflictions are listed in Table 6, with indications of the tissue source of the problems. Table 7 adds pathophysiological terms used to describe the expressions of disease to the lexicon. Irrespective of their fundamental tissue origins, most diseases fan out and involve other tissue components. Inflammation and skin eruption are common sequelae. The nature and developing pattern of a skin eruption become the determinants of its diagnosis. There are subtleties, and it often takes a dermatologist to make a proper differential diagnosis.

The pharmacist will, from time to time, be called upon to examine an eruption or condition and make recommendation for treatment. If and only if the condition is unmistakable in origin, delimited in area, and of modest intensity should the pharmacist recommend an over-the-counter remedy for its symptomatic relief. Physicians neither need nor want to see inconsequential cuts, abrasions, or mosquito bites or unremarkable cases of chapped skin, sunburn, or poison ivy eruption, and so on. However, if infection is present and at all deep-seated or if expansive areas of the body are involved, otherwise minor problems can pose a serious threat and physician referral is mandatory. Patients should also be directed to counsel with a physician whenever the origins of a skin problem are in question.

B. Surface Effects

Of the many possible dermatological targets mentioned above, the skin surface is clearly the easiest to access. Surface treatment begins at the fringe of cosmetic practice. Special cosmetics are available to hide unsightly blemishes and birthmarks. These lessen self-consciousness and are psychologically uplifting. Applying a protective layer over the skin is sometimes desirable. For example, zinc oxide pastes are used to create a barrier between an infant and its diaper that adsorbs irritants found in urine, ameliorating diaper rash. These same pastes literally block out the sun and at the same time hold in moisture, protecting the ski enthusiast from facial sunburn and windburn on the high slopes. Transparent films containing ultraviolet light–absorbing chemicals are also used as sunscreens. Lip balms and like products lay down occlusive (water-impermeable) films over the skin, preventing dehydration of the underlying stratum corneum and thereby allaying dry skin and chapping. The actions of calamine lotion and other products of the kind are limited to the skin's surface. The suspended matter in these purportedly binds urushiol, the hapten (allergen) found in poison ivy and oak. However, these may best benefit the patient by drying up secretions, relieving itchiness. In all these instances where the film itself is therapeutic, bioavailability has little meaning.

Table 6 Common Afflictions: Brief Outline of Common Dermatological Disorders and Other Common Skin Problems

Skin problems	Examples
I. General involvements	
A. Physical damage	
1. Blunt instrument	Contusion, bruise
2. Sharp instrument	Cut, nick, animal bite
3. Scraping, rubbing	Abrasion, blister
4. Heat	Burns (1°, 2°, 3°), blister
5. Ultraviolet radiation	Sunburn
6. Insects	Mosquito bite, bee sting, ticks, mites (chiggers), lice, crab lice
B. Chemical damage	
1. Contact dermatitis	Poison ivy, poison oak
2. Contact allergy	Cosmetic dermatitis
3. Solvent extraction	"Dishpan hands"
II. Abnormalities of the epidermis	
A. Stratum corneum	
1. Tardigrade sloughing and thickening	Ichthyosis
2. Hyperdryness	Chapping, windburn
3. Hyperproliuerative thickening, abnormal structural organization	Psoriasis
B. Viable epidermis	
1. Cell damage and inflammation	Eczema, general dermatitis
2. Fluid collection	Blister
3. Abnormal cell growth (not division)	Keratosis
4. Thickening of granular layer	Lichen planus
5. Hyperproliferation, incomplete keratinization	Psoriasis
6. Malignancy	Epithelioma
III. Abnormalities of the dermis and dermal epidermal interface	
A. Melanocyte abnormalities	
1. Hyperfunction	Tanning, chloasma, freckles
2. Hypofunction	Vitiligo
3. Abnormal growth	Mole
4. Malignancy	Melanoma
B. Dermal/epidermal interface	
1. Lifting of the epidermis	Dermatitis hypetiformis
2. Overgrowth of papillary layer	Warts
C. Dermis	
1. Vascular reactions	Urticaria, hives
2. Abnormal growth of fibrinocyte	Scar, keloid
3. Abnormal polymerization	Scieroderma, lupus erythematosus
IV. Abnormalities of the glands (appendages)	
A. Hair follicle	
1. Hyperactivity	Hirsutism
2. Hypoactivity	Alopecia, baldness
B. Sebaceous glands	
1. Hyperactivity	Seborrhea
2. Occlusion	Acne, pimples
C. Eccrine sweat gland	
1. Hyperactivity	Hyperhidrosis
2. Occlusion, inflammation	Miliaria (pricky heat, heat rash)
V. Infectious diseases	
A. Bacterial	Carbuncles (boils)
B. Fungal	Athlete's foot, ringworm
C. Viral	Chickenpox, herpes simplex (cold sores)
D. Protozoal	Topical amebiasis

Source: Refs. 16 and 19.

Table 7 Pathophysiological Terms: Brief Definitions of Select Pathophysiological Terms

Term	Definition
Acne	Inflammatory disease of the sebaceous glands characterized by papules, comedones, pustules, or a combination thereof
Alopecia	Deficiency of hair
Bulla	Large blister or vesicle filled with serous fluid
Chloasma	Cutaneous discoloration occurring in yellow-brown patches and spots
Comedo (pl. comedones)	Plug of dried sebum in the sebaceous duct; blackhead
Dermatitis	Inflammation of the skin
Dermatitis herpetiformis	Dermatitis marked by grouped erythematous, papular, vesicular, pustular, or bullous lesions occurring in varied combinations
Eczema	An inflammatory skin disease with vesiculation, infiltration, watery discharge, and the development of scales and crusts
Hirsutism	Abnormal, heavy hairiness
Ichthyosis	A disease characterized by dryness, roughness, and scaliness of the skin caused by hypertrophy of the stratum corneum
Infiltration	An accumulation in a tissue of a foreign substance
Keloid	Growth of the skin consisting of whitish ridges, nodules, and plates of dense tissue
Keratosis	Any horny growth
Lichen planus	Inflammatory skin disease with wide, flat papules occurring in circumscribed patches
Lupus erythematosus	A superficial inflammation of the skin marked by disklike patches; with raised reddish edges and depressed centers, covered with scales or crusts
Miliaria	An acute inflammation of the sweat glands, characterized by patches of small red papules and vesicles, brought on by excessive sweating
Nodule	Small node that is solid to the touch
Papilla	Small, nipple-shaped elevation
Psoriasis	A skin disease characterized by the formation of scaly red patches, particularly on the extensor surfaces of the body (elbows, knees)
Pustule	Small elevation of the skin filled with pus
Scleroderma	A disease of the skin in which thickened, hard, rigid, and pigmented patches occur with thickening of the dermal connective tissue layer
Seborrhea	A disease of the sebaceous glands marked by excessive discharge
Urticaria	Condition characterized by the appearance of smooth, slightly elevated patches, whiter than the surrounding skin
Vesicle	Small sac containing fluid; a small blister
Vitiligo	A skin disease characterized by the formation of light-colored (pigment-free) patches

Bioavailability does matter with topical antiseptics and antibiotics even though these also act mainly at the skin's surface. These anti-infectives are meant to stifle the growth of surface microflora, and thus formulations that penetrate into the cracks and fissures of the skin where the microorganisms reside are desirable. The extent to which the surface is sanitized then depends on uptake of the anti-infective by the microbes themselves. Slipshod formulation can result in a drug being entrapped in its film and inactivated. For instance, little to no activity is to be expected when a drug is placed in a vehicle in which it is highly insoluble. Ointment bases that contain salts of neomycin, polymyxin, and bacitracin are suspect in this regard in that hydrocarbon vehicles are extremely poor solvents for such drugs. Inunction (rubbing in) may release such drugs, but pharmacist should seek evidence that such formulations are effective before recommending them.

Deodorants are also targeted to the skin surface to keep microbial growth in check. They slow or prevent rancidification of the secretions of apocrine glands found in and around the axillae (armpits) and the anogenital regions. Medicated soaps also belong in this family.

C. Stratum Corneum Effects

The stratum corneum is the most easily accessed part of the skin itself, and there are two actions targeted to this tissue, namely emolliency, the softening of the horny tissue, which comes about through remoisturizing it, and keratolysis, the chemical digestion and removal of thickened or scaly horny tissue. Tissue needing such removal is found in calluses, corns, and psoriasis and as dandruff. Common agents such as salicylic acid and, to a lesser extent, sulfur cause lysis of the sulfhydral linkages holding the keratin of the horny structure together, leading to its disintegration and sloughing.

It has been mentioned that elasticity of the stratum corneum depends on its formation and on the presence of adequate natural lipids, hygroscopic substances, and moisture [19,20]. Simply occluding the surface and blocking insensible perspiration can induce remoisturization (emolliency). However, it is best accomplished by lotions, creams, and/or waxy formulations (e.g., lip balms), which replenish lost lipid constituents of the stratum corneum. The fatty acids and fatty acid esters these contain in part fill the microscopic cracks and crevices in the horny layer, sealing it off, stabilizing its bilayer structures, allowing it to retain moisture. Many emollient products also contain hygroscopic glycols and polyols to replenish and augment natural moisturizing factors of this kind, also assisting the stratum corneum in retaining moisture.

The introduction of moisturizing substances into the stratum corneum is ordinarily a straightforward process. Deposition of keratolytics, on the other hand, is not as easily achieved, as these agents must penetrate into the horny mass itself. Some salicylic acid–containing corn removers are therefore made up as concentrated nonaqueous solutions in volatile solvents. As these volatile solvents evaporate, drug is concentrated in the remaining vehicle and thereby thermodynamically driven into the tissue. These many examples illustrate the fact that when the therapeutic target is at the skin's surface or is the stratum corneum, the therapeutic rationale behind the treatment usually involves enhancing or repairing or otherwise modulating barrier functions (Table 5).

D. Drug Actions on the Skin's Glands

A few products moderate operation of the skin's appendages. These include antiperspirants (as opposed to deodorants), which use the astringency of chemicals such as aluminum chloride to reversibly irritate and close the orifices of eccrine glands [21] to impede the flow of sweat. Astringents also decimate the population of surface microbes, explaining their presence in deodorants. The distinction between antiperspirants and deodorants is legally significant because antiperspirants alter a body function and are regulated as drugs while deodorants are classified as cosmetics. Thus, the antiperspirant action has to be scientifically proven before it can be claimed for a product. Nevertheless, given the similarities in the compositions of deodorants and antiperspirants, they are likely functionally equivalent. Since eccrine glands are mediated by cholinergic nerves, sweating also can be shut off by anticholinergic drugs administered systematically [22] or topically. However, such drugs are too toxic for routine use as antiperspirants even when administered topically.

Acne is a common glandular problem arising from hyperproliferative closure of individual glands in the unique set of pilosebaceous glands located in and around the face and across the upper back. Irritation of cells lining the ducts of such glands initiates the formation of lesions. Sheets of sloughed, sebum-soaked, keratinized cells that grow out from the walls surrounding the sebaceous duct are what clog the duct. Still forming sebum is then trapped behind the obstruction, often bulging out the skin and giving rise to an observable lesion (papule). This may become infected and fill with a purulent exudate (pustule), or, after infection has set in, it may internally rupture and thereby begin the processes that lead to ulceration and scarring. Alternatively, the buildup of concentric sheets of sloughed cells may widen the glandular opening, with melanin in the widening plug darkening to the point of being black (blackhead).

Soap and water is considered a therapeutic treatment in acne when it is used to unblock the pores. Sebum is emulsified and it and other debris is removed. Alcoholic solvents, often packaged as moistened pledgets, are used for the same purpose. With either treatment care must be exercised not to dry out and further irritate the skin. Both local and systemic antibiotics and antiseptics suppress the formation of lesions. It is believed these attenuate the population of anerobic microorganisms that are deep-seated in the gland, the metabolic byproducts of which irritate the lining of the gland, setting off lesion formation. Mild cases of acne improve and clear under the influence of astringents, possibly for the same reason. Retinoids, oral and topical, reset the processes of epidermal proliferation and differentiation. Through such dramatic influences on cell growth patterns, they actually prevent the formation of lesions. However, because of concerns over toxicity, they tend to be used only in the most severe cases of acne and thus are prescribed for those patients whose acne lesions progress to cysts.

Hair is a product of the pilosebaceous apparatus and in this sense is glandular. It often grows out visibly in places where such display is unwanted. It may be shaved, but chemical hair removers (depilatories) along with other products are also used to remove it. In the main, the use of depilatories is cosmetic rather than therapeutic. However, depilatories may be prescribed in hirsutism, where the existence of coarse, dark facial hair is psychologically distressing to the female patient for whom shaving is an anathema. Hair, like the stratum corneum, is composed of layers of dead, keratinized cells. However, its keratin is more susceptible to the action of keratolytics because it is structured in ways that make it more chemically pervious. Thioglycolate-containing, highly alkaline creams generally dissolve hair in short order without doing great harm to surrounding tissues. Facial skin is delicate, however, and depilatories must be used carefully here.

E. Effects in Deep Tissues

Local, Regional, and Systemic Delivery

When the target of therapy lies beneath the stratum corneum, topical drug delivery is more difficult and becomes more uncertain. Therefore, many potentially useful drugs find no place in topical therapy due to their inability to adequately penetrate the skin. Nevertheless, a number of pathophysiological states can be controlled through local administration and subsequent percutaneous absorption. For example, most skin conditions are accompanied by inflammation of the skin; topical corticosteroids and nonsteroidal anti-inflammatory drugs alike are used to provide symptomatic relief in such instances. Corticosteroids are also used in psoriasis where, in addition to suppressing inflammation, they somehow act on the basal epidermal layer to slow proliferation and restore the skin's normal turnover rhythm [23]. Pain originating in the skin can be arrested with locally applied anesthetics. Over-the-counter (OTC) benzocaine and related prescription drugs are used for this purpose. Hydroquinone is applied to the skin to lighten excessively pigmented skin by oxidizing melanin deep within the surface. Another treatment that involves percutaneous absorption is the application of 5-fluorouracil (5-FU) for the selective eradication of premalignant and basal cell carcinomas of the skin [22]. In all of these examples the key to success is the ability we have to get therapeutic amounts of the drugs through the stratum corneum and into the viable tissues.

Systemic actions of some drugs can also be achieved via local application, in which case their delivery is known as transdermal delivery. The application of warmed, soft masses of medicated bread meals and clays over wounds or aching parts of the body dates to antiquity. However, few such plasters and poultices (cataplasms) have survived into modern medicine. Just past the middle of the twentieth century improvements in analytical instrumentation made it possible to measure the exceedingly low circulating levels of drugs that build up in the body during the course of therapy. It was at this time that serious research was begun on the ways drugs might be delivered to lower their risk and extend their duration of action. Novel delivery systems involving nontraditional routes of administration were subsequently conceived, constructed, and put to the test. Transdermal delivery with adhesive patches evolved as one of the innovations.

The possibilities for transdermal delivery might have been seen long ago in the systemic toxicities of certain topically contacted chemicals. As long as a century ago it was known that munitions workers who handle nitroglycerine suffer severe headaches and ringing in the ears (tinnitus). These same effects are experienced to a degree by those taking nitroglycerine to alleviate angina. The association between therapy and the inadvertent percutaneous absorption of nitroglycerine was finally made in the 1970s and a nitroglycerine ointment was introduced, producing peak blood levels comparable to those attained upon sublingual administration of traditional tablet triturates, but levels that were also sustained. Since the permeability of human skin is highly variable and since patient needs themselves vary, patients using nitroglycerine ointments were (and are) instructed to gradually lengthen the ribbon of ointment expressed from the tube and rubbed into the skin until tinnitus and headache were experienced. They were then counseled to back off from this dosage. The lasting nature of nitroglycerine's clinical action when administered in this fashion helped free patients from the fear they had of waking in the middle of the night with a heart attack (angina). Consequently, a nitroglycerine ointment became the first commercially successful, therapeutically proven transdermal delivery system. But ointments are greasy and suffer variability in their dosing, even with dose titration, as a result of the fact that different patients apply semisolids more or less thinly and therefore over lesser or greater areas.

Since about 1980, sophisticated adhesive patches for transdermal delivery of scopolamine (motion sickness), nitroglycerine (anginal symptoms), clonidine (regulation of blood pressure), β-estradiol (menopausal symptoms), fentanyl (cancer pain), nicotine (smoking cessation), and testosterone (hypogonadism) have been introduced into medicine [24–26]. These patches, affixed to an appropriate body location, deliver drug continuously for periods ranging from about half of a day (nitroglycerine) to a week (clonidine, β-estradiol). To achieve a long duration of delivery, a patch must contain a reservoir of its respective drug. In one early type of system, nitroglycerine was formulated into a liquid-filled sponge that was held in intimate contact with the skin by an adhesive band around the periphery of the patch. In more recent patch designs a membrane is placed over the delivery surface of the patch. Adhesive covering this membrane anchors the patch to the skin over the entire contact area of the patch. This interfacing membrane can be turned into a rate-controlling membrane to regulate delivery and prevent dose dumping should the patch be inadvertently placed over a site of inordinately high permeability. Actually, this rate-controlling concept was used in the design of the first patch, the scopolamine transdermal system. The development of transdermal patches for yet other drugs is an active research area.

It is obvious from the above that the skin is a formidable barrier irrespective of whether therapy is to be local, regional or systemic, and the first concern in topical delivery is sufficiency of delivery. With local therapy, the aim is to get enough drug into the living epidermis or its surroundings to effect a pharmacological action there without producing a systemically significant load of the drug. The latter is actually a rare occurrence except when massive areas of application are involved. Regional therapy involves effects in musculature and joints deep beneath the site of application. To be successful, this requires a greater delivery rate because an enormous fraction of the drug that passes through the epidermis is routed systemically via the local vasculature. Indeed, the levels of drug reached in deep local tissues have proven to be only a few multiples higher than those obtained upon systemic administration of the drug [27]. Even more drug has to be delivered per unit area to transdermally effectuate a systemic action.

Factors Affecting Functioning of the Skin Barrier

A matter of considerable consequence in topical delivery is variability in skin permeability between patients, which may be as much as 10-fold. The underlying sources of this high degree of variability are thought to be many and diverse. Humans differ in age, gender, race, and health, all of which are alleged to influence barrier function. Yet, insofar as can be told, a full-term baby is born with a barrier-competent skin, and, barring damage or disease, the skin remains so through life. There is little convincing evidence that senile skin, which tends to be dry, irritable, and poorly vascularized, is actually barrier compromised [28]. However, premature neonates have inordinately permeable skins. The incubators used to sustain such infants provide a humidified environment, which abates insensible perspiration, and a warm one, conditions that not only make the baby comfortable but that also forestall potentially lethal dehydration and hypothermia [29].

Gender, too, affects the appearance of human skin. Nevertheless, there is little evidence that the skin of males and females differs greatly in permeability. However, there are established differences in the barrier properties of skin across the races of humans. While the horny layers of Caucasians and Blacks are of equal thickness, the latter has more cell layers and is measurably denser [30]. As a consequence, black skin tends to be severalfold less permeable [30,31].

Humidity and temperature also affect permeability. It has long been known that skin hydration, however brought about, increases skin permeability. Occlusive wrappings are therefore placed over applications on occasion to seal off water loss, hydrate the horny layer, and increase drug penetration. In the absence of such intervention, the state of dryness of the stratum corneum is determined by the prevailing humidity, explaining why a dry skin condition is exacerbated in the winter months in northern climes.

Temperature influences skin permeability in both physical and physiological ways. For instance, activation energies for diffusion of small nonelectrolytes across the stratum corneum have been shown to lie between 8 and 15 kcal/mole [4,32]. Thus thermal activation alone can double the rate skin permeability when there is a 10°C change in the surface temperature of the skin [33]. Additionally, blood perfusion through the skin in terms of amount and closeness of approach to the skin's surface is regulated by its temperature and also by an individual's need to maintain the body's 37°C isothermal state. Since clearance of percutaneously absorbed drug to the systemic circulation is sensitive to blood flow, a fluctuation in blood flow might be expected to alter the uptake of chemicals. No clear-cut evidence exists that this is so, however, which seems to teach us that even the reduced blood flow of chilled skin is adequate to efficiently clear compounds from the underside of the epidermis.

Above all else, the health of the skin establishes its physical and physiological condition and thus its permeability. Consequences attributable to an unhealthy condition of skin can be subtle or exaggerated. Broken skin represents a high permeability state, and polar solutes are several log orders more permeable when administered over abrasions and cuts. Irritation and mild trauma tend to increase the skin's permeability even when the skin is not broken, but such augmentation is far less substantial. Sunburn can be used to illustrate many of the barrier-altering events that occur in traumatized skin. Vasodilation of the papillary vasculature with marked reddening of the skin is among the first signs that a solar exposure has been overdone. In its inflamed state, the skin becomes warm to the touch. After a day or two, epidermal repair begins in earnest and the tissue is hyperproliferatively rebuilt in its entirety. It doubles in thickness and a new stratum corneum is quickly laid down [34]. Because the newly formed stratum corneum's anchorage to existing tissues is faulty, the preexisting horny layer often eventually peels. Of more importance, hyperplastic repair leads to a poorly formed horny structure of increased permeability to water (as measured by transepidermal water loss) and presumably other substances. Given these events surrounding irritation, since many chemicals found in the workplace and home are mildly irritating, including the soaps we use to bathe and the detergents we use to clean house and cloths, is it really any wonder that the permeability of human skin is so demonstrably variable?

Some chemicals have prompt, destructive effects on the skin barrier. Saturated aqueous phenol, corrosive acids, and strong alkalis instantly denature the stratum corneum and destroy its functionality even as their corrosive actions stifle the living cells beneath. Though the stratum corneum may appear normal following such damage, the skin may be only marginally less permeable than denuded tissue [35]. Furthermore, permeability remains high during the full duration of wound repair and until a competent stratum corneum is laid down over the injured surface. Other chemicals are deliberately added to formulations to raise the permeability of skin and improve drug delivery. For obvious reasons, these are referred to as skin penetration enhancers. More will be said of these later.

Thermal burning produces comparably high states of permeability immediately following burning providing that the surface temperature of the skin is raised above 80°C, a temperature on the lower side of temperatures able to denature keratin [36]. However, burning temperatures below 75°C, though fully capable of deep tissue destruction in seconds, leave the structure of the stratum corneum itself relatively unscathed. Burn wounds of this kind remain impermeable until tissue repair and restructuring processes get under way and the necrotic tissue with its horny capping is sloughed. The increased permeability of severely burned skin immediately following the trauma can be highly consequential in terms of drug delivery. In the instance of deep burns obtained at lower than keratin-denaturing temperatures, topical delivery of antibiotics and antiseptics into a wound, as may be necessary to control wound sepsis, remains difficult for as long as the stratum corneum over the wound stays in place, and aggressive use of antiseptics is warranted. In the other extreme there is risk of toxic systemic accumulation of the antiseptics and antibiotics, particularly in major burns covering 20% or more of the body surface area. Conservative treatment is warranted. Since burns are rarely well characterized with respect to their permeability dimension, attending physicians and pharmacists need to monitor antiseptic usage carefully to control wound sepsis without poisoning the patient. Finally, if not surgically debrided, the necrotic tissue is eventually walled off, enzymatically digested, loosened, and sloughed, producing a denuded, open, granulating surface.

Small full-thickness wounds are closed and sealed off quickly by reconstruction of the epidermis from the edges of the wound. Large full-thickness injuries take too long to heal by this process and require grafting. All such wounds remain highly permeable until covered over again with a healthy, fully differentiated epidermis.

As with burns, physical disruption of the stratum corneum opens the skin in proportion to the extent of damage. Cuts and abrasions are associated with high permeability at and around such injuries. Eruption of the skin in disease has a similar effect to the extent that the stratum corneum's integrity is lost. The skin over eczematous lesions should be regarded as highly permeable. Not all skin diseases raise permeability, however. The states of permeability of ichthyosiform, psoriatic, and lichenified skin have not been well characterized but in all likelihood are low for most drugs. It has been proven difficult to get potent corticosteroids through psoriatic plaque, for instance, and occlusive wrapping is often called for.

Percutaneous Absorption—the Process

The process of percutaneous absorption can be described as follows. When a drug system is applied topically, the drug diffuses passively out of its carrier or vehicle and, depending on where the molecules are placed down, it partitions into either the stratum corneum or the sebum-filled ducts of the pilosebaceous glands. Inward diffusive movement continues from these locations to the viable epidermal and dermal points of entry. In this way a concentration gradient is established across the skin up to the outer reaches of the skin's microcirculation where the drug is swept away by the capillary flow and rapidly distributed throughout the body. The volume of the epidermis and dermis beneath a 100 cm^2 area of application, roughly the size of the back of the hand, is approximately 2 cm^3. The total aqueous volume of a 75 kg ($\sim$165 lb) person is about 50,000 cm^3, yielding a systemic-to-local dilution factor well in excess of 10,000. Consequently, systemic drug levels are usually low and inconsequential. Thus selectively high epidermal concentrations of some drugs can be obtained. However, if massive areas of the body ($\geq$20% of the body surface) are covered with a topical therapeutic, systemic accumulation can be appreciable. For instance, corticosteroids have produced serious systemic toxicities on occasion when they have been applied over large areas of the body [37]. Moreover, as has already been pointed out, if the stratum corneum is not intact, many chemicals can gain systemic entrance at alarming rates. Together these factors may place a patient at grave risk and should always be taken into account when topical drugs are put in use. The pharmacist should therefore carefully measure how topical systems are to be applied and be on the alert for untoward systemic responses when body coverages are unavoidably extensive.

The events governing percutaneous absorption following application of a drug in a thin vehicle film are illustrated in Fig. 2. The important processes of dissolution and diffusion within the vehicle are cataloged. These will be discussed later. Two principal absorption routes are indicated in the figure: (a) the transepidermal route, which involves diffusion directly across the stratum corneum, and (b) the transfollicular route, where diffusion is through the follicular pore. Much has been written concerning the relative importance of these two pathways. Claims that one or the other of the routes is the sole absorption pathway are groundless since percutaneous absorption is a spontaneous, passive diffusional process that takes the path of least resistance. Therefore, depending on the drug in question and the condition of the skin, either or both routes can be important. There are temporal dependencies to the relative importance of the routes as well. Corticosteroids breach the stratum corneum so slowly that clinical responses to them, which are prompt, are reasoned to be due to follicular diffusion [4].

Sight should not be lost of the fact that the chemical barrier of the skin actually consists of all skin tissues between the surface and the systemic entry point. While it is true that the stratum corneum is a source of high diffusional resistance to most compounds and thus the skin's foremost barrier layer, exceptional situations exist where it is not the only or even the major resistance to be encountered. For example, extremely hydrophobic chemicals have as much or more trouble passing across the viable tissues lying immediately beneath the stratum corneum and above the circulatory bed because such drugs have little capacity to partition into these tissues. Backing for the latter assertion comes from extensive clinical experience as well as from physical modeling of percutaneous absorption. Consider that ointments can be used safely over open wounds because their hydrocarbon constituents are not transported significantly across even denuded skin. Similarly, the skin is considerably more impermeable to octanol and higher alkanols than is the stratum corneum alone because of the presence of the viable tissue layer beneath.

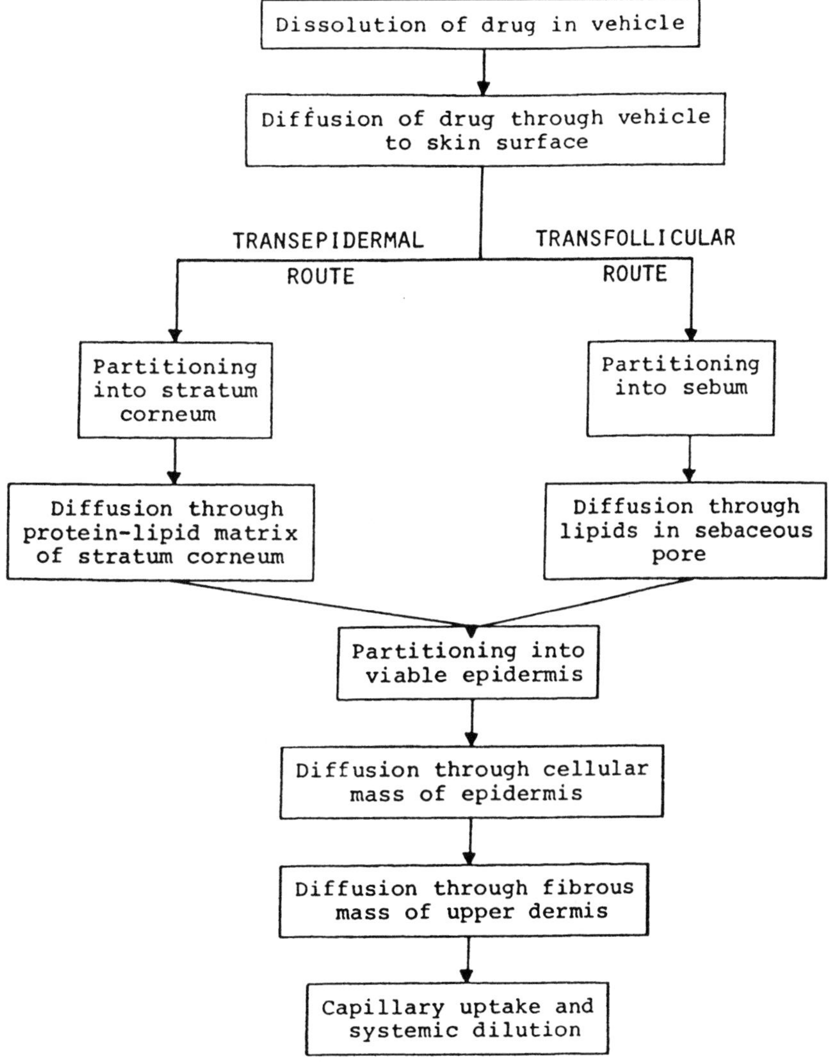

Fig. 2 Events governing percutaneous absorption.

Model of the Skin Barrier

The percutaneous absorption picture can be qualitatively clarified by considering Fig. 3, where the schematic skin cross section is placed side by side with a simple model for percutaneous absorption patterned after an electrical circuit. In the case of absorption across a membrane, the current or flux is in terms of matter or molecules rather than electrons, and the driving force is a concentration gradient (technically, a chemical potential gradient) rather than a voltage drop [38]. Each layer of a membrane acts as a diffusional resistor. The resistance of a layer is proportional to its thickness (*h*), inversely proportional to the diffusive mobility of a substance within it as reflected in a diffusion coefficient (*D*), inversely proportional to the capacity of the layer to solubilize the substance relative to all other layers as expressed in a partition coefficient (*K*), and inversely proportional to the fractional area of the membrane occupied by the diffusion route (*f*) if there is more than one route in question [39]. In general, an individual resistance in a set may be represented by:

$$R_i = \frac{h_i}{f_i \cdot D_i \cdot K_i} = \frac{[\text{thickness}]}{[\text{fractional area}][\text{diffusion coefficient}][\text{partition coefficient}]} \qquad (1)$$

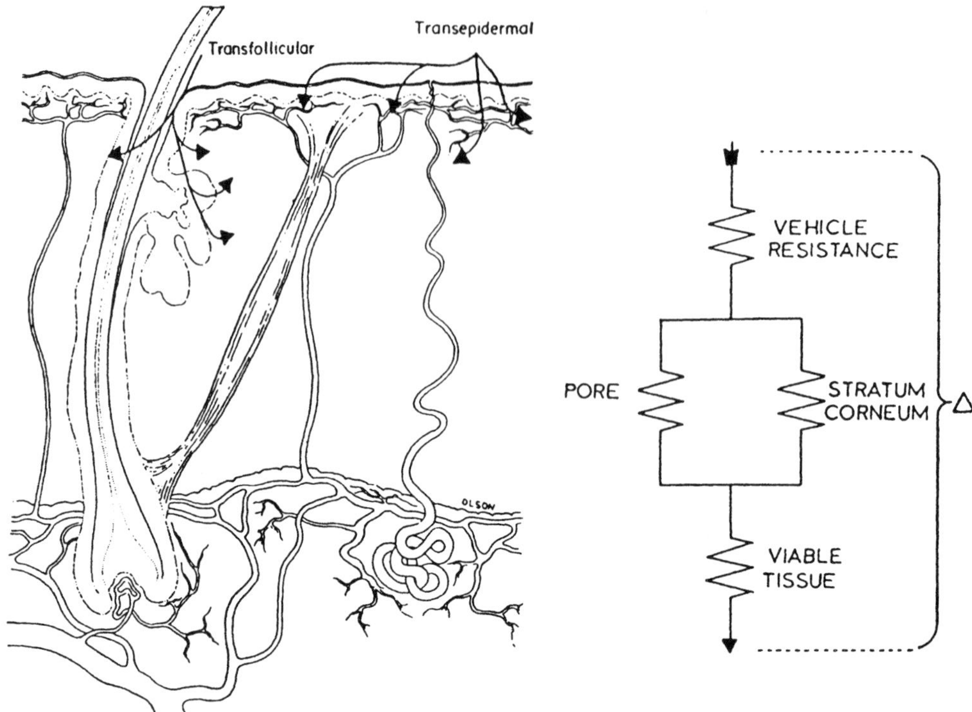

Fig. 3 Skin cross section beside a simple model.

The overall phenomenon of percutaneous absorption is describable upon recognizing that the resistances of phases in series (phases encountered serially) are additive and that diffusional currents (fluxes) through routes in parallel (differing routes through a given phase) are additive. Such considerations applied to skin allow one to explain, in semi-quantitative terms, why percutaneous absorption through intact skin is slow for most chemicals and drugs and why disruption of the horny covering of the skin profoundly increases permeability of the ordinary run of solutes.

First, consider the transepidermal route. The fractional area of this route is virtually 1.0, meaning the route constitutes the bulk of the area available for transport. Molecules passing through this route encounter the stratum corneum and then the viable tissues located above the capillary bed. As a practical matter, the total stratum corneum is considered a singular diffusional resistance. Because the histologically definable layers of the viable tissues are also physicochemically indistinct, the set of strata represented by viable epidermis and dermis is handled comparably and treated as a second diffusional resistance in series.

Estimated diffusion coefficients in the stratum corneum are up to 10,000 times smaller than found anywhere else in the skin, reflecting in part the considerable density of this tissue. If diffusion is almost exclusively through the intercellular lipid regime within the horny tissue as most experts believe, then the estimates, which range between 1×10^{-13} cm^2/s to a low of 1×10^{-9} cm^2/s, have to be tempered with the knowledge that path tortuosity (nonlinearity) and excluded volume were not taken into account. In any case, such low values still speak to the high resistance of the horny tissue [4], particularly given that the thickness of the stratum corneum is only about 1×10^{-3} cm (10 μm). The parameter exhibiting the most variability relative to the stratum corneum's diffusion resistance is the partition coefficient, K_{sc}. The partition coefficient can take values several log orders less than one with highly polar molecules, e.g., glucose, or values several log orders greater than one for hydrophobic molecules, e.g., β-estradiol. The wedge of living tissue lying between the stratum corneum and the capillaries is on the order of 100 μm thick (1×10^{-2} cm). Permeation of this element of the barrier is facile and without great molecular selectivity. Where measured, diffusion coefficients through this cellular mass have proven to be no less than one tenth of the magnitude of those found for the same compounds passing through water [40].

The follicular route can be analyzed similarly. The fractional area available for penetration by this route is on the order of one one-thousandth [4], clearly a restricting factor. Here partitioning is into sebum and the distance that has to be traveled through sebaceous medium filling the follicular duct can only be guessed at, but it has to be greater than the thickness of the stratum corneum. Fifty μm seems a reasonable estimate, the actual value almost certainly being within a factor of two of this value. Diffusion coefficients in the quasi-liquid sebum can be guessed to be from a hundred to a thousand times greater than found for the stratum corneum [4,10]. Since sebum is lipoidal, partition coefficients associated with passage through this route must exhibit wide-ranging values even as found for the stratum corneum. A thickness of viable tissue perhaps comparable to that found along the transepidermal route also lies within this pathway to the microcirculation.

Net chemical penetration of the skin is simply the sum of the accumulations by each of the mentioned routes and by other routes, for instance eccrine glands, where these contribute. The latter tiny glands are ubiquitously distributed over the body but are generally discounted in importance due to the limited fractional area they occupy and their unfavorable physiological states, either empty or profusely sweating.

All the salient features described here can be incorporated into a quantitative framework that takes into account stratification within the tissues and the parallel pathways [39]. It is instructive to consider a simple model based on these descriptions that embodies only transepidermal and transfollicular barrier elements. We can assume that each distinct tissue acts as a homogeneous phase, a gross distortion of reality but an assumption that nevertheless leads to a useful conceptual description. The resistance by the transepidermal route would be:

$$R_{\text{TransEpidermal}} = R_{\text{stratum corneum}} + R_{\text{viable tissues transepidermally}}$$

or

$$R_{\text{TE}} = R_{\text{sc}} + R_{\text{vt-TE}} \tag{2}$$

Similarly, the transfollicular resistance would be:

$$R_{\text{TF}} = R_{\text{seb}} + R_{\text{vt-TF}} \tag{3}$$

Since these routes are in parallel, the total resistance on combining them is:

$$R_{\text{total}} = \frac{1}{\frac{1}{R_{\text{sc}}+R_{\text{vt-TE}}} + \frac{1}{R_{\text{seb}}+R_{\text{vt-TF}}}} \tag{4}$$

The mass transfer coefficient (permeability coefficient) of a route is the reciprocal of the resistance of that route, and thus we can amend Eq. (4) to read:

$$R_{\text{total}} = \frac{1}{P_{\text{TE}} + P_{\text{TF}}} \tag{5}$$

Similarly, the overall permeability coefficient is the reciprocal of the total resistance and thus P_{total} is:

$$P_{\text{total}} = P_{\text{TE}} + P_{\text{TF}} \tag{6}$$

For reasons that need not be elaborated here, water is invariably the solvent medium used to experimentally access permeability coefficients. Accordingly, water is assumed to be the vehicle used to apply a drug to the skin. This choice of vehicle effectively sets the partition coefficients between the aqueous tissues and the vehicle roughly to unity. Choosing water as the vehicle of consideration does not in any way invalidate insights that can be drawn from the model as long as saturated solutions, which operate at the thermodynamic activity of the solid drug, are brought into the analysis. Barring specific solvent-induced changes in the physical chemistry of the tissue, from the thermodynamic perspective all saturated solutions should deliver drug at the same rate. Substituting fractional areas, thicknesses, partition coefficients, and diffusion coefficients for all the phases while recognizing that partition coefficients between water and the viable tissues functionally assume values of unity leads to the following expression for the overall permeability coefficient:

$$P_{\text{total}} = f_{\text{TE}}\left(\frac{D_{\text{sc}}K_{\text{sc/w}}D_{\text{vt}}}{D_{\text{sc}}K_{\text{sc/w}}h_{\text{vt-TE}} + D_{\text{vt}}h_{\text{sc}}}\right) + f_{\text{TF}}\left(\frac{D_{\text{seb}}K_{\text{seb/w}}D_{\text{vt}}}{D_{\text{seb}}K_{\text{seb/w}}h_{\text{vt-TF}} + D_{\text{vt}}h_{\text{seb}}}\right) \tag{7}$$

Finally, a general expression describing the steady state flux across a membrane, $\partial M/\partial t$ can be written as:

$$\frac{\partial M}{dt} = A \cdot P_{\text{total}} \cdot \Delta C \tag{8}$$

This equation teaches us that the total stead-state flux (total rate of permeation across a membrane in the steady state of permeation), $\partial M/dt$, is proportional to the involved area (A) and the concentration differential expressed across the membrane, ΔC. In an experiment, flux is the experimentally measured parameter while A and ΔC are fixed in value when setting up an experiment. The value of the permeability coefficient, P_{total}, is what is calculated upon completion of an experiment using Eq. (8). The permeability coefficient, besides having the specific attributes ascribed to it, is the number that converts the combined area and concentration proportionalities of flux to an equality (an equation containing an equal sign). The permeability coefficient takes units of distance over time (cm/h) and can be regarded as the average velocity of molecules penetrating a membrane irrespective of the complexity of the membrane. Its magnitude depends on the properties of the vehicle, membrane, and permeant. Moreover, when the membrane consists of several phases, the permeability coefficient is also dependent on the juxtaposition of the phases. We can now write for the skin:

$$\frac{\partial M}{dt} = A\left\{ f_{\mathrm{TE}}\left(\frac{D_{\mathrm{sc}}K_{\mathrm{sc/w}}D_{\mathrm{vt}}}{D_{\mathrm{sc}}K_{\mathrm{sc/w}}h_{\mathrm{vt\text{-}TE}} + D_{\mathrm{vt}}h_{\mathrm{sc}}}\right) + f_{\mathrm{TF}}\left(\frac{D_{\mathrm{seb}}K_{\mathrm{seb/w}}D_{\mathrm{vt}}}{D_{\mathrm{seb}}K_{\mathrm{seb/w}}h_{\mathrm{vt\text{-}TF}} + D_{\mathrm{vt}}h_{\mathrm{seb}}}\right)\right\}\Delta C \quad (9)$$

where A is the involved area of the skin and the term ΔC is the permeant's concentration differential across the skin. In clinical situations ΔC is usually well approximated by the actual concentration in the topical vehicle because dilution by way of systemic absorption of the permeant is so great. In many real instances ΔC reflects saturation of a drug in its vehicle.

Equation (9) defines the steady state in flux in terms of physically meaningful parameters. In other words, it is an anatomically based mathematical representation (model) of the skin barrier. The upper collection of terms in the greater parentheses defines the role of the transepidermal route. The second group of terms below in the greater parentheses characterizes the transfollicular pathway. To breathe life into the model, values for the parameters of Eq. (9) that are representative have to be plugged into the equation. Some parameter estimates are given in Table 8. The listed fractional areas, diffusion coefficients, and strata thicknesses reported in Table 8 are based on the best information available. All the values are approximations; some are no more than best guesses. Regardless, the impressions drawn from the model when they are plugged into it are consistent with known percutaneous absorption behavior.

To illustrate the above point, take the set of largest values given for the diffusion coefficients found in Table 8, that is, 10^{-9} cm^2/s for the stratum corneum, 10^{-7} cm^2/s for sebum, and 10^{-6} cm^2/s for the viable tissue, and convert them to cm^2/h. Conversion of these from reciprocal seconds to reciprocal hours eventually leads to permeability coefficients that are more easily compared with literature values (P in units of cm/h) When these values are substituted into Eq. (7) along with

Table 8 Representative Parameters to Probe Model

	Diffusion coefficient, D (cm^2/s)[a] [4,8]
Stratum corneum	10^{-9}–10^{-13}
Water	$\simeq 10^{-9}$
n-Alkanols (hydrated tissue)	$\simeq 10^{-9}$
n-Alkanols (dry tissue)	$\simeq 10^{-10}$
Small nonelectrolytes	10^{-9}– 10^{-10}
Progesterone	$\simeq 10^{-11}$
Cortisone	$\simeq 10^{-12}$
Hydrocortisone	$\simeq 10^{-13}$
Follicular pore (sebum)	10^{-7}– 10^{-9}
Viable tissue	$\simeq 10^{-6}$
	Tissue thickness, h (μm) [2,8,11]
Stratum comeum	
Dry (normal state)	~10
Hydrated (as by occlusion) state	20–30
Pore diffusional length	Approximately two to five times greater than the stratum corneum thickness
Viable tissue stratum	150–2000[b] (200)
	Fractional area of the routes, F [4,8]
Transepidermal	~1
Transfollicular	$\sim 10^{-3}$
Transeccrine	$< 10^{-4}$[c]
	Tissue/vehicle partition coefficient, K
Stratum corneum	From < 1 to $\gg 1$[d]
Sebum	From $\ll 1$ to $\gg 1$[d]
Viable tissue	
Aqueous vehicle	~1
Nonaqueous vehicle	From $\ll 1$ to $\gg 1$[d]

[a]These diffusivities are estimates obtained by in vitro experiment (stratum corneum) or by comparison with small tissues in which diffusivities have been measured (all others). They do not account for regional variations across the body surface, so on both counts must be considered highly approximate.
[b]Highly approximate and variable, depending on blood flow patterns.
[c]This is sufficiently small to discount transeccrine diffusion contributions in the general treatment.
[d]All depend on the physiocochemical nature of the drug and vehicle as well as the physicochemical nature of the respective tissues.

the estimated thicknesses of the respective tissues (cm) and the fractional areas of the routes, the steady-state flux through the transepidermal route is projected to be

30 times greater than through the follicular pores, everything else being equal.* The suggestion is strong here that high sebum diffusivity by itself is insufficient to offset the small fractional area of the follicular route. Clearly, partitioning tendencies favoring one or the other of these routes will magnify or shrink this multiple. Unfortunately, there is no a priori way to estimate the relative magnitudes of the operative partition coefficients.

Some scientists, including this author, believe that the stratum corneum harbors a minor polar (aqueous pore) pathway† mostly because of evidence that suggests that the stratum corneum offers higher fluxes to polar solutes such as methanol, ethanol, propylene glycol, glycerol, and glucose than one would otherwise expect. In this regard, it is also relevant that ions diffuse through the stratum corneum with deceptive ease considering their solution attributes. Sebum is not well characterized as a diffusion medium, but it is generally taken to be an oily composite. If the latter portrayal is apt, then sebum would have a thermodynamically limited ability to dissolve polar compounds. On these admittedly flimsy grounds, an argument can be mounted that the transepidermal route dominates the transfollicular route with respect to the permeation of small, polar nonelectrolytes and ions [4,8,10].

It is thought that both the stratum corneum and sebum are, to first good approximations, lipoidal routes. Consequently, drug substances of diminishing polarity should partition out of water into the key transport regimes within these routes to increasing extents. Homologs formed by extending the length of an alkyl chain provide a means for testing this hypothesis due to the fact that oil/water (o/w) partition coefficients of alkyl homologs grow exponentially. One can therefore probe the fundamental physical behaviors of lipid membranes as long as (in the permeability domain where) permeability coefficients are directly related to o/w partitioning. The slope of log(partition coefficient) against alkyl chain length plot indicates the sensitivity of partitioning between the phases in question to the addition of a methylene (CH_2) group. The value of $d[\log(K_{o/w})]/dn$, the slope, is referred to as the π-value for the partitioning system in question. The π-value for the partitioning of homologs between octanol and water is very close to 0.5. Thus, regardless of the homologous series in question, octanol/water partition coefficients, increase by a factor of about 10 for every two methylene units added to an alkyl chain. With a π-value of greater than 0.6, hexane/water partitioning evidences an even greater lipoidal sensitivity. Based on permeation of *n*-alkanols through human skin (and the permeability partitioning relationship), human stratum corneum appears have a π-value slightly less than 0.3 [4]. The low partitioning sensitivity to the addition of a methylene group suggests that the stratum corneum's lipoidal phase is considerably more polar than the reference organic solvents. If the substance of the sebaceous gland were more hydrophobic than the polar lipids found between the cell platelets of the stratum corneum, as is thought, then its methylene partitioning sensitivity would be greater than the stratum corneum's, though almost certainly less than seen with the organic solvents. This means, all else being equal, that partition coefficients would increase more rapidly by this route. It also suggests that the region of direct partitioning dependency of permeability by this route would be narrower than found for the transdermal pathway [41,42]. It doesn't appear that these combined effects should lead to a sizable shift in the relative importance of the routes as judged through modeling. This is because by the time $K_{seb/w}$ takes a value of one, passage through the transfollicular route is already approaching the point where the resistance of the viable tissue within the route is reaching a magnitude comparable to that offered by the sebum plug. Consequently, further increases in $K_{seb/w}$ would not lead to increased permeation via this pathway. On the other hand, according to the model, the value of $K_{sc/w}$ has to approach 50 before the viable tissue becomes the rate-controlling element in the transepidermal route. Perhaps by coincidence, 50 is the published partitioning value for octanol, which actually does appear to be at the threshold of viable tissue control of its permeation [4].

Model interpretation takes a different bent when minimum values for the respective diffusion coefficients are incorporated in the steady-state model, i.e., $10^{-13}\,cm^2/s$ for the stratum corneum and $10^{-9}\,cm^2/s$ for the follicular shunt route. Inserting these values, everything else held constant, suggests there should be a substantial upgrading of the importance of the transfollicular contribution. Data with steroids seem to indicate, however, that the transepidermal route retains a dominant position in the steady state even in this case.

In the main, to this point, the permeation model represented by Eq. (9) can be considered esoteric. The value of the model to practicing pharmacists stems substantially from what the model teaches us about barrier damage. To measure the result of extreme barrier damage, one only needs to use zero for

*Everything else equal here means $K_{sc/water}$ would be equal to $K_{seb/water}$.

†This supposition is hotly debated in scientific circles.

the value of h_{sc}, an operation equivalent to removing the stratum corneum. Under this circumstance, the permeability coefficient via the expansive transepidermal route takes the simplified value, $D_{vt}/h_{vt\text{-}TE}$. $D_{vt}/h_{vt\text{-}TE}$ can be as much or more that 1000-fold larger for polar compounds than found when the stratum corneum is present. However, for compounds at the extreme of nonpolarity, negligible increases in permeability are projected because $K_{sc/w}$, which appears in reciprocal in the statement of the stratum corneum's resistance, is so large that the stratum corneum is not of much consequence even when it is intact. It follows then that the level of increased permeability resulting from skin damage depends on exactly how lipophilic a compound is. The bottom line, however, is that many compounds that are safe to apply to normal skin experience up to a 1000-fold increases in their skin permeability and become very dangerous when in contact with skin. This is especially true when large areas of contact, A in the model equation, are involved. There are many cases of lethal systemic poisonings resulting from contact of chemicals with barrier-compromised skin in the literature. Pharmacists must understand and take cognizance of the kind of danger outlined here when counseling patients on the use of topical medications.

So far only steady-state conditions for permeation have been considered. But in all phenomena involving the mass transport of substances across membranes, one also has to consider the time it takes for gradients to be set up across the membranes by molecules moving randomly within the substance of the membranes. This early period of permeation is referred to as the nonstationary state period. The duration of this period is characterized by a lag time, as illustrated in Fig. 4*. The nonstationary-state period may be of some importance in the instance of skin permeation [43]. Where independent parallel pathways exist, as they seem to do through the stratum corneum, compounds may gain access to underlying tissues far more readily by one pathway than by the other. We can consider this point in terms of the lag time, t_L, that one expects to obtain for a compound diffusing through a simple isotropic field of a membrane:

$$t_L = \frac{h^2}{6 \cdot D} \tag{10}$$

*The lag time is the intercept that results by extrapolating the steady-state line of a plot of cumulative amount of drug penetrated versus time to the time axis.

where h identifies the membrane's thickness and D is the compound's diffusion coefficient. The equation teaches us that the lag times for parallel routes should differ to the extents that h and D are different for the routes. We can crudely estimate the respective lag times for the transepidermal and transfollicular routes from the diffusion coefficient and thickness estimates tabulated in Table 8. Taking this approach, lag times for the transepidermal route are projected to range from minutes for small nonelectrolytes to multiple days for molecules of the size and properties of the corticosteroids. On the other hand, the lag times for breaching the transfollicular route should range from seconds to minutes. Though relatively few molecules reach the living tissues via the transfollicular route due to the limited fractional area of this pathway, it appears that the first molecules to reach the viable epidermis actually get there via this path. This comparison has led scientists to suggest that the early clinical responses seen with drugs as large as steroids are the result of follicularly transported molecules. However, if the lag time for passage directly through the stratum corneum is also very brief, the follicular shunt diffusion is far less likely to be clinically meaningful. These nonstationary-state considerations do not apply at all when the horny barrier is impaired. Under this circumstance transepidermal lag times can be so brief that they cannot be easily measured.

Equations (8) and (9) point to the fact that the amount of drug delivered through the skin is proportional to the area of application of a topical dosage form or a transdermal patch. Nitroglycerine and other patches are available in different sizes (areas) to take advantage of this proportionality in dosing. Pharmacists have to be cognizant of this area dependency for another important reason, this being that the systemic accumulations, and thus systemic toxicities, of topically applied drugs are proportional to application area. Indeed, excessive area of application is the most frequent cause of the untoward systemic actions seen with topically applied drugs. Tiny infants have been fatally poisoned following too liberal applications of borate-containing talcum powders. As a result, borates are no longer used as lubricants in powder formulations. Babies have also been poisoned upon bathing them with a hexachlorophene-containing soap. Bathing, of course, is virtually synonymous with whole body coverage. Hexachlorophene is no longer used as an antiseptic soap. Diaper dermatitis tends to be expressed over large areas. Anti-inflammatory corticosteroids have occasionally been used too liberally to remedy this condition, again eventuating in serious

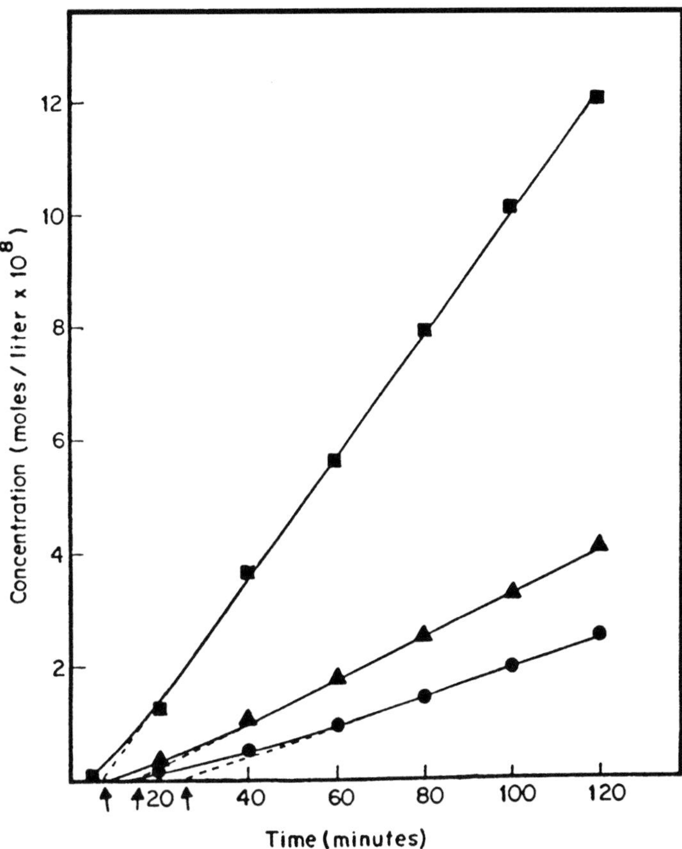

Fig. 4 Generalized permeation profile. From left to right the data are for n-butanol permeating hairless mouse skin at 20°, 25°, and 30°C respectively. Increasing temperature raises the flux (slope) and shortens the lag time.

toxicity. And systemic toxicities have at times accompanied the application of salicylic acid, a keratolytic agent or substance that breaks down keratin, to large psoriatic lesions. There are documented cases of abuse of transdermal patches, including a case in which a patient, confused about the manner of usage, succumbed to fentanyl by wearing four patches simultaneously. A pharmacist must realize that in the instance of topical therapy, area is dose!

Phenomenological Considerations in Percutaneous Delivery

While the model helps us understand the chemical structure dependencies of skin permeability, it isn't all that useful for calculating permeability coefficients because of the many iffy assumptions it contains. A different tack has to be taken to gain a sense of the limits, especially the upper limit, of cutaneous drug delivery. There is no lower limit. Even proteins penetrate intact skin to some extent. Some idea of the upper limit can be gained upon examining the rates of delivery of nitroglycerine and like facile penetrants of the skin. Nitroglycerine, a liquid at room temperature, is a lipophilic nonelectrolyte of 227 dalton molecular weight. These physical properties make this drug about as good a skin penetrant as can be found. It is formulated in transdermal systems virtually as a neat liquid and thus near its upper attainable thermodynamic activity. It diffuses through the skin at between 0.02 and 0.04 mg/cm^2/h from the transdermal reservoirs it is placed in. These rates equate with a delivery of 0.5–1.0 mg/cm^2/day [24]. Consequently, 20 cm^2 patches provide a daily delivery of between 10 and 20 mg of the drug [24]. Nicotine, another low molecular weight, substantially hydrophobic, liquid compound at 25°C, permeates human skin from its transdermal delivery systems with comparable ease. Selegiline is yet another drug with properties like these that is a facile skin penetrant. Putting all of this together, it appears that a percutaneous delivery rate of about 1 mg/cm^2/day is near the upper achievable limit for "skin delivery."

Now it is true that water diffuses out through the skin far faster than any of these compounds diffuse in the reverse direction. To be specific, we typically lose about 0.5 mg/cm^2/h of water through the skin into a dry external atmosphere, a flux that exceeds those of the referenced compounds by more than an order of magnitude. However, water is a very unique molecule both with respect to its size and its interactions within the horny layer. It appears that its diffusion is not constrained to the intercellular domain of the stratum corneum, but, rather, some water almost certainly works its way into and up through keratin amassed in the intracellular space. A major fraction of insensible perspiration exits the skin this way. By way of contrast, permeation of nitroglycerine and the other drugs mentioned is thought to mainly take place through the intercellular domain of the stratum corneum.

If all nonpolar drugs were as skin permeable as nitroglycerine, many more transdermal delivery systems might exist. Why are there so few transdermally delivered drugs? The crystallinity of compounds is one important answer, for, in a general way, the level of crystallinity sets a limit on solubility and thus the activity gradient that can be expressed across the skin. Superimposing crystallinity on nitroglycerine illustrates this point. By thermodynamic derivation, the activity of a crystalline compound relative to the activity of its pure liquid state (its supercooled liquid state) is given by:

$$\ln a_2 = \frac{\Delta H_f(T_f - T)}{RT_fT} \tag{11}$$

where a_2 is the activity of a solid, ΔH_f is its heat of fusion, T_f is its melting point (temperature of fusion), T is the experimental temperature (nominally 25°C), and R is the gas constant (1.987 in cal/mol/degree units). Upon hypothetically superimposing a melting point of 100°C and a heat of fusion of 5000 cal/mol (about 20,000 J/mol) on nitroglycerine, the activity of the compound is seen to drop about fivefold. It would now only be possible to deliver 200 μg/cm^2/day of the drug or only about 4 mg of it from a 20 cm^2 patch. If it were that nitroglycerine melted at 200°C, all else being equal, its activity would be only 4% of that of its neat liquid. At 40 μg/cm^2/day, the dose achievable using a 20 cm^2 patch would now be roughly 1 mg. Since most drugs are quite crystalline, the delivery of 1 mg of drug per day through a 20 cm^2 area (roughly the area of a Ritz cracker) can be feat. This is one of the main reasons only exceptionally potent drugs are taken seriously for transdermal delivery. The dose limit results from the fact that, irrespective of solvent, drug solubilities are lowered over what they would otherwise be by crystallinity. Referring back to the model, the impact of lowered solubility is experienced in the term ΔC. This is so because, barring supersaturation, the largest value ΔC can take turns out to be the solubility of the compound. In other words, a drug's solubility ordinarily sets the upper limit on a drug's driving force and therefore on its achievable dose. It is particularly important to give serious weight to the crystallinity factor when selecting compounds for topical or transdermal purposes from the many that may be available. Everything else being equal, low melting compounds are far easier to deliver in therapeutically adequate amounts.

The solubility of a drug in any specified particular solvent is also determined by its interactions within the solvent. The activity of a dissolved solute is related to its concentration through an activity coefficient, i.e.:

$$a_2 = X_2 \cdot \gamma_2 \tag{12}$$

where X_2 is the mole fraction concentration of the solute in a saturated solution. Mole fraction concentration is specified in lieu of molar or percentage concentration because it fits better in theoretical developments that lead up to Raoult's law. γ_2 is the drug's activity coefficient on the mole fraction scale. The activity coefficient is simply a number that is needed turn the proportionality that exists between activity and concentration into an equality. Combining equations, one can now write

$$\ln X_2 = -\frac{\Delta H_f(T_f - T)}{RT_fT} - \ln \gamma_2 \tag{13}$$

The right-hand side of Eq. (13) teaches us that the solubility of a drug in a specified solvent depends on the drug's melting parameters in the same way activity does. However, the drug's solubility also depends on its activity coefficient in the solvent in question as indicated by the second term on the right side of Eq. (13) If the solute's solution phase interactions are strong (energetic), the activity coefficient will take a value less than one. Consequently, the solubility of the compound in this circumstance exceeds that of an ideal solution (where $\gamma_2 = 1.0$ and $a_2 = X_2$. Relatively weak interactions between the solute and solvent, on the other hand, result in activity coefficients greater than unity. In this case, solubilities are lower than ideal. The bottom line of all of this is that a high level of crystallinity is associated with low activity and vice versa. This factor is set apart from solute-solvent interactions. It is differing solute-solvent interactions that cause a compound to express different solubilities in different solvents. However and importantly, the thermodynamic activity of a drug is identical across all its saturated solutions as long as its crystallinity is independent of the solvents it is placed in. This does not necessarily mean that the delivery of a drug has to be the same from every one of its saturated solutions regardless of solvent, for kinetic (as opposed to thermodynamic) factors can exert their influences. Consider, for example, the situation where dissolution of drug particles suspended in a particular vehicle cannot keep up with release of the drug into the skin. The thermodynamic activity of the drug will necessarily drop below that of a saturated solution even when suspended drug is still present. And when skin is the membrane, the differing abilities of various media to alter the physicochemical attributes of the conduit phases of the stratum corneum and thereby enhance permeation have to be taken into account.

Crystallinity aside, the two physical attributes of a drug that most control its skin permeability are its physical size and its lipophilicity [44,45]. When all extant human permeability coefficients (at the time over 90 compounds) were subjected to multiple linear regression by Potts and Guy using the following semi-empirical equation [45]:

$$\log 10(P) = \log 10\left(\frac{D^\circ}{h}\right) + \alpha \cdot \log 10(K_{oct/w}) - \beta \cdot (\mathrm{MW}) \qquad (14)$$

they found that almost 70% of the variation exhibited by human skin permeability coefficients is explained by differences in their molecular sizes and partitioning coefficients. D° in equation 14 is the hypothetical diffusivity of a molecule having zero molecular volume (the molecular size influence appears in the molecular weight term). As before, h is meant to represent the length of the diffusion pathway. $K_{oct/w}$ is the octanol/water partition coefficient of each compound. The octanol/water partition coefficient is a general measure of the relative lipophilicity of each compound and also something of a surrogate for a compound's stratum corneum/water partition coefficient, $K_{sc/w}$. α is a proportionality factor relating $K_{sc/w}$ to $K_{oct/w}$, while β is a constant arising from the dependency of diffusion coefficients on molecular size. The computer-determined expression that best fit all the permeability coefficient data is [44]:

$$\log 10(P) = -6.3 + 0.71(K_{oct/w}) - 0.0061 \cdot (\mathrm{MW}) \qquad (15)$$

Equation (15) ostensibly allows one to estimate permeability coefficients in units of cm/s. However, as with any parameter calculated from statistically drawn relationships, such estimates have to be "taken with a grain of salt," because the absolute error of estimation for a single compound can be large.

V. UNIQUE PHYSICOCHEMICAL SYSTEMS USED TOPICALLY

As one scans the products at the drug counter, one finds an enormous variety of formulation types available for topical therapy or for cosmetic purposes. Solutions are commonly found. They come in packages that allow them to be rubbed on, sprayed on by aerosol and atomizers, painted on, rolled on, swabbed on by premoistened pledgets, and dabbed on from applicators. Assorted medicated soaps are available for a range of purposes. Emulsions for the skin are found in the form of shampoos and as medicated lotions. Powders to soothe and lubricate are placed in sprinkling cans, while others containing drugs are formulated into aerosols to be sprayed on the skin. There are numerous fluid suspensions to be used as makeup or for therapeutic purposes. Clear and opaque gels are also to be found in both cosmetic and therapeutic spheres, as are assorted semisolid creams, ointments, and pastes. The physical natures of these latter systems range from soft semisolids that are squeezed out of tubes to hardened systems suitable for application in stick form. There are therapeutic and cosmetic oils for the bath. The list of products and formulation types is nearly endless.

Of all these formulations, it is the diverse semisolids that stand out as being uniquely topical. Semisolid systems fulfill a special topical need as they cling to the surface of the skin to which they are applied, generally until being washed off or worn off. In contrast, fluid systems have poor substantivity and readily streak and run off the desired area. Similarly, powders have poor staying properties. Importantly, the fundamental physicochemical characteristics of solutions, liquid emulsions and suspensions, and powders are independent of their route of application, and are discussed adequately elsewhere in this text and need not be reconsidered. This is not to say the compositions of such systems cannot be uniquely topical, for there are chemicals that can be safely applied to the skin which are unsafe to use systemically. It is necessary to elaborate upon the properties of semisolids.

A. General Behavior of Semisolids

The term semisolid infers a unique rheological character. Like solids, such systems retain their shape until acted upon by an outside force, whereupon, unlike solids, they are easily deformed. Thus, a finger drawn through a semisolid mass leaves a track that does not fill up when the action is complete. Rather, the deformation made is for all practical purposes permanent, an outcome physically characterized by saying semisolids deform plastically. Their overall rheological properties allow them to be spread over the skin to form films that cling tenaciously.

To be semisolid, a system must have a three-dimensional structure that is sufficient to impart solid-like character to the undistributed system that is easily broken down and realigned under an applied force. The semisolid systems used pharmaceutically include ointments and solidified w/o emulsion variants thereof, pastes, o/w creams with solidified internal phases, o/w creams with fluid internal phases, gels, and rigid foams. The natures of the underlying structures differ remarkably across all these systems, but all share the property that their structures are easily broken down, rearranged, and reformed. Only to the extent that one understands the structural sources of these systems does one understand them at all.

B. Ointments

Unless expressly stated otherwise, ointments are hydrocarbon-based semisolids containing dissolved or suspended drugs. They comprise fluid hydrocarbons, C_{16} to perhaps C_{30} straight chain and branched, entrapped in a fine crystalline matrix of yet higher molecular weight hydrocarbons. The high molecular weight fraction precipitates out substantially at room temperature, forming interlocking crystallites [46]. The extent and specific nature of this structure determine the stiffness of the ointment. It follows directly from this that hydrocarbon-based ointments liquefy upon heating when the crystallites melt. Moreover, when cooled very slowly, they assume a fluidity much greater than when rapidly cooled because slow cooling leads to fewer and larger crystallites and therefore less total structure. Ordinary white and yellow petrolatum are examples of such systems.

Several alternative means of forming hydrocarbon ointments illustrate their structural properties. Ointments can be made by incorporating high melting waxes into mineral oil (liquid petrolatum) at high temperature. Upon cooling, interlocking wax crystallites form and the system sets up. Polyethylene too can gel mineral oil if dissolved into this vehicle at high temperature and the solution is then force cooled [47]. A network of polyethylene crystallites provides the requisite solidifying matrix. This polyethylene gelled system is more fluid on the molecular level than are the semisolid petroleum distillates while at the same time macroscopically behaving as an ointment. Consequently, diffusion of drugs through this vehicle is more facile and drug release is somewhat greater than in petrolatum-based systems [48]. Plastibase (Squibb) is the commercially available base of polyethylene gelled mineral oil. It is useful for the extemporaneous preparation of ointments by cold incorporation of drugs. Pharmacists should not melt down this base to incorporate drugs because its gelled state cannot be restored without special processing equipment.

If a material other than a hydrocarbon is used as the base material of an ointment-like system, the ointment bears the name of its principal ingredient. There are silicone ointments that contain polydimethylsiloxane oil in large proportion. These reportedly act as excellent water barriers and superior emollients. Some are actually used to protect skin from the undesirable effects of long immersion in water.

Ointments of the specific kinds mentioned above are taken to be good vehicles to apply to dry lesions but not to moist ones. All are also greasy and stain clothes. The principal ingredients forming the systems, hydrocarbons and silicone oils, are generally poor solvents for most drugs, seemingly setting a low limit on the drug-delivery capabilities of the systems. This solubility disadvantage can be offset somewhat if hydrocarbon miscible solvents are blended into the systems to raise solvency. Alternatively, they can be made over into emulsions to increase their abilities to dissolve drugs. Along these lines, absorption bases are conventional ointments that contain w/o emulsifiers in appreciable quantity. A w/o emulsion is formed when an aqueous medium, perhaps containing the drug in solution, is worked into the base. Such emulsions are still ointments, as structurally defined, for it is the external phase of the formed emulsion that imparts the structure, and this retains its ointment-like character. It is important to note that the term "absorption base" refers to a water-incorporation capacity and infers nothing about bioavailability. This is not to say that it is not better to have water-soluble drugs emulsïfied than as suspended solids in such systems from a bioavailabi1ity standpoint. In this regard, for optimum results, the internal, presumably aqueous phase should be close to saturated. Diverse additives are used to emulsify water into these systems, including cholesterol, lanolin (which contains cholesterol and cholesterol esters and other emulsifiers), semi-synthetic lanolin derivatives, and assorted ionic and nonionic surfactants singularly or in combination.

Polyethylene glycol *ointment* is a water-soluble system that contains fluid, short-chain polyoxyethylene polymers (polyethylene glycols) in a crystalline network of high-melting, long-chain polyoxyethylene polymers (Carbowaxes, Union Carbide). The structure formed is totally analogous to that of the standard ointment. In one variation, this system functions well as a suppository base. Liquid polyethylene glycols are fully miscible with water, and many drugs that are insoluble in petroleum vehicles readily dissolve in the polar matrix of this base. In fact, with some drugs, delivery (bioavailability) can be compromised by an excessive capacity of the base to dissolve substances, resulting in poor vehicle-into-skin partitioning. Since polyethylene glycols are highly water soluble, bases formed from them literally dissolve off the skin when placed under a stream of running water.

C. Pastes

Pastes are basically ointments into which a high percentage of insoluble particulate solids have been added—as much or more than 50% by weight in some instances. This extraordinary amount of particulate matter stiffens the systems through direct interactions of the dispersed particulates and by adsorbing the liquid hydrocarbon fraction within the vehicle onto the particle surfaces. Insoluble ingredients such as starch, zinc oxide, calcium carbonate, and talc are used as the dispersed phase. Pastes make particularly good protective barriers when placed on the skin for, in addition to forming an unbroken film, the solids they contain can absorb and thereby neutralize certain noxious chemicals before they ever reach the skin. This explains why they are used to ameliorate diaper rash, for when spread over the baby's bottom they absorb irritants (ammonia, others?) formed by bacterial action on urine. Like ointments, pastes form an unbroken, relatively water-impermeable film on the skin surface and thus are emollients; unlike ointments, the film is opaque and therefore an effective sun block. Thus, skiers apply pastes around the nose and lips to gain dual protection. Pastes are actually less greasy than ointments because of the adsorption of the fluid hydrocarbon fraction onto the particulates.

D. Creams

Creams are semisolid emulsion systems having a creamy appearance as the result of reflection of light from their emulsified phases. This contrasts them with simple ointments, which are translucent. Little agreement exists among professionals as to what constitutes a cream, and thus the term has been applied both to absorption bases containing emulsified water (w/o emulsions) and to semisolid o/w systems, which are physicochemically totally different, strictly because of their similar creamy appearances. Logically, classification of these systems should be based on their physical natures, in which case absorption bases would be ointments and the term "cream" could be reserved exclusively for semisolid o/w systems, which in all instances derive their structures from their emulsifiers and internal phases.

The classical o/w cream is vanishing cream that contains only 15% stearic acid or its equivalent as the internal phase. Vanishing cream and its variants are first prepared as ordinary liquid emulsions at high temperature; the structure that gives them their semisolid character forms as the formed emulsions cool. Both the aqueous and stearic acid phases are heated above the point where the waxy components liquefy and then are emulsified. Sufficient emulsifier is either formed in situ or added in to create a substantial micellar phase to exist in equilibrium with the liquefied internal phase of the hot emulsion. In the instance of the classical vanishing cream, about 20% of the stearic acid it contains is neutralized with strong alkali to form the surfactant. Portions of the waxy alcohols and/or undissociated waxy acids are solubilized within such micelles. As these systems are then cooled, their emulsion droplets solidify and the micellar structures linking all together take on a liquid crystalline character [49]. The latter three-dimensional matrix has been referred to as *frozen micelles* and is what actually solidifies such creams. The compositions and amounts of both the internal phase and emulsifiers determine the extent and qualities of the structure. Creams like this are more or less stiff, depending on the level of micellar solubilization and the melting properties of the internal waxy component [49]. Within the family of such creams, the internal phase ranges in composition from about 12 to 40% by weight.

Stiff o/w emulsions can also result from droplet interactions of the internal phase, but this requires emulsifying such a huge amount of internal phase that the droplets exceed close spherical packing. In this state the emulsified particles are squashed together, losing their spherical shape, producing large interfacial areas of contact at the sites where the droplets come into contact. A fragile structure is obtained, somewhere between that of a highly viscid liquid and a true semisolid. This cream type is far less common than systems built around frozen micellar structures.

A semisolid cream of the o/w type containing a solidified, liquid crystalline internal phase is an elegant topical system preferred by many for general purposes. Such o/w systems are readily diluted with water and thus easily rinsed off the skin and are generally nonstaining. Upon application, volatile components of the cream, which may comprise as much as 80% of the total system, evaporate, and the thin application shrinks down into an even thinner layer. Stearic acid creams are particularly interesting in this regard. The small amount of internal phase they contain causes them to evaporate down to near nothingness. The dry, nontacky, translucent nature of the stearic acid crystals left on the skin contributes to the sense of their lack of discernibility. Most hand lotions and creams and foundation creams used to make face powders adherent to the face are variants of the vanishing cream formula.

Through evaporation, the drug in a cream is concentrated in its forming film, a process that can be orchestrated to program drug delivery. If no thought is given to the consequences attending drying out of the formulation, however, the drug is just as likely to precipitate out, in which instance drug delivery comes to an abrupt stop. One must therefore ensure that the formed film has some capacity to dissolve its drug. To this end, low-volatility, water-miscible solvents such as propylene glycol are added to many cream formulations. When ingredients like water and alcohol evaporate, the film left upon applying such creams becomes a rich concentrate of drug, internal phase, and its less volatile external phase components. One strives to add just enough co-solvent to keep the drug solubilized in the equilibrium film but also near saturation. It should be kept in mind that, unless the internal phase liquefies at body temperature, the waxy constituents cannot act as a solvent for the drug and thus do not lend the film much capacity for delivery.

The typical cream, a soft, emulsified mass of solidified particles in an aqueous, micelle-rich medium, does not form a water-impermeable (occlusive) film on the skin. Nevertheless, creams contain lipids and other moisturizers that replace substances lost from the skin in the course of everyday living. Creams thus make good emollients because, by replenishing lipids and in some instances also polar, hygroscopic substances, they restore the skin's ability to hold onto its own moisture.

The oleaginous phases of creams differ compositionally from hydrocarbon ointments. Many, but not all, creams are patterned after vanishing cream and contain considerable stearic acid. In lieu of some or all of the stearic acid, creams sometime contain long-chain waxy alcohols (cetyl, C_{16}; stearyl, C_{18}), long-chain esters (myristates, C_{14}; palmitates, C_{16}; stearates, C_{18}), other long-chain acids (palmatic acid), vegetable and animal oils, and assorted other waxes of both animal and mineral origin.

Properly designed o/w creams are elegant drug-delivery systems, pleasing in both appearance and feel post application. They are nongreasy and are easily rinsed off of the skin. They are good for most topical purposes and are considered particularly suited for application to oozing wounds.

E. Gels (Jellies)

Gels are semisolid systems in which a liquid phase is trapped within an interlocking, three-dimensional polymeric matrix of a natural or synthetic gum. A high degree of physical or chemical cross-linking of the polymer is involved. It only takes 0.5–2.0% of the most commonly used gelants to set up the systems. Some of these systems are as transparent as water, an aesthetically pleasing state. Others are turbid because the polymer is present in colloidal aggregates that disperse light. Clarity of the latter ranges from slightly hazy to a whitish translucence not unlike that observed with petrolatum.

Agarose gels admirably illustrate the properties and to an extent the structural characteristics of most gels. Agarose solutions are water-thin when warm but solidify near room temperature to form systems that are soft to rubbery, depending on the source and concentration of the agarose. A three-dimensional structure arises from the entwining of the ends of polymer strands into double helices. Kinks in the polymer mark the terminal points of these windings. Because individual polymer strands branch to form multiple endings, a three-dimensional array of physically cross-linked polymer strands is formed. The process of physical cross-linking is actually a crystallization phenomenon tying polymeric endings together, fixing the strands in place, yielding a stable, yet pliant structure [50]. Less extensive structure than that found in agar growth media results in a spreadable semisolid suitable for medical application. The structure should persist to temperatures exceeding body temperature for the gelled systems to be the most useful. It is important to note that gelation is never a result of mere physical entanglement of polymer strands, otherwise the systems would be highly viscid. The polymers used to prepare pharmaceutical gels include natural gums such as tragacanth, pectin, carrageen, agar, and alginic acid and synthetic and semi-synthetic materials such as methylcellulose, hydroxyethylcellulose, carboxymethylcellulose, and carboxypolymethylene (carboxy vinal polymers sold under the name Carbopol, B. F. Goodrich).

Gels or jellies are used pharmaceutically as lubricants and also as carriers for spermacidal agents to be used intravaginally with diaphragms as an adjunctive means of contraception. Since the fluid phase of a gel does not have to be strictly water, gels offer a wide range of uses; by blending solvents, it is possible to form films that exhibit a range of evaporation rates, solvency, and other release-determining attributes [51]. Gel products containing anti-inflammatory steroids are used to treat inflammations of the scalp because this is an area of the body where creams and ointments are too greasy for patient acceptance.

F. Rigid Foams

Foams are systems in which air or some other gas is emulsified in a liquid phase to the point of stiffening. As spreadable topical systems go, medicated foams tend towards the fluid side, but like some shaving creams, they can be stiffer and approximate a true semisolid. Like the second type of o/w emulsion that only borders on semisolidity, these derive structure from an internal phase, bubbles of an entrapped gas so voluminous that it exceeds close spherical packing. Consequently, the bubbles interact with their neighbors over areas rather than points of contact. The interactions are sufficient in many cases to provide a resistance to deformation and something approaching semisolid character. Whipped cream is a common example of this type of system. Here air is literally beaten into the fluid cream until it becomes stiff. Aerosol shaving creams and certain medicated quick-breaking antiseptic foams are examples of the foams currently found in cosmetic and therapeutic practice. These are supplied in pressurized cans that have special valves capable of emulsifying a gas into the extruded preparations.

G. Common Constituents of Dermatological Preparations

So many materials are used as pharmaceutical necessities and as vehicles in topical systems that they defy thorough analysis. The pharmacist should nevertheless make some effort to learn about the more common constituents and their principal functions. The compositions of formulations as presented on product labels are the main source of such information. The compositions presented in Table 9 offer a glimpse into the compositional natures of semisolids.

Due to the large number of materials that are used in topical preparations and the diversity of their physical properties, the formulation of topical dosage forms tends to be something of an art perfected through experience. Only by making myriad recipes does one eventually gain insight into the materials and their use in designing new formulations. Such insight allows the experienced formulator to manipulate the properties of existing formulations to gain a desired characteristic. Often one finds good recipes to use as starting points for formulations in the trade literature. Two factors have to be kept in mind when borrowing the compositions of such trade formulations. First, the trade recipes (recipes supplied with advertising material touting specific components) are often inadequately tested in terms of long-term stability. Second, the dominant features used in judging the merits of trade-promoted formulas tend to be their initial appearances and overall elegance. Little to no attention can be paid to the drug-delivery attributes of the prototypical systems when they are first prepared in the suppliers' laboratories because the drug-delivery attributes are so compound specific. Thus it is left up to the pharmacist (industrial research pharmacist) to make adjustments in the formulas that are consistent with good delivery of specific drugs. Each drug requires unique adjustments in accord with its singular physicochemical properties.

H. General Methods of Preparation of Topical Systems

Irrespective of whether the scale of preparation is large or small, ointments, pastes, and creams tend to be produced by one or the other of two general methods. Some are made at high temperature by blending liquid and melted solid components together and then dispersing all other ingredients within the hot, oily melt. Alternatively, drug and/or adjuvants can be dispersed or dissolved within one of the phases or a fraction of one of the phases of an emulsion prior to forming the emulsion. The drug can be mixed into a freshly formed, still molten emulsion while it is still warm. Finally, a drug can be incorporated into an already solidified base via cold incorporation. As pointed out earlier, the

Table 9 Prototype Formulations

I. Ointment (white ointment, USP)	
White petrolatum	95% (w/v)
White wax	5%
Melt the white wax and add the petrolatum; continue heating until a liquid melt is formed. Congeal with stirring. Heating should be gentle to avoid charring (steam is preferred), and *air incorporation* by too vigorous stirring is to be avoided.	
II. Absorption ointment (hydrophilic petrolatum, USP)	
White petrolatum	86% (w/w)
Stearyl alcohol	3%
White wax	8%
Cholesterol	3%
Melt the stearyl alcohol, white wax, and cholesterol (steam bath). Add the petrolatum and continue heating until a liquid melt is formed. Cool with stirring until congealed.	
III. Water-washable ointment (hydrophilic ointment, USP)	
White petrolatum	25% (w/w)
Stearyl alcohol	25%
Propylene glycol	12%
Sodium lauryl sulfate	1%
Methylparaben	0.025%
Propylparaben	0.015%
Purified water	37%
Melt the stearyl alcohol and white petrolatum (steam bath) and warm to about 75°C. Heat the water to 75°C and add the sodium lauryl sulfate, propylene glycol, methylparaben, and propylparaben. Add the aqueous phase and stir until congealed.	
IV. Water-soluble ointment (polyethylene glycol ointment, USP 14)	
Polyethylene glycol 4000 (Carbowax 4000)	50%
Polyethylene glycol 400	50%
Melt the PG 4000 and add the liquid PG 400. Cool with stirring until congealed.	
V. Cream base, w/o (rose water ointment, NF 14)	
Oleaginous phase	
Spermaceti	12.5%
White wax	12.0%
Almond oil	55.58%
Aqueous phase	
Sodium borate	0.5%
Stronger rose water, NF	2.5%
Purified water, USP	16.5%
Aromatic	
Rose oil, NF	0.02%
Melt the spermaceti and white wax on a steam bath. Add the almond oil and continue heating to 70°C. Dissolve the sodium borate in the purified water and stronger rose Water, warmed to 75°C. Gradually add the aqueous phase to the oil phase with stirring. Cool to 45°C with stirring and incorporate the aromatic (rose oil).	
Note: This is a typical cold cream formulation. The cooling effect comes from the slow evaporation of water from the applied films. The aromatic is added at as low a temperature as possible to prevent its loss by volatilization during manufacture.	
VI. Cream base, o/w (general prototype)	
Oleagenous phase	
Stearyl alcohol	15%
Beeswax	8%
Sorbitan monooleate	1.25%
Aqueous phase	
Sorbitol solution, 70% USP	7.5%
Polysorbate 80	3.75%

Table 9 (*Continued*)

Methylparaben	0.025%
Propylparaben	0.015%
Purified water, q.s. ad	100%
Heat the oil phase and water phase to 70°C. Add the oil phase slowly to the aqueous phase with stirring to form a crude emulsion. Cool to about 55°C and homogenize. Cool with agitation until congealed.	
VII. Cream base, o/w (vanishing cream)	
Oleagenous phase	
Stearic acid	13%
Stearyl alcohol	1%
Cetyl alcohol	1%
Aqueous phase	
Glycerin	10%
Methylparaben	0.1%
Propylparaben	0.05%
Potassium hydroxide	0.9%
Purified water, q.s. ad	100%
Heat the oil phase and water phase to about 65°C. Add the oil phase slowly to the aqueous phase with stirring to form a crude emulsion. Cool to about 50°C and homogenize. Cool with agitation until congealed.	
Note: In this classic preparation, the stearic acid reacts with the alkaline borate to form the emulsifying stearate soap.	
VIII. Paste (zinc oxide paste, USP)	
Zinc oxide	25%
Starch	25%
Calamine	5%
White petrolatum, q.s. ad	100%
Titrate the calamine with the zinc oxide and starch and incorporate uniformly in the petrolatum by levigation in a mortar or on a glass slab with a spatula. Mineral oil should *not* be used as a levigating agent, since it would soften the product. A portion of the petrolatum can be melted and used as a levigating agent is so desired.	
IX. Gel (lubricating jelly)	
Methocel 90 H.C. 4000	0.8%
Carbopol 934	0.24%
Propylene glycol	16.7%
Methylparaben	10.015%
Sodium hydroxide, q.s. ad	pH 7
Purified water, q.s. ad	100%
Disperse the Methocel in 40ml of hot (80°–90°C) water. Chill overnight in a refrigerator to effect solution. Disperse the Carbopol 934 in 20ml of water. Adjust the pH of the dispersion to 7.0 by adding sufficient 1% sodium hydroxide solution (about 12 ml is required per 100 ml) and bring the volume to 40 ml with purified Water. Dissolve the methylparaben in the propylene glycol. Mix the Methocel, Carbopol 934, and propylene glycol fractions using caution to avoid the incorporation of air.	

first of these methods is commonly used to make o/w creams of the vanishing type. The fusion method is used to prepare many ointments as well. Cold incorporation comes into play in large-scale manufacture when the systems in preparation contain heat-labile drugs. In this instance the drug is first crudely worked into an ointment or cream base using by serial dilution and then distributed uniformly with the aid of a roller mill. Cold incorporation is also necessary when a base is destroyed by heat, as happens with Plastibase (Squibb).

In the fusion method for ointments, mineral oil, petrolatum, waxes, and other ingredients that belong in the formulation are heated together to somewhere between 60 and 80°C, depending on the components, and mixed to a uniform composition while in the fluidized state. Cooling is then effected using some sort of heat exchanger. To prevent decomposition, drugs and certain delicate adjuvants are added sometime during the cooling process. If insoluble solids need to be dispersed, the system is put through a milling process (colloid mill, homogenizer, ultrasonic mixer, etc.) to disperse them fully. A hand homogenizer works well at the prescription counter for small-volume, extemporaneously prepared systems. Systems in preparation are always cooled with mild stirring until they are close to solidification. The rate of cooling is important, for rapid cooling, as mentioned, imparts a finer, more rigid structure. Stirring should be set to minimize vortexing and thereby prevent air incorporation into the solidifying system. Representative formulations with more system-specific, detailed directions are given in Table 9 for ointments and the other semisolid systems of note.

The fusion method for preparing creams is a bit more complex. In this instance the aqueous and oil phases are heated separately to somewhere between 60 and 80°C. As a general rule the oil phase is heated to 5°C above the melting point of the highest-melting waxy ingredient and the water phase is heated to 5°C above the temperature of the oil phase, the latter to prevent premature solidification during the emulsification process. Water-soluble ingredients are dissolved in the heated aqueous phase and oil-soluble ingredients are dissolved in the oily melt, but only as long as they are heat stable and not too volatile. If an o/w system is to be made, the emulsifiers are added to the aqueous phase and the emulsion is formed by slow addition of the oil phase. In the industry the crude emulsion is then passed through a high-shear mixer to form a finely divided emulsion state. Following this, the emulsion is cooled with gentle stirring until congealed, again taking care not to whip air into the formulation. Typically, the emulsions solidify between 40 and 50°C. If a w/o emulsion is to be made, the addition steps are usually reversed. Therefore and generally, the discontinuous phase is added to the continuous, external phase containing the emulsifier. However, methods vary here, and for a particular formula the reverse order of addition may work best. Any means that reliably leads to a good emulsion is obviously acceptable.

A solid can be incorporated directly into an already congealed system in several ways. This is accomplished on a small scale by levigating the solid with a small portion of the total base it is to be suspended in to obtain a paste-like mass. The drug is worked into the base on a glass plate with the aid of a spatula or is triturated in using a mortar and pestle. After the initial mix is smooth, a portion of the vehicle roughly equal in bulk to that of the pasty mass is added and blended in. This latter procedure is repeated several times (geometric dilution) until the drug is uniformly dispersed throughout its total vehicle. In large-scale manufacture, solids are crudely dispersed into the base using a blender and then roller mills, in which a film of the formulation is passed from one roller to another and so on, in each passage with kneading and mixing, are used to obtain fine dispersion. As outlined when discussing absorption bases, the drug may also be dissolved in water to form a solution to be levigated into an ointment base or cream. Such addition softens creams even to the point of converting them to thick lotions. The chosen vehicle, of course, must have an inherent capacity to emulsify or otherwise take up the solution. Aromatic materials such as essential oils, perfume oils, camphor, and menthol, which volatilize if added when the base is hot, are incorporated into these semisolids while they are still being mixed but near the temperature where a particular system starts to congeal. Volatile materials are often introduced into the formulation as hydroalcoholic solutions.

The preparation of gels can also involve high-temperature processing. It is easier to disperse methylcellulose in hot than in cold water, for instance. The polymer then goes into solution and thickens or sets up as the temperature is lowered. Adding the hot methylcellulose dispersion to ice water gets one quickly to the final equilibrium state. Tragacanth gels, on the other hand must be prepared at room temperature due to the extreme heat lability of this natural gum. A little alcohol or propylene glycol can be mixed into this gum before adding water to it to facilitate wetting of the gum prior to its dispersion. By way of contrast, Carbopol-containing systems are gelled by neutralizing the medium they have been dispersed in with alkali. Neutralization induces carboxyl groups found on the polymer backbone to ionize, instantaneously drawing these polymers into solution. Organic solvents can be gelled with Carbopol polymers as well, in such instances using soluble amines for the neutralization step.

Several prototype gel formulations are given in Table 9 to illustrate general compositional requirements and manufacturing methods. The design of specific systems tailored to meet predetermined, demanding performance criteria, particularly with respect to bioavailability, generally requires modification of published formulations or a totally original approach.

VI. PERFORMANCE OF TOPICAL THERAPEUTIC SYSTEMS

Topical preparations, like all other dosage forms, must be formulated, manufactured, and packaged in a manner that assures that they meet general standards of bioavailability, physical (physical system) stability, chemical (ingredient) stability, freedom from contamination, and elegance. Like all other pharmaceuticals, these factors must remain essentially invariant over the stated shelf life of the product and they must be reproducible from batch to batch.

A. Bioavailability

Chemical Structure, Delivery, Clinical Response

Much has already been said concerning the chemical structural dependencies of skin permeation. However, the goal of all treatment is successful therapy, not delivery per se, and consequently the intrinsic activities of the drugs must also be taken into account when selecting compounds for dermatological and transdermal development. The pharmacological response depends on delivering sufficient drug of a given activity to the target zone. Clearly, the more potent a compound is, the less of it that needs to be delivered. Since topical delivery is difficult at best, potency often dictates which of the compounds found within a family of drugs should be developed, for the highly potent analog, reasonably formulated, offers the best chance of obtaining clinically sufficient delivery. Conversely, marginally potent analogs, even when expertly formulated, often fail because of inadequate delivery. An excellent example of this principle is found with the narcotic analgesics. Because of its extraordinary potency, fentanyl, with a daily palliative requirement of 1 mg, and not morphine, which requires between 60 and 120 mg to alleviate pain over the course of a day, has made it way into transdermal use. The fact that fentanyl is also physicochemically more suited to transdermal delivery than is morphine does not controvert this axiom.

Unlike mass transport across membranes, which relates to chemical structure in predictable ways, the potencies of drugs as seen in pharmacological, pharmacodynamic, or other tests are highly structurally specific within a class of drugs and are without commonality across classes. A drug's activity involves a complex merging of these separate structural influences, with bioavailability always one of the concerns. Such concern is minimal when a truly superficial effect is involved, however. For example, the most potent antiseptic as measured in the test tube is likely to have near the highest topical potency as well. The intrinsic activities of compounds may be poor indicators of relative topical potentials when deep skin penetration is required, however, because the structural features benefiting the biological response are often distinct from than those that favor permeation. Thus, tissue permeability can be an important and sometimes a dominant factor in the clinical structure-activity profile.

We have seen that the determinants of skin permeation are the activity (concentration) of a drug in its vehicle, the drug's distribution coefficients between the vehicle and the skin and across all phases of the skin, and the drug's diffusion coefficients within the skin strata. Congeners, if comparably sized, exhibit little variance in their diffusion coefficients. However, the structural differences seen within congeneric families profoundly affect the solubility, partitioning, and in transit binding tendencies of the family members in addition to determining their binding with receptors. Drug delivery and resulting clinical effectiveness are a function of the former phenomena [52]. For example, the 21-ester of hydrocortisone is more hydrophobic than its parent, its ether/water partition coefficient being about 18 times that of hydrocortisone [53]. Given the strong parallels in partitioning behaviors that exist across partitioning systems, it stands to reason that similar order-of-magnitude increases exist with respect to the acetate's stratum corneum/water and sebum/-water partition coefficients. At the same time, acetylating hydrocortisone at the 21-position increases the melting point 12°C. Consequently, not only does derivatization drop the aqueous solubility precipitously, but it depresses solubility in all other solvents as well [54]. While the increase in partition coefficient raises the permeability coefficient relative to hydrocortisone, this impact is more than offset by reduced solubility, and far less of the acetate derivative can be delivered through the skin from respective saturated solutions [55]. However, as the alkyl chain length of the ester is methodically extended (C_3, C_4,...,C_7), the growing bulkiness of the alkyl group increasingly interferes with crystalline packing. Consequently, melting points fall incrementally from the 224°C peak of the acetate ester to 111°C when a chain length of seven, the heptanoate ester, is reached [54]. An especially sharp drop of 69°C is experienced between chain lengths five and six. Because of declining crystallinity beyond the chain length of two, solubilities of the esters in organic solvents rise markedly. Moreover, aqueous solubilities, though methodically depressed by increasing hydrophobicity, remain many times higher than they otherwise would

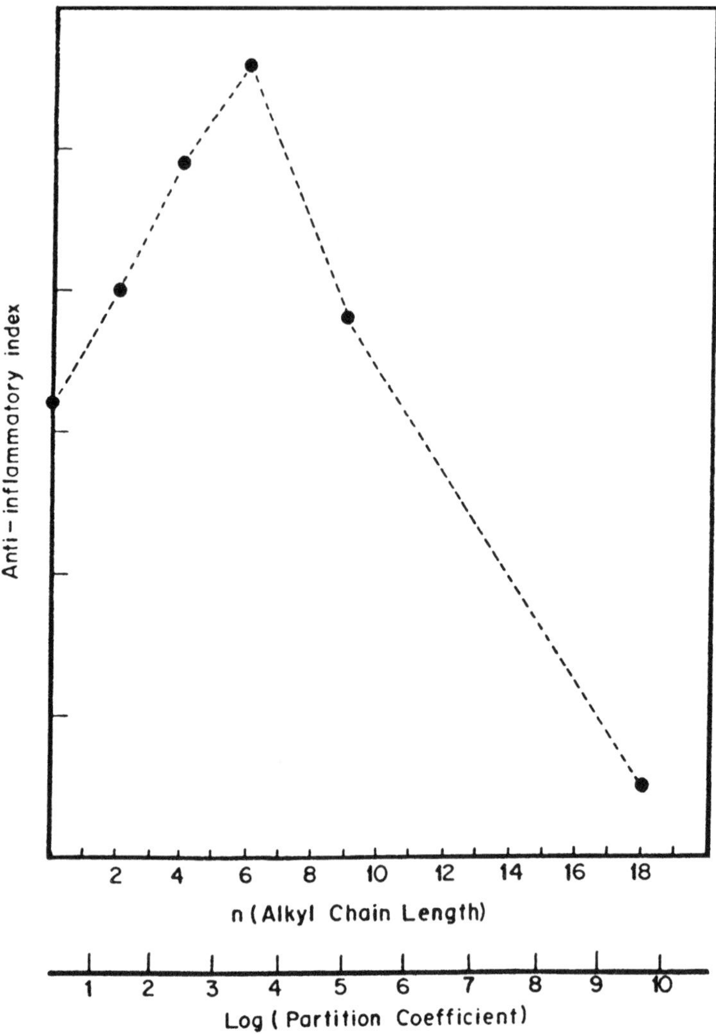

Fig. 5 Ability of hydrocortisone esters to suppress inflammation.

be. The net effect of these concerted forces is that the hexanoate and heptanoate esters of hydrocortisone are well over an order of magnitude more skin permeable than hydrocortisone when they are administered as saturated solutions [54,55].

Armed with the above insight, we can examine the pharmacological ramifications of esterifying hydrocortisone. In Fig. 5 the ability of hydrocortisone esters to suppress inflammation induced by tetrahydrofurfural alcohol, which acts simultaneously as irritant and vehicle, is shown as a function of the alkyl chain length of the esters [56]. An optimum chain in effect is seen at an alkyl chain length of six (hexanoate), with substantially longer and shorter esters being measurably less effective. The behavior is exactly what would be predicted from partitioning and solubility considerations. That this is not an isolated behavioral pattern with corticosteroids can be seen in Fig. 6, where vasoconstriction data of McKenzie and Atkinson for three betamethasone ester families, 21-esters, 17,21-*ortho*-esters, and 17-esters, are shown as functions of the ether/water partition coefficients of the compounds [57]. Vasoconstriction, blanching of the skin under the site of steroid application, is a proven index of a steroid's combined potency and ability to permeate through skin. Maxima are apparent in the

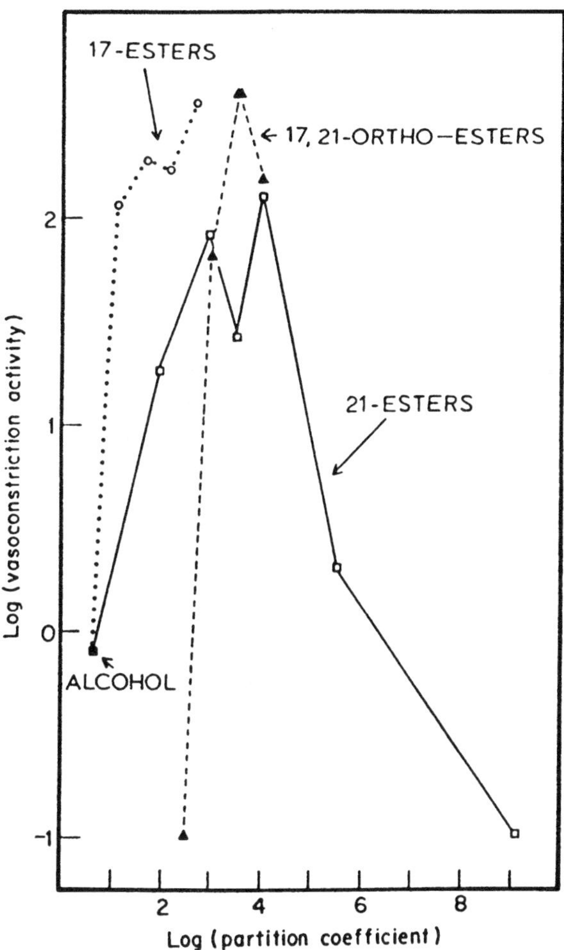

Fig. 6 Vasoconstriction data of betamethasone family.

data for the first two of these series, and the indications are that the 17-ester series is also peaking. Both maxima lie between ether/water partition coefficients of 1000 and 10,000 [53], as, interestingly and probably significantly, does the optimum ether/water partition coefficient of the hydrocortisone esters. The differing shapes and heights of the curves are not readily quantitatively explained but reflect differences in intrinsic vasomotor activities of each ester type. The coincidence of the maxima on the partitioning scale, on the other hand, seemingly relates to an optimum lipophilicity for delivery.

The decline in activity at the longer chain lengths (Fig. 6) also has a plausible explanation. Two factors are reasoned to be operative here: declining solubilities coupled with changes in the absorption mechanism associated with stratification of the barrier. Aqueous solubilities of homologs exponentially decline as alkyl chain length is extended [58,59]. While melting points are negatively impacted and depressed early in the series, the crystalline structure eventually accommodates the alkyl chain, whereupon further increases in chain length reverse the trend, reducing all solubilities [59]. Through all of this, o/w partition coefficients, which are unaffected by crystallinity, increase exponentially, which has the effect of exponentially increasing the ability of the stratum corneum and sebum phases to transport the steroids relative to that of the viable tissue layer. In other words, the resistance of the stratum corneum drops precipitously without a commensurate drop in the resistance of the viable tissue layer. As a result, the latter takes control of the permeation process [10,37,60]. Once this change in mechanism is manifest, the permeation of homologs from their saturated solutions mirrors the downward trend in aqueous solubilities, with further increases in chain length (hydrophobicity) marked with exponential declines in steady-state fluxes. The homologs quickly become inactive [60]. In effect, the homologs become so insoluble in water that they are thermodynamically restrained from partitioning into the viable tissues upon breaching the stratum corneum (or pore lipids). These features are in total agreement with expectations drawn from the earlier presented skin permeability model.

Clearly the physicochemical properties of a drug are a decisive factor in its overall activity. Where possible, molecular structures should be optimized to obtain best clinical performance. Rarely does an oral drug have physicochemical features suitable for topical or transdermal therapy, and it can take a great deal of systematic research to identify where the best balance of activity and permeability lies. Experience with corticosteroids suggests that as much as a 100-fold improvement in clinical activity may be attainable through molecular design, for today's most potent topical corticosteroids are more active than hydrocortisone by a factor at least this large.

Vehicle Properties and Percutaneous Absorption

The role solubility plays relative to maximal flux across membranes is clear from the preceding paragraphs. To kinetically reach the skin's surface, an appreciable fraction of a drug must also be in solution in the vehicle designed around it. Otherwise, diffusion of the drug through the vehicle to its interface with the skin may not completely compensate for drug lost through partitioning into the skin, kinetically dropping the drug's activity within this critical juncture of formulation and skin below saturation, lowering the drug's release into the surface tissues. Taken to an extreme, low vehicle solubility sets up a situation in which drug dissolution within and diffusion through the vehicle becomes delivery rate controlling [61,62]. In instances where a drug's pharmacological activity depends on getting as much drug as possible into the tissues, this is a problem. The outcome is similar when the drug is formulated in a highly unsaturated state in the first place. Again, it will not partition into the skin to the fullest possible extent, resulting in less than maximal bioavailability. Assuming maximal delivery is the goal, the optimum between these extremes is achieved by adjusting the solvency of the vehicle so that all or most of the drug is in solution but at the same time the vehicle is saturated or close thereto. This has the effect of balancing the kinetic and thermodynamic factors. It is for this reason that solvents like propylene glycol are added to topical formulations. Slowly evaporating propylene glycol provides a chemical environment in which drugs dissolve or remain dissolved, facilitating delivery. Therefore, one frequently finds propylene glycol (5–15%) in topical corticosteroid creams and other formulations.

These principles, which have been clinically validated, establish the critical role the vehicle plays in a drug's activity. While pharmacists do not have the wherewithal to actually test products at the dispensing counter, they nevertheless should be aware of these principles in order to select and dispense products from manufacturers who can demonstrate that such formulation factors have been given due consideration. These delivery dependencies also stand to caution the pharmacist. Extemporaneous mixing of commercial products, for example, one containing a steroid and another an antibiotic, and the diluting of products with homemade vehicle are suspect practices because the compositional changes associated with such blending are likely to adversely affect the delivery attributes of otherwise carefully designed systems [63,64].

There is another way vehicles can influence percutaneous absorption, which is by altering the physicochemical properties of the stratum corneum. In the main modification of the barrier results in increased skin permeability, but a buttressing effect is also achievable with substances having the capacity to solidify the horny structure. To repeat a point, simply hydrating the stratum corneum promotes absorption. This may be accomplished by covering the skin with a water-impermeable bandage or other wrapping (an occlusive dressing). The blockage of evaporative water loss leads to hydration of the stratum corneum, softening it and increasing the diffusive mobility of chemicals through it. The occlusive covering also prevents evaporation of volatile vehicle components, compositionally stabilizing a spread film, maintaining its solvency for the drug. It is estimated that occlusive hydration increases percutaneous absorption from 5-to 10-fold, enlargements that are often clinically significant [65]. The technique has been used with corticosteroids in refractory dermatoses such as psoriasis.

The following interesting phenomena associated with the occlusion of corticosteroids are enlightening. When applied under an occlusive dressing corticosteroids induce vasoconstriction at lower concentrations than when applied in the open. When the dressing is removed, vasoconstriction subsides in a few hours. However, as many as several days later blanching can sometimes be restored simply by rewrapping the area of application [66]. This suggests that steroid molecules somehow bottled up in the stratum corneum are released when occlusion is reestablished. It appears that as the stratum corneum dehydrates and returns to its normal state, substances such as the corticosteroids that may be present are entrapped within one of its physical domains, freezing them in place until either the stratum corneum is sloughed or until occlusive hydration is reinstated. The phenomenon is referred to as the skin's *reservoir effect*. The application of drugs dissolved in volatile solvents like acetone and ethanol also creates reservoirs in the stratum corneum for, as the solvents evaporate, the concentrating drug is driven into the skin's surface. Certain solvents also momentarily increase the solvency of the stratum corneum [67].

A few water-miscible organic solvents are taken up by the stratum corneum in amounts that soften its liquid crystalline, lipoidal domain [67], particularly when applied in concentrated form. If used very liberally (under laboratory conditions), these so-called skin penetration enhancers even elute interstitial lipids and denature keratin [68,69]. Under admittedly artificial research conditions, the increases in percutaneous absorption resulting from their actions can be dramatic. Dimethylsulfoxide (DMSO), dimethylacetamide (DMA), and diethyltoluamide (DEET) are key examples. DMSO has long been touted as a skin penetration enhancer. Experimental studies indicate that it reversibly denatures keratin, opening up the protein matrix, facilitating permeation [68,69]. DMSO also extracts lipids from the skin when applied liberally. Even when used sparingly, neat DMSO is imbibed to a degree by the stratum corneum, increasing the ability of the tissue to dissolve substances of all kinds [70].

This favors the absorption of drugs by allowing more drug to dissolve in the tissue, steepening diffusion gradients that are expressed across the tissue. Moreover, opposing flows of DMSO (inward) and water (outward) are set up when concentrated DMSO is placed over the skin that delaminates the stratum corneum, apparently with a pooling of solvent between the separated layers. Of all the possible actions of DMSO, the latter two seem to be the most important because extraction of skin lipids and denaturation of keratin require far more DMSO than found in a topical application of ordinary thickness (20–30 μm). These collective factors, in the extreme, effectively chemically remove the stratum corneum as a contributing part of the skin barrier [33]. In reality, however, the limited amounts of enhancer actually applied limit enhancement. Moreover, much of the enhancement capacity is lost if the solvents are in any way diluted. Thus, the use of neat organic solvents as skin penetration enhancers is an infrequent practice.

It has long been known that certain surfactants (e.g., sodium lauryl sulfate) are skin irritants, even in relatively dilute states, in part because they impair the barrier function of the stratum corneum, facilitating their own absorption. Concern about irritation precludes serious consideration of agents like this as enhancers. However, certain weaker amphiphilic substances (e.g., methyl oleate, glyceryl monolaurate, proplyene glycol monolaurate), some of which have long been used as ingredients in cosmetics if not therapeutic systems, are showing they have an unrealized potential as enhancers. Of special importance, surface-active (amphiphilic) substances are effective in the small amounts that can actually be applied to skin in spread films. Amphiphilic molecules penetrate into and blend with the stratum corneum's own lipids, which themselves are polar, amphiphilic substances. Thermoanalytical and spectroscopic evidence indicates that, in doing so, they relax the ordered structure of the stratum corneum's natural lipids, facilitating diffusion through existing channels and perhaps freeing up new channels [71–73]. Moreover, the reduction in liquid crystallinity invariably increases the capacity of the stratum corneum to dissolve substances, further magnifying the effect. It appears that relatively short alkyl chains (C_{10}, C_{12}) and a relatively weak polar end groups favor enhancement.

These emerging structural requirements of enhancement have launched a quest for new, even more powerful enhancers. Several potent amphiphilic compounds have surfaced from this pursuit that, at their worst, are only mildly tissue provocative, key examples being *N*-dodecylazacycloheptan-2-one (Azone®) and methyl decyl sulfoxide. Each of these compounds contains a short alkyl chain (Azone $= C_{12}$; decyl methyl sulfoxide $= C_{10}$) attached to a highly water-interactive but nonionic head group. Neither compound is at all water soluble, indicating that neither has the amphiphilic balance to form its own micelles. Of the two compounds, Azone has been the most scrutinized. It promotes the absorption of polar solutes at surprisingly low percentage concentrations. Its effects on animal skins have been especially profound; up to several hundred-fold improvements in the in vitro permeation rates of highly polar cyclic nucleosides through hairless mouse skin have been reported [74], for example. Azone does not appear to be comparably effective on human skin, but those actions it has are effected at low concentration [75]. As with any agent of the kind, its actions are dependent on formulation and how this affects the thermodynamic activity of the enhancer in the delivery system. Concern over toxicity and the availability of alternative substances with established safety pedigrees have become impediments to the introduction enhancers having new, totally unfamiliar chemical structures.

The effects of skin penetration enhancers on the stratum corneum may or may not be lasting, depending on the degree of chemical alteration of the stratum corneum that is experienced. Irreversibility is a perceived problem to the extent that the skin is left vulnerable to the absorption of other chemicals that come in contact with the conditioned area for as long at the area remains highly permeable. The fear is that such vulnerability will stay high until the greater part of the stratum corneum is renewed through mitosis, which minimally takes several days. Moreover, the enhancing solvents are themselves absorbed to some degree, another source of toxicological concern. DMSO, for instance, is known to increase intraocular pressure. DMA has been associated with liver damage. Azone may irritate, but its real liability is that its chemical structure is totally novel and without toxicological precedent. While worry over toxicity may be out of proportion with actual degrees of exposure attending the ordinary circumstances of clinical use of dermatological products, concern is nevertheless warranted given the occasional use of products over expansive areas.

Transdermal Delivery—Attributes of Transdermal Delivery Systems

We are learning more and more that the conditions of use of topical delivery systems have a profound influence on their performance. In this regard, transdermal systems, specifically the adhesive patches that are used to treat systemic disease, and dermatological products are subject to very different operating environments and conditions [76]. Transdermal delivery is aimed at achieving systemically active levels of a drug. A level of percutaneous absorption that leads to appreciable systemic drug accumulation is absolutely essential. Ideally one would like to avoid any build-up of a drug within the local tissues, but build-up is nevertheless unavoidable, for the drug is driven through a relatively small diffusional area of the skin defined by the contact area (absorption window) of the application. Consequently, high accumulations of drug in the viable tissues underlying the patch are preordained by the nature of the delivery process. Irritation and sensitization can be associated with such high levels, and therefore careful testing is done to rule out these complications before a transdermal delivery system gets far along in development.

Table 10 outlines general expectations associated with transdermal delivery. The water-impermeable backing materials of present and presumably most future transdermal systems cause make them occlusive. There is good reason for this. Foremost is again the fact that occlusion facilitates drug delivery. In labs where these systems are designed it has been learned that occlusion is often essential to achieving adequate rates of delivery. Furthermore, transdermal drugs such as nitroglycerin and nicotine are themselves relatively volatile compounds. While they can be packaged in a fashion that prevents drug loss, a backing material that is substantially impermeable is also needed to prevent these compounds from evaporating off into space after placing patches containing them on the skin. Impermeable polymer or foil backings also block the diffusive transport of body water to the atmosphere by way of the patch. Insensible perspiration at the site of the patch is thus held in check, but not without creating a substantially moist environment at the interface of the patch with the skin. Consequently, if given enough time, organisms already in the skin can colonize within this interface.

Table 10 Norms of Operation of Transdermal Patches

Occluded applications
Composition relatively invariant in use
System size (area) predetermined
Specific site prescribed for application
Application technique highly reproducible
Delivery is sustained
Generally operate at unit drug activity, at least operate at steady activity
Delivery is zero-order
Serum levels related to product efficacy
Bioequivalency based on pharmacokinetic (blood level) endpoint
Unavoidable local tissue levels consequential only to system toxicity
Individual dose interruptable
Whole system removed when spent
Delivery efficiency is low (only a fraction of drug content is delivered)

Other than possibly for the insensible perspiration they absorb, transdermal patches tend to operate as thermodynamically static systems, meaning as compositionally fixed systems, from the moment they are applied until their removal. Marketed ethanol-driven estradiol and fentanyl patches are exceptions because they meter out ethanol and drive it into the stratum corneum to propel the absorption process. Compositional steadfastness is still the rule, however, and it is this feature that bestows the zero-order delivery attribute on the ordinary transdermal patch. Drug is present within the patches in reservoir amounts whether or not the reservoir compartment is easily distinguished, for there must be enough drug to sustain delivery over the full course of patch wear.

In some prototypes, e.g., the nitroglycerin transdermal systems, huge excesses of drug are placed in the patch to assure that the drug's activity remains essentially level. Only a small fraction of the drug, well under 50% of the patch's total content, is actually delivered during the prescribed time the patch is to be worn. In situations where the drug is prohibitively expensive or prone to abuse (e.g., fentanyl), efficiencies have to be raised to the maximum physically achievable, and the fractional delivery of formulated drug has been made to approach or exceed 50%. The inherent stability of the delivery environment of patches results partly from their main materials of construction are polymers, fabricating laminates, and adhesives, all of which tend to be chemically robust. Solubilizing solvents (e.g., ethanol) and skin penetration enhancers (e.g., propylene glycol monolaurate) may also be present and their absorption into the skin may change patch compositions, but even here the processes are carefully orchestrated to gain a stable delivery environment over the long term.

A transdermal patch is a self-contained system that is applied as it is packaged, with its only manipulation being removal of the release liner to expose and ready its adhesive surface. The size of a patch, meaning its area of contact with the skin, is determined before it is made. All of this area or only an inner portion of it may actually be involved in drug delivery, but, either way, the area is fixed. Since absorption is proportional to area, to meet the differing drug requirements of individual patients, patches of different sizes are generally made available. The application site is also a constant of therapy in that a specific site or sites are recommended for use (not always for scientifically supportable reasons, e.g., nitroglycerine patches are worn over the heart!). Users tend to follow such dictates. Beyond this, the manner of application is also highly reproducible. Thus there is as tight a control over absorption area and application site variables here as can be found in all of therapy. The only variability not customarily controlled for is that associated with the skin's permeability itself, but even here some systems have been made to operate with high delivery precision by incorporating a rate-controlling membrane into them. Altogether the manner of use of the systems is highly reproduced from one application to the next.

Measures of function of transdermal systems distinguish them among the systems we use topically. Since systemic actions are sought, blood levels of the drug in question must reach and remain within therapeutic bounds. More often than not the requisite blood level is known from a drug's use by other routes of administration. Thus, a clear systemic target level usually exists, and an absolute rate of delivery commensurate with reaching this is a built-in feature of the patch. The requisite delivery rate can be estimated in several ways even before an attempt is made to design a transdermal system. For instance, once an upper size limit is set for the patch, the total daily oral requirement of the drug can be used to calculate the minimal delivery rate in $mg/cm^2/h$. This is done after making an appropriate downward adjustment in the transdermal dose to account for oral drug losses attributable to first-pass metabolism. Alternatively, the rate can be estimated from an established blood level and a known rate of systemic clearance (as the product of these). Comparing performances of transdermal delivery systems is a straightforward matter too. Bioequivalency of different systems built around a specific drug are easily measured in terms of the blood levels they produce. And if therapy isn't going well, one can bring delivery to a reasonably abrupt halt by simply removing a patch.

Topical Delivery—Attributes of Topical Delivery Systems

Topical delivery systems fill an important niche in therapy. Despite the fact that often less than 1% and almost never more than 15% of the drug in a dermatological application is systemically absorbed (systemically recoverable), topical delivery nevertheless allows one to achieve drug levels in local tissues far in excess of those that can be achieved by other means of administration. At the same time, systemic toxicities of the drug are rarely encountered with topical administration, with the exceptions occurring when dermatological formulations are used liberally over extensive areas. Because only small amounts of a drug are ordinarily applied topically, in most instances the amounts absorbed are so limited that one has trouble even measuring them. Thus, albeit imprecise, topical therapy actually represents a brute force form of drug targeting and has been discussed in this context. The principal drug-delivery systems for this purpose are of course ointments, creams, and gels, with miscellaneous other powder, liquid, and semisolid vehicles sometimes being employed. The *norms* of topical delivery, which are in striking contrast to the *norms* of transdermal delivery, are outlined in Table 11.

We tend to think of them being much the same, but the functioning of semisolid dermatological products stands in stark contrast with that of transdermal delivery systems. To begin with, most topical applications

Table 11 Norms of Operation of Dermatological Formulations

Open application
Experience profound compositional shifts in use
May experience phases changes in use
Site in the disease's location
Operate at variable drug activity
Highly nonstationary state kinetics
Application technique and amount are highly individualized
Applications short-acting
Local tissue levels tied to efficacy
Used on diseased, damaged skin
No easy bioequivalency endpoint
Systemic absorption absolutely undesirable, but some unavoidable
Therapy interruptable by washing off application
System removal inadvertent—wear and tear
Delivery efficiency is low (only a small fraction of drug is delivered)

are left open to the atmosphere. Amounts applied per unit area depend on the individual making the application. Of singular importance with respect to system function, extraordinary physicochemical changes accompany the evaporative concentration of these formulations, possibly including the precipitation of the drug or other substances that were comfortably in solution at the moment of their application. Evaporative concentration can also upset the oil-to-water balance of emulsions, destabilizing them, at times causing them to break or invert. In a matter of hours, if not just minutes, a surface film or dry residue having a totally different delivery faculty than the bulk formulation may be all that is left of the application. Such precipitous changes, if out of control, can bring drug delivery to an abrupt halt.

The amounts of ointments and creams people apply are highly individualized. So are the techniques of application. Some patients vigorously rub semisolid formulations into the skin, while others just spread films until they are more or less uniform over the desired area. While pharmacokinetic assessments of a system's delivery attributes is ordinarily done using normal skin (in vitro) or on healthy volunteers (in vivo), the site of its clinical deployment is usually anything but normal. Rather, it is determined by the skin condition to be treated. Clearly, the manufacturer is without control over how a disease is expressed in a particular patient. For many diseases, disease manifestation can be anywhere on the body. Moreover, from individual to individual it varies in intensity and vastness. Thus, more area may be involved in one case than in another, and the barrier function of the skin may be more or less intact in any instance. This creates a set of imponderables with respect to delivery, efficacy, and safety.

The removal of the dermatological application is rarely deliberate. Rather, some substance is usually transferred to clothing, etc., some is absorbed, some evaporates, and some is inadvertently removed by activities such as bathing. Of course, applications can be deliberately washed from the skin if one wishes to terminate therapy. Partly because of their temporal, inhabitancy, local applications tend to be short acting relative to transdermal delivery systems. Other factors are the finite doses that are actually administered and the often rapid evaporative concentration of such films to compositions that cease supporting dissolution of the drug and its diffusion to the skin's surface. Consider that the application of a topical product to the skin in a representative, 20 μm thick layer places only 20 μg of drug over each cm^2 of skin when the drug is formulated at the relatively high concentration of 1%. Roughly 10 mg of stratum corneum covers each cm^2 of skin, enough for 20 μg of drug to effectively get lost in. Consequently, only a fraction of the drug that does enter the skin actually reaches the live tissues. Such finite doses do not sustain delivery, and thus delivery wanes after several hours irrespective of the wearability of the application or processes attending its evaporative shrinkage. Since all these attending processes defy quantification, there is precious little existing information to guide one concerning a fitting regimen of application for most topical dosage forms. Rather, dosing regimens evolve historically from collective clinical experience. All in all, topical therapy is an extraordinarily complex operation.

Compositional changes following the application of certain topical systems are unavoidable. Many o/w creams contain as much as 80–85% external phase, usually primarily water. Lotions and gels also contain volatile constituents in large proportion. All rapidly evaporate after their application, and, consequently, the drug-delivery system is the formed, concentrated film that develops on the skin and not the medium as packaged in the tube, jar, or bottle. Ingredients should be chosen to assure that compositional changes as invariably occur interfere as little as possible with delivery and therapy. In this regard, the rate at which the volatile components evaporate to form the equilibrium film can itself be a factor in bioavailability [77]. It has been reported, for instance, that a thinly applied corticosteroid preparation produced greater vasoconstriction than did thicker applications of the same material [78]. Though the total amounts of drug per unit area were greater with the thick films, responses were less in their case because evaporative concentration of the steroid in the applied medium proceeded more slowly. Even without knowing the mechanistic details, we can conclude from this that less steroid was driven into the skin from the thick applications in the course of the test. It has also been demonstrated that vasoconstriction is more pronounced at low concentrations when steroid is applied in volatile ethanol than when applied in propylene glycol [56]. While differences in solvency play a role here, it is also clear that the rapid evaporation of solvents like ethanol drives drug into the skin. Such observations emphasize the importance of distinguishing between the system as packaged and the transitional system following application. Unfortunately, this distinction is not always made and much topical delivery research aimed at assessing the relative abilities formulations have to deliver drug has been performed by placing extraordinarily thick layers of formulation over the skin. Such thick applications do not even remotely simulate the clinical release situation, especially when it comes to creams and gels. This area of drug delivery is in need of much research.

Formulators can use the tendency of creams, gels, and other systems to evaporatively concentrate to advantage. Solvents are chosen and blended so that the drug remains soluble in the formed film long after application is made. This can be accomplished by replacing a fraction of the water or other highly volatile solvent found in these systems with solvents of far lower volatility. As previously pointed out, 5–15% propylene glycol is found in many topical corticosteroid creams and lotions just for this reason.

In summary, the way a topical drug is formulated has a great deal to do with its clinical effectiveness, not a surprising conclusion given what is known about the relationships between bioavailability and formulation for other modes of administration. Yet in the area of topical drug performance, antiquated concepts and approaches to system design linger. In days when topical bioavailability was little understood and therefore ignored, formulators concentrated on vehicle elegance and stability. Attempts were made to design vehicles compatible with all types of drugs, so-called universal vehicles. Universal vehicles are still discussed in many standard texts. Today's technology and science clearly indicate that the universal vehicle is akin to a unicorn, beautiful but totally mythical. In the real world, each system must be designed around the drug it contains to optimize the clinical potential of the active ingredient. The duration of action will depend on how long the drug remains appreciably in solution within its spread film. These matters are carefully examined when a drug-delivery system, topical or not, reaches the FDA as an Investigational New Drug (IND), New Drug Application (NDA) or Abbreviated New Drug Application (ANDA) [79].

B. Aspects of Physical and Chemical Stability

Concern for the physical and chemical integrity of topical systems is no different than for other dosage forms. However, there are some unique and germane dimensions to stability associated with semisolid systems. A short list of some of the factors to be evaluated for semisolids is given in Table 12. All factors must be acceptable initially (within prescribed specifications), and all must remain so over the stated lifetime for the product (the product's shelf life).

Table 12 Factors for Evaluation of Semisolids

Stability of the active ingredient(s)
Stability of the adjuvants
Visual appearance
Color
Odor (development of pungent odor or loss of fragrance)
Viscosity, extrudability
Loss of water and other volatile vehicle components
Phase distribution (homogeneity or phase separation, bleeding)
Particle size distribution of dispersed phases
pH
Texture, feel upon application (stiffness, grittiness, greasiness, tackiness)
Particulate contamination
Microbial contamination and sterility (in the unopened container and under conditions of use)
Release and bioavailability

The chemical integrities of drugs, preservatives, and other key adjuvants must be assessed as a function of time to establish a product's useful shelf life from a chemical standpoint. Semisolid systems present two special problems in this regard. First, semisolids are chemically complex to the point that just separating drug and adjuvants from all other components is an analyst's nightmare. Many components interfere with standard assays, and therefore difficult separations are the rule before anything can be analyzed. Also, since semisolids undergo phase changes upon heating, one cannot use high-temperature kinetics for stability prediction. Thus, stability has to be evaluated at the storage temperature of the formulation, and this of course takes a long time. Under these circumstances problematic stability may not be evident until studies have been in progress for a year or more. Be this as it may, stability details are worked out in the laboratories of industry, the pharmacist ordinarily accepting projected shelf lives as fact. Some qualitative indicators of chemical instability that the pharmacist might look for are the development of color (or a change in color and/or its intensity) and the development of an off-odor. Often products yellow or brown with age as the result of oxidative reactions occurring in the base. Discolorations of the kind are commonly seen when natural fats and oils, e.g., lanolins, are used to build the vehicle. Extensive oxidation of natural fatty materials (rancidification) is accompanied by development of a disagreeable odor. One may also notice phase and texture changes in a suspect product. Pharmacists should take note of the appearances of the topical products they dispense, removing all those from circulation that exhibit color changes or become fetid. Changes in product pH also indicate chemical decomposition, most probably of a hydrolytic nature, and, if somehow detected, are reason to return a product.

Time-variable rheological behavior of a semisolid may also signal physical and/or chemical change. However, measures such as spreadability and feel upon application are probably unreliable indicators of a changing rheology, and more exacting measurements are necessary. A pharmacist does not ordinarily have the tools at hand to make accurate rheological assessments, but the equipment to do so is generally available and used within the development labs of the industry. Here one may find exquisitely sensitive plate and cone research viscometers that in principle precisely quantify viscosity and also utilitarian rheometers that put viscosities on a relative scale. The latter include extrusion rheometers, which measure the force it takes to extrude a semisolid through a narrow orifice, penetrometers, which characterize viscosity in terms of the penetration of a weighted cone into a semisolid, and Brookfield viscometers with spindle and helipath attachments. The latter measure the force it takes to drive a spindle helically through a semisolid. As used with semisolids, the utilitarian rheometers only provide relative, although quite useful, measures of viscosity. Increases (or decreases) in viscosity by any of these measuring tools indicate changes in the structural elements of the formulation. The gradual transformations in semisolid structure that take place are more often than not impermanent, in which case the systems are restored to their initial condition simply by mixing them. Substantial irreversible rheological changes are a sign of poor physical stability.

Changes in the natures of individual phases of or phase separation within a formulation are reasons to discontinue use of a product. Phase separation may result from emulsion breakage, clearly an acute instability. More often it appears more subtly as bleeding—the formation of visible droplets of an emulsion's internal phase in the continuum of the semisolid. This problem is the result of slow rearrangement and contraction of internal structure. Eventually, here and there, globules of what is often clear liquid internal phase are squeezed out of the matrix. Warm storage temperatures can induce or accelerate structural crenulation such as this; thus, storage of dermatological products in a cool place is prudent. The main concern with a system that has undergone such separation is that a patient will not be applying a medium of uniform composition application after application. Due to unequal distribution between phases (internal partitioning), one phase will invariably have a higher concentration of the drug than the other. Therefore, since semisolid emulsions, unlike liquid emulsions, cannot be returned to an even distribution by shaking, formulations exhibiting separation are functionally suspect and should be removed from circulation.

Pharmacists should also take a dim view of changes in the particle size, size distribution, or particulate nature of semisolid suspensions. They are the consequence of crystal growth, changes in crystalline habit, or the reversion of the crystalline materials to a more stable polymorphic form. Any crystalline alteration can lead to a pronounced reduction in the drug-delivery capabilities and therapeutic utility of a formulation. Thus, products exhibiting such changes are seriously physically unstable and unusable.

A more commonly encountered change in formulations is the evaporative loss of water or other volatile phases from a preparation while it is in storage. This can occur as the result inappropriate packaging or a flaw made in packaging. Some plastic collapsible tubes allow diffusive loss of volatile substances through the container walls. One will find this phenomenon occasionally in cosmetics that are hurried to the marketplace without adequate stability assessment, but rarely in ethical pharmaceuticals, which are time-tested. However, a bad seal may occur in any tube or jar no matter what its contents, with eventual loss of volatile ingredients around the cap or through the crimp. Such evaporative losses cause a formulation to stiffen and become puffy and its application characteristics change noticeably. There is corresponding weight loss. Under this influence the contents of a formulation may shrink and pull away from the container wall. These phenomena are most likely to be seen in creams and gels due the high fractions of volatile components that characterize them. Problems here are exacerbated when products are stored in warm locations.

Gross phase changes are detectable by eye upon close inspection of products. The package of course gets in the way of such analysis, but if a product is truly suspect, it should be closely examined by opening and inspecting the full contents of the container. A jar can be opened and its contents probed with a spatula without ruining the container. Close inspection of the contents of a tube requires destruction of the package, however. The easy way to do this is to cut off the seal along the bottom of the tube with scissors and then make a perpendicular cut up the length of the tube to the edge of the platform to which the cap is anchored. Careful further trimming a quarter of the way around the platform in each direction creates left and right panels that can be pealed back with tweezers to expose the tube's contents. Textural changes such as graininess, bleeding, and other phase irregularities are easily seen on the unfolded, flat surface. Normally it takes a microscope to reveal changes in crystalline size, shape and/or distribution, but palpable grit is a sure sign that a problem exists. Weight loss of a product, which is easily checked at the prescription counter, clearly indicates the loss of volatile ingredients (the weight of a suspect tube can be directly compared to the weight of a fresh tube, etc.). On the rare occasions when deterioration like this is noted by a pharmacist in the course of handling products or is reported to the pharmacist by a knowledgeable patient, the suspect package should be removed from circulation and the manufacturer informed of the action. If a problem seems general rather than isolated (i.e., to a single bad package), the FDA should be notified as well to safeguard the public. This agency will determine if a product has gone bad and a general recall is warranted.

C. Freedom from Contamination

Particulates

Numerous topical preparations contain finely dispersed solids. Pastes, for example, contain as much as or more than 50% solids dispersed in an ointment medium. Powders themselves are used topically. Many dermatological liquids and semisolids contain suspended matter. However present, the particles should be impalpable, i.e., incapable of being individually perceived by touch, so that the formulations don't feel gritty. The palpability of a particle is a function of its hardness, shape, and size. The pharmacist can only manipulate the latter, and thus it is important to prepare or use finely subdivided solids when making topical dosage forms. Individual particles greater than 50 μm in their longest dimension can be individually perceived by touch. The surface of the eye is substantially more sensitive, and a 10 μm particle can be distinguished here. Clearly, the presence of hard, palpable particulates in semisolids makes them abrasive, particularly when applied to disease- or damage-sensitized skin. Severe eye irritation is possible if ophthalmic ointments contain them. One particularly troublesome source of particulate contamination is flashings (tiny metal slivers and shavings) left over from the production tin and aluminum collapsible tubes. These often adhere electrostatically and tenaciously to tubing walls following cutting of the containers down to a particular size. Some escape removal by the washing and rinsing done to cleanse the empty containers. Consequently, a jet of exceedingly high-velocity air is blown into the open end of tubes just prior to their filling to remove all particulates. If this precaution is not taken, tiny metal slivers may be packaged with the product, posing the threat that they will become dislodged and instilled into the eye while the product is in use. For these reasons, the United States Pharmacopoeia/National Formulary (USP/NF) has a particulate test for ophthalmic ointments. In this test the ointments are liquefied in a petri dish at high temperature (85°C) for 2 hours and then solidified by cooling. Particles that have settled to the bottom of the shallow glass container are counted by microscopic scanning at 30 times magnification. The requirements are met is the total number of particles 50 μm or larger in any dimension does not exceed 50 in the 10 tubes tested and if not more than 8 particles are found in a single tube. Products that are put into the distribution channels have to meet this test. Nevertheless, the pharmacist should be on the lookout for particulate problems associated with commercial products. The pharmacist must also take measures to ensure that extemporaneously compounded formulations are free of particulates. Particular attention must be paid to the cleaning of collapsible tubes and other package parts prior to their use.

Microbial Specifications and Sterility

As of the USP XIX, ophthalmic ointments must be prepared and dispensed as sterile products (until opened for use). Presently in the United States, non-ophthalmic topical preparations do not need to be sterile, although they cannot contain pathogens and must have low microbe counts. The reasons ophthalmic sterility requirements were broadened to cover ointments are enlightening. In the mid-1960s there was an outbreak of extremely serious *Pseudomonas* eye infections in the Scandinavian block of countries, in some instances resulting in loss of sight. The source of the contamination was traced to antibiotic-containing ophthalmic ointments made by a regional manufacturer known for its high standards of manufacturing and quality control [80]. Pathogenic *Pseudomonas* organisms were found in both the products and the manufacturing facilities where the ointments were prepared. It was widely believed up until this time that pathogens could not and would not survive and grow in ointments and similar media. The presence of antibiotics in the preparations could only have added to the false sense of security this company had. This incident sent shock waves throughout the pharmaceutical world and spawned revisions in all world compendia. In the United States ophthalmic ointments must be sterile when dispensed. In Europe dermatological products which are to be used over broken skin must also be sterile.

The foregoing incident has special meaning to the dispensing pharmacist. Unopened ophthalmic ointments should be dispensed for each condition and should be given very short shelf-life datings. Patients should be advised to discard unused quantities of old preparations and to return for fresh supplies if and when chronic symptoms reappear. Similar advice and precautions are good practice with dermatological products like ointments that do not ordinarily contain microbial preservatives. Lotions, creams, and topical solutions that contain preservatives tend to remain pathogen-free after their packages have been opened, providing an extra measure of safety.

Preservatives have an important purpose in topical medications. Systems containing them tend to remain aseptic. Even if a few organisms subsist in the presence of the preservatives, these tend to be nonvegetative. Importantly, no pathogenic forms survive to cause problems. Preservatives are necessary for systems that have an aqueous phase, because water offers an environment that is particularly conducive to microbial growth. Therefore, all emulsions and aqueous solutions and suspensions should be preserved. However, choosing a preservative is no easy task, for the physical systems tend to be compositionally complex and polyphasic, affording many possible means for specific preservatives to be inactivated. In mass-produced products the effectiveness of the preservation system of formulations is checked by the USP preservative challenge test.

D. Pharmaceutical Elegance

A number of attributes of topical drug systems that may be classified as cosmetic can make patients more or less willing to use their medications (compliant). These include ease of application, the feel of the preparation once it is on the skin, and the appearance of the applied film. Ideally, the application should be undetectable to the eye and neither tacky nor greasy. Certain items, such as ointments and pastes, are, of course, intrinsically greasy, and suspensions of all types tend to leave an opaque, easily detectable film. Thus the extent to which the cosmetic features can be idealized is dependent on the nature and purpose of the dosage form.

The ease of application and method of application of a formulation depend on the physicochemical attributes of the system involved. Solutions and other highly fluid systems may be swabbed on, sprayed on, or rolled on. A cotton pledget or other applicator is often necessary to obtain an even application. Soft semisolid systems, on the other hand, may be spread evenly and massaged into the skin with the fingers, a procedure technically referred to as inunction. The spreadability is a rheological quality related to the nature and degree of internal structure of the formulation. Formulations such as pastes that are very stiff tend to be hard to apply; their application over broken or irritated skin can be disagreeable. The stiffness of a preparation can be upregulated or downregulated by manipulating the amounts of structure-building components of a vehicle and in some instances by adjusting the phase/volume ratio of semisolid emulsions. Thus, for ointments, increased spreadability can be obtained by decreasing the ratio of the waxy components (waxes and petrolatum) to fluid vehicle components (mineral oil, fixed oils). Greasiness of such preparations goes in the opposite direction. For o/w creams, decreasing the ratio of the internal phase to the external phase tends to make the systems more fluid. Substitution of more liquid oils for some of the high-melting waxy components of creams achieves the same end.

Tackiness and greasiness are determined by the physicochemical properties of the vehicle constituents that comprise the formed film on the skin. A sticky film is extremely uncomfortable, and, generally, considerable effort is directed to minimizing this inelegant feature. Where creams are concerned, waxy ingredients such as stearic acid and cetyl alcohol produce noticeably nontacky films. Stearic acid is the principal internal phase component of vanishing creams, systems that are virtually undetectable visually or by touch after inunction. On the other hand, propylene glycol, which may be added to creams and gels to solubilize a drug, tends to make systems tacky. The synthetic and natural gums used as thickening and suspending agents in gels and lotions tends to increase their tackiness, and, therefore, these materials are used as sparingly as function allows.

Creams tend to be invisible on the skin. The same is true for ointments, although the oiliness of ointments causes them to glisten to an extent. Whatever opacity creams and ointments have is due primarily to the presence of insoluble solids. These often imbue applications with a powdery or even crusty appearance. Dispersed solids are usually functional, as in calamine lotion, zinc sulfide lotion, zinc oxide paste, and so on, and are an implacable feature of these preparations. However, at times insoluble solids are added as tints to match the color of the skin and to impart opacity. Since individual skins vary widely in hue (pigmentation) and texture, tinting to a single color and texture is generally unsuccessful.

Evaluation of the cosmetic elegance of topical preparations can be accomplished scientifically, but it is questionable whether physical experiments on system rheology and the like offer appreciable advantage over the subjective evaluations of the pharmacist, the formulator, or other experienced people. Persons who use cosmetics are particularly adept and helpful as evaluators.

E. Skin Sensitivity—A Specific Toxicological Concern

One further problem of topical formulations associated with many ingredients and of special concern with preservatives is the development of skin sensitivity [81]. The skins of some individuals are particularly susceptible to an allergic conditioning to chemicals known as Type IV contact hypersensitivity. Haptens (chemicals like urushiol found in poison ivy) are absorbed through the skin and, while in the local tissues, chemically react with local proteins. Langerhans cells, the local cells involved in immunological surveillance, identify these now denatured proteins as foreign (nonhost). The Langerhans cells then leave the dermis by way of the lymphatics and enter the draining lymph node, where they complete the sensitization process by passing the allergen message on to resident lymphocytes (antigen presentation). Once sensitized, subsequent contact with the offending chemical (hapten) leads to inflammation and skin eruption. Many of the preservatives used in pharmacy are phenols and comparably reactive substances, compounds that have a high propensity to sensitize susceptible individuals. The pharmacist should be alert to this possibility and prepared to recommend discontinuing therapy and physician referral when allergic outbreak is evident or suspected. Moreover, the pharmacist should be ready to recommend alternative products that do not contain an allergically offending substance once it has been identified, assuming of course that therapeutically suitable alternatives exist.

Allergic incidents are widespread, and, from an allergy standpoint, it is useful that the ingredients of dermatological medications are listed on the package or in the package insert. This allows the pharmacist to screen products for their suitability for individuals with known sensitivities. Over-the-counter medications and cosmetics also contain a qualitative listing of their ingredients. The pharmacist thus has access to critical information he or she needs to safeguard patients relative to their known hypersensitivity.

REFERENCES

1. A. P. Lemberger, in *Handbook of Non-Prescription Drugs*, American Pharmaceutical Association, Washington, DC, 1973, p. 161.
2. G. L. Wilkes, I. A. Brown, and R. H. Wildnauer, CRC Crit. Rev. Bioeng., Aug., 453 (1973).
3. K. F. Rushmer, K. J. K. Buettner, J. M. Short, and G. F. Odland, Science, 154, 343 (1966).
4. R. J. Scheuplein and I. H. Blank, Physiol. Rev., 51, 762 (1971).
5. W. Montagna, *The Structure and Function of Skin*, 3rd ed., Academic Press, New York,1974.
6. P. M. Elias, S. Grayson, M. A. Lampe, M. L. Williams, and B. E. Brown, in *Stratum Corneum* (R. Marks and G. Plewig, eds.), Springer-Verlag, New York, 1983, pp. 53–67.
7. J. W. Tingstad, D. E. Wurster, and T. Higuchi, J. Am. Pharm. Assoc., 47, 187 (1958).
8. R. J. Scheuplein, J. Invest. Dermatol., 47, 334 (1965).
9. H. Baker and A. M. Kligman, Arch. Dermatol., 96, 441 (1967).
10. R. J. Scheuplein, J. Invest. Dermatol., 48, 79 (1967).
11. R. T. Woodburne, *Essentials of Human Anatomy*, Oxford University Press, New York, 1965, p.6.
12. S. Rothman, *Physiology and Biochemistry of the Skin*, University of Chicago Press, Chicago, 1954, p. 26.
13. A. E. McKenzie, Arch. Dermatol., 86, 611 (1962).
14. R. B. Stoughton, Southern Med. J., 55, 1134 (1962).
15. G. Sazbo, Adv. Biol. Skin, 3, 1 (1962).
16. M. Katz and B. J. Poulsen, in *Handbook of Experimental Pharmacology, New Series*, Vol. 28 (B. B. Brodie and J. Gillette, eds.), Springer-Verlag, New York, 1972, p. 103.
17. S. M. Peck and W. R. Russ, Arch. Dermatol. Syphilol., 56, 601 (1947).
18. M. R. Liggins, Patient Care, July 1, 56 (1974).
19. B. Idson, J. Soc. Cosmet. Chem., 24, 1972 (1973).
20. K. Laden, Am. Perfum. Cosmet., 82, 77 (1967).
21. J. N. Robinson, in *Handbook of Non-Prescription Drugs*, American Pharmaceutical Association, Washington, DC, 1973, p. 209.
22. R. B. Stoughton, Clin. Pharmacol. Ther., 16, 869 (1974).

23. J. J. Voorhees, E. A. Duell, M. Stawiski, and E. R. Harrell, Clin. Pharmacol. Ther., 16, 919 (1973).
24. W. R. Good, Med. Device Diag. Ind., Feb., 35 (1986).
25. G. W. Cleary, in *Medical Applications of Controlled Release*, Vol. 1 (R. S. Langer and D. L. Wise eds.), CRC Press, Boca Raton, FL, 1983, pp. 203–251.
26. Y. W. Chien, *Novel Drug Delivery Systems*, Marcel Dekker, New York, 1982, pp. 149–217.
27. J. P. Marty, R. H. Guy, and H. I. Maibach, *Percutaneous Absorption*, 2nd ed. (R. L. Bronaugh and H. I. Maibach, eds.), Marcel Dekker, New York, 1989, pp. 511–529.
28. C. R. Behl, N. H. Bellantone, and G. L. Flynn, in *Percutaneous Absorption* (R. L. Bronaugh and H. I. Maibach, eds.), Marcel Dekker, New York, 1985, pp. 183–212.
29. L. B. Fisher, in *Percutaneous Absorption*, 2nd ed. (R. L. Bronaugh and H. I. Maibach, eds.), Marcel Dekker, New York, 1989, pp. 213–222.
30. D. A. Weingand, C. Haygood, J. R. Gaylor, and J. H. Anglin, Jr., in *Current Concepts in Cutaneous Toxicity* (V. A. Drill and P. Lazar, eds.), Academic Press, New York, 1980, pp. 221–235.
31. D. A. Weingand, C. Haygood, and J. R. Gaylor, J. Invest. Dermatol., 62, 563 (1974).
32. H. H. Durrheim, G. L. Flynn, W. I. Higuchi, and C. R. Behl, J. Pharm. Sci., 69, 781 (1980).
33. G. L. Flynn, E. E. Linn, T. Kurihara-Bergstrom, S. K. Govil, and S. Y. E. Hou, in *Transdermal Delivery of Drugs*, Vol. 2, CRC Press, Boca Raton, FL, 1987.
34. C. G. T. Mathias, in *Dermatotoxicology*, 2nd ed. (F. N. Marzulli and H. I. Maibach, eds.), Hemisphere Publishing, New York, 1983, pp. 167–183.
35. M. S. Roberts, A. A. Anderson, J. Swarbrik, and D. E. Moore, J. Pharm. Pharmacol., 30, 486 (1978).
36. H. P. Bader, L. A. Goldsmith, and L. Bonar, J. Invest. Dermatol., 60, 215 (1971).
37. J. A. Keipert, Med. J. Aust., 1, 1021 (1971).
38. G. L. Flynn, in *Percutaneous Absorption: Mechanism—Methodology—Drug Delivery*, 2nd ed. (R. Bronaugh and H. I. Maibach, eds.), Marcel Dekker, New York, 1989, pp. 27–51.
39. G. L. Flynn, S. H. Yalkowsky, and T. J. Roscman, J. Pharm. Sci., 63, 479 (1974).
40. R. J. Scheuplein and R. L. Bronaugh, in *Biochemistry and Physiology of the Skin*, Vol. 2 (L. A. Goldsmith, ed.), Oxford University Press, New York, 1983, pp. 1255–1295.
41. T. Higuchi and S. S. Davis, J. Pharm. Sci., 59, 1376 (1970).
42. S. S. Davis, T. Higuchi, and J. H. Rytting, Adv. Pharm. Sci., 4, 73 (1974).
43. R. J. Scheuplein, I. H. Blank, G. J. Brauner, and D. J. MacFarlane, J. Invest. Dermatol., 52, 63 (1969).
44. G. L. Flynn, in *Principles of Route-to-Route Extrapolation for Risk Assessment* (T. R. Gerrity and C. J. Henry, eds.), Elsevier, New York, 1990, pp. 93–128.
45. R. O. Potts and R. H. Guy, Pharm. Res., 9, 663 (1992).
46. N. Z. Erdi, M. M. Cruz, and O. A. Battista, J. Colloid Interface Sci., 28, 36 (1968).
47. P. Thau and C. Fox, J. Soc. Cosmet. Chem., 16, 359 (1965).
48. S. Foster, D. E. Wurster, T. Higuchi, and L. W. Busse, J. Am. Pharm. Assoc. (Sci. Ed.), 40, 123 (1951).
49. B. W. Barry, J. Pharm. Pharmacol., 21, 533 (1969).
50. S. Amott, A. Fulmer, W. E. Scott, I. C. M. Dea, R. Moorhouse, and D. A. Rees, J. Mol. Biol., 90, 269 (1974).
51. *Physician's Desk Reference*, 28th ed., Medical Economics, Oradell, NJ, 1974, p. 1460.
52. G. L. Flynn and T. J. Roseman, J. Pharm. Sci., 60, 1778 (1971).
53. G. L. Flynn, J. Pharm. Sci., 60, 345 (1971).
54. T. A. Hagen, *Physicochemical Study of Hydrocortisone and Hydrocortisone n-Alkyl-21-Esters*, thesis, University of Michigan, 1979.
55. W. M. Smith, *An Inquiry into the Mechanism of Percutaneous Absorption of Hydrocortisone and its n-Alkyl Esters*, thesis, University of Michigan, 1982.
56. C. A. Schlagel, Adv. Biol. Skin, 12, 339 (1972).
57. A. W. McKenzie and R. M. Atkinson, Arch. Dermatol., 89, 741 (1964).
58. G. Saracco and B. Spaccamella-Marcheti, Ann. Chem., 48, 1357 (1958).
59. S. H. Yalkowsky, G. L. Flynn, and T. G. Slunick, J. Pharm. Sci., 61, 852 (1972).
60. G. L. Flynn and S. H. Yalkowsky, J. Pharm. Sci., 61, 838 (1972).
61. D. E. Wurster, Am. Perfum. Cosmet., 80, 21 (1965).
62. T. Higuchi, J. Soc. Cosmet. Chem., 11, 85 (1960).
63. K. H. Burdick, B. J. Poulsen, and V. A. Place, JAMA, 211, 462 (1970).
64. H. Schaefer and T. E. Redelmeier, *Skin Barrier—Principles of Percutaneous Absorption*, Karger, Basel, 1996, pp. 213–223.
65. A. W. McKenzie and R. B. Stoughton, Arch. Dermatol., 86, 608 (1962).
66. C. F. H. Vickers, Adv. Biol. Skin, 12, 177 (1972).
67. R. B. Stoughton, Arch. Dermatol., 91, 657 (1965).
68. R. J. Scheuplein and L. Ross, J. Soc. Cosmet. Chem., 21, 853 (1970).
69. S. G. Elfbaum and K. Laden, J. Soc. Cosmet. Chem., 19, 163 (1968).
70. R. Jones, Excipient effects on topical drug delivery paper presented at the Industrial Pharmaceutical Technology Section Symposium, 121st Annual Meeting of the American Pharmaceutical Association, Chicago, Abstracts, Vol. 4, p. 24.
71. M. Goodman and B. W. Barry, in *Percutaneous Absorption*, 2nd ed. (R. L. Bronaugh and

H. I. Maibach, eds.), Marcel Dekker, New York, 1989, pp. 567–593.
72. W. Abraham and D. T. Downing, in *Prediction of Percutaneous Absorption* (R. C. Scott, R. H. Guy, and J. Hadgraft, eds.), IBC Technical Services, London, 1990, pp. 110–122.
73. B. D. Anderson, W. I. Higuchi, and P. Raykar, Pharm. Res., 5, 566 (1988).
74. W. I. Higuchi, W. W. Shannon, J. L. Fox, G. L. Flynn, W. F. H. Ho, R. Vaidyanathan, and D. C. Baker, in *Recent Advances in Drug Delivery Systems* (J. M. Anderson and S. W. Kim, eds.), Plenum Press, New York, 1984, pp. 1–7.
75. S. Y. E. Hou and G. L. Flynn, Pharm. Res., 3(Suppl.), 525 (1986).
76. G. L. Flynn and N. D. Weiner, in *Dermal and Transdermal Delivery—New Insights and Perspectives* (R. Gurny, ed.), APV, Stuttgart, 1993, pp. 33–65.
77. M. Goldman, B. J. Poulsen, and T. Higuchi, J. Pharm. Sci., 58, 1098 (1969)
78. B. J. Poulsen, E. Young, V. Coquilla, and M. Katz, J. Pharm. Sci., 57, 928 (1968).
79. V. P. Shah, T. M. Ludden, S. V. Dighe, J. P. Skelly and R. L. Williams, in *Topical Drug Bioavailability, Bioequivalence, and Penetration* (V. P. Shah and H. I. Maibach, eds.), Plenum Press, New York, 1993, pp. 414–424.
80. L. O. Killings, O. Ringerts, and L. Silverstolpe, Acta Pharm. Suec., 3, 219 (1966).
81. A. A. Fisher, E. Pascher, and N. B. Kanot, Arch. Dermatol., 104, 286 (1971).

Chapter 9

Disperse Systems

Wandee Im-Emsap and Juergen Siepmann

Freie Universität Berlin, Berlin, Germany

Ornlaksana Paeratakul

Srinakharinwirot University, Nakhonnayok, Thailand

I. INTRODUCTION

A disperse system is defined as a heterogenous, two-phase system in which the internal (dispersed, discontinuous) phase is distributed or dispersed within the continuous (external) phase or vehicle. Various pharmaceutical systems are included in this definition, the internal and external phases being gases, liquids, or solids. Disperse systems are also important in other fields of application, e.g., processing and manufacturing of household and industrial products such as cosmetics, foods, and paints.

This chapter describes the basic principles involved in the development of disperse systems. Emphasis is laid on systems that are of particular pharmaceutical interest, namely, suspensions, emulsions, and colloids. Theoretical concepts, preparation techniques, and methods used to characterize and stabilize disperse systems are presented. The term "particle" is used in its broadest sense, including gases, liquids, solids, molecules, and aggregates. The reader may find it useful to read this chapter in conjuction with Chapters 8, 12, and 14, since they include some of the most important applications of disperse systems as pharmaceutical dosage forms [1].

A. Classification

Disperse systems can be classified in various ways. Classification based on the physical state of the two constituent phases is presented in Table 1. The dispersed phase and the dispersion medium can be either solids, liquids, or gases. Pharmaceutically most important are suspensions, emulsions, and aerosols. (Suspensions and emulsions are described in detail in Secs. IV and V; pharmaceutical aerosols are treated in Chapter 14.) A suspension is a solid/liquid dispersion, e.g., a solid drug that is dispersed within a liquid that is a poor solvent for the drug. An emulsion is a liquid/liquid dispersion in which the two phases are either completely immiscible or saturated with each other. In the case of aerosols, either a liquid (e.g., drug solution) or a solid (e.g., fine drug particles) is dispersed within a gaseous phase. There is no disperse system in which both phases are gases.

Another classification scheme is based on the size of the dispersed particles within the dispersion medium (Table 2). The particles of the dispersed phase may vary considerably in size, from large particles visible to the naked eye, down to particles in the colloidal size range, and particles of atomic

Table 1 Classification Scheme of Disperse Systems on the Basis of the Physical State of the Dispersed Phase and the Dispersion Medium

Dispersed phase	Dispersion medium		
	Solid	Liquid	Gas
Solid	Solid suspension (zinc oxide paste, toothpaste)	Suspension (tetracycline oral suspension USP, bentonite magma NF)	Solid aerosol (epinephrine bitartrate inhalation aerosol USP, smoke)
Liquid	Solid emulsion (hydrophilic petrolatum USP, butter)	Emulsion (mineral oil emulsion USP, Milk)	Liquid aerosol (nasal sprays, fog)
Gas	Solid foam Foamed plastics Pumice	Foam Effervescent salts in water Carbonated beverages	None

Pharmaceutical and other examples are given in parentheses.

and molecular dimensions. Generally, three classes are distinguished: molecular, colloidal, and coarse dispersions. Molecular dispersions are homogeneous in character and form true solutions. Colloidal dispersions are intermediate in size between true solutions and coarse dispersions. The term "colloidal" is usually applied to systems in which the particle size of the dispersed phase is in the range of 1–1000 nm and where the dispersion medium is a liquid. Nanoparticles distributed within a liquid and aqueous polymer dispersions for pharmaceutical coating applications are examples of colloidal systems. (Colloidal dispersions are described in more detail in Sec. VI.) Dispersions containing larger dispersed phases, usually 10–50 μm in size, are referred to as "coarse dispersions," which include most pharmaceutical suspensions and emulsions.

The defined size ranges and limits are somewhat arbitrary since there are no specific boundaries between the categories. The transition of size ranges, either from molecular dispersions to colloids or from colloids to coarse dispersions, is very gradual. For example, an emulsion may exhibit colloidal properties, and yet the average droplet size may be larger than 1 μm. This is due to the fact that most disperse systems are heterogeneous with respect to their particle size [1–2].

Table 2 Classification Scheme of Disperse Systems on the Basis of the Particle Size of the Dispersed Phase

Category	Range of particle size	Characteristics of system	Examples
Molecular dispersion	< 1.0 nm	Particles invisible by electron microscopy; pass through semipermeable membranes; generally rapid diffusion	Oxygen molecules, potassium and chloride ions dissolved in water
Colloidal dispersion	1.0 nm–1.0 μm	Particles not resolved by ordinary microscope but visible by electron microscopy; pass through filter paper but not semipermeable membranes; generally slow diffusion	Colloidal silver sols, surfactant micelles in an aqueous phase, aqueous latices and pseudolatices
Coarse dispersion	> 1.0 μm	Particles visible by ordinary microscopy; do not pass through normal filter paper or semipermeable membranes	Pharmaceutical emulsions and suspensions

In colloid science, colloidal systems are commonly classified as being lyophilic or lyophobic, based on the interaction between the dispersed phase and the dispersion medium. In lyophilic dispersions, there is a considerable affinity between the two constituent phases (e.g., hydrophilic polymers in water, polystyrene in benzene). The more restrictive terms hydrophilic and oleophilic can be used when the external phase is water and a nonpolar liquid, respectively. In contrast, in lyophobic systems there is little attraction between the two phases (e.g., aqueous dispersions of sulfur). If the dispersion medium is water, the term hydrophobic can be used. Resulting from the high affinity between the dispersed phase and the dispersion medium, lyophilic systems often form spontaneously and are considered as being thermodynamically stable. On the other hand, lyophobic systems generally do not form spontaneously and are intrinsically unstable.

The number of the constituent phases of a disperse system can be higher than two. Many commercial multiphase pharmaceutical products cannot be categorized easily and should be classified as complex disperse systems. Examples include various types of multiple emulsions and suspensions in which solid particles are dispersed within an emulsion base. These complexities influence the physicochemical properties of the system, which, in turn, determine the overall characteristics of the dosage forms with which the formulators are concerned.

Disperse systems can also be classified on the basis of their aggregation behavior as molecular or micellar (association) systems. Molecular dispersions are composed of single macromolecules distributed uniformly within the medium, e.g., protein and polymer solutions. In micellar systems, the units of the dispersed phase consist of several molecules, which arrange themselves to form aggregates, such as surfactant micelles in aqueous solutions.

B. Pharmaceutical Applications

Disperse systems have found a wide variety of applications in pharmacy [2]. Liquid dispersions, such as emulsions and suspensions, have the advantage of being easily swallowed and flexibly dosed compared to solid dosage forms. This is particularly important in the case of infants, children, and elderly patients (patient compliance). In addition, the small particle size of the drug present in disperse systems results in a large specific surface area. This leads to a higher rate of drug dissolution and possibly a superior bioavailability compared to solid dosage forms containing larger drug particles [3–7]. This can be of major importance in the case of poorly soluble drugs.

A suspension dosage form is often selected if the drug is insoluble in aqueous vehicles at the dosage required and/or when the attempts to solubilize the drug through the use of cosolvents, surfactants, and other solubilizing agents would compromise the stability or the safety of the product or, in the case of oral administration, its organoleptic properties [8–11]. The bitter or unpleasant tastes of dissolved drug molecules can often be improved by the selection of an insoluble form of the drug.

Colloidal systems have been used extensively in pharmacy, and their applications have grown rapidly over the last decades. Colloids have been employed in nuclear medicine as diagnostic and therapeutic aids (e.g., colloidal ^{198}Au, ^{99m}Tc, and sulfur); as adjuvants enhancing the immune effect of various agents (e.g., toxins adsorbed onto a colloidal carrier); and as anticancer agents (e.g., colloidal copper) [12]. Certain drugs show improved therapeutic effects when formulated in a colloidal state [13]. Colloidal silver chloride, silver iodide, and silver protein are effective germicides and do not cause irritation that is characteristic of ionic silver salts. More advanced applications of colloids include a variety of drug-delivery systems, the development of polypeptide chemotherapeutic agents, and the utilization of colloidal systems as pharmaceutical excipients, product components, vehicles and carriers. Colloidal drug-delivery systems, administered topically, orally, parenterally, or by inhalation, have been prepared for the purposes of drug targeting, controlled release, and/or protection of the drugs [14–18]. Naturally occurring plant macromolecules are capable of existing in the colloidal state and have been used for medical purposes, for example, hydroxyethyl starch (HES) has been used widely as plasma extender. Aqueous polymer latexes and pseudolatexes based on cellulosic and acrylic polymers have replaced organic solvent–based systems in a wide range of pharmaceutical coatings and controlled release technologies [19–22].

Patient acceptance is probably the most important reason why emulsions are popular oral and topical dosage forms. Oils and drugs having an objectionable taste or texture can be made more palatable for oral administration by formulating into emulsions [23–28]. As a result, mineral oil–based laxatives, oil-soluble vitamins, vegetable oils, high-fat nutritive preparations for enteral feeding, and certain drugs such as valproic acid, are formulated frequently in an oil-in-water (O/W) emulsion form. With topically applied emulsions, the formulation scientist can control the viscosity, appearance, and degree of greasiness of cosmetic and dermatological products. O/W emulsions are most useful as water-washable bases, whereas water-in-oil (W/O) emulsions are used widely for the treatment of dry skin and emollient applications to provide an occlusive effect. Semisolid preparations, such as ointments and creams, represent the dispersions of liquids in solids that are used topically. Emulsions are also employed in many other clinical applications as radio-paque emulsions, parenteral emulsions, and in blood replacement therapy [29–36].

Solid dispersions are disperse systems where both phases, the dispersed phase as well as the dispersion medium, are in the solid state. The drug can, for example, be present in the form of very fine particles or molecules distributed within an inert water-soluble carrier. This type of system is frequently used to enhance the dissolution rate and oral absorption of poorly water-soluble drugs [2,37]. Several techniques have been used to prepare such solid dispersions. The drug may be dissolved in the molten carrier. After cooling, a mixture of drug and carrier or a solid solution of the drug in the carrier results. Another method is to dissolve the drug and the carrier in a suitable organic solvent, followed by evaporation of the solvent and subsequent co-precipitation of the drug and carrier.

A solid or a liquid aerosol can be defined as a solid/gas or liquid/gas disperse system [38,39]. The main purpose of this dosage form is to deliver the drug to body surfaces or cavities, such as nasal passages or the respiratory tract. Pharmaceutical dosage forms include aerosol sprays, inhalations, and insufflations. Another type of the dispersion involving gas is the foam product, in which air or a propellant is emulsified within a liquid phase. Such preparations containing drugs (e.g., antibiotics or steroids) are often used topically. Foams containing spermicides are used for topical application within the vagina. Others have also been used widely for cosmetic purposes.

From a technical point of view, disperse systems are often involved in various steps of pharmaceutical manufacturing processes. The principles of colloid science govern many practices and operations in industrial pharmacy, such as particle size reduction (e.g., milling of pharmaceuticals), coating of pharmaceutical solids/solid dosage forms, microencapsulation, solubilization, and complexation of drugs. Solutions of water-soluble polymers act as viscosity-imparting agents, thus permitting the improvement of the physical stability of emulsions and suspensions. Organic polymer solutions or aqueous polymer dispersions are used as coating materials for solid dosage forms to achieve controlled drug release, to improve chemical stability, to provide taste masking and/or the identification of the product. Dispersions of surfactants provide a means of enhancing the solubility of a drug via micellar solubilization.

II. FUNDAMENTAL PROPERTIES

A. Particle Properties

The most significant characteristics of a dispersion are the size and shape of the dispersed particles. Both properties depend largely on the chemical and physical nature of the dispersed phase and on the method used to prepare the dispersion. The mean particle diameter as well as the particle size distribution of the dispersed phase have a profound effect on the properties of the dosage forms, such as product appearance, settling rate, drug solubility, resuspendability, and stability. Clinically important, the particle size can affect the drug release from the dosage forms that are administered orally, parenterally, rectally, and topically. Thus, these parameters have to be taken into account when formulating pharmaceutical products with good physical stability and reproducible bioavailability. This section discusses the basic principles of micromeritics, the science and technology of small particles. (Further information on the techniques and equipment currently used in the determination of particle size can be found in Sec. VIII.A.)

Particle Shape

Insoluble particles of drugs or pharmaceutical excipients obtained from various sources and manufacturing processes are seldom uniform spheres even after size reduction and classification. For example, precipitation and mechanical comminution generally produce randomly shaped particles unless the solids possess pronounced crystal habits or the solids being ground possess strongly developed cleavage planes. Primary particles may exist in various shapes, ranging from simple to irregular geometries. Their aggregation behavior produces an even greater variety of shapes and structures. The terminology and definitions of different particle shapes have been described previously [40]. Most common shapes found with pharmaceutical solids are spheres, cylinders, rods, needles, and various crystalline shapes.

Emulsification processes produce spherical droplets of the internal phase to minimize the interfacial area between the two phases. For example, the particles of true polymer latexes are spherical because they are typically prepared by emulsion polymerization, and the polymerization of solubilized monomer is initiated inside the spherical, swollen surfactant micelles [21,41]. Polymeric particles of pseudolatexes prepared from preformed polymers by either solvent evaporation or inverse emulsification processes are also spherical or near-spherical in shape for analogous reasons. Various pharmaceutical excipients exhibit characteristic particle morphologies determined by their molecular structure and the arrangement of the molecules. Some clay particles have plate-like structures possessing straight edges and hexagonal angles, e.g., bentonite and kaolin, while other clays may have lath-shaped or rod-shaped particles.

Characterization of the particle shape is generally described by the deviation from sphericity, as in the case of ellipsoids where the ratio of the two radii is the measure of deviation. The surface and volume are important properties affected by the overall shape of a particle. A more complicated relationship for particle characterization was described by Heywood, who introduced shape coefficients such as surface and volume coefficients and elongation and flatness ratios [42].

The information on particle shape is particularly important for the understanding of the behavior of suspensions during storage. The particle shape of the suspended particles (suspensoids) may have an impact on the packing of sediment (e.g., packing density and settling characteristics) and thus the product's resuspendability and stability. Packing density is defined as the weight-to-volume ratio of the sediment at equilibrium. Goodarznia and Sutherland [43] reported that the deviations from spherical shape and/or size uniformity can affect the packing density of suspensions containing cubes and spheroids. A wide particle size distribution often results in a high-density suspension, whereas widely differing particle shapes (e.g., plates, needles, filaments, and prisms) often produce low-density slurries. Symmetrical barrel-shaped particles of calcium carbonate were found to produce stable suspensions without caking upon storage, while asymmetrical needle-shaped particles formed a tenacious sediment cake, which could not be easily redispersed [44].

The viscosity of colloidal dispersions is affected by the shape of the dispersed phases. Sphero-colloids form dispersions of relatively low viscosity, while systems containing linear particles are generally more viscous. The relationship of particle shape and viscosity reflects the degree of solvation of the particles. In a good solvent, a colloidal particle unrolls and exposes its maximum surface area due to an extensive interaction between the dispersed phase and the dispersion medium. In contrast, in a poor solvent, the particle tends to coil up to assume a spherical shape, and the viscosity drops accordingly. Properties such as flow, sedimentation, and osmotic pressure are also affected by the changes in the particle shape of colloids.

Particle Size and Size Distribution

The particle size and size distribution of the dispersed phase represent a very important part of the knowledge required for a thorough understanding of any disperse system. The particle size can significantly affect the absorption behavior of a drug [6,7,45]. Certain types of dosage forms require specific size ranges, for example, suspension aerosols delivering drugs into the respiratory tract should contain particles in the order of 1–5 μm and no particles larger than 10 μm.

The size of a spherical particle is readily expressed in terms of its diameter. With asymmetrical particles, an equivalent spherical diameter is used to relate the size of the particle to the diameter of a perfect sphere having the same surface area (surface diameter, d_s), the same volume (volume diameter, d_v), or the same observed area in its most stable plane (projected diameter, d_p) [46]. The size may also be expressed using the Stokes' diameter, d_{st}, which describes an equivalent sphere undergoing sedimentation at the same rate as the sample particle. Obviously, the type of diameter reflects the method and equipment employed in determining the particle size. Since any collection of particles is usually polydisperse (as opposed to a monodisperse sample in which particles are fairly uniform in size), it is necessary to know not only the mean size of the particles, but also the particle size distribution.

The particle size data can be presented by graphical and digital methods. When the number or weight of particles lying within a certain size range is plotted against the size range or mean particle size, a bar graph (histogram) or a frequency distribution curve is obtained [13]. Alternatively, the cumulative percentage over or under a particular size can be plotted against the particle size. This results in a typical sigmoidal curve called a cumulative frequency plot. From these data, the mean particle size, standard deviation, and the extent of polydispersity may be determined.

Various theoretical distribution functions have been proposed, such as normal or Gaussian distribution and the log-normal distribution. The simplest case is described by the normal distribution equation with a specific mean value and standard deviation. However, for most pharmaceutical disperse systems, the normal equation is usually not adequate and the log-normal equation is commonly applied. For example, the log-normal distributions are often used to describe the particle size distributions of ground drug powders [40,47].

Special attention must be paid to the interpretation of particle size data presented in terms of either weight or number of particles. Particle weight data may be more useful in sedimentation studies, whereas number data are of particular value in surface-related phenomena such as dissolution. Values on the basis of number can be collected by a counting technique such as microscopy, while values based on weight are usually obtained by sedimentation or sieving methods. Conversion of the estimates from a number distribution to a weight distribution, or vice versa, is also possible using adequate mathematical approaches, e.g., the Hatch-Choate equations.

B. Surface Properties and Interfacial Phenomena

One of the most obvious properties of a disperse system is the vast interfacial area that exists between the dispersed phase and the dispersion medium [48–50]. When considering the surface and interfacial properties of the dispersed particles, two factors must be taken into account: the first relates to an increase in the surface free energy as the particle size is reduced and the specific surface increased; the second deals with the presence of an electrical charge on the particle surface. This section covers the basic theoretical concepts related to interfacial phenomena and the characteristics of colloids that are fundamental to an understanding of the behavior of any disperse systems having larger dispersed phases.

The Interface

An interface is defined as a boundary between two phases. The solid/liquid and the liquid/liquid interfaces are of primary interest in suspensions and emulsion, respectively. Other types of interfaces such as liquid/gas (foams) or solid/gas interfaces also play a major role in certain pharmaceutical dosage forms, e.g., aerosols.

A large surface area of the dispersed particles is associated with a high surface free energy that renders the system thermodynamically unstable. The surface free energy, ΔG, can be calculated from the total surface area, ΔA, as follows:

$$\Delta G = \gamma_{SL} \cdot \Delta A \qquad \text{or} \qquad \Delta G = \gamma_{LL} \cdot \Delta A \tag{1}$$

where γ_{SL} and γ_{LL} are the interfacial tension between the solid particles and the liquid medium and the liquid/liquid interfacial tension, respectively.

Very small dispersed particles are highly energetic. In order to approach a stable state, they tend to regroup themselves in order to reduce the surface free energy of the system. An equilibrium will be reached when $\Delta G = 0$. This condition may be accomplished either by a reduction of the interfacial tension or by a decrease of the total surface area.

Particle Interactions

The interactions between similar particles, dissimilar particles, and the dispersion medium constitute a complex but essential part of dispersion technology. Such interparticle interactions include both attractive and repulsive forces. These forces depend upon the nature, size, and orientation of the species, as well as on the distance of separation between and among the particles of the dispersed phase and the dispersion medium, respectively. The balance between these forces determines the overall characteristics of the system.

The particles in a disperse system with a liquid or gas being the dispersion medium are thermally mobile and occasionally collide as a result of the Brownian motion. As the particles approach one another, both attractive and repulsive forces are operative. If the attractive forces prevail, agglomerates result indicating an instability of the system. If repulsive forces dominate, a homogeneously dispersed or stable dispersion remains.

Various types of attractive interaction are operating: (a) dipole-dipole or Keesom orientation forces, (b) dipole-induced dipole or Debye induction forces, (c) induced dipole–induced dipole or London dispersion forces, and (d) electrostatic forces between charged particles. The strongest forces are the electrostatic interactions between charged particles. These forces, either attractive or repulsive, are effective over a relatively long range and are dependent on the ionic charge and size of the particle. Forces that are weaker and effective over a shorter distance include other types of electrostatic forces such as ion-dipole, ion-induced dipole, and (a)–(c). The group of these last three forces are often referred to as van der Waals forces, which result from the interaction of electromagnetic dipoles within the particles. They produce a short-range type of interaction, varying inversely with r^6, where r is the interparticle distance. Even though they are relatively weak, van der Waals forces coupled with hydrogen bond interactions are significant factors describing the behavior of most nonionic compounds in liquids and other dispersion media. These various types of attractive interparticulate forces can lead to the instabilities of disperse systems described in Sec. II.C.

Electrical Properties of the Interfaces

Most insoluble materials, either solids or liquids, develop a surface charge when dispersed within an aqueous medium. These surface charges of particles may arise from several mechanisms. For example, the ionization of functional groups present at the surface of the particle, such as carboxylic acid or amine groups, can be involved. The charge is then dependent on the extent of ionization and is a function of the pH of the dispersion medium. Furthermore, surface charges can be developed due to the adsorption or desorption of protons. A variety of colloidal systems (e.g., polymers, metal oxides) fall into this group. For example, the surface hydroxyl groups of aluminum hydroxide gel can adsorb protons and become positively charged or may donate protons to become negatively charged. An important property of such systems is the point of zero charge (PZC), which represents the pH at which the net surface charge is zero. More general, surface charges of dispersed particles may be caused by preferential adsorption of specific ions onto the surface. Surface charges can also be introduced by ionic surfactants. For example, oil globules in an O/W emulsion exhibit a surface charge if anionic or cationic surface-active agents are used. The surfactant molecules are oriented at the oil/water interface so that the charged hydrophilic groups are directed towards the water phase. Ion deficiencies in the crystal lattice or interior of the particles may also cause surface charges. Many mineral clays exhibit a negative surface charge because of isomorphic substitution, e.g., an Al^{3+} ion occupies a site that is usually occupied by a Si^{4+} ion, resulting in a deficit of charge. Similarly, antacid magaldrate exhibits a positive surface charge: Mg^{2+} ions in the crystal lattice are partially substituted by Al^{3+} ions.

When a charged particle is dispersed within a dispersion medium containing dissolved cations and anions, the surface charges of the particle interact with the dissolved ions in solution. For a detailed description of the occurring phenomena, the reader is referred to the literature [13]. Roughly, the electric distribution at the interface is equivalent to a double layer of charge: a first layer being tightly bound, and a second layer that is more diffusive. The zeta (ζ) potential is defined as the potential at the shear plane (interface separating layers that move with the particle from layers that do not move with the particle) and can be regarded as the "apparent" or "active" charge of the particle.

Derjaguin, Landau, Verwey, and Overbeek developed a theory giving insight into the energy of interaction between suspended particles [51–53]. This theory is thus often referred to as the DLVO theory. It relates the stability of a disperse system to the electrolyte content in the continuous phase and provides an insight into the factors responsible for controlling the rate at which particles in disperse systems come into contact or aggregate. The process of aggregation subsequently accelerates particle sedimentation and affects redispersibility of the disperse systems. In general, the DLVO theory is applicable to pharmaceutical dosage forms [54–56] such as colloids, suspensions, and O/W emulsions. In the case of W/O systems, it must be applied with extreme caution. Figure 1 [13] shows typical potential energy curves for the interaction of two charged particles as a function of interparticle distances: the attractive energy curve (V_A), the repulsive energy curve (V_R), and the net or total potential energy curve (V_T). The total energy of interaction,

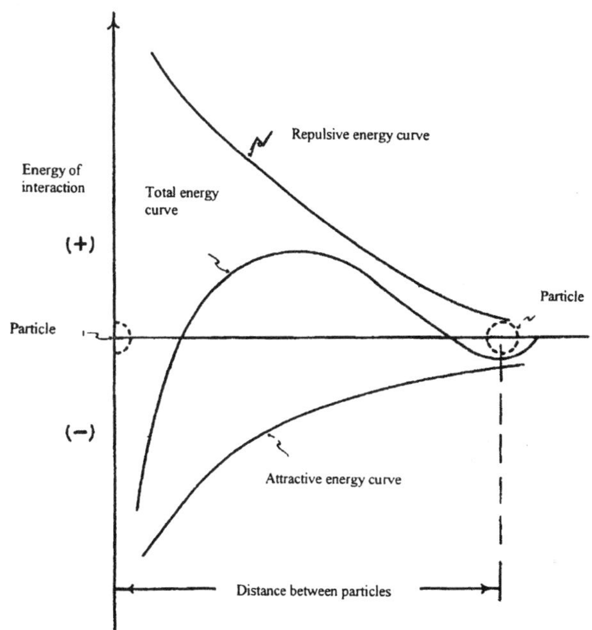

Fig. 1 Illustration of the DLVO theory: interaction of two charged particles as a function of the interparticle distance (attractive energy curve, V_A; repulsive energy curve, V_R; and net or total potential energy curve, V_T).

V_T, between two particles is defined as the sum of the attraction and repulsion energies:

$$V_T = V_A + V_R \tag{2}$$

From these curves, it is evident that the attractive potential is predominant at short distances, and the net interaction is attraction in the deep potential energy minimum, V_p. At greater distances, the electrostatic repulsion energy falls off more rapidly with increasing separation distance than the van der Waals attraction energy, and the net interaction is attraction in the shallow secondary minimum, V_s. At intermediate distances, the electrostatic repulsion predominates and the net interaction is repulsion with the maximum potential, $V_{\max}$. The stability of a disperse system is indicated by the height of the maximum in the potential energy curve, $V_{\max}$. This potential energy barrier must be surmounted if the particles are to approach each other sufficiently closely to fall into the deep primary energy minimum of irreversible coagulation. To gain information about the stability of a disperse system, it is important to compare the total energy of the particles with the kinetic energy of the particles, kT, where k is the Boltzmann constant and T is the absolute temperature. The value of $V_{\max}$ necessary to prevent the irreversible contact of particles is considered to be about 10–20 kT, which correponds to a zeta potential of approximately 50 mV [41]. If the secondary minimum is deep enough (about 5 kT or greater), the particles might associate to form a cluster that is loose and reversible, called floc or floccule. Such flocculation in the secondary minimum, however, does not occur with small colloidal particles since the energy minimum is of the same order as the thermal energy of the particles, and the aggregation is easily reveresed by Brownian motion.

According to the DLVO theory, disperse systems become unstable whenever their kinetic energy is sufficient to overcome the potential energy barrier, $V_{\max}$. Thus, the instability of disperse systems increases when decreasing the height of this energy barrier and when increasing the kinetic energy of the particles. The reduction of $V_{\max}$ can result from the addition of substances that (a) neutralize the surface particle charge or cause the loss of the hydration layer, (b) compress the double layer, and/or (c) cause adsorbed species (e.g., surfactants) to desorb from the particle surface. The primary factor determining the thickness of the electric double layer is the potential energy drop-off. The potential gradient strongly depends on the concentration and charge of any electrolyte present in the dispersion medium. In water at room temperature, the thickness of the electric double layer ranges from 1 to 1000 Å, depending on the concentration of ions in the bulk phase. Increasing electrolyte concentrations lead to compressed double layers (decreasing double layer thicknesses). Thus, the particles can approach each other more closely, and the attractive forces become more important. The concentration of foreign electrolytes required to cause flocculation decreases as the valence of the coagulating ion increases. For example, fewer Al^{3+} ions are required to flocculate a suspension than Na^+ ions. This has been observed in many instances and is known as the Schulze-Hardy rule [13]. It has been shown that the quantity of electrolyte required to cause flocculation decreases by a factor of 10 when a monovalent electrolyte, e.g., Na^+, is replaced by a divalent electrolyte, e.g., Mg^{2+}. Furthermore, the efficiency of electrolytes in precipitating a dispersion depends on how extensively the electrolytes are hydrated. The Hofmeister or lyotropic series arranges ions in the order of increasing hydration and increasing efficiency in causing the instability. For example, the series for monovalent cations is $Cs^+ < Rb^+ < NH_4^+ < Na^+ < Li^+$ and for divalent ions is $Ba^{2+} < Sr^{2+} < Ca^{2+} < Mg^{2+}$.

Wetting

The wetting process is a primary concern, particularly in the preparation of a liquid disperse system in which the internal phase is a solid (suspension). A solid material to be suspended must first be separated into single particles, and the particles must be individually wetted by the dispersion medium to achieve a homogeneous distribution of the internal phase. Upon wetting, the air at the solid surface is replaced by the liquid medium. Obviously, the tendency of a solid to be wetted by a liquid is primarily determined by the interaction between the three phases. Experimentally, the degree of wetting of a powder can be evaluated by observing the contact angle, θ, which is defined by the boundaries of the solid surace and the tangent to the curvature of the liquid drop. The contact angle results from an equilibrium involing three interfacial tensions: those acting at the liquid/gas, solid/liquid, and solid/gas interfaces. A contact angle of 0° indicates an extensive interaction between the solid and the liquid phase. Thus, the solid is completely wetted by the liquid. Partial wetting occurs when the contact angles are between 0 and 90°. In contrast, contact angles greater than 90°are classified as nonwetting situations in which the liquid cannot spread over the solid surface spontaneously. If the angle is close to 180°, the solid substance is considered to be unwettable by the liquid.

Hydrophilic substances are readily wetted by water or other polar liquids due to the good interfacial interaction resulting in small contact angles. Once dispersed, they may significantly increase the viscosity of the liquid system. On the other hand, hydrophobic substances repel water but can easily be wetted by nonpolar liquids. They usually do not alter the viscocity of aqueous systems. In pharmaceutical dosage forms, aqueous vehicles or hydroalcoholic mixtures are often used. Thus, proper wetting of hydrophobic drugs is a necessary first step when preparing suspensions. Hydrophobic materials are often extremely difficult to disperse because of poor wetting or presence of entrained air pockets, minute quantities of grease, and other contaminants. The powder may just float on the surface of the liquid despite its higher density. Fine powders are particularly susceptible to this effect, and they may fail to become wetted even when mechanically forced below the surface of the suspending medium. To overcome this problem, to improve the wetting characteristics of hydrophobic drug powders, often anionic or nonionic surfactants are used. These substances decrease the solid/liquid interfacial tension, thus facilitating the wetting process. The mechanism of surfactant action involves the preferential adsorption of the hydrophobic part of the surfactant onto the hydrophobic surface of the particle. The polar part of the surfactant is directed towards the aqueous medium.

Different experimental methods have been developed to provide a measure for the efficiency of a wetting agent. For example, narrow lyophobic troughs can be used, in which one end holds the powder while a solution of a wetting agent is placed in the other end. The rate of penetration is observed and measured as the degree of wettability. Another technique involves measuring the relative ability of solutions of different wetting agents to carry a drug powder through a gauze when the solutions are dropped onto the gauze supporting a powder. Good wetting agents are able to carry greater amounts of powder through the gauze than poor wetting agents. Also for nonaqueous systems, different methods have been developed to compare the efficiency of wetting agents (e.g., for certain lanolin derivatives). In the paint industry two techniques are often used that could also be applied to pharmaceutical systems: the so-called wet and flow point methods. In the first case, the amount of vehicle required to wet a known amount of powder is measured, whereas in the second case, the amount of vehicle needed to prepare a pourable system is measured.

Adsorption

Adsorption is the tendency of atoms, molecules, ions, etc. to locate at a particular surface/interface in a concentration different from the concentrations in the surrounding bulk media. The adsorption process occurs as a result of the unequal distribution of the forces at the interfaces. The adsorbing species may be gases, solvents, or solutes, and the interfaces may be solid/solid, solid/liquid, solid/gas, liquid/liquid, or liquid/gas interfaces. Adsorption is termed "positive" if the concentration of adsorbed species at the interface is greater than that in the bulk and "negative" when the opposite is true. According to the nature of interaction, adsorption can be divided into two main classes: (a) physical adsorption or physisorption, where the forces and processes are reversible, nonspecific, and of relatively low energy, and (b) chemisorption, where the forces and processes of adsorption are specific, irreversible, and of higher energy.

Of special interest in liquid dispersions are the surface-active agents that tend to accumulate at air/liquid, liquid/liquid, and/or solid/liquid interfaces. Surfactants can arrange themselves to form a coherent film surrounding the dispersed droplets (in emulsions) or suspended particles (in suspensions). This process is an oriented physical adsorption. Adsorption at the interface tends to increase with increasing thermodynamic activity of the surfactant in solution until a complete monolayer is formed at the interface or until the active sites are saturated with surfactant molecules. Also, a multilayer of adsorbed surfactant molecules may occur, resulting in more complex adsorption isotherms.

Adsorption of species onto a particle surface is responsible for many resultant properties of the system. The adsorption of surfactants alters the properties at the interface and promotes wetting of the dispersed phase in suspensions. The reduction of the interfacial tension can effectively decrease the resulting surface free energy and hence the tendency for coalescence or aggregation. Thus, the formation and stabilization of the disperse systems can be significantly facilitated. An additional effect promoting stability is the presence of a surface charge, which causes electrostatic repulsion between adjacent particles. The adsorption of ionic surfactants generally increases the charge density on the surface of the dispersed particles, thus improving the stability of the dispersion.

Protective colloids or polymeric materials can be adsorbed onto the surface of the dispersed phase. Polymer adsorption can be accomplished simply by adding a solution of adsorbable polymeric species into a slurry of the dispersed particles. Then, adequate time must be provided for the system to equilibrate and complete the interaction between the adsorbent and the adsorbate. The mode of adsorption strongly depends on the number of sites and functional groups of the polymer chains available for the interaction with the particle surface. Most nonelectrolyte polymers promote steric stabilization, generally the result of either entropic stabilization or osmotic repulsion [41]. Entropic stabilization arises when two opposing adsorbed polymer layers of adjacent particles overlap, resulting in compression and interpenetration of their chain segments. The restriction of the movements of the polymer chains in the overlap region leads to a negative entropy change. Thus, the reverse process of disentanglement of the two adsorbed layers occurs and is energetically more favorable. This mechanism predominates when the concentration of polymer in the adsorbed layer is low. The osmotic repulsion is operative in cases where more polymer segments are involved and become crowded in the overlap regions. The increase in polymer concentration within these areas causes a local increase in osmotic pressure and results in an influx of water. This influx pushes the particles apart.

C. Instabilities and Stabilization Concepts

Content uniformity and long-term stability of a pharmaceutical product are required for a consistent and accurate dosing. Aggregation of dispersed particles and resulting instabilities such as flocculation, sedimentation (in suspensions), or creaming and coalescence (in emulsions) often represent major problems in formulating pharmaceutical disperse systems.

Instabilities

As discussed above, an instability of a dispersion may result from the tendency of the system to reduce its surface free energy, ΔG. Unfortunately, the terminology used in the literature to describe the occurring phenomena is not uniform. Flocculation is generally understood as a process in which particles are allowed to come together and form loosely bound clusters having an open structure. Unlike coalescence, the total surface area is not reduced during the flocculation process. Deflocculation is the opposite, i.e., breakdown of clusters into individual particles. Some authors differentiate between the terms aggregates and agglomerates: in aggregates the particles are more strongly bound than in flocculates, thus these systems are more difficult to be redispersed. The term agglomerates is then used as a general expression covering both flocculates and aggregates. Other authors use the terms aggregates and agglomerates as synonyms. In the case of coalescence, the total surface area of the particles is reduced. (For a more detailed description of the instabilities of emulsions and suspensions, the reader is referred to Secs. IV and V, respectively)

Although disperse systems are thermodynamically unstable, certain systems can remain "stable" over a prolonged period of time. Thermodynamically driven changes to a lower energy state may be reversible or irreversible. The type and kinetics of these changes determine the usefulness of a product, as indicated, for example, by its shelf life. A disperse system remains stable as long as the repulsive forces are sufficiently strong to outweigh the van der Waals and/or other attractive forces. These repulsive forces are generally acquired through one or both of the following mechanisms: (a) electrostatic repulsion, which arises from the presence of an ionic charge on the surface of the dispersed particles; (b) steric repulsion, which arises from the presence of uncharged molecules on the surface of the particles.

Stabilization by Electrostatic Repulsion

The electrostatic stabilization of disperse systems can be described by the DLVO theory (see above). The electrostatic repulsive forces can prevent the dispersed particles having surface charges of the same sign from approaching each other, thus stabilizing the dispersion against interparticle attraction or coagulation. As long as the height of the potential energy barrier, V_{max}, exceeds the kinetic energy, the approaching particles do not come sufficiently close to each other to establish important attractive forces (van der Waals forces), but move away from each other due to steric or electrostatic effects. A net positive potential energy of about $20\,kT$ is usually sufficient to keep the particles apart, rendering the dispersion permanently stable. At $T = 298\,K$, this equals 1×10^{-12} erg or 1×10^{-5} J. Correspondingly, moderate physical stability is achieved when the zeta potential is between ± 30 and ± 60 mV, and good to excellent physical stability is achieved when the zeta potential is between ± 60 and ± 100 mV. However, when the size of the dispersed particles exceeds 1 μm and the density is greater than $1.0\,g/cm^3$, the effect of the zeta potential becomes less significant.

Ionic solids with surface layers containing the ionic species in near proper stoichiometric balance and most water-insoluble organic compounds have relatively low surface charge densities. They may adsorb ionic, equally charged surfactants from solutions, which increases their surface charge densities and the magnitude of their ζ potentials, resulting in an enhanced electrostatic stabilizing effect. In suspensions, the addition of ions that are adsorbed onto the surface of the dispersed particles generally creates strong repulsion forces between suspended particles and stabilizes the system. In contrast, the addition of water-miscible solvents (e.g., alcohols, glycerin, or propylene glycol) to aqueous dispersions can lower the dielectric constant of the medium. This results in a reduction of the thickness of the electric double layer and the magnitude of the potential energy barrier. Thus, the addition of these solvents tends to cause instability or makes the system more sensitive to coagulation.

Stabilization by Steric Repulsion

When a strongly hydrated hydrophilic polymer is adsorbed onto the surface of a hydrophobic solid particle surrounded by an aqueous medium, the affinity of the polymer for water can exceed the attractive forces between the suspended particles. For example, a hydrophilic polymer such as gelatin can increase the strength of the protective hydration layer formed around the dispersed particles. Water-soluble polymers whose adsorption stabilizes dispersions and protects them against coagulation are also called protective colloids. The hydrated, protective shell becomes an integral part of the particles' surface. Adsorption of nonionic polymers (e.g., gums or water-soluble cellulosic derivatives) or surfactants (e.g., polysorbate 80) of sufficient chain length can create steric hindrance between adjacent particles. A polymer can be adsorbed in the forms of loops, tails, and trains. Parts of the long-chain molecules are adsorbed onto the surface of the particles (e.g., trains), whereas other parts extend into the bulk liquid (e.g., tails) [57]. Some molecules are adsorbed onto the solid surfaces in the form of loops projecting into the aqueous phase rather than lying flat against the solid substrate. The stabilizing efficiency of the adsorbed macromolecules depends on the presence of sufficiently long tails or loops. The adsorbed species usually form multi- rather than monomolecular films at the interface.

Two mechanisms of steric stabilization can be distinguished: entropic stabilization and osmotic repulsion. Entropic stabilization arises when two opposing adsorbed polymer layers of adjacent particles overlap, resulting in compression and interpenetration of their chain segments. The restriction of the movements of the polymer chains in the overlap region leads to a negative entropy change. Thus, the reverse process of disentanglement of the two adsorbed layers occurs and is energetically more favorable. This mechanism predominates when the concentration of polymer in the adsorbed layer is low. The osmotic repulsion mechanism is operative in cases where more polymer segments are involved and become crowded in the overlap regions. The increase in polymer concentration within these areas causes a local increase in osmotic pressure and results in an influx of water. This influx pushes the particles apart.

Steric stabilization is particularly useful and widely applied during emulsification processes. One major advantage compared to electrostatic stabilization is the relative insensitivity towards added electrolytes. An auxiliary effect promoting dispersion stability is the significant viscosity increase of the dispersion medium.

D. Rheological Properties

Rheology is the study of flow and deformation of materials under the influence of external forces. It involves the viscosity characteristics of powders, liquids, and semisolids. Rheological studies are also important in the industrial manufacture and applications of plastic materials, lubricating materials, coatings, inks, adhesives, and food products. Flow properties of pharmaceutical disperse systems can be of particular importance, especially for topical products. Such systems often exhibit rather complex rheological properties, and pharmaceutical scientists have conducted fundamental investigations in this area [58–64].

Newton's Law and Newtonian Flow

To characterize rheological behavior of materials, some basic terms need to be defined. Consider a liquid material that is subjected to a shearing force as illustrated in Fig. 2. The liquid is assumed to consist of a series of parallel layers with the surface area A, the bottom layer being fixed. When a force is applied on the top layer, the top plane moves at a constant velocity, whereas each lower layer moves with a velocity directly proportional to its distance from the stationary bottom layer. The velocity gradient (dv/dr, the difference in velocity, dv, between the top and bottom planes of liquid separated by the distance, dr) is also called the rate of shear, G:

$$G = \frac{dv}{dr} \tag{3}$$

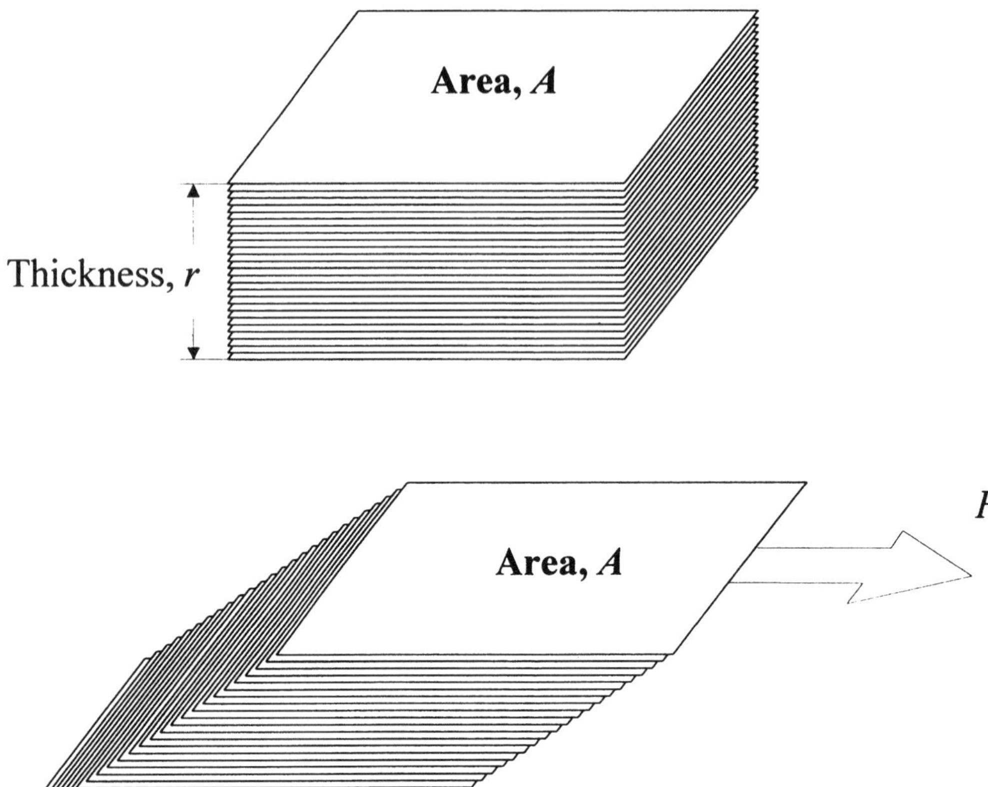

Fig. 2 Model of a liquid material that is subjected to a shearing force. The liquid is assumed to consist of a series of parallel layers, the bottom layer being fixed.

The force per unit area, F'/A, required to cause flow is called the shearing stress (F):

$$F = \frac{F'}{A} \tag{4}$$

The rate of shear, G, is directly proportional to the shearing stress, F, and the relationship can be expressed as:

$$\frac{F'}{A} = \eta \frac{dv}{dr} \quad \text{or} \quad \eta = \frac{F}{G} \tag{5}$$

where η is the coefficient of viscosity, or viscosity.

A plot of F vs. G yields a rheogram or a flow curve. Flow curves are usually plotted on a log-log scale to include the many decades of shear rate and the measured shear stress or viscosity. The higher the viscosity of a liquid, the greater the shearing stress required to produce a certain rate of shear. Dividing the shear stress by the shear rate at each point results in a viscosity curve (or a viscosity profile), which describes the relationship between the viscosity and shear rate. The unit of viscosity is poise, which is the shearing force required to produce a velocity of 1 cm/s between two parallel planes of liquid, each 1 cm^2 in area and separated by a distance of 1 cm. The most often used unit is centipoise, or cp (equivalent to 0.01 poise). Another term, fluidity, ϕ, is defined as the reciprocal of viscosity:

$$\phi = \frac{1}{\eta} \tag{6}$$

In addition, the U.S. Pharmacopoeia includes the explanation of kinematic viscosity [units in stoke (s) and centistoke (cs)], defined as the absolute viscosity divided by the density of the liquid at a definite temperature, ρ:

$$\text{Kinematic viscosity} = \frac{\eta}{\rho} \tag{7}$$

For simple Newtonian fluids (e.g., pure water), a plot of rate of shear against shearing stress gives a straight line, thus the slope (η) is constant (Fig. 3a, curve A) [65]. In other words, the viscosity is constant, depending on neither the shear rate nor time. However, pharmaceutical disperse systems rarely exhibit simple Newtonian flow, and their viscosity is not constant but changes as a function of shear rate and/or time. The rheological properties of such systems cannot be defined simply in terms of one value. These non-Newtonian phenomena are either time-independent or time-dependent. In the first case, the systems can be classified as pseudoplastic, plastic, or dilatant, in the second case as thixotropic or rheopective.

Pseudoplastic Flow

Many fluids show a decrease in viscosity with increasing shear rate. This behavior is referred to as "shear thinning," which means that the resistance of the material to flow decreases and the energy required to sustain flow at high shear rates is reduced. These materials are called "pseudoplastic" (Fig. 3a and b, curves B). At rest the material forms a network structure, which may be an agglomerate of many molecules attracted to each other or an entangled network of polymer chains. Under shear this structure is broken down, resulting in a shear

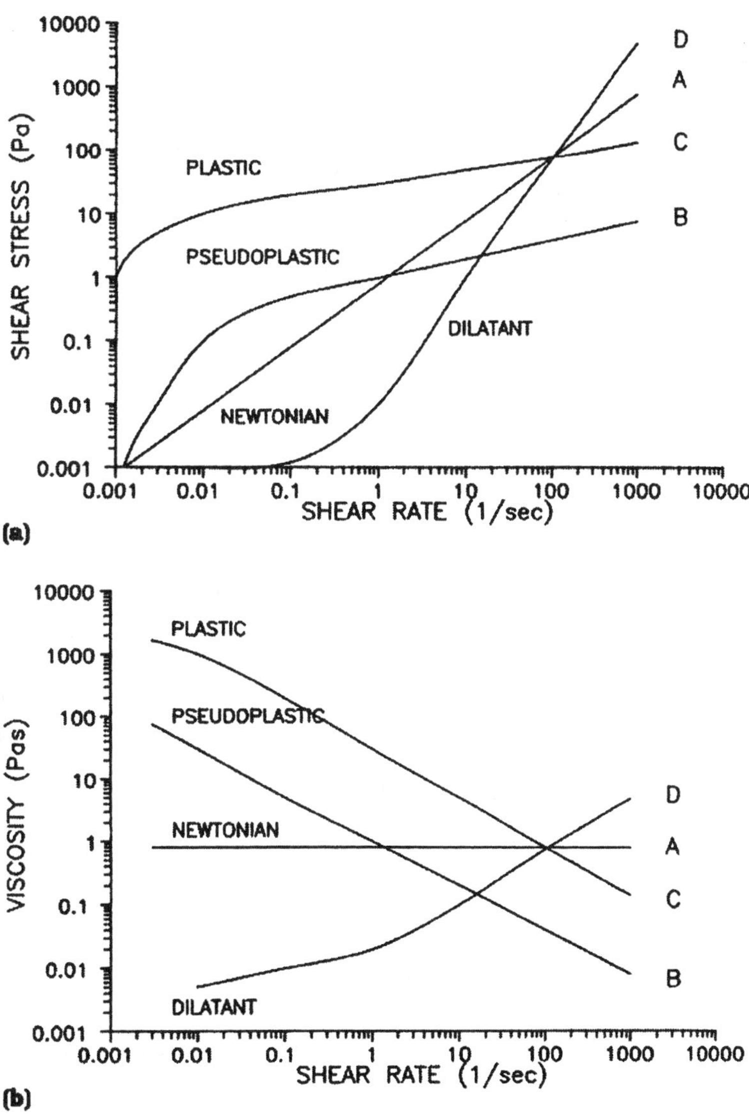

Fig. 3 Newtonian and non-Newtonian behaviours as a function of shear rate: (a) flow profile; (b) viscosity profile. (From Ref. 65.)

thinning behavior. With linear polymers, it is speculated that the axes of such molecules become more oriented in the direction of flow as shearing stress is increased. Pseudoplastic flow can be found in emulsions, suspensions, as well as various pharmaceutical thickening agents, e.g., polymer solutions.

Plastic Flow

Plastic fluids are Newtonian or pseudoplastic liquids that exhibit a "yield value" (Fig. 3a and b, curves C). At rest they behave like a solid due to their interparticle association. The external force has to overcome these attractive forces between the particles and disrupt the structure. Beyond this point, the material changes its behavior from that of a solid to that of a liquid. The viscosity can then either be a constant (ideal Bingham liquid) or a function of the shear rate. In the latter case, the viscosity can initially decrease and then become a constant (real Bingham liquid) or continuously decrease, as in the case of a pseudoplastic liquid (Casson liquid). Plastic flow is often observed in flocculated suspensions.

Dilatant Flow

In some cases, the viscosity increases with increasing shear rate. The system appears to become more structured and more viscous with increasing shear stress. This flow behavior is called "dilatant" (Fig. 3a and b, curves D). Examples include pastes containing plasticizers, ionic polymers, suspensions with high solids content, highly pigmented systems, and quicksand.

Thixotropy and Rheopexy

Thixotropy is a phenomenon that occurs frequently in dispersed systems. It is defined as a reversible, time-dependent decrease in viscosity at a constant shear rate. Generally, a dispersion that shows an isothermal gel-sol-gel transformation is a thixotropic material. The mechanism of thixotropy is the breakdown and reforming of the gel structure.

An example for a rheogram of a thixotropic material is given in Fig. 4 [13]. Here, the rate of shear, G, is plotted as a function of the shearing stress, F. Due to the time dependence of the viscosity, a hysteresis loop results: the up curve (early times) is not identical with the down curve (late times). The up curve shows the rate of shear when increasing the shearing stress; the down curve shows the rate of shear when subsequently decreasing the shearing stress. As the shear rate decreases, the structure rebuilds and viscosity is restored to its original value. If the recovery is fast, as in many water-based systems, the down curve is superimposed on the up curve. If the rearrangement is slow, as in

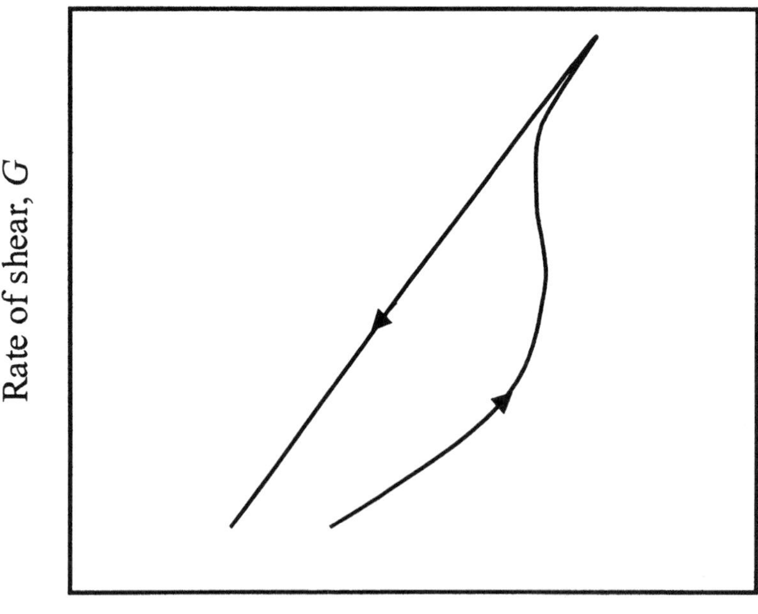

Fig. 4 Flow curves of a system exhibiting thixotropy.

many organic solvent–based systems, it may take longer for the fluid to regain its initial properties after shearing, and therefore the down curve will be above the up curve. The hysteresis area between the up curve and the down curve defines the energy required to break down the network structure of the material; its dimensions are energy/volume.

If, in contrast, the viscosity *in*creases with time while the material is being sheared and recovers its original viscosity when allowed to rest, the material is called "rheopective." In this case the down curve is positioned below the up curve.

III. FORMULATION ADDITIVES

A. Surfactants

According to the colloid scientist Winsor, surfactants are defined as compounds "which possess in the same molecule distinct regions of hydrophilic and lipophilic character." For example, in the oleate ion there is an alkyl chain that is basically hydrophobic (lipophilic tail) and a COO^- headgroup that is hydrophilic (lipophobic). Being amphiphilic in nature, surfactants have the ability to modify the interface between various phases [66]. Their effects on the interface are the result of their ability to orient themselves in accordance with the polarities of the two opposing phases. The polar part can be expected to be oriented towards the more polar (hydrophilic, aqueous) phase, whereas the nonpolar tails should direct towards the nonpolar (lipophilic, oil) phase.

Surfactants are useful in formulating a wide variety of disperse systems. They are required not only during manufacture but also for maintaining an acceptable physical stability of these thermodynamically unstable systems. Besides the stabilizing efficiency, the criteria influencing the selection of surfactants for pharmaceutical or cosmetic products include safety, odor, color, and purity.

When the variation of any colligative property of a surfactant in aqueous solution is examined, two types of behavior are apparent. At low concentrations, properties approximate those to be expected from ideal behavior. However, at a concentration value that is characteristic for a given surfactant system (critical micelle concentration, CMC), an abrupt deviation from such behavior is observed. At concentrations above the CMC, molecular aggregates called micelles are formed. By increasing the concentration of the surfactant, depending on the chemical and physical nature of the molecule, structural changes to a more orderly state than micellar structure in the molecular assembly of amphiphiles occur. These are, generally, hexagonal, cubic, and lamellar liquid crystalline structures; their occurrence relates mostly to the concentration of the surfactant in the system. Liquid crystals have been known for more than a century and have been formulated as parts of many creams, lotions, and cosmetic products.

Surfactants can be classified according to their functionality and their natures of hydrophilic and hydrophobic portions. A typical functional scheme was developed in the CTFA (Cosmetic Ingredient Handbook) by creating six functional categories for surfactants: cleansing agents, emulsifying agents, foam boosters, hydrotropes, solubilizing agent, and suspending agents. Another means for classification is based on the nature of the hydrophobic portions of surfactants. Such a classification would create groups based on the presence of hydrophobes derived from paraffinic, olefinic, aromatic, cycloaliphatic, or heterocyclic hydrophobes. This type of classification is of particular interest in comparing surfactants' characteristics with regard to their physiological effects related to the origin of the lipophilic constituents.

The most useful and widely accepted classification is based on the nature of the hydrophilic head groups. This classification system has universal acceptance and has been found to be practical throughout the surfactant industry. This approach creates four large groups of surfactant structures: anionics, cationics, amphoterics (zwitterionics), and nonionics. Anionic surfactants carry negative charges and include a large group of surfactants used in pharmaceutical products, such as soaps, sulfates, and sulfonates. Soaps can be prepared in situ by a reaction between a fatty acid and an alkali. Cationic surfactants, carrying positively charged head groups, are of special pharmaceutical interest since they often possess antimicrobial activity. Examples include quaternary ammonium compounds and cetyltrimethylammonium bromide. Cationic surfactants should not be used in the same formulation with anionic surfactants, since they will interact. Amphoteric surfactants possess both positive and negative charges in their structures and include substances like lecithin and *N*-dodecyl-*N*,*N*-dimethylglycine. Nonionic surfactants are not dissociated and, thus, are not charged. Unlike the anionic and cationic types, they are not susceptible to pH changes and to the presence of electrolytes. *N*-Alkyl polyoxyethylene surfactants, of general formula $CH_3(CH_2)_n(OCH_2CH_2)_mOH$, where n is often between 10 and 18 and m between 6 and 60, are good examples of nonionic surfactants.

Particularly useful is the physical classification of surfactants based on the hydrophile-lipophile balance (HLB) system [67,68] established by Griffin [69,70]. More than 50 years ago he introduced an empirical scale of HLB values for a variety of nonionic surfactants. Griffin's original concept defined HLB as the percentage (by weight) of the hydrophile divided by 5 to yield more manageable values:

$$\mathrm{HLB} = \frac{\text{wt\% hydrophile}}{5} \tag{8}$$

Griffin studied primarily ethylene oxide (EO) adducts and routinely substituted "% EO" for "% hydrophile." Since that time, the HLB system has become very popular, especially to characterize emulsifying agents. (The reader is referred to sec. V.B. for a more detailed discussion of the use of the HLB system for the identification of adequate emulsifiers and combinations thereof.)

Finely divided solid particles that are wetted to some degree by both oil and water can also act as emulsifying agents. This results from the fact that they can form a particulate film around dispersed droplets, preventing coalescence. Powders that are wetted preferentially by water form O/W emulsions, whereas those more easily wetted by oil form W/O emulsions. The compounds most frequently used in pharmacy are colloidal clays, such as bentonite (aluminum silicate) and veegum (magnesium aluminum silicate). These compounds tend to be adsorbed at the interface and also increase the viscosity of the aqueous phase. They are frequently used in conjunction with a surfactant for external purposes, such as lotions or creams.

The common concentration of a surfactant used in a formulation varies from 0.05 to 0.5% and depends on the surfactant type and the solids content of the dispersion. In practice, very often combinations of surfactants rather than single agents are used to prepare and stabilize disperse systems. The combination of a more hydrophilic surfactant with a more hydrophobic surfactant leads to the formation of a complex film at the interface. A good example for such a surfactant pair is the Tween-Span system of Atlas-ICI [71].

B. Protective Colloids and Viscosity-Imparting Agents

Protective colloids can be divided into synthetic and natural materials. Table 3 classifies the pharmaceutical gums, thickeners, and other hydrophilic polymers according to their origins [72]. Protective colloids of natural origin, such as gelatin, acacia, and tragacanth, have been used for years as emulsifying agents [73,74]. Gelatin and serum albumin are preferred protective colloids for stabilizing parenteral suspensions because of their biocompatibility. These two polymers, as well as casein, dextrin, and plant gums, can be metabolized in the human body. Dispersing a natural gum within water yields a thick, viscous liquid called a mucilage. Mucilages are used primarily to aid in suspending insoluble substances within liquids because their colloidal character and viscosity can help to prevent sedimentation. However, the drawbacks of mucilages include their sensitivity to pH change, addition of electrolytes, and/or heat, which adversely affect viscosity. Mucilages of vegetable gums are prone to microbial decomposition and show appreciable decrease in viscosity upon storage.

Besides these naturally derived protective colloids, several synthetic, water-soluble substances are widely used at appropriate concentrations as mucilage substitutes, suspending agents, emulsifying agents, and/or viscosity-imparting agents. Synthetic cellulose derivatives include sodium carboxymethylcellulose, hydroxypropylcellulose, hydroxypropyl methyl cellulose, and methyl cellulose. The resulting viscosity depends on the concentration and specification (e.g., molecular weight) of the polymers. Many of these substances are used as protective colloids at low concentrations ($<0.1\%$) and as viscosity builders at relatively high concentrations ($>0.1\%$). Since these agents do not reduce the surface and interfacial tension significantly, it is often advantageous to use them in combination with surfactants. Unlike many natural polymers, cellulose derivatives and most synthetic protective colloids are not biotransformed. When administered orally, they are not absorbed, but excreted intact.

When polymeric substances and hydrophilic colloids are used as suspending agents, it is recommended that appropriate tests be performed to show that the agent does not interfere with the drug and does not modify the resulting therapeutic effect. With regard to the raw material selection, protective colloids may be chosen according to their abilities to aid in stabilizing a dispersion as well as other factors, such as cost, toxicity, and resistance to chemical and/or microbial attack. Although many natural substances are nontoxic and relatively inexpensive, they often show considerable batch-to-batch variations and a relatively high risk for microbial contamination.

C. pH-Controlling Agents

A properly formulated disperse system should exhibit an acceptable physical stability over a wide range of

Table 3 Classification of Protective Colloids (gums, thickeners, and polymers) According to Their Origins

Classification		Origin	Products
Natural	Plant	Tree and shrub exudates	Karaya gum
			Tragacanth gum
			Gum acacia
		Seed extracts	Guar gum
			Locust bean gum
			Psyllium seed
			Quince seed
		Seaweed extracts	Carrageenan
			Alginates
			Agar
		Tree extracts	Larch gum
		Fruit extracts	Pectins
		Grains and roots	Starches
	Microbial	Exocellular polysaccharides	Xanthan gum
			Dextran
	Animal	Milk protein	Casein
		Skin and bones	Gelatin
			Keratin
		Insect secretion	Shellac
Modified natural	Plant	Wood pulp and cotton	Cellulose derivatives: methylcellulose, sodium carboxymethylcellulose
		Seed extracts	Guar derivatives
Synthetic		Petroleum based	Acrylic acid polymers
			Polyacrylamides
			Alkylene/alkylene oxide polymers
Inorganic		Clays	Smectite hydrophilic and organoclays
		Amorphous silicon dioxide	Hydrated silica
			Fumed silica

Source: Ref. 72.

pH values. If a specific pH is required, the system can be maintained at the desired pH value using an adequate buffer. This is especially important for drugs that possess ionizable acidic or basic groups in which the pH of the vehicle often influences the stability and/or solubility. These buffering salts or electrolytes must be used with extreme caution since small changes in electrolyte concentration can alter the surface charge of the dispersed phase and, thus, affect the overall stability of the system. Osmotic active salts (e.g., sodium chloride) and/or stabilizers (e.g., disodium edetate) may be replaced by organic nonelectrolytes, such as dextrose, mannitol, or sorbitol, in order to avoid possible destabilization. Adjustments in osmolarity or tonicity are generally required when preparing ophthalmic or injectable disperse systems.

For suspensions primarily stabilized by a polymeric material, it is important to carefully consider the optimal pH value of the product since certain polymer properties, especially the rheological behavior, can strongly depend on the pH of the system. For example, the viscosity of hydrophilic colloids, such as xanthan gums and colloidal microcrystalline cellulose, is known to be somewhat pH- dependent. Most disperse systems are stable over a pH range of 4–10 but may flocculate under extreme pH conditions. Therefore, each dispersion should be examined for pH stability over an adequate storage period. Any changes in the pH values could be indicative of a potential instability problem.

D. Preservatives

Preservation against microbial growth is an important aspect of disperse systems, not only with respect to the primary microbiological contamination, but also in terms of the physical and chemical integrity of the system [75]. Aqueous liquid products are prone to microbial contamination because water in combination with excipients derived from natural sources (e.g., polypeptides, carbohydrates) serves as an excellent medium for the growth of microorganisms. Besides the pathogenic hazards, microbial contamination can result in discoloration or cracking (separation into two bulk phases) of the products. The evolution of carbon dioxide gas may result in the explosion of containers. Colloidal dispersions and systems prepared by a controlled flocculation may become unstable and deflocculate due to a decrease in the zeta potential in the absence of adequate preservation.

The types of microorganisms found in various products are *Pseudomonas* species, including *Pseudomonas aeruginosa*, *Salmonella*, species, *Staphylococcus aureus*, and *Escherichia coli*. The USP and other pharmacopoeias recommend certain classes of products to be tested for specified microbial contaminants, e.g., natural plant, animal, and some mineral products for the absence of *Salmonella* species, suspensions for the absence of *E. coli*, and topically administered products for the absence of *P. aeruginosa* and *S. aureus*. Emulsions are especially susceptible to contamination by fungi and yeasts. Consumer use may also result in the introduction of microorganisms. For aqueous-based products, it is therefore mandatory to include a preservative in the formulation in order to provide further assurance that the product retains its pharmaceutically acceptable characteristics until it is used by the patient.

Substances that have been used as preservatives for disperse systems include chlorocresol, chlorobutanol, benzoates, phenylmercuric nitrate, parabens, and others [76,77]. The use of cationic antimicrobial agents such as quaternary ammonium compounds (e.g., benzalkonium chloride) is contraindicated in many cases because they may be inactivated by other formulation components and/or they may alter the charge of the dispersed phase. Clay suspensions and gels should be adequately preserved with nonionic antimicrobial preservatives. The use of preservatives is generally limited to products that are not intended for parenteral use. Intravenous injectable preparations should be prepared according to stringent sterile conditions from pyrogen-free raw materials and normally be terminally sterilized by either autoclaving or aseptic filtration.

In emulsions, partitioning of the incorporated preservative can occur between the aqueous and the oil phase. A lipophilic preservative may pass into the oil phase so that a significant portion is removed from the aqueous phase. Since it is the latter in which microorganisms tend to grow, the use of water-soluble preservatives can be more effective, especially for O/W emulsions. For most emulsion systems, the esters of *p*-hydroxybenzoic acid (parabens) appear to be the most satisfactory. Since microorganisms can also reside within the oil phase, it is further recommended that a pair of preservatives having different oil and water solubilities be used in order to ensure appropriate concentrations in both phases.

The major criteria for the selection of an appropriate preservative include efficiency against a wide spectrum of microorganisms, stability (shelf life), toxicity, sensitizing effects, compatibility with other ingredients in the dosage form, and taste and odor. Other specific factors to be considered may include the application site (e.g., external, ophthalmic, parenteral), pH of the dispersion medium, solubility in the vehicle, partitioning into an oil phase (in emulsions), and adsorption onto the solid phase (in suspensions) or onto the packaging materials [78]. Finally, the establishment of microbiological standards for raw materials and strict adherence to the Good Manufacturing Practice (GMP) protocols during industrial-scale production can efficiently reduce the severity of the contamination problem.

E. Antioxidants

Many pharmaceutical products undergo oxidative deterioration upon storage because the therapeutic ingredients or adjuvants oxidize in the presence of atmospheric oxygen. Vitamins, essential oils, and almost all fats and oils can be oxidized readily. The decomposition can be particularly significant in disperse systems, such as emulsions, because of the large area of interfacial contact and because the manufacturing process may introduce air into the product. Many drugs commonly incorporated into emulsions are subjected to autooxidation and subsequent decomposition. Traces of oxidation products are undesirable because they are generally easily noticed by their smell or taste. The term autooxidation is used when the ingredient(s) in the product react(s) with oxygen without drastic external interference. Series of autooxidative reactions involve the initiation step or the formation of a free radical, the propagation step where the free radical is regenerated and reacts with more oxygen, followed by the termination step as the free radicals react with each other resulting in the inactive products.

Antioxidants are classified into three main groups. The first group, comprising the true antioxidants, probably inhibits oxidation by reacting with free radicals, thus blocking the chain reaction. Examples include tocopherols, alkyl gallates, butylated hydroxyanisole (BHA), and butylated hydroxytoluene (BHT). They are commonly used at concentrations ranging from 0.001 to 0.1%. Antioxidants of the second group, comprising the reducing agents, have a lower redox potential than the drug or other substances that they should protect and are therefore more readily oxidized. They may also react with free radicals. Examples are ascorbic and isoascorbic acids and the potassium or sodium salts of sulfurous acid. The latter group, such as sodium metabisulfite, has been reported to produce sensitivity reactions. The third group comprises the antioxidant synergists, including sequestering and chelating agents, which possess little antioxidant effect themselves but enhance the action of a true antioxidant by reacting with heavy metal ions that catalyze oxidation. The synergist class includes citric acid, tartaric acid, disodium edetate, and lecithin.

The selection of an appropriate antioxidant depends on factors such as stability, toxicity, efficiency, odor, taste, compatibility with other ingredients, and distribution phenomena between the two phases. Antioxidants that give protection primarily in the aqueous phase include sodium metabisulfite, ascorbic acid, thioglycerol, and cysteine hydrochloride. Oil-soluble antioxidants include lecithin, propyl gallate, ascorbyl palmitate, and butylated hydroxytoluene. Vitamin E has also been used, but its virtue as a natural antioxidant has been the subject of some controversy.

IV. SUSPENSIONS

A suspension is defined as a disperse system in which the dispersed phase is in the solid state, whereas the dispersion medium is in the liquid state. For example, the internal phase (suspensoid, suspended phase) can be uniformly distributed throughout the suspending medium (suspending vehicle) in which it exhibits a minimum degree of solubility. The internal phase consists of a homogeneous or heterogeneous distribution of solid particles having a specific range of size. Coarse suspensions contain suspended particles, which are larger than about 1 μm in size with the practical upper limit of about 75 μm. The particle diameter of most good pharmaceutical suspensions lies between 1 and 50 μm. When one or more of the ingredients constituting the internal phase are pharmaceutically useful and/or pharmacologically active, the system is called a pharmaceutical suspension.

Suspensions have several advantages as a dosage form. They allow the development of a liquid product containing an appropriate quantity of the active ingredient in a reasonable volume. Resistance to hydrolysis and oxidation is generally good in suspensions when compared with that in respective aqueous solutions. In such a case, a suspension would insure chemical stability while permitting liquid therapy. Suspensions can also be used for taste-masking purposes. A disagreeable taste of certain drugs when given in solution form can be overcome when administered as undissolved particles in an oral suspension. A number of chemical derivatives of many poor-tasting drugs, such as chloramphenicol, have been specifically developed for their insolubility in a desired vehicle for the purpose of preparing a palatable liquid dosage form.

On the other hand, there are a number of disadvantages of suspensions that should be noted. The content uniformity and dosage accuracy of suspensions are unlikely to compare favorably with that obtainable by the use of tablets, capsules, or solutions. Sedimentation and compaction of sediment, so-called caking, frequently cause problems that are not always easy to solve. In addition, the product is liquid and relatively bulky compared to solid dosage forms. These properties are disadvantageous for both pharmacists and patients. However, the above-mentioned advantages can, under certain circumstances, outweigh the disadvantages of this type of dosage forms.

A. Sedimentation and Stokes' Law

The control of sedimentation is required to ensure a sufficient and uniform dosage. Sedimentation behavior of a disperse system depends largely on the motion of the particles which may be thermally or gravitationally induced. If a suspended particle is sufficiently small in size, the thermal forces will dominate the gravitational forces and the particle will follow a random motion owing to molecular bombardment, called "Brownian motion." The distance moved or displacement, D_i, is given by:

$$D_i^2 = \frac{RTt}{3N\pi\eta r} \tag{9}$$

where R is the universal gas constant, T is the absolute temperature, t is the time, N is the Avogadro's number, η is the viscosity, and r is the particle radius. Note that the displacement, D_i, decreases with increasing radius of the particle, r. For any given system, one can define a "no sedimentation diameter" (NSD), below which value the Brownian motion will be sufficient to keep particles from sedimentation. The value of NSD obviously depends on the density and viscosity of the respective system.

Increasing the radius of the suspended particles, Brownian motion becomes less important and sedimentation becomes more dominant. These larger particles therefore settle gradually under gravitational forces. The basic equation describing the sedimentation of spherical, monodisperse particles in a suspension is Stokes' law. It states that the velocity of sedimentation, v, can be calculated as follows:

$$v = \frac{2gr^2(\rho_1 - \rho_2)}{9\eta} = \frac{gd^2(\rho_1 - \rho_2)}{18\eta} \tag{10}$$

where r is the particle radius, d is the particle diameter, ρ_1 and ρ_2 are the densities of the particle and dispersion medium, respectively, g is the acceleration caused by gravity, and η is the viscosity of the medium.

The settling velocity is proportional to the second power of the particle radius or particle diameter. It is apparent that agglomerates and flocculates settle more rapidly than individual particles. Since both gravity and buoyancy are operating simultaneously on the particle, either upward movement or downward movement results. Suspensions generally undergo sedimentation upon storage while emulsions may exhibit either upward creaming (O/W type) or downward creaming (W/O type). The determining factor is the difference in the densities of the internal and the external phases.

Stokes' law is rigorously applicable only for the ideal situation in which uniform and perfectly spherical particles in a very dilute suspension settle without turbulence, interparticle collisions, and without chemical/physical attraction or affinity for the dispersion medium [79]. Obviously, the equation does not apply precisely to common pharmaceutical suspensions in which the above-mentioned assumptions are most often not completely fulfilled. However, the basic concept of the equation does provide a valid indication of the many important factors controlling the rate of particle sedimentation and, therefore, a guideline for possible adjustments that can be made to a suspension formulation.

Since the sedimentation rate increases with increasing particle size, it is apparent that particle size reduction is beneficial to the stability of suspensions. However, one should avoid reducing the particle to an extreme degree of fineness since very fine particles have the tendency to form compact cakes upon storage. The rate of sedimentation may also be appreciably reduced by increasing the viscosity of the continuous phase. But this can only be achieved within a practical limit. From Stokes' law, it can also be seen that if the density difference of both phases is eliminated, sedimentation can be entirely prevented. However, it is seldom if ever possible to increase vehicle density above about 1.3. In addition, a product having a too high viscosity is not desirable because of its poor pourability and difficulty of redispersion. A wide variety of suspending agents are available. Some excipients, such as cellulose derivatives, have a pronounced effect on the viscosity, but hardly any on density. Others, such as sorbitol, can modify both density and viscosity.

Generally, the physical stability of a pharmaceutical suspension can be appropriately adjusted by an alteration in the dispersed phase rather than by significant modifications in the dispersion medium. These adjustments are mainly concerned with particle size, uniformity of particle size, and separation of the particles so that they are not likely to become larger or to form a solid cake upon standing.

B. Flocculation and Deflocculation Phenomena

The zeta potential is a measurable indication of the apparent particle charge in the dispersion medium. When its value is relatively high, the repulsive forces usually exceed the attractive forces. Accordingly, the particles are individually dispersed and are said to be "deflocculated." Thus, each particle settles separately, and the rate of sedimentation is relatively small. The settling particles have plenty of time to pack tightly by falling over one another to form an impacted bed. The sedimentation volume of such a system is low, and the sediment is difficult to redisperse. The supernatant remains cloudy even when settling is apparent.

Controlled flocculation is the intentional formation of loose agglomerates of particles held together by comparatively weak bonding forces. This can be achieved by the addition of a preferentially adsorbed ion whose charge is opposite in sign to that of the zeta potential–determining ions. Thus, the apparent active charge of the particles is progressively lowered. At certain concentration of the added ion, the forces of repulsion are sufficiently small that the forces of attraction start to predominate. Under these conditions the particles may approach each other closely and form loose agglomerates, termed "flocs," "flocculates," or "floccules" ("flocculated" system). When compared to the deflocculated particles, the flocs settle rapidly and form a higher sedimentation volume. The loose structure permits the flocculates to break up easily and distribute uniformly with only a small amount of agitation. Controlled flocculated systems usually develop a clear supernatant solution above the loose sediment. Thus, they might look less uniform upon standing, even though they provide easy redispersion and better dose uniformity than many other types of suspensions.

Flocculating agents can be simple electrolytes that are capable of reducing the zeta potential of suspended charged particles. Examples include small concentrations (0.01–1%) of monovalent ions (e.g., sodium chloride, potassium chloride) and di- or trivalent ions (e.g., calcium salts, alums, sulfates, citrates or phosphates) [80–83]. These salts are often used jointly in the formulations as pH buffers and flocculating agents. Controlled flocculation of suspensions can also be achieved by the addition of polymeric colloids or alteration of the pH of the preparation.

A caking diagram, described by Martin [81], shows the flocculation of a bismuth subnitrate suspension by means of the flocculating agent monobasic potassium phosphate. The addition of the negatively charged phosphate ions to the suspended drug particles causes the positive zeta potential to decrease. Upon further phosphate addition, the zeta potential falls to zero and then becomes negative. Microscopic examination reveals that maximum flocculation occurs and persists until the zeta potential becomes sufficiently negative for deflocculation. The onset of flocculation coincides with the maximum sedimentation volume determined.

The controlled flocculation method may be used in conjunction with the addition of a polymeric material to form a structured vehicle. After the formation of the flocs, an aqueous solution of polymeric material, usually negatively charged, such as carboxymethylcellulose or carbopol, is added. The concentration employed depends on the consistency desired for the suspension, which also relates to the size and density of the dispersed phase. Care must be taken to ensure the absence of any incompatibility between the flocculating agent and the polymer used for the formation of the structured vehicle.

When formulating a deflocculated system, a number of materials may be used as dispersion aids. Deflocculating agents include polymerized organic salts of sulfonic acid of both types—alkyl-aryl and aryl-alkyl—that can alter the surface charge of the particles by physical adsorption. Unlike surfactants, these agents do not lower surface and interfacial tension appreciably; hence, they have little or no tendency to create foam or wet particles. Most deflocculants are not generally considered safe for internal use; the only acceptable dispersant for parenteral products is lecithin.

C. Crystal Growth and Polymorphism

The growth in time of unprotected slightly soluble drug solids and subsequent changes in their particle size distribution in suspension have been reviewed by several researchers [84–89]. The crystal growth in disperse systems may be attributed to one or more of the following mechanisms: Ostwald ripening, temperature changes, and polymorphic transformation.

Ostwald ripening is the growth of large particles at the expense of smaller ones as a result of a difference in the solubility of the particles of varying sizes. The surface free energy of small particles is greater than that of large particles. Therefore, small particles can be appreciably more soluble than larger ones. A concentration gradient results, with higher drug concentrations in the area of small particles and lower drug concentrations in the area of large particles. Thus, according to Fick's law of diffusion, the dissolved particle molecules diffuse from the environment of the smaller particles to the environment of the larger particles. An increase in the concentration in the area of the large particles leads to crystallization and particle growth. Thus, small particles become smaller, whereas large particles become larger upon storage. Small fluctuations in temperature can accelerate this effect. Small particles dissolve to a greater extent when the temperature increases and then recrystallize on the surface of existing larger particles as the temperature drops. The suspension becomes coarser, and the mean particle size spectrum shifts to higher values. This effect can be expressed by the following relationship:

$$\log \frac{S}{S_o} = \frac{k}{2.303 \cdot r} \tag{11}$$

where S is the initial solubility rate of small particles; S_o is the solubility rate of large particles at equilibrium, r is the particle radius in cm, and k is a constant that includes surface tension, temperature, molar volume, and thermodynamic terms ($k = 1.21 \times 10^{-6}$). Thus, it can be seen that the increase in solubility rate of a 0.2 μm particle is 13%, 1% for a 2 μm particle, and negligible for particles of 20 μm and larger.

Crystal growth due to temperature fluctuations during storage is of importance especially when the suspensions are subjected to temperature cycling of 20°C or more. These effects depend on the magnitude of temperature change, the time interval, and the effect of temperature on the drug's solubility and subsequent recrystallization process. At each crystal contact point there exists a thin layer of supersaturated solution that facilitates crystal growth. The type of inherent crystal form is determined by the factors governing the rate of crystal growth. The degree of supersaturation is dependent on the rate of cooling, the extent and degree of agitation, and the size and number of nuclei available for the particle nucleation. Other factors include pH, solvent effects, and the impurities present.

As crystal growth generally increases with an increase in particle solubility, the excipients that tend to increase the particle solubility should be kept to a minimum. Many pharmaceutical gums can absorb onto the surfaces of drug crystals and, thus, can be used to inhibit the crystal growth. In a dilute suspension, crystal growth increases with the degree of agitation because the mass transfer in the bulk fluid is increased (conventional transport). If sedimentation occurs, the local increase in particle concentration decreases the mean free diffusion path of the solute molecules and may thus promote the particle growth.

Polymorphism refers to the different internal crystal structures of a chemically identical compound. Drugs may undergo a change from one metastable polymorphic form to a more stable polymorphic form. Also, the crystal habit might change due to the degree of solvation or hydration. The formation of distinct new crystalline entities during storage is possible. For example, an originally anhydrous drug in a suspension may rapidly or slowly form a hydrate. These various forms may exhibit different solubilities, melting points, and x-ray diffraction patterns. In the preparation of suspensions using precipitation methods, the solvent and the rate of cooling are important factors determining the type of polymorph(s) obtained.

Various drugs are known to exist in different polymorphic forms (e.g., cortisone and prednisolone). The rate of conversion from a metastable into the stable form is an important criteria to be considered with respect to the shelf life of a pharmaceutical product. Polymorphic changes have also been observed during the manufacture of steroid suspensions. When steroid powders are subjected to dry heat sterilization, subsequent rehydration of anhydrous steroid in the presence of an aqueous vehicle results in the formation of large, needle-like crystals. A similar effect may be produced by subject finished suspensions to moist heat sterilization in an autoclave.

Higuchi showed that crystal growth may also arise when the more energetic amorphous or glassy forms of a drug exhibit significantly greater initial solubility in water than their corresponding crystalline forms [84]. In addition, size reduction by crushing and grinding can produce particles whose different surfaces exhibit high or low dissolution rates. This effect can be correlated to differences in the free surface energy introduced during comminution.

To prevent crystal growth and possible changes in particle size distribution, one or more of the following procedures and techniques may be employed [9,89]: (a) selection of particles with a narrow size range; (b) selection of a more stable crystalline form of the drug; (c) avoidance of the use of high-energy milling during particle size reduction; (d) incorporation of a wetting agent (e.g., surfactant) and/or a protective colloid (e.g., cellulose derivatives forming film barriers around the particles); (e) increase of the viscosity of the vehicle to retard particle dissolution and subsequent crystal growth; and (f) avoidance of temperature extremes during storage.

D. Pharmaceutical Suspensions

In the preparation of physically stable pharmaceutical suspensions, a number of formulation components can be incorporated to maintain the solid particles in the dispersed state. These substances can be classified as (a) components of the suspending system, including wetting agents, dispersants or deflocculating agents, flocculating agents, and thickeners, and (b) components of the suspending vehicle (external phase), including pH-control agents and buffers, osmotic agents, coloring/flavoring agents, preservatives, and liquid vehicles. The components of each category are individually selected for their use in the preparation of orally, topically, or parenterally administered suspensions.

Orally administered suspensions containing a wide class of active ingredients (e.g., antibiotics, antacids, radiopaque agents) are of major commercial importance. The solids content of an oral suspension may vary considerably. For example, antibiotic preparations may contain 125–500 mg solid drug per 5 mL or a teaspoonful dose, while a drop concentrate may provide the same amount of drug in only 1–2 mL. Antacid or radiopaque suspensions also contain relatively high amounts of suspended material for oral administration. The suspending vehicle can, for example, be a syrup, sorbitol solution, or gum-thickened water with added artificial sweeteners. Taste and mouthfeel are important considerations when formulating oral suspensions.

Many antibiotic drugs are unstable in the presence of an aqueous vehicle and, therefore, are frequently supplied as dry powder mixtures for reconstitution at the time of dispensing. Generally, this type of product is either a powder mixture or a completely/partially granulated product, which upon dilution and agitation with a specified quantity of vehicle (e.g., water) results in the formation of a suspension suitable for administration [90]. The preparation is typically designated in the USP by a title of the form "For Oral Suspension," whereas the ready-to-use suspension preparations are simply designated as "Oral Suspension." The dry mix products often contain drugs, colorants, flavorants, sweeteners (e.g., sucrose or sodium saccharin), stabilizing agents (e.g., citric acid, sodium citrate), suspending agents (e.g., guar gum, xanthan gum, methylcellulose), and preservatives (e.g., parabens, sodium benzoate).

The formulation of oral sustained-release suspensions has resulted in only limited success due to the difficulty in maintaining the stability of sustained-release particles when present in liquid systems. Formulation techniques, such as coated beads, drug-impregnated wax matrix, microencapsulation, and ion-exchange resins, have been used for this purpose [91–93]. The combination of an ion-exchange resin complex with particle coating has resulted in a commercial product, the so-called Pennkinetic system. By this technique, ionic drugs are complexed with ion-exchange resins, and the drug-resin complex particles are then treated with an impregnating polymer such as polyethylene glycol 4000 followed by coating with a sustaining polymer, such as ethyl cellulose [94,95]. In liquid suspension (the dispersion medium being free of ions that could replace drug ions in the resin complex), the drug remains absorbed to the resin. However, upon swallowing ions from the gastrointestinal liquid can penetrate the particles and replace the drug ions, which subsequently diffuse out of the system (at a controlled, slow rate). Drug release from these systems depends on the type of drug-resin complex, on the ionic environment (e.g., pH and electrolyte concentration within the GI tract), as well as on properties of the resin. Most ion-exchange resins currently employed in sustained-release products contain sulfonic acid groups that exchange cationic drugs possessing amine functionality. An example is hydrocodone polistirex [Tussionex® Pennkinetic Extended-Release Suspension (Pennwalt)].

Topical suspensions are intended to be applied externally. Shake lotion and calamine lotion are good examples of historical products in this class. Because safety and toxicity are dealt with in terms of dermatological acceptability, many useful new suspending agents have been introduced in topical formulations. The protective action and cosmetic properties of topical lotions usually require the use of high concentrations of disperse phase.

In contrast, parenteral suspensions have relatively low solids contents, usually between 0.5 and 5%, with the exception of insoluble forms of penicillin in which concentrations of the antibiotic may exceed 30%. These sterile preparations are designed for intramuscular, intradermal, intralesional, intraarticular, or subcutaneous injection. Syringeability is an important factor to be taken into consideration with injectable dosage forms. The viscosity of a parenteral suspension should be sufficiently low to facilitate injection. Common suspending vehicles include preserved isotonic saline solution or a parenterally acceptable vegetable oil. Ophthalmic and optic suspensions that are instilled into the eye/ear must also be prepared in a sterile manner. The vehicles are essentially isotonic and aqueous in composition. The reader should refer to Chapter 12 for further discussion on parenteral products.

E. Methods of Evaluating Suspensions

Suspensions are generally evaluated with respect to their particle size, electrokinetic properties (zeta potential), and rheological characteristics. A detailed discussion on the methods/techniques and relevant instrumentation is given in Sec. VII. A number of evaluating methods done specifically with suspension dosage forms, such as sedimentation volume, redispersibility, and specific gravity measurements, will be treated in this section.

The sedimentation volume of a pharmaceutical suspension can be evaluated using simple, inexpensive, graduated, cylindrical graduates (100–1000 mL). It is defined as the ratio of the equilibrium volume of sediment, V_u, to the total volume of the suspension, V_o.

$$F = \frac{V_u}{V_o} \tag{12}$$

The value of F ranges between 0 and 1 and increases as the volume of suspension that appears occupied by the sediment increases. For example, if 100 mL of a well-shaken test formulation is placed in a graduate cylinder and the final height of the sediment is at the 20 mL line, then F is 0.2. It is normally found that the greater the value of F, the more stable the product.

When $F = 1$, no sediment is apparent and caking is absent, and the suspension is considered esthetically pleasing. This method of evaluation is quite useful in determining the physical stability of suspensions. It can be used to determine the settling rates of flocculated and deflocculated suspensions by making periodic measurement of sedimentation height. Tingstad [96] indicated that a flocculated suspension that settles to a level that is 90% of the initial suspension height ($F = 0.9$) and no further is probably satisfactory.

The degree of flocculation, β, is defined as the ratio of the sedimentation volume of the flocculated suspension, F, to the sedimentation volume of the suspension when deflocculated, F_∞. It is expressed as:

$$\beta = \frac{F}{F_\infty} \tag{13}$$

The degree of flocculation, therefore, is an expression of the increased sediment volume resulting from flocculation. For example, if β has a value of 5.0, this means that the volume of sediment in the flocculated system is five times that in the deflocculated state. As the value of β approaches unity, the degree of flocculation decreases.

Great care must be exercised when using graduated cylinders because decreases in the diameter of small containers can produce a "wall effect," which often affects the settling rate or ultimate sedimentation volume of flocculated suspensions. Such small containers have a tendency to hold up the suspensions due to adhesive forces acting between the container's inner surface and the suspended particles.

If a pharmaceutical suspension produces a sediment upon storage, it is essential that it should be readily dispersible so that uniformity of dose is assured. The amount of shaking required to achieve this end should be minimal. Various redispersibility tests have been described. For example, the test suspension is placed in a 100 mL graduated cylinder, which, after storage and sedimentation, is rotated through 360° at 20 rpm. The endpoint is taken when the inside of the base of the graduated cylinder is clear of sediment. The ultimate test of redispersibility is the uniformity of suspended drug dosage delivered from a product, from the first to the last volumetric dose out of the bottle, under one or more standard shaking conditions.

V. EMULSIONS

An emulsion is a two-phase system consisting of at least two immiscible liquids (or two liquids that are saturated with each other), one of which is dispersed as globules (internal or dispersed phase) within the other liquid phase (external or continuous phase), generally stabilized by an emulsifying agent [81,97]. Emulsions have been widely used in many areas of application: in industries [98–100], agricultures [101,102], food technologies [103–109], pharmaceutics [110–114], and cosmetics [115–119]. Very frequently emulsions are used in cosmetic products as topical vehicles for dermal application since they have high patient/consumer acceptance. Pharmaceutical emulsions are currently used internally for the administration of nutrients, drugs, and diagnostic agents. Emulsions discussed in this chapter include macroemulsions, multiple emulsions, microemulsions, liposomes, and a special emulsion type: in situ forming microparticle (ISM) systems.

A. Types of Emulsions

Macroemulsions

Based on the nature of the dispersed phase and the dispersion medium, two types of macroemulsions can be distinguished. If the continuous phase is an aqueous solution and the dispersed phase an oil, the system is called an oil-in-water emulsion. Such an O/W emulsion is generally formed if the aqueous phase constitutes more than 45% of the total weight and a hydrophilic emulsifier is used. Conversely, when the aqueous phase is dispersed within the oil, the system is called a water-in-oil emulsion. W/O emulsions are generally formed when the aqueous phase constitutes less than 45% of the total weight and a lipophilic emulsifier is used. Generally, O/W emulsions are more popular than W/O emulsions in the pharmaceutical field, especially when they are designed for oral administration. In the cosmetic industries, lotions or creams are of either the O/W or the W/O type, depending on their applications. O/W emulsions are most useful as water-washable drug bases and for general cosmetic purposes, while W/O emulsions are employed more widely for the treatment of dry skin and emollient applications. It is important for a pharmacist to know the type of emulsion, since it can significantly affect its properties and performance. There are several methods of determining the emulsion type, as summarized in Table 4 [120].

Multiple Emulsions

Multiple emulsions are more complex systems. If a simple emulsion is further dispersed within another continuous phase, these systems are called

Table 4 Methods to Determine Type of Macroemulsion (W/O or O/W)

Test	Method/Observation
Phase dilution test	Place two emulsion droplets on a glass slide and add a droplet of one component to each emulsion droplet, stir, and observe under a microscope. This test is based on the principle that an emulsion can only be diluted with the liquid that constitutes the continuous phase.
Dye solubility test	A colored dye soluble in only one component is added to the emulsion. If the color spreads throughout the whole emulsion, the phase in which the dye is soluble is the continuous phase.
Conductivity test	Immerse a pair of electrodes connected to an external electric source in the emulsion. If the external phase is water, a current passes through the emulsion. If the oil is the continuous phase, the emulsion fails to carry the current.

multiple emulsions. Figure 5 presents schematically the preparation of a W/O/W emulsion [122,123]. In step 1 an aqueous phase is added to an oily phase, containing a lipophilic surfactant. Upon mixing, a W/O emulsion is formed. In the second step, this W/O emulsion is then poured into a second aqueous solution, containing a hydrophilic surfactant. Upon mixing, the multiple W/O/W emulsion is formed.

Water-in-oil-in-water (W/O/W) and oil-in-water-in-oil systems (O/W/O) are the two basic types of multiple emulsions. Recently multiple emulsions have been developed with the purpose of prolonging the release of incorporated drugs. This technology has gained particular interest for the microencapsulation of peptides/proteins and hydrophilic drugs [124]. To increase the encapsulation efficiency of hydrophilic compounds W/O/W, O/W/O, W/O/O, and W/O/O/O emulsions have been used [125]. Cosmetically interesting is the application of multiple emulsions as supermoisturizing product bases, combining the benefits of O/W and W/O emulsions.

Microemulsion

In 1959, J. H. Schulman introduced the term "microemulsion" for transparent-solutions of a model four-component system [126]. Basically, microemulsions consist of water, an oily component, surfactant, and co-surfactant. A three phase diagram illustrating the area of existence of microemulsions is presented in Fig. 6 [24]. The phase equilibria, structures, applications, and chemical reactions of microemulsion have been reviewed by Sjöblom et al. [127]. In contrast to macroemulsions, microemulsions are optically transparent, isotropic, and thermodynamically stable [128, 129]. Microemulsions have been subject of various investigations because their unique properties allow a wide range of potential practical applications [130–132]. However, there is still substantial controversy concerning the exact nature of these systems and the appropriateness of the terminology. Terms as transparent emulsions, micellar solutions, solubilized systems, and swollen micelles have all been applied to the same or similar systems. Nonetheless, emulsions and microemulsions may be differentiated on the basis of particle size: microemulsions contain particles in the nanometer size range (typically 10–100 nm), whereas conventional emulsions (or macroemulsions, coarse emulsions) contain particles in the micrometer range.

Liposomes

Liposomes are vesicular lipid systems with diameter ranging between 50 nm and a few μm. They are composed of membrane-like lipid layers surrounding aqueous compartments. The lipid layers consist of phospholipids, making liposomes biocompatible and biodegradable. The phospholipids have a hydrophilic head and a lipophilic tail. Different preparation methods for liposomes have been described by Vemuri et al. [133], leading to different types of vesicular structures (Fig. 7) [134]. Nowadays, liposomes are widely used for drug delivery and drug targeting [135–137]. For a detailed description of this type of drug delivery system, the reader is referred to Chapters 15 and 16.

In Situ Forming Microparticle Systems

ISM systems were first introduced by Bodmeier and coworkers [138–140]. They are included in this chapter as special disperse systems because these

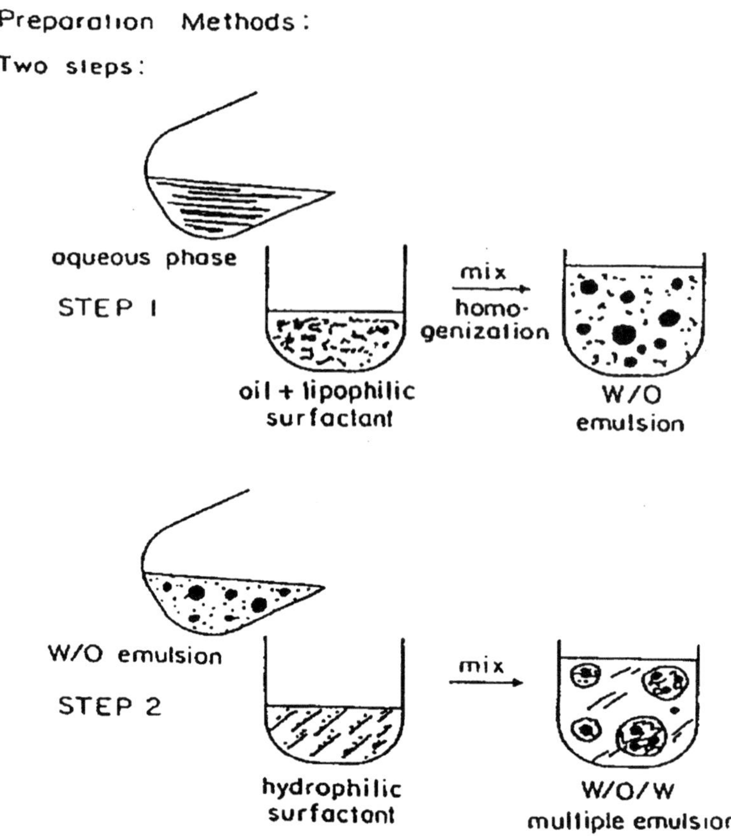

Fig. 5 Schematic of a two-step procedure to produce a W/O/W emulsion. (From Ref. 28.)

formulations are based on O/O or O/W emulsions. Being liquids, the ISM systems can easily be injected intramuscularly or subcutaneously and subsequently form microparticles within the human body upon contact with physiological fluids. The ISM system is composed of a drug and biodegradable polymer, which are co-dissolved in a water-miscible, biocompatible solvent. This solution is emulsified into an external, either oily or aqueous phase containing an emulsion stabilizer to form O/O or O/W emulsions. Upon contact with aqueous physiological fluids, the polymer solvent dissipates, leading to polymer solidification and hardening of the emulsion droplets. Thus, the microparticle formation occurs *in situ*. The resulting microparticles are regular in shape and reproducible. Furthermore, drug release can be prolonged and controlled during desired periods of time. The major advantages of this new technology over implants and the classical solvent evaporation method used to prepare microparticles are the ease of preparation and the avoidance of surgical insertion or removal of empty remnants.

B. Formulation and Preparation Techniques for Emulsions

The preparation techniques for emulsions can be divided into laboratory-scale productions and large-scale productions. Details on the latter are given in the manufacturing and equipment part of this chapter (see Sec. IX). Each method requires that energy be introduced into the system, either by trituration, homogenization, agitation or heat. The production of satisfactory stable emulsions requires adequate formulations and preparation techniques. It has been suggested that the formulator first determine the physical and chemical characteristics of the drug, which include the structure formula, melting point, solubilities in different media, stability, dose, and specific chemical incompatibilities. This information is essential for the selection of the appropriate type of emulsion. Then the required emulsifying agent(s) and its (their) concentration(s) should be identified. The choice of materials to be used largely depends on the purpose for which the emulsion is designed.

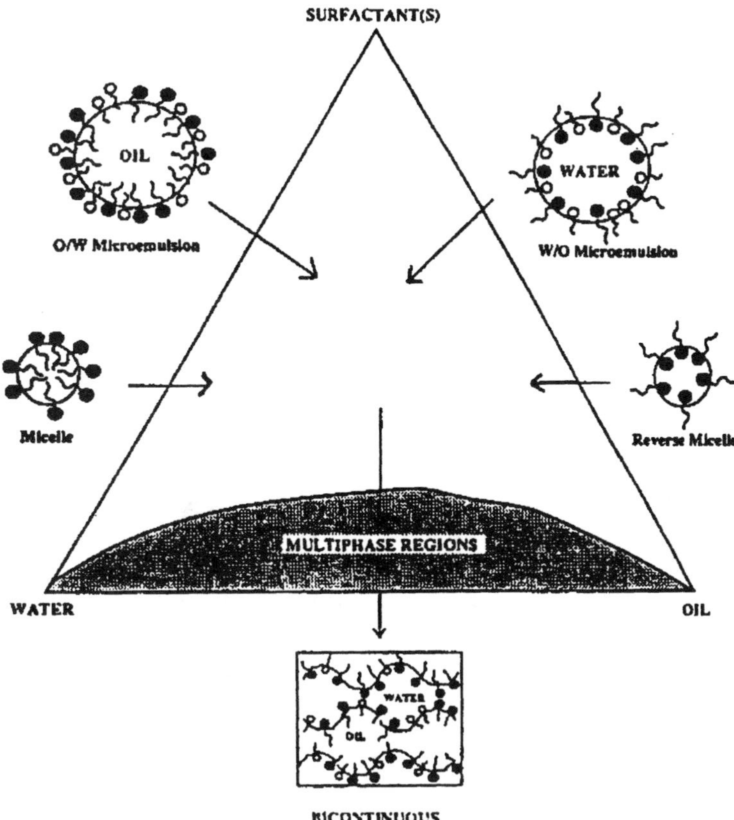

Fig. 6 Three-phase diagram illustrating the area of existence of microemulsions. (From Ref. 24.)

Phase Volume Ratio

The ratio of volume of disperse phase to volume of the dispersion medium greatly influences the characteristics of an emulsion. The choice of the phase volume ratio depends on a number of factors, including the requested consistency. It is generally difficult to formulate emulsions containing less than about 25% of disperse phase due to their susceptibility to severe creaming or sedimentation problems. However, a combination of proper emulsifying agents and suitable processing technology makes it possible to prepare emulsions with only 10% disperse phase without considerable stability problems. Conversely, products containing a high percentage of disperse phase (more than about 70%) are likely to exhibit phase inversion (the disperse phase becomes the dispersion medium).

Emulsifying Agents

Emulsions are thermodynamically unstable systems. However, using appropriate emulsifying agents (emulsifiers) to decrease the interfacial tension, the stability of these systems can be significantly increased. A satisfactory emulsifier should have a reasonable balance between its hydrophilic and hydrophobic groups, produce a stable emulsion (both initially and during storage), be stable itself, be chemically inert, be nontoxic and cause no irritation upon application, be odorless, tasteless, and colorless, and be inexpensive. Emulsifying agents can be classified into the following three groups:

1. Surfactants that are adsorbed at oil/water interfaces to form monomolecular films and reduce interfacial tension.
2. Natural macromolecular materials, which form multimolecular films around the disperse droplets of O/W emulsions. They are frequently called auxiliary emulsifying agents and have the desirable effect of increasing the viscosity of the dispersion medium. However, they often suffer from the disadvantages of being subject to hydrolysis and sensitive to variations in pH.

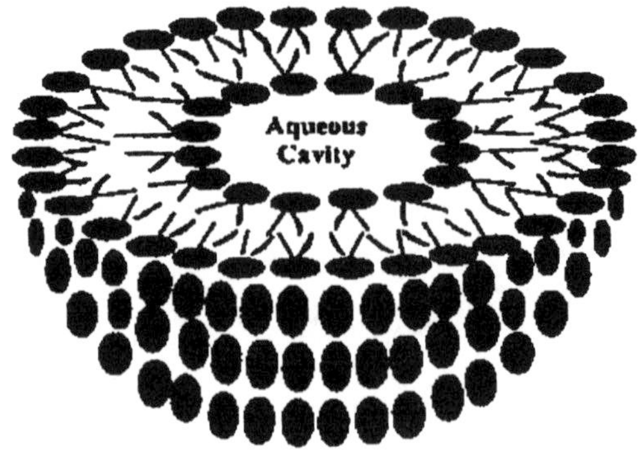

Liposome model

DENOMINATION	Large unilamellar vesicles LUV	Multi- or Oligolamellar vesicles MLV/OLV	Small unilamellar vesicles SUV
DIAMETER (nm)	80-1000	100-4000	20-80

Fig. 7 Different types of vesicular structures of liposomes. (From Ref. 134.)

3. Very finely disperse solids, which are adsorbed at the liquid/liquid interfaces, forming films of particles around the disperse globules. Certain powders can very effectively stabilize against coalescence. The solid's particle size must be very small compared with the emulsion droplet size and must exhibit an appropriate angle of contact at the three-phase (oil/water/solid) boundary [141].

The selection of a suitable emulsifying agent and its appropriate concentration are matters of experience and of trial and error. It is not necessary to use emulsifier amounts above the required quantities to produce complete interfacial films, unless an increase in the viscosity of the dispersion medium is intended. Reducing the interfacial tension makes emulsification easy but does not by itself prevent coalescence of the particles and resultant phase separation. Frequently, combinations of two or more emulsifying agents are used [2] to (a) adequately reduce the interfacial tension, (b) produce a sufficiently rigid interfacial film, and (c) achieve the most suitable viscosity of the external phase. Care must be taken to ensure the compatibility between the different emulsifiers. For example, charged emulsifying agents of opposite sign are likely to interact and coagulate when combined.

As described in Sec. III, surfactants can be classified using the hydrophile-lipophile balance (HLB) system [142], established by Griffin (see Sec. III.A) The HLB system provides a scale of surfactant hydrophilicity (HLB values range from 0 to 20, 20 corresponding to the highest possible hydrophilicity) that simplifies emulsifier selection and blending. In Table 5 the HLB values of some pharmaceutically relevant surfactants are listed. Surfactants with a low HLB value (<6) tend to provide stable W/O emulsions; those with a high HLB value (>8) tend to stabilize O/W emulsions. Table 6 gives an overview of the classical use of surfactants in the preparation of pharmaceutical dosage forms depending on their HLB value.

The HLB values required for the emulsification of commonly used oils and waxes in pharmaceutical applications are given in Table 7 [143]. To obtain a

Table 5 HLB Values of Surfactants Commonly Used in Pharmaceutical Products

Surfactant	HLB
Nonionic	
Sorbitan monolaurate (Span 20)	8.6
Sorbitan monopalmitate (Span 40)	6.7
Sorbitan monostearate (Span 60)	4.7
Sorbitan monooleate (Span 80)	4.3
Sorbitan trioleatem (Span 85)	1.8
Polyoxyethylene (20) sorbitan monolaurate (Tween 20)	16.7
Polyoxyethylene (20) sorbitan monopalmitate (Tween 40)	15.6
Polyoxyethylene (20) sorbitan monostearate (Tween 60)	14.9
Polyoxyethylene (20) sorbitan monooleate (Tween 80)	15.0
Polyoxyethylerie-polyoxypropylene block copolymers (Pluronics or Poloxamer)	29.0
Amphoteric	
Lecithin (from egg yolk or soybean)	7–10
Hydrogenated lecithin	7–10
Anionic	
Sodium doecyl sulfate	40.0
Bile salts	20–25

desired HLB value, lipophilic and hydrophilic surfactants can also be mixed. The following equation allows the calculation of the resulting HLB value of a mixture of two surfactants (A and B):

$$\text{HLB(blend)} = f \times \text{HLB(A)} + (1 - f) \times \text{HLB(B)} \tag{14}$$

where f is the fraction of surfactant A in the blend. For example, a mixture of 30% Span 80 (HLB = 4.3) and 70% Tween 80 (HLB = 15) has an overall HLB value of HLB = (0.3 × 4.3) + (0.7 × 15) = 11.8.

Table 6 Relationship Between the Use of Surfactants in the Preparation of Pharmaceutical Dosage Forms, Their Dispersibility in Water and Their HLB Values

HLB	Dispersibility in water	Suitable application
1–4	Nil	
3–6	Poor	W/O emulsifier
6–8	Milky dispersion on agitation	Wetting agent
8–10	Stable milky dispersion	Wetting agent; O/W emulsifier
10–13	Translucent to clear dispersion	O/W emulsifier
>13	Clear solution	O/W emulsifier; solubilizing agent

Viscosity-Imparting Agents

The viscosity of an emulsion can be of crucial importance for its stability, especially the viscosity of the external phase. A high viscosity reduces creaming and also lessens the tendency of particles to coalescence and produce phase separation. Examples of the widely used viscosity-imparting agents are alginates, bentonite, carboxymethylcellulose, polyvinyl pyrrolidone, hydroxypropylcellulose, and carbomer.

Emulsification Techniques

Techniques of emulsification of pharmaceutical products have been reviewed by Block [27]. The location of the emulsifier, the method of incorporation of the phases, the rates of addition, the temperature of each phase, and the rate of cooling after mixing of the phases considerably affect the droplet size distribution, viscosity, and stability of the final emulsion. Roughly four emulsification methods can be distinguished:

1. Addition of the internal phase to the external phase, while subjecting the system to shear or fracture.
2. Phase inversion technique: the external phase is added to the internal phase. For example, if an O/W emulsion is to be prepared, the aqueous phase is added to the oil phase. First a W/O emulsion is formed. At the inversion point, the

Table 7 Required HLB Values for the Emulsification of Oils and Waxes Commonly Used in Pharmaceutical Applications

Compound	HLB	Compound	HLB
O/W emulsions			
Isostearic acid	15–16	Ethyl benzoate	13
Linoleic acid	16	Isopropyl myristate	12
Oleic acid	17	Isopropyl palmitate	12
Ricinoleic acid	16	Kerosene	12
Cetyl alcohol	16	Lanolin, anhydrous	12
Stearyl alcohol	15–16	Mineral oil, aromatic	12
Tridecyl alcohol	14	Mineral oil, paraffinic	10
Beeswax	9	Mink oil	9
Carbon tetrachloride	16	Paraffin wax	10
Carnaubawax	15	Patrolatum	7–8
Caster oil	14	Pine oil	16
Coco butter	6	Rapeseed oil	7
Corn oil	8	Safflower oil	7
Cottonseed oil	6	Soyabean oil	6
W/O emulsion			
Mineral oil	6	Stearyl alcohol	7

Source: Adapted from Ref. 143.

addition of more water results in the inversion of the emulsion system and the formation of an O/W emulsion. The phase inversion technique allows the formation of small droplets with minimal mechanical action and attendant heat. A classical example is the so-called *dry gum* technique, which is a phase inversion technique when hydrophilic colloids are part of the formulation. First the dry hydrocolloid (e.g., acacia, tragacanth, methyl cellulose) is dispersed within the oil phase. Then water is added until the phase inversion occurs to form a O/W emulsion.

3. Mixing both phases after warming each. This method is frequently used in the preparation of ointments and creams.
4. Alternate addition of the two phases to the emulsifying agent. In this method, the water and oil are added alternatively, in small portions, to the emulsifier. This technique is especially suitable for the preparation of food emulsions.

C. Emulsion Stability

Types of Instability

Four major phenomena are associated with the physical instability of emulsions: flocculation, creaming, coalescence, and breaking (Fig. 8) [144]. *Flocculation* is best defined as the association of particles within an emulsion to form large aggregates, which can easily be redispersed upon shaking (see also sec. IV.B). Flocculation is generally regarded as a precursor to the irreversible process of coalescence. It differs from coalescence primarily in that the interfacial film and individual droplets remain intact. The reversibility of flocculation depends mainly on the strength of the interaction between the droplets and on the phase volume ratio. The relationship of droplet deformation, surfactant transfer, and interfacial rheology for emulsion stability has been discussed by Ivanov et al. [145]. *Creaming* occurs when the disperse droplets or floccules separate from the disperse medium under the influence of gravitational force. Generally, a creamed emulsion can be restored to its original state by gentle agitation. According to Stokes' law, the direction in which the droplet moves depends on the relative values of the densities of the two phases. Furthermore, larger droplets cream more rapidly than smaller droplets. Reducing the droplet sizes and thickening the continuous phase can minimize the rate of creaming. *Coalescence* is a much more serious type of instability. It occurs when the mechanical or electrical barrier is insufficient to prevent the formation of progressively larger droplets (Fig. 9) [144], which can finally lead to *breaking* (complete phase separation). Coalescence can be avoided by the formation of thick interfacial films consisting of macromolecules or particulate solids.

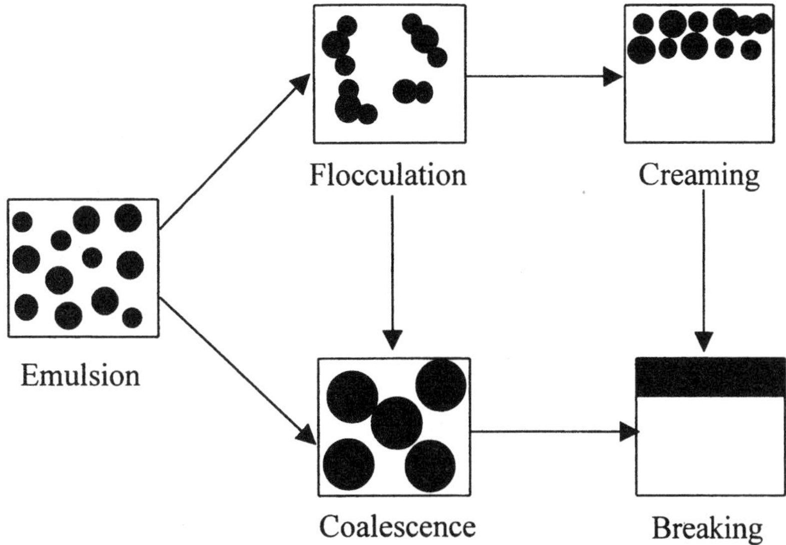

Fig. 8 Schematic illustration of different types of instability of emulsions.

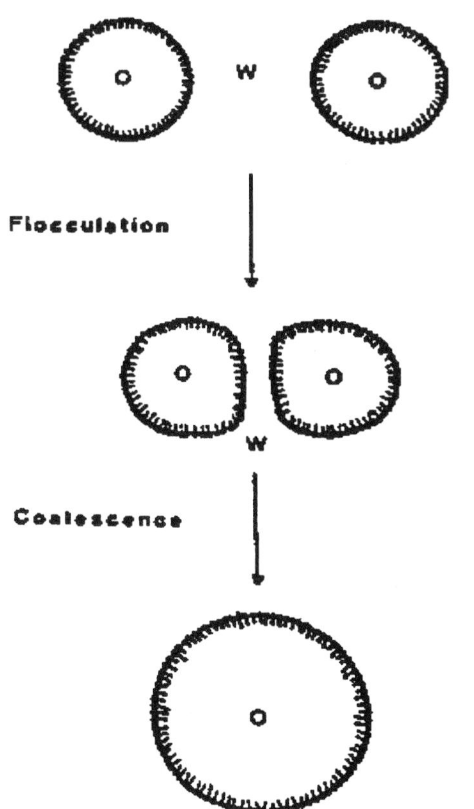

Fig. 9 Schematic presentation of flocculation and coalescence of emulsion droplets. (From Ref. 144.)

Stress Tests

The primary objective when studying the stability of emulsions is to predict the shelf life of these systems under normal storage conditions. The problem of stability assessment studies under normal storage conditions is that they last long periods of time. To shorten the time, many types of stress tests and stress conditions are used to provide a basis for the prediction of the stability of an emulsion. These methods can provide valuable information, but one should always be aware of the risk that changes occurring under stress conditions must not necessarily occur under normal market conditions. Steps should be taken so that the accelerated conditions do not introduce new and unanticipated mechanisms of instability, especially those bearing little relationship to what happens long-term. Stress conditions normally employed for evaluating the stability of emulsions include thermal stress and gravitational stress.

Thermal Stress. The Arrhenius equation states that a 10°C increase in the temperature doubles the rate of most chemical reactions. However, this approach is generally only useful to predict a product's shelf life if the instability of the emulsion is due to a chemical degradation process. Furthermore, this degradation must be identical in mechanism but different in rate at the investigated temperatures. Thus, the instability of emulsion systems seldom obeys the Arrhenius equation. Emulsion systems are often more complex; their instability might include phenomena such as (a) temperature-dependent solubilities and phase distributions of emulsifiers, (b) degradation reactions occurring only at higher temperatures, (c) temperature-induced phase changes, resulting in composition changes and altered rheological behavior, and (d) structural deformations and reformations, which may markedly vary with time and temperature [144]. It is considered reasonable to use the time for destabilization at 40°C multiplied by 4 to give an estimate shelf life at room temperature [134]. In addition, low temperature may also cause the precipitation of the emulsifiers and thus accelerate emulsion instability [142].

Gravitational Stress. Gravitational stress such as centrifugation may allow phase separation to occur quickly. Although this technique has been considered in a casual manner in the evaluation of emulsion stability, prediction of emulsion shelf life from this method was not much investigated until the use of ultracentrifuges [141]. Becher [120] indicates that centrifugation at 3750 rpm in a 10 cm radius centrifuge for a period of 5 hours is equivalent to the effect of gravity for about one year. It has been reported that the logarithm of the root mean cube diameter of particles after being centrifuged at 20,000 rpm produced a linear relationship to the centrifuging time [142]. In general, centrifugation is a useful tool to predict the emulsion shelf life, but the technique may not be suitable for very viscous or semisolid products.

Evaluation of Emulsion Stability

The most useful parameters commonly measured to assess the effect of stress conditions on emulsions include phase separation, rheological property determination, electrical property measurements, and particle size analysis.

Phase Separation. An approximate estimation of phase separation may be obtained visually. In general, creaming, flocculation, and coalescence have occurred before phase separation is visible, thus sometimes making quantitative evaluations more difficult. Accelerating the separation by centrifugation followed by appropriate analysis of the specimens may be useful to quantitatively determine the phase separation. Details on mechanisms of creaming and phase separation as well as some advances in the monitoring techniques of emulsion stability have been reviewed by Robins [146].

Rheological Property Determination. The rheology of an emulsion is often an important factor in determining its stability. Any variation in droplet size distribution, degree of flocculation, or phase separation frequently results in viscosity changes. Since most emulsions are non-Newtonian, the cone-plate type device should be used to determine their viscosity rather than the capillary viscometer.

Electrical Property Measurements. The surface charge and zeta potential (measure of the apparent, active charge) of emulsified droplets is often an important indicator for the stability of the system because electrostatic repulsion can significantly contribute to the avoidance of flocculation and coalescence (see also Sec. II.C). Recently, a new method to determine the creaming state of an emulsion has been established [147, 148]. The conductivity of the emulsion at different heights of the storage cell and at different times is measured, and the values are converted into volume fraction of the disperse phase. The creaming profile of O/W emulsions was described based on a kinetic model to extrapolate for the long-term stability prediction [149, 150].

Particle Size Measurement. The best way to evaluate an emulsion's stability is probably to measure its particle size distribution. A number of methods are available for droplet size determination (see Sec. VIII.A). Optical microscopy, although a time-consuming technique, is a direct way of measuring droplets larger than 1 μm. Nowadays, laser light-scattering, diffraction, and transmission methods are becoming popular for routine determination of particle size [151, 152].

VI. COLLOIDS AND COLLOIDAL DISPERSIONS

A colloid is defined as a system consisting of discrete particles in the size range of 1 nm to 1 μm, distributed within a continuous phase [153]. On the basis of the interaction of particles, molecules, or ions of the disperse phase with molecules of the dispersion medium-, colloidal systems can be classified as being lyophilic or lyophobic. In lyophilic systems, the disperse phase molecules are dissolved within the continuous phase and in the colloidal size range or spontaneously form aggregates in the colloidal size range (association systems). In lyophobic systems, the disperse phase is very poorly soluble or insoluble in the continuous phase. During the last several decades, the use of colloids in the pharmaceutical sciences has gained considerable attention. These systems have been investigated primarily for site-specific drug delivery, for controlled drug delivery, and also for the enhancement of the dissolution rate/bioavailability of poorly water-soluble drugs. Applications of colloidal materials in the preparation of pharmaceutical dosage forms are presented in Table 8 [12]. In this section two types of colloidal systems, namely drug-free aqueous colloidal polymeric dispersions (latices and pseudolatices) and drug-loaded nanoparticles, will be discussed.

A. Latices and Pseudolatices

An aqueous colloidal polymeric dispersion by definition is a two-phase system comprised of a disperse phase and a dispersion medium. The disperse phase consists of spherical polymer particles, usually with an average diameter of 200–300 nm. According to their method of preparation, aqueous colloidal polymer dispersions can be divided into two categories: (true) latices and pseudolatices. True latices are prepared by controlled polymerization of emulsified monomer droplets in aqueous solutions, whereas pseudolatices are prepared starting from already polymerized macromolecules using different emulsification techniques.

To prepare (*true*) latices, the monomers are emulsified in water with stirring and addition of emulsifiers, which help stabilize the monomer droplets. The molecular weight of the polymer molecules in the resultant latex can be controlled by the concentration and decomposition rate of added polymerization initiators. The residual monomer content can be reduced by optimizing the polymerization conditions and can also later be eliminated by steam distillation.

For the preparation of *pseudolatices*, the following three methods are commonly used [41]:

1. Direct emulsification: A solution of the polymer within a volatile, water-immiscible organic solvent (or mixture of solvents), or a polymer melt is emulsified within a surfactant-containing aqueous phase. If used, the organic solvent is then removed by steam distillation to obtain the pseudolatices.
2. Inverse emulsification: A solution of the polymer within a volatile, water-immiscible organic solvent (or mixture of solvents) or a polymer melt is compounded with a long-chain fatty acid (e.g., oleic acid) using conventional rubber-mixing equipment and mixed slowly with a dilute aqueous phase to give a W/O emulsion, which then inverts to an O/W emulsion upon further addition of the aqueous phase. If used, the organic solvent is then removed by steam distillation to obtain the pseudolatices [154, 155].
3. Self-emulsification: The polymer molecules are modified chemically by the introduction of basic (e.g., amino) or acidic (e.g., carboxyl) groups in such concentration and location that the polymer undergoes self-emulsification without surfactant after dispersion in an acidic or basic solution.

Latices and pseudolatices are widely used for the coating of solid pharmaceutical dosage forms such as tablets, capsules, and pellets. The major advantage compared to conventional coating techniques is the avoidance of organic solvents.

B. Nanoparticles

As indicated by the name, nanoparticles are colloidal particles in the size range of 1 to 1000 nm. The term nanoparticles encompasses both nanocapsules and nanospheres. Nanocapsules have a core-shell structure (reservoir system), while nanospheres represent matrix systems. Analogously to the above-described latices and pseudolatices (which are spherical, drug-free, aqueous, polymeric, nanoparticulate dispersions with a narrow size distribution), the techniques used to prepare polymeric nanoparticles can be classified in two groups. Nanoparticles are prepared either from preformed polymers or through various polymerization reactions of lipophilic or hydrophilic monomers. The choice of a particular preparation method and a suitable polymer depends on the physicochemical properties of the drug, the desired release characteristics, the therapeutic goal, the route of administration, the biodegradability/biocompatibility of the carrier material and regulatory considerations. From a technological point of view, the successful selection of a preparation method is determined by the ability to achieve high drug loadings, high encapsulation efficiencies, high product yields, and the potential for an easy scale-up.

Nanoparticles Based on Water-Insoluble Polymers

To prepare nanoparticles based on water-insoluble polymers, a solution of the polymer in an organic solvent can be emulsified within an aqueous phase. This O/W emulsion is then homogenized under high shear with an appropriate homogenization equipment

Table 8 Examples of Colloidal Materials Used in the Preparation of Pharmaceutical Dosage Forms

Colloidal materials	Uses
Acacia	Emulsifier, microcapsule wall material, suspending agent
Ailgnic acid	Microcapsule wall material, viscosity-imparting agent, disintegration, binder
Bentonite	Stabilizer, gelling agent, suspending agent, viscosity-imparting agent
Calcium carbonate	Diluent
Carbomer	Emulsifier, gelling agent, suspending agent
Carboxymethyl cellulose	Emulsifier, gelling agent, suspending agent, disintegrant, binder
Cellulose acetate phthalate	Enteric-coating agent
Cellulose	Binder, disintegrant, filler
Dextrin	Stabilizer, viscosity-imparting agent, adhesive, binder, plasticizer, sugar coating agent
Ethylcellulose	Viscosity-imparting agent, microcapsule wall material, binder
Gelatin	Microcapsule wall material, suspending agent, binder, coating agent
Guar gum	Viscosity-imparting agent, stabilizer, binder
Hydroxypropylcellulose	Viscosity-imparting agent, microcapsule wall material, granulating agent
Methylcellulose	Emulsifier, viscosity-imparting agent, gelling agent, suspending agent, binder, disintegrant, sugar coating agent
Poloxamer 188	Emulsifier, stabilizing agent, gelling agent base material for suppositories, coating agent
Polyethylene glycols	Gelling agent, base material for suppositories, coating agent, lubricant, plasticizer
Polymethacrylate	Film coating material, granulating binder
Silicon dioxide	Lubricant for capsules and tablets, viscosity-imparting agent, drying agent for powder
Starch	Binder, disintegrant
Tragacanth	Emulsifier, viscosity-imparting agent, suspending agent

Source: Adapted from Ref. 12.

(e.g., microfluidizer, sonication) prior to the precipitation of the polymer to further reduce the particle size of the internal organic phase into the colloidal size range [156–159]. The high pressure emulsification–solvent evaporation method is limited to water-insoluble drugs. Unless specific binding exists, water-soluble drugs are difficult to encapsulate because of partitioning into the external aqueous phase during emulsification. The particle size of the solidified nanoparticles is determined by the size of the emulsified polymer–drug–solvent droplets and hence depends on the homogenization equipment. Nanoparticles have been prepared with conventional laboratory homogenizers [12], by ultrasonication [157–159], and by microfluidization [159]. With the microfluidizer, the particle size decreases with increasing operating pressure and increasing number of cycles [159]. The particle size of the nanoparticles is also affected by the type of surfactant and surfactant concentration, the viscosity of the organic polymer solution, and the phase ratio of the internal to the aqueous phase [159, 160].

A similar technique, the so-called spontaneous emulsification solvent diffusion method, is derived from the solvent injection method to prepare liposomes [161]. Kawashima et al. [162] used a mixed-solvent system of methylene chloride and acetone to prepare PLGA nanoparticles. The addition of the water-miscible solvent acetone results in nanoparticles in the submicrometer range; this is not possible with only the water-immiscible organic solvent. The addition of acetone decreases the interfacial tension between the organic and the aqueous phase and, in addition, results in the perturbation of the droplet interface because of the rapid diffusion of acetone into the aqueous phase.

Nanocapsules of biodegradable polymers, such as PLA and PLA copolymers or poly (ε-caprolactone), have been prepared by an "interfacial polymer deposition mechanism" [163–166]. An additional component, a water-immiscible oil, is added to the drug-polymer-solvent mixture. A solution of the polymer, the drug, and a water-immiscible oil in a water-miscible solvent such as acetone is added to an external aqueous phase. This technique results in nanocapsules with a core-shell structure. The drug must have a high solubility in the oil-solvent mixture in order to obtain nanoparticles with high drug loadings.

An interesting modification of the solvent evaporation method is the "salting-out procedure" [167–172]. The nanoparticles are prepared by adding an aqueous phase saturated with an electrolyte or nonelectrolyte to a solution of the polymer and drug in a water-miscible organic solvent under agitation until an O/W emulsion forms. Saturating the aqueous phase reduces the miscibility of acetone and water by a salting-out process and allows the formation of an O/W emulsion from the otherwise miscible phases. The major advantages of the salting-out method are the avoidance of chlorinated solvents and surfactants commonly used with the conventional solvent evaporation method.

Nanoparticles Based on Hydrophilic Polymers

Nanoparticles based on hydrophilic polymers (e.g., albumin, chitosan, gelatin, or carbohydrates) can be prepared by W/O emulsification techniques. This process has been developed for the preparation of albumin microspheres [173–176]. However, the use of high-shear homogenization equipment or ultrasonication has allowed the formation of emulsions in the nanometer size range. Basically, an aqueous polymer solution is emulsified into an external, water-immiscible phase, such as an oil or organic solvent, followed by homogenization. Upon water removal, the polymer droplets solidify. Insoluble nanoparticles can be obtained by further hardening/insolubilizing the polymer through chemical cross-linking with aldehydes or other cross-linking agents or through denaturation at elevated temperatures. In order to obtain high encapsulation efficiencies, the drug must be insoluble in the external phase. Gelatin nanoparticles have been prepared by emulsifying a concentrated gelatin solution (30%) into hydrogenated castor oil containing proper emulsifying agents above the gelation temperature of the gelatin solution [177]. The W/O emulsion is then cooled in order to gel the aqueous gelatin droplets. Chitosan is one of the few naturally derived polysaccharides carrying basic functional groups. Since it is only soluble in acidic media, chitosan micro-nanoparticles are prepared by emulsifying aqueous solutions of chitosan in acetic acid into an external oil phase [178]. The cross-linking agent can be added to the aqueous chitosan solution prior to the emulsification. The polysaccharides chitosan and sodium alginate form gels with counterions such as tripolyphosphate or calcium chloride. Nanoparticles can be prepared by emulsifying an aqueous polysaccharide solution into the oil phase followed by emulsification of an aqueous solution of the counterion solution.

The drawbacks of the W/O emulsification method include the use of large amounts of oils as the external phase, which must be removed by washing with organic solvents, heat stability problems of drugs, possible interactions of the cross-linking agent with the drug, and, as with all nanoparticles prepared by emulsification techniques, a fairly broad particle size distribution.

Gelatin and albumin nanoparticles have been prepared through desolvation of the dissolved macromolecules by either salts (e.g., sodium sulfate or ammonium sulfate) or ethanol [179–182]. This is, in principle, similar to a simple coacervation method. The particles can then be insolubilized through cross-linking with an optimum amount of aldehydes. These phase separation methods avoid the use of oils as the external phase.

Alginate nanoparticles have been prepared by the addition of an optimized amount of calcium chloride to a sodium alginate solution [183]. This so-called "microgel" can be crosslinked with the oppositely charged polymer, poly-*l*-lysine, to form nanospheres. This technique uses the well-known gelification phenomenon of sodium alginate with calcium ions, but at much lower concentrations than normally used for gel formation. Again, since only one phase is used, high drug loadings are difficult to obtain unless specific binding of the drug to the anionic polymeric carrier occurs.

VII. PARENTERAL DISPERSE SYSTEMS

During the past 30 years, there have been significant developments of parenteral disperse formulations. The use of parenteral emulsions can overcome the problems of low aqueous solubility and water hydrolysis of many drugs [184, 185]. Such formulations can avoid the use of conventional co-solvent systems and the undesirable effects caused by precipitation of drugs at the injection site. Recent developments of parenteral disperse formulations have the potential to provide sustained release and targeting of drugs [186–189].

A. Parenteral Emulsions

Like all parenteral products, parenteral emulsions are required to be sterile, isotonic, nonpyrogenic, nontoxic, and stable. Unique to parenteral emulsions are the requirements for droplet size and surface charge [190], since the parameters have a direct effect on both toxicity and stability.

Particle Size

The British Pharmacopoeia (1980) states that the diameter of emulsion globules for intravenous administration may not exceed 5 μm. Emulsion globules larger than 4–6 μm are known to increase the incidence of emboli and may cause changes in blood pressure [32, 190]. However, lipid particles larger than 7.5 μm have been reported to deform and pass through the pulmonary vasculature without difficulty [191]. In general, emulsions that contain globules 200–500 nm in size tend to be most physically stable. Smaller emulsions are utilized by the body more rapidly than larger ones [190].

Surface Charge

A reduction in the electrical charge is known to increase the flocculation and coalescence rates. Sufficient high zeta potential (> − 30 mV) ensures a stable emulsion by causing repulsion of adjacent droplets. The selection of suitable surfactants can help to optimize droplet surface charges and thus enhance emulsion stability. Lipid particles with either positive or negative surface charges are more stable and are cleared from the bloodstream more rapidly than those with neutral charge [192, 193].

Ingredients

Oils. Among many investigated oils, soy oil, middle-chain triglycerides (MCT), safflower oil, and cottonseed oils are favoured for use as the oil phase due to their low incidence of toxic reactions. Purity is regarded as an important criterion for parenteral use. Undesirable contaminants such as hydrogenated oil, saturated fatty materials, pigments, or oxidative decomposition products should be minimized.

Emulsifiers. Natural lecithin is one of the most widely used emulsifiers because it is metabolized in the body. However, type I allergic reaction to soybean lecithin emulsified in lipid solutions has been observed [195]. Among the synthetic emulsifying agents, block copolymers of polyoxyethylene-polyoxypropylene (poloxamer) have attracted increasing interest for parenteral emulsions. Other examples of emulsifiers commonly found in parenteral formulations are given in Table 9 [190].

Table 9 Most Commonly Used Emulsifiers in Parenteral Emulsions

Emulsifiers	Range
Egg lecithin	1–3% w/w
Soyabean lecithin	1–3% w/w
Phosphatidylcholine	Approximately 50%
Glycerol/propylene glycol	30–70% w/w individually
Glyceryl fatty acid esters	3% w/w
Pluronic F68, 88, 108	1.5–10%
Poloxamer 401 (Pluronic L121)	5%
Polysorbate 80	4%

Source: Adapted from Ref. 190.

Additives. Additives are used to adjust the tonicity and pH of emulsions and to increase emulsion stability. Glycerol is a commonly used isotonic agent for parenteral emulsions. The pH of the emulsion should be also adjusted close to a physiological pH of 7–8 by adding aqueous solutions of NaOH or HCl. Tocopherols and oleic acid may be added as antioxidants and stabilizer, respectively. Some commercially available fat emulsions and their compositions are listed in Table 10 [144].

Sterilization

Autoclaving can be used for the sterilization of parenteral emulsions, provided the required sterilization conditions do not lead to significant product degradation. Alternatively, parenteral emulsions can be

Table 10 Compositions of Some Commercially Available Fat Emulsions

Trade name (company)	Oil phase	Emulsifier	Other components
Intralipid	Soybean oil	Lecithin	Glycerol
(Kabi-Vitrum)	10–20%	1.2%	2.5%
Lipofundins	Soyabean oil	Soyabean lecithin	Xylitol
(Braun)	10–20%	0.75–1.2%	5%
Lipofundins	Cottonseed oil	Soyabean lecithin	Sorbitol
(Braun)	10%	0.75%	5%
Liposyn	Safflower oil	Lecithin	Glycerol
(Abbot)	10–20%	1.2%	2.5%
Travemulsion	Soybean protein	Lecithin	Glycerol
(Travenol)	10–20%	1.2%	2.5%

Source: Ref. 144.

sterilized by filtration if the emulsion globules can pass through the filter. For thermolabile products and/or products in which sterile filtration is almost impossible, terminal gamma irradiation may be useful. However, restrictions in the use of gamma sterilization differ from country to country, and in some cases changes in the product might occur. Most desirable in terms of stability, is aseptic processing in clean rooms, but there is also a high risk of contamination in the final product.

B. Parenteral Suspensions

Parenteral suspensions are heterogeneous systems consisting of a solid phase that is disperse within a liquid phase. The requirements for and limitations involved in preparing parenteral suspensions include microbiological control, ingredient allowance, and mechanical flow properties [196–198]. Excipients used in parenteral suspensions should be nonpyrogenic, nontoxic, and chemically inert. Flocculating and wetting agents are important ingredients to maintain product stability and good mechanical properties. Water for injection is the most widely used solvent in parenteral formulations but is sometimes not applicable to lipophilic compounds. Nonaqueous solvents can be used to promote solubility and stability. Examples of nonaqueous solvents used in parenteral products include benzyl benzoate, glycofurol, ethyl lactate, polyethylene glycols, glycerin, and ethanol [199]. The basic sterilization methods for solid materials used in parenteral suspensions are recrystallization, spray-drying, lyophilization, ethylene oxide gas, dry heat, and gamma irradiation.

Due to particle sizes in the micrometer range, parenteral suspensions are generally limited to either subcutaneous or intramuscular routes of administration. However, ultrafine suspensions can be approached by high-pressure homogenization [200]. The particle size obtained from this technique is in the 100–500 nm range, thus intravenous administration is possible [201]. General information on parenteral formulations is given in Chapter 12.

VIII. CHARACTERIZATION OF DISPERSE SYSTEMS

A. Particle Size Analysis

Particle size is a major characteristic of a disperse system. Particle size measurements provide the evaluation of possible particle aggregation or crystal growth, and particle size distribution data are often employed as fundamental quality control standards for pharmaceutical disperse systems. A broad particle size distribution is known to promote uneven settling in suspensions and coalescence in emulsions.

Various techniques and equipment are available for the measurement of particle size, shape, and volume. These include for microscopy, sieve analysis, sedimentation methods, photon correlation spectroscopy, and the Coulter counter or other electrical sensing devices. The specific surface area of original drug powders can also be assessed using gas adsorption or gas permeability techniques. It should be noted that most particle size measurements are not truly direct. Because the type of equipment used yields different equivalent spherical diameter, which are based on totally different principles, the particle size obtained from one method may or may not be compared with those obtained from other methods.

Microscopy

Microscopic or optical methods range in complexity and cost from a simple laboratory microscope to refined pieces of automated equipment. The microscope provides a direct observation of the sample and allows the evaluation of particle diameters. An ordinary microscope generally measures the particle size in the range of 0.2 μm to about 100 μm. With this method, a diluted or undiluted sample, e.g., an emulsion or suspension, is mounted on a slide or ruled cell and placed on a mechanical stage. The microscope eyepiece is fitted with a micrometer or a graticule by which the linear dimension of the particles may be estimated. The field can be photographed or projected onto a screen to ease the process of particle measurements. Electronic scanners and video recording equipment have been developed to remove the necessity of measuring particles by visual observation.

To obtain a value for the dimensions of an irregular particle, several measurement approaches can be used: Martin's diameter (defined as the length of a line that bisects the particle image), Feret's diameter (or end-to-end measurement, defined as the distance between two tangents on opposite sides of the particle parallel to some fixed direction), and the projected area diameter (defined as the diameter of a circle having the same area as that of the particle observed perpendicular to the surface on which the particle rests). With any technique, a sufficiently large number of particles is required in order to obtain a statistically valid conclusion. This is best accomplished by using a sampling procedure such as quartering or a device that riffles the samples.

One advantage of the optical method is to obtain information about the particle shape and presence of particle aggregations, e.g., degree and character of aggregations. A disadvantage is that the diameter is obtained from only two (of the three) dimensions of the particle, e.g., length and breadth; no information on the thickness or depth is available. The large number of particles that must be counted (300–500) in order to obtain a good estimation of the distribution makes the method rather slow and tedious.

Electron microscopes are high-resolution equipment used to visualize the samples having particle sizes below the limit of resolution of an optical microscope. The radiation source is a beam of high-energy electrons having wavelengths in the region of 0.1 Å. With current instrumentation, this results in smallest distances by which two objects are separated and remain distinguishable of approximately 5 Å. Scanning electron microscopy (SEM) finds wide application in the field of pharmaceutical technology followed by transmission electron microscopy (TEM) [202].

Sieve Analysis

Sieve analysis, based on either vibratory or suction principle, uses a series of standard sieves calibrated by the National Bureau of Standards. The method is generally used for screening coarse particles down to a material as fine as 44 μm (No. 325 sieve). Sieves produced by photoetching and electroforming techniques are now available with apertures from 90 down to 5 μm.

A typical testing procedure involves several steps. First, the selected number and size of sieves are stacked upon one another, with the largest openings (inversely related to mesh per inch) being at the top of the stack, and beneath that a pan to collect the particles finer than the smallest sieve. The known amount of powder to be analyzed is then placed on the top sieve and the set is vibrated in a mechanical device for a predetermined time period. The results are obtained by weighing the amount of material retained on each sieve and on the collecting pan. The suction method uses one sieve at a time and examines the amount retained on the screen. In both methods the data are expressed as frequency or cumulative frequency plots, respectively.

Sieving errors can arise from a number of variables, including sieve loading and duration and intensity of agitation [203]. Sieving can also cause attrition and, thus, size reduction of granular pharmaceutical materials. Standard sieving protocols must be employed in order to ensure reproducible particle size distributions between different batches of raw materials.

Sedimentation Method

This method is based on Stokes' law (see Sec. IV.A.). Practical techniques include simple sedimentation methods such as the Anderson pipette and the Cahn sedimentation balance. The Andreason pipette involves measuring the percentage of solids that settle with time in a graduated sedimentation vessel. Samples are withdrawn from the bottom of the vessel using a pipette, and the amount of solids is determined by drying and weighing. The Cahn sedimentation balance electronically records the amount of disperse powder settling out as a function of time. One advantage of this method is that the mass of particles is recorded continuously. Both methods are appropriate when the particle size is generally larger than 5 μm. In case particles smaller than 5 μm are to be evaluated, a centrifugal method is often employed to speed up the data collection by overcoming the effects of convection and diffusion. The method involves a photosedimentation device in which the light transmittance is measured through a cell filled with a dispersion of interest. An ultracentrifuge can also be used in such cases in order to increase the sedimentation rate of colloidal particles.

Coulter Counter and Electrical Sensing Devices

Counters, such as the Coulter Counter, determine the number of particles in a known volume of an electrolyte solution. The device employs the electrolyte displacement method and measures the equivalent spherical volume diameter, d_v. This type of equipment is used primarily to obtain the particle size distribution of the sample. It measures the change in an electrical sensing zone that occurs when a particle passes through an orifice positioned between two electrodes. The dispersion is drawn through a small orifice that has an electrode on either side. The disperse particles interfere with the current flow, causing the resistance to change. The resistance changes are related to the particle volumes and, when amplified as voltage pulses, may be counted. The instrument is capable of counting particles at a rate of approximately 4000 per second, and so both gross counts and particle size distributions are obtained in a relatively short period of time. Electronic pulse counters are also useful in studying particle growth, dissolution, and particulate contamination. Examples are the Coulter Counter and the Electrozone Counter. Coulter Electronics also manufactures a submicrometer particle sizing instrument, the Coulter Model N4, for analyzing particles in the size range of 0.003–0.3 μm. The instrument also provides molecular weights and diffusion coefficients.

Light Scattering

The quasi-elastic light-scattering technique (QELS), also called photon correlation spectroscopy (PCS), is based on the principle of light scattering and has been employed to determine the mean particle diameter and size distribution (polydispersity). Light scattering depends on the Faraday-Tyndall effect and is used widely in the determination of molecular weight, size, and shape of colloidal particles. Scattering may be described in terms of the turbidity, τ, the fractional decrease in intensity due to scattering as the incident light passes through a solution. When the particle is asymmetrical, the intensity of scattered light varies with the angle of observation, permitting an estimation of the shape and size of the particle. Light scattering has been used to study proteins, synthetic polymers, association colloids, and lyophobic sols.

Racey et al. [204, 205] applied QELS that uses laser light to determine diffusion coefficients and particle sizes as the Stokes' diameters. It consists of a laser light source, a temperature-controlled sample compartment, and a photomultiplier to detect the scattered light at a certain angle (usually 90°). QELS has been used in the examination of heparin aggregates in commercial preparations. The method is applicable for measuring the particle size ranging from 5 nm to approximately 3 μm. In this size range, the particles exhibit Brownian motion as a result of collisions with the molecules of surrounding liquid medium, which causes fluctuation in the intensity of scattered light. PCS, however, cannot characterize systems having broadly distributed particles. This problem has been overcome by combining sedimentation field-flow fractionation and QELS, which presents a detailed record of the particle size at each size interval.

Hydrodynamic Chromatography

This method is used particularly for colloids. A colloidal dispersion is forced through a long column packed with nonporous beads with an approximate radius of 10 μm. Particles of different particle size travel with different speeds around the beads and are thus collected in size fractions.

B. Determination of Electrical Properties

The movement of a charged particle with respect to an adjacent liquid phase is the basic principle underlying four electrokinetic phenomena: electrophoresis, electroosmosis, sedimentation potential, and streaming potential.

Electrophoresis involves the movement of a charged particle through a liquid under the influence of an applied potential difference. A sample is placed in an electrophoresis cell, usually a horizontal tube of circular cross section, fitted with two electrodes. When a known potential is applied across the electrodes, the particles migrate to the oppositely charged electrode. The direct current voltage applied needs to be adjusted to obtain a particle velocity that is neither too fast nor too slow to allow for errors in measurement and Brownian motion, respectively. It is also important that the measurement is taken reasonably quickly in order to avoid sedimentation in the cell. Prior to each measurement, the apparatus should be calibrated with particles of known zeta potential, such as rabbit erythrocytes.

The velocity of particle migration, v, across the field is a function of the surface charge or zeta potential and is observed visually by means of an ultramicroscope equipped with a calibrated eyepiece and a scale. The movement is measured by timing the individual particles over a certain distance, and the results of approximately 10–15 timing measurements are then averaged. From the measured particle velocity, the electrophoretic mobility (defined as v/E, where E is the potential gradient) can be calculated.

Electroosmosis is essentially opposite in principle to that electrophoresis. In this case, the particles are rendered immobile by forming a capillary or a porous plug. The liquid now moves through this plug or membrane, across which a potential is applied. The rate of flow of liquid through the plug is then determined under standard conditions. Electroosmosis provides another method for obtaining the zeta potential. Streaming potential differs from electroosmosis in that the potential is created by forcing a liquid to flow through a plug or bed of particles. Sedimentation potential measures the potential generated when the particles undergo sedimentation.

The determination of the zeta potential of particles in a disperse system provides useful information concerning the sign and magnitude of the charge and its effect on the stability of the system (see Sec. II.B) [56, 206–208]. It can be of value in the development of pharmaceutical suspensions, particularly if the controlled aggregation approach is used. The use of the zeta potential to evaluate the electrophoretic properties of other dosage forms such as liposomes and microcapsules has also been reported [209, 210].

A number of semi-automated or fully automated instruments are currently used for studying the electrokinetic properties. These include the electrophoretic mass transport analyzer (Zeta Potential Analyzer, Micrometrics Instrument Corp.), the streaming current detector (Hydroscan, Leeds and Northrup Co.), the electrokinetic sonic amplitude device (Matec Instruments, Inc.), and the instruments that determine zeta potential by measuring the electrophoretic mobility of the disperse particles in a charged electric field (Zeta Reader, Komline-Sanderson; Zeta Meter, Laser Zee Meter, Pen Kem Co.). The first three devices are suitable for determining the average zeta potential of coarse suspensions in systems having high solids contents, whereas the latter three are more useful for the measurement of colloidal particles in systems with low solids contents.

C. Rheological Measurements

Rheological evaluations can be simple or complex, depending on the nature of the product. They feature important quality control of all disperse systems. For example, the adequacy of hydration and quality control of the gums used as viscosity-imparting agents in the products is best confirmed by a rheological test. These natural or synthetic gums are polymers of varying molecular weights from lot to lot, which directly affect the product's viscosity. In addition, the degree of dispersion, particle size, and size distribution influence the viscosity and dispersion consistency. Also, formulation additives, such as sweeteners, surfactants, and flocculating agents, influence the rheological properties of the dispersions. Viscosity characteristics of a suspension may be altered not only by the vehicle used but also by the solids content. Increasing amounts of solid particles lead to increased viscosities of the disperse system. The viscosity of lyophobic dispersions is not much higher than that of the original liquid because of minimal interaction between the internal and external phases. The viscosity of lyophilic systems, especially polymer solutions, is much higher because of the interaction between the two phases. As a result of this interaction, dispersions possessing both Newtonian and non-Newtonian properties are formed. Highly viscous or rigid gels can be formed at higher polymer concentrations.

A wide variety of viscometers (ranging from simple to sophisticated) has been designed to evaluate the rheological properties of various disperse systems. It is necessary to select one suitable for the viscosity ranges encountered in a given application. The instrument should provide the required rheological data over the desired range of shear, time under shear, time and temperature. Viscometers are classified as those that operate at a single shear rate and those that allow more than one rate of shear to be examined. The simplest qualitative measurement of viscosity may be obtained by bubble, cup, falling-ball, falling-rod, and capillary viscometers. These simple devices provide a one-point measurement and are widely used for Newtonian fluids and dilute solutions. The glass capillary Cannon-Fenske, Ubbelohde, and Ostwald viscometers are the most popular instruments based on this method.

Most rheometers in use to date are based on rotating the samples and measuring its response to the applied stress by a variety of sensors. The advantages of rotational viscometers are that the shear rate can be varied over a wide range, and that continuous measurements at a given shear rate or shear stress can be made for extended periods of time, allowing the evaluation of time-dependency and shear-dependency properties. Viscometers of this type are routinely found in many pharmaceutical laboratories. Simple rotational viscometers are the Stormer viscometer, the ICI viscometer, and the Brookfield viscometer. A Brookfield viscometer with the helipath attachment is a valuable piece of rheological equipment for measuring the settling behavior and structure of pharmaceutical suspensions. The instrument consists of a slowly rotating T-bar spindle, which is lowered into an undisturbed sample. The dial reading of the viscometer measures the resistance to flow that the spindle encounters from the structure at various levels in the sediment. Taking rheograms at various time intervals, under standard conditions, gives a description of the suspension and its physical stability. The technique is most useful for viscous suspensions high in solids that develop sufficient shear stress for measurement. The instrument is also excellent for characterizing flocculated systems. To simulate the situation illustrated in Fig. 2, coaxial-cylinder viscometers have been designed in which the plates are bent to form cylindrical surfaces, one of which is stationary and the other is rotating. There are two types of concentric cylinder viscometers, namely, the Searle system and the Couette system.

In the Couette type, the material is contained in an annular gap between the inner cylindrical bob or spindle and the outer, concentric cylindrical cup. In the Stormer viscometer or the more advanced Haake Rotovisco, the cup is stationary. Cone-and-plate and parallel-plate rheometers are designed to handle small-quantity samples, from about 0.2 to 5 mL. The plate may be stationary while the cone is rotating, or vice versa. The angle between the cone and the plate has to be extremely small, usually 0.1–3°. Since the sample size is very small, this method is very sensitive to sample drying and temperature changes. Another disadvantage of this method is the loss of material due to slinging from the gap and sample heating, especially at high shear rates.

D. Temperature and Gravitational Stress Tests

Disperse systems can be subjected to cyclic temperature testing, e.g., to conditions of repeated freezing and thawing (e.g., −50°C to +40 °C in 24 h) exposing them to elevated temperatures (>40 °C) for short periods of storage to test for the physical stability. The value of such a stress test procedure may be questionable since the exposure to elevated temperatures often results in a drastic change in the drug's solubility. Significant amounts of drug may go into solution and reprecipitate upon subsequent cooling. Most suspension systems contain surfactants and protective colloids to prevent crystal growth, and, thus, inducing crystal growth during stress testing may be of limited value. The use of stressful aging tests, however, has one advantage. If a given suspension is able to withstand exposure to extreme temperatures, it is safe to assume that the product will have good physical stability during prolonged storage at ambient temperature. On the other hand, failure of any preparations to meet such stringent testing procedures should not be considered a bar to further testing, since many marketed pharmaceutical suspensions would have been rejected from further consideration on this basis alone.

The use of stress tests to study the stability of emulsions has been described in Sec. V.C.

IX. MANUFACTURING AND EQUIPMENT

The preparation of satisfactory disperse systems consists of three main steps: preparing the internal phase in the proper size range, dispersing the internal phase in the dispersion medium, and, finally, stabilizing the resultant product. These three steps may be done sequentially, but in many cases (e.g., emulsions), they are usually done simultaneously.

Suspensions can be prepared by either dispersing finely divided powders in an appropriate vehicle or causing precipitation within the vehicle. For most pharmaceutical preparations, the proper size of the internal phase is obtained by a mechanical breakdown of the solid material. One of the most rapid, convenient, and inexpensive methods of producing fine drug powders about 10–50 μm in size is micropulverization. Micropulverizers are high-speed attrition or impact mills, which are efficient in reducing powders to the size acceptable for most oral and topical suspensions. For finer particles, fluid energy grinding, sometimes referred to as jet-milling or micronizing, is quite effective. By this process, the shearing action of high-velocity compressed air streams on the particles in a confined chamber produces the desired ultra-fine or micronized particles. The particles are accelerated to high velocities by the sonic and supersonic velocity of turbulent air streams and collide with one another, resulting in fragmentation and size reduction. These micronized drugs are often employed in parenteral and ophthalmic preparations. Particles of extremely small dimension may also be produced by spray-drying techniques [211]. This method results in a porous, free flowing, easily wetted, monodisperse microcrystalline powder. Other equipment for particle size reduction include colloid mills, ball mills, ultrasonic generators, or homogenizers.

The precipitation (condensation, aggregation) method is more complex and has been used to create particles of suitable size by permitting the atoms or molecules of the material to gather together. In this process, the material is dissolved in a suitable solvent, then a miscible nonsolvent is added and a precipitate is formed. For example, fine sulfur particles can be obtained when water (nonsolvent) is added into an alcoholic solution of sulfur. Suspensions can be prepared by controlled crystallization wherein a supersaturated solution is cooled rapidly with constant agitation to obtain a large number of small, uniform drug crystals. Microcrystals can also be conveniently produced by bubbling liquid nitrogen through a saturated solution of solute prior to solvent freezing. Other methods for obtaining fine particles include phase change such as sublimation and pH adjustment. Shock cool methods can offer a possible solution to the electrostatic charge problems associated with dry particle milling. Chemical reactions, such as double decomposition, have also been used for certain pharmaceutical preparations, e.g., White lotion.

The second step is to disperse the particles within the dispersion medium. In emulsions, this step is accomplished at the same time that particle reduction occurs (Sec. V.B. gives more details on the commonly applied techniques to obtain pharmaceutically relevant emulsions). Surfactants are usually added in order to promote both particle size reduction and uniform dispersion. Suspensions may be prepared by dispersing the particles resulting from the mechanically breakdown process, along with an addition of a surfactant to aid the wetting process. Alternatively, both size reduction and dispersion processes can take place simultaneously in a manner similar to that for emulsions. Homogenization is normally required when various other additives are incorporated. On a laboratory scale, an ultrasonic generator may be used, whereas a conventional colloid mill is more suitable for an industrial-scale production. The most important techniques to prepare nanoparticles are described in Sec. VI.B.

For the production of emulsions on a large scale, the oil and water phases are often heated separately in large tanks. When waxes are present, both phases must be heated at a temperature above the highest melting point of any one component. One phase is then pumped into the tank containing the second phase with constant agitation throughout the time of addition. After cooling, the product is once again homogenized and then packaged. Semisolid preparations, such as creams and ointments, are prepared using appropriate mixing machinery. Often the dispersion step is carried out with colloid mills or homogenizers at elevated temperatures to reduce the viscosity of waxy constituents. On a small scale, a mortar and pestle may be used for communition, and dispersion may be done either sequentially or simultaneously (see Sec. V.B.). Once a satisfactory R&D laboratory-scale formulation has been developed, the problem of pilot- and manufacturing-scale production must be solved. In this scale-up step, formulators may encounter problems of mixing and dispersion not found in a small-scale production [212, 213].

REFERENCES

1. SE Tabibi, CT Rhodes. Disperse systems. In: GS Banker, CT Rhodes, eds. *Modern Pharmaceutics*, 3rd ed. New York: Marcel Dekker, 1996, pp 299–331.
2. JG Nairn. Disperse systems. In: J Swarbrick, JC Boylan, eds. *Encyclopedia of Pharmaceutical Technology*, Vol. 4. New York: Marcel Dekker, 1992, pp 107–120.
3. RB Pates, IJR Patel, MC Roggle, VP Shah, VK Prasad, A Selen, PG Welling. Bioavailability of hydrochlorothiazide from tablets and suspensions. J Pharm Sci 73:359–365, 1984.
4. PJ Stout, SA Howard, JW Mauger. Dissolution of pharmaceutical suspensions. In: J Swarbrick, JC Boylan, eds. *Encyclopedia of Pharmaceutical Technology*, Vol. 4. New York: Marcel Dekker, 1992, pp 169–192.
5. MD Donovan, DR Flanagan. Bioavailability of disperse dosage form. In: HA Lieberman, MM Rieger, GS Banker, eds. *Pharmaceutical Dosage Forms: Disperse Systems*, Vol. 1. 2nd ed. New York: Marcel Dekker, 1996, pp 315–376.
6. JW Mauger, SA Howard, K Amin. Dissolution profiles for finely divided drug suspensions. J Pharm Sci 72(2):190–193, 1983.
7. K Hirano, H Yamada. Studies on the absorption of practically water-insoluble drugs following injection VI: subcutaneous absorption from aqueous suspensions in rats. J Pharm Sci 71(5):500–505, 1982.
8. RA Nash. Pharmaceutical suspensions. In: HA Lieberman, MM Rieger, GS Banker, eds. *Pharmaceutical Dosage Forms: Disperse Systems*, Vol. 1. New York: Marcel Dekker, 1988, pp 151–198.
9. NK Patel, L Kennon, RS Levinson. Pharmaceutical suspensions. In: L Lachman, HA Lieberman, JL Kanig, eds. *The Theory and Practice of Industrial Pharmacy*, 3rd ed. Philadelphia: Lea & Febiger, 1986, pp 479–501.
10. J Swarbrick. Coarse dispersions. In: AR Gennaro, ed. *Remington: The Science and Practice of Pharmacy*, 19th ed. Easton, Pennsylvania: Mack Publishing Co., 1995, pp 278–291.
11. MJ Falkiewicz. Theory of suspensions. In: HA Lieberman, MM Rieger, GS Banker, eds. *Pharmaceutical Dosage Forms: Disperse Systems*, Vol. 1. New York: Marcel Dekker, 1998, pp 13–48.
12. DJ Burgess. Colloids and colloid drug delivery systems. In: J Swarbrick, JC Boylan, eds. *Encyclopedia of Pharmaceutical Technology*, Vol. 3. New York: Marcel Dekker, 1992, pp 31–64.
13. A Martin. *Physical Pharmacy*, 4th ed. Philadelphia: Lea & Febiger, 1993, pp 393–422.
14. MJ Alonso. Nanoparticulate drug carrier technology. In: S Cohen, H Bernstein, eds. *Microparticulate Systems for the Delivery of Proteins and Vaccines*. New York: Marcel Dekker, 1996, pp 203–242.
15. R Bodmeier, P Maincent. Polymeric dispersions as drug carriers. In: HA Lieberman, MM Rieger, GS Banker, eds. *Pharmaceutical Dosage Forms: Disperse Systems*, Vol. 3. 2nd ed. New York: Marcel Dekker, 1998, pp 87–128.
16. F Jaeghere, E Doelker, R Gurny. Nanoparticles. In: E Mathiowitz, ed. *Encyclopdia of Controlled Drug Delivery*, Vol. 2. New York: John Wiley & Sons, 1999, pp 641–664.
17. JS Lucks, BW Müller, RH Müller. Polymeric and emulsion carriers—interaction with antiflocculants and ionic surfactants. Int J Pharm 63:183–188, 1990.
18. RH Müller, BHL Böhm. Nanosuspensions. In: RH Müller, S Benita, BHL Böhm, eds. *Emulsions and*

Nanosuspensions for the Formulation of Poorly Soluble Drugs. Stuttgart: Medpharm Scientific Publishers, 1998, pp 149–174.

19. TA Wheatley, CR Steuernagel. Latex emulsions for controlled drug delivery. In: JW McGinity, ed. *Aqueous Polymeric Coatings for Pharmaceutical Dosage Forms*,
2nd ed. New York: Marcel Dekker, 1997, pp 1–54.
20. MR Harris, I Ghebre-Sellassie. Aqueous polymeric coating for modified release oral dosage forms. In: JW McGinity, ed. *Aqueous Polymeric Coatings for Pharmaceutical Dosage forms*, 2nd ed. New York: Marcel Dekker, 1997, pp 81–100.
21. KOR Lehmann. Chemistry and application properties of polymethacrylate coating systems. In: JW McGinity, ed. *Aqueous Polymeric Coatings for Pharmaceutical Dosage forms*, 2nd ed. New York: Marcel Dekker, 1997, pp 101–176.
22. J Wang, I Ghebre-Sellassie. Aqueous polymer dispersions as film formers. In: HA Lieberman, MM Rieger, GS Banker, eds. Pharmaceutical Dosage Forms: Disperse Systems, Vol. 3. 2nd ed. New York: Marcel Dekker, 1998, pp 129–161.
23. B Idson. Pharmaceutical emulsions. In: HA Lieberman, MM Rieger, GS Banker, eds. *Pharmaceutical Dosage Forms: Disperse Systems*, Vol. 1. New York: Marcel Dekker, 1988, pp 199–244.
24. GM Eccleston. Emulsions. In: J Swarbrick, JC Boylan, eds. *Encyclopedia of Pharmaceutical Technology*, Vol. 5. New York: Marcel Dekker, 1992, pp 137–188.
25. BA Mulley. Medicinal emulsions. In: KJ Lissant, ed. *Emulsions and Emulsion Technology, Part I*. New York: Marcel Dekker, 1974, pp 291–350.
26. MM Rieger. Emulsions. In: L Lachman, HA Lieberman, JL Kanig, eds. *The Theory and Practice of Industrial Pharmacy*, 3rd ed. Philadelphia: Lea & Febiger, 1986, pp 502–532.
27. LH Block. Pharmaceutical emulsions and microemulsions. In: HA Lieberman, MM Rieger, GS Banker, eds. *Pharmaceutical Dosage Forms: Disperse Systems*, Vol. 2. New York: Marcel Dekker, 1996, pp 47–110.
28. N Garti. Double emulsions-scope, limitations and new achievements. Colloids Surfaces A: Physicochem Eng Aspects 123–124:233–246, 1997.
29. SH Klang, M Parnas, S Benita. Emulsions as drug carriers – possibilities, limitations and future perspectives. In: RH Müller, S. Benita, BHL Böhm, eds. *Emulsions and Nanosuspensions for the Formulation of Poorly Soluble Drugs*. Stuttgart: Medpharm Scientific Publishers, 1998, pp 31–78.
30. B Lundberg. Preparation of drug-carrier emulsions stabilized with phosphatidylcholine-surfactant mixtures. J Pharm Sci 83(1):72–75, 1994.
31. DP Bluhm, RS Summers, MMJ Lowes, HH Durrheim. Lipid emulsion content and vitamin A stability in TPN admixtures. Int J Pharm 68:277–280, 1991.
32. JB Boyett, CW Davis. Injectable emulsions and suspensions. In: HA Lieberman, HA, MM Rieger, GS Banker, eds. *Pharmaceutical Dosage Forms: Disperse Systems*, Vol. 2, New York: Marcel Dekker, 1989, pp 379–416.
33. PJ Breen, DT Wasan, Y-H Kim, AD Nikolov, CS Shetty. Emulsions and emulsion stability. In: J Sjöblom, ed. *Emulsions and Emulsion Stability*. New York: Marcel Dekker, 1996, pp 23–286.
34. MJ Parnham. Safety and tolerability of intravenously administered phospholipids and emulsions. In: RH Müller, S Benita, BHL Böhm, eds. *Emulsions and Nanosuspensions for the Formulation of Poorly Soluble Drugs*. Stuttgart: Medpharm Scientific Publishers, 1998, pp 131–140.
35. M Rosoff. Specialized pharmaceutical emulsions. In: HA Lieberman, MM Rieger, GS Banker, eds. *Pharmaceutical Dosage Forms: Disperse Systems*, Vol. 3, 2nd ed. New York: Marcel Dekker, 1998, pp 1–42.
36. K Westesen, T Wehler. Physicochemical characterization of a model intravenous oil-in-water emulsion. J Pharm Sci 81(8):777–786, 1992.
37. C Leuner, J Dressman. Improving drug solubility for oral delivery using solid dispersions. Eur J Pharm Biopharm 50(1):47–60, 2000.
38. JJ Sciarra. Aerosols. In: AR Gennaro, ed. *Remington: The Science and Practice of Pharmacy*, 19th ed. Easton, Pennsylvania: Mack Publishing Co., 1995, pp 1676–1692.
39. MJ Clarke, MJ Tobyn, TN Staniforth. Physicochemical factors governing the performance of nedocromil sodium as a dry powder aerosol. J Pharm Sci 89(9):11601–1169, 2000.
40. T. Allen. Particle size measurement. In: JC Williams, ed. *The Powder Technology Series*. London: Chapman and Hall, 1975.
41. JW Vanderhoff, MS El-Aasser. Theory of colloids. In: HA Lieberman, MM Rieger, GS Banker, eds. *Pharmaceutical Dosage Forms: Disperse Systems*, Vol. 1, 2nd ed. New York: Marcel Dekker, 1996, pp 91–152.
42. H Heywood. Symposium on particle size analysis. Inst Chem Eng Supp 25:14–24, 1947.
43. I Goodarznia, DN Sutherland. Floc simulation: Effects of particle size and shape. Chem Eng Sci 30:407–412, 1975.
44. A Heyd, D Dhabhar. Particle shape effect on caking of coarse granulated antacid suspensions. Drug Cosmet Ind 125:42–45. 1979.
45. M Bisrat, C Nyström. Physicochemical aspects of drug release. VIII. The relation between particle size and surface specific dissolution rate in agitated suspensions. Int J Pharm 47:223–231, 1988.
46. A Martin. *Physical Pharmacy*, 4th ed. Philadelphia: Lea & Febiger, 1993, pp 423–452.
47. DP McNamara, ML Vieira, JR Crison. Dissolution of pharmaceuticals in simple and complex systems. In: GL Amidon, PI Lee, EM Topp, eds. *Transport Processes in*

Pharmaceuticl Systems. New York: Marcel Dekker, 2000.

48. PC Hiemenz. *Principles of Colloid and Surface chemistry,* 2nd ed. New York: Marcel Dekker, 1986.
49. T Handa, Y Maitani, K Miyazima, M Nakagaki. Interfacial phenomena. In: J Swarbrick, JC Boylan, eds. *Encyclopedia of Pharmaceutical Technology*, Vol. 8, New York: Marcel Dekker, 1993, pp 131–174.
50. G Zografi. Interfacial phenomena. In: AR Gennaro, ed. *Remington: The Science and Practice of Pharmacy*, 19th ed. Easton, Pennsylvania: Mack Publishing Co., 1995, pp 241–251.
51. EJW Verwey, JThG Overbeek. *Theory of the Stability of Lyophobic Colloids*. Amsterdam: Elsevier, 1948.
52. B Derjaguin, L Landau. Acta Physica Chim, USSR 14:663, 1941.
53. B Derjaguin, L Landau. J Exp Theor Physics, USSR 11:802, 1941.
54. BA Matthews, CT Rhodes. Use of the Derjaguin, Landau, Verwey and Overbeek theory to interpret pharmaceutical suspension stability. J Pharm Sci 59:521–525, 1970.
55. JB Kayes. Pharmaceutical suspensions: relation between zeta potential, sedimentation volume and suspension stability. J Pharm Pharmacol 29:199–204, 1977.
56. A Delgado, V Gallardo, A Parrera, F González-Caballero. A study of the electrokinetic and stability properties of nitrofurantoin suspensions. II: Flocculation and redispersion properties as compared with theoretical interaction energy curves. J Pharm Sci 79:709–718, 1990.
57. ThF Tadros. Polymeric surfactants:, stabilization of emulsions and dispersions. In: E Desmond Goddard, JV Gruber, eds. *Principles of Polymer Science and Technology in Cosmetics and Personal Care*. New York: Marcel Dekker, 1999, pp 73–112.
58. RJ Meyer, L Cohen. Rheology of natural and synthetic hydrophilic polymer solutions and related to suspending ability. J Soc Cosmet Chem 10:1–11, 1959.
59. P Sherman. The flow properties of emulsions. J Pharm Pharmacol 16:1–25, 1964.
60. JT Carstensen. *Theory of Pharmaceutical Systems*, Vol. 2, *Heterogeneous Systems*. New York: Academic Press, 1973, pp 1–89.
61. DE Deem. Rheology of dispersed systems. In: HA Lieberman, MM Rieger, GS Banker, eds. *Pharmaceutical Dosage Forms: Disperse Systems*, Vol. 1, New York: Marcel Dekker, 1988, pp 367–514.
62. MA Ramadan, R Tawashi. Effect of surface geometry and morphic features on the flow characteristics of microsphere suspensions. J Pharm Sci 79:929–933, 1990.
63. PE Miner. Emulsion rheology: creams and lotions. In: D Laba, ed. *Rheological Properties of Cosmetics and Toiletries*. New York: Marcel Deklcer, 1993, pp 313–370.
64. CD Vaughan. Predicting stability in rheologically modified systems. In: D Laba, ed. *Rheological Properties of Cosmetics and Toiletries*. New York: Marcel Dekker, 1993, pp 371–401.
65. HN Naé. Introduction to rheology. In: D Laba, ed. *Rheological Properties of Cosmetics and Toiletries*. New York: Marcel Dekker, 1993, pp 9–33.
66. MM Rieger. Surfactants. In: HA Lieberman, MM Rieger, GS Banker, eds. *Pharmaceutical Dosage Forms: Disperse Systems*, Vol. 1, 2nd ed. New York: Marcel Dekker, 1996, pp 211–286.
67. RG Laughlin. HLB, from a thermodynamic perspective. J Soc Cosmet Chem 32:371–378, 1981.
68. H Schott. Solubility parameter and hydrophilic lipophilic balance of nonionic surfactants. J Pharm Sci 73:790–792, 1984.
69. WC Griffin. Classification of surface-active agents by "HLB". J Soc Cosmet Chem 1:311–326, 1949.
70. WC Griffin. Emulsions. In: RE Kirk, DF Othmer, eds. *Encyclopedia of Chemical Technology*, Vol. 5, New York: Interscience, 1950, pp 692–718.
71. Atlas Booklet. A Guide to Formulation of Industrial Emulsions with Atlas Surfactants, Wilmington: Atlas Powder Co., 1953.
72. MT Clarke. Rheological additives. In: D Laba, ed. *Rheological Properties of Cosmetics and Toiletries*. New York: Marcel Dekker, 1993, pp 55–152.
73. JL Zatz, JJ Berry, DA Alderman. Viscosity-imparting agents in disperse systems. In: HA Lieberman, MM Rieger, GS Banker, eds. *Pharmaceutical Dosage Forms: Disperse Systems*, Vol. 2, New York: Marcel Dekker, 1989, pp 171–204.
74. JA Ranucci, IB Silverstein. Polymeric pharmaceutical excipients. In: HA Lieberman, MM Rieger, GS Banker, eds. *Pharmaceutical Dosage Forms: Disperse Systems*, Vol. 3, 2nd ed. New York: Marcel Dekkter, 1998, pp 243–289.
75. CB Anger, D Rupp, P Lo, H Takuri. Preservation of dispersed systems. In: HA Lieberman, MM Rieger, GS Banker, eds. *Pharmaceutical Dosage Forms: Disperse Systems*, Vol. 1, 2nd ed. New York: Marcel Dekker, 1996, pp 377–435.
76. TE Haag, DF Loncrini. Esters of para-hydroxybenzoic acid. In: JJ Kabara, ed. *Cosmetic and Drug Preservation*. New York: Marcel Dekker, 1984, pp 63–77.
77. WB Hugo. Phenols as preservatives for pharmaceutical and cosmetic products. In: JJ Kabara, ed. *Cosmetic and Drug Preservation*. New York: Marcel Dekker, 1984, pp 109–113.
78. TJ McCarthy. Formulated factors affecting the activity of preservatives. In: JJ Kabara, ed. *Cosmetic and Drug Preservation*. New York: Marcel Dekker, 1984, pp 359–388.
79. KS Alexander, J Azizi, D Dollimore, V Upaala. Interpretation of the hindered settling of calcium carbonate

suspensions in terms of permeability. J Pharm Sci 79:401–406, 1990.

80. RDC Jones, BA Matthews, CT Rhodes. Physical stability of sulfaguanidine suspensions. J Pharm Sci 59:518–520, 1970.
81. A Martin. *Physical Pharmacy*, 4th ed. Philadelphia: Lea & Febiger, 1993, pp 477–511.
82. JL Zatz, L Schnitzer, P Sarpotdar. Flocculation of sulfamerazine suspensions by a cationic polymer. J Pharm Sci 68(12):1491–1494, 1979.
83. GC Jeffrey, RH Ottewill. Reversible aggregation Part reversible flocculation monitored by turbidity measurements. Colloids Polymer Sci 266:173–179, 1988.
84. T Higuchi. Some physical chemical aspects of suspension formulation. J Am Pharm Assoc, Sci Ed 47:657–660, 1958.
85. KJ Frederick. Performance and problems of pharmaceutical suspensions. J Pharm Sci 50:531–535, 1961.
86. BA Matthews. The use of the Coulter counter in emulsion and suspension studies. Can J Pharm Sci 6:29–34, 1971.
87. JE Carless. Dissolution and crystal growth in aqueous suspension of cortisone acetate. J Pharm Pharmacol 10:630–639, 1968.
88. SA Young, G Buckton. Particle growth in aqueous suspensions: the influence of surface energy and polarity. Int J Pharm 60:235–241, 1990.
89. NB Shah, BB Sheth. Effect of polymers on dissolution from drug suspensions. J Pharm Sci 65(11):1618–1623, 1976.
90. CM Ofner III, RL Schnaare, JB Schwartz. Reconstitutable suspensions. In: HA Lieberman, MM Rieger, GS Banker, eds. *Pharmaceutical Dosage Forms: Disoerse Systems*, Vol. 2, New York: Marcel Dekker, 1989, pp 317–334.
91. R Bodmeier, O Paeratakul. Suspensions and dispersible dosage forms of multiparticulates. In: I Ghebre-Sellassie, ed. *Multiparticulate Oral Drug Delivery*. New York: Marcel Dekker, 1994, pp 143–157.
92. Y Kawashima, T Iwamoto, T Niwa, H Takeuchi. Preparation and characterization of a new controlled release ibuprofen suspension for improving suspendability. Int J Pharm 75:25–36, 1991.
93. R Sjöqvist, C Graffner, I Ekman, W Sinclair, JP Woods. In vivo validation of the release rate and palatability of remoxipride-modified release suspension. Pharm Res 10(7):1020–1026, 1993.
94. Y Raghunathan (to Pennwalt Corporation). U.S. Patent 4,221,778 (1980).
95. Y Raghunathan, L Amsel, O Hinsvark, W Bryant. Sustained-release drug delivery system I: coated ion-exchange resin system for phenylpropanolamine and other drugs. J Pharm Sci 70:379–384, 1981.
96. JE Tingstad Physical stability testing of pharmaceuticals. J Pharm Sci 53(8):955–962, 1964.
97. TF Tadros, B Vincent. Emulsion stability. In: P Becher, ed. *Encyclopedia of Emulsion Technology*. Vol. 1, New York: Dekker, 1983, pp 129–285.
98. J Mikula, VA Munoz. Characterization of emulsions and suspensions in the petroleum industry using cryo-SEM and CLSM. Colloids Surfaces A: Physicochem Eng Aspects, 174(1–2):23–36, 2000.
99. DBR Kumar, MR Reddy, VN Mulay, N Krishnamurti. Acrylic co-polymer emulsion binders for green machining of ceramics. Eur Polym J 36(7):1503–1510, 2000.
100. M Chappat. Some applications of emulsions. Colloids Surfaces A: Physicochem Eng Aspects 9:57–77, 1994.
101. Z Ju, Y Duan, Z Ju. Plant oil emulsion modifies internal atmosphere, delays fruit ripening and inhibits internal browning in Chinese pears. Postharvest Biol and Tech 20(3):243–250, 2000.
102. Y Sela, S Magdassi, N Garti. Release of markers from the inner water phase of W/O/W emulsions stabilized by silicone based polymeric surfactants. J Control Release 33(1):1–12, 1995.
103. D Rousseau. Fat crystals and emulsion stability—a review. Food Res Inter 33(1):3–14, 2000.
104. K Heinzelmann, K Franke. Using freezing and drying techniques of emulsions for the microencapsulation of fish oil to improve oxidation stability. Colloids Surfaces B: Biointerfaces 12(3–6):223–229, 1999.
105. P Paquin. Technological properties of high pressure homogenizers: the effect of fat globules, milk proteins and polysaccharides. Int Dairy J 9(3–6):329–335, 1999.
106. SM Joscelyne, G Traegardh. Food emulsions using membrane emulsification: conditions for producing small droplets. J Food Eng 39(1):59–64, 1999.
107. HD Goff. Colloidal Aspects of Ice Cream-A Review, Int Dairy J 7(6–7):363–373, 1997.
108. DJ McClements. Advances in the application of ultrasound in food analysis and processing. Trends Food Sci Tech 6(9):293–299, 1995.
109. D Peressini, A Sensidoni, B de Cindio. Rheological Characterization of Traditional and light mayonnaises. J Food Eng 35(4):409–417, 1998.
110. A M. Lipid emulsions in parenteral nutrition. Ann Nutr Metab 43(1):1–13, 1999.
111. S Ding. Recent developments in ophthalmic drug delivery. Pharm Sci Tech Today 1(8):328–335, 1998.
112. CA Gogos, F Kalfarentzos. Total parenteral nutrition and immune system activity: A review. Nutrition 11(4):339–344, 1995.
113. H Okochi, M Nakano. Preparation and evaluation of W/O/W type emulsions containing vancomycin. Adv Drug Del Rev 45(1):5–26, 2000.
114. F Nielloud, G Marti-Mestres, JP Laget, C Fernandez, H Maillols. Emulsion formulations:study of the influence of parameters with experimental designs. Drug Dev Ind Pharm 22(2):159–166, 1996.

115. M Gallarate, ME Carlotti, M Trotta, S Bovo. On the stability of ascorbic acid in emulsified systems for topical and cosmetic use. Int J Pharm 188(2):233–241, 1999.
116. C Gallegos, JM Franco. Rheology of food, cosmetics and pharmaceuticals. Curr Opin Colloid Interf Sci 4(4):288–293, 1999.
117. D Miller, EM Wiener, A Turowski, C Thunig, H Hoffmann. O/W emulsions for cosmetic products stabilized by alkyl phosphates rheology and storage tests. Colloids Surfaces A: Physicochem Eng Aspects 152(1–2):155–160, 1999.
118. R Clark. Cosmetic emulsions. In: HW Hibbott, ed. *Handbook of Cosmetic Science*. New York: Pergamon Press, 1963, pp 175–204.
119. BW Barry. *Dermatological Formulations*. New York: Marcel Dekker, 1983, pp 296–350.
120. P Becher. Testing of emulsion properties. In: *Emulsions Theory and Practice*, 2nd ed. New York: Reinhold Publ. Co., 1957, pp 381–429.
121. P Couvreur, MJ Blanco-Prieto, F Puisieux, B Roques, E Fattal. Multiple emulsion technology for the design of microspheres containing peptides and olegopeptides. Adv Drug Del Rev 28:85–96, 1997.
122. N Garti, A Aserin. Double emulsions stabilized by macromolecular surfactants. Advances in colloid and interfaces science 65:37–69, 1996.
123. N Garti. Double emulsions-scope, limitations and new achievements. Colloids Surfaces A: Physicochem Eng Aspects 123–124:233–246, 1997.
124. J Herrmann, R Bodmeier. Biodegradable somatostatin acetate containing microspheres prepared by various aqueous and non-aqueous solvent evaporation method. Eur J Pharm Biopharm 45(1):75–82, 1998.
125. PB O'Donnell, JW McGinity. Preparation of microspheres by the solvent evaporation technique. Adv Drug Del Rev 28(1):25–42, 1997.
126. FB Rosevear. Liquid crystals: The mesomorphic phases of surfactant compositions. J Soc Cosmet Chem 19:581, 1968.
127. J Sjöblom, R Lindberg, SE Friberg. Microemulsions-phase equilibria characterization, structures, applications and chemical reactions, Adv Colloid Interf Sci 65:125–287, 1996.
128. HN Bhargava, A Narurkar, LM Lieb. Using microemulsions for drug delivery. Pharm Tech 11:46–54, 1987.
129. H Wennerström, O Söderman, U Olsson, B Lindman. Macroemulsions versus microemulsions. Colloids Surfaces A: Physicochem Eng Aspects 123–124:13–26; 1997.
130. WA Ritschel. Microemulsions for improved peptide absorption from the gastrointestinal tract. Methods Find Exp Clin Pharmacol 13:205–220, 1991.
131. A Haße, S Keipert. Development and characterization of microemulsions for ocular application. Eur J Pharm Biopharm 43(2): 179–183, 1997.
132. MB Charro, GI Vilas, TB Méndez, MAL Q, JP Marty, RH Guy. Delivery of a hydrophilic solute through the skin from novel microemulsion systems. Eur J Pharm Biopharm 43(1):37–42, 1997.
133. S Vemuri, CT Rhodes. Preparation and characterization of liposomes as therapeutic delivery systems: a review. Pharm Acta Helv 70(2):95–111, 1995.
134. A Bochot, P Couvreur, E Fattal. Intravitreal administration of antisense oligonucleotides: potential of liposomal delivery. Prog Retin Eye Res 19(2):131–147, 2000.
135. C Nastruzzi, R Cortesi, E Esposito, R Gambari, M Borgatti, N Bianchi, G Feriotto, C Mischiati. Liposomes as carriers for DNA PNA hybrids. J Control Rel 68(2):237–249, 2000.
136. C Welz, W Neuhuber, H Schreier, R Repp, W Rascher, A Fahr. Nuclear gene targeting using negatively charged liposomes. Int J Pharm 196(2):251–252, 2000.
137. C Mader, S Küpcü, UB Sleytr, M Sára. S-layer-coated liposomes as a versatile system for entrapping and binding target molecules. Biochem Biophys Acta Biomembranes 1463(1):142–150, 2000.
138. R Bodmeier. Multiphase system. Int Patent Application WO 98/55100 (1998).
139. W Im-Emsap, GA Brazeau, JW Simpkins, R Bodmeier. Sustained drug delivery of 17-β estradiol from injectable biodegradble in situ forming microparticles (ISM) system. AAPS PharmSci Supplement 2(4), AAPS Annual Meeting Abstracts, 2000.
140. W Im-Emsap, R Bodmeier. In vitro drug release from in situ forming microparticle (ISM)-systems with dispersed drug. AAPS PharmSci Supplement 2(4), AAPS Annual Meeting Abstracts, 2000.
141. SE Friberg, LS Quencer, ML Hilton. Theory of emulsions. In: HA Lieberman, MM Rieger, GS Banker, eds. *Pharmaceutical Dosage Forms: Disperse Systems*, 2nd ed. Vol. 1, New York: Marcel Dekker, 1996, pp 53–90.
142. ER Garrett. Stability oil-in-water emulsions. J Pharm Sci 54(11):1557–1570, 1965.
143. K Shinoda, H Kunieda. Phase properties of emulsions: PIT and HLB. In: P Becher, ed. *Encyclopedia of Emulsion Technology*, Vol. 1, New York: Dekker, 1983, pp. 337–368.
144. N Garti, A Aserin. Pharmaceutical emulsions double emulsions and microemulsions. In: S Benita, ed. *Microencapsulation-Methods and Industrial Applications*. New York: Marcel Dekker, 1996, pp 411–534.
145. IB Ivanov, KB Danov, PA Kralchevsky. Flocculation and coalescence of micron-size emulsion droplets. Colloids Surfaces A: Physicochem Eng Aspects 152:161–168, 1999.
146. MM Robins. Emulsions-creaming phenomena. Curr Opin Colloid Interf Sci 5:265–272, 2000.

147. M Bury. J Gerhards, W Erni. Monitoring sedimentation processes by conductivity measurements. Int J Pharm 76:207–217, 1991.
148. M Bury, J Gerhards, W Erni, A Stamm. Application of a new method based on conductivity measurements to determine the creaming stability of O/W emulsions. Int Pharm 124(2):183–194, 1995.
149. KI Al-Malah , MOJ Azzam, RM Omari. Emulsifying properties of BSA in different vegetable oil emulsions using conductivity technique. Food Hydrocolloids 14:485–490, 2000.
150. F Babick, F Hinze, S Ripperger. Dependence of ultrasonic attenuation on the material properties. Colloids Surfaces A: Physicochem Eng Aspects 172:33–46, 2000.
151. WD Bachalo. Method for measuring the size and velocity of spheres by dual-beam light-scatter interferometry. Apply Opt 19:73–83, 1980.
152. DL Black, MQ McQuay, MP Bonin. Laser-based techniques for particle-size measurement: a review of sizing methods and their industrial applications. Prog Energy Combustion Sci 22(3):267–306, 1996.
153. E Dikinson, G Stainsby. *Colloidals in Food.* New York: Applied Sci Publ., 1982.
154. RK Chang, C Hsiao, JR Robinson. A review of aqueous coating techniques and preliminary data on release from a theophylline product. Pharm Technol 11(3):56–68, 1987.
155. KL Moore. Physicochemical properties of Opadry®, Coateric®, and Surelease®. In: JW Mcginity, ed. *Aqueous Polymeric Coatings for Pharmaceutical Dosage Forms.* New York: Marcel Dekker, 1989, pp 303–315.
156. R Gurny, NA Peppas, DD Harrington, GS Banker. Development of biodegradable and injectable latices for controlled release of potent drugs. Drug Dev Ind Pharm 7:1–25, 1981.
157. HJ Krause, A Schwarz, P Rohdewald. Polylactic acid nanoparticles, a colloidal drug delivery system for lipophilic drugs. Int J Pharm 27: 145–155, 1985.
158. F Koosha, RH Müller, SS Davis, MC Davies. The surface chemical structure of poly (β-hydroxybutyrate) microparticles produced by solvent evaporation process. J Control Rel 9:149, 1989.
159. R Bodmeier, H Chen. Indomethacin polymeric nanosuspensions prepared by microfluidization. J Control Rel 12:223–233, 1990.
160. PD Scholes, AGA Coombes, L Illum, SS Davis, M Vert, MC Davies. The preparation of sub-200 nm poly (lactide-co-glycolide) microspheres for site-specific drug delivery. J Control Rel 25:145–153, 1993.
161. S Batzri, ED Korn. Single bilayer liposomes prepared without sonication. Biochem Biophys Acta 443:629–634, 1973.
162. T Niwa, H Takeuchi, T Hino, N Kunou, Y Kawashima. Preparations of biodegradable nanospheres of water-soluble and insoluble drugs with d,l-lactide/glycolide copolymer by a novel spontaneous emulsification solvent diffusion method, and the drug release behavior. J Control Rel 25:89–98, 1993.
163. H Fessi, F Puisieux, JP Devissaguet. Procede de preparation de systemes colloidaux dispersibles d'une substance, sous forme de nanocapsules. European patent 274, 961 (1987).
164. N Ammoury, H Fessi, JP Devissaguet, M Allix, M Plotkine, RG Boulu. Effect on cerebral blood flow of orally administered indomethacin-loaded poly (isobutylcyanoacrylate) and poly(d,l-lactide) nanocapsules. J Pharm Pharmacol 42:558–561, 1990.
165. N Ammoury, H Fessi, JP Devissaguet, M Dubrasquet, S Benita. Jejunal absorption, pharmacological activity, and pharmacokinetic evaluation of indomethacin-loaded poly(d,l-lactide) and poly(-isobutyl-cyanoacrylate) nanocapsules in rats. Pharm Res 8:101–105, 1991.
166. N Ammoury, H Fessi, JP Devissaguet, F Puisieux, S Benita. In vitro release kinetic pattern of indomethacin from poly (d,l-lactide) nanocapsules. J Pharm Sci 79(9):763–767, 1990.
167. C Bindschaedler, R Gurny, E Doelker. Process for preparing a powder of water insoluble polymer which can be redispersed in a liquid phase, the resulting powder and utilization thereof. Swiss Patent 1497/88 (1988).
168. H Ibrahim, C Bindschaedler, E Doelker, P Buri, R Gurny. 1991. Concept and development of opthalmic pseudo-latices triggered by pH. Int J Pharm 77:211–219, 1991.
169. H Ibrahim, C Bindschaedler, E Doelker, P Buri, R Gurny. Aqueous nanodispersions prepared by a salting-out process. Int J Pharm 87:239–246, 1992.
170. E Allemann, R Gurny, E Doelker. Preparation of aqueous polymeric nanodispersions by a reversible salting-out process, influence of process parameters on particle size. Int J Pharm 87:247–253, 1992.
171. E Allemann, JC Leroux, R Gurny, E Doelker. In *vitro* extended-release properties of drug loaded poly (dl-lactic acid) nanoparticles produced by a salting-out procedure. Pharm Res 10(12):1732–1737, 1993.
172. E Allemann, E Doelker, R Gurny. Drug loaded poly (lactic acid) nanoparticles produced by a reversible, salting-out process: purification of an injectable dosage form. Eur J Pharm Biopharm 39:13–18, 1992.
173. B Ekman, I Sjöholm. Incorporation of macromolecules in microparticles: preparation and characteristics. Biochem 15:5115, 1976.
174. AFJr Yapel. Albumin microspheres: heat and chemical stabilization. In: KJ Widder, R Green, eds. *Methods in Enzymology:* Part A, *Drug and Enzyme Targeting.* Orlando: Academic Press, 1985, pp 3–18.

175. WE Longo, EP Goldberg. Hydrophilic albumin microspheres. In: KJ Widder, R Green, eds. *Methods in Enzymology:* Part A, *Drug and Enzyme Targeting*. Orlando: Academic Press, 1985, pp 18–26.
176. E Tomlinson, JJ Burger. Incorporation of water-soluble drugs in albumin microspheres. In: KJ Widder, R Green, eds. *Methods in Enzymology:* Part A, *Drug and Enzyme Targeting*. Orlando: Academic Press, 1985, pp 27–43.
177. T Yoshioka, M Hashida, S Muranishi, H Sezaki. Specific delivery of mitomycin C to the liver, spleen, and lung: Nano-and microspherical carriers of gelatin. Int J Pharm 8:131–141, 1981.
178. EE Hassan, RC Parish, JM Gallo. Optimized formulation of magnetic microspheres containing the anticancer agent, oxantrazole. Pharm Res 9:390–397, 1992.
179. JJ Marty, RC Oppenheim, P Speiser. Nanoparticles-a new colloidal drug delivery system. Pharm Acta Helv 53:17–22, 1978.
180. M El-Samaligy, P Rohdewald. Triamcinolone diacetate nanoparticles, a sustained release drug delivery system suitable for parenteral administration. Pharm Acta Helv 57:201, 1982.
181. M El-Samaligy, P Rohdewald. Reconstituted collagen nanoparticles, a novel drug carrier delivery system. J Pharm Pharmacol 35:537–539, 1983.
182. RC Oppenheim. Solid colloidal drug delivery systems: nanoparticles. Int J Pharm 8:217–234, 1981.
183. M Rajanorivony, C Vauthier, G Couarraze, F Puisieux, P Couvreur. Development of a new drug carrier made from alginate. J Pharm Sci 82(9):912–917, 1993.
184. WR Perkins, I Ahmad, X Li, DJ Hirsh, GR Masters, CJ Fecko, JK Lee, S Ali, J Nguyen, J Schupsky, C Herbert, AS Janoff, E Mayhew. Novel therapeutic nano-particles (lipocores): trapping poorly water soluble compounds. Int J Pharm 200(1):27–39, 2000.
185. DF Driscoll, MN Bacon, BR Bistrian. Physicochemical stability of two types of intravenous lipid emulsion as total nutrient admixtures. J Parent Enteral Nutr 24(1):15–22, 2000.
186. HS Yoo, JE Oh, KH Lee, TG Park. Biodegradable nanoparticles containing doxorubicin-PLGA conjugate for sustained release. Pharm Res 16(7): 1114–1118, 1999.
187. RH Müller, K Mäder, S Gohla. Solid lipid nanoparticles (SLN) for controlled drug delivery-A review of the state of the art. Eur J Pharm Biopharm 50(1): 161–177, 2000.
188. S Harnisch, RH Müller. Adsorption kinetics of plasma proteins on oil-in-water emulsions for parenteral nutrition. Eur J Pharm Biopharm 49(1):41–46, 2000.
189. PP Constantinides, KJ Lambert, AK Tustian, B Schneider, S Lalji, W Ma, B Wentzel, D Kessler, D Worah, SC Quay. Formulation development and antitumor activity of a filter-sterilizable emulsion of paclitaxel. Pharm Res 17(2):175–182, 2000.
190. AG Floyd. Top ten considerations in the development of parenteral emulsions. Pharm Sci Tech Today 2(4):134–143, 1999.
191. VS Koster, PFM Kuks, R Langer, H Talsma. Particle size in parenteral fat emulsions, what are the true limitations? Int J Pharm 134:235–238, 1996.
192. G Chansiri, RT Lyons, MV Patel, SL Hem. Effect of surface charge on the stability of oil/water emulsions during steam sterilization. J Pharm Sci 88(4):453–458, 1999.
193. V Labhasetwar, C Song, W Humphrey, R Shebuski, RJ Levy. Arterial uptake of biodegradable nanoparticles: effect of surface modifications. J Pharm Sci 87(10): 1229–1234, 1998.
194. M Jumaa, BW Müller. The effect of oil components and homogenization conditions on the physicochemical properties and stability of parenteral fat emulsions. Int J Pharm 163(1–2):81–89, 1998.
195. Y Kawano, T Noma. Inhibition by lecithin-bound iodine (LBI) of inducible allergen-specific T lymphocytes' responses in allergic diseases. Int J Immunopharmacol 18(4):241–249, 1996.
196. GC Na, HJ Stevens, BO Yuan, N Rajagopalan. Physical stability of ethyl diatrizoate nanocrystalline suspension in steam sterilization. Pharm Res 16(4):569–574, 1999.
197. K Westesen, B Siekmann. Investigation of the gel formation of phospholipid-stabilized solid lipid nanoparticles. Int J Pharm 151(1):35–45, 1997.
198. J Mewis. Flow behaviour of concentrated suspensions: predictions and measurements. Int J Miner Proc 44–45:17–27, 1996.
199. AJ Spiegel, MM Noseworthy. Use of nonaqueous solvents in parenteral products. J Pharm Sci 52(10):917–927, 1963.
200. RH Müller, K Peters. Nanosuspensions for the formulation of poorly soluble drugs I.Preparation by a size-reduction technique. Int J Pharm 160(2):229–237, 1998.
201. K Peters, S Leitzke, SE Diederichs, K Borner, H Hahn, RE Müller, S Ehlers. Preparation of a clofazimine nanosuspension for intravenous use and evaluation of its therapeutic efficacy in murine Mycobacterium avium infection. J Antimicrobial Chemother 45(1):77–83, 2000.
202. PC Schmidt. Secondary electron microscopy in pharmaceutical technology, In: J Swarbrick, JC Boylan, eds. *Encyclopedia of Pharmaceutical Technology*, Vol. 19. New York: Marcel Dekker, 2000, pp 311–356.
203. JW Mullin. Sieving of pharmaceuticals. In: J Swarbrick, JC Boylan, eds. *Encyclopedia of Pharmaceutical Technology*, Vol. 14. New York: Marcel Dekker, 1996, pp 63–86.
204. TJ Racey, P Rochon, DVC Awang, GA Neville. Aggregation of commercial heparin samples in storage. J Pharm Sci 76: 314–318, 1987.

205. TJ Racey, P Rochon, F Mori, GA Neville. Examination of a possible role of dermatan sulfate in the aggregation of commercial heparin samples. J Pharm Sci 78:214–218, 1989.
206. JB Kayes. Pharmaceutical suspensions: microelectrophoretic properties. J Pharm Pharmacol 29:163–168, 1977.
207. V Gallardo, L Zurita, A Ontiveros, JDG Durán. Interfacial properties of barium sulfate suspensions. Implications in their stability. J Pharm Sci 89:1134–1142, 2000.
208. K Thode, RH Müller, M Kresse. Two-time window and multiangle photon correlation spectroscopy size and zeta potential analysis—highly sensitive rapid assay for dispersion stability. J Pharm Sci 89:1317–1324, 2000.
209. DJA Crommelin. Influence of lipid composition and ionic strength on the physical stability of liposomes. J Pharm Sci 73:1559–1563, 1984.
210. H Takenaka, Y Kawashima, SY Lin. Electrophoretic properties of sulfamethoxazole microcapsules and gelatin-acacia coacervates. J Pharm Sci 70:302–305, 1981.
211. MJ Killeen. Spray drying and spray congealing of pharmaceuticals. In: J Swarbrick, JC Boylan, eds. *Encyclopedia of Pharmaceutical Technology*, Vol. 14. New York: Marcel Dekker, 1996, pp. 207–222.
212. LH Block. Scale-up of disperse systems: Theoretical and practical aspects. In: HA Lieberman, MM Rieger, GS Banker, eds. *Pharmaceutical Dosage Forms: Disperse Systems*, Vol. 3, 2nd ed. New York: Marcel Dekker, 1998, pp 363–394.
213. RA Nash. Validation of disperse systems. In: HA Lieberman, MM Rieger, GS Banker, eds. *Pharmaceutical Dosage Forms: Disperse Systems*, Vol. 3, 2nd ed. New York: Marcel Dekker, 1998, pp 473–512.

Chapter 10

Tablet Dosage Forms

Mary Kathryn Kottke

Cubist Pharmaceuticals, Inc., Lexington, Massachusetts

Edward M. Rudnic

Advancis Pharmaceutical Corp., Gaithersburg, Maryland

I. INTRODUCTION

During the past four decades, the pharmaceutical industry has invested vast amounts of time and money in the study of tablet compaction. This expenditure is quite reasonable when one considers how valuable tablets, as a dosage form, are to the industry. Because oral dosage forms can be self-administered by the patient, they are obviously more profitable to manufacture than parenteral dosage forms that must be administered, in most cases, by trained personnel. This is reflected by the fact that well over 80% of the drugs in the United States that are formulated to produce systemic effects are marketed as oral dosage forms. Compared to other oral dosage forms, tablets are the manufacturer's dosage form of choice because of their relatively low cost of manufacture, package, and shipment; increased stability and virtual tamper resistance (most tampered-with tablets either become discolored or disintegrate).

II. DESIGN AND FORMULATION OF COMPRESSED TABLETS

A. General Considerations

The most common solid dosage forms in contemporary use are tablets, which may be defined as unit forms of solid medicaments prepared by compaction. Most consist of a mixture of powders that are compacted in a die to produce a single rigid body. The most common types of tablets are those intended to be swallowed whole and then disintegrate and release their medicaments in the gastrointestinal tract (GIT). A less common type of tablet that is rapidly gaining popularity in the United States is formulated to allow dissolution or dispersion in water prior to administration. Ideally, for this type of tablet all ingredients should be soluble, but frequently a fine suspension has to be accepted. Many tablets of this type are formulated to be effervescent, and their main advantages include rapid release of drug and minimization of gastric irritation.

Some tablets are designed to be masticated (i.e., chewed). This type of tablet is often used when absorption from the buccal cavity is desired or to enhance dispersion prior to swallowing. Alternatively, a tablet may be intended to dissolve slowly in the mouth (e.g., lozenges) so as to provide local activity of the drug. A few tablets are designed to be placed under the tongue (i.e., sublingual) or between the teeth and gum (i.e., buccal) and rapidly release drug into the bloodstream. Buccal or sublingual absorption is often desirable for drugs liable to extensive hepatic metabolism by the first-pass effect (e.g., nitroglycerin, testosterone). Recently, a lozenge on a stick, or "lollipop," dosage form of fentanyl was developed for preoperative sedation in pediatric patients (Oralet®) and breakthrough cancer pain in adults (Actiq®). Active ingredient is released from the lozenge into the bloodstream from the oral mucosa.

There are now many types of tablet formulations that provide for the release of drug to be delayed or control the rate of the drug's availability. Some of these preparations are highly sophisticated and are rightly referred to as complete "drug-delivery systems." Since the concepts of controlled drug delivery are the subjects of Chapter 15, the strategies of these systems will not be discussed here. However, solid dosage formulators must be aware of the various options available to them.

For example, when prolonged release of a water-soluble drug is required, water-insoluble materials must be co-formulated with the drug. If the dose of the drug is high and it exhibits poor compactibility, purely hydrophobic agents, such as waxes, will exacerbate the inability of the material to form a compact. In such cases, formulators need to turn to other types of water-insoluble materials, such as polymers, to achieve both drug release and tableting goals.

Some tablets combine sustained-release and rapid disintegration characteristics. Products such as K-Dur® (Key Pharmaceuticals) combine coated potassium chloride crystals in a rapidly releasing tablet. In this particular instance, the crystals are coated with ethylcellulose, a water-insoluble polymer, and are then incorporated into a rapidly disintegrating microcrystalline cellulose (MCC) matrix. The purpose of this tablet is to minimize GI ulceration, commonly encountered by patients treated with potassium chloride. This simple but elegant formulation is an example of a solid dosage form strategy used to achieve clinical goals.

Thus, the single greatest challenge to the tablet formulator is in the definition of the purpose of the formulation and the identification of suitable materials to meet development objectives. In order to do this properly, the formulator must know the properties of the drug, the materials to be co-formulated with the drug, and the important aspects of the granulation, tableting, and coating processes.

Pharmaceutical compressed tablets are prepared by placing an appropriate powder mix, or granulation, in a metal die on a tablet press. At the base of the die is a lower punch, and above the die is an upper punch. When the upper punch is forced down on the powder mix (single station press) or when the upper and lower punches squeeze together (rotary or multiple station press), the powder is forced into a tablet. Despite the fact that powder compaction has been observed for hundreds of years, scientists still debate the exact mechanisms behind this phenomenon.

Perhaps the most significant factor in the tableting of materials for use as drug products is the need to produce tablets of uniform weight. This is achieved by feeding constant volumes of homogeneous material to the dies. Such an approach is necessary because direct weighing at rates commensurate with modern tablet press operation is impossible. This requirement immediately places demands on the physical characteristics of the feed and on the design of the tablet press itself. In the case of the former, precompression treatment of the granulation is one of the most common ways of minimizing difficulties arising from this source.

The great paradox in pharmaceutical tableting is the need to manufacture a compact of sufficient mechanical strength to withstand the rigors of processing and packaging that is also capable of reproducibly releasing the drug. In most cases, the release of the drug is produced by the penetration of aqueous fluids into the fine residual pore structure of the tablet and the contact of these fluids with components that either swell or release gases.

The selected precompression treatment, if any, markedly affects the manufacture of tablets. In particular, one must determine whether a mixture of powdered ingredients is to be tableted directly or if an intervening wet granulation step is to be introduced. This decision is influenced by many factors, including the stability of the drug to heat and moisture; the flow properties of the granulation; and the tendency of the granulation to segregate. At the present time there are also two conflicting considerations that tend to play a major role in this choice. These are the reluctance to change methods employed traditionally by the company versus the economic advantages of omitting complete stages in the production sequence.

In wet granulation, the components of the formulations are mixed with a granulating liquid, such as water or ethanol, to produce granules that will readily compress to give tablets. Wet granulation methods predominate in the manufacture of existing products, while the trend for new products is to use direct compression procedures. Although many steps are eliminated when using direct compression, some formulators have found that wet granulated products are more robust and able to accommodate variability in raw materials and tableting equipment. Thus, for some companies, the trend is reverting to the formulation of tablets by wet granulation.

B. Desirable Properties of Raw Materials

Most formulations are composed of one or more medicaments plus a variety of excipients. Irrespective of the type of tablet, general criteria for these raw materials are necessary. In order to produce accurate, reproducible dosage forms, it is essential that each component be uniformly dispersed within the mixture and that any tendency for component segregation be minimized. In addition, the processing operations demand that the mixture be both free-flowing and cohesive when compressed.

Particle Size

In general, the tendencies for a powder mix to segregate can be reduced by maintaining similar particle size distribution, shape, and, theoretically, density of all the ingredients. Flow properties are enhanced by using regular-shaped, smooth particles with a narrow size distribution together with an optimum proportion of "fines" (particles 50 μm). If such conditions cannot be met, then some form of granulation should be considered.

Particle size distribution, and hence surface area of the drug itself, is an important property that has received considerable attention in the literature. For many drugs, particularly those whose absorption is limited by the rate of dissolution, attainment of therapeutic levels may depend upon achieving a small particle size [1]. In fact, it has been suggested that for such drugs, standards for specific surface areas and the number of particles per unit weight should be developed. However, the difficulty in handling very fine powders, as well as the possibility of altering the material in other ways, has shifted the emphasis towards producing an optimum, rather than a minimum, particle size. For instance, several researchers have found that decreasing particle size produces tablets of increased strength that also have a reduced tendency for lamination [2–5]. This is probably due to the minimization of any adverse influences that a particular crystal structure may have on the bonding mechanism. On the other hand, samples of milled digoxin crystals prepared by a number of size-reduction techniques have been reported to elicit different equilibrium solubilities [1]. This suggests that the method of grinding may well affect the dissolution behavior of certain drugs.

The effect of particle size on the compaction characteristics of two model sulfonamide drugs, one exhibiting brittle fracture and the other being compressed chiefly by plastic deformation, has been reported [3]. In particular, it was shown that the tensile strength of tablets made from the brittle material were more sensitive to the drug's particle size than that of tablets made from the plastically deforming material. In addition, larger granules possess better flow, while small aggregates deform during compaction (e.g., spray-dried lactose) [6].

An alternative approach aimed at reducing the segregation tendencies of medicaments and excipients involves milling the former to a small particle size and then physically absorbing it uniformly onto the surface of the larger particles of an excipient substrate. By these means "ordered," as opposed to "random," mixing is realized and dissolution is enhanced as a result of the fine dispersion [7].

Moisture Content

One of the most significant parameters contributing to the behavior of many tablet formulations is the level of moisture present during manufacture as well as that residual in the product. In addition to its role as a granulation fluid and its potentially adverse effects on stability, water has some subtle effects that should not be overlooked. For example, there is increasing evidence to suggest that moisture levels may be very critical in minimizing certain faults, such as lamination, that can occur during compression. Moisture levels can also affect the mechanical strength of tablets and may act as an internal lubricant. For example, Fig. 1 illus-

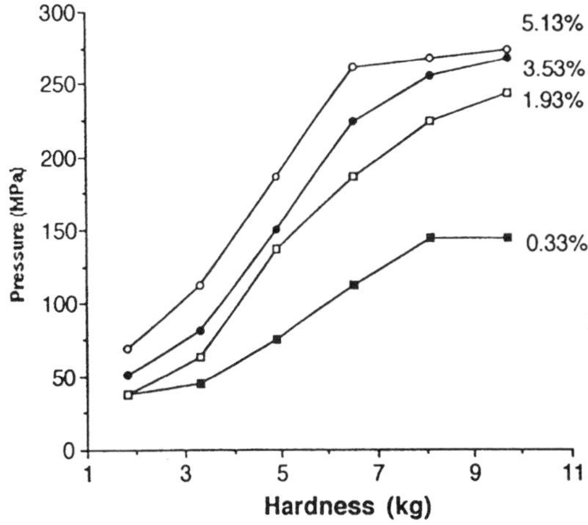

Fig. 1 The effect of moisture content on the compactibility of anhydrous beta lactose tablets. (From Ref. 8.)

trates the effect of moisture content on the compactibility of anhydrous lactose [8]. As the moisture content increases, it is adsorbed by the lactose, thereby converting it from the anhydrous to the hydrous form. During this transformation, the β-form of lactose most probably changes to the α-form and thus produces changes in compactibility.

Accelerated aging and crystal transformation rates have also been traced to high residual moisture content. Ando et al. studied the effect of moisture content on the crystallization of anhydrous theophylline in tablets [9]. Their results also indicate that anhydrous materials convert to hydrates at high levels of relative humidity. In addition, if hygroscopic materials (e.g., polyethylene glycol 6000) are also contained in the formulation, needle-like crystals form at the tablet surface and significantly reduce the release rate of the theophylline.

In many products it seems highly probable that there exists a narrow range of optimum moisture contents that should be maintained. More specifically, the effect of moisture on MCC-containing tablets has been the subject of an investigation that demonstrates the sensitivity of this important excipient to moisture content [10]. These researchers found that differences exist in both the cohesive nature and the moisture content to two commercial brands of MCC. A very useful report on the equilibrium moisture content of some 30 excipients has been compiled by a collaborative group of workers from several pharmaceutical companies and appears in the *Handbook of Pharmaceutical Excipients* [11,12].

Crystalline Form

Selection of the most suitable chemical form of the active principle for a tablet, while not strictly within our terms of reference here, must be considered. For example, some chloramphenicol esters produce little clinical response [13]. There is also a significant difference in the bioavailability of anhydrous and hydrated forms of ampicillin [14]. Furthermore, different polymorphic forms, and even crystal habits, may have a pronounced influence on the bioavailability of some drugs due to the different dissolution rates they exhibit. Such changes can also give rise to manufacturing problems. Polymorphism is, of course, not restricted to active ingredients, as shown, for example, in an evaluation of the tableting characteristics of five forms or sorbitol [15].

Many drugs have definite and stable crystal habits. Morphological changes rarely occur in such drugs as the formulation process is scaled up. However, some drugs exhibit polymorphism or have different identifiable crystal habits. Chan and Doelker reviewed a number of drugs that undergo polymorphic transformation when triturated in a mortar and pestle [16]. Some of their conclusions are listed in Table 1 and illustrated in Fig. 2. In addition, a number of researchers have concluded that both polymorph and crystal habit influence the compactibility and mechanical strength to tablets prepared from polymorphic materials [16–21]. York compared the compressibility of naproxen crystals that had been spherically agglomerated with different solvents and found that significant differences existed between the various types of agglomerates (see Fig. 3) [21]. Other investigators have found that, in some instances, there is a correlation between the rate of reversion to the metastable form during dissolution and the crystal growth rate of the stable form [22]. These polymorphic changes may have a profound effect on tablet performance in terms of processing, in vitro dissolution and in vivo absorption. Thus, formulators of solid dosage forms must be aware of a subject compound's propensity for polymorphic transition so that a rational approach to formulation can be followed.

Table 1 Some Drugs That Undergo Polymorphic Transition When Triturated

Drug	Number of polymorphs before trituration	Number of polymorphs after trituration
Barbitone	2	1
Caffeine	2	1
Chlorpropamide	3	2
Clenbuterol HCl	2	3
Dipyridamole	2	1
Maprotiline HCl	3	1
Mebendazole	4	5
Nafoxidine HCl	4	3
Pentobarbitone	3	2
Phenobarbitone	2	1
Sulfabenzamide	2	1

Source: Ref. 16.

Hiestand Tableting Indices

Materials that do not compress well produce soft tablets. In addition, brittle crystalline materials will yield brittle tablets. Hiestand was the first pharmaceutical scientist to quantify rationally the compaction properties of pharmaceutical powders [23–28]. The results

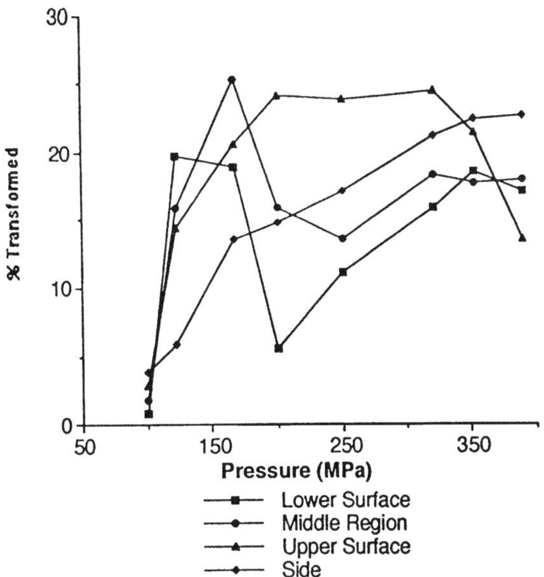

Fig. 2 Percentage of caffeine "form A" transformed vs. applied pressure. (From Ref. 16.)

of this work are three indices known as the Hiestand Tableting Indices. The strain index (SI) is a measure of the internal entropy, or strain, associated with a given material when compacted. The bonding index (BI) is a measure of the material's ability to form bonds and

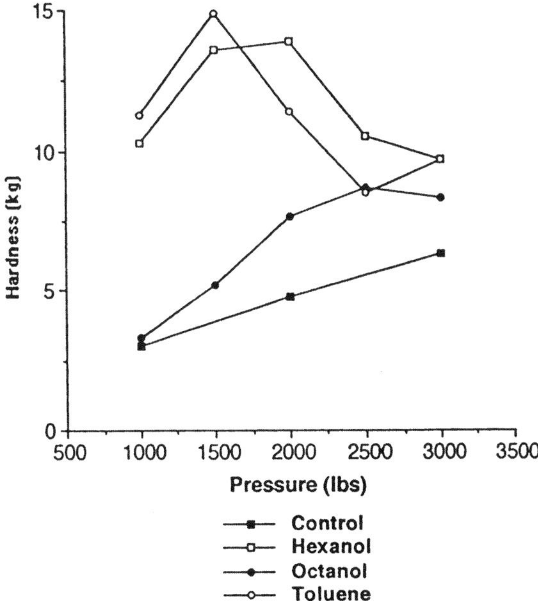

Fig. 3 Intrinsic compressibility of nonagglomerated naproxen (control) and of naproxen that has been spherically agglomerated with different solvents. (From Ref. 21.)

undergo plastic transformation to produce a suitable tablet. The third index, the brittle fracture index (BFI), is a measure of the brittleness of the material and its compact. Table 2 lists these indices for a number of drugs and excipients. For most materials, the strength of the tablet is a result of competing processes. For example, erythromycin is a material known for its tendency to cap and laminate when tableted. On the basis of its BI value, one might expect relatively good bonding. However, the very high strain index associated with this drug appears to overcome its bonding abilities. MCC, on the other hand, has very high strain index, but its bonding index is exceptionally high and compensates for this effect.

Other investigators have evaluated the potential for these indices. In their studies, Williams and McGinnity have concluded that evaluation of single-material systems should precede binary or tertiary powder systems [29]. A full discussion of compaction mechanisms is given later in this chapter.

Variability

The effect of raw material variability on tablet production [2,30,31] and suggestions for improving tableting quality of starting materials [21] has been the subject of several publications. Table 3, which lists the characteristics of different sources of magnesium stearate, clearly illustrates the variability of this material [32]. Phadke and Eichorst have also confirmed that significant differences can exist between different sources, and even different lots, of magnesium stearate [33]. Given the fact that the effectiveness of magnesium stearate is due, in large part, to its large surface area, these variations should not be overlooked. In addition, studies assessing raw material variability emphasize the need for physical as well as chemical testing of raw materials to ensure uniformity of the final product.

Purity

Raw material purity, in general, must also be given careful attention. Apart from the obvious reasons for a high level of integrity, as recognized by the regulatory requirements, one should be aware of more subtle implications that are perhaps only just beginning to emerge. For instance, small proportions of the impurity acetylsalicylic anhydride have been shown to reduce the dissolution rate of aspirin itself (see Fig. 4) [34].

Another area of interest is that of microbiological contamination of solid dosage forms, which is thought to arise chiefly from raw materials rather than the

Table 2 Hiestand Compaction Indices for Some Drugs and Excipients

Material	Bonding index	Brittle fracture index	Strain index
Aspirin	1.5	0.16	1.11
Caffeine	1.3	0.34	2.19
Croscarmellose sodium NF	2.7	0.02	3.79
Dicalcium phosphate	1.3	0.15	1.13
Erythromycin dihydrate	1.9	0.98	2.13
Hydroxypropyl cellulose	1.6	0.04	2.10
Ibuprofen			
A	1.9	0.05	0.98
B	1.8	0.57	1.51
C	2.7	0.45	1.21
Lactose USP			
Anhydrous	0.8	0.27	1.40
Hydrous Fast-Flo	0.4	0.19	1.70
Hydrous bolted	0.6	0.12	2.16
Hydrous spray process	0.6	0.45	2.12
Spray-dried			
A	0.6	0.18	1.47
B	0.5	0.12	1.81
Mannitol			
A	0.8	0.19	2.18
B	0.5	0.15	2.26
Methenamine	1.6	0.98	0.84
Methyl cellulose	4.5	0.06	3.02
Microcrystalline cellulose NF			
Avicel PH 102 (coarse)	4.3	0.04	2.20
Avicel PH 101 (fine)	3.3	0.04	2.37
Povidone USP	1.7	0.42	3.70
Sorbitol NF	0.9	0.16	1.70
Starch NF			
Corn	0.4	0.26	2.48
Pregelatinized	1.8	0.14	2.02
Pregelatinized compressible	1.2	0.02	2.08
Modified (starch 1500)	1.5	0.27	2.30
Sucrose NF			
A	1.0	0.35	1.45
B	0.8	0.42	1.79
C	0.5	0.53	1.55

Source: Refs. 23–28.

manufacturing process [35,36]. Ibrahim and Olurinaola monitored the effects of production, environment and method of production, as well as microbial quality of starting materials, on the microbial load during various stages of tablet production [35]. Although high levels of contamination were present during the wet granulation process, these levels were significantly reduced during the drying process. The investigators also found that products derived from natural origins, such as gelatins and starch, can be contaminated heavily.

Table 3 Average Particle Data for Different Sources of Magnesium Stearate

Source	Size (μm)	Surface area (m^2/g)	Pore radius (Å)
United States	1.5–3.2	13.4	50
Great Britain	2.1–5.2	12.2	68
Germany	4.1–6.9	7.4	61
Italy	5.5–9.1	4.6	36

Source: Ref. 32.

Compatibility

One final area that should be considered when choosing the excipients to be used in the tablet formulation is that of drug-excipient interactions. There is still much debate as to whether excipient compatibility testing should be conducted prior to formulation [37–39]. These tests most often involve the trituration of small amounts of the active ingredient with a variety of excipients. Critics of these small-scale studies argue that their predictive value has yet to be established and indeed do not reflect actual processing conditions [37]. Instead, they suggest a sound knowledge of the chemistry of the materials used in conjuncture with "mini-formulation" studies as a preferable method for investigation of drug-excipient interactions.

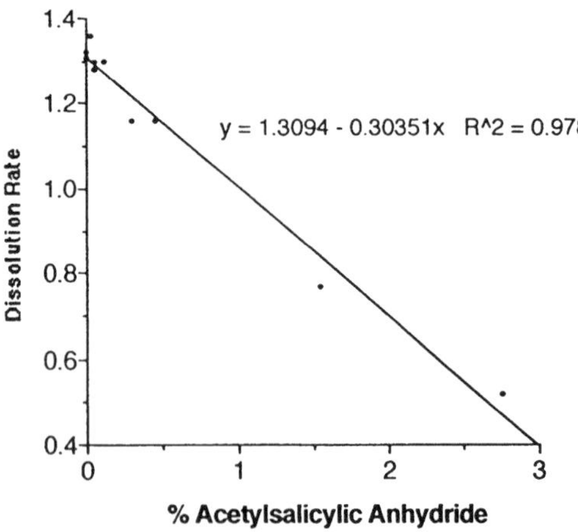

Fig. 4 Effect of acetylsalicylic anhydride impurity on the dissolution rate of aspirin tablets. (From Ref. 34.)

C. Tablet Components

Conventional solid dosage forms can be divided into two classes: those that disintegrate and those that do not. Disintegrating dosage forms release drug by breaking down the physical integrity of the dosage from, usually with the aid of solid disintegrating agents or gas-releasing effervescent agents. Nondisintegrating tablets are usually made of soluble drugs and excipients that will rapidly dissolve in the mouth or GIT upon ingestion.

With the advent of prolonged-release dosage forms, some pharmaceutical scientists have begun to regard conventional disintegrating dosage forms as "non–controlled-release." This term is a misnomer since, with the aid of "super-disintegrants" and other excipients, the disintegration of these dosage forms can be controlled, both quantitatively and qualitatively. Moreover, there are still many drugs in which rapid attainment of therapeutic levels, rather than controlled release, is required. Analgesics, antibiotics, and drugs for the acute treatment of angina pectoris are prime examples. These tablets need to be designed so that the drug is liberated from the dosage form in such a manner that dissolution of the drug is maximized. Very often, this means that disintegration of the tablet must be followed by granular disintegration (see Fig. 5) to promote rapid dissolution and, hence, absorption.

The ingredients, or excipients, used to make compressed tablets are numerous. They can be classified by their use, or function, as in Table 4. Keep in mind, however, that formulations need not contain all the types of ingredients listed in this table. Certain excipients, such as antioxidants and wetting agents, are used only in situations where they are expressly needed to assure the stability and solubility of the active ingredients. Other excipients, such as dissolution modifiers, are used primarily in controlled-release formulations. In fact, by reducing the number of ingredients in a formulation, one will generally be reducing the number of problems that can arise in the manufacturing process. Hence, many formulators adhere to the motto "Keep it simple."

Because of the nature of modern pharmaceutical systems, formulators have made more complete investigations of the materials they use. This interest has identified several materials that may have more than one use in tableted systems. The type of effect that an excipient will produce is often dependent upon the concentration in which it is used. For example, Table 5 lists some "multiuse" excipients and the corresponding concentration ranges required for their various applications.

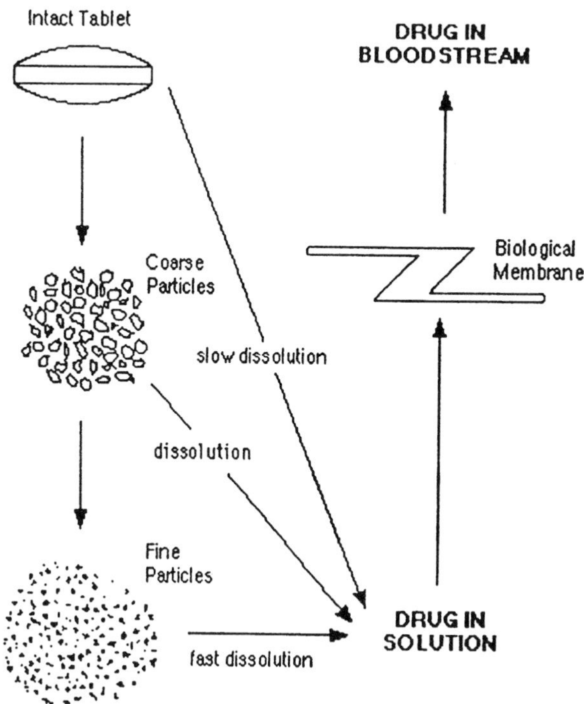

Fig. 5 Absorption of a drug from an intact tablet.

A relatively new class of "co-processed" excipients now exists. These excipients are essentially a "preblend" of two or more excipients that are commonly used in conjunction with each other.

Active Ingredients

The dose of the drug to be administered has a profound effect on the design and formulation of a dosage form. Content uniformity and drug stability become very important issues when dealing with highly potent compounds that are delivered in very small doses (e.g., oral contraceptives). However, the effect of the drug's properties on the tablet, in this case, is minimal. In general, as the dosage increases, so does the effect of the drug's attributes on the tablet.

Table 4 Ingredients Used in Tablet Formulation

Active ingredient (drug)	Dissolution modifiers
Fillers	Absorbents
Binders (dry and wet)	Flavoring agents
Disintegrants	Coloring agents
Antifrictional agents	Wetting agents
Lubricants	Antioxidants
Glidants	Preservatives
Antiadherants	

Table 5 Some Multiple-Use Excipients for Tablet Formulation

Excipient/concentration in formula	Use
Ethylcellulose	
1–3%	Wet or dry binder
1–3%	Controlled-release coating
Glyceryl palmitostearate	
0–5%	Lubricant
10–50%	Controlled-release excipient
Hydroxypropylmethyl cellulose (HPMC), low viscosity	
2–5%	Wet or dry binder
2–10%	Film former
5–25%	Controlled-release excipient
Magnesium aluminum silicate	
2–10%	Binder
2–10%	Disintegrant
Microcrystalline cellulose (MCC)	
0–8%	Improve adhesion of film coat to core
0.2–0.5%	Glidant
5–20%	Antiadherant
5–20%	Disintegrant
5–95%	Binder/filler
Polyethylene glycol	
0–10%	Lubricant
0–15%	Thermoplastic filler/binder
5–40%	Controlled-release excipient
Poly(methacrylates)	
2–10%	Film former
5–20%	Controlled-release excipient
10–50%	Filler
5–10%	Coating excipient
Poly(vinyl pyrrolidone) (Povidone, PVP)	
5–15%	Wet binder
5–10%	Coating excipient
5–30%	Disintegrant
10–35%	Controlled-release excipient
Starch	
3–15%	Intragranular binder/disintegrant
5–25%	Wet binder
5–20%	Disintegrant

Sometimes processing can affect the particle morphology of the active ingredient. This in turn may lead to adverse effects on mixing and tableting operations. In particular, micronization of a drug may cause crystals to change their shape even though polymorphism is not evidenced.

Fillers

An increasing number of drugs are highly potent and are thus used in very low dosages. In order to produce tablets of a reasonable size (i.e., minimum diameter of 3 mm), it is necessary to dilute the drug with an inert material. Such diluents should meet important criteria, including low cost and good tableting qualities. It may be possible, in some instances, to combine the role of diluent with a different property, such as disintegrant or flavoring agent.

Commonly used fillers and binders and their comparative properties are listed in Table 6. As can be seen by this list, both organic and inorganic materials are used as fillers and binders. The organic materials used are primarily carbohydrates because of their general ability to enhance the product's mechanical strength as

Table 6 Comparative Properties of Some Directly Compressible Fillers[a]

Filler	Compactibility	Flowability	Solubility	Disintegration	Hygroscopicity	Lubricity	Stability
Dextrose	3	2	4	2	1	2	3
Spray-dried lactose	3	5	4	3	1	2	4
Fast-Flo lactose	4	4	4	4	1	2	4
Anhydrous lactose	2	3	4	4	5	2	4
Emdex (dextrates)	5	4	5	3	1	2	3
Sucrose	4	3	5	4	4	1	4
Starch	2	1	0	4	3	3	3
Starch 1500	3	2	2	4	3	2	4
Dicalcium phosphate	3	4	1	2	1	2	5
Avicel (MCC)	5	1	0	2	2	4	5

[a]Graded on a scale from 5 (good/high) down to 1 (poor/low); 0 means none.

well as their freedom from toxicity, acceptable taste, and reasonable solubility profiles.

One of the most commonly used carbohydrates in compressed tablets is lactose. Work by Bolhuis and Lerk [40] and Shangraw et al. [6] has demonstrated that all lactoses are not equivalent as determined by chemical, physiochemical, and functional measurements. In addition to the various particle-size grades of normal hydrous lactose, one can purchase spray-dried lactose, which is an agglomerate of α-lactose monohydrate crystals with up to 10% amorphous material. Spray-dried lactose has very good flow properties, but its poor compression characteristics require the addition of a binder such as MCC. However, one particular brand of spherical crystalline/amorphous agglomerate, Fast-Flo (NF hydrous), possesses superior compressibility and dissolution characteristics. The spherical nature of the crystals make them more compressible than spray-dried agglomerates of lactose [41]. Anhydrous lactose has also been used as a diluent, particularly in direct compression formulations where low moisture content is desirable, since it has very good stability and a reduced tendency to color upon aging. Another advantage in the use of anhydrous lactose is that its insensitivity to temperature changes allows it to be reworked with relative ease. Unfortunately, its flow properties are not particularly good and its compressibility is inferior to other forms of lactose. One must also give attention, though, to this component's stability, as aging may adversely affect these properties.

Some other sugars are now being produced in special grades to meet the needs of the pharmaceutical industry. Most of these products contain combinations of sucrose with invert sugar or modified dextrins and are of particular value in the formulation of chewable tablets. In addition, crystalline maltose and directly compressible grades of fructose are currently available and have gained a large degree of acceptance in the "nutraceutical" industry [41a].

Starch is often cited as a filler, but it is more commonly used in its dry state as a disintegrating agent. However, modified starches such as StaRx 1500 and National 1551 (partially hydrolyzed, or pregelatinized starch) are marketed for direct compression and appear to offer the advantage of substantial mechanical strength and rapid drug release.

Certain inorganic salts are also used as fillers. Some common examples are listed in Table 7 together with their comparative properties. Among the most popular

Table 7 Comparative Properties of Some Inorganic Fillers[a]

Filler	Availability	Mechanical	Solubility	Absorbency	Acid/base	Abrasiveness	Lubricity
Calcium carbonate	2	4	0	3	Base	2	1
Dicalcium phosphate	2	2	0	4	Base	2	0
Calcium triphosphate	3	2	0	5	Base	2	0
Magnesium carbonate	2	2	0	4	Base	1	1
Sodium chloride	5	5	5	1	Neutral	3	2

[a]Graded on a scale from 5 (good/high) down to 1 (poor/low); 0 means none.

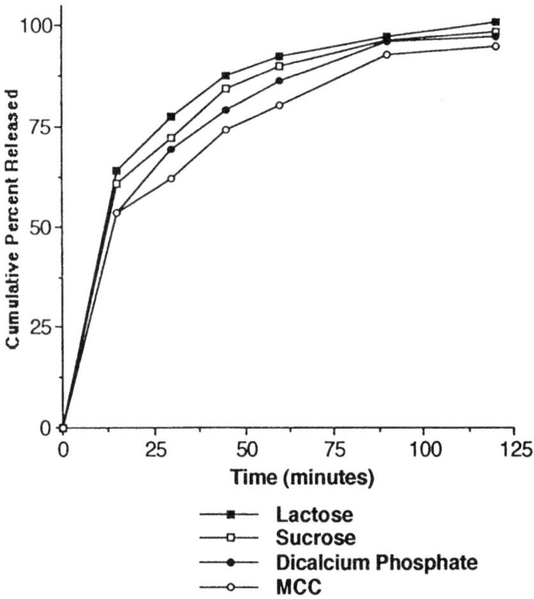

Fig. 6 Dissolution of digoxin tablets containing different fillers (in simulated gastric fluid at 37°C). (From Ref. 45.)

is dicalcium phosphate dihydrate, a comparatively low-cost insoluble diluent with good powder flow potential but inherently poor compression characteristics [41]. It is important to note that this material is slightly alkaline and thus must not be used where the active ingredient is sensitive to pH values of 7.3 or above. Fuji has recently introduced an anhydrous grade of dibasic calcium phosphate (DCPA) as Fujicalin. Investigators have found that DCPA is highly compressible and promotes rapid dissolution, most likely due to its anhydrous nature [41b]. Special formulations in which unmilled dicalcium phosphate is the main ingredient are available under the trade name Emcompress® and contain 5–20% of other components designed to improve compaction and disintegration performance [6,40,42]. In accelerated stability studies, Shah and Arambulo [43] found Emcompress to be unsuitable for use with ascorbic acid and thiamine hydrochloride due to deteriorating hardness and disintegration characteristics evidenced, as well as the chemical degradation of ascorbic acid. In addition, calcium salts present in dibasic calcium phosphate may adversely affect the absorption profile of certain drugs [44].

The influence of the actual manufacturing process can also affect the contribution of the diluent to the final characteristics of the product. For instance, Shah et al. [45] demonstrated that the release of drug from tablets formulated with soluble excipients may be more prompt than those formulated with insoluble excipients (see Fig. 6). However, they also found that the method of preparing the triturates was also very significant. In this example, ball or Muller milling gave the best overall results.

Few tablets intended for oral administration are totally soluble in aqueous media, but if such a product is needed, then soluble excipients are employed. These include dextrose, lactose, mannitol, and sodium chloride, with the last of these sometimes acting as its own lubricant. Urea may also be used, but due to its known pharmacological effects, it is less desirable than the other soluble compounds cited.

Binders and Granulating Fluids

Most binders used in wet granulation tend to be polymeric in nature. The binders most commonly used are natural in source, such as starch or cellulose derivatives. Typically, these agents are dispersed or dissolved in water or a hydro-alcoholic medium. The binders can be sprayed, poured, or admixed into the powders to be agglomerated. The methods of incorporating these materials can be classified into low-shear, high-shear, atomization, and extrusion methods. As illustrated in Fig. 7, one can see that the concentration of binder used and its method of addition (as a dry powder or as a granulating fluid) can affect significantly affect granule size [46]. Moreover, some researchers have found that increasing the amount of

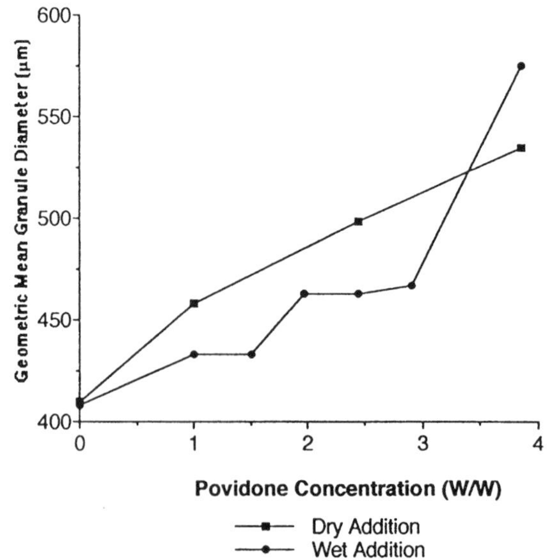

Fig. 7 Effect of binder concentration and method of addition on granule size. (From Ref. 46.)

granulating fluid used can have profound effects on a tablet's mechanical strength and disintegration time [47]. Some commonly used binders are listed in Table 8.

Seager et al. [48] showed that a binder can be useful for a given process but may not be universally useful. They studied gelatin in granulations made by roller-compaction, conventional wet granulation, and spray-drying. These researchers found spray drying to be the preferred method of granulation for gelatin-granulated acetaminophen. They hypothesized that this was due to the improved distribution of the binder in this system. Studies evaluating the influence of PVP-based granulating methods on granules of lactose and MCC found that MCC granules (plastically deformable) were highly dependent on granulating method while brittle lactose granules were not (brittle) [48a]. Chowhan showed that considerable variability often occurs when scale-up of a granulation takes place. He demonstrated that a major factor in scale-up is the drug itself, which may require more or less granulating fluid and binder to make a suitable tablet. He also found that this may impact the drug release and thus bioavailability of the dosage form [49].

Iyer et al. [50] investigated the effects of roto-granulation on the performance of hydroxypropyl methylcellulose (HPMC), gelatin, and poly(-vinylpyrrolidone) (Povidone, PVP). In this process, all three binders produced similar results. However, HPMC was preferred due to prolonged drug release profiles, smaller particle size, and better content uniformity.

The use of hydroxypropyl cellulose (HPC), a binder, has increased in recent years [50a–50c]. This material has been shown to reduce the incidence of capping when compared with MCC, PVP, and starch [50a]. In addition, low substituted grades of HPC can also be used as a filler/ binder [50b].

York, reviewed the solid-state properties of solids and showed that both intrinsic and induced properties can have a profound effect on wettability and processing [51]. In addition, Lerk et al. [52,53] investigated the surface characteristics of a number of drugs and showed that the contact angles can vary greatly depending on the drug (see Table 9). Of interest is the difference in wettability of different crystalline forms of the same drug [52,53]. These properties will have a profound effect on the ability of various binders to function as well as change the processing parameters needed to effect proper granulation.

Disintegrants

For most tablets, it is necessary to overcome the cohesive strength introduced into the mass by compression. It is therefore common practice to incorporate an excipient, called a disintegrant, which induces this process. Several types, acting by different mechanisms, may be distinguished: (a) those that enhance the action of capillary forces in producing a rapid uptake of aqueous liquids, (b) those that swell on contact with water, (c) those that release gases to disrupt the tablet

Table 8 Some Commonly Used Wet Binders and Granulating Fluids

Name	Strength (%)	Comments
Acacia mucilage[a]	1–5	Produces hard, friable granules
Cellulose derivates[a]	5–10	HPMC[b] is most common
Ethanol		Applied to easily hydratable material
Gelatin solutions	10–20	Gels when cold, therefore use warm; strong adhesive; used in lozenges; less suitable in warm moist climates
Glucose syrups	25–50	Strong adhesive; tablets may soften in high humidity
Povidone	5–15	Different MW grades give varying results
Starch mucilage[a]	5–10	One of best general binders; better when used warm
Sucrose syrups[a]	65–85	Strongly adhesive; tablets may soften in high humidity
Tragacanth mucilage[a]	10–20	Produces hard, friable granules
Water		Applied to easily hydratable material

[a]May also be added as dry powder to the formulation, but this is less efficient than liquid preparation.
[b]Hydroxypropylmethylcellulose.

Table 9 Contact Angles for Some Powders

Material	Contact angle (ϕ)
Acetylsalicylic acid	74
Aminophylline	47
Ampicillin, anhydrous	35
Ampicillin, trihydrate	21
Calcium stearate	115
Chloramphenicol	59
Chloramphenicol palmitate (α-form)	122
Chloramphenicol palmitate (β-form)	108
Diazepam	83
Digoxin	49
Indomethacin	90
Lactose	30
Magnesium stearate	121
Phenylbutazone	109
Prednisolone	43
Prednisone	63
Stearic acid	98
Sulfacetamide	57
Theophylline	48
Tolbutamide	72

Source: Refs. 52 and 53.

structure, and (d) those that destroy the binder by enzymatic action.

The method of addition has also received attention. In particular, during wet granulation, the addition of the disintegrant before (intragranular) or after (extragranular) the granulation process has been investigated (see Figs. 8 and 9) [54]. The extragranular portion ensures rapid disintegration, while the intragranular fraction leads to harder tablets and a finer size distribution on dispersion. The consensus of the published papers on this topic appears to be that there are advantages to be gained in dividing the disintegrant into both extra- and intragranular portions, with between 20 and 50% being external. For example, 2.5% intragranular and 12.5% extragranular disintegrant produced the best overall performance in tablets of calcium orthophosphate [55].

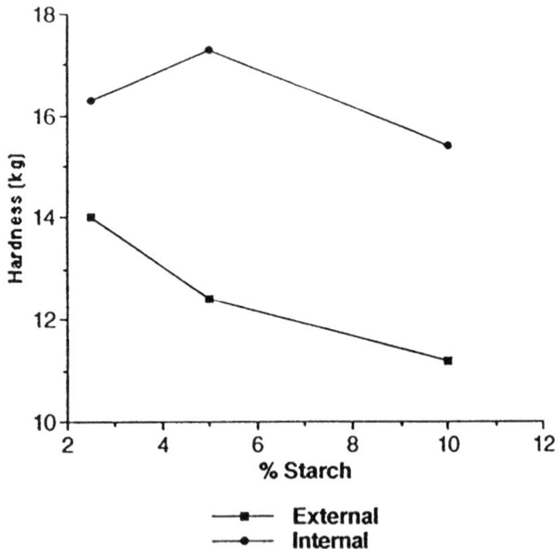

Fig. 8 Effect of starch concentration and location on tablet hardness. (From Ref. 54.)

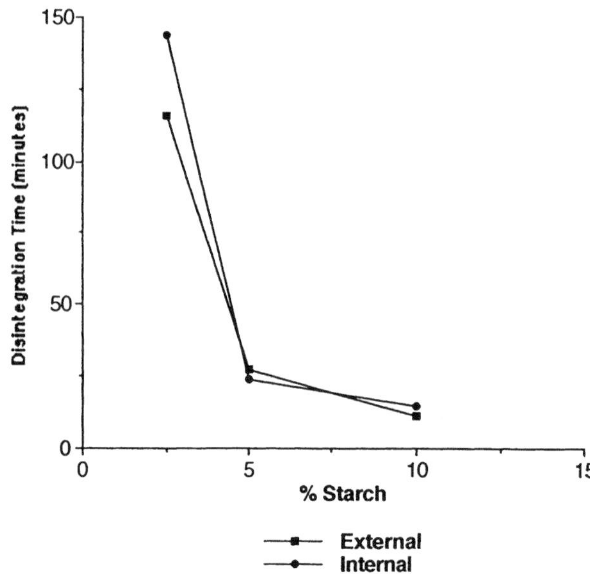

Fig. 9 Effect of starch concentration and location on tablet disintegration time. (From Ref. 54.)

Water Uptake. There is evidence to suggest that water uptake caused by capillary forces is the crucial factor in the disintegration process of many formulations. In such systems the pore structure of the tablet is of prime importance and any inherent hydrophobicity of the tablet mass will adversely affect it. Therefore, disintegrants in this group must be able to maintain a porous structure in the compressed tablet and show a low interfacial tension towards aqueous fluids. Rapid penetration by water throughout the entire tablet matrix to facilitate its breakup is thus achieved. Concentrations of disintegrant that ensure a continuous matrix of disintegrant are desirable and levels of between 5 and 20% are common.

Water uptake has been implicated as a mechanism of action for tablet disintegrants. Khan and Rhodes studied the adsorption and absorption properties of various disintegrants [56]. They concluded that the ability of particles to draw water into the porous network of a tablet (wicking) was essential for efficient disintegration. Work conducted by Mitrevej and Hollenbeck substantiates these claims [57]. A sophisticated method of determining water uptake was developed by Nogami et al. [58]. Their study further supports the theory that the rate of wetting is responsible, at least in part, for the disintegrant action.

Starch was the first disintegrant used in tablet manufacture and still enjoys wide use today [59–66]. Its mode of action is probably through the induction of water uptake into the tablet rather than by the swelling action previously ascribed to it [57–63]. Other workers [67] still consider that the hydration of the hydroxyl groups causes them to move apart, yet it appears that starch swells little in water at body temperature. There is some evidence to suggest that the fat content of starch can also influence its performance as a disintegrant. In addition, since starch possesses poor binding characteristics, once the tablets containing it become thoroughly wetted they break up easily [62,63,65]. Varieties of starch containing large grains are preferred for other reasons, but in the present context a large particle size may provide the optimum pore size distribution within the tablet and thus promote capillary action (e.g., potato starch).

Some forms of MCC have been shown to be highly porous, with strong "wicking" tendencies, thereby making them good disintegrants. This is a fortuitous finding since they also serve as excellent binders and are able to improve significantly the mechanical strength of some weak formulations. One disadvantage of using MCC, however, is that dissolution performance may be adversely affected at higher compression forces. Another disintegrant group, the insoluble cationic exchange resins, typified by polyacrylin, exhibits better dissolution characteristics when subjected to higher pressures. Comparisons of disintegrant action, however, will only be valid if carried out under the same controlled conditions.

Some disintegrants propagate capillary effects but also swell and/or dissolve to enhance disintegration behavior. Sodium starch glycolate and insoluble cationic exchange resins are two examples that have been extensively studied by Khan and Rhodes [56,68], who demonstrated their superiority to sodium carboxymethylcellulose and corn starch. Their results correlated will with the comparative release patterns of a dye from tablets containing these materials. In addition, they were able to show the long-term deterioration in hardness and disintegration time when the tablets containing the more effective disintegrants were subjected to high humidities. A comparative evaluation of sodium starch glycolate against cross-linked carboxymethylcellulose and sodium glycine carbonate has been carried out by Bavitz et al. [69], who determined that cross-linked carboxymethylcellulose compared very favorably with sodium starch glycolate in formulations of four different actives over long test periods. Colloidal silicon dioxide has been investigated as a disintegrant, and, although capable of absorbing approximately nine times more water than starch, the process is several times slower; the hindered action offsets much of the advantage of its greater absorbency.

Swelling. Perhaps the more widely accepted general mechanism of action for tablet disintegrants is swelling. Almost all disintegrants swell to some extent, and swelling has been reported quite universally in the literature [6,70,71]. Historically, sedimentation volumes of the disintegrant in a slurry have been used as measures of swelling. This test is a fair appraisal of swelling capacity but does not provide for the dynamic measurement of the swelling itself. As a result, many disintegrants studied by this method do not show a correlation between sedimentation volumes and disintegrant efficiency. Nogami et al. developed a reliable test to measure swelling and water uptake simultaneously with the aid of two graduated columns connected by a rubber tube [58]. This apparatus was later refined by several research groups [72–74]. Figure 10 illustrates the essential features of this apparatus, which is very useful for the quantification of swelling and hydration rates for many excipients and polymers.

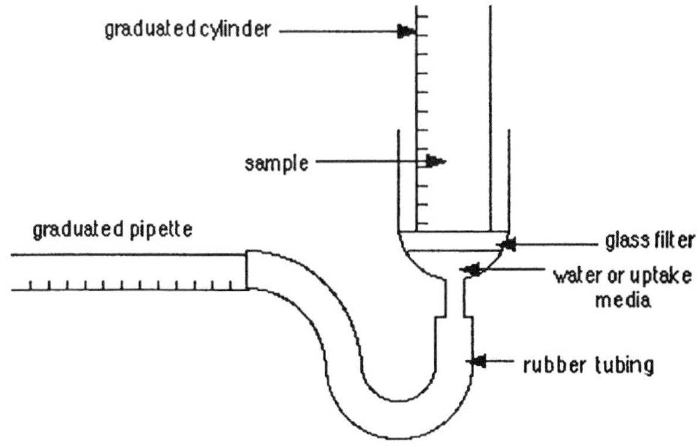

Fig. 10 Bulk swelling and water uptake apparatus.

Both sedimentation volumes and swelling rates were evaluated by Rudnic et al., who found a poor correlation between the static test (sedimentation) and disintegrant efficiency [74]. In addition, they found that swelling tests, such as those reported above, are dependent upon a number of variables including water transport through a gel layer and rates of hydration. These investigators developed methods to evaluate intrinsic swelling through the use of high-speed cinemicroscopy in conjunction with computerized image analysis. Although their method allowed for more accurate and precise measure of swelling, they concluded that both bulk swelling and intrinsic swelling produced similar rank order disintegrant swelling rates.

All of the investigations described above have placed importance not only on the extent of swelling, but also on the rate at which swelling develops. In addition, it is important to understand that, as particles swell, there must be little or no accommodations by the tablet matrix to that swelling. If the matrix yields elasticity to the swelling, little or no force will be expended on the system and disintegration will not take place. If the matrix is rigid and does not accommodate swelling, however, deaggregation or disintegration will occur.

One general problem with this group of disintegrants is that upon swelling, many disintegrants produce a sticky or gelatinous mass that resists breakup of the tablet, making it particularly important to optimize the concentration present within the granulation. For example, some powdered gums, such as agar, karaya, or tragacanth, swell considerably when wet, but their pronounced adhesiveness limits their value as disintegrants and restricts the maximum concentration to which they can be effectively used to approximately 5% of tablet weight. Because these substances are nonsynthetic, they also exhibit considerable lot-to-lot variability, are liable to microbiological contamination, and can be quite expensive. However, alginic acid and its sodium salt have sufficient swelling with minimum stickiness, and concentrations as low as 4 or 5% are often adequate. The small levels of alginates required compensate for the somewhat high cost of these materials.

Although untreated starches do not swell sufficiently, certain modified forms, such as sodium starch glycolate, do swell in cold water and are better as disintegrants. Various cellulose derivatives, including methylcellulose and carboxymethylcellulose, have been used in this role, but with limited success due to the marked increase in viscosity they produce around the dispersing tablet mass.

Gas Production. Gas-producing disintegrants are used when especially rapid disintegration or a readily soluble formulation is required [70]. They have also been found to be of value when poor disintegration characteristics have resisted other methods of improvement. Their main drawback is the need for more stringent control over environmental conditions during the manufacture of tablets made with these materials. In particular, gas-producing disintegrants are quite sensitive to small changes in humidity levels. For this reason, these disintegrants are often incorporated immediately prior to compression, when the moisture content can be controlled more easily and/or they can be added to two separate fractions of the formulation. Composition is based upon the same principles as those used for effervescent tablets, the most common being mixtures of citric and tartaric acids plus carbonates or bicarbonates.

In many instances, lower concentrations of gas-producing disintegrants can be used than are required by other disintegrating agents. This is a distinct point in their favor. Certain peroxides that release oxygen have been used for this purpose, but they do not perform as well as those releasing carbon dioxide.

Enzymes. Where tablets are not naturally very cohesive and have thus been manufactured by a wet granulation process involving one of the binders listed in Table 8, addition of small quantities of appropriate enzyme may be sufficient to produce rapid disintegration. It has also been proposed that disintegration action might result from expansion of the entrapped air due to generation of "heat of wetting" when the tablet is placed in a fluid. This concept has received little attention.

Other Factors

DEFORMATION. The existence of plastic deformation under the stress of tableting has been reported for many years. Hess determined that disintegrant particles deform when compressed during the tableting process with the aid of scanning electron micrographs [64]. He found that the deformed particles returned to their normal shapes when exposed to water. Work completed by Fuhrer yielded similar results [75]. In some cases, the swelling capacity of starch granules was improved when the granules were extensively deformed during compression. Obviously, the role of deformation and rebound under actual production conditions need to be studied in more detail before the full effect of this phenomenon can be understood.

PARTICLE REPULSION THEORY. Another theory of tablet disintegration attempts to explain the swelling of tablets made with "nonswellable" starch. Guyot-Hermann and Ringard have proposed a particle repulsion theory based upon the observation that particles that do not seem to swell may still disintegrate tablets [66]. In their study they altered the dielectric constant of the disintegrating media in an effort to identify electric repulsive forces as the mechanism of disintegration and concluded that water is required for tablet disintegration. These investigators espoused repulsion, secondary to wicking, as the primary mechanism of action for all tablet disintegrants.

HEAT OF WETTING. Matsumaru was the first to propose that the heat of wetting of disintegrant particles could be a mechanism of action [76]. He observed that starch granules exhibit slight exothermic properties when wetted and reported that this was the cause of localized stress resulting from capillary air expansion. This explanation, however, is limited to only a few types of disintegrants and cannot describe the action of most modern disintegrating agents. List and Muazzam [77] studied this phenomenon and also found disintegrants where significant heat of wetting is generated. However, in these cases there is not always a corresponding decrease in disintegration time.

PARTICLE SIZE. Physical characteristics of disintegrants, such as particle size, also have some bearing on the mechanisms of disintegration (e.g., swelling and water uptake). Several authors have attempted to relate the particle size of disintegrants to their relative efficiency. Smallenbroek et al. [78] evaluated the effect of particle size of starch grains on their ability to disintegrate tablets. They concluded that starch grains with relatively large particle sizes were more efficient disintegrants than the finer grades. These authors theorized that this behavior resulted from increased swelling pressure. Investigations made by Rudnic et al. [74,79] confirm these results. They also found a correlation between the rate of swelling and the amount of water uptake of sodium starch glycolate and have thus postulated that particle size plays a key role in the overall efficiency of commercial sources of this material.

MOLECULAR STRUCTURE. In their attempts to identify the mechanism(s) of action of tablet disintegrants, researchers recently have turned their attention to the molecular structure of disintegrants. Schwartz and Zelinskie [65] published one of the first such reports in which they examined the two corn starch fractions amylose and amylopectin. They concluded that the linear polymer amylose was responsible for the disintegrant properties of starch while the amylopectin fraction was primarily responsible for the binding properties associated with starches (see Fig. 11). Because of the work by Schwartz and Zelinskie, tablet formulators can now select from a range of specialty starches that represent different ratios of amylose and amylopectin content to solve disintegrant/dissolution problems encountered in tablet formulation.

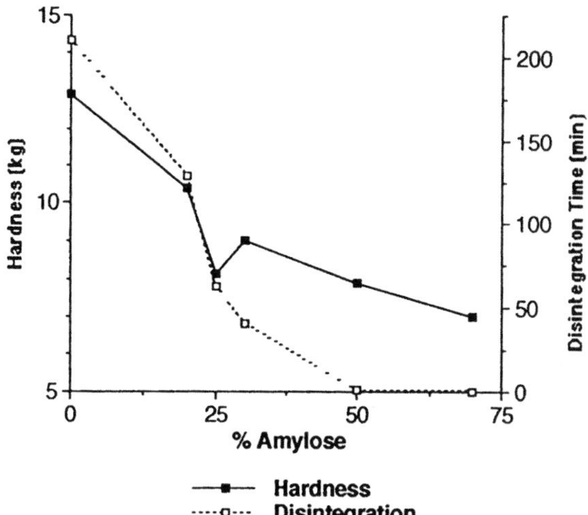

Fig. 11 Effect of amylose on the hardness and disintegration of dicalcium phosphate tablets. (From Ref. 62.)

Super Disintegrants. Shangraw et al. identified three major groups of compounds that have been termed superdisintegrants [6]. Many of these so-called superdisintegrants are substituted and cross-linked polymers. One group—the sodium starch glycolates—has enjoyed widespread popularity due to its exceptional ability to disintegrate tablets as well as the relative ease with which this type of compound can be processed into tablet formulations.

Sodium starch glycolate is manufactured by cross-linking and carboxymethylating potato starch. It provides an excellent opportunity to measure the relationship between molecular structure and disintegrant efficiency by altering the degree of substitution and the extent of cross-linking. Optimization of one sodium starch glycolate was performed using both direct compression and wet granulation methods.

These studies showed that the swelling to the disintegrant particles was inversely proportional to the level of substitution [80].

A number of published studies have described the use of various substances as tablet disintegrants. Reviews by Lowenthal and Kanig and Rudnic have been published on the various agents used to bring about tablet disintegration [70,71]. Shangraw et al. reviewed the modern so-called superdisintegrants and compared their relative morphological properties [6]. Most published studies have attempted to explain mechanisms that relate to observed efficiency of the disintegrating agent, and some have explored secondary attributes within the disintegrants themselves. None have succeeded, however, in advancing an explanation of disintegration that approaches a universal understanding applicable to all disintegrants. It now seems obvious that no single mechanism is applicable to all tablet disintegrants. In fact, a combination of mechanism may be operative.

Antifrictional Agents

Insoluble Lubricants. Lubricants act by interposing an intermediate layer between the tablet constituents and the die wall. The smaller the amount of stress needed to shear the material, the better its lubricant properties will be. Since they are primarily required to act at the tooling/material interface, lubricants should be incorporated in the final mixing step after all granulation and preblending is complete. In this way, overmixing is less likely to occur.

A common mistake in the design of tablet operations is adding both the disintegrant and lubricant together in one mixing step. This causes the disintegrant to become coated with lubricant and often results in both a decrease in the disintegrant's porosity and a decrease in the efficiency of the disintegrant. Rather than add the disintegrant and lubricant simultaneously, a better approach is to add these excipients sequentially, with a disintegrant being first.

The surface area of the lubricant may be the most important parameter to monitor, in terms of lubricant efficiency. Substantial decreases in both ejection forces and tablet hardness are noted when using brands of magnesium with larger surface areas. Lubricants with high surface areas may also be more sensitive to changes in mixing time than lubricants with low surface areas. Thus, if a particular drug or formulation is deleteriously affected by prolonged mixing of lubricants, adequate characterization of monitoring of a lubricant surface area should be an integral part of product development and quality control.

Some of the more common antifrictional agents are listed in Table 10. Many of these are hydrophobic and may consequently affect the release of medicament. Therefore, lubricant concentration and mixing time should be kept to the absolute minimum. Lubricants may also reduce significantly the mechanical strength of the tablet (see Fig. 12) [29,81]. Stearic acid and its magnesium and calcium salts are widely used, but the

Table 10 Some Commonly Used Antifrictional Agents

Soluble lubricants	Insoluble lubricants
Adipic acid	Calcium, magnesium, and zinc salts of stearic acid
d, *l*-Leucine	Glyceryl monostearate
Glyceryl triacetate	Glyceryl palmitostearate
Magnesium lauryl sulfate	Hydrogenated vegetable oils
PEG 400, 6000, and 8000	Hydrogenated castor oil
Polyoxyethylene monostearates	Light mineral oil
Sodium benzoate	Paraffins
Sodium lauryl sulfate	Polytetrafluoroethylene
Sucrose monolaurate	Sodium stearyl fumarate
Glidants	Stearic acid
Calcium silicate	Talc
Colloidal silicon dioxide	Waxes
Magnesium carbonate	Antiadherants
Magnesium trisilicate	Most lubricants
Starch	Starch
Talc	Talc

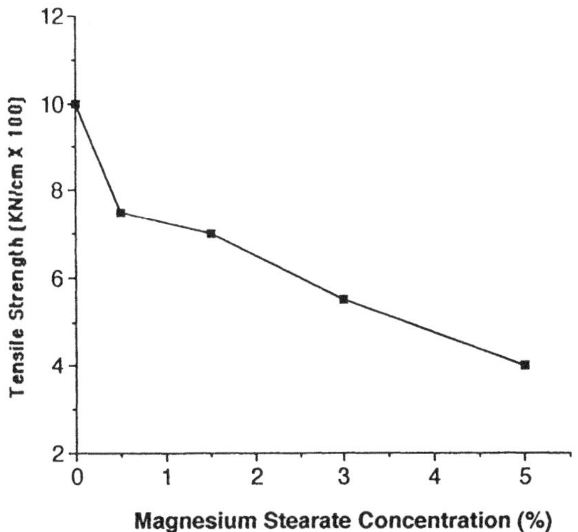

Fig. 12 Tensile strength of calcium sulfate tablets as a function of magnesium stearate concentration (solid fraction = 0.57). (From Ref. 29.)

latter can be sufficiently alkaline to react with certain amine salts such as aminophylline, resulting in the release of free base and discoloration of the tablet. Published formulas show levels of these lubricants between 1 and 4%, but there is evidence to show that, in many cases, they can be reduced to as little as 0.25% without significantly affecting the lubrication of the system.

Liquid paraffins, particularly those of low viscosity, have been used and are said to be of value for colored tablets, and even the use of modified vegetables has been attempted. However, they appear, in general, to offer little advantage over solid lubricants, and their incorporation into the precompression mixture is more difficult, requiring solution in a volatile liquid that is then sprayed onto the unlubricated material. Due to handling and EPA requirements, these materials are often rejected in the preformulation stage.

Isolated references in the literature describe the use to talc as a lubricant, but this material is better regarded as a glidant [82–85]. It has several disadvantages, including its insolubility in body fluids and the abrasiveness found when using all but the finest grades of this material. Finally, it loses some of its effectiveness after compression so that tablets containing talc cannot be readily reworked without extra quantities of it being added to the formulation.

Soluble Lubricants. Because of the association of lubricant properties with lipophilic materials (and hence poor aqueous solubility), alternative, more hydrophilic materials have been investigated. Soluble lubricants do not appear to be as efficient in lubricating tablet systems as their insoluble counterparts [82]. Receiving increasing attention in this context is a group of soluble, if less effective, lubricants that also possess surfactant qualities and are typified by the lauryl sulfates. For example, when tablets lubricated with sodium lauryl sulfate were compared to those lubricated with magnesium stearate, the tablets containing sodium lauryl sulfate exhibited a significantly higher rate of dissolution. Physical mixtures of the lubricant with stearates can lead to the best compromise in terms or lubricity, tablet strength, and disintegration. Recently, magnesium lauryl sulfate has been found to have an attractive balance of these properties, although requiring a concentration of 5% to provide the same lubricating efficiency as 2% magnesium stearate.

Some of the synthetic, soluble, wax-like polymers, typified by the high molecular weight polyethylene glycols (PEGs), have also been used as soluble lubricants. PEG 4000 and 6000 have been investigated, but their lubricant efficiency is less than that of magnesium stearate. In attempts to find the optimum lubricant from all standpoints, combinations of polymers such as polyoxyethylene monostearates and polyoxethylene lauryl sulfates have undergone limited trials, with some encouraging results, but more information is required.

Glidants. Glidants are added to the formulation in order to improve the flow properties of the material to be fed into the die and sometimes aid in particle rearrangement within the die during the early stages of compression [6,85]. They may act by interposing their particles between those of the other components and so, by virtue of their reduced adhesive tendencies, lower the overall interparticulate friction of the system. In addition, there may be adsorption of glidant into the irregularities of the other materials. It follows that, like lubricants, they are required at the surface of feed particles and that they should be in a fine state of division and appropriately incorporated in the mix.

Starches remain a popular glidant, in particular those with the larger grain sizes such as potato starch, possibly because of their additional value as a disintegrant in the formulation. Concentrations up to 10% are common, but it should be appreciated that excess may result in exactly the opposite effect of that desired (i.e., flow properties may worsen). Talc is also widely used and has the advantage that it is superior to starches in minimizing any tendency for material to stick to the punch faces, a property sometimes classified as antiadherent. Because of its totally insoluble nature, and hence potential retardant effect of dissolution, concentration must be strictly limited and should rarely exceed 5%. In fact, the best overall compromise may be realized by using a mixture of starch and talc.

Several silaceous materials have been used successfully to induce flow. Among those quoted in the literature are pyrogenic silica in concentrations as low as 0.25% and hydrated sodium silioaluminate in concentrations of around 0.75%. The former has the additional property of being able to scavenge moisture, which might otherwise contribute to restricted flow characteristics.

Phyllosilicates, in addition to talc and silica, have recently been evaluated for their use as tableting excipients. These compounds include the smectites, palygorskites, and sepiolites [85a]. Although they show some promise, current levels of metallic impurities are currently too high for use in pharmaceutical preparations.

Antiadherents. Some materials strongly adhere to the metal of the punches and dies. Although not a frictional effect, this results in material preferentially sticking to the punch faces and gives rise to tablets with rough surfaces. This effect, called picking, can also arise in formulations containing excess moisture.

Normally, the lubricants present in the tableting mass also act as antiadherents, but in the worst cases it may be necessary to add more starch or even talc to overcome the defect. So by judicious choice of a combination of excipients, all of these undesirable effects of the tableting process can be minimized.

Table 11 Some Commonly Used Controlled-Release Excipients

Hydrophilic
Acrylic acid
Acrylic acid derivatives/esters
Carboxymethyl cellulose (CMC)
Ethylcellulose (EC)
Hydroxypropylcellulose (HPC)
Hydroxypropylmethylcellulose (HPMC)
Methylcellulose (MC)
Poly(acrylic acid) (PAA)
Poly(aminobutyl glycolic acid) (PAGA)
Poly(caprolactone) (PCL)
Poly(lactic acid) (PLA)
Poly(lactic co-glycolic acid) (PLGA)
Poly(vinyl acetate) (PVAc)
Poly(vinyl alcohol) (PVA)
Poly(vinyl pryrrolidone) (Povidone, PVP)
Polyethylene glycol (PEG)
Hydrophobic
Carnauba wax
Glyceryl monostearate
Glyceryl palmitostearate
Hydrogenated vegetable oil
Paraffin
White wax
pH-dependent
Cellulose acetate phthalate (CAP)
Hydroxypropylmethyl cellulose phthalate (HPMCP)
Poly(methacrylates)
Poly(vinyl acetate phthalate) (PVAP)
Shellac
Zein
Surface-active
Pluronics

Dissolution Modifiers

This topic is the subject of Chapter 15, but some of the materials that are used in these systems have other uses as well (Table 5). Materials used to modify dissolution can be incorporated in the formulation on either a dry or wet basis. Table 11 lists some of the more commonly used controlled release excipients.

Absorbents

Some tablet formulations call for the inclusion of a small amount of semisolid, or even semiliquid, ingredient. It is highly desirable that any such component should be adsorbed onto, or absorbed into, one of the powders. In cases where none of the other excipients in the formulation is able to act as a carrier, an absorbent may have to be included. When oily substances, such as volatile-favoring agents, are involved, magnesium oxide and magnesium carbonate have been found to be suitable for this purpose. Natural earths, such as kaolin, bentonite, and Fuller's earth, have also been used and possess pronounced absorbent qualities. In general, they tend to reduce tablet hardness and may be abrasive. Therefore, fine, grit-free grade must be specified.

An absorbent may also be necessary when the formulation contains a hygroscopic ingredient, especially when absorption of moisture produces a cohesive powder that will not feed properly to the tablet press. In such instances, silicon dioxide has been found to be of particular value.

One special problem in the tableting of volatile medicaments, like nitroglycerin, is the loss of activity through evaporation. This effect can be reduced by fixing agents such as PEG 400 or 4000 in concentrations of 85%. Alternatively, cross-linked povidone can also be used to enhance the stability of this particular drug.

Flavoring Agents

Making a formulation palatable enough to be chewed may result in enhanced availability of the drug. In addition, for patients who are unable to swallow a tablet whole (e.g., children), such a tablet may be the only reasonable alternative. Sweetening agents such as dextrose, mannitol, saccharin, and sucrose are widely used as flavoring agents (see Table 12). When choosing a flavoring agent, however, one must carefully assess potential incompatibilities that may exist between the agent and the active ingredient. Perhaps the most extensively documented examples concern nitroglycerin tablets, which at one time were formulated in a chocolate base containing nonalkalized cocoa. Unfortunately, the cocoa affected the product's stability and has since been replaced by mannitol.

Flavoring agents proper are commonly volatile oils that have been dissolved in alcohol and sprayed onto the dried granules or have simply been adsorbed onto another excipient (e.g., talc). They are added immediately prior to compression to avoid loss through volatilization. In some cases they may even have some lubricating activity. If the oil normally contains terpenes, a low terpene grade is better so as to avoid possible deterioration in taste due to terpene oxidation products. When an oil flavoring is prone to oxidation, it may be protected by a special type of encapsulation involving spray drying or an aqueous emulsion containing the flavor. The emulgent used in spray-dried products may be starch or acacia gum giving rise to the so-called dry flavors.

Table 12 Some Commonly Used Sweetening Agents

Bulk
Compressible sugar
Confectioner's sugar
Dextrose
Glycerin
Lactose
Liquid glucose
Maltitol solution
Mannitol
Sorbitol
Sucrose
Xylitol
Intense
Acesulfame potassium
Aspartame
Saccharin
Saccharin sodium
Sodium cyclamate

Pharmaceutical Colors

Colorants do not contribute to therapeutic activity, nor do they improve product bioavailability or stability. Indeed, they increase the cost and complication of the manufacturing process. Their main role is to facilitate identification and to enhance the esthetic appearance of the product. In common with all material to be ingested by humans, solid dosage forms are severely restricted in the coloring agents that are allowable. This situation is complicated by the lack in international agreement on an approved list of colorants suitable for ingestion.

Colorants are available as either soluble dyes (i.e., giving a clear solution) or insoluble pigments that must be dispersed in the product (see Table 13). There is an increasing tendency to use dyes in the form of special pigments termed "lakes." The pigment in this case is adsorbed onto some inert substrate, usually aluminum hydroxide. These pigments can be directly incorporated into tablets. In such cases it is often preferable to mix the lake with an extendor prior to incorporation into the tablet blend to minimize any mottling. Ordinary starch or modified starches, such as StaRx 1500, or sugars can be used for this purpose. In addition, mottling is less evident in pastel shades and colors in the center of the visible spectrum.

For tablet coating there are distinct advantages to using pigments rather than dyes. Color development is more rapid and hence processing time is shorter. Since the final color is a function of the quantity of dye in the coating suspension, rather than the number of coats applied, there will be less operator influence and a better chance of achieving uniformity within and between batches. There may also be a reduced risk of interaction between the drug and other ingredients.

All dyes, and to a lesser extent lakes, are sensitive to light to varying degrees, and their color may be affected by other ingredients in the formulation. For example, since many colorants are sodium salts of organic acid, they may react in solution with cationic drugs (e.g., antihistamines). In addition, nonionic surfactants may adversely effect color stability. This is more prevalent when using natural colorants, which also tend to have a higher degree of batch-to-batch

Table 13 Differences Between Lakes and Dyes

Characteristics	Lakes	Dyes
Solubility	Insoluble in most solvents	Soluble in water, propylene glycol, and glycerin
Method of coloring	By dispersion	By solution
Pure dye content	10–40%	Primary colors: 90–93%
Rate of use	0.1–0.3%	0.01–0.03%
Particle size	< 0.5 μm	12–200 mesh
Stability		
Light	Better	Good
Heat	Better	Good
Coloring strength	Not proportional to dye content	Directly proportional to pure dye content
Shades	Varies with pure dye content	Constant

Source: Warner Jenkinson Pamphlet on Lake Pigments, September 1990.

variability. However, unlike artificial dyes, natural colors do not require FDA certification prior to use in drug products. Some of the more common synthetic colorants are listed in Table 14 together with their important properties.

Wetting Agents

Wetting agents have been used in tablets containing very poorly soluble drugs in order to enhance their rate of dissolution [86–89]. Surfactants are often chosen for this purpose, with sodium lauryl sulfate being the most common. Paradoxically, some ionic surfactants have recently been formulated with oppositely charged drugs to produce a sustained release complex [90–92]. Thus, one might want to consider using an uncharged surfactant, such as polysorbate 80 (Tween 80), which has less likelihood of interacting with charged molecules.

Co-processed Excipients

It is now possible to commercially obtain co-processed excipients (see Table 15). These excipients are essentially a "preblend" of two or more excipients that are commonly used in conjunction with each other [92a–92d]. Advantages to using co-processed excipients include a reduction in the number of raw materials and processing time required for a given formulation and a potential for improved batch-to-batch consistency. In addition, investigators found that tablets prepared from silified MCC (co-processed MCC and colloidal silicon dioxide) exhibited improved tablet strength, improved retention of compressibility after granulation, and superior flow properties when compared to tablets made from these MCC and colloidal silicon dioxide added as individual components [92d].

III. TABLET MANUFACTURE

Thus far in this chapter, the emphasis has been on the material rather than on the processes involved in tablet manufacture, but the latter are of equal importance. The pharmaceutical industry is highly regulated and must comply with current Good Manufacturing Practices (cGMPs). In terms of equipment, this translates into preparing products in totally enclosed systems by processes that minimize the handling and transfer of materials. Irrespective of the particular production route—wet granulation or direct compression—the first stage is likely to involve the intimate mixing together of several powdered ingredients.

A. Powder Mixing

The successful mixing together of fine powder is acknowledged to be one of the more difficult unit operations because, unlike the situation with liquid, perfect homogeneity is practically unattainable. All that is possible is to realize a maximum degree of randomness in the arrangement of the individual components of the mix. In practice, problems also arise because of the inherent cohesiveness and resistance to movement between the individual particles. The process is further complicated in many systems by the presence of significant segregative influences in the powder mix. These arise due to difference in particle size, shape, and density of the component particles.

Table 14 Some Commonly Used Pharmaceutical Colorants (Synthetic)

		Solubility (g/100 mL at 25°C)				Stability to					
FD&C color	Common name	Water	Glycerin	Propylene glycol	25% Ethanol	Light	Oxidation	pH 3	pH 5	pH 7	pH 8
Red[a]	Erythrosine	9.0	20.0	20.0	8.0	Poor	Fair	Insol	Insol	NNC	NNC
Red 40	Allura red AC	22.0	3.0	1.5	9.5	Good	Fair	NNC[b]	NNC	NNC	NNC
Yellow 5	Tartrazine	20.0	18.0	7.0	12.0	V. Good	Fair	NNC	NNC	NNC	NNC
Yellow 6	Sunset Yellow	19.0	20.0	2.2	10.0	Mod	Fair	NNC	NNC	NNC	NNC
Blue 1	Brilliant blue	20.0	20.0	20.0	20.0	Fair	Poor	S. fade[c]	V.S. fade[d]	V.S. fade	V.S. fade
Blue 2	Indigotine	1.6	1.0	0.1	1.0	V. poor	Poor	A. fade[c]	A. fade	A. fade	C. fade[f]
Green 3	Fast green	20.0	14.0	20.0	20.0	Fair	Poor	S. fade	V.S. fade	V.S. fade	S. fade

[a]Note: FD&C Red 3 lake has been delisted by FDA as of January 29, 1990.
[b]No noticeable change.
[c]Slight fade.
[d]Very slight fade.
[e]Appreciable fade.
[f]Completely fades.
Source: Warner-Jenkinson Pamphlet of Certified Colors, September 1990.

Table 15 Several Co-Processed Excipients

Excipient	Components	Manufacturer
Advantose FS	Fructose, pregelatinized starch	DMV
Avicel CE-15	MCC, guar gum	FMC
Cellactose	MCC, α-lactose monohydrate	Meggle GmbH
Ludipress	α-Lactose monohydrate, povidone, crospovidone	BASF
LustreClear	MCC, carrageenan	FMC
Microcelac	MCC, α-lactose monohydrate	Meggle GmbH
Pharmatose DCL	Anhydrous lactose, lactitol	DMV
ProSolv SMCC	MCC, colloidal silicon dioxide	Penwest

MCC, Microcrystalline cellulose.

It is not possible here to present a full account of the interactions between these effects, so the reader is referred to standard texts dealing with this important topic [93]. However, there may be an optimum mixing time and in such cases, prolonged mixing may result in an undesired product. In the special case of mixing in a lubricant, which is required at the granule surface, overmixing can be particularly detrimental.

Powder mixers vary widely in their ability to produce adequately mixed powders and the time needed to accomplish it. For intimate mixing of powders, energy must be supplied at a high enough rate to overcome the inherent resistance to differential movement between particles. Older mixers attempt to supply sufficient energy to mix the entire batch at once, but modern designs tend to be based on mechanisms for sequentially feeding a proportion of the total mix to a region of high-energy mixing potential. Typical examples of the general design of such mixers are shown diagrammatically in Fig. 13. Mixing is achieved by means of a main impeller, which feeds material to a high-speed "chopper," producing an intense shear mixing zone.

With all mixers, however, it is necessary to establish that an acceptable degree of homogeneity has been reached. Quantitative methodologies for establishing an "index of mixing" or "efficiency of mixing" are reported in the literature [94].

Direct Compression

For obvious reasons, the possibility of compressing mixed powders into tablets without an intermediate granulating step is an attractive one. For many years,

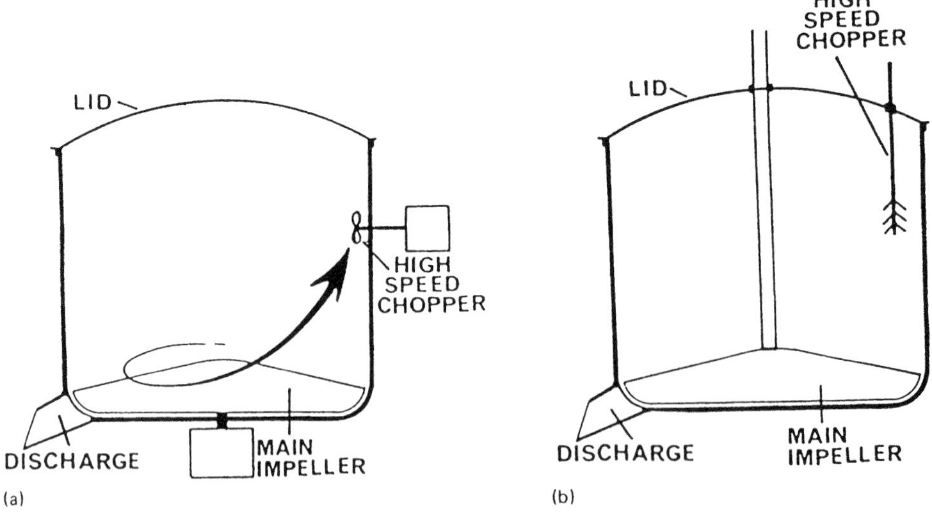

Fig. 13 High-shear mixers: (a) underdriven; (b) overdriven.

several widely used drugs, notably aspirin, have been available in forms that can be tableted without further treatment. Recently, there has been a growing impetus to develop so-called direct compression (DC) formulations, and the range of excipients, especially diluents, designed for this specific role has expanded dramatically.

It is possible to distinguish two types of DC formulations: (a) those where a major proportion is an active ingredient, and (b) those where the active ingredient is a minor component (i.e., $<10\%$ of the compression weight). In the former case, the inherent characteristics of the drug molecule, in particular the ability to prepare a physical form that will tablet directly, will have profound effects on the tablet's characteristics.

It may sometimes by necessary to supplement the properties of the drug so that it compresses more easily, and these needs have been realized by several manufacturers of excipients. Materials described as "compression aids" are now commercially available. Ideally, such adjuvants should develop mechanical strength while improving, or at least not adversely affecting, release characteristics. Among the most successful at meeting both these needs have been the microcrystalline celluloses (partially acid-hydrolyzed forms of cellulose). A number of grades are available based upon particle size and distribution.

Most other DC excipients really belong in the second category, where the drug is present in low concentration. In such cases, the use of an inexpensive DC diluent is warranted. Before considering some of these, certain generalizations are worth noting since there seems to have arisen an erroneous belief that DC is always a simpler formulation route. For instance, many DC fillers, such as spray-dried lactose, should not be reworked because this affects their compressibility. In addition, those diluents with a large particle size may give rise to mixing problems due to segregation unless an optimum proportion of fine material is present. More often, one is faced with the problem of an excessively narrow particle size distribution so that flow, in general, and uniform feeding to the dies, in particular, are difficult. Sometimes batch-to-batch variation is more prevalent in soluble DC fillers, such as sugars. Unlike wet granulation, DC has little ability to mask inherent tableting deficiencies in an ingredient. In addition, there will be little possibility for prior wetting of a hydrophobic drug and subsequent dissolution enhancement, which is a proven effect of wet granulation. On the other hand, DC formulations are likely to be more stable, show fewer aging effects, and, in specific cases, offer the only workable production method.

Wet Granulation

Although many existing products continue to be processed by a lengthy wet granulation that includes blending of dry ingredients, wet massing, screening, and then tray or fluidized bed drying, there is a trend toward using machines that can carry out the entire granulation sequence in a single piece of equipment or single-pot processor [95]. Formulators must be aware, however, that the type of granulation procedure used can have a profound impact on the granules produced. Thus, a formulation that produces adequate granules by conventional planetary mixing may produce suboptimal product if transferred to a single-pot processor.

It is generally agreed that there will exist an optimum range of granule sizes for a particular formulation, and therefore, certain generalizations are worthy to note here. Within limits, smaller granules will lead to higher and more uniform tablet weight and higher tablet crushing strength, with subsequent longer disintegration time and reduced friability. The strength of granules has also been shown to influence the tensile strength of the tablets prepared from them, with stronger granules leading, in general, to harder tablets [96].

One important finding with widespread implications arises from work by Chaudry and King [97], who demonstrated that migration of a soluble drug during moist granulation was responsible for uneven content uniformity of tablets of warfarin. A modified base (containing dibasic calcium phosphate, alginic acid, and acacia), developed from experiments to assess migration-retarding ability, enhanced tablet performance.

B. Powder Compaction

For simplicity, the physics of tablet compaction discussed here will deal with the single punch press, where the lower punch remains stationary. Initially, the powder is filled into the die with the excess being swept off. When the upper punch first presses down upon the powder bed, the particles rearrange themselves to achieve closer packing. As the upper punch continues to advance upon the powder bed, the rearrangement becomes more difficult and deformation of particles at points of contact begins. At first the particle will undergo elastic deformation, which is a reversible process, but as continual pressure is applied, the particle begins to deform irreversibly. Irreversible deformation can be due either to plastic deformation, which is a major factor attributing to the tablet's mechanical strength, or to brittle fracture, which produces poor quality compacts that crumble as the tablets are ejected [25,98]. In general, as increasing pressure is applied to a compact, its porosity will be reduced.

The surface area of the individual particles themselves changes during the compaction process. Initially, an increase in surface area is noted due to the fracture as compression force increases. Eventually, the surface area decreases due to bonding and consolidation of particles at higher compression forces [25,98]. Higuchi et al. [98] postulated that an additional increase in surface area occurs after this point and that this effect may cause lamination of the tablet due to extensive rebound at decompression. In other words, at the tablet punch powder interface, there may be zones of high density during compression, but upon decompression these zones have elastic rebound and are pulled apart from the rest of the tablet that did not contain this high density.

The major forces involved in the formation of a tablet compact are illustrated in Fig. 14 (a single-ended model) and are notated as follows: F_A represents the axial pressure, which is the force applied to the compact by the upper punch, F_L is the force translated to the lower punch, and F_D is the force lost to the die wall. If one remembers that for every force there must be an equal and opposite force, the following relationship is obvious:

$$F_A = F_L + F_D$$

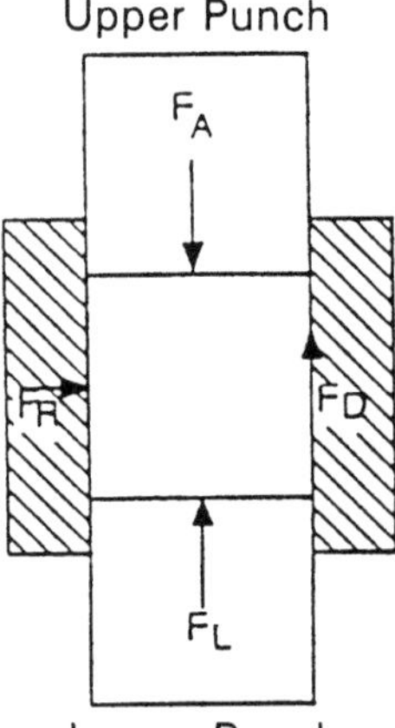

Fig. 14 Forces developed in the formation of a tablet compact. ▨, die wall; F_A, axial pressure applied by upper punch; F_D, force lost to die wall; F_R, radial die wall; □, tablet compact.

F_R is the radial die wall force that develops because the powder is in a confined environment (i.e., not able to spread outward as pressure is applied down upon it because it is residing within the die). The coefficient of friction at the die wall, μ_W, is due to the shearing adhesion that occurs along the die a as the powder is made more dense and compressed. The following relationship between and F_D, μ_W, and F_R is found to exist:

$$F_D = \mu_W F_R$$

The force of tablet ejection from the die, F_E, is a function of both and the residual die wall force, $RDWF$, that exists after decompression. As the friction decreases, one will obviously see a corresponding drop in F_E. It is important to remember here that it is desirable for F_E to be as low as possible so that minimal damage is imparted to both the tablet and the tooling.

The first applications of this technique [99] were directed to developing a more sensitive assessment of lubricant efficiency than that offered by the traditional "coefficient of lubrication", or R-value (i.e., $F_L : F_A$ ratio). Since then, its use has been extended to provide predictive information on formulation performance [100,101]. Lammens et al. [102] have stressed the importance of ensuring precision and accuracy in such measurements for correct interpretation of the data so produced.

Although the choice of precise tablet geometry may be more the prerogative of the marketing department than of the pharmaceutical formulation or production department, certain general technical observations must be taken into account. Bearing in mind that most tablets are cylindrical in shape, diameters between 3 and 12 mm are preferred, with either beveled edges or biconvex profile. Low height-to-diameter ratios, consistent with adequate tablet strength, are desirable so as to minimize die-wall fractional effects, which can consume a significant amount of the total energy required in tableting. In addition, the internal stress differences will be minimized if a biconvex profile is selected, although the tablet's shape may affect the release of the drugs in matrix tablets [103]. The effect of punch face geometry and lubricant compression on tablet properties has been reported by Mechtersheimer and Zucker [104].

As a generalization, increasing compressional force will retard dispersion on administration, and therefore, levels should be kept as low as possible, consistent with achieving acceptable mechanical properties. With some excipients there is a critical compressional force range required to achieve minimum disintegration times.

This has been demonstrated for starch-containing formulations and was thought to be linked to production of an optimum pore size distribution that allowed rapid uptake of water without providing large internal air spaces to accommodate the swelling starch grains [105]. The importance of press speed must also be taken into account, particularly where plastic deformation is thought to play a major role in tablet formation. The effect of this rate of compaction has been demonstrated quantitatively in a report by Roberts and Rowe [106].

IV. TABLETING EQUIPMENT

A. Granulators

Originally, wet granulation involved the hand process of preparing a wet mass and forcing it through a screen onto trays that was placed into a convection oven where the granules were dried. With increasing batch sizes, the need for bulk granulation procedures became necessary. Many of these procedures involved mixing the powdered ingredients in a special ribbon blender, which could also accomplish the wet massing process. The moistened materials were then usually granulated by forcing them through a screen, using oscillating blades of a modified comminuting mill, onto trays that were then transferred to an oven for drying. Current granulating methods can be classified into the following categories: (a) traditional methods as detailed above; (b) high-shear mixing; (c) fluid-bed granulation; and (d) single-pot processing.

High shear mixers, which make use of both a high-speed mixing blade and chopper, have largely replaced traditional planetary mixing. This process can reduce granulation time and produces dense granules. Material processed in a high-shear mixer is discharged from the unit and transferred to a drying unit, with or without an intermediate screening step.

Fluidized beds have been expanded from their original use as dryers to encompass granulation as well. Granulation in a fluidized bed is achieved by suspending the powder in the air of the fluidized bed and then spraying a liquid binder from nozzles that are positioned above or below the powder bed. In general, top-spray operation produces porous granules while bottom-spray granules are dense and highly spherical. When using fluidized beds in the granulation/drying mode, the process conditions, such as drying temperature and length of the drying cycle, must be optimized, and it may be necessary to adopt a different approach to formulation than would have been used with the more traditional equipment. For example, granulating fluid is sprayed into the bed of mixed powder at a given temperature; its volatility and viscosity under these conditions will influence the characteristics of the final product. The important parameters governing the performance of fluidized beds used as MGDs has been studied by Worts and Schoefer [107]. They concluded that in addition to the inlet air temperature, the type of binder solution and its flow rate and droplet size were critical variables that had to be controlled. These investigators also found that the residual moisture levels of granulations are a major factor contributing to the *in vitro* dissolution and friability of tablets made from them.

Single-pot processors that can are capable of mixing, granulation, drying, and even pelletization and coating are now commercially available from a number of sources. The first of these processors were simply granulation units that had been retrofitted for drying and did not provide significant advantages over traditional granulation and drying methods. With the advent of microwave- and gas-assisted vacuum-drying techniques, drying times were drastically reduced, thereby making these units more viable as commercial equipment [95]. In addition to time savings that can be realized when using single-pot processors, these systems offer the following advantages over conventional methods: (a) improved yield due to minimization of product loss during transfer; (b) closed unit operation, minimizing product contamination and environmental exposure to high potent substances; and (c) reduced risk of explosion due to near absence of oxygen in the closed unit [95].

Granulation by preliminary compression, originally performed in heavy-duty tablet machines, when it was called "slugging," has been used for a small number of products for many years. This approach has been further developed in machines that are essentially roll compactors, squeezing the material to produce agglomerates. In addition, most high-output tablet presses are now equipped with precompression rollers that perform the "slugging" of the granulation prior to its "true" compaction (see Fig. 15).

Another method of producing materials to be tableted is pelletization. Pellets are typically larger and more spherical in nature than granules and possess high bulk density and excellent flow properties. Pellets can be prepared by several methods, including (a) layering active material onto an inert core (nonpariel), (b) extruding a wet mass through a large number of small orifices and then rotating the "strands" in a special bowl capable of spheronizing the granules, or

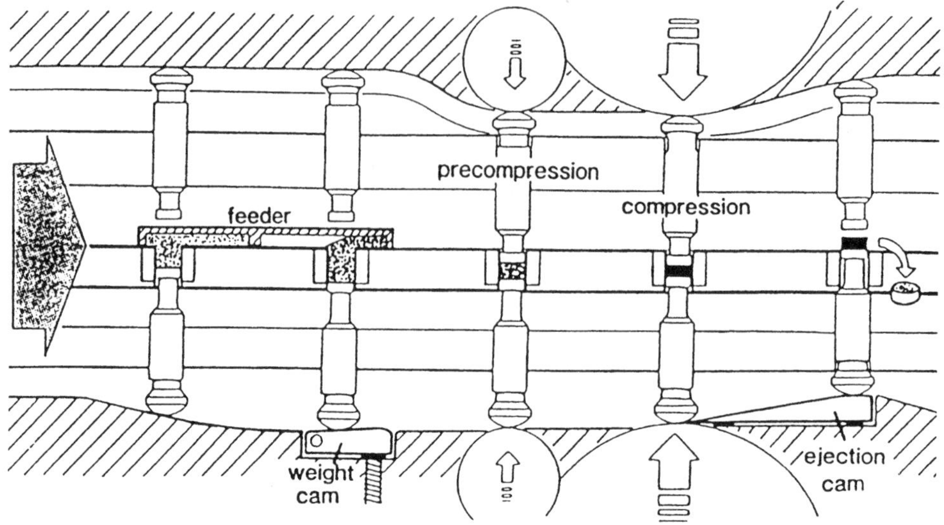

Fig. 15 Multistation press cycle.

(c) mixing the active substance and binder powders together and then heating to a temperature above the melting point of the binder. Pelletization by extrusion and spheronization, or marumerization, is the most common of these methods. The parameters controlling this process have been studied by Malinowski [108] and the effect on the tablet produced from it evaluated.

B. Tablet Presses

With the exception of presses designed to produce coated or layered tablets, the development of tableting equipment has been one largely of continuing evolution. In many areas, the incentives have come from the pharmaceutical industry, rather than the tablet press manufacturers, as a result of certain trends in tableting operations. These include (a) increased rate of production, (b) direct compression of powders, (c) stringent standards for cleanliness to comply with cGMPs, and (d) automation, or at least continuous monitoring of the process. However, there is now evidence to suggest that we may be approaching inherent limits to further development of some press variables on existing lines.

At present, and in the immediate future, one can anticipate the continual vying of one manufacturer with another over relatively minor improvements, with possibly significant advances in instrumentation, automation, and hygiene. However, several easy-to-clean high-output presses are currently manufactured. Most Kikisui models are "self-cleaning" and allow for the entire turret area to be filled with solvents and cleaned by running the press.

All tableting presses employ the same basic principle—they compress the granular or powdered mixture of ingredients in a die between two punches with the die and its associated punches being called a "station of tooling." Tablet machines can be divided into two distinct categories:

1. Those with a single set of tooling—"single station" (or "single-punch") or "eccentric" presses
2. Those with several stations of tooling—"multistation" (or "rotary") presses

Figures 15 and 16 provide a summary of the compression cycles for rotary and single-punch tablet presses. The formation of the tablet compact in these two types of presses mainly differs in the compaction mechanism itself, as well as the much greater speeds achieved with rotary type presses. The single punch basically uses a hammering type of motion (i.e., the upper punch moves down while the lower punch remains stationary), while rotary presses make use of an accordion-type compression (i.e., both punches move toward each other). The former find their primary use as an R&D tool, whereas the latter, having higher outputs, are used in most production operations.

Single Station Presses

All commercial types of single station presses have essentially the same basic operating cycle (see Fig. 16), where filling, compression, and ejection of tablets from the die is accomplished by punch movement utilizing cam actions. Material is fed to the die from the hopper

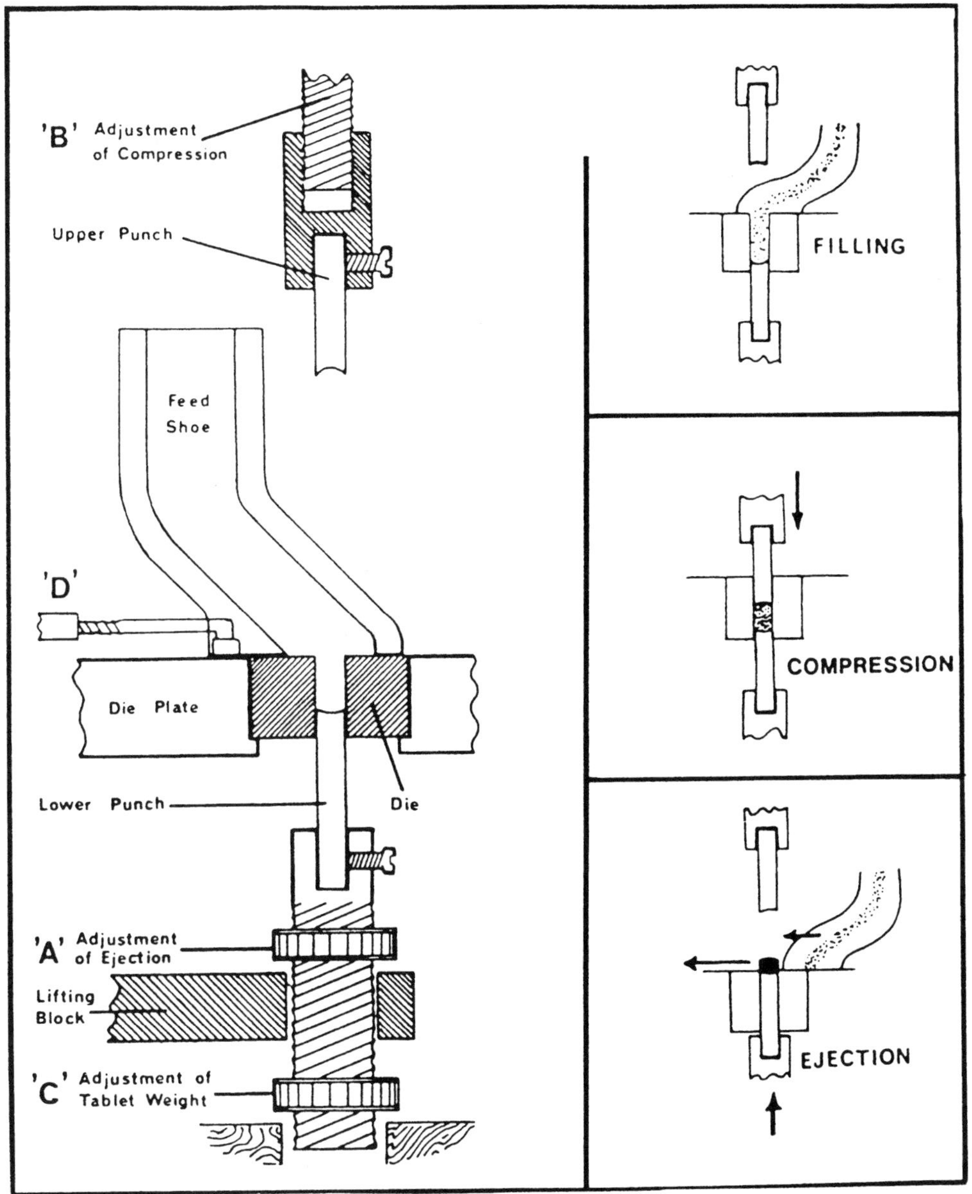

Fig. 16 Single station press cycle.

via an oscillating feed shoe; the position of the lower punch at this point determines the tablet weight. The feed shoe then moves away and the upper punch descends into the die to compress the tablet, with the extent of this movement controlling the level of compression force. As the upper punch moves upward, the lower punch rises and in so doing ejects the tablet from the die. At this point, the feed shoe moves in and knocks the tablet out of the machine as the lower punch moves to its bottom position ready for the next press cycle.

The largest single-punch machines are capable of making tablets up to 22 mm in diameter at rates of about 80 tablets per minute (TPM) and exerting maximum forces on the order of 40 kN (see Table 16). In isolated cases tablets can only be made on this type of machine, probably because their mode of operation gives the material a longer "dwell time" under compression. Although the table output rate from single station presses can be increased by use of multitip tooling, the rotary machine remains the method of choice for production purposes.

Table 16 Approximate Specifications of Some Small Single-Station Laboratory Presses

Manufacturer: Model Number:	Fette Exacta 1	Kilian SP300	Korsch EK-O/DMS	Manesty F3
Maximum output (tabs/min)	75	80	60	85
Maximum tablet diameter (mm)	15	18	20	22
Maximum fill (mm)	16	16	20	17
Maximum applied force (kN)	15	25	30	40
Motor (HP)	0.75	1.1	0.5	2.0
Weight (kg)	250	300	200	476
Approximate dwell time (ms)	133	125	100	118

Multistation Presses

In this type of machine the operating cycle and methods of filling, compression, and ejection are different from those of single-station presses and are summarized in Fig. 15. More specifically, the dies and punches are mounted on a rotating turret.

All operations take place simultaneously in different stations. Sixteen stations were commonly used in earlier machines with outputs between 500 and 1000 TPM and tablet diameters up to 15 mm. Presses with outputs orders of magnitude greater than the above are now widely available. The dies are filled as they pass beneath a stationary feed frame, which may be fitted with paddles to aid material transfer. The die cavities are completely filled and excess ejected prior to compression. Compression involves the movement of both punches between compression rolls, in contrast to single station operations where only the upper punch effects compression. Ejection occurs as both punches are moved away from the die on cam tracks until the tablet is completely clear of the die, at which point it hits the edge of the feed frame and is knocked off the press. Tooling pressure may be exerted hydraulically, rather than through the use of mechanical camming actions, as is the case with machines produced by Courtoy.

The ways in which individual manufacturers of tableting equipment have sought to achieve higher output fall into four groups:

1. Increasing the effective number of punches (i.e., multitipped)
2. Increasing the number of stations
3. Increasing the number of points of compression
4. Increasing the rate of compression (i.e., turret speed)

Each of these approaches has its own particular set of advantages and disadvantages. In addition, all make demands on other aspects of press design and certain general inherent characteristics of die compaction have to be taken into account.

Generally, the high-speed machines consist of "double-rotary" presses where the cycle of operation is repeated twice in one revolution of the turret carrying the tooling, although one press (Magna, Vector Corp.) has four cycles per revolution (the Magna is no longer manufactured due to the small demand required for these very high-output machines). Most high-output tablet presses have odd numbers of stations, with up to 101 in the largest presses (see Table 17). Double-rotary presses have also been modified to produce layered tablets, whereas other machines have been adapted to produce coated tablets by a "dry" compression technique.

C. Tablet Machine Instrumentation

In order to produce an adequate tablet formulation, certain requirements, such as sufficient mechanical strength and desired drug release profile, must be met. At times this may be a difficult task for the formulator to achieve, due to poor flow and compactibility characteristics of the powdered drug. This is of particular importance when one only has a small amount of active material to work with and cannot afford to make use of trial-and-error methods. The study of the physics of tablet compaction through the use of instrumented tableting machines (ITMs) enables the formulator to systematically evaluate his formula and make any necessary changes.

ITMs provide a valuable service to all phases of tablet manufacture, from research to production and quality control [109–111]. As a research tool, ITMs allow in-depth study of the mechanism of tablet compaction by measuring the forces that develop during formation, ejection, and detachment of tablets. ITMs can also provide clues about how materials bond,

Table 17 Comparative Specifications of Some High-Output Tablet Presses

Manufacturer: Model:	Fette PT3090	Kikusi Gemini	Korsch PH 800	Manesty Rotapress
Maximum output (tabs/min)	16,750	10,720	18,360	13,360
Number of stations	79	67	85	75
Maximum turret speed (rpm)	106	80	108	89
Maximum tablet diameter (mm)	34	25	34	25
Maximum fill depth (mm)	18	16	22	20.6
Maximum compression force (kN)	100	80	80	100
Precompression (kN)	100	80	80	10
Net weight (kg)	4500	3900	4000	3700

deform, and react to frictional effects. The formulator himself is able to monitor the effects of additives in the overall tableting process, as well as the effects of operation variables in the manufacture and performance of the dosage form. As stated above, this markedly reduces the formulator's reliance on empiricism in formulation design. In the area of product and quality control, ITMs are able to monitor tablet weight and punch and machine wear and damage. More recently, ITMs have been used to characterize unique "typical batches" of materials so that one has a baseline for troubleshooting formulations or a basis for quality control [109–111].

ITMs in Research and Development

The tableting process involves two phenomena: (a) a reduction in the bulk volume of the tablet mass by elimination of air, referred to as "compression," and (b) an increase in the mechanical strength of the mass due to particle-particle interactions, which is termed "consolidation." This latter process results from utilization of the free surface energies of the particles in bond formation, referred to as "cold welding," plus intermolecular interactions via van der Waals forces, for example. The process is enhanced by generation of large areas of clean surface, which are then pressed together; such a mechanism is feasible if appreciable brittle fracture and plastic deformation can be introduced into the system. Therefore, the manner in which the various components compress will be significant.

It is also important to appreciate that the behavior on decompression can markedly affect the characteristics of the finished tablets, because the structure must be strong enough to accommodate the recovery- and ejection-induced stresses. Indeed, tablet strength is a direct function of the number of "surviving bonds" in the finished tablet. In addition, ability to monitor ejection forces leads to valuable information on lubricant efficiency.

Analysis of Data Obtained from ITMs

Measurement of the punch and die forces plus the relative displacement of the punches can provide raw data which, when suitably processed and interpreted, facilitate the evaluation of many tableting parameters. Many of the workers first involved in instrumenting tablet presses concentrated on deriving relationships between the applied force (F_A) and the porosity (E) of the consolidating mass.

Heckel proposed that a correlation exists between yield strength and an empirically determined constant, K, which is a measure of the ability of the compact to deform [28,112]. He discovered that, indeed, K is inversely proportional to yield strength. Further, he derived an equation expressing the relationship between the density of a compact and the compressional force applied. This relationship is based on the assumption that decreasing void space (i.e., decreasing porosity) of a compact follows a first order rate process:

$$\frac{dD}{dP} = K(1 - D)$$

where

D = relative density
P = pressure
$(1 - D)$ = pore fraction
K = proportionality constant

By integrating and rearrange this equation, one obtains the following linear relationship:

$$\ln\left(\frac{1}{1 - D}\right) = KP + A$$

where

$$A = \ln\left(\frac{1}{1 - D_0}\right) + B$$

and B is a measure of particle rearrangement.

It has been claimed [113] that the presentation of data in the form of Athy-Heckel plots [112,114], as illustrated in Figure 17, facilitates assessment of the relative proportions of brittle fracture and plastic deformation present. Each set of curves within a plot represents the same formulation, with decreasing particle size fractions. If the curves remain discrete, as in Fig. 17a, one can assume that plastic deformation is the predominant mechanism because all formulations have sufficient time to rearrange (n.b., plastic deformation is a time-dependent process). In contrast, Fig. 17b illustrates the behavior of a material that primarily deforms by brittle fracture. Here, the original particle size distribution is rapidly destroyed and the curves become superimposed. Additionally, the slope of the lines, which represents K, is approximately unity. Higher slopes (i.e., low yield pressure) are found when evaluating plastically deforming materials. Subsequent studies [115,116] have cast doubts on the universality of this claim, and conflicting data have been reported. In addition, several adaptations have been made to correct for inconsistencies present in Heckel's model [116a,116b].

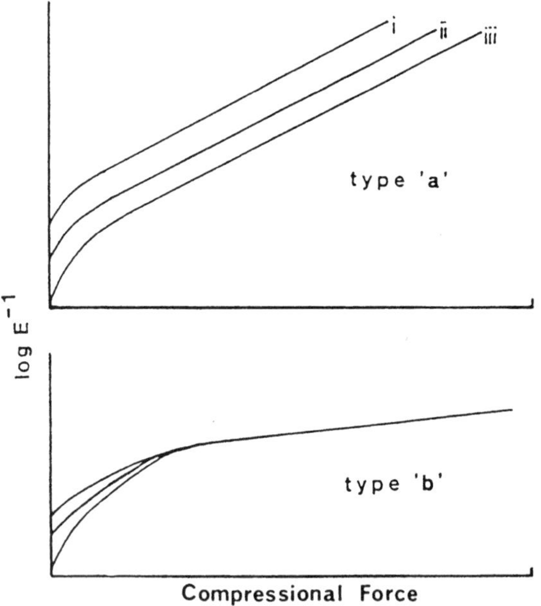

Fig. 17 Athy-Heckel plots: (a) material undergoing plastic deformation; (b) material undergoing brittle fracture.

Applied force and displacement measurements have also been used to generate force versus displacement curves (F-D plots) [99]. Such information can be used to estimate the energy necessary to form a compact in the following manner:

$$W = F \int dD$$

where

$W =$ work
$F =$ force
$D =$ distance

When one plots force vs. displacement, the area under the curve thus represents work. In practice, the compression/decompression data take the form shown in Fig. 18. The area under the upward line represents the work done on the tableting mass during compaction, while that under the downward line arise from the fact work is done on the punch by the tablet as a result of the latter's elastic recovery on decompression.

In single-station presses a further subdivision of work can be made by considering the force transmitted to the lower punch during the compression. This will be less than that registered by the upper punch due to frictional effects at the die wall. Three components to the total work can therefore be distinguished; W_F, the work done in overcoming die wall friction, W_D, the work of elastic recovery, and W_N, the net work involved in forming the tablet. Interpretation of F-D curves, on single-station presses, has proved to be particularly attractive, as demonstrated by the work of Travers and Cox [117].

Some researchers have extended the monitoring of work to the determination of the rate of doing work, or power [116], as illustrated in the following equation:

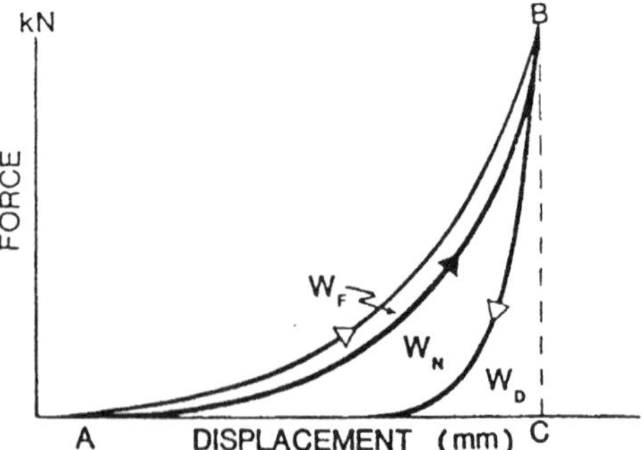

Fig. 18 A typical force-displacement curve. $W_F =$ work done overcoming die wall friction; W_D, work of elastic recovery; W_N, net work involved in tablet compact formation.

$$\frac{dW}{dt} = power$$

The rationale behind this approach is that due to the varying degrees of bond formation, different materials require a greater, or lesser, amount of energy to compress them to a given degree. In a tablet press running at a given speed, the rate of doing work must therefore be different and may be related to tablet strength. In addition, since plastic deformation is a time-dependent phenomenon, power, which takes time into account, may be indicative of the contribution of this mechanism.

The compressive behavior of the material is also reflected in that proportion of the axial force (F_A) that is transmitted radially to the die wall (F_R) during compression and decompression. Therefore, monitoring the ratio of these two forces during the entire machine operation can provide valuable data referred to as the "compaction profile." As shown in Fig. 19, this normally takes the form of a hysteresis loop, the area of which is a function of the departure of the material from purely elastic behavior. Other features of the profile provide valuable guidelines as to tablet strength, likely levels of lubrication required, and predominant type of deformation. The line OA is represented as a dotted line because this region is due to repacking, which can be quite variable. At point A, elastic deformation becomes dominant and continues until the yield stress, at point B, is reach. At this point, the deformation of the compact is due to plastic deformation and brittle fracture. This process continues to point C, at which time force is removed and decompression begins. From point C to D, the material is elastically recovering. If a second yield point, D, is reached, the material has become plastically deformed of brittley fractured. To sum up all of these processes:

Slope AB = function of elastic deformation
Slopes BC and DE = function of plastic deformation and brittle fracture
Slopes BC′and CD = function of elastic recovery
Lines OC′and OE = function of (residual die wall force) RDWF

One should note that BC′ represents a highly elastic material as little plastic deformation or brittle fracture has occurred. Also, sharp differences between the slope CD and DE are indicative of weak, or failed, tablet structures. The *RDWF* estimated from these plots can provide a good indication of the ejection force. More detailed treatments of such studies are now in the open literature, to which the interested reader is referred [118–120].

Another approach to determining the contribution being made by each of the possible compression/decompression mechanisms involves monitoring the degree and rate of relaxation in tablets immediately after the point of maximum applied force has been reached. Once a powder bed exceeds a certain yield stress, it behaves as a fluid and exhibits "plastic flow" [121,122]. Certain investigators [122] have studied plastic flow in terms of viscous and elastic elements and have derived the following equation:

$$\ln F_1 = \ln F_0 - kt$$

where

F = compressional force in viscoelastic region
t = time
k = degree of plastic flow

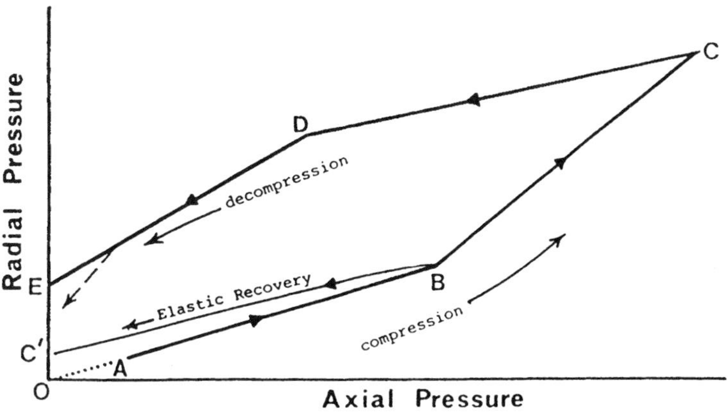

Fig. 19 Compaction profile.

which can be integrated and rearranged to yield the linear equation:

$$\ln F_1 = \ln F_0 - kt$$

Thus, if one plots log(F) vs. time, one only needs to calculate the slope of the line so plotted to determine the plastic flow, k. Materials with higher values of k (i.e., more plastic flow) tend to form stronger tablets than those with low k values.

Compaction Simulators

In 1972, Rees et al. [123] developed the compaction simulator that, in oversimplified terms, is a hydraulic press capable of accurately mimicking the action of any high-speed rotary press. This is an overwhelming achievement in the study of compaction physics when one reflects upon the various disadvantages associated with single punch and rotary presses that this system can overcome. For instance, single punch measurements, while providing a baseline for formulation development, do not accurately reflect the forces incurred at the production level; the lower punch remains stationary rather than moving in single punch systems, and the dwell time, which influences the extent of plastic deformation, is significantly increased due to the low speed of manufacture. On the other hand, rotary presses require relatively large amounts of granulation and therefore are inappropriate for the initial phases of formulation when only small amounts of material are available. Also, the rate of applying and removing forces varies appreciably from machine to machine depending on the way the machine is operated, the punches used, etc. The compaction simulator is able to compensate for all of these disadvantages so that production level conditions can exist for small amounts of material. Additionally, the compaction simulator is capable of reproducing the variables associated with each machine and thereby providing adequate means for transferring a formulation from one machine to another. Until the 1990s, there were only two compaction simulators in use in the United States: one at SmithKline Beecham and the other, used by a consortium of companies in the U.S., at Rutgers College of Pharmacy. Several commercial "simulators" are now available, including the PCS-1 from AC Computing, the Presster from Metropolitan Computing Corp. and the P1200 G/TSC Galenic Version from Fette International.

Several reviews of the mechanisms involved in the compaction process and interpretation of the large amount of data generated from such studies have been published [124,125]. The solution to this complex process is still incomplete and provides continuing research opportunities for the pharmaceutical scientist. The actual mechanics of instrumenting presses has also been reviewed [111], and a recently published book [126] is devoted entirely to this subject. Instrumentation typically involves the use of piezoelectric transducers or strain gauges and requires that modifications be made to either the tablet punches or the die table. However, Yeh et al. have described the use of finite element analysis (FEA) that does not require die table modification [126a]. Guo et al. have also developed a noninvasive technique that relies on the use of confocal laser scanning microscopy [126b]. Another new development is the use of calorimeters to directly evaluate the thermodynamic properties of compression [126c].

There has also been significant growth in the number of press manufacturers offering instrumentation packages for use with high-speed multistation machines to control tablet weight variation and, in some cases, divert out-of-tolerance tablets to a reject container. The more sophisticated systems result in a fully automated press operation with minimal operator intervention required (see Fig. 20).

V. COATED TABLETS

The coating of pharmaceutical tablets may be divided conveniently into the traditional sugar, or pan-coating procedures, and contemporary techniques that include film coating and compression coating. Coating methods were developed for a variety of reasons, including the need to mask an unpleasant taste or unsightly appearance of the uncoated tablet, as well as to increase patient acceptability. Protection of an ingredient from degradation effects due to exposure to moisture, air, and light were further incentives. The newer techniques have extended the usefulness of coating to include the facilitation of controlled-release characteristics and the ability to co-formulate inherently incompatible materials.

A. Sugar Coating

The sugar coating process involves building up layers of coating material on the tablet cores as they are tumbled in a revolving pan by repetitively applying a coating solution or suspension and drying off the solvent. Traditionally, the cores were made using tooling with deep concave geometry so as to reduce the problems associated with producing a sufficiently thin coat around the tablet's edge, as illustrated in Fig. 21.

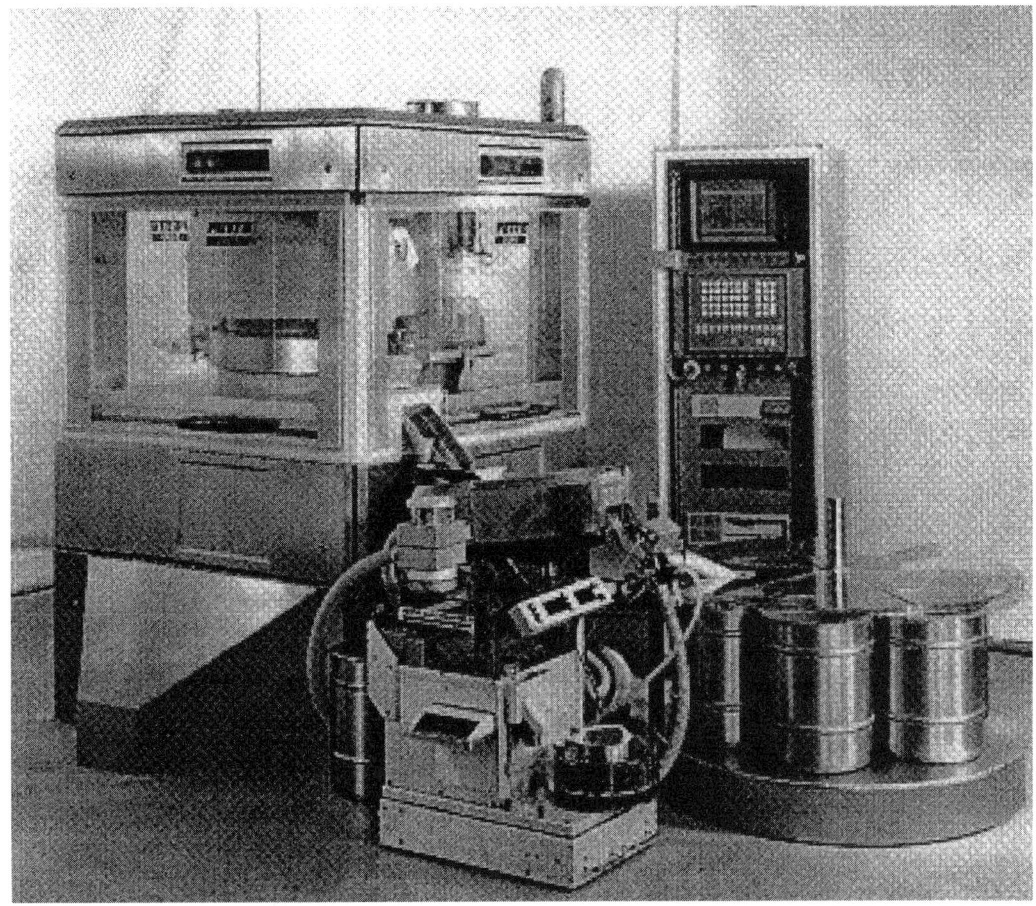

Fig. 20 Automated high-output rotary tablet press. (Courtesy of Fette America.)

However, it has been shown that this shape may not be ideal for all products due to the inherent softer crown region exhibited in tablets manufactured from such tooling. In addition, deep concave tooling often produces tablets of poor mechanical strength [127]. Core mechanical strength, in particular friability, must be adequate enough to withstand the abrasive effects of the tumbling action while retaining the dissolution characteristics of an uncoated tablet. Large tablets, in particular, sometimes require higher compressional forces than are necessary for uncoated tablets of the same size. Care must also be exercised to minimize penetration of coating solutions into the core itself, although the coat should, of course, adhere well to the tablet surface. It will also be important to maintain a smooth, uniform surface and to provide careful control of the environment within the coating pan. Because of these requirements, the process may best be described by means of a generalized example.

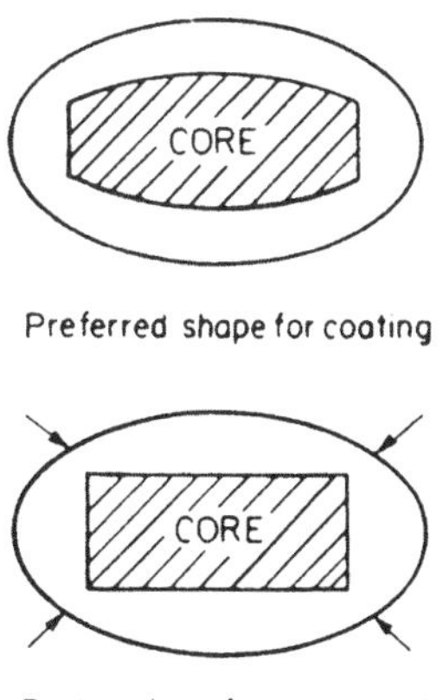

Fig. 21 Tablet-coating geometry.

In the past, the initial layers of coating (the sealing coat) were achieved by applying one or two coats of shellac. However, due to the variability between batches of this material, PVP-stabilized types of shellac or other polymeric materials, such as cellulose acetate phthalate (CAP) and poly(vinyl acetate phthalate) (PVAP), are now more popular. It should be appreciated that a fine balance must exist between minimizing the thickness of the sealing coat and providing an adequate moisture barrier.

The next stage is to build up a subcoat that will provide a good bridge between the main coating and the sealed core, as well as rounding off any sharp corners. This is normally a two-step procedure. The first step involves the application of a warm subcoat syrup (containing acacia and/or gelatin) that rapidly distributes uniformly over the tablets and eventually becomes partially dry and tacky. At this point, a subcoat powder (containing material such as calcium carbonate, talc, kaolin, starch, and acacia) is dusted evenly over the tablets, after which the pan is allowed to rotate until the coat is hard and dry. This subcoat cycle is usually repeated three or four times, taking care to avoid the production of rough surfaces, which would be difficult to eradicate later on, and ensuring that each coat is absolutely dry before the next is applied.

The step that follows is known as "smoothing" or "grossing." It produces the bulk of the total coating weight and involves the application of a suspension of starch, calcium carbonate, or even some of the subcoat powder, in syrup. Each application is dried and the process repeated until the desired build-up has been realized. The last few applications may be made with a syrup free from suspended powders, so as to produce a smooth surface. If the tablets are to be colored, colorants are normally added in these clear syrup layers. It is important that the tablet surfaces be smooth before this is attempted, otherwise uneven coloring may result. The final finishing stage is accomplished by again applying one or two layers of clear syrup, taking care not to overdry between coats and stopping while the final coat is still slightly damp. Jogging (i.e., pan stationary apart from intermittent rotation through a small angle) is then carried out until the tablets appear dry.

The tablets are then left for several hours and are transferred to the polishing pan, which is usually of cylindrical design with canvas side walls. The polish is a dilute wax solution (e.g., carnauba or beeswax in petroleum spirit) applied sparingly, following which the tablets are left to roll until a high luster is produced. They are the normally "racked" to allow any traces of solvent to evaporate before being sent to the inspection and packing operations.

There are as many variations in coating procedures as there are tablet coaters, and so the account given here is only a guide. Nevertheless, it illustrates the complexity and time-consuming nature of the process, and the reader will realize why efforts have been made to develop alternate coatings, equipment, and methods that permit at least some degree of automation.

B. Film Coating

Film coating has increased in popularity for a number of reasons. The film process is simpler, and therefore easier to automate. It is also more rapid than sugar coating, since weight gains of only 2–6% are involved, as opposed to more than 50% with sugar coating. In addition, moisture involvement can be avoided, if necessary, through the use of nonaqueous solvents. Moreover, distinctive identification tablet markings are not obscured by film coats.

There are now many synthetic polymeric materials available for film coating, many of which meet all the requirements of a good film former. These include lack of toxicity and a suitable solubility profile for film application and upon ingestion, together with the ability to produce a tough, yet elastic film even in the presence of powdered additives such as pigments. The film must, of course, be stable to heat, light, and moisture and be free from undesirable taste or odor.

Some of the more commonly used materials meeting these criteria are listed in Table 18 together with some important properties. Two major groups may be distinguished: (a) materials that are nonenteric and for the most part cellulose derivatives and (b) materials that can provide an enteric effect and are commonly esters of phthalic acid. Within both groups it is general practice to use a mixture of materials to give a film with the optimum range of properties. They may contain a plasticizer that, as the name implies, prevents the film from becoming brittle with consequent risk of chipping [128]. Some popular choices are shown in Table 19. Because they essentially function by modifying polymer-to-polymer molecular bonding, the choice of plasticizer is dependent upon the particular film polymer. Like so many other facets of tablet coating, there is no substitute for properly designed experimental trials in developing a robust procedure.

The nature of the solvent system may markedly influence the quality of the film [129], and, to optimize the various factors, mixed solvents are usually necessary. More specifically, the rate of evaporation, and hence the time for the film to dry, has to be con-

Table 18 Some Commonly Used Film-Coating Materials

Full name	Abbreviation	Soluble in	Comments
Nonenteric			
Methylcellulose	MC	Cold water, GI fluids, organic solvents	Useful polymer for aqueous films; low-viscosity grade best
Ethylcellulose	EC	Ethanol, other organic solvents	Cannot be used alone as is totally insoluble in water and GI fluids; employed as a film toughner
Hydroxyethylcellulose	HEC	Water and GI fluids	Properties similar to MC, but gives clear solutions
Methylhydroxyethylcellulose	MHEC	GI fluids	Similar properties to HPMC, but less soluble in organic systems
Hydroxypropylcellulose	HPC	Cold water, GI fluids, polar organics such as anhydrous lower alcohols	Difficulty in handling due to tackiness while drying
Hydroxypropylmethylcellulose	HPMC	Cold water, GI fluids, methanol/methylene chloride, alcohol/fluorohydrocarbons	Excellent film former and readily soluble throughout GIT; low-viscosity grades to be preferred, e.g., Methocel HG (Dow)
Sodium carboxymethylcellulose	Na-CMC	Water and polar organic solvents	Main use where presence of moisture in solvent not a problem
Povidone	PVP	Water, GI fluids, alcohol, and IPA	Care needed in use due to tackiness during drying; best used in mixtures to increase adhesion; is hydroscopic if used alone
Polyethylene	PEGs	Water, GI fluids, some organic solvents	Low molecular weight grades used mainly as film modifiers, particularly plasticizers[a]
Enteric			
Shellac		Aqueous if pH 7.0	May delay release too long; high batch-to-batch variability
Cellulose acetate	CAP	Acetone, ethyl acetate/IPA, alkalies, if pH 6.0	Dissolves in distal end of duodenum; requires presence of plasticizer such as triacetin or castor oil; is somewhat hygroscopic
Polyvinyl acetate phthalate	PVAP	As above, if $pH > 5.0$	Dissolves along whole length of duodenum
Hydroxypropylmethylcellulose phthalate	HPMCP	As above, if $pH > 4.5$	Dissolves in proximal end of duodenum
Poly(methacrylates)		Eudragit L[b] $pH > 6$ Eudragit S[b] $pH > 7$	Solubilized in alkaline media; mixtures of "L" and "S" can provide enteric coating plus sustained release

[a]High molecular weight grades are less hygroscopic and give tough coating.
[b]Rohm Pharma.

Table 19 Some Commonly Used Film Plasticizers

Phthalate esters	Propylene glycol
Citrate esters	Polyethylene glycol
Triacetin	Glycerin

trolled within fine limits if a uniform smooth coat is to be produced. The solvent mixture must be capable of dissolving the required amount of coating material, yet give rise to a solution within a workable range of viscosity. Until relatively recently, alcohols, esters, chlorinated hydrocarbons, and ketones were among the most frequently used types of solvents.

However, as a result of increasing regulatory pressures against undesirable solvents, there has been a pronounced trend towards aqueous film coating. Many of the same polymers can be used, but it may be necessary to employ lower molecular weight grades due to their high viscosity in aqueous systems. Alternatively, water-insoluble polymers may be dispersed as a latex (emulsion) or pseudo-latex (suspension) in an aqueous media. This approach permits a high solids content without attendant high viscosity problems. However, acceptable film forming in these systems is dependent upon coalescence or agglomeration. In the case of pseudo-latices, this agglomeration requires a soft particle, and thus a high concentration of plasticizer in the system, to ensure formation of a continuous film.

In a four-part article, Porter [130] provided a comprehensive review of tablet coating technology, with emphasis on contemporary practice. More specifically, a recent review [131] discusses characterization techniques for the aqueous film coating process and provides a useful "influence matrix" between process variables and final product attributes.

Due to the need to develop a uniform color, with minimum application, the colorants used in film coating are more likely to be lakes than dyes. In "lakes" the colorant has been adsorbed onto the surface of an insoluble substrate. This gives both opacity and brightness to the pigments that are formulated with other materials so as to be easily dispersed while retaining the desired film-forming capabilities of the polymeric film former. Complete, matched coloring systems are now available as fine powders that can be readily suspended in organic solvents or aqueous systems and, as such, provide a very convenient colorant source.

C. Modified Release Coatings

A coating may be applied to a tablet to modify the release pattern of the active ingredient from it. There are two general types of modified release coatings: enteric and controlled-release. The former are insoluble in the low pH environment of the stomach but dissolve readily on passage into the small intestine with its elevated pH. They are used to minimize irritation of the gastric mucosa by certain drugs and to protect others that are degraded by gastric juices. Controlled-release coatings are reviewed in Chapter 15.

The most common mode of action of enteric coating is pH-related solubility (i.e., insoluble at gastric pH but soluble at some pH above $\sim$4.5). A list of the most widely used enteric coatings is given in Table 18. A less popular alternative has been the use of materials that are affected by the changing enzymatic activity on passage from the stomach to the small intestine. Since their performance is dependent upon the digestion of the coating, the intrinsic in vivo variability of this action makes this type of enteric coating less predictable.

D. Coating Equipment

Conventional coating pans are subglobular, pear-shaped, or even hexagonal (see Fig. 22) with a single front opening through which materials and processing air enter and leave. Their axis is normally inclined at approximately 45° to the horizontal plane, and they are rotated between 25 and 40 rotations per minute (rpm), the precise speed depending, most often, on the product involved. One modification of the normal pan has been the substitution of a cylindrical shape, rotated horizontally with regions of the walls perforated by small holes or slots. This design permits a one-way air flow through the pan as shown in Fig. 23. This figure also illustrates the ways in which vendors have chosen to modify the basic concept. In the Accela-Cota (Manesty) and Hi-Coater (Vector Corp.) (Fig. 24), the flow of air is through the tablet bed and out through the perforated wall of the pan. In the Driacoater (Driam) the air flows from the perforated pan wall through the tablet and into the central region (i.e., countercurrent to the direction of the coating spray). The Glatt-Coater (Glatt Air Techniques) permits either co- or countercurrent air flow to suit particular products.

The traditional method of ladling the coating solutions into the rotating bed of tablets has given way to systems capable of spraying material, with or without the assistance of an air jet. More specifically, two general types are available: those that rely entirely on hydraulic pressure to produce a spray when material is forced through a nozzle (airless spraying) and those in which atomization of the spray is assisted by turbulent

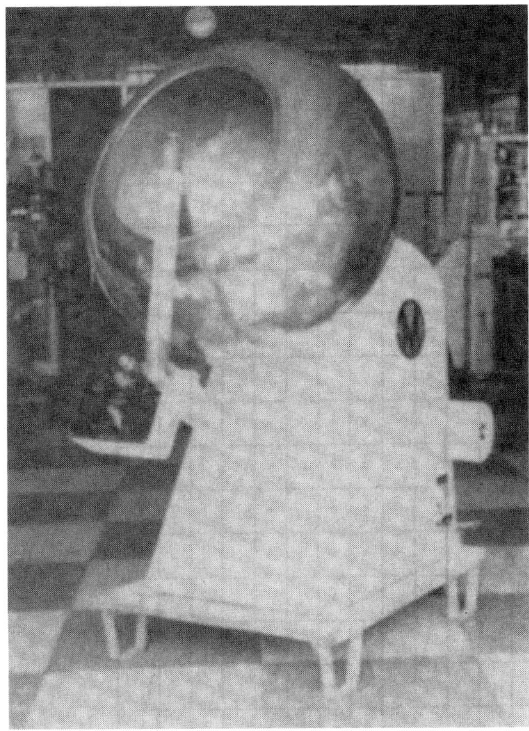

Fig. 22 Conventional coating pan.

jets of air introduced into it. The latter type tends to produce a more easily controlled spray pattern and is therefore better for small-scale operations, although both are capable of giving the flat jet profile preferred for pan operation. Other important parameters include the distance from nozzle to bed surface and whether continuous or intermittent spraying is utilized. One interesting development in this area has been the introduction of a special plough-shaped head, which is immersed in the tumbling bed of tablets and through which both coating solutions and air can be delivered into the bed.

The film-coating process can be carried out in conventional pans, although operation variables such as speed of pan rotation, angle of pan axis, and temperature and humidity control may be more critical. Newer pans with one-way air flow through the tablet bed offer an even better alternative, because the pan environment can be controlled within finer limits.

Coating in Fluidized Beds

Fluidized beds, in general, and the air-suspension technique patented by Wurster, in particular, now offer an attractive alternative to pan coating. The basic principle underlying their operation is to suspend the tablets in an upward moving stream of air so that they are no longer in contact with one another.

An atomizer introduces spray solution into the stream and onto the tablets, which are then carried away from the spraying region where the coating is dried by the fluidized air. In the Wurster process, the design is such that the tablets are sprayed at the bottom of the coating column and move upwards centrally, being dried as they do so. They then leave the top of the central region and return down the periphery of the column to be recycled into the coating zone, as shown in Fig. 25. The process can be controlled by careful adjustment of the air and rate of coating solution delivery and monitoring of the exiting air temperatures.

Compression Coating

A method has been described [132] for compressing a coating around a tablet "core" using specially designed presses. The process involves preliminary compression of the core formulation to give a relatively soft tablet, which is then transferred to a large die already containing some of the coating material. After centralizing the core, further coating granulation is added and the whole compressed to form the final product. From a formulation point of view, this requires a core material that develops reasonable strength at low compressional loads and a coating material in the form of fine free-flowing granules with good binding qualities.

Perhaps the best known commercial presses developed for this work are the Drycota (Manesty) and the Prescoter (Killian). Due to the small number of applications in which it can be used, Manesty no longer manufactures the Drycota. The Prescoter, however, is in the process of being updated (Model S250M) for the first time since its introduction 15 years ago. The Prescoter uses cores produced on another machine and, for this reason, requires somewhat harder cores capable of withstanding the additional handling that may result in weaker bonding between core and coating.

Incompatible drugs may be co-formulated by this method by incorporating one drug in the core and the other in the coating formulation. The possibility of having a dual-release pattern of the same drug (e.g., a rapidly released fraction in the coat and an extended release component in the core) is perfectly feasible. Compression of an enteric coating around a tablet, and even a second layer of coating, have been attempted, but not widely adopted. A machine developed for this purpose, the Bicota (Manesty), is no longer commercially available.

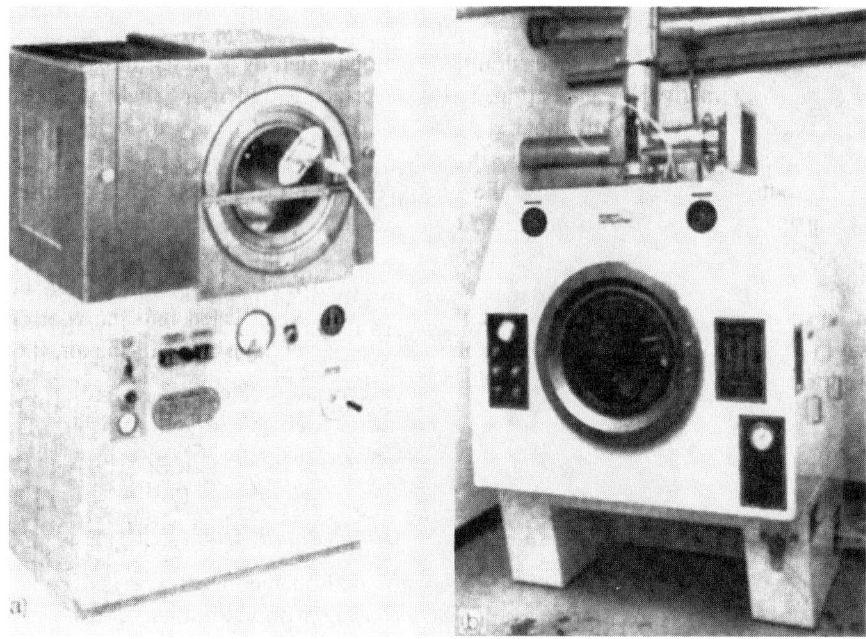

Fig. 23 Typical side-vented pan.

Layered Tablets

In a search for novelty as much as functionality, tablets have been produced on presses capable of compressing a second (or even third) layer on top of the original material. Indeed, the standard double-rotary machines require little modification in order to achieve this goal. Such tableting procedures facilitate the co-formulation of incompatible materials and design of complex release patterns, as well as adding a new dimension to ease of identification. A considerable amount of expertise is needed to formulate and consistently manufacture these tablets to meet the strict regulatory requirements now demanded. Several high-output tablet presses designed to produce two- or three-layered tablets are commercially available.

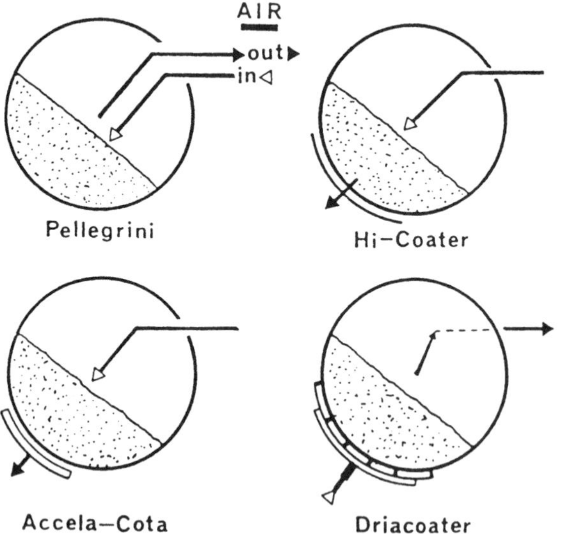

Fig. 24 Coating pan air configurations.

VI. EVALUATION OF TABLETS

Under this heading it will be convenient to divide the types of test procedures into two major categories: those that are requirements in an official compendium and those that, though unofficial, are widely used in commerce. In certain cases it will also be of value to consider specialized evaluative procedures that have perhaps a more academic background.

Several "all-in-one" tablet testers are currently available that measure weight, thickness, diameter, and hardness of tablets. In addition these instruments provide digital storage and calculation of statistical parameters and allow for rapid feedback during the tableting process so that the tableting equipment can be adjusted accordingly with minimal "downtime."

A. Official Standards

The discussion will be restricted to those tests that are mandatory in The United States Pharmacopoeia (USP)

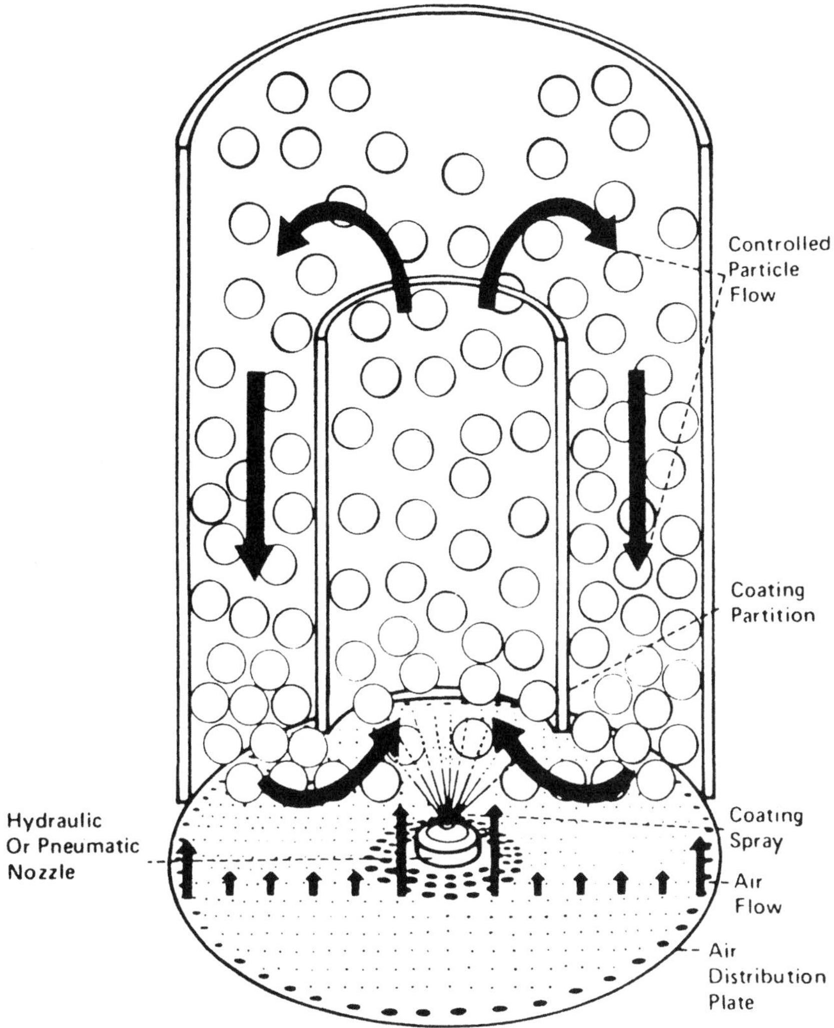

Fig. 25 Diagram of Wurster coating chamber.

and The National Formulary (NF), although reference to the monographs of other compendia is included where appropriate. Tests concerned with dissolution rate determinations are discussed in Chapter 20, and assay procedures are omitted as they are essentially analytical methods pertaining to a particular drug.

Uniformity of Dosage Units

The dose uniformity of tablets can be determined by two different general approaches: the weight variation between a specified number of tablets or the extent of drug content uniformity. The USP permits the latter approach in all cases. Moreover, drug content uniformity must be measured for coated tablets because the tablet coat, which does not usually contain the active ingredient(s), may vary significantly from tablet to tablet. The use of weight uniformity as a singular means of quantifying uniformity of dosage units is only permitted in cases where the tablet is uncoated and contains 50 mg or more of a single active ingredient that comprises 50% or more of the total tablet weight.

Most pharmacopoeias include a simple weight test on a specified number of tablets that are weighed individually. The arithmetic mean weight and relative standard deviation (i.e., mean divided by standard deviation) of these tablets is then calculated. Only a specified number of test tablets may lie outside the prescribed limits. These specifications vary depending upon the type of tablet and amount of active present.

Content uniformity is a USP test is designed to establish the homogeneity of a batch. Ten tablets are assayed individually after which the arithmetic mean and relative standard deviation (RSD) are calculated. USP criteria are met if the content uniformity lies within 85–115% of the label claim and the RSD is not greater than 6%. Provision is included in the compendium for additional testing if one or more units fail to meet the standards.

Disintegration Testing

Determination of the time for a tablet to disintegrate when immersed in some test fluid has been a requirement in most compendia for many years. For many years, it was the only test available to evaluate the release of medicaments from a dosage unit. We now recognize the severe limitations of such tests in assessing this property—hence, the introduction of dissolution rate requirements.

The USP disintegration test is typical of most and is described in detail in a monograph of that volume. Briefly, it consists of an apparatus in which a tablet can be introduced into each of six cylindrical tubes, the lower end of which is covered by a 0.025 in.^{2} wire mesh. The tubes are then raised and lowered through a distance of 5.3–5.7 cm at a rate of 29–32 strokes per minute in a test fluid maintained at $37 \pm 2°C$. Continuous agitation of the tablets is ensured by this stroking mechanism and by the presence of a specially designed plastic disk, which is free to move up and down in the tubes.

The tablets are said to have disintegrated when the particles remaining on the mesh (other than fragments of coatings) are soft and without palpable core. A maximum time for disintegration to occur is specified for each tablet, and at the end of this time the aforementioned criteria must be met. The disintegration media required varies depending on the type of tablet to be tested. Apparatus meeting the official specification is available from several sources. Several modifications of the official method have been suggested in the literature, including a basket insert as an alternative to the disks [133].

The disintegration time may be markedly affected by the amount of disintegrant used as well as the tablet process conditions. In particular, a log/linear relationship between disintegration time and compressional force has been suggested by several authors [134–136]. Mufrod and Parrot concluded that although disintegration is affected by changes in compression pressure, these changes do not significantly alter the product's dissolution profile [137].

B. Unofficial Tests

Mechanical Strength

The mechanical strength of tablets is an important property of this form of drug presentation and plays a significant role in both product development and control. It has been described by various terms, including friability [138], hardness [139], fracture resistance [140], crushing strength [141], and flexure, or breaking strength [142].

Even in tablets of the simplest geometry, interpretation of this property is less straightforward than it first might appear. Some degree of anisotropy is almost certain to be present, and the ideal test conditions, employing closely defined uniform stresses, are rarely met. The mechanical strength of the tablet is primarily due to two events that occur during compression: the formation of interparticulate bonds and a reduction in porosity resulting in an increased density.

Crushing Strength

Many crushing strength testers are described in the literature [133,138–141]. In industry, mechanical strength is most often referred to as the tablet's hardness or, more precisely, its crushing strength. Brook and Marshall described crushing strength as "the compressional force that, when applied diametrically to a tablet, just fractures it" [141]. In most cases, the tablet is placed upon a fixed anvil and the force is transmitted to it by means of a moving plunger. Many testers of this type are commercially available, including the Stokes (or Monsanto), Strong-Cobb, Pfizer, and Erweka and Schleuniger (or Heberlein). Based upon the particular tester's design, the plunger is moved either manually or electronically. Comparisons between the different types of testers has proved that the electronic testers produce results that are much more reproducible than those obtained from the manual testers [130,141,143–145]. This is due, in large part, to the constant rate of loading achieved with electronic testers [123] (see Fig. 26).

In general, the load is applied at 90° to the longest axis (i.e., across the tablet's diameter) (see Fig. 27). In such cases, the load required to break the tablet is referred to as the diametrical strength. The load can also be applied across the tablet's thickness, in which case it is referred to as flexure or breaking strength [140,142]. The tensile strength, σ, can be calculated once the load required to fracture the tablet has been determined. The precise calculation of tensile strength depends upon the method used to break the tablet. When using a diametrical, or diametral, test the calculation is as follows:

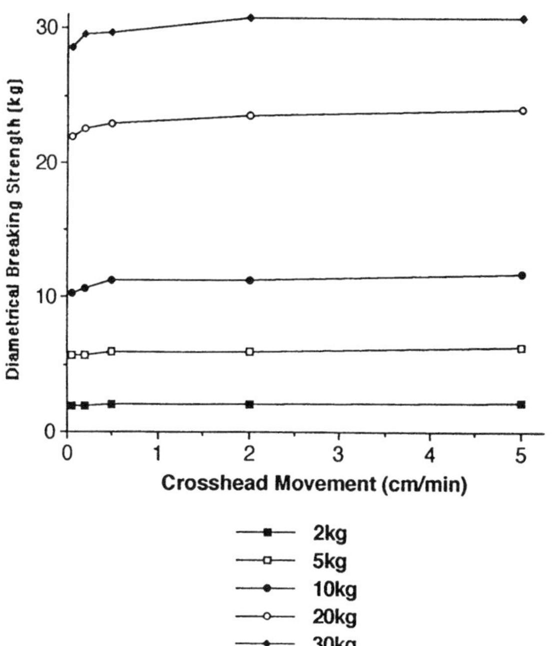

Fig. 26 Effect of loading rate on the diametrical breaking strength of tablets compressed at different levels. (From Ref. 123.)

$$\sigma_d = \frac{2F_d}{\pi DH}$$

where

σ_d = tensile strength
F_d = load required to fracture tablet
D = tablet diameter
H = tablet height

From a test of the tablet's flexure, tensile strength (σ_f) is calculated from the following equation:

$$\sigma_f = \frac{3F_f D'}{4DH^2}$$

where

σ_f = tensile strength
F_f = load required to fracture tablet
D = tablet diameter
D = distance from fulcrum to fulcrum
H = tablet height

In their evaluation of flexure and diametral testing, David and Augsburger found the tensile strength to be the same regardless of the method used as long as the appropriate calculation was employed [142].

Two types of inherent error may be present: that associated with an incorrect zero and a scale that does not accurately indicate the actual load being applied. In some models there is the additional problem of a variable rate of loading. Moreover, when using unpadded flat anvils the failure may involve some compression. Thus, it is essential to realize what is being measured in a particular instrument.

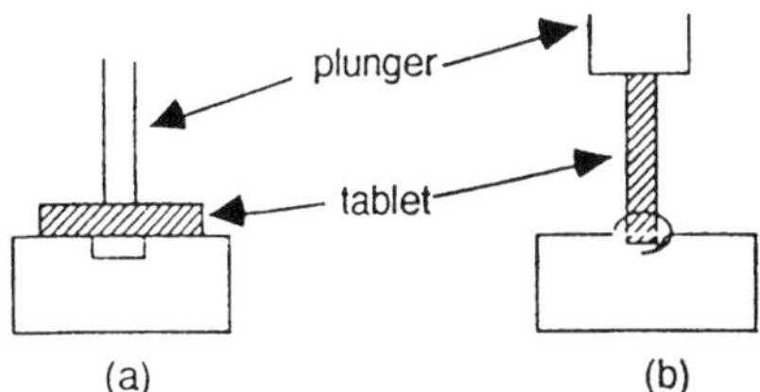

Fig. 27 Methods of evaluating tablet crushing strength: (a) bending or flexure strength; (b) diametrical compression. (From Ref. 145.)

The Stokes and Pfizer testers apply force through a coil spring, which after long periods of use shows signs of fatigue and may also show some loss of load due to frictional effects [141,145]. The rate of loading is not controlled in these types or in the Strong-Cobb tester, which applies force through hydraulic pressure. The scale of this machine registers air pressure, and comparison of results with other instruments is therefore only possible if these readings are converted to compressional load.

The Erweka and Schleuniger testers operate on a counterweight principle that eliminates fatigue, if not frictional, losses. The latter of these two devices is supplied calibrated and a "mechanical tablet" is available for periodic recalibration. More recently, testers have been introduced that measure the load being applied to the tablet by means of load cells and therefore facilitate direct electronic digital readout. This eliminates the two major sources of error referred to above and permits recording of production of hard copies of the test results.

Comparative reports in the literature confirm the necessity of employing some calibration procedure if results from testers are to be compared or reduced to actual units of force. This is particularly true where the information is being used to determine relationships between crushing strength to other tablet properties.

It can be argued that the crushing strength of a tablet is more closely related to the compressional process, and the results may not give the best indication of how the tablet will behave during handling. If information in this respect is required, then the groups of instruments in the following paragraphs are more relevant.

One might anticipate that the crushing strength (F) of a tablet is a function of the pressure (P) employed during its compaction [134]. For example the following relationship may hold true:

$$F = k \log P + k_1$$

where k and k_1 are constants. However, deviation from this logarithmic relationship at compressional pressure values, above 150 MPa has been reported [81,135]. In addition, the crushing strength has been related to certain physical properties of the compact. For example:

$$F = kE^{-1} + k_1$$

where E, the porosity, has values between 5 and 20%. The most obvious use of crushing strength measurements has been to give indications of possible disintegration times (t_p), i.e.,

$$F = kt_p + k_1$$

Abrasion

While the crushing strength of a tablet gives some indication of its mechanical robustness, it does not truly measure the ability of the tablet to withstand the handling it will encounter during processing and shipping. Tests designed to assess the resistance of the surface regions to abrasion or other forms of general "wear and tear" may be more appropriate in this regard.

Many tests to assess abrasion are quoted in the literature [138,146,147]. Most measure the weight loss on subjecting tablets to a standard level of agitation for a specified time. The choice of agitation should be based on knowledge of the likely level during use or manufacture.

More specifically a certain weight of tablets, W_0, is subjected to a well-defined level of agitation in a fixed-geometry, closed container for a specific time. They are then reweighed, W. The measure of abrasion resistance or friability, B, is usually expressed as a percentage loss in weight:

$$B = 100 \cdot \left[1 - \frac{W}{W_0}\right]$$

It might be advantageous to relate friability to unit time or number of falls.

The Roche Friabilator is one of the most common methods used to test for resistance to abrasion [147]. In this case, a minimum of 6 g (often 20 tablets) of dedusted and weighed tablets are placed in a 12 in. high drum, which is then rotated for 100 revolutions. A shaped arm lifts the tablets and drops them half the height of the drum during each revolution. At the end of this operation, the tablets are removed, dedusted, and reweighed. Should any tablet break up, the test is rejected. Values of B from 0.8 to 1.0% are frequently quoted as the upper level of acceptability for pharmaceutical products [147].

Indentation hardness using modified tests based on "Brinell" hardness measurements have been used by some researchers [148] to provide information on the surface hardness of tablets. In addition, these tests are capable of providing a measure of a tablet's plasticity or elasticity. For the most part, such tests have been confined to basic research applications in a few laboratories, but their value is beginning to be more widely recognized.

Porosity

The bioavailability of drugs from tablets can be markedly influenced by the rate and efficiency of the initial disintegration and dissolution process. Unfortunately, one is faced with a compromise situation — a structure that has both a durable structure prior to administration and the ability to readily break down when placed in the in vivo environment. One of the major factors affecting both these properties is the structure of the tablet, in particular its density (or porosity) and the pore structure. Study of the significance of such measurements and interpretation of the results is a relatively recent field of interest.

Determination of the porosity of a tablet presents the classic problem of defining the appropriate volume to be measured. The displacement medium may be able to penetrate the most minute crevices, as is the case for helium. Other displacement media, such as mercury, are unable to enter the smallest tablet crevices and thus produce different porosity values. Standardization of displacement media is therefore necessary for comparative evaluations.

Pore Structure and Size

The relationship between applied pressure (P) and the diameter of the smallest circular pore penetrated (d) by a liquid gas is given by the equation:

$$d = \frac{4\pi\gamma \cos\beta}{P}$$

where γ is the surface tension of the liquid and β is the contact angle solid and liquid.

Originally, the method of porosimetry was only of interest to those involved with the high-pressure techniques associated with pore analysis. However, with the increasing availability of sophisticated porosimeters, the technique of porosimetry is being used on a frequent basis to investigate tablet structure. High-pressure mercury intrusion porosimeters are capable of assessing a wide range of pore radii. A typical example of the application of such an instrument to evaluate wet and dry techniques of precompression treatment is reported by Ganderton and Selkirk [149]. These authors found that lactose granulations resulted in a wider pore size distribution than ungranulated lactose.

This technique has also been used in combination with nitrogen absorption to study the pore structure of some excipients, particularly MCC in both the powdered and compacted state. The intraparticulate porosity of MCC has been shown to be unaffected by tableting; the interparticular pores, however, are gradually reduced in size [38]. Recently this method has been used to evaluate the internal structure of tablets prepared from microcapsules [150].

Liquid Penetration

The rate at which selected liquids penetrate into tablets can be used to study their pore structure. A knowledge of the rate of liquid penetration should also provide information on the disintegration/dissolution behavior of a tablet on administration. Such investigations are capable of forming a valuable link between physicomechanical characteristics and in vivo performance.

Evaluation of Bioadhesive Tablets

With the advent of increasingly sophisticated tableted delivery systems comes the task of assessing these systems. Bioadhesive tablets, in particular, present an interesting problem to the formulator. Although such tablets are not currently marketed in the U.S., they are currently being evaluated in many laboratories as an alternative means for providing sustained release of drug. The sustained-release characteristic of bioadhesive tablets is afforded through their ability to adhere to the intestinal mucosa. Thus, an estimation of their adhesiveness is a key factor in their in vitro evaluation.

Ishida et al. were some of the first investigators to propose a method for investigating the adhesive properties of tablets [151]. Their method involved placing a tablet onto a membrane under constant pressure for one minute and then measuring the force required to remove it. Most methods published since that time involve essentially the same principle, with variations in the type of membrane used and the manner in which the adhesive force is measured [152,153]. An excellent review of these methods has been published by Duchene et al. for those interested in the precise details of such tests [154].

Jimenez-Castellanos et al. developed a method to measure both the adhesional and frictional forces involved in the attachment of such tablets to mucosa. These researchers found that a good correlation existed between the maximal adhesion strength and polymer content of the tablets tested [155].

Near-Infrared Spectroscopy

In the late 1990s researchers began to evaluate the use of near-infrared (NIR) spectroscopy in pharmaceutical analyses [156–158]. NIR analyses are particularly useful because they are both rapid and nondestructive to the sample. Morisseau and Rhodes reviewed the application of NIR in the pharmaceutial industry and determined that it has been used to measure sample composition and identification, moisture content, content uniformity, homogeneity of mixing, degradation products, and particle size [156]. Recently its potential to differentiate between compression force used during tableting and to assess moisture profile during the granulation process has been evaluated [157,158]. As researchers become more familiar with this method, its applications will undoubtedly grow.

VII. RECENT DEVELOPMENTS IN TABLETING

A. Rapidly Disintegrating Tablets

The trend toward formulation of dispersible tablets is evident in Europe [159–162] and is becoming more commonplace in the United States with over-the-counter preparations available in the form of the following technologies: Zydis® (Scherer DDS), Lyoc® (Farmalyoc), WOW® Tab (Yamanouchi), FlashDose® (Fuisz Technologies), OraSolv® (CIMA), and DuraSolv® (CIMA). These tablets are either placed in the mouth where they quickly dissolve or are placed in a glass of water prior to ingestion and provide consumers with a dosage form that is both potable and easy to swallow.

A challenge faced by formulators designing dispersible tablets is the ability to develop a formulation that rapidly disintegrates and is able to withstand shipping processes. In addition, this type of tablet should form a uniform and somewhat stable suspension when dispersed in water. An interesting answer to this challenge is the design of a "porous table" [163–165], in which a volatizable solid (e.g., urethane or ammonium bicarbonate) is added to a standard, directly compressible formulation. After the tablets have been compressed, the volatilizable solid is removed by a freeze-drying or heating process. Water easily penetrates through the pores and promotes rapid disintegration of the tablets produced in this manner. Thus, these tablets are able both to maintain their mechanical strength and to provide rapid disintegration or dispersion of product. Lyoc and Zydis tablets both use freeze-drying technologies.

B. Three-Dimensional Printing Tablets

For years, formulators have been searching for a means to accurately and consistently deliver a specified level of coating onto a tablet. The answer may have been found in the three-dimensional printing (3DP) of tablets. The process involves the computer-controlled preparation of tablets by building layer upon layer of powder that are joined by a binder solution dispersed by a printing head [166,167]. Several modes of release have successfully been implemented in 3DP tablets, including (a) immediate- and extended-release tablets with two drug-containing components whose release with pH-dependent release, (b) breakaway tablets composed an interior fast-eroding section that separates two drug-containing components, (c) enteric dual pulsatory tablets comprised of a continuous enteric excipient with two drug-containing sections, and (d) immediate- and extended-release tablets with two drug-containing components with erosion-dependent release [166].

C. Web System

A system was developed at Roche Laboratories whereby a sheet (or "web") was coated with a drug/binder mixture. The solid dosage units were then punched from the web [168]. This system was very flexible and amenable to immediate release and sustained-release technologies. However, due to the impracticality of the system, it was abandonned in the mid-1980s and is only of historical significance.

VIII. FUTURE DIRECTIONS

Tablets were a viable dosage form well before William Brockendon's patent for a tablet machine in 1843. His invention only made them easier to produce. As tablet presses and production-monitoring systems developed, these dosage forms have become the most economical of any ever developed. It will be hard to improve on their efficiency, but several attempts, like three-dimensional printing, have been made recently.

Newer technologies may become available, but it is unlikely that any new tableting technology will render the old technology obsolete any time soon. Processing technologies such as high-shear mixing and microwave drying seem to be having the most impact on processing times and efficiency. Coating technologies are becoming more controllable, and they offer the most hope for efficiency improvements.

Another new development has been the application of oral absorption promoters. These materials are designed to enhance the oral bioavailability of many compounds and improve variable absorption. However, many of these compounds are hydrophobic in nature and cause difficulty during tableting itself. The challenge for formulators is to arrive at clever solutions to the process problems while retaining material performance.

The ultimate challenge for tablet formulators in the twenty-first century is to achieve a true understanding of material properties and material science. Those who can quickly conceive a compatible, functional formulation will be irreplaceable as large companies shrink their R&D resources and the public sector demands better efficiency.

REFERENCES

1. A. T. Florence, E. G. Salole, and J. B. Stenlake, J. Pharm Pharmacol., 26, 479 (1974).
2. P. Timmins, I. Browning, A. M. Delargy, J. W. Forrester, and H. Sen, Drug Dev. Ind. Pharm., 12, 1293 (1986).
3. N. Kaneniwa, K. Imagawa, and J.-I. Ichikawa, Chem. Pharm. Bull., 36, 2531 (1988).
4. B. M. Hunter, J. Pharm. Pharmacol., 26, 58P (1974).
5. S. Vesslers, R. Boistelle, A. Delacourte, J. C. Guyot, and A. M. Guyot-Hermann, Drug Dev. Ind. Pharm., 18, 539 (1992).
6. R. F. Shangraw, J. W. Wallace, and F. M. Bowers, Pharm. Tech., 11, 136 (1987).
7. J. W. McGinity, C.-T. Ku, R. Bodmeier, and M. R. Harris, Drug Dev. Ind. Pharm., 11, 891 (1985).
8. A. J. Shukla, and J. C. Price, Drug Dev. Ind. Pharm., 17, 2067 (1991).
9. H. Ando, M. Ishii, M. Kayano, and H. Ozawa, Drug Dev. Ind. Pharm., 18, 453 (1992).
10. P. W. S. Heng, and J. N. Staniforth, J. Pharm. Pharmacol., 40, 360 (1988).

11. J. C. Callahan, G. W. Cleary, M. Elefant, G. Kaplan, T. Tensler, and R. A. Nash, Drug Dev. Ind. Pharm., 8, 355 (1982).
12. A. Wade and P. J. Weller (eds.), Handbook of Pharmaceutical Excipients, 2nd ed., The Pharmaceutical Press, Washington, DC, 1994.
13. C. M. Anderson, Aust. J. Pharm., 47, S44 (1966).
14. J. W. Poole and C. K. Bahal, J. Pharm. Sci., 57, 1945 (1968).
15. O. Weis-Fogh and T. Dansk, Farm. Suppl., 11, 276 (1956).
16. H. K. Chan and E. Doelker, Drug Dev. Ind. Pharm., 11, 315 (1985).
17. S. Kopp, C. Beyer, E. Graf, F. Kubel, and E. Doelker, J. Pharm. Pharmacol., 41, 79 (1989).
18. M. Otsuka, T. Matsumoto, and N. Kaneniwa, J. Pharm. Pharmacol., 41, 667 (1989).
19. T. Matsumoto, N. Kaneniwa, S. Higuchi, and M. Otsuka, J. Pharm. Pharmacol., 43, 74 (1991).
20. C. R. Lerk and H. Vromans, Acta Pharm. Suec., 24, 60 (1987).
21. P. York, Drug Dev. Ind. Pharm., 18, 677 (1992).
22. W. I. Higuchi, P. D. Bernardo, and S. C. Mehta, J. Pharm. Sci., 56, 200 (1967).
23. E. N. Hiestand, J. Bane, and E. Strzelinski, J. Pharm. Sci., 60, 758 (1971).
24. E. N. Hiestand and C. B. Peot, J. Pharm. Sci., 63, 605 (1974).
25. E. N. Hiestand, J. E. Wells, C. B. Peot, and J. F. Ochs, J. Pharm. Sci., 66, 510 (1977).
26. E. N. Hiestand and D. Smith, Powder Technol., 38, 145 (1984).
27. E. N. Hiestand, J. Pharm. Sci., 74, 768 (1985).
28. E. N. Hiestand, Pharm. Tech., 10, 52 (1986).
29. R. O. Williams, and J. W. McGinnity, Drug Dev. Ind. Pharm., 14, 1823 (1988).
30. A. J. Romero, G. Lukas, and C. T. Rhodes, Pharm. Acta Helv., 66, 34 (1991).
31. D. Q. M. Craig, C. T. Davies, J. C. Boyd, and L. B. Hakess, J. Pharm. Pharmacol., 43, 444 (1991).
32. H. G. Brittain, Drug Dev. Ind. Pharm., 15, 2083 (1989).
33. D. S. Phadke, and J. L. Eichorst, Drug Dev. Ind. Pharm., 17, 901 (1991).
34. H. Bundgaard, J. Pharm. Pharmacol., 26, 535 (1974).
35. Y. K. E. Ibrahim and P. R. Olurinaola, Pharm. Acta Helv., 66, 298 (1991).
36. H. L. Avallone, Pharm. Tech., 16, 48 (1992).
37. D. C. Monkhouse, and A. Maderich, Drug Dev. Ind. Pharm., 15, 2115 (1989).
38. H. Nyquist, Drug Dev. Ind. Pharm., 12, 953 (1986).
39. Z. T. Chowhan and L.-H. Chi, J. Pharm. Sci., 75, 534 (1986).
40. G. K. Bolhuis and C. F. Lerk, Pharm. Weekblad., 108, 469 (1973).
41. J. W. Wallace, J. T. Capozzi, and R. F. Shangraw, Pharm. Tech., 7, 95 (1983).
41a. K. B. Mulderrig, Pharm. Tech., 24(5), 34 (2000).
41b. Y.-E. Zhang and J. B. Schwartz, Drug Dev. Ind. Pharm., 26(7), 761 (2000).
42. J. T. Carstensen and C. Ertell, Drug Dev. Ind. Pharm., 16, 1121 (1990).
43. D. H. Shah and A. S. Arambulo, Drug Dev. Ind. Pharm., 1, 495 (1974–1975).
44. K. A. Khan and C. T. Rhodes, Chemist Druggist, 159, 158 (1973).
45. N. Shah, R. Pytelewski, H. Eisen, and C. I. Jarowski, J. Pharm. Sci., 63, 339 (1974).
46. G. D. D'Alonzo and R. E. O'Connor, Drug Dev. Ind. Pharm., 16, 1931 (1990).
47. O. Shirakura, M. Yamada, M. Hashimoto, S. Ishimaru, K. Takayama, and T. Nagai, Drug Dev. Ind. Pharm., 18, 1099 (1992).
48. H. Seager, P. J. Rue, I. Burt, J. Ryder, and J.K. Warrack, Int. J. Pharm. Tech Prod. Mfr., 2(2), 41 (1981).
48a. E. Horisawa, K. Danjo, and H. Sunada,
49. Z. Chowhan, Pharm. Tech., 12(2), 26 (1988).
50. R. M. Iyer, L. L. Augsburger, and D. M. Parikh, Drug, Dev. Ind. Pharm., 19(9), 981 (1993).
50a. S. K. Joneja, W. W. Harcum, G. W. Skinner, P. E. Barnum, and J.-H. Guo, Drug Dev. Ind. Pharm., 25(10), 1129 (1999).
50b. C. Alvarez-Lorenzo, J. L. Gomez-Amoza, P. Martinez-Pacheco, C. Souto, and A. Concheiro, Int. J. Pharm., 197(1–2), 107 (2000).
51. P. York, Int. J. Pharm., 14, 1 (1983).
52. C. F. Lerk, M. Lagas, J. P. Boelstra,, and P. Broersma, J. Pharm. Sci., 66, 1480 (1977).
53. C. F. Lerk, M. Lagas, J. T. Fell, and P. Nauta. J. Pharm. Sci., 67, 935 (1978).
54. E. Shotton and G. S. Leonard, J. Pharm. Pharmacol., 24, 798 (1972).
55. M. H. Rubinstein and D. M. Bodey, J. Pharm. Pharmacol., 26, 104P (1974).
56. K. A. Khan and C. T. Rhodes, J. Pharm. Sci., 64, 166 (1975).
57. A. Mitrevej and R. G. Hollenbeck, Pharm. Tech., 6, 48 (1982).
58. H. Nogami, T. Nagai, E. Fukuoka, and T. Sonobe, Chem. Pharm. Bull., 17, 1450 (1969).
59. R. F. Shangraw, Manuf. Chem., 57, 22 (1986).
60. H. Burlinson and C. Pickering, J. Pharm. Pharmacol., 2, 630 (1950).
61. L. C. Curlin, J. Am. Pharm. Assn., Sci. Ed., 44, 16 (1955).
62. N. R. Patel and R. E. Hopponen, J. Pharm. Sci., 55, 1065 (1966).
63. K. S. Manudhane et. al., J. Pharm. Sci., 58, 616 (1969).
64. H. Hess, Pharm. Tech., 11, 54 (1987).

65. J. B. Schwartz and J. A. Zelinskie, Drug Dev. Ind. Pharm., 4, 463 (1978).
66. A. M. Guyot-Hermann and J. Ringard, Drug Dev. Ind. Pharm., 7, 155 (1981).
67. W. Lowenthal and J. H. Wood, J. Pharm. Sci., 62, 287 (1973).
68. K. A. Khan and C. T. Rhodes, J. Pharm. Pharmacol., 23, 261A (1971).
69. J. F. Bavitz, N. R. Bohidar, and F. A. Restaino, Drug Dev. Comm., 1, 331 (1974–1975).
70. W. Lowenthal, J. Pharm. Sci., 61, 1695 (1972).
71. J. L. Kanig and E. M. Rudnic, Pharm. Tech., 8, 50 (1984).
72. D. Gissinger and A. Stamm, Drug Dev. Ind. Pharm., 6, 511 (1980).
73. P. V. Marshall, D. G. Pope, and J. T. Carstensen, J. Pharm. Sci., 80(19), 899 (1991).
74. E. M. Rudnic, C. T. Rhodes, S. Welch, and P. Bernardo, Drug Dev. Ind. Pharm., 8, 87 (1982).
75. C. Fuhrer, Informationsdienst APV, 20, 58 (1964).
76. H. Matsumaru, Yakugaku Zashi, 79, 63 (1959).
77. P. H. List and V. A. Muazzam, Drugs Made in Germany, 22, 161 (1979).
78. A. J. Smallenbroek, G. K. Bolhuis, and C. F. Lerk, Pharm. Weekblad Sci. Ed., 3, 172 (1981).
79. E. M. Rudnic, J. M. Lausier, R. N. Chilamkurti, and C. T. Rhodes, Drug Dev. Ind. Pharm., 6, 291 (1980).
80. E. M. Rudnic, J. L. Kanig, and C. T. Rhodes, J. Pharm. Sci., 74, 647 (1985).
81. E. Shotton and C. Lewis, J. Pharm. Pharmacol., 16, 111T (1964).
82. H. C. Caldwell and W. J. Westlake, J. Pharm. Sci., 61, 984 (1972).
83. Y. Matsuda, Y. Minamida, and S.-I. Hayashi, J. Pharm. Sci., 65, 1155 (1976).
84. J. Kikuta and N. Kitamori, Durg Dev. Ind. Pharm., 11, 845 (1985).
85. S. Dawoodbhai and C. T. Rhodes, Drug Dev. Ind. Pharm., 16, 2409 (1990).
85a. C. Viseras, A. Yebra, and A. Lopez-Galindo, Pharm. Dev. Technol., 5(1), 53 (2000).
86. P. W. S. Heng, L. S. C. Wan, and T. S. H Ang, Drug Dev. Ind. Pharm., 16, 951 (1990).
87. L. S. C. Wan and P. W. S. Heng, Pharm. Acta Helv., 62, 169 (1987).
88. L. S. C. Wan and P. W. S. Heng, Pharm. Acta Helv., 61, 157 (1986).
89. H. Schott, L. C. Kwan, and S. Feldman, J. Pharm. Sci., 71, 1038 (1982).
90. M. L. Wells and E. L. Parrott, Drug Dev. Ind. Pharm., 18, 175 (1992).
91. M. L. Wells and E. L. Parrott, Drug Dev. Ind. Pharm., 18, 265 (1992).
92. M. L. Wells and E. L. Parrott, J. Pharm. Sci., 81, 453 (1992).
92a. L. Flores, R. Arellano, and J. Esquivel, Drug Dev. Ind. Pharm., 26(3), 297 (2000).
92b. L. Flores, R. Arellano, and J. Esquivel, Drug Dev. Ind. Pharm., 26(4), 465 (2000).
92c. R. Heinz, H. Wolf, H. Schuchmann, L. End, and K. Kolter, Drug Dev. Ind. Pharm., 26(5), 513 (2000).
92d. G. Buckton and E. Yonemochi, Eur. J. Pharm. Sci., 10(1), 77 (2000).
93. J. T. Carstensen, *Theory of Pharmaceutical Systems*, Vol. 2, Academic Press, New York, 1973.
94. J. A. Hersey, J. Pharm. Pharmacol., 63, 1685 (1967).
95. H. Stahl, Pharm. Tech. Yearbook 2000, 32–40 (2000).
96. P. J. Jarosz and E. L. Parrott, J. Pharm. Sci., 72, 530 (1983).
97. I. A. Chaudry and R. E. King, J. Pharm. Sci., 61, 1121 (1972).
98. T. Higuchi, E. Nelson, and L. W. Busse, J. Am. Pharm. Assn. Sci. Ed., 43, 344 (1954).
99. J. Polderman and C. J. DeBlaey, Farm. Aikak., 80, 111 (1971).
100. C. J. DeBlaey and J. Polderman, Pharm. Weekblad, 105, 241 (1970).
101. C. J. DeBlaey, A. B. Weekers-Anderson, and J. Polderman, Pharm. Weekblad, 106, 893 (1971).
102. R. F. Lammens, J. Polderman, and C. J. DeBlaey, Int. J. Pharm. Tech. Prod. Mfr., 1, 26 (1979).
103. J. Cobby, M. Mayersohn, and G. C. Walker, J. Pharm. Sci., 63, 725,732 (1974).
104. B. Mechtersheimer and H. Zucker, Pharm. Tech., 38 (1986).
105. T. Higuchi, L. N. Elow, and L. W. Busse, J. Am. Pharm. Assn. Sci. Ed., 43, 688 (1954).
106. R. J. Roberts and R. C. Rowe, J. Pharm. Pharmacol., 38, 567 (1986).
107. O. Worts and T. Schoefer, Arch. Pharm. Chem. Sci. Ed., 6, 1 (1978).
108. H. J. Malinowski, Ph.D. dissertation, Philadelphia College of Pharmacy, 1973.
109. J. J. Williams and D. M. Stiel, Pharm. Tech., 8, 26 (1984).
110. J. B. Schwartz, Pharm. Tech., 5, 102 (1981).
111. K. Marshall, Pharm. Tech., 7, 63 (1983).
112. R. W. Heckel, Trans. Met. Soc. AIME, 221, 671,1001 (1961).
113. J. A. Hersey and J. E. Rees, Nature, 230, 96 (1971).
114. L. F. Athy, Bull. Am. Assn. Petrol. Geologist, 14, 1 (1930).
115. R. J. Rue and J. E. Rees, J. Pharm. Pharmacol., 30, 642 (1978).
116. M. Celik and K. Marshall, Drug Dev. Ind. Pharm., 15, 759 (1989).
116a. F. Nicklasson and G. Alderborn, Pharm. Res., 17(8), 949 (2000).
116b. M. Krumme, L. Schwabe, and K. Fromming, Eur. J. Pharm. Biopharm., 49(3), 275 (2000).

117. D. N. Travers and M. Cox, Drug Dev. Ind. Pharm., 4, 157 (1978).
118. S. Leigh, J. E. Carless, and B. W. Burt, J. Pharm. Sci., 56, 888 (1967).
119. E. Shotton and B. A. Obiorah, J. Pharm. Pharmacol., 25, 37P (1973).
120. J. T. Carstensen, J.-P. Marty, F. Puisieux, and H. Fessi, J. Pharm. Sci., 70, 222 (1981).
121. E. G. Rippie and D. W. Danielson, J. Pharm. Sci., 7, 476 (1981)
122. S. T. David and L. L. Augsburger, J. Pharm. Sci., 66, 155 (1977).
123. J. E. Rees, J. A. Hersey, and E. T. Cole, J. Pharm. Pharmacol., 22, 64S (1970).
124. I. Krycer and D. G. Pope, Drug Dev. Ind. Pharm., 8, 307 (1982).
125. I. Krycer, D. G. Pope, and J. A. Hersey, Int. J. Pharm., 12, 113 (1982).
126. P. Ridgeway-Watt, *Tablet Machine Instrumentation in Pharmaceutics*, J. Wiley & Sons, New York, 1988.
126a. C. Yeh, S. A. Altaf, and S. W. Hoag, Pharm. Res., 14(9), 1161 (1997).
126b. H. X. Guo, J. Heinamaki, and J. Yliruusi, Int. J. Pharm., 186(2), 99 (1999).
126c. M. T. DeCrosta, J. B. Schwartz, R. J. Wigent, and K. Marshall, Int. J. Pharm., 198(1), 113 (2000).
127. H. Seager, P. J. Rue, I. Burt, J. Ryder, J. K. Warrack, and M. Gamlen, Int. J. Pharm. Tech. Prod. Mfr., 6, 1 (1985).
128. S. M. Blaug and M. R. Gross, Drug Standards, 27, 100 (1959).
129. G. S. Banker, J. Pharm. Sci., 55, 81 (1966).
130. S. C. Porter, Drug Cosmet. Ind., 130, 46 (May); 131, 44 (June) (1981).
131. L. K. Mathur and S. J. Forbes, Pharm. Tech., 42 (1984).
132. R. C. Whitehouse, Pharm. J., 172, 85 (1954).
133. L. L. Kaplan and J. A. Kish, J. Pharm. Sci., 51, 708 (1962).
134. T. Higuchi, A. N. Rao, L. W. Busse, and J. V. Swintosky, J. Am Pharm. Assn. Sci. Ed., 42, 194 (1953).
135. T. Higuchi, L. N. Elowe, and L. W. Busse, J. Am. Pharm. Assn. Sci. Ed., 43, 685 (1954).
136. K. C. Kwan, F. O. Swart, and A. M. Mattocks, J. Am. Pharm. Assn., 46, 236 (1957).
137. Mufrod and E. L. Parrot, Drug Dev. Ind. Pharm., 16, 1081 (1990).
138. A. Nutter-Smith, Pharm. J., 163, 194 (1949).
139. A. McCallum, J. Buchter, and R. Albrecht, J. Am. Pharm. Assn. Sci. Ed., 44, 83 (1955).
140. C. J. Endicott, W. Lowenthal, and H. M. Gross, J. Pharm. Sci., 50, 343 (1961).
141. D. B. Brook and K. Marshall, J. Pharm. Sci., 57, 481 (1968).
142. S. T. David and L. L. Augsburger, J. Pharm. Sci., 63, 933 (1974).
143. H. J. Fairchild and F. Michel, J. Pharm. Sci., 50, 966 (1961).
144. J. F. Bavitz, N. R. Bohidar, J. I. Karr, and F. A. Restaino, J. Pharm. Sci., 62, 1520 (1973).
145. F. W. Goodhardt, J. R. Draper, D. Dancz, and F. C. Ninger, J. Pharm. Sci., 62, 297 (1973).
146. H. Burlinson and C. Pickering, J. Pharm. Pharmacol., 2, 630 (1950).
147. E. G. E. Shafer, E. G. Wollish, and C. E. Engel, J. Am. Pharm. Assn. Sci. Ed., 45, 114 (1956).
148. K. Ridgway, M. E. Aulton, and P. H. Rosser, J. Pharm. Pharmacol., 22, 70S (1970).
149. D. Ganderton and A. B. Selkirk, J. Pharm. Pharmacol., 22, 345 (1970).
150. H. Yuasa, Y. Kanaya, and K. Omata, Chem. Pharm. Bull., 38, 752 (1990).
151. M. Ishida, Y. Machida, N. Nambu, and T. Nagai, Chem. Pharm. Bull., 29, 810 (1981).
152. G. Ponchel, F. Touchard, D. Duchene, and N. A. Peppas, J. Controll. Rel., 5, 129 (1987).
153. V. S. Chitnis, V. S. Malshe, and J. K. Lalla, Drug Dev. Ind. Pharm., 17, 879 (1991).
154. D. Duchene, F. Touchard, and N. A. Peppas, Drug Dev. Ind. Pharm., 14, 283 (1988).
155. M. R. Jimenez-Castellanos, H. Zia, and C. T. Rhodes, Int. J. Pharm., 89, 223 (1993).
156. K. M. Morisseau and C. T. Rhodes, Pharm. Technol. Yearbook. 1997, 6 (1997).
157. J. Rantanen, O. Antikainen, J.-P. Mannermaa, and J. Yliruusi, Pharm. Dev. Tech., 5(2), 209 (2000).
158. J.-H. Guo, G. W. Skinner, W. W. Harcum, J. P. Malone, and L. G. Weyer, Drug Dev. Ind. Pharm., 25(12), 1267 (1999).
159. E. Norris and M. Guttadauria, Eur. J. Rheumatol. Inflamm., 8(1), 94 (1987).
160. T. Ishikawa, Y. Watanabe, N. Utoguchi, and M. Matsumoto, Chem. Pharm. Bull. (Tokyo), 47(10), 1451 (1999).
161. Y. Bi, Y. Yonezawa, and H. Sunada, J. Pharm. Sci., 88(10), 1004 (1999).
162. Y. X. Bi, H. Sunada, Y. Yonezawa, and K. Danjo, Drug Dev. Ind. Pharm., 25(5), 571 (1999).
163. S. Corveleyn and J. P. Remon, Drug Dev. Ind. Pharm., 25(9), 1005 (1999).
164. S. Corvelyn and J. P. Remon, Int. J. Pharm., 166, 65 (1997).
165. S. Corvelyn and J. P. Remon, Int. J. Pharm., 173, 149 (1998).
166. C. W. Rowe, W. E. Katstra, R. D. Palazzolo, B. Giritlioglu, P. Teung, and M. J. Cima, J. Control. Release, 66(1), 11 (2000).
167. W. E. Katstra, R. D. Palazzolo, C. W. Rowe, B. Giritlioglu, P. Teung, and M. J. Cima, J. Control. Release, 66(1), 1 (2000).
168. A. Sturzeneggar, A. R. Mlodozeniec, and E. S. Lipinsky, United States Patent 4,197,289 (8 April 1980).

Chapter 11

Hard and Soft Shell Capsules

Larry L. Augsburger

School of Pharmacy, University of Maryland, Baltimore, Maryland

I. HISTORICAL DEVELOPMENT AND ROLE AS A DOSAGE FORM

Capsules are solid dosage forms in which the drug substance is enclosed within either a hard or soft soluble shell. The shells generally are formed from gelatin. The capsule may be regarded as a "container" drug-delivery system that provides a tasteless/odorless dosage form without the need for a secondary coating step, as may be required for tablets. Swallowing is easy for most patients, since the shell is smooth and hydrates in the mouth, and the capsule often tends to float upon swallowing in the liquid taken with it. Their availability in a wide variety of colors makes capsules aesthetically pleasing. There are numerous additional advantages to capsules as a dosage form, depending on the type of capsule employed.

Capsules may be classified as either hard or soft depending on the nature of the shell. Soft gelatin capsules (sometimes referred to as "softgels") are made from a more flexible, plasticized gelatin film than hard gelatin capsules. Most capsules of either type are intended to be swallowed whole; however, some soft gelatin capsules are intended for rectal or vaginal insertion as suppositories. The majority of capsule products manufactured today are of the hard gelatin type. One survey [1] has estimated that the utilization of hard gelatin capsules to prepare solid dosage forms exceeds that of soft gelatin capsules about 10-fold.

The first capsule prepared from gelatin was a one-piece capsule, which was patented in France by Mothes and DuBlanc in 1834 [2]. Although the shells of these early capsules were not plasticized, such capsules would be classified today as "soft gelatin capsules" on the basis of shape, contents, and other features. Intended to mask the taste of certain unpleasant tasting medication, they quickly gained popularity primarily as a means for administering copaiba balsam, a drug popular at the time in the management of venereal disease [2]. These capsules were made one at a time by hand by dipping leather molds in a molten gelatin mixture, filled with a pipette, and sealed with a drop of molten gelatin [3]. Today, soft gelatin capsules may be prepared from plasticized gelatin by means of a plate process or, more commonly, by a rotary die process in which they are formed, filled, and sealed in a single operation. With few exceptions, soft gelatin capsules are filled with solutions or suspensions of drugs in liquids that will not solubilize the gelatin shell. They are a completely sealed dosage form: the capsule cannot be opened without destroying the capsule. Because liquid contents can be metered with high-quality pumps, soft gelatin capsules are the most accurate and precise of all solid oral dosage forms. Depending on the machine tooling, a wide variety of sizes and shapes is possible. Typical shapes include spherical, oval, oblong, tube, and suppository types; size may range from 1 to 480 minims (16.2 minims = 1 mL) [3].

Although the patent holders at first sold both filled and empty soft gelatin capsules, the sale of empty shells was discontinued after 1837 [2]. However, the demand that had been created for the empty capsules led to several attempts to overcome the patents, which, in turn, resulted in the development both of the gelatin-coated pill and the hard gelatin capsule [2]. The first hard gelatin capsule was invented by J. C. Lehuby, to whom a French patent was granted in 1846 [2]. It resembled the modern hard gelatin capsule in that it consisted of two telescoping cap and body pieces. In Lehuby's patent, the capsule shells were made of starch or tapioca sweetened with syrup, although later additions to the patent claimed carragheen (1847) and mixtures of carragheen with gelatin (1850) [2]. The first person to describe a two-piece capsule made from gelatin was James Murdock, who was granted a British patent in 1848 and who is often credited as the inventor of the modern hard gelatin capsule. Becuase Murdock was a patent agent by profession, it has been suggested that he was actually working on behalf of Lehuby [2].

Unlike soft gelatin capsules, hard gelatin capsules are manufactured in one operation and filled in a completely separate operation. Originally they were made by hand-dipping greased metal pin-like molds into a molten gelatin mixture, drying the resultant films, stripping them from the pins, and joining the same two pieces together [2]. Today they are manufactured in a similar manner by means of a completely automated process. For human use, hard gelatin capsules are supplied in at least eight sizes ranging in volumetric capacity from 0.13 to 1.37 mL. Typically they are oblong shaped; however, some manufacturers have made modest alterations in that shape to be distinctive.

In further contrast to soft gelatin capsules, hard gelatin capsules typically are filled with powders, granules, or pellets. Modified-release granules or pellets may be filled without crushing or compaction, thus avoiding disruption of barrier coats or other possible adverse effects on the release mechanism. Although many manufacturers of hard capsule filling equipment also have developed modifications to their machines that would permit the filling of liquid or semi-solid matrices, there currently are few commercial examples.

Filled hard gelatin capsules are held together by interlocking bumps and grooves molded into the cap and body pieces, and the capsules are usually additionally sealed by a banding process, which places a narrow strip of gelatin around the midsection of the capsule where the two pieces are joined.

Although capsules made from gelatin predominate, recent years have seen an increased interest in and availability of nongelatin capsules. Such alternative shell compositions may satisfy religious, cultural, or vegetarian needs to avoid animal sources. Hard shell capsules made from starch were developed by Capsugel (Div. Pfizer, Inc.). These consist of two fitted cap and body pieces that are made by injection molding the glassy mass formed when starch containing 13–14% water is heated and then dried [4]. Temperatures in the range of 140–190°C reportedly produce masses that flow satisfactorily without degradation. The two parts are formed in separate molds. Unlike hard gelatin capsules, which are supplied with the caps and bodies prejoined, the two parts are supplied separately. The caps and bodies do not interlock and must be sealed together at the time of filling to prevent their separation. Capsugel has licensed the technology for the manufacture and filling of these capsules to West Pharmaceutical Services (Lionville, PA), which uses the starch capsule in their TARGIT® technology for site-specific delivery to the colon. TARGIT is based on the application of enteric polymer coatings to the starch capsules.

Shells manufactured from hydroxypropylmethylcellulose (HPMC) are also available (Shionogi Qualicaps Co., LTD, Whitsett, NC; Capsugel Div. Pfizer, Greenwood, SC; Vegicaps Technologies, Div. American Home Products and Whitehall-Robins, Springfield, UT). HPMC capsules can be made using a dipping technology similar to that used with gelatin. HPMC capsules generally have lower equilibrium moisture contents than gelatin capsules and may show better physical stability on exposure to extremely low humidities.

Additional advantages and attributes of both hard and soft shell capsules are discussed in the following sections.

II. HARD GELATIN CAPSULES

A. Advantages

Hard shell capsules have often been assumed to have better bioavailability than tablets. Most likely this assumption derives from the fact the gelatin shell rapidly dissolves and ruptures, which affords at least the potential for rapid release of the drug, together with the lack of utilization of a compaction process comparable to tablet compression in filling the capsules. However, capsules can be just as easily malformulated as tablets. A number of cases of bioavailability problems with capsules have been reported [5–8].

Hard shell capsules allow for a degree of flexibility of formulation not obtainable with tablets: often they are easier to formulate because there is no requirement that the powders be formed into a coherent compact that will stand up to handling. However, the problems of powder blending and homogeneity, powder fluidity, and lubrication in hard capsule filling are similar to those encountered in tablet manufacture. It is still necessary to measure out an accurate and precise volume of powder or pellets, and the ability of such dry solids to uniformly fill into a cavity (often comparable to a tablet die) is the determining factor in weight variation and, to a degree, content uniformity.

Modern filling equipment offers flexibility by making possible the multiple filling of diverse systems, e.g., beads/granules, tablets, powders, semi-solids, in the same capsule, which offers many possibilities in dosage form design to overcome incompatibilities by separating ingredients within the same capsule or to create modified or controlled drug delivery. Indeed, capsules are ideally suited to the dispensing of granular or bead-type modified release products since they may be filled without a compression process that could rupture the particles or otherwise compromise the integrity of any controlled-release coatings.

Hard gelatin capsules are uniquely suitable for blinded clinical tests and are widely used in preliminary drug studies. Bioequivalence studies of tablet formulations may be conveniently "blinded" by inserting tablets into opaque capsules, often along with an inert filler powder. Even capsule products may be disguised by inserting them into larger capsules.

B. Disadvantages

From a pharmaceutical manufacturing point of view, there perhaps is some disadvantage in the fact that the output of even the fastest automatic capsule-filling machines is about one-fifth that of typical modern high-speed production tablet presses. Generally, hard gelatin capsule products tend to be more costly to produce than tablets; however, the relative cost-effectiveness of capsules and tablets must be judged on a case-by-case basis. This cost disadvantage diminishes as the cost of the active ingredient increases or when tablets must be coated [9]. Furthermore, it may be possible to avoid the cost of a granulation step by choosing encapsulation in lieu of tableting.

Highly soluble salts (e.g., iodides, bromides, chlorides) generally should not be dispensed in hard gelatin capsules. Their rapid release may cause gastric irritation due to the formation of a high drug concentration in localized areas. A somewhat related concern is that both hard gelatin capsules and tablets may become lodged in the esophagus where the resulting localized high concentration of certain drugs (doxycycline, potassium chloride, indomethacin, and others) may cause damage [10]. Marvola [10] measured the force required to detach various dosage forms from isolated pig esophagus mounted in an organ bath and found that capsules tended to adhere more strongly than tablets. However, the detachment forces were greatly reduced for both after a water rinse (to simulate drinking) or when there was a slow continuous flow of artificial saliva. In an in vivo study, Hey et al. [11] studied the esophageal transit of barium sulfate tablets and capsules radiologically in 121 healthy volunteers. The subject's position (standing or lying down) and the volume of water taken (25 or 100 mL) during swallowing were considered. The majority (60%) of the volunteers had some difficulty in swallowing one or more of the preparations: many preparations were shown to adhere to the esophagus and to begin to disintegrate in the lower part of the esophagus. Delayed transit time occurred more frequently with large round tablets than with small tablets or capsules. In contrast to tablets, patient position or the volume of water taken had less influence on the passage of capsules. Despite their findings, Hey et al. preferred not to use capsules because of their potential for esophageal adhesion. In general it was recommended that patients should remain standing 90 seconds or more after taking tablets or capsules and that they should be swallowed with at least 100 mL of water. In a study considering only the esophageal transit of barium sulfate–filled hard gelatin capsules, Channer and Virjee [12] found that 26 of 50 patients exhibited sticking; however, only 3 of these patients were aware that a capsule had lodged in their esophagus. These investigators also concluded that drugs should be taken with a drink while standing. Evans and Roberts [13] compared barium sulfate tablets and capsules and found a greater tendency for esophageal retention with tablets than with capsules. Fell [14] has pointed to the large difference in density between barium sulfate and typical pharmaceutical preparations as a complicating factor in drawing conclusions about any differences in esophageal retention between tablets and capsules.

C. The Manufacture of Hard Gelatin Capsules

The three producers of hard gelatin capsules in North America are Shionogi Qualicaps™ (Whitsett, NC) Capsugel Div. Pfizer, Inc. (Greenwood, SC), and R.P. Scherer Hardcapsule (Windsor, Ontario). In all cases, the shells are manufactured by a dipping process in which sets of stainless steel mold pins are dipped into gelatin solutions and the shells are formed by gelatin on the pin surfaces. The basic mechanical design of the equipment was developed about 50 years ago by Colton [15].

Shell Composition

Gelatin is the most important constituent of the dipping solutions, but other components may also be present.

Gelatin

Gelatin is prepared by the hydrolysis of collagen obtained from animal connective tissue, bone, skin, and sinew. This long polypeptide chain yields on hydrolysis 18 amino acids, the most prevalent of which are glycine and alanine. Gelatin can vary in its chemical and physical properties depending on the source of the collagen and the manner of extraction. There are two basic types of gelatin. Type A, which is produced by an acid hydrolysis, is manufactured mainly from pork skin. Type B gelatin, produced by alkaline hydrolysis, is manufactured mainly from animal bones. The two types can be differentiated by their isoelectric points (4.8–5.0 for Type B and 7.0–9.0 for Type A) and by their viscosity-building and film-forming characteristics.

Either type of gelatin may be used, but combinations of pork skin and bone gelatin are often used to optimize shell characteristics [15,16]. Bone gelatin contributes firmness, whereas pork skin gelatin contributes plasticity and clarity.

The physicochemical properties of gelatin of most interest to shell manufacturers are the bloom strength and viscosity. Bloom strength is an empirical gel strength measure, which gives an indication of the firmness of the gel. It is measured in a Bloom Gelometer, which determines the weight in grams required to depress a standard plunger a fixed distance into the surface of a $6\frac{2}{3}\%$ w/w gel under standard conditions. Those gelatins that are produced from the first extraction of the raw materials have the highest bloom strength. Bloom strengths in the range of 150–280 g are considered suitable for capsules.

The viscosity of gelatin solutions is vital to the control of the thickness of the cast film. Viscosity is measured on a standard $6\frac{2}{3}\%$ w/w solution at 60°C in a capillary pipette and generally the range of 30–60 millipoise is suitable.

Colorants

Commonly, various soluble synthetic dyes ("coal tar dyes") and insoluble pigments are used. Commonly used pigments are the iron oxides.

Colorants not only play a role in identifying the product, but may also play a role in improving patient compliance. Thus, the color of a drug product may be selected in consideration of the disease state for which it is intended. For example, Buckalew and Coffield [19] found in a panel test that four colors were significantly associated with certain treatment groups—white, analgesia; lavender, hallucinogenic effects; orange or yellow, stimulants and antidepressants.

Opaquing Agents

Titanium dioxide may be included to render the shell opaque. Opaque capsules may be employed to provide protection against light or to conceal the contents.

Preservatives

When preservatives are employed, parabens are often selected.

Water

Hot, demineralized water is used in the preparation of the dipping solution. Initially, a 30–40% w/w solution of gelatin is prepared in large stainless steel tanks. Vacuum may be applied to assist in the removal of entrapped air from this viscous preparation. Portions of this stock solution are removed and mixed with any other ingredients, as required, to prepare the dipping solution. At this point, the viscosity of the dipping solution is measured and adjusted. The viscosity of this solution is critical to the control of the thickness of the capsule walls.

Shell Manufacture

The Colton machine illustrated in Fig. 1 is a fully automatic implementation of the dipping process. The steps are as follows:

1. Dipping (Fig. 2)—Pairs of stainless steel pins are dipped into the dipping solution to simultaneously form the caps and bodies. The pins are lubricated with a proprietary mold release agent. The pins are at ambient temperature (about 22°C), whereas the dipping solution is maintained at a temperature of about 50°C in a heated, jacketed dipping pan. The length of time to cast the film has been reported to be about 12 seconds, with larger capsules requiring longer dipping times [16].
2. Rotation—After dipping, the pins are withdrawn from the dipping solution, and as they are done so, they are elevated and rotated $2\frac{1}{2}$ times until they are facing upward. This rotation

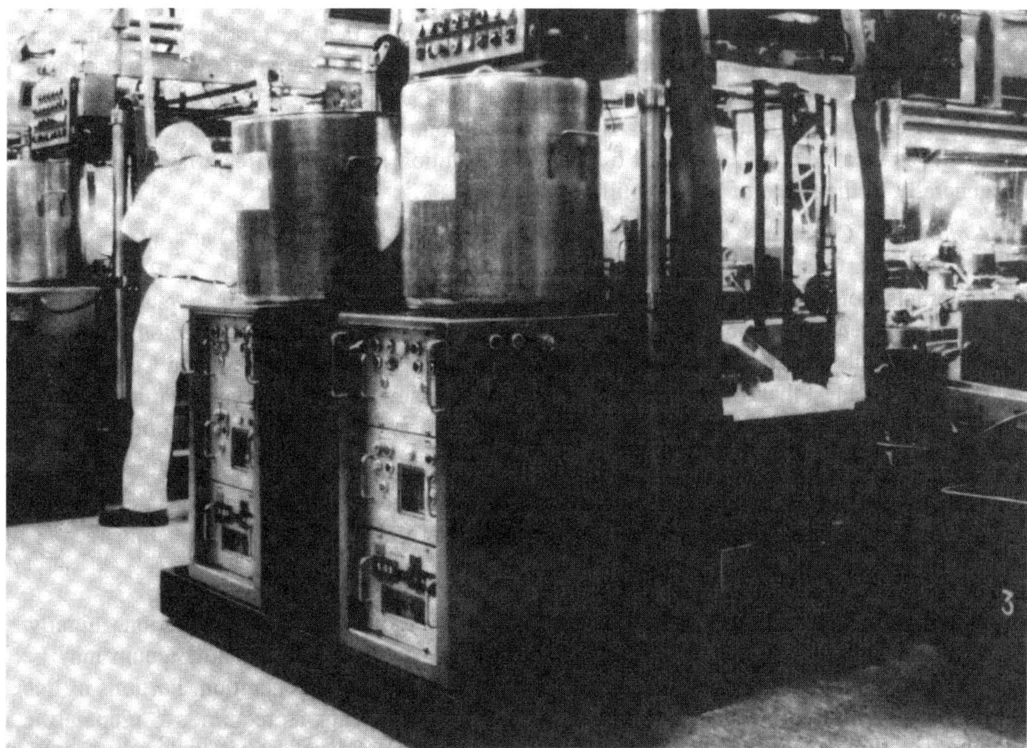

Fig. 1 View of a hard gelatin capsule manufacturing machine. (Courtesy of Elanco Qualicaps, formerly a Division of Eli Lilly Co., Indianapolis, IN)

helps to distribute the gelatin over the pins uniformly and to avoid the formation of a bead at the capsule ends. After rotation they are given a blast of cool air to set the film.

3. Drying—The racks of gelatin-coated pins then pass into a series of four drying ovens. Drying is done mainly be dehumidification by passing large volumes of dry air over the pins. Only a temperature elevation of a few degrees is permissible to prevent film melting. Drying also must not be too rapid to prevent "case hardening." Overdrying must be avoided as this could cause films to split on the pins due to shrinkage or at least make them too brittle for the later trimming operation. Underdrying will leave the films too pliable or sticky for subsequent operations.
4. Stripping—A series of bronze jaws (softer than stainless steel) strip the cap and body portions of the capsules from the pins.
5. Trimming (Fig. 3)—The stripped cap and body portions are delivered to collets in which they are firmly held. As the collets rotate, knives are brought against the shells to trim them to the required length.
6. Joining (Fig. 4)—The cap and body portions are aligned concentrically in channels, and the two portions are slowly pushed together.

The entire cycle takes about 45 minutes, about two thirds of which is required for the drying step alone.

Sorting

The moisture content of the capsules as they are ejected from the machine will be in the range of 15–18% w/w. Additional adjustment of moisture content toward the final desired specification will occur during the sorting step. During sorting, the capsules passing on a lighted moving conveyor are examined visually by inspectors. Any defective capsules spotted are thus manually removed. Defects are generally classified according to their nature and potential to cause problems in usage. The most serious of these are those that could cause stoppage of a filling machine, such as imperfect cuts, dented capsules, or capsules with holes. Other

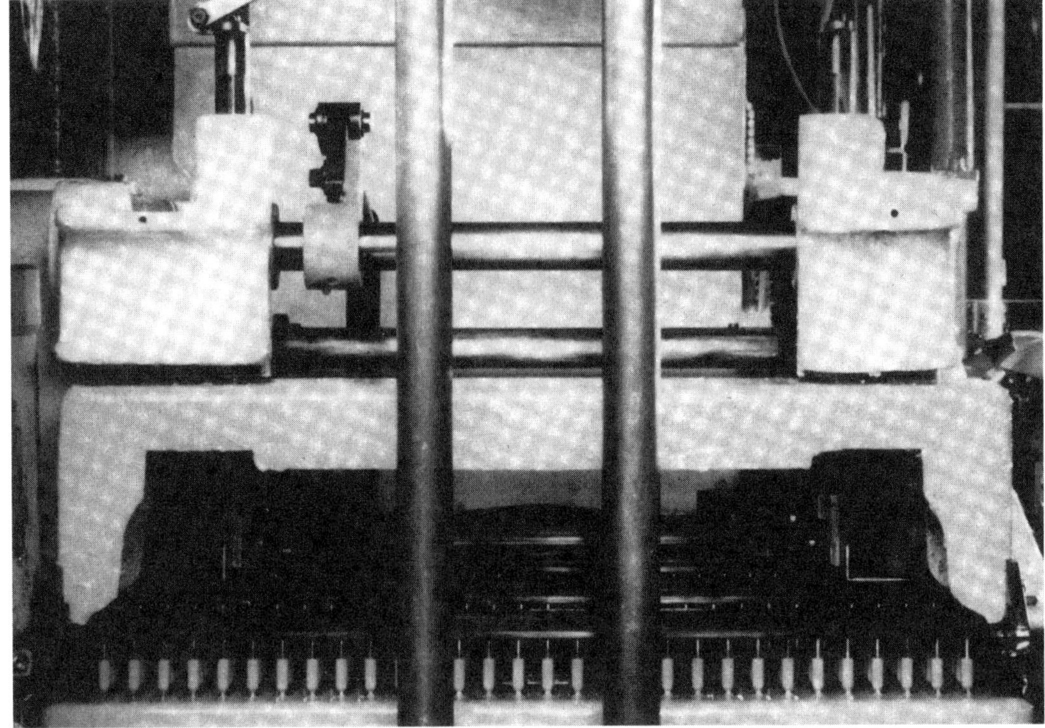

Fig. 2 Dipping of pins in the manufacture of hard gelatin capsules. (Courtesy of Elanco Qualicaps, formerly a Division of Eli Lilly and Co., Indianapolis, IN)

defects may cause problems on usage, e.g., capsules with splits, long bodies, or grease inside. Many less important cosmetic faults that only detract from appearance may also occur (small bubbles, specks in the film, marks on the cut edge, etc.)

Printing

In general, capsules are printed prior to filling. Empty capsules can be handled faster than filled capsules, and should there be any loss or damage to the capsules during printing, no active ingredients would be involved [15]. Generally, printing is done on offset rotary presses having throughput capabilities as high as $\frac{3}{4}$ million capsules per hour [15]. Available equipment can print either axially along the length of capsules or radially around the circumference of capsules.

Sizes and Shapes

For human use, empty gelatin capsules are manufactured in eight sizes, ranging from 000 (the largest) to 5 (the smallest). The volumes and approximate capacities for the traditional eight sizes are listed in Table 1.

The largest size normally acceptable to patients is a No. 0. Size 0 and size 00 hard gelatin capsules having an elongated body (e.g., 0E and 00E) also are available that provide greater fill capacity without an increase in their respective diameters. Three larger sizes are available for veterinary use: Nos. 10, 11, and 12, having approximate capacities of 30, 15, and 7.5 g, respectively.

Although the standard shape of capsules is the traditional, symmetrical, generally cylindrical shape, some manufacturers have employed distinctive proprietary shapes. Lilly's Pulvule^{R} is designed with a characteristic body section that tapers to a bluntly pointed end. Smith Kline Beacham's Spansule^{R} capsule exhibits a characteristic taper at both the cap and body ends.

Sealing and Self-Locking Closures

Positive closures help prevent the inadvertent separation of capsules during shipping and handling. Such safeguards have become particularly important with the advent of high-speed filling and packaging equipment. This problem is particularly acute in the filling of noncompacted, bead, or granular formulations.

Hard gelatin capsules are made self-locking by forming indentations or grooves on the inside of the

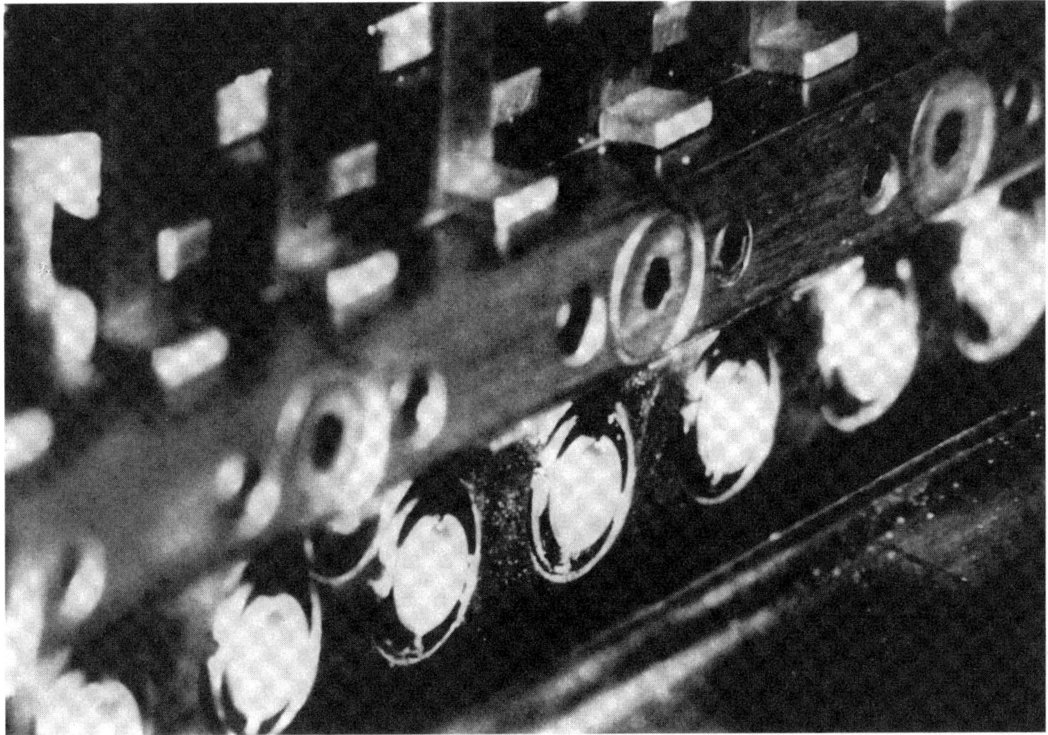

Fig. 3 Trimming the newly cast and dried shells to proper length. (Courtesy of Elanco Qualicaps, formerly a Division of Eli Lilly and Co., Indianapolis, IN)

cap and body portions. Thus, when they are fully engaged, a positive interlock is created between the cap and body portions. Indentations formed further down on the cap provide a prelock, thus preventing accidental separation of the empty capsules. Examples include Posilok^R (Shionogi Qualicaps), Coni-Snap^R (Capsugel, Div. Pfizer Inc.), and Loxit^R (R.P. Scherer Hardcapsule). The rim of the body portion of Coni-Snap capsules is tapered to help guide the cap onto the body. In high-speed automatic capsule-filling machines, this feature can reduce or eliminate snagging or splitting of capsules. The Coni-Snap principle and prelock feature are illustrated in Fig. 5.

Capsugel has also developed the Coni-Snap Supro^R capsule (Fig. 6). Similar to Coni-Snap in regard to locking mechanism and tapered body edge, this capsule differs in that it is short and squat and the cap overlaps the body to a greater degree [21].

Hard gelatin capsules may be made hermetically sealed by the technique of banding wherein a film of gelatin, often distinctively colored, is laid down around the seam of the cap and body. Parke Davis' Kapseal^R is a typical example. In the Quali-Seal^R process (Shionogi Qualicaps), two thin layers are applied, one on top of the other. Banding currently is the single most commonly used sealing technique. Banded capsules can provide an effective barrier to atmospheric oxygen [22].

Spot welding was once commonly used to lock the cap and body sections of bead-filled capsules together. In the thermal method, two hot metal jaws are brought into contact with the area where the cap overlaps the filled body [23].

Capsugel had proposed a low-temperature thermal method of hermetically sealing hard gelatin capsules [23]. The process involved immersion of the capsules for a fraction of a second in a hydroalcoholic solvent, followed by rapid removal of excess solvent, leaving traces in the overlapping area of the cap and body (held by capillary forces). Finally, the capsules are dried with warm air. A more recent adaptation of this approach involves the spraying of a mist of the hydroalcoholic solution onto the inner cap surface immediately prior to closure in filling machines. Such a process is also used to seal starch capsules together. In the wake of several incidents of tampering with over-the-counter (OTC) capsules, sometimes with fatal consequences, much thought was given as to how to make capsules safer [23]. Attention was focused on sealing techniques as possible

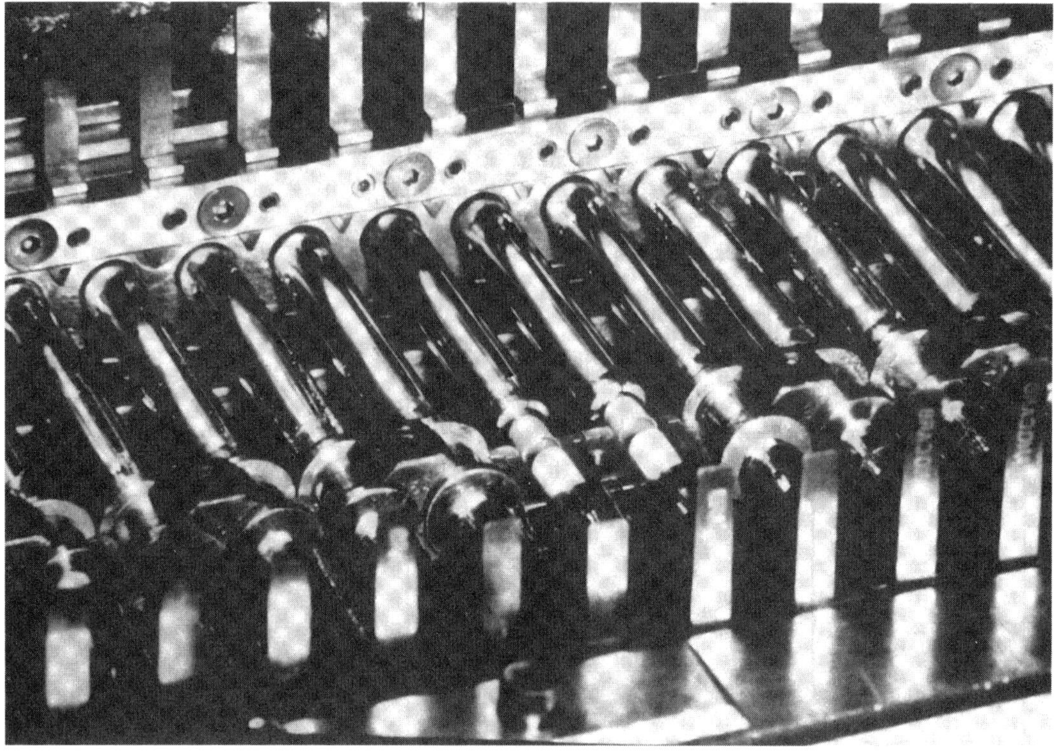

Fig. 4 Joining caps and bodies. (Courtesy of Elanco Qualicaps, formerly a Division of Eli Lilly and Co., Indianapolis, IN.)

means of enhancing the safety of capsules by making them tamper evident, i.e., so that they could not be tampered with without destroying the capsule or at least causing obvious disfigurement.

Storage, Packaging, and Stability Considerations

Finished hard gelatin capsules normally contain an equilibrium moisture content of 13–16%. This moisture is critical to the physical properties of the shells since at lower moisture contents (<12%) shells become too brittle; at higher moisture contents (>18%) they become too soft [24,25]. It is best to avoid extremes of temperature and to maintain a relative humidity of 40–60% when handling and storing capsules.

Table 1 Capsule Volumes

Size	Volume (mL)	Fill weight (g) at powder density of 0.8 g/cm^3
000	1.37	1.096
00	0.95	0.760
0	0.68	0.544
1	0.50	0.400
2	0.37	0.296
3	0.30	0.240
4	0.21	0.168
5	0.13	0.104

Source: Ref. 20

The bulk of the moisture in capsule shells is physically bound, and it can readily transfer between the shell and its contents, depending on their relative hygroscopicity [26,27]. The removal of moisture from the shell could be sufficient to cause splitting or cracking, as has been reported for the deliquescent material, potassium acetate [28]. Sodium cromoglycate has been reported to act as a "sink" for moisture in that moisture was continuously removed from hard gelatin shells, especially at higher temperatures [29]. Conditions that favor the transfer of moisture to powder contents may lead to caking and retarded disintegration or other stability problems. It may be useful to first equilibrate the shell and its contents to the same relative humidity within the acceptable range [30,31].

One issue that has received substantial attention in recent years is the loss of water solubility of shells, apparently as a result of exposure to high humidity

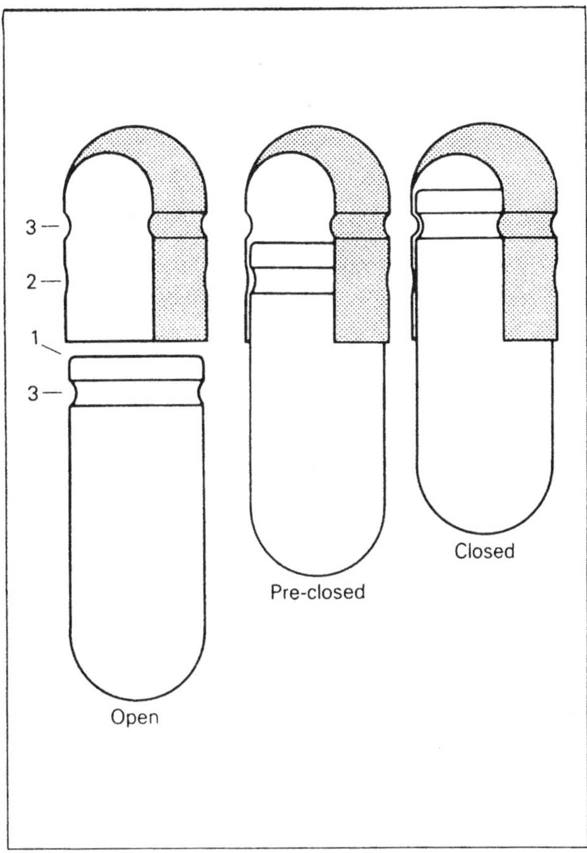

1 The tapered rim prevents faulty joins
2 These indentations prevent the pre-closed capsule from opening too early
3 These groovs lock the two halves together after filling (SNAP-FIT™ principle)

Fig. 5 Coni-Snap mechanically locking capsule showing prelock feature. (Courtesy of Capsugel, a Division of Warner-Lambert Co., Greenwood, SC.)

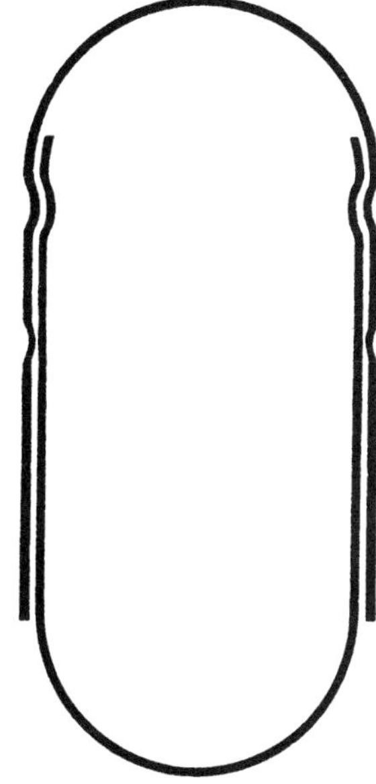

Fig. 6 Coni-Snap Supro. (Courtesy of Capsugel, a Division of Warner-Lambert Co., Greenwood, SC.)

and temperature or to trace reactive aldehydes [32]. Such capsules frequently develop a "skin" or pellicle during dissolution testing, exhibit retarded dissolution, and may fail to meet USP drug dissolution specifications. This insolubilization of gelatin capsules is presumed to be the result of "gelatin cross-linking." In one example, photoinstability compounded by humidity has been suggested as the explanation for the retarded dissolution of model compounds from hard gelatin capsules containing certified dyes, particularly when FD&C Red No. 3 was incorporated in both the cap and the shell [33,34]. The problem also has been attributed to the presence of trace aldehydes in excipients [35] as well as to the liberation of furfural from the rayon stuffing in packages [32]. These results point to the need for appropriate storage conditions and moisture-tight packaging, as well as to the need to exclude aldehydes. The issue is not new, nor is it a capsule issue per se; rather, it is a gelatin issue. The loss of water solubility on exposure of gelatin to elevated temperature and humidity was reported in 1968 to be "particularly disadvantageous in the case of gelatin desserts" [36]. The phenomenon also has been reported to occur with gelatin-coated acetaminophen tablets [37]. The inclusion of gastric enzymes in dissolution media tends to negate these effects [34,37,38]; thus, the phenomenon may have little physiological significance.

In 1992, the U.S. Food and Drug Administration (FDA) formed the Gelatin Capsule Working Group to address this gelatin solubility problem [39]. Composed of members of pharmaceutical industry trade associations, gelatin capsule manufacturers, the United States Pharmacopieia Conventions, Inc. (USP), and academia, the Working Group developed a protocol to use stressed and unstressed capsules to determine if these in vitro changes in dissolution were reflected in in vivo performance. Both hard gelatin and soft gelatin capsules were stressed by exposure to formaldehyde. Bioequivalence studies comparing stressed and unstressed capsules of acetaminophen indicated that moderately stressed capsules that failed to meet dissolution specifications without enzymes were bioequivalent to unstressed capsules. Overstressed capsules that failed dissolution specifications with and without enzymes in the dissolution medium failed the bioequivalence test. Based on these data, the Working Group recommended a second step (tier) be added to standard USP or New Drug Application/Abbreviated New Drug Application dissolution tests. The second tier incorporates enzymes in the dissolution medium. Thus, if the product fails the dissolution test in the absence of enzymes but passes the test when enzymes are added to the dissolution medium, the product's performance is considered acceptable.

D. The Filling of Hard Gelatin Capsules

The several types of filling machines in use in the pharmaceutical industry have in common the following operations:

1. Rectification: The empty capsules are oriented so that all point the same direction, i.e., body end downward. In general, the capsules pass one at a time through a channel just wide enough to provide a frictional grip at the cap end. A specially designed blade pushes against the capsule and causes it to rotate about its cap end as a fulcrum. After two pushes (one horizontally and one vertically downward), the capsules will always be aligned body end downward regardless of which end entered the channel first.
2. Separation of caps from bodies: This process also depends on the difference in diameters between cap and body portions. Here, the rectified capsules are delivered body end first into the upper portion of split bushings or split filling rings. A vacuum applied from below pulls the bodies down into the lower portion of the split bushing. The diameter of the caps is too large to allow them to follow the bodies into the lower bushing portion. The split bushings are then separated to expose the bodies for filling.
3. Dosing of fill material: Various methods are employed, as described below.
4. Replacement of caps and ejection of filled capsules: The cap and body bushing portions are rejoined. Pins are used to push the filled bodies up into the caps for closure and to push the closed capsules out of the bushings. Compressed air also may be used to eject the capsules.

These machines may be either semi-automatic or fully automatic. Semi-automatic machines such as the Type 8 machines (e.g., Capsugel's Cap 8 machine) require an operator to be in attendance at all times. Depending on the skill of the operator, the formulation, and the size of the capsule being filled, these machines are capable of filling as many as 120,000–160,000 capsules in an 8-hour shift. This output contrasts sharply with the output of fully automatic machines, some models of which are rated to fill that many capsules in one hour. Some representative automatic capsule-filling machines are listed in Table 2. Automatic capsule filling machines may be classified as either intermittent or continuous motion machines. Intermittent machines exhibit an interrupted filling sequence as indexing turntables must stop at various stations to execute the basic operations described above. Continuous motion machines execute these functions in a continuous cycle. The elimination of the need to decelerate and accelerate from one station to the next makes greater machine speeds possible with continuous motion machines [40]. Although capsule-filling machines may vary widely in their engineering design, the main difference between them from a formulation point of view is the means by which the formulation is dosed into the capsules.

Powder Filling

Capsule-filling equipment has been the subject of several reviews [18, 40–45]. Four main dosing methods may be identified for powder filling:

Table 2 Selected Automatic Capsule-Filling Machines

Make/Model	Dosing principle	Motion	Rated[a] capacity (capsules/hr)
Bosch	Dosing Disc[b]		
GKF 400S		I	24,000
GKF 2000S		I	150,000
GKF 3000		I	180,000
IMA[c]	Dosator		
Zanasi 6		I	6000
Zanasi 40		I	40,000
Matic 60		C	60,000
Matic 120		C	120,000
MG2[d]	Dosator		
Futura		C	48,000
G60		C	60,000
G120		C	120,000

[a] Based on manufacturer/distributor literature
[b] Bosch-TL Systems Corp., Minneapolis, MN
[c] IMA North America, Inc., Fairfield, CT
[d] MG America, Inc., Fairfield, NJ
I, Intermittent
C, Continuous

Auger Fill Principle

At one time nearly all capsules were filled by means of semi-automatic equipment wherein the powder is driven into the capsule bodies by a rotating auger, as exemplified by the Type 8 machines (see Fig. 7). The empty capsule bodies are held in a filling ring, which rotates on a turntable under the powder hopper. The fill of the capsules is primarily volumetric. Because the auger mounted in the hopper rotates at a constant rate, the rate of delivery of powder to the capsules tends to be constant. Consequently, the major control over fill weight is the rate of rotation of the filling ring under the hopper. Faster rates produce lighter fill weights because bodies have a shorter dwell time under the hopper. Ito et al. [46] compared an experimental flat-blade auger with an original screw auger and found that the screw auger provided greater fill weight (30–60% greater for a test lactose formulation) and smaller coefficients of weight variation (up to 50% smaller at the two fastest ring speeds). The formulation requirements of this type of machine have been the subject of a limited number of reports. In general, the flow properties of the powder blend should be adequate to assure a uniform flow rate from the hopper. Glidants may be helpful. Ito et al. [46] studied the glidant effect of a colloidal silica using a Capsugel Type 8 filling machine. They found that there was an optimum concentration for minimum weight variation (approximately 0.5% for lactose capsules; approximately 1% for corn starch capsules). Using a similar Elanco machine, Reier et al. [47] reported that the presence of 3% talc reduces weight variation compared to 0% talc in a multivariate study involving several fillers. These investigators analyzed their data by multiple stepwise regression analysis and concluded that the mean fill weight was dependent on machine speed, capsule size,

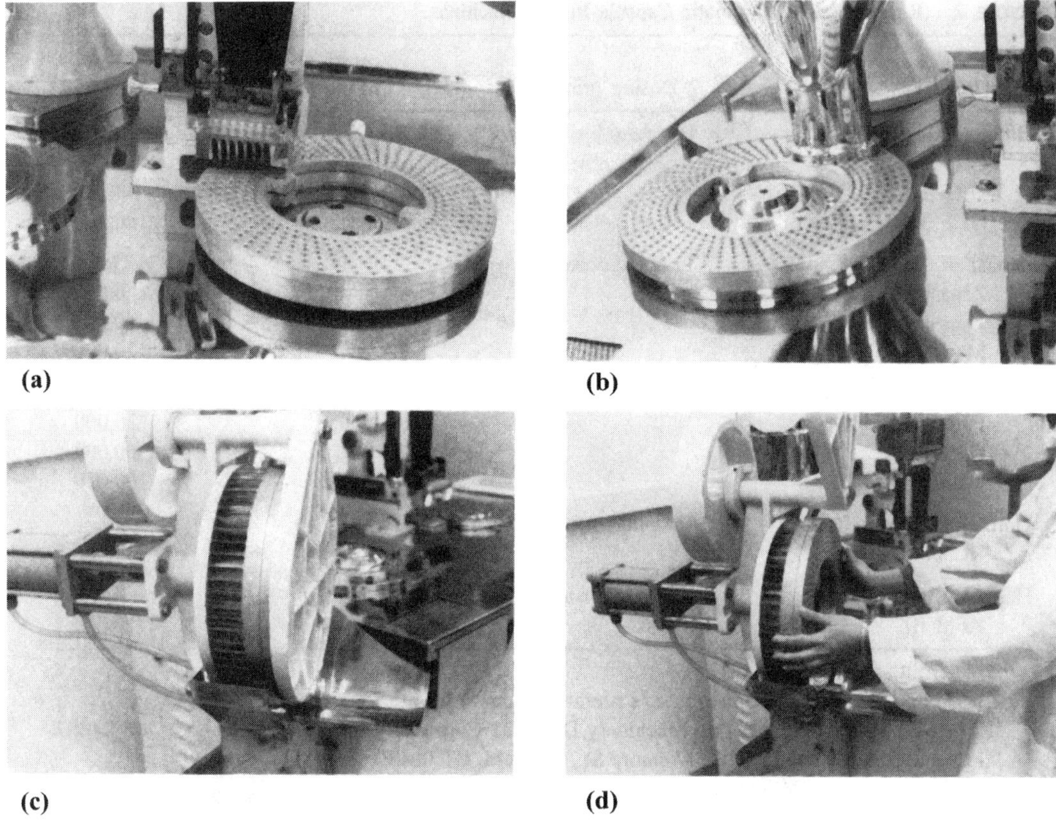

Fig. 7 Type 8 semiautomatic capsule-filling machine. (a)"Sandwich" of cap and body rings positioned under rectifier to receive empty capsules. Vacuum is pulled from beneath the rings to separate caps from bodies. (b) Body ring is positioned under foot of powder hopper for filling. (c) After filling the bodies, the cap and body rings are rejoined and positioned in front of pegs. A stop plate is swung down in back of rings to prevent capsule expulsion as the pneumatically driven pegs push the bodies to engage the caps. (d) The plate is swung aside and the pegs are used to eject the closed capsules.

and the formulation specific volume, in that order. Weight variation was found to be a function of machine speed, specific volume, flowability, and the presence of glidant but was independent of capsule size.

Lubricants such as magnesium stearate and stearic acid are also required. These facilitate the passage of the filling ring under the foot of the powder hopper and help prevent the adherence of certain materials to the auger.

Vibratory Fill Principle

The Osaka machines (Fig. 8) utilize a vibratory feed mechanism [48,49]. In this machine, the capsule body passes under a feed frame, which holds the powder in

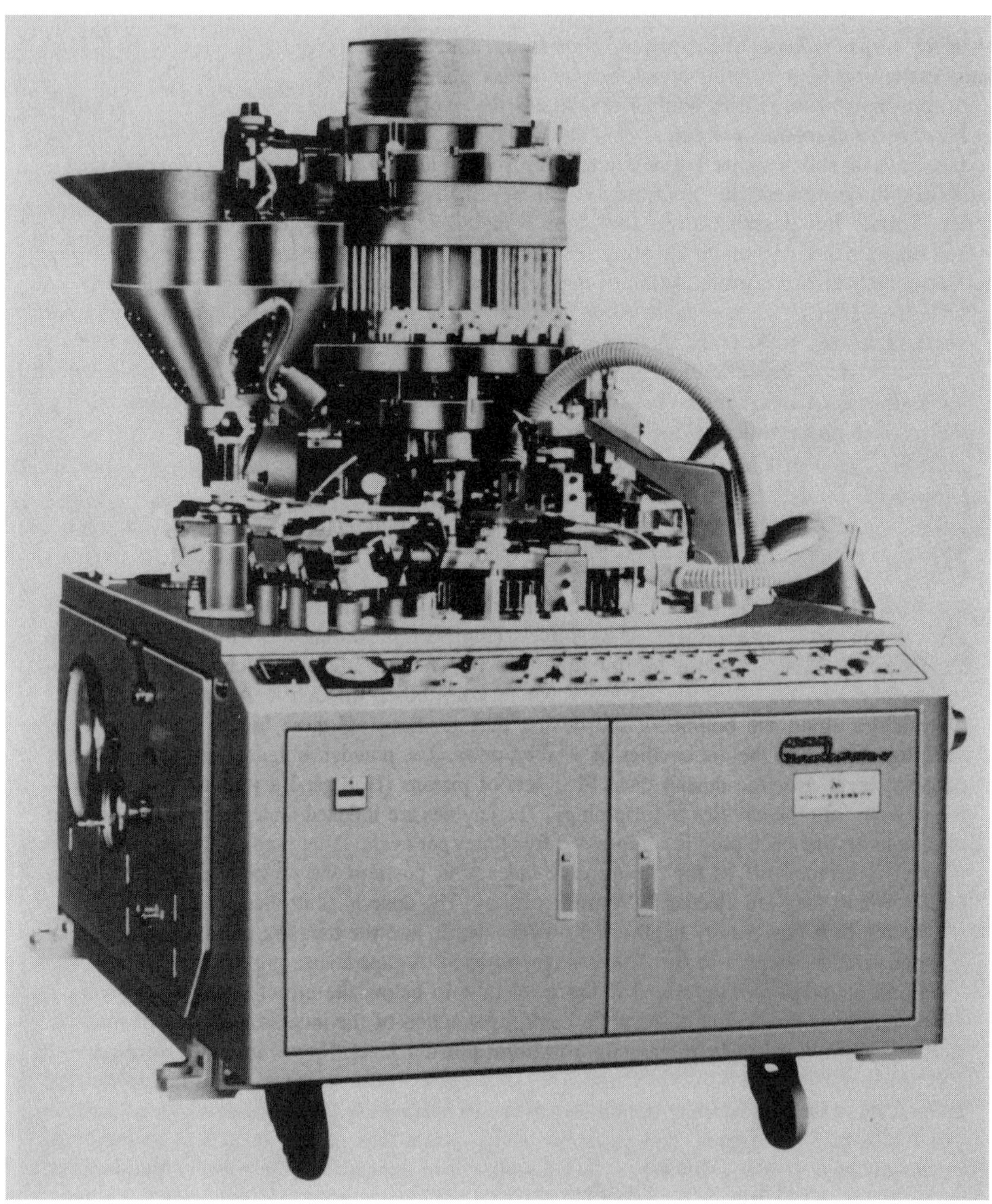

Fig. 8 Osaka model R-18O automatic capsule-filling machine. (Courtesy of Sharpley-Stokes Division, Pennwalt Corp., Warminster, PA)

the filling section. In the powder, a perforated resin plate is positioned that is connected to a vibrator. The powder bed tends to be fluidized by the vibration of the plate, and this assists the powder to flow into the bodies through holes in the resin plate [49]. The fill weight is controlled by the vibrators and by setting the position of the body under the feed frame. Much like the fill mechanism of a tablet press, there is overfill and then adjustment with scrape-off of the excess material as the capsule bodies pass under the feed frame. The capsule bodies are supported on pins in holes bored through a disc plate. While they pass under the feed area, the pins may be set to drop the bodies to below the level of the disc, thereby causing "overfill". However, before their passage is completed under the feed frame, the capsules are eventually pushed up so their upper edges become level with the surface of the disc plate. When this occurs, the excess powder is forced out and eventually scraped off by the trailing edge of the feed frame. This process affords some light compression of the powder against the resin plates and offers the opportunity to modify the fill weight. Weight variation has been related to the formulation flow properties. Kurihara and Ichikawa [48] reported that the fill weight variation with Model OCF-120 was more closely related to the minimum orifice diameter than to the angle of repose. Apparently the minimum orifice diameter is a better analogy of the flowing of powder into capsule bodies than the static angle of repose. No studies of the formulation requirements for this machine have been reported; however, typical stearate lubricants may be indicated to prevent the binding of push rods and guides.

Piston-Tamp Principle

Most capsules are filled on piston-tamp machines. These are fully automatic fillers in which pistons or tamping pins lightly compress the individual doses of powders into plugs (sometimes referred to as "slugs") and eject the plugs into the empty capsule bodies. The compression forces are low, often in the range of 50–200 N, or about 50–100-fold less than typical tablet compression forces. Hence, the plugs frequently will have the consistency of very soft compacts and will not be able to be recovered intact from the filled capsule.

There are two types of piston-tamp fillers: dosator machines and dosing-disc machines. In a recent survey of equipment used in production, it was found that dosator machines are used slightly more frequently than dosing disc machines, with about 18% of the companies responding reporting that they use both types of filling machines [50].

Dosing-Disc Machines. This type of machine is exemplified by the Bosch GKF models (formerly Hofliger-Karg) and the Harro-Hofliger KFM models (see Fig. 9). The dosing-disc filling principle has been described [51,52] and is illustrated in Fig. 10. The dosing disc, which forms the base of the dosing or filling chamber, has a number of holes bored through it. A solid brass "stop" plate slides along the bottom of the dosing-disc to close off these holes, thus forming openings similar to the die cavities of a tablet press. The powder is maintained at a relatively constant level over the dosing disc. Five sets of pistons (Bosch GKF machines) compress the powder into the cavities to form plugs. The cavities are indexed under each of the five sets of pistons so that each plug is compressed five times per cycle. After the five tamps, any excess powder is scraped off as the dosing disc indexes to position the plugs over empty capsule bodies where they are ejected by transfer pistons. The dose is controlled by the thickness of the dosing disc (i.e., cavity depth), the powder level, and the tamping pressure. The flow of powder from the hopper to the disc is auger assisted. A capacitance probe senses the powder level and activates an auger feed if the level falls below the preset level. The powder is distributed over the dosing disc by the centrifugal action of the indexing rotation of the disc. Baffles are provided to help maintain a uniform powder level. However, working with a GKF model 330, Shah et al. [52] noted that a uniform powder bed height was not maintained at the first tamping station because of its nearness to the scrape-off device.

Kurihara and Ichikawa [48] reported that variation in fill weight was closely related to the angle of repose of the formulation; however, a minimum point appeared in the plots of the angle of repose vs. coefficient of variation of filling weight. Apparently at higher angles of repose, the powders did not have sufficient mobility to distribute well under the acceleration of the intermittent indexing motion. At lower angles of repose, the powder was apparently too fluid to maintain a uniform bed. However, these investigators did not appear to make use of powder compression through tamping, and this complicates the interpretation of their results.

In a more recent study running model formulations having different flow properties on a GKF 400 machine, Heda [50] found that Carr Compressibility Index (CI) values should be $18 < CI\% < 30$ to maintain low weight variation. Poorly flowing powders ($CI\% > 30$) were observed to dam up around the

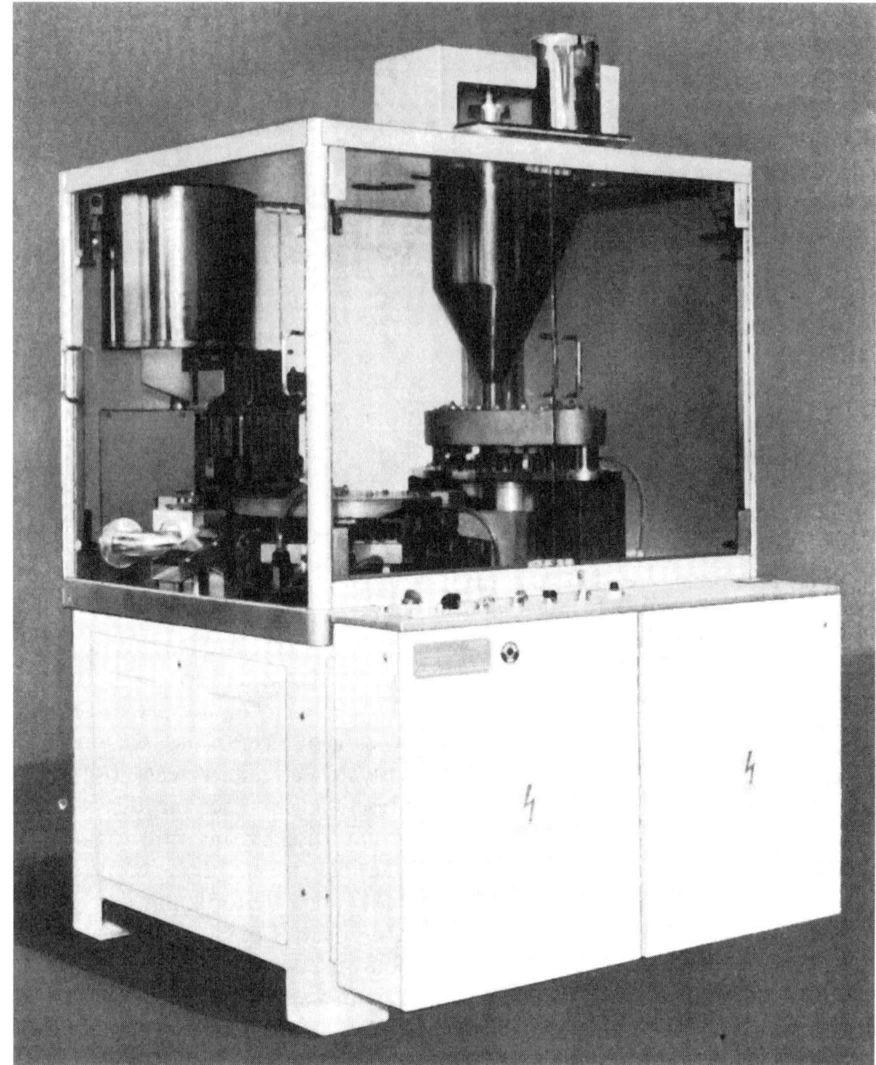

Fig. 9 Hofliger Karg model GKF 1500 automatic capsule-filling machine. (Courtesy of Robert Bosch Corp., Packaging Machinery Division, South Plainfield, NJ.)

ejection station. The Carr Compressibility Index is calculated from the loose and tapped bulk density as follows [53]:

$$CI\% = \frac{\rho_{Tapped} - \rho_{Loose}}{\rho_{Tapped}} \times 100 \tag{1}$$

where ρ_{Tapped} and ρ_{Loose} are the tapped and loose bulk densities, respectively. Relatively higher values indicate that the interparticulate cohesive and frictional interactions that interfere with powder flow are relatively more important. Thus, flowability is inversely related to the CI% value.

Dosing-disc machines generally require that formulations be adequately lubricated for efficient plug ejection, to prevent filming on pistons, and to reduce friction between any sliding components that powder may come in contact with. Some degree of compactibility is important as coherent plugs appear to be desirable for clean, efficient transfer at ejection. However, there may be less of a dependence on formulation compactibility than exists for dosator machines [43].

The Harro-Hofliger machine is similar to Bosch GKF machines, except that it employs only three tamping stations. However, at each station, the powder in the dosing cavities is tamped twice before rotating a

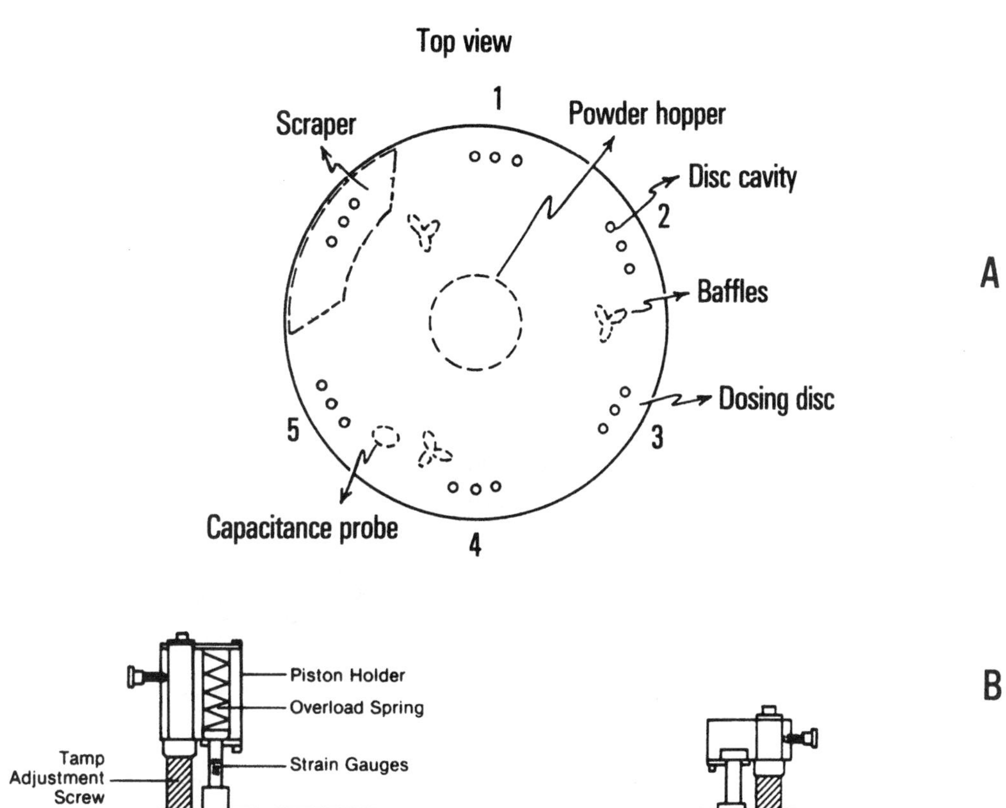

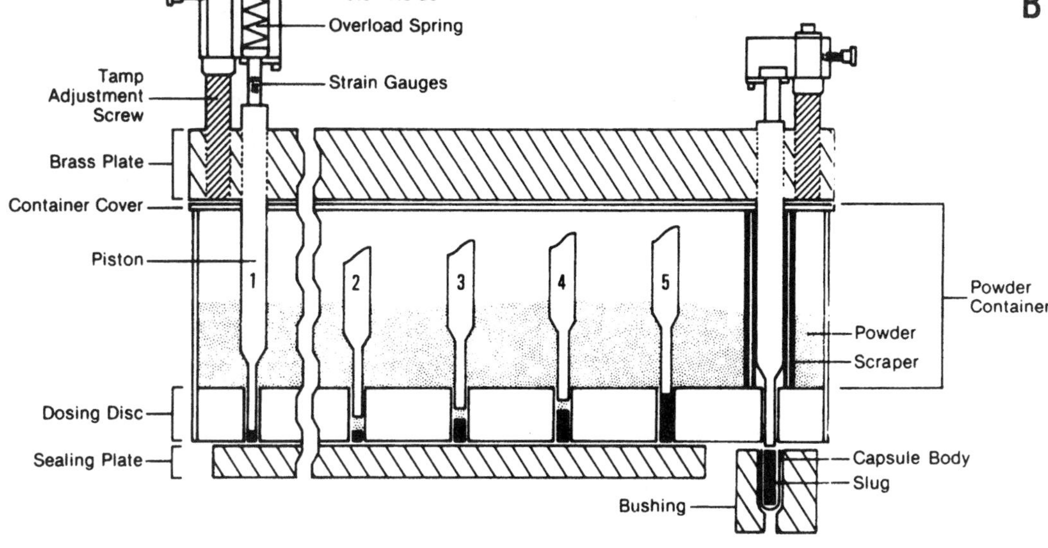

Fig. 10 Illustration of the dosing–disk filling principle: (A) view looking down on the dosing disk; (B) side view (projected) showing progressive plug formation. Note the placement of strain gauges on the piston to measure tamping and plug ejection forces (see text). (From Ref. 37.)

quarter turn to the next station. One other difference is that the powder in the filling chamber is constantly agitated to help in the maintenance of a uniform powder bed depth.

Dosator Machines. The dosator machines are exemplified by the Zanasi and MG2 pictured in Fig. 11 and 12. Figure 13 illustrates the basic dosator principle, which has been previously described [54,55]. The dosator consists of a cylindrical dosing tube fitted with a movable piston. The end of the tube is open and the position of the piston is preset to a particular height to define a volume (again,

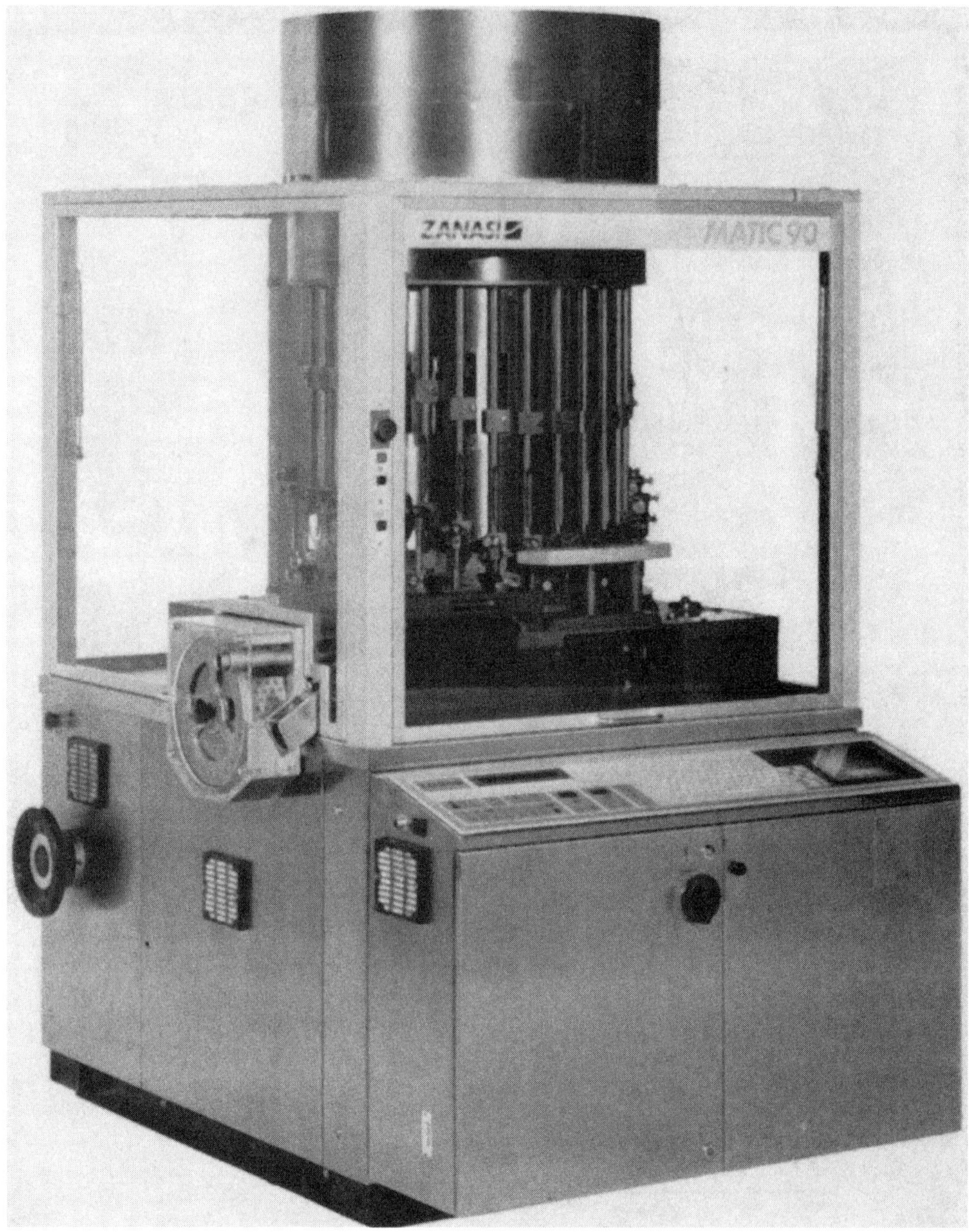

Fig. 11 Zanasi Matic 90 automatic capsule-filling machine. (Courtesy of IMA North America, Inc., Fairfield, CT.)

comparable to a tablet press "die cavity"), which would contain the desired dose of powder. In operation, the dosator is plunged down into a powder bed maintained at a constant preset level by agitators and scrapers. The powder bed height is generally greater than the piston height. Powder enters the open end and is slightly compressed against the piston (sometimes termed "precompression" [54]). The piston then gives a tamping blow, forming the powder into a plug. The dosator, bearing the plug, is withdrawn from the powder hopper and is moved over to the empty capsule body where the piston is pushed downward to eject the plug. In certain machines, such as the Macofar machines, the body bushing is rotated into position under the dosator to receive the ejected plug [56]. The primary

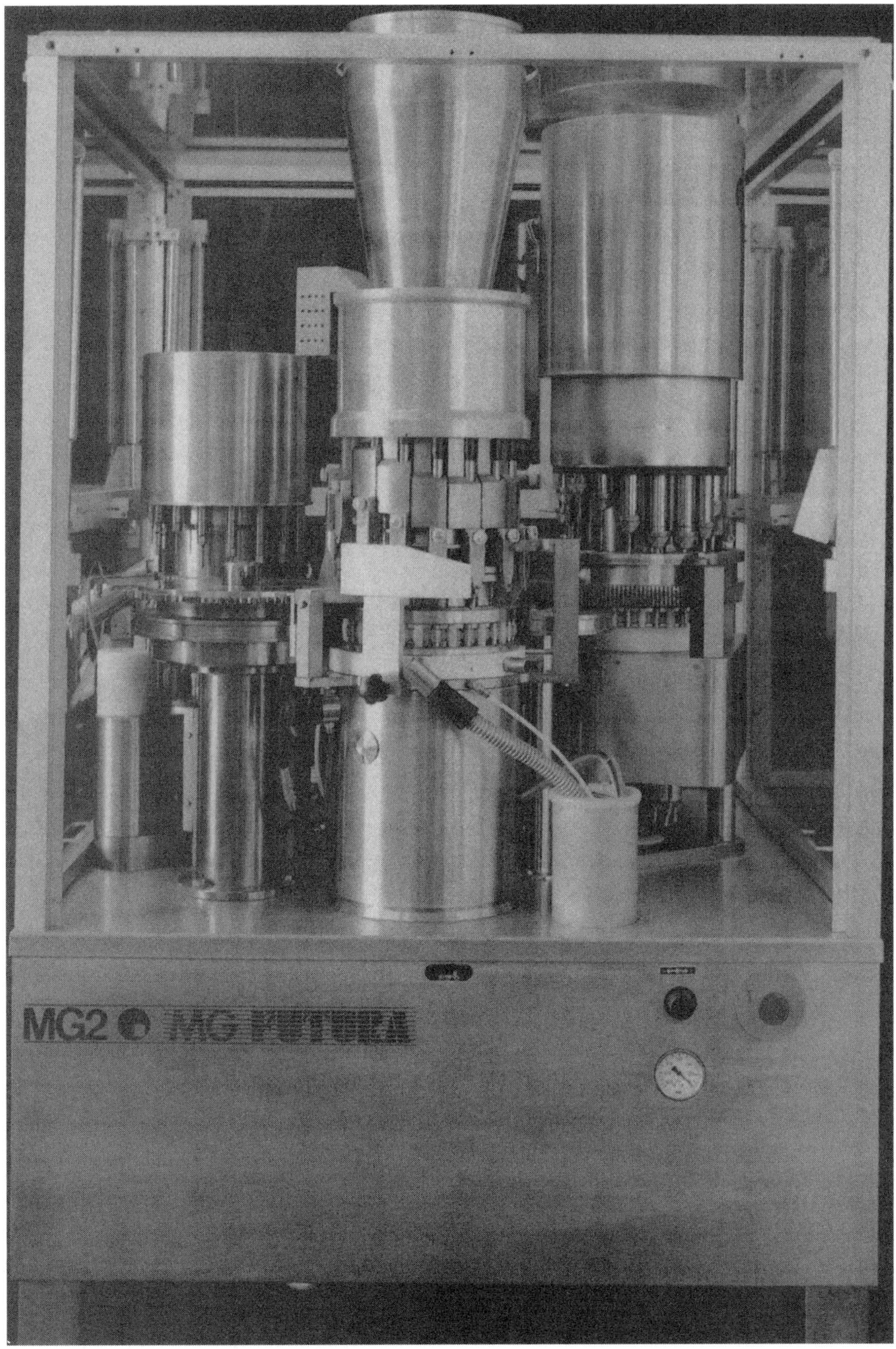

Fig. 12 MG2 Futura automatic capsule-filling machine. (Courtesy of MG America, Inc., Fairfield, NJ.)

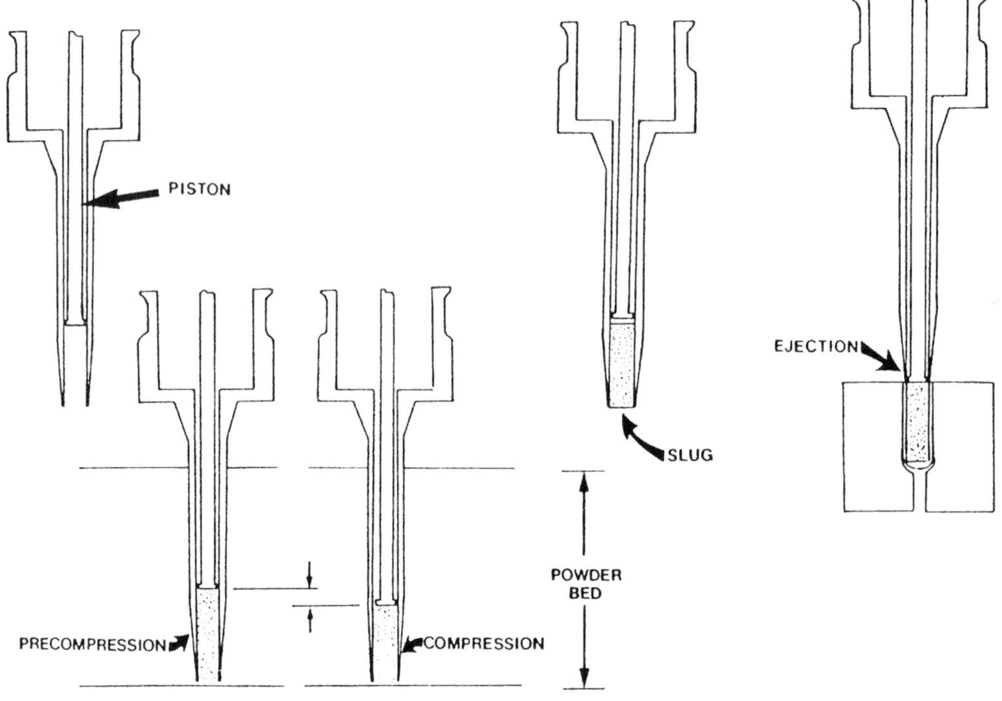

Fig. 13 Dosator filling principle. (From Ref. 48.)

control over fill weight (for a given set of tooling) is the initial piston height in the dosing tube. A secondary control of weight is the height of the powder bed into which the dosator dips.

In one of the earliest reports evaluating the Zanasi machine, Stoyle [55] suggested that formulations should have the following characteristics for successful filling:

1. Fluidity is important for powder feed from the reservoir to the dipping bed and also to permit efficient closing in of the hole left by the dosator.
2. A degree of compactibility is important to prevent loss of material from the end of the plug during transport to the capsule shell.
3. Lubricity is needed to permit easy and efficient ejection of the plug.
4. Formulations should have a moderate bulk density. It was suggested that low bulk density materials or those that contain entrapped air may not consolidate well and that capping similar to that which occurs in tableting may result.

The relationship between formulation flow properties and weight variation on Zanasi machines has been studied. For example, Irwin et al. [57] compared the weight variation of capsules filled on a Zanasi LZ-64 machine with formulations composed of different diluents and lubricants. The formulations had different flow properties, as judged in a recording flow meter. Generally, it was found that the better the rate of flow, the more uniform the capsule fill weight was. Chowhan and Chow [58] compared the powder consolidation ratio with the coefficient of variation (relative standard deviation) of capsule weight and found a linear relationship for a test formulation containing 5% or 15% drug, 10% starch, 0.5% magnesium stearate, and lactose q.s. The capsules were filled on a Zanasi machine. Powder flow characteristics were inferred from the volume reduction (consolidation), which occurs when a series of loads are applied to the surface of the loosely packed powder bed in cylindrical containers. The powder consolidation ratio was the intercept of the plot of:

$$\log \frac{V_0 - V}{V} \text{ vs. } \frac{P}{P_0} \tag{2}$$

where V_0 = initial powder volume, V = powder volume at a given surface pressure, P = surface pressure, and $P_0 = l$ kg/cm^2. Further work to assess the usefulness and limitations of this approach appears warranted.

The effect of machine variables on fill weight and its uniformity were evaluated by Miyake et al. [59] using a Zanasi Z-25. In general, they found that the filling mechanism was a compaction process. The following relationship was found to apply:

$$r = a(i) \log P_r + b(i) \quad (3)$$

where r = density ratio, $a(i)$ and $b(i)$ are constants, and P_r = compression ratio = $(H - L)/L$, where H = powder bed height and L = piston height (within the dosator).

The quantitative retention of powder within the dosator during transfer from the powder bed to the capsule shell is essential to a successful filling operation. Applying hopper design theory, Jolliffe et al. [60,61] reported that powder retention requires a stable powder arch be formed at the dosator outlet which depends on the angle of wall friction. In general, there is an optimum angle of wall friction for which the compression force needed to ensure a stable arch is a minimum. Obviously, that angle will be dependent on the finish of the inner surface of the dosing tube as well as the properties of the powder. For example, more freely flowing powders will require larger minimum compressive stresses, and these minimum stresses occur at smaller angles of wall friction. In this case, smaller angles of wall friction promote the transmission of stress to the region where the arch forms. Jolliffe and Newton presented experimental data comparing a more freely flowing larger particle size fraction of lactose to a smaller size fraction that agreed with this theory [61]. Comparing two different finishes of the inner surface of a dosing tube, they also showed that the rougher surface promoted the formation of a stable arch by different size fractions of lactose by reducing the cohesive strength required within the powder plug for arching [61].

Heda [50] found that the optimum Carr Index value (CI%) for minimum weight variation for a Zanasi LZ-64 machine was between 25 and 35. Powders with high CI% values (> 30) produced stronger plugs with lower weight variation. For more freely flowing powders having CI% values < 20, higher compression force (150–200 N) may be required to improve powder retention in the dosator tube.

Nonpowder Filling

Modern automatic capsule-filling machines offer enormous flexibility in terms of what can be filled into hard shell capsules. In addition to powder dosing, filling devices also are available that can feed beads or pellets, microtablets, tablets, and liquid or pasty materials into capsules. Often these can be installed at different filling stations of the same machine such that capsules may be dosed from several different filling devices as they pass by each station before closure and ejection. Such arrangements could, for example, permit the dosing of several different tablets, different batches of beads (perhaps immediate release and modified release beads), or combinations of tablets, powder plugs, and beads into the same capsule.

Beads, pellets, etc. may be poured directly into the capsule body via gravity feed devices, which rely on the free-flowing nature of such materials. In this approach, capsules are filled to their volumetric capacity, and partial fills for multiple dosing are not possible. Modern automatic filling machines circumvent this issue by employing various indirect filling methods, i.e., the required quantity of beads, granules, etc. are first fed to a separate, volumetric metering chamber, and then the measured volume of material is transferred to the capsule body. The metering chamber is usually filled by gravity (e.g., Bosch GKF); however, in certain machines (e.g., Zanasi), the chamber is a modified dosator that draws and holds the beads into its open end by means of vacuum. In general, the dose is determined by the size of the metering chamber. If blends are being dispensed, the uniformity of the dose dispensed depends upon the size and shape of the granules or pellets, since differences in these properties may cause pellet segregation. The development of electrostatic charges on beads or pellets may also cause separation of individual beads as well as problems in flowing and transferring from chambers.

Typically, tablets are fed to the bodies through a tube and are simply released in the required number as the body passes beneath. Pumpable liquid fills are dosed by conventional liquid-dispensing devices.

E. Instrumentation of Capsule-Filling Machines and Their Role in Formulation Development

A major development in pharmaceutical technology has been the application of instrumentation techniques to tablet presses. The ability to monitor the forces that develop during the compaction, ejection, and detachment of tablets has brought about new insights into the physics of compaction, facilitated formulation development, and provided a means for the in-process control of tablet weight in manufacturing [62,63]. In most cases, automatic capsule filling is carried out on dosator or dosing-disc machines, which resemble tableting in that there are compression and ejection events. Given this similarity to tableting and the benefits that have accrued from instrumented tablet machines, it was only logical that similar instrumentation techniques be applied to these capsule-filling machines. Although both types of machines have been instrumented, most reports have been concerned with dosator machines [64].

Cole and May [65,66] were the first investigators to report the instrumentation of an automatic capsule-filling machine. They bonded strain gauges to the piston of a Zanasi LZ-64 dosator. Because of dosator rotation, this machine required modification by installation of a planetary gear system to prevent the continuous twisting of the output cable during operation. Their work demonstrated for the first time that compression and ejection forces could be recorded during plug formation. They reported (a) an initial compaction force as the plug was being formed by the dosator dipping into the powder bed, (b) a partial retention of this force during passage to the ejection station, and (c) an ejection force as the plug was pushed out of the dosator.

Small and Augsburger [54] also reported on the instrumentation of the same model Zanasi with strain gauges. Twisting of the output cable was avoided by connecting it to a low-noise mercury contact swivel mounted over the capsule hopper. This was a simpler arrangement than that employed by Cole and May [66] in that it permitted electrical contact to be maintained during experimental runs without the need for a planetary gear system or any other machine modification. Figures 14 and 15 illustrate the instrumented piston and the mounting of the mercury swivel. In contrast to Cole and May [66], Small and Augsburger [54] reported a two-stage plug formation trace: (a) a precompression force, which occurs when the dosator dips into the powder bed, and (b) compression of the powder by the tamping of the piston at the bottom of dosator travel in the powder bed. Apparently the earlier workers did not make use of the piston compression feature of the Zanasi filling principle. Like Cole and May, Small and Augsburger also reported retention and ejection forces. The retention force, which apparently is a result of elastic recovery of the plug against the piston, was observed by Small and Augsburger only when running unlubricated materials under certain conditions. This phenomenon was not observed in any lubricated runs, apparently because the lubricant permits the plug to more readily slip to relieve any residual pressure [54]. It is interesting to note that both teams of investigators reported

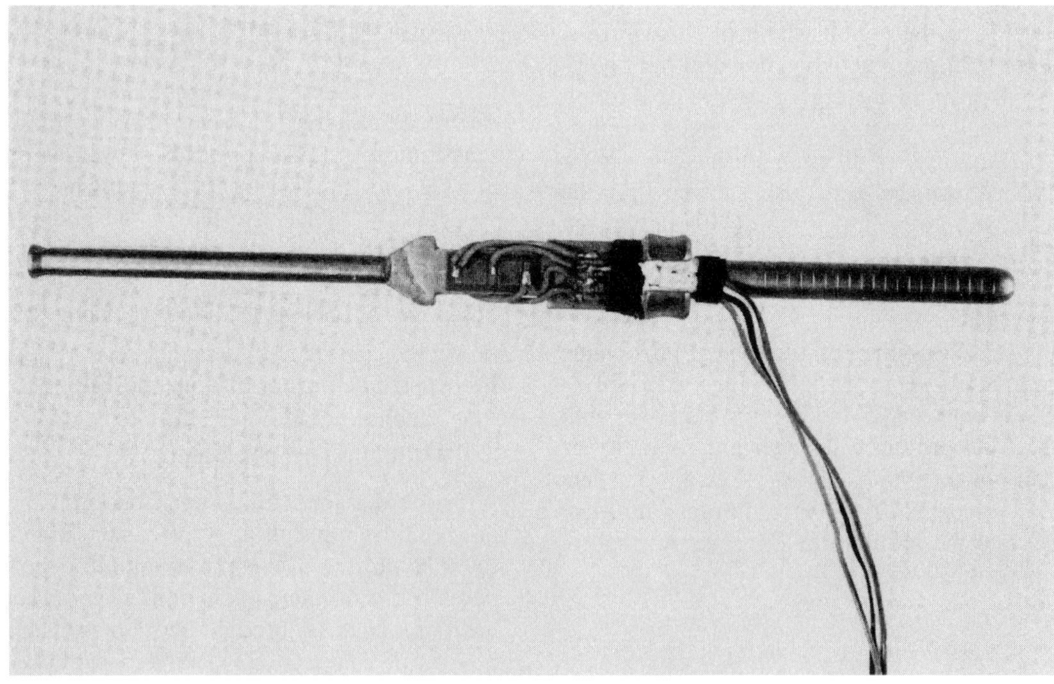

Fig. 14 Strain gauges bonded to Zanasi piston. (From Ref. 38.)

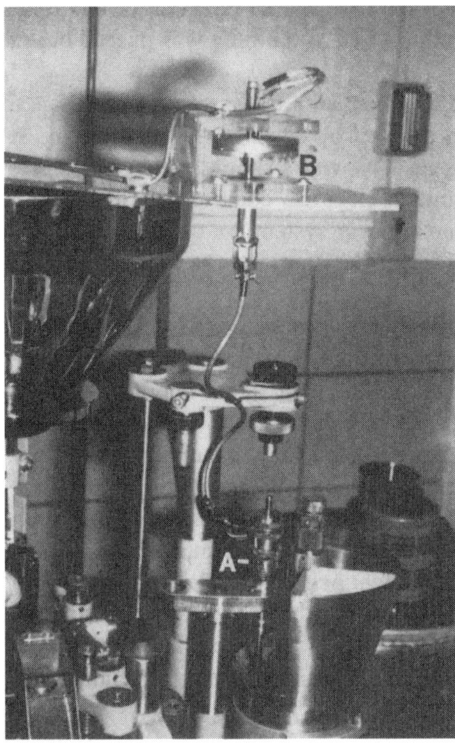

Fig. 15 Instrumented Zanasi LZ-64 showing mercury swivel for signal removal: (A) dosator containing strain-gauged piston; (B) mercury swivel. (From Ref. 38.)

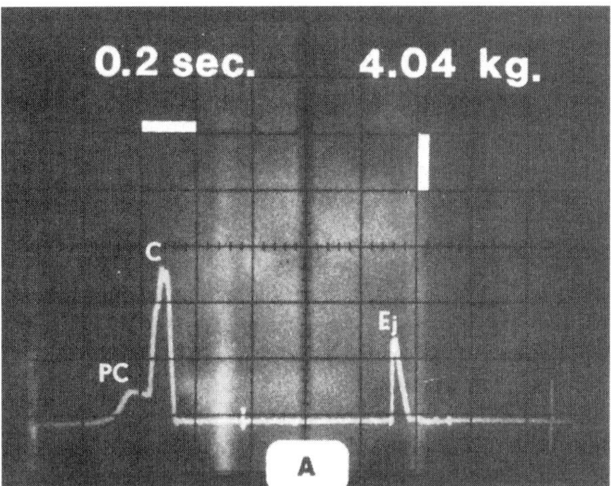

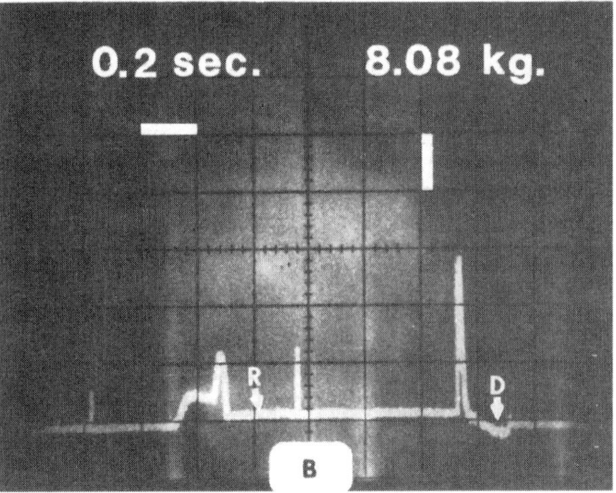

Fig. 16 Typical force–time trace from an instrumented Zanasi LZ-64 automatic capsule-filling machine. PC, precompression resulting from dipping of dosator into the powder bed; C, compression resulting from actual piston tamping; R, retention force; Ej, ejection; D, drag force developing during retraction of piston. (From Ref. 38.)

instances of drag on the piston as it returns to the original position after ejection, which may be due to inadequate lubrication. This was manifested by the appearance of a negative force (i.e., a trace below the baseline) during retraction of the piston. Sample traces from Small and Augsburger appear in Fig. 16.

Using this instrumentation, Small and Augsburger [67] later reported a detailed study of the formulation lubrication requirements of the Zanasi LZ-64. Three fillers were studied (microcrystalline cellulose, pregelatinized starch, and anhydrous lactose). Powder bed height, piston height, compression force, and lubricant type and concentration were varied to determine their effects on ejection force. In general, anhydrous lactose exhibited higher lubrication requirements than either pregelatinized starch or microcrystalline cellulose. Comparing several concentrations of magnesium stearate, minimum ejection forces were recorded at 1% with anhydrous lactose, 0.5% with microcrystalline cellulose, and 0.1% with pregelatinized starch. Magnesium lauryl sulfate compared favorably with magnesium stearate in the starch filler but was not as efficient as magnesium stearate for the other two fillers. It was also found that the magnitude of the ejection force was affected by machine operating variables. After precompression, ejection force was found to increase with the compression force. However, at a given compression force, ejection force also increases with an increase in either the piston height or the powder bed height. Figure 17 is typical. These results suggest the possibility of manipulating machine operating variables to reduce formulation lubricant requirements.

Mehta and Augsburger [68] later reported the mounting of a linear variable displacement transducer (LVDT) on the previously instrumented Zanasi LZ-64 machine [54] to allow the measurement of piston

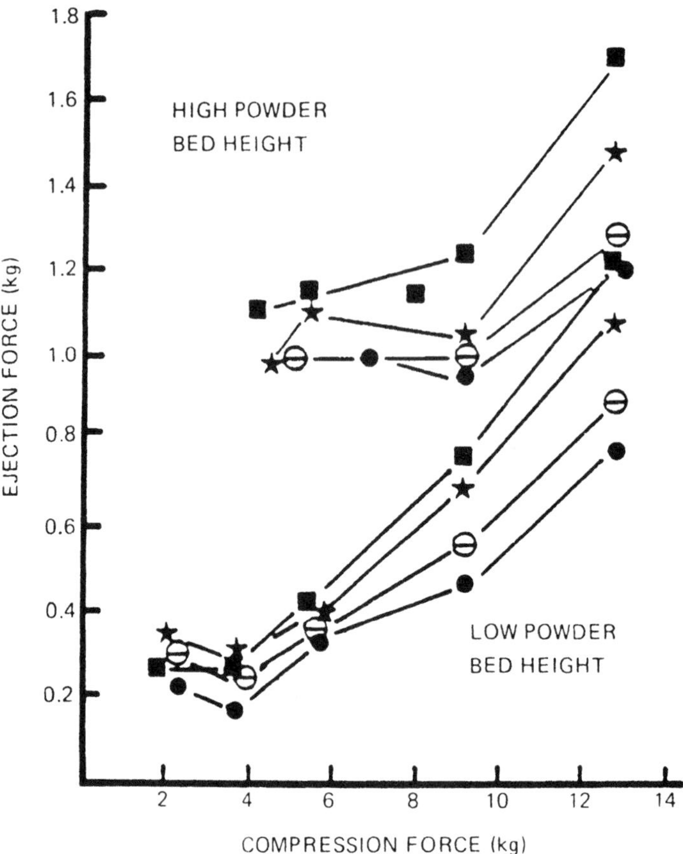

Fig. 17 Effect of powder bed height, piston height, and compression force on plug ejection force in an instrumented Zanasi LZ-64 automatic capsule-filling machine (pregelatinized starch lubricated with 0.005% magnesium stearate). Note that the first point of each curve is precompression. Piston height (mm): ■, 15; ★, 14; ⊖, 13; ●, 12. Powder bed height (mm); heavy line, 30; light line, 50. (From Ref. 51.)

movement during compression and ejection. The work of ejection, calculated from force-displacement profiles, was found to be different for several formulations having comparable peak ejection forces [69].

Following the approach of Small and Augsburger [54], Greenberg [70] used strain gauges to instrument a larger Zanasi machine (model AZ-60). This intermittent motion machine employs three groups of eight dosators. Two instrumented pistons were installed in two dosators in one group. The system was unique in that a high quality 10-pole slip ring was used to avoid twisting of the cables. Botzolakis [71] described the successful replacement of the previously reported mercury swivel with a 10-pole gold-contact slip ring assembly.

Piezoelectric transducers have also been used to instrument automatic capsule filling machines. Mony et al. [72] instrumented a Zanasi RV/59 by fitting a piezoelectric load cell to the upper end of a piston. This system can only register a force when the upper end of the piston is in actual contact with the compression or ejection knobs. Although this instrumentation provides a measure of overall compression and ejection forces, it does not permit the detection of precompression, retention, or piston retraction drag forces. Moreover, this instrumentation adds the force required to compress the piston retraction spring to any forces measured. No attempt to correct their data for this variable was reported. Rowley et al. [73] reported the mounting of a small piezoelectric load cell to the ejection knob of a Zanasi LZ-64 machine to monitor ejection force. This approach suffers from the same disadvantages as that of Mony et al. [72]. However, these latter investigators did report subtracting out the force required to compress the dosator spring from their measurements. This correction was obtained by making a "blank" run with an empty dosator.

The instrumentation of a dosing-disc machine was first reported by Shah et al. [52]. Two pistons of a GKF 330 (Hofliger and Karg) filling machine were instrumented using strain gauges to enable simultaneous monitoring of either two of the tamping stations or one tamping station and ejection (Fig. 10, 18). This preliminary study revealed the complexity of the interaction of the various tamping stations on the final fill weight. Using additional instrumented pistons and microprocessor controlled data acquisition techniques, Shah et al. [74] later evaluated seven compaction parameters and concluded that, aside from station #l, all tamping stations and all piston positions within a station contribute equally to plug formation. The nearness of station #l to the scrape-off bar results in nonuniform powder bed height and a high degree of compression force variability. Model calculations suggesting that fill weight could be achieved with only three tamps were supported by experiments in which fill weight was determined as a function of tamping force and the number of tamps for typical lubricated fillers. The effect of tamping force and multiple tamping on drug dissolution was also investigated using this equipment [75]. Cropp et al. [76] later installed displacement transducers on the machine previously instrumented by Shah et al. [74] to further study the multiple tamping effect and to assess the role of overload spring tension on fill weights obtained. More recently, Podczeck [77] reported the instrumentation of a Bosch GKF 400S dosing-disc machine using a prototype pneumatic tamping head fitted with a piezoelectric force transducer. The pneumatic system, which replaces the overload springs normally mounted over the tamping pins, is fitted with a feedback switch valve and provides a potential means for feedback control of fill weight during continuous running of the machine. Further development of this prototype will be required before the system can be adapted to full industrial use.

Instrumentation has also been developed to measure the mechanical strength of plugs. Greenberg [70] was the first investigator to report the measurement of plug "hardness." A pneumatically driven piston, moving at a controlled rate, was brought against the plug held in a narrow channel. A ring indicator registered the highest force developed as the plug fails. Hardness values were generally under 0.1 N. Later, others reported measuring the maximum bending resistance of plugs in a three-point flexure test [74,78,79]. In this test, the plug is supported at each end, and a

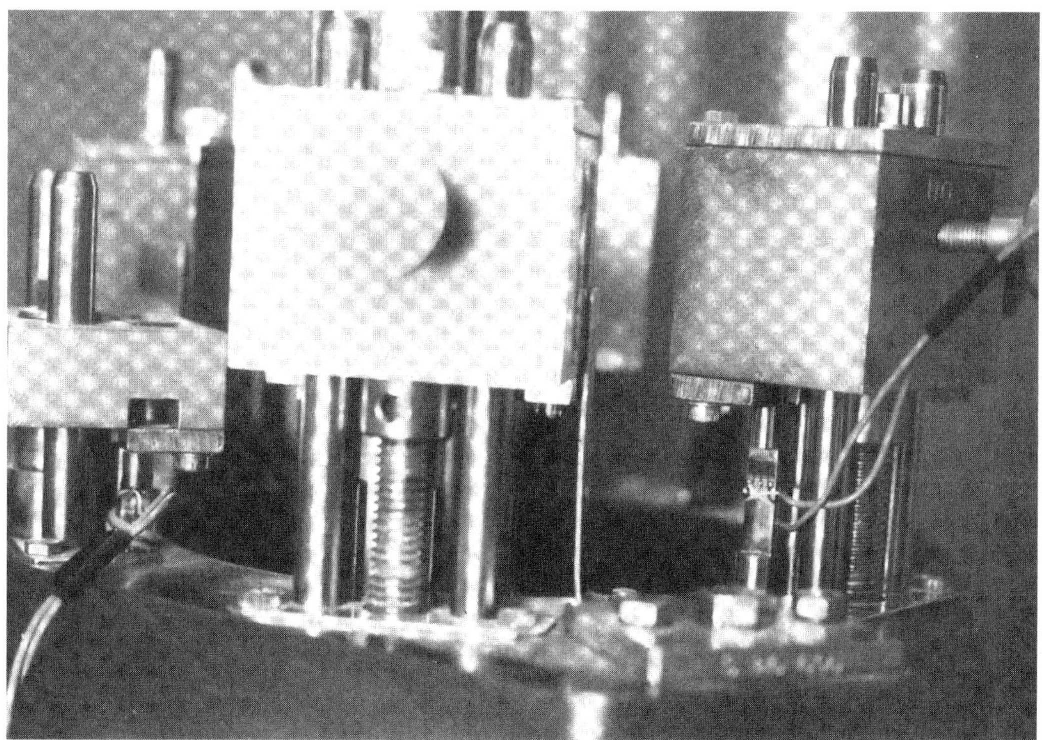

Fig. 18 Strain-gauged pistons mounted in a Hofliger Karg model 330 automatic capsule-filling machine. (From Ref. 37.)

blunt edge blade mounted on the moving head of a bench type tensile strength tester is lowered at a slow, controlled rate against the unsupported midpoint of the plug. When tested in this manner, the maximum force required for plug failure is generally up to 1 N.

F. Capsule-Filling Machine Simulation

The development of programmable compaction simulators was a significant development in tablet research. Since they can be programmed to simulate the action of different rotary tablet presses at their operating speeds under controlled laboratory conditions, require only small quantities of material, and provide independent control over compressive force, punch position and punch speed, compaction simulators offer substantial advantages over instrumented tablet presses in research and development [80]. Clearly, the programmable simulation of automatic capsule-filling machines also would be advantageous in the design and development of capsule formulations, and researchers have taken the first steps toward that end.

It could be argued that researchers have been simulating capsule filling under laboratory conditions for a number of years. Generally this simulation involved using the dosing mechanism that had been removed from an actual machine to make plugs. Such approaches allow for the convenient study of plug formation using small quantities of material, but programmability to simulate the action of different machines at their operating speeds is not possible. For example, Stewart et al. [81] reported research using a Zanasi dosator fitted to a moveable crosshead. Veski and Marvola [82] reported the use of an MG-2 dosing tube mounted on a digital balance with piston fitted to a manually operated lever system.

Jolliffe et al. [83] reported the development of an MG2 capsule-filling simulator. The simulator employs the filling turret of a model G-36 machine and a drive mechanism, which allows the normal up-and-down motion of the dosators but without the usual turret rotation. One dosator was employed that was instrumented by bonding strain gauges to the piston. Additionally, displacement transducers were fitted to permit registration of piston movement relative to the dosator and dosator movement relative to the turret. Using this device, Jolliffe and Newton [84] studied the effects of changes in the compression ratio on fill weight variation and the resultant compression and ejection stresses for four size fractions of lactose. In general, it was found that the ranges of compression ratio over which uniform weights could be obtained with minimum tamping pressure was far greater for finely divided, cohesive powders than for the coarser, freely flowing size fractions. Fine, cohesive powders have greater void volumes and, therefore, are capable of greater volume reduction than free-flowing powders. This system was later used by Jolliffe and Newton to study the role of dosator nozzle inner wall texture on plug retention [85]. Tan and Newton also used this system to study the relationship between flow parameters, fill weight, and weight variation [86] to explore further the relationship between powder retention and dosator inner wall texture [87–89] and to study the effect of compression setting on fill weight and weight variability [90] and plug density [91].

Britten and Barnett [92] fitted the dosator mechanism from a Macofar MT13-2 capsule-filling machine with pneumatic cylinders. One pneumatic cylinder brings the bowl bearing the powder bed to the dosator (simulating the dipping action leading to precompression), and separate pneumatic cylinders provide piston compression and plug ejection. The speeds of these three cylinders are adjustable through flow control valves. LVDTs monitor the movement of the bowl and piston. Semiconductor strain gauges are mounted on the piston and on the outer surface of the dosator tube to measure both the tamping pressure and the radial pressure on the plug. The analog signals from the transducers are digitized and stored by a microprocessor-controlled data acquisition system, and the data are downloaded to a PC for further manipulation [93]. Capable of maximum dosator and pistons speeds of 500 mm/s and 600 mm/s, respectively [93], this system is only able to attain about 75% of the full range of speeds attainable with the Macofar MT13-2. However, this range nearly covers the full range of speeds of the Zanasi AZ-20, a machine that employs a similar dosator mechanism [93]. Using this system, Britten et al. [94] were the first to report the direct measurement of residual radial plug pressures.

More recently, Heda et al. reported the simulation of plug formation using a programmable tablet compaction simulator [79]. The simulator was fitted with tooling made to match No. 1 tamping pins and a special deep die to accommodate capsule plugs of different length. Although the simulator was capable of running at much higher speeds, tamping pin speed was limited to100 mm/s in this preliminary study, a speed that slightly exceeds the reported tamping pin movement of a GKF 330 dosing-disc machine. This study revealed that certain compression equations available for tableting can be applied to plug formation and demonstrated the potential for programmable capsule machine simulation.

G. Design of Hard Gelatin Capsule Formulations for Powder Fill

Like any dosage form, the capsule can be viewed as a *drug-delivery system* since the choice of excipients and the principles involved in the design of the dosage form can affect the rate and amount of drug delivered to the site of action. Clearly, the initial design criterion of the dosage form must be to make the drug optimally available for absorption in a manner consistent with intended use (e.g., immediate release or modified release). However, the dosage form also must be designed to meet a number of other criteria. These include stability, manufacturability, and patient acceptability. Both the shell and its contents must exhibit physical and chemical stability. Not only must the drug substance be stable, but the rate and extent of drug release must be stable for an extended period of time. The formulation also should allow for efficient, cost-effective production of the required batch sizes and provide for accuracy and uniformity of drug content from one capsule to the next within acceptable limits. Patient acceptability is also an important design criterion as this encourages patent compliance with the prescribed dosing. As much as possible, the dosage form should have an attractive appearance, including color, be of a size easily swallowed, and not have and unpleasant odor or taste. As discussed previously, the capsule easily meets this criterion. However, as much as possible, capsule sizes that are difficult to swallow should be avoided.

Often these design criteria involve *competitive requirements*. What is best for meeting one criterion may be counterproductive in meeting another. For example, certain excipients such as the hydrophobic stearate lubricants are important for efficient manufacture, yet they have the potential to retard the release of drug from an immediate-release formulation. The design of a dosage form thus frequently requires the optimization of formulation and process variables in a way that best meets all design criteria.

This section addresses the design of immediate-release powder formulations for hard gelatin capsules. In general, powder formulations for encapsulation should be developed in consideration of the particular filling principle involved. The requirements imposed on the formulation by the filling process, such as lubricity, compressibility and/or compactibility, and fluidity can vary between machine types. Furthermore, the interplay between formulation variables and process variables may be expected to influence drug release. This seems particularly evident in the case of those machines which form compressed plugs.

When immersed in a dissolution fluid at 37°C, hard gelatin capsules can be seen to rupture first at the shoulders of the cap and body where the gelatin shell is thinnest [95,96]. As the dissolution fluid penetrates the capsule contents, the powder mass begins to disintegrate and deaggregate from the ends to expose drug particles for dissolution. It is apparent that the efficiency with which the drug will be released will depend on the wettability of the powder mass, how rapidly the dissolution fluid penetrates the powder, the rate of disintegration and deaggregation of the contents, and the nature of the primary drug particles. These processes, in turn, can be significantly affected by the design of the formulation and the mode of filling. Such factors as the amount and choice of fillers and lubricants, the inclusion of disintegrants or surfactants, and the degree of plug compaction can have a profound effect on drug release.

Active Ingredient

The dose of the drug and its solubility are important considerations in the design of the formulation. The amount and type of active ingredient influences capsule size and the nature and amount of excipients to be used in the formulation. Larger-dose drugs that must be granulated to produce tablets may be more easily direct-filled into hard shell capsules with proper choice of excipients.

The dissolution of the drug in gastrointestinal fluids must occur before absorption can occur, and drugs having high water solubility generally exhibit few formulation problems. For drugs of low water solubility, the absorption rate may be governed by the dissolution rate. In such cases, if dissolution occurs too slowly, absorption efficiency may suffer. Drug stability in gastrointestinal fluids is another concern for slowly dissolving drugs, which can affect their bioavailability.

The solubility of a drug should be considered together with its dose. Even a poorly soluble drug can completely dissolve under physiological conditions if its dose is sufficiently small. Thus, a *dose solubility volume*, i.e., the volume required to dissolve the dose of the drug, is a more useful tool to judge potential solubility problems than the equilibrium solubility of the drug alone. Amidon et al. [97] defined a drug as having "high solubility" if the largest human dose is soluble in 250 mL (or less) of water throughout the physiological pH range of 1–8 at 37°C. A drug is considered a "low-solubility" drug if more than 250 mL of water is required to dissolve the largest dose at any pH within that range at 37°C. The reference volume estimate of 250 mL is the assumed minimum initial gastric volume available. This volume is based on the volume of water recommended for ingestion during the administration of a dosage form in a typical bioequivalence study protocol [98].

Bioavailability depends not only on having the drug in solution, but also on the drug's permeability. A jejunal permeability of at least $2\text{–}4 \times 10^{-4}$ cm/s, measured in human subjects by intubation, is considered high [97]. For many drugs and other substances, this permeability corresponds to a fraction absorbed of 90% or better. Amidon et al. [97] thus proposed a Biopharmaceutics Classification System (BCS) for drugs based on the above definitions of these two parameters. Table 3 defines the BCS and includes some drugs representative of each class.

The BCS makes an important contribution to the rational formulation of both drug products and regulatory policy. Since the BCS gives formulation scientists the ability to estimate the likely contribution of dissolution rate, solubility, and intestinal permeability to oral drug absorption, it provides a basis for estimating the risk of encountering bioavailability problems. Because of their high solubility and permeability, Class I drugs are expected to exhibit few bioavailability problems. However, Class II drugs (low solubility and high permeability) are prone to exhibit dissolution rate–limited absorption. On the other hand, Class III drugs (high solubility and low permeability) are likely to exhibit permeation rate–limited absorption. Class IV drugs (low solubility and low permeability) present serious obstacles to bioavailability, and some may best be formulated in solubilized form, such as a parenteral or a liquid-filled or semisolid–filled soft or hard gelatin capsule formulation. Clearly the early recognition of the BCS class into which the drug falls will provide important guidance in making formulation decisions.

The U.S. Food and Drug Administration (FDA) applied the BCS in a regulatory guidance entitled "Immediate Release Solid Oral Dosage Forms; Scale-Up and Post Approval Changes: Chemistry, Manufacturing, and Controls; *In Vitro* Dissolution Testing; *In Vivo* Bioequivalence Documentation" [104]. Also known as SUPAC-IR, this guidance defines levels of postapproval changes and recommends tests and other requirements needed to document that product quality and performance had not changed after certain minor changes in manufacturing (batch size, equipment, process, or site) or product composition (levels of excipients) were made to an approved product. Postapproval changes are often needed to update processes through the use of newer, more efficient equipment and methods, to change site of manufacture as a result of mergers and acquisitions, or to change scale of manufacture in response to product demand. SUPAC-IR deals with these changes by defining three levels of change. Level I changes are those that are unlikely to have any detectable impact on product quality and performance. Level 2 changes are those that could have significant impact on product quality and performance. Level 3 changes are those that are likely to have significant impact on quality and performance. As the level changes from 1 to 3, the rigor of testing and filing requirements needed to justify the change increases. For certain changes, the tests and filing requirements depend on the biopharmaceutic classification of the drug. Along with certain other requirements, dissolution

Table 3 Biopharmaceutics Classification System

	High permeability (fraction absorbed $\geq 90\%$)	Low permeability (fraction absorbed $< 90\%$)
High solubility (≤ 250 mL required to dissolve largest dose in pH range 1–8 at 37°)	I Metoprolol tatrate Propranolol HCl	II Piroxicam Naproxen
Low solubility (> 250 mL required to dissolve largest dose in pH range 1–8 at 37°C)	III Ranitidine Cimetidine	IV Furosemide Hydrochlorothiazide

Source: Ref. 97–103.

testing may be used to justify Level 1 and 2 compositional changes, i.e., drug dissolution from the changed product and the original product should be similar. However, the rigor of the dissolution test to be used depends on the risk of bioavaialbility problems as represented by the drug's BCS class (Class IV excluded). High solubilityhigh permeability drugs require the least rigorous dissolution test. More rigorous dissolution testing is required for high solubilitylow permeability drugs, and the most rigorous dissolution testing is required for low solubilityhigh permeability drugs. Level 3 composition and process changes require human bioequivalence tests to justify the change. In a more recent guidance [103] that addresses BCS, FDA broadened this policy. This latter guidance permits the use of dissolution testing as a surrogate for human bioavailability testing for any rapidly dissolving immediate-release products of highly soluble and highly permeable drugs that are not considered by FDA to be narrow therapeutic index drugs. That guidance also changed the pH range in which to determine the drug's solubility volume to 1–7.5. For the purposes of this guidance, "*rapidly dissolving*" is defined as not less than 85% of labeled content dissolving in not more than 30 minutes in 900 mL (or less) of each of three vehicles: Simulated Gastric Fluid USP (without enzymes), pH 4.5 buffer and pH 6.8 buffer or Simulated Intestinal Fluid USP (without enzymes). Either USP dissolution Apparatus I at 100 rpm or USP Apparatus II at 50 rpm may be used.

Drugs of low water solubility are usually micronized to increase the dissolution rate. Particle size reduction increases the surface area per unit weight of the drug, thereby increasing the surface area available from which dissolution can occur. For instance, Fincher et al. [105] studied the different particle size fractions of sulfathiazole administered in capsules to dogs and found that the smallest particle size gave the highest blood level. Also, Bastami and Groves [106] reported that reducing the particle size of sodium phenytoin improved the dissolution rate from capsules containing 100 mg of the drug and 150 mg of lactose. There are, however, practical limitations to this approach. Micronized particles with high surface-to-mass ratios may tend to aggregate owing to surface cohesive interaction, thereby reducing the surface area effectively available for dissolution. Newton and Rowley [107] found that at equivalent bed porosities, larger particle size fractions of a poorly soluble drug, ethinamate, gave better dissolution from capsules of the pure drug than smaller particle sizes. They attributed this result to the smaller particle size fractions having reduced effective surface area for dissolution owing to aggregation. The compaction of fine particles into capsules also reduces the bed permeability and generally retards dissolution [107].

From a manufacturing point of view, a compromise may have to be struck between small particle size and good flow properties. Small particles in general are more poorly flowing than larger particles. Surface cohesive and frictional interactions, which oppose flow properties, are more important in smaller particle size powders because of their larger specific surface areas. One possible way to both reduce the effects of aggregation of fine particles and enhance flow properties is granulation. When micronized ethinamate was granulated in a simple moist process with isopropanol, bed permeability and drug dissolution from capsules were greatly enhanced compared to the micronized powder [107]. (see below for additional comments on the role of granulation in capsules).

Fillers

Fillers (diluents) are often needed to increase the bulk of the formulation. The most common capsule diluents are starch and lactose. Inorganic salts appearing in capsule formulations include, among others, magnesium and calcium carbonate and calcium phosphate. Modification of fillers that enhances their flowability and compactibility is particularly advantageous in developing formulations for automatic capsule filling machines. Examples include pregelatinized starch (Starch 1500[R]; Colorcon Inc., West Point, PA), spray processed lactose (Fast-Flo[R] Lactose; Foremost, Div. Wisconsin Dairies, Baraboo, WI), and unmilled dicalcium phosphate dihydrate (Ditab[R]; Rhone-Poulenc Basic Chemicals Co., Shelton, CT; Emcompress[R]; Penwest Co., Patterson, NY).

Formulations intended to be run on dosator machines may sometimes benefit from the greater compactibility of microcrystalline cellulose (Avicel[R]; FMC Corp., Food and Pharmaceutical Products Div., Philadelphia, PA, Emcocel[R]; Penwest Co., Patterson, NY), particularly when the drug dosage is large. In these machines it is essential to prevent powder loss from the end of the cylinder during the transfer from the powder bed to ejection into the capsule body. The failure to have a cohesive plug may also cause a "blow off" of powder as the plug is ejected into the shell. As previously pointed out, a degree of compactibility is also important in formulations for dosing-disc machines. Using a Zanasi AZ5 dosator machine, Patel and Podceck [108] studied several microcrystalline celluloses and concluded that medium and coarse particle size grades can be considered "good" excipients for capsules. Of the 8 sources and types tested, Avicel PH 101, PH103, Microcel, and Emcocel appeared the most suitable sources for capsule filling.

From a drug dissolution point of view, formulators may need to consider the solubility of both the filler and the drug. For instance, Newton et al. [109] demonstrated that the dissolution of poorly soluble ethinamate from capsules improved greatly when the concentration of lactose in the formulation was increased to 50%. However, with the soluble drug chloramphenicol, Withey and Mainville [110] found that the inclusion of 80% lactose in the formulation severely retarded drug dissolution from capsules. There was little or no effect on dissolution when up to 50% lactose was included. It was suggested that dissolution of the lactose occurs more rapidly and that chloramphenicol dissolution is retarded because of the high concentration of lactose already in solution. The effect of the filler on bioavailability was graphically illustrated [111] when Australian physicians noted an increase in the number of patients exhibiting phenytoin toxicity while using a particular sodium phenytoin capsule product. This occurrence coincided with the manufacturer changing the filler from calcium sulfate to lactose and was the result of increased bioavailability when lactose was the filler. In this case, the effect may not be solely due to the greater solubility of lactose. Bastami and Groves [106] reported that the in vitro dissolution of phenytoin may not be complete in the presence of calcium sulfate and suggested the formation of an insoluble calcium salt of the drug. It has also been reported that lactose at a concentration of 50% enhanced the dissolution of phenobarbital from capsules but had no effect on the dissolution of the water-soluble sodium phenobarbital [112]. On the other hand, corn starch at 50% slowed the dissolution of sodium phenobarbital and improved the dissolution of the free acid; however, the effect in either case was dependent on the moisture content of the starch [112]. The t_{50} (time required for 50% drug dissolution) for 50:50 phenobarbital/corn starch capsules decreased from 28 to 9 minutes as the starch moisture content increased from 1.2 to 9.5% w/w. This compares to a t_{50} of 25 minutes for the drug alone. Drug dissolution also improved in the 50:50 sodium phenobarbital/corn starch mixtures with increased moisture; however, even at the highest moisture content (13.5%), t_{50} was still about double that of the drug alone (4.9 vs. 2.5 minutes).

The intrinsic dissolution rates of selected fillers are compared in Table 4. Anhydrous lactose, which is predominantly the more soluble β-lactose, exhibits nearly twice the intrinsic dissolution rate of the α-lactose monohydrate. Of particular interest is the pH-dependent solubility of some fillers, which show dramatically reduced intrinsic dissolution rates under less acidic conditions. Such fillers are of potential concern for populations that exhibit achlorhydria, such as the elderly. In such cases, disintegration and dissolution could be substantially delayed.

Table 4 Intrinsic Dissolution Rates of Selected Fillers (mg min^{-1} cm^{-2} at 37°C)

Anhydrous lactose
Purified water — 21.9
Lactose monohydrate
Purified water — 12.4
Dicalcium phosphate, dihydrate
0.1 M HCl — 6.27
0.01 M HCl — 0.90
Anhydrous dicalcium phosphate
0.1 M HCl — 5.37
0.01 M HCl — 0.69
Calcium sulfate dihydrate
0.1 M HCl — 1.15
0.01M HCl — 0.75

Source: Ref. 113.

Glidants

Glidants are finely divided dry powders added to formulations in small quantities to improve their flow properties. Glidant particles of sufficiently fine particle size have been observed to adsorb onto the surfaces of the bulk powder particles. Glidants are thought to enhance the fluidity of the formulation (or bulk powder) by one or more of several possible mechanisms [114,115]: (a) reducing roughness by filling surface irregularities, (b) reducing attractive forces by physically separating the bulk powder particles, (c) modifying electrostatic charges, (d) acting as moisture scavengers, and (e) serving as ball bearings between bulk powder particles. Usually there is an optimum concentration for best flow. For the colloidal silicas, this is often less than 1%. The optimum concentration varies with the glidant and may be related to the concentration just needed to coat the host particles [114,116]. Exceeding this concentration will usually result in no further improvement in flow or, possibly, a worsening of flow. Glidants include the colloidal silicas, cornstarch, talc, and magnesium stearate. York [115] reported the following order of effectiveness for two powder systems: fine silica>magnesium stearate>purified talc.

Lubricants

Capsule formulations usually require lubricants just as do tablet formulations. Lubricants ease the ejection of plugs, reduce filming on pistons and adhesion of powder to metal surfaces, and reduce friction between sliding surfaces in contact with powder. The same lubricants are used in both tablet and capsule formulations.

The most effective lubricants are the hydrophobic stearates, such as magnesium stearate, calcium stearate, and stearic acid. Magnesium stearate is the most widely used lubricant [117,118]. Lubricants proposed as being less hydrophobic such as hydrogenated vegetable oils, polyethylene glycols, and sodium stearyl fumarate are less effective in this application [118].

Increasing the concentration of hydrophobic lubricants such as magnesium stearate is generally understood to retard drug release by making formulations more hydrophobic [109,119–121]. Laminar lubricants (magnesium stearate, calcium stearate) are "mixing sensitive." Under the rigors of mixing, the particles delaminate, i.e., shear readily when subjected to a tangential force, to form a film on the surfaces of host particles [122–124]. If blended for a sufficient length of time, even a low level of addition of a laminar lubricant can retard wetting and drug dissolution [121]. Generally, the appropriate level of lubricant is added last and blended for a minimum amount of time, usually 2–5 minutes.

Mixing and delamination of lubricants like magnesium stearate do not end when a blender is stopped. The powder-handling mechanism of the filling machine can cause additional mixing and shearing of the formulation. For example, Desai et al. [125] reported over mixing of magnesium stearate in the hopper of an MG2 dosator machine. During operation of the machine, the powder in the hopper is continuously mixed with a rotating blade. Compared to initial dissolution profiles (before running the machine), the dissolution of three drugs was markedly reduced after running the machine for 30 minutes when the magnesium stearate level was 1%. When the level of magnesium stearate was reduced to 0.25%, lubrication was adequate and dissolution was satisfactory over the 30-minute filling run. Replacement of magnesium stearate with the more hydrophilic lubricants Stear-O-Wet (magnesium stearate coprocessed with sodium lauryl sulfate) and sodium stearyl fumarate also resulted in satisfactory dissolution. Ullah et al. [126] encountered a related problem when scaling up cefadroxil monohydrate capsules. The formulation was initially developed on a small-scale Zanasi LZ-64 dosator machine with a blend containing 1% magnesium stearate. Upon scale-up to a GKF 1500 production dosing-disc machine, the capsules exhibited significantly slower dissolution than those produced on the Zanasi machine. Further study suggested that shearing during the tamping step resulted in increased coating of the drug particles with magnesium stearate. Using a laboratory-scale mixer/grinder to simulate the shearing action of the filling machine, a level of 0.3% magnesium stearate was selected for scale-up to 570 and 1100 kg (full production) size batches. Dissolution for both scale-up batches was found satisfactory.

Interestingly, exceptions are possible. Stewart et al. [81] reported that the effect of magnesium stearate concentration on the dissolution of a model low-dose drug, riboflavin, from capsules was dependent in some manner on the type of filler. Soluble fillers exhibited the anticipated prolonged times with increasing lubricant levels. However, the trends with insoluble fillers were less predictable. In some cases insoluble fillers were only slightly affected by the concentration of magnesium stearate. For others, such as microcrystalline cellulose, there appeared to be an ideal intermediate concentration of lubricant at which the dissolution rate was maximized.

In a follow-up of this work, Mehta and Augsburger [78] suggested that the mechanical strength of plugs produced in a dosator may be reduced by the amount of lubricant used and that this could have a beneficial effect on drug dissolution. As previously described, plug "hardness" was assessed by measuring their breaking load in a three-point flexure test. Using hydrochlorothiazide as the tracer drug for dissolution, these investigators compared the time for 60% of the drug content to dissolve (t_{60}) and plug breaking force for two fillers lubricated with 0.05–0.75% magnesium stearate and compressed at the same 22 kg compression force. With microcrystalline cellulose, t_{60} decreased from 55 to 12 minutes. Paralleling this observation was a dramatic decrease in plug breaking force from 84 to about 2.0 g. With lactose, t_{60} increased with the lubricant level from 12 to 18 minutes. while plug breaking force decreased slightly, although not significantly ($p = 0.05$), from 18 to 13 g. For the microcrystalline cellulose case, it was suggested that the increase in hydrophobicity due to increased lubricant concentration initially was more than offset by reduced plug cohesiveness, which probably enhances moisture penetration and promotes deaggregation in the dissolution medium. This dual effect of magnesium stearate has also been noted in a study of the dissolution of rifampicin from hard gelatin capsules [127].

Disintegrants

Although tablet disintegrants are being used in some capsule formulations, until recently the role they play in capsules has been a relatively unexplored area. The few studies that had been reported only produced mixed results and usually involved hand-filled capsules [120,128,129]. Capsules filled by methods that afford little compression of contents (e.g., auger method) are much looser than tablets, and there is little structure for disintegrants to swell against to effect disintegration. However, the advent in recent years of filling machines that actually compress capsule contents, together with the development of newer disintegrants that have superior swelling and/or moisture absorbing properties, appear to warrant serious consideration of disintegrants in modern capsule formulations. These newer disintegrants, which have been called "super disintegrants" [130,131], include croscarmellose sodium, Type A (AcDiSol[R]; FMC Corp., Food and Pharmaceutical Products, Philadelphia, PA), sodium starch glycolate (Primojel[R]; Generichem Corp., Totowa, NJ; Explotab[R]; Penwest Co., Patterson, NY) and crospovidone (Polyplasdone[R] XL; ISP Corp., Wayne, NJ). For instance, Botzolakis et al. [132] compared various levels of these newer disintegrants against 10% starch and 0% disintegrant as controls in dicalcium phosphate–based capsules filled on an instrumented Zanasi LZ-64 at a uniform compression force. In most cases, the dissolution rate of hydrochlorothiazide was dramatically enhanced (Fig. 19). Disintegrant efficiency was concentration dependent. Although the typical use levels of these disintegrants in tablets is 2–4%, the most effective disintegrants required 4–6% for fast dissolution. The importance of drug solubility or magnesium stearate level was also clear. When magnesium stearate was reduced (from 1% to 0.5%) or when a more soluble drug (acetaminophen) was substituted for hydrochlorothiazide, less croscarmellose was needed to exert a similar effect on dissolution (Fig. 20 and 21) [132].

In a later study [133] the effect of disintegrants on hydrochlorothiazide dissolution from both soluble (anhydrous lactose) and "insoluble" (dicalcium phosphate) fillers was compared for different lubricant levels and tamping forces (instrumented Zanasi LZ-64 machine). Statistical analysis of this multivariable study revealed all main factors and their interactions to

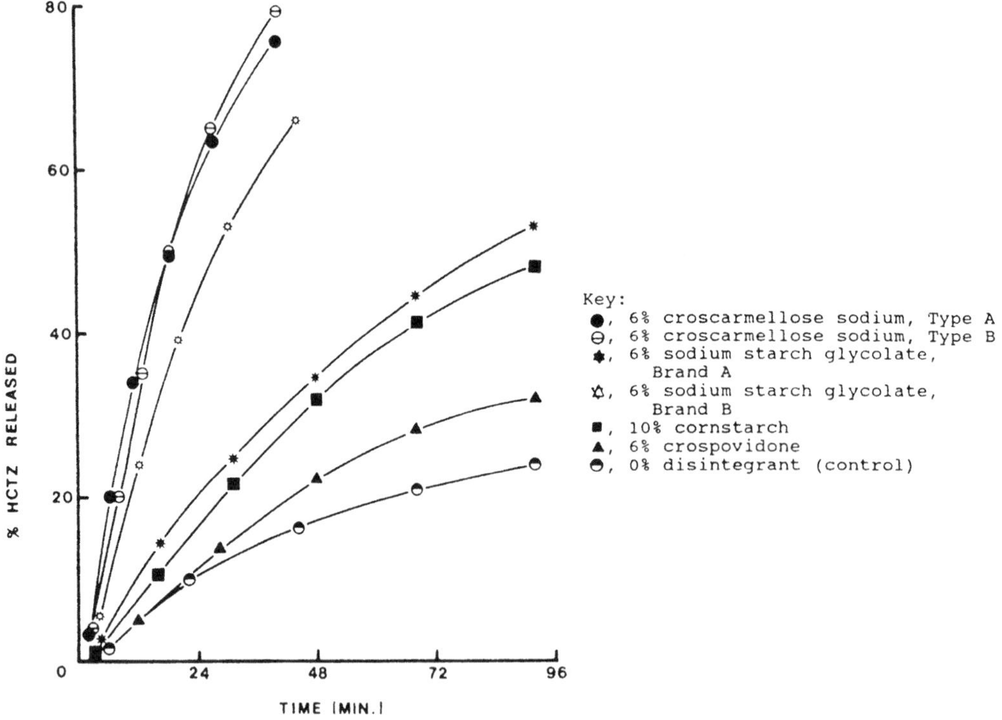

Fig. 19 Effect of disintegrants on hydrochlorothiazide dissolution from hard gelatin capsules (filler, dicalcium phosphate; lubricant, 1% magnesium stearate). (From Ref. 132.)

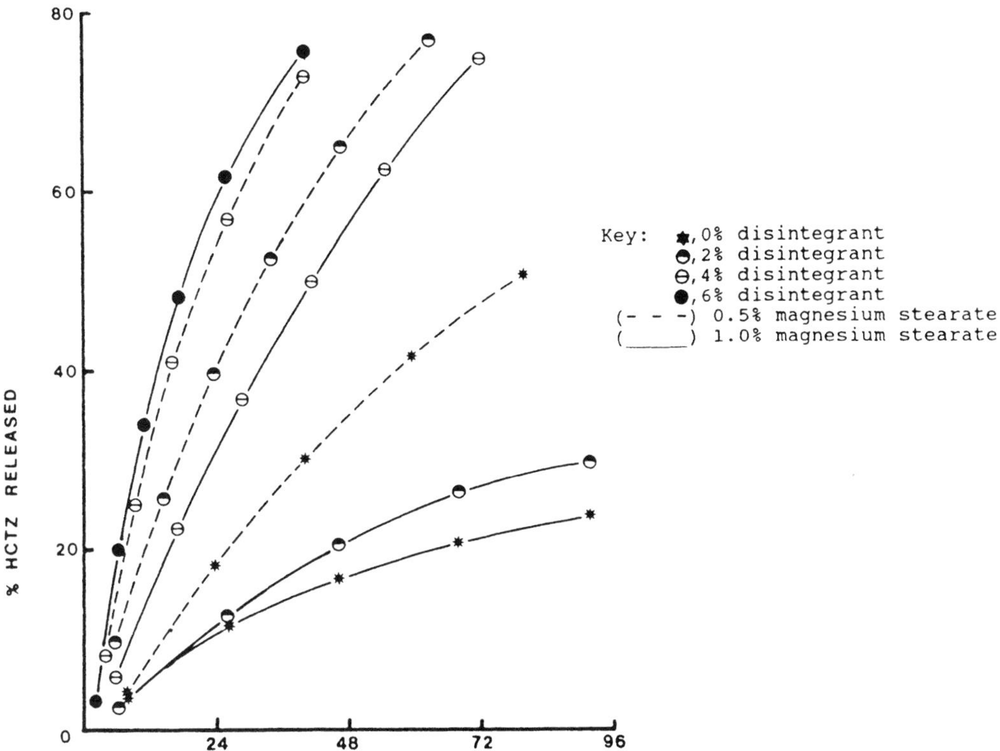

Fig. 20 Effect of lubricant level on hydrochlorothiazide dissolution from hard gelatin capsules (filler, dicalcium phosphate; disintegrant, croscarmellose sodium, type A). (From Ref. 132.)

be significant. However, by averaging the results for each factor over all conditions, the relative magnitude of each main factor could be assessed, as in Fig. 22 and 23. Although the disintegrants were effective in promoting drug dissolution from both fillers, the effect was much less dramatic with lactose. This finding is not surprising since the lactose-based capsule without disintegrant is already a fast-releasing formulation. Soluble fillers tend to dissolve rather than disintegrate. A beneficial effect of increasing the tamping force also was much more evident with the dicalcium phosphate–based capsules. As compression force increases, plug porosity may decrease, possibly making more effective the swelling action of disintegrants. Again, the retardant effect on dissolution of the hydrophobic lubricant is evident; however, it is apparent that the soluble lactose-based formulation is much less profoundly affected.

Surfactants

Surfactants may be included in capsule formulations to increase the wetting of the powder mass and enhance drug dissolution. The "water-proofing" effect of hydrophobic lubricants may be offset by the use of surfactants. Numerous studies have reported the beneficial effects of surfactants on disintegration and deaggregation and/or drug dissolution [107,109, 119,129]. Botzolakis [71] demonstrated enhanced liquid uptake into capsule plugs due to surfactants. Common surfactants employed in capsule formulations are sodium lauryl sulfate and sodium docusate. Levels of 0.1–0.5% are usually sufficient (Fig. 24).

Ong et al. [134] found that several hydrophilic anionic, non ionic, or cationic surfactants can alleviate the deleterious effect of magnesium stearate over-mixing on dissolution from capsules when added with the lubricant in a ratio as low as 1:5 (w/w). These successful surfactants were sodium *N*-lauroyl sarcosinate, sodium stearoyl-2-lactylate, sodium stearate, poloxamer 188, cetylpyridinium chloride, and sodium lauryl sulfate. The lipophilic surfactant glyceryl monostearate did not alleviate the magnesium stearate mixing effect. A reduction in thier particle size was shown to enhance effectiveness, particularly in the case of surfactants with low solubility and slow dissolution rate.

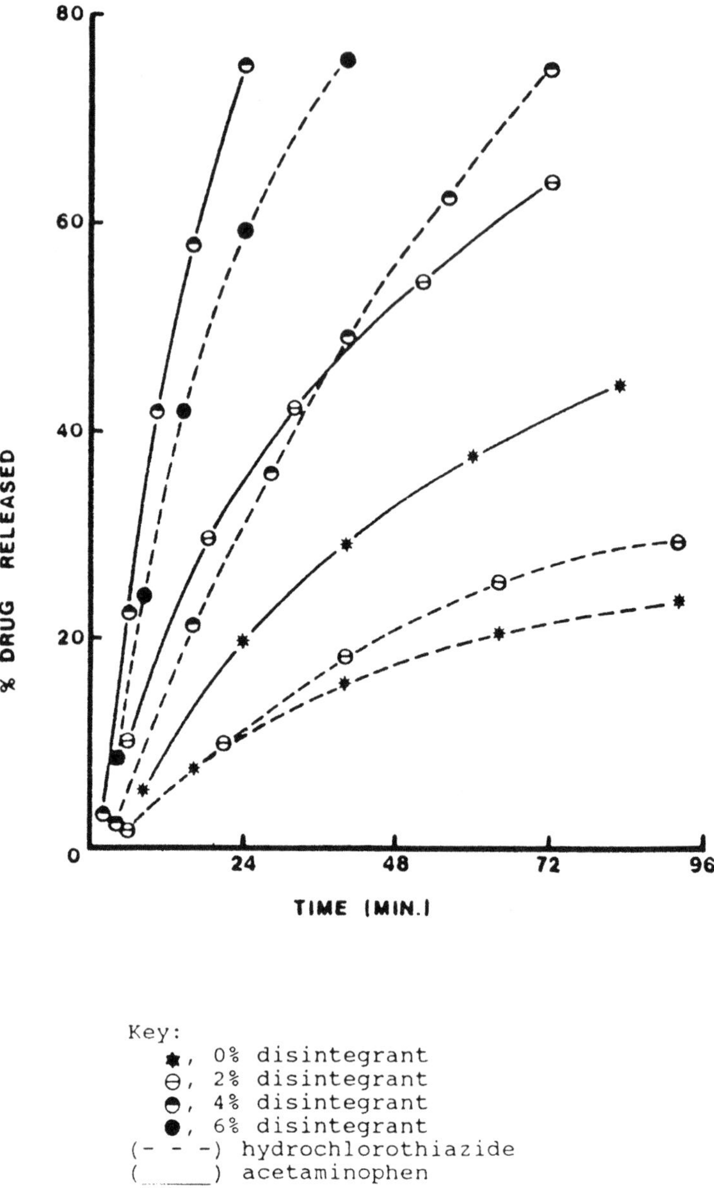

Fig. 21 Effect of croscarmellose sodium (type A) on drug dissolution from hard gelatin capsules (filler, dicalcium phosphate; lubricant, 1% magnesium stearate). (From Ref. 132.)

The effectiveness of surfactants in overcoming the hydrophobic effect of magnesium stearate may not be a result solely of an increase in the wetting properties of the bulk phase. Compared to putting the surfactant in the dosage form, Botzolakis [71] and Wang and Chowhan [135] found that adding an equivalent amount of surfactant to the dissolution medium was not effective. The possible impact of the surfactant at particle surfaces in the microenvironment around the dissolving particles where local concentrations are high should be considered. In addition to the wetting effect, at concentrations exceeding the critical micelle concentration surfactants can increase drug solubility, thereby resulting in a greater effective concentration gradient. The situation is complex, since drug solubilization within micelles reduces the effective rate of

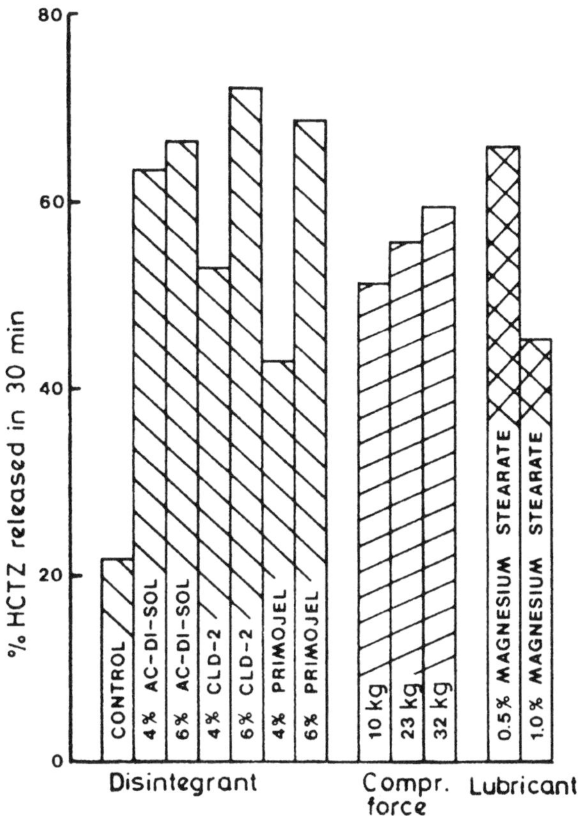

Fig. 22 Averaged effect of disintegrant, lubricant, and compression force on hydrochlorothiazide dissolution from dicalcium phosphate-based capsules. (From. Ref. 133.)

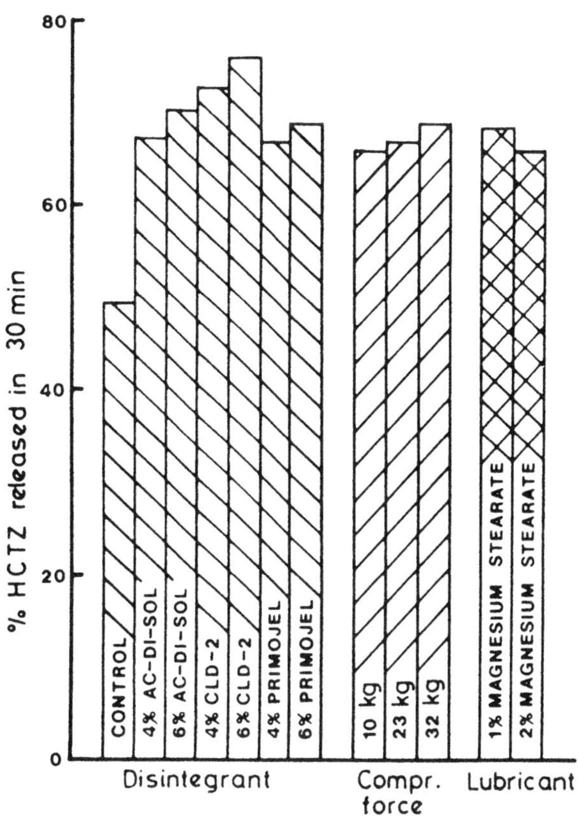

Fig. 23 Averaged effect of disintegrant, lubricant, and compression force on hydrochlorothiazide dissolution from anhydrous lactose-based capsules. (From Ref. 133.)

diffusion [136]. Another, perhaps contributing mechanism for surfactants has been proposed by Ong et al. [134] and Wang and Chowhan [135]. Based on order-of-mixing studies and scanning electron microscopy of powder mixtures, these investigators suggest that surfactants and magnesium stearate may interact strongly enough with each other to inhibit the magnesium stearate and drug-excipient interactions that cause reduced dissolution.

Hydrophilization and Granulation

Another approach to improving the wettability of poorly soluble drugs is to treat the drug with a solution of a hydrophilic polymer. Lerk et al. [137] reported that both wettability of the powder and the rate of dissolution of hexobarbital from hard gelatin capsules could be greatly enhanced if the drug were treated with methylcellulose or hydroxyethylcellulose. In this process, called hydrophilization, a solution of the hydrophilic polymer was spread onto the drug in a high shear mixer and the resultant mixture dried and screened. No benefit accrued when the drug and polymer were merely dry blended. No other excipients were included, and the capsules were loosely packed by hand. Lerk et al. [138] later treated phenytoin by hydrophilization with methylcellulose and compared the pure and treated drug compressed into plugs at 120 N to simulate a tamping machine. The plugs were manually filled into hard gelatin capsules. The treated phenytoin was found to dissolve and be absorbed (in humans) considerably faster than the untreated drug. However, no lubricants or fillers, etc. were included in these capsules as may be required for actual filling. The beneficial effect of hydrophilization on disintegration of benylate from hard gelatin capsules was demonstrated in vivo in Humans by external scintigraphy [139].

The benefits of hydrophilization can be expected whenever powders are wet granulated with typical

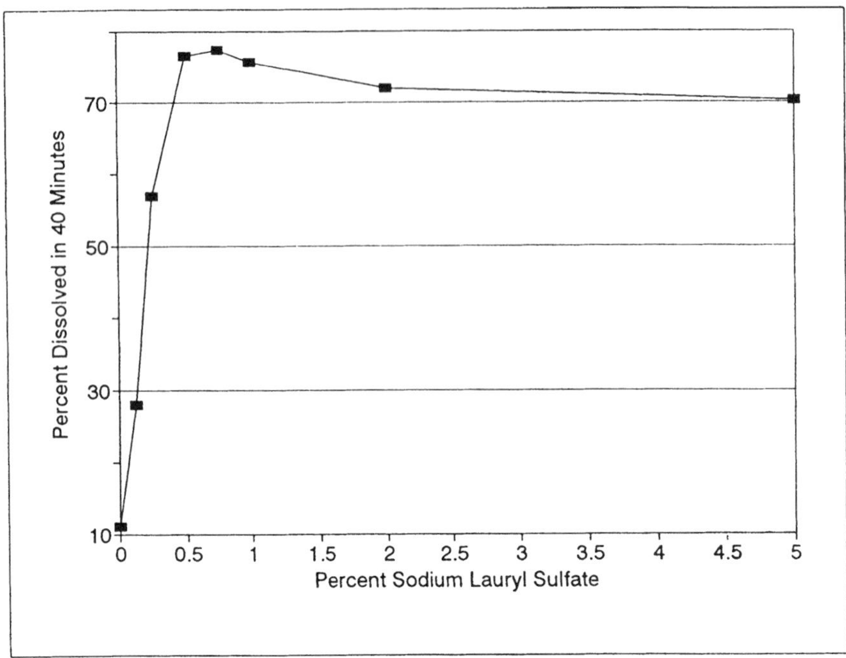

Fig. 24 The effect of percentage of sodium lauryl sulfate in the formulation on the dissolution of hydrochlorothiazide from capsules containing dicalcium phosphate as filler, 0.75% magnesium stearate, and filled on a dosator machine with 300 N tamping force (*USP* method 2, 900 mL 0.1 N HCl, 50 rpm). (Adapted from Ref. 71.)

binders such as pregelatinized starch, hydroxpropylmethylcellulose, and polyvinyl pyrrolidone, which form a hydrophilic film on surfaces. Powders for encapsulation may be granulated to reduce bulk, enhance flow, reduce agglomeration of fine particles or their adhesion to metal surfaces, and improve the content uniformity of low-dose drugs. Wet granulation provides for the addition of a liquid phase (binder solution or solvent) in which a very-low-dose drug may be dissolved and which facilitates its uniform dispersion throughout the mass. When the moist agglomerates formed by the granulation process are dried, the drug is "locked" in the granules, thereby preventing its segregation in subsequent handling steps. Granulation is thus a form of ordered mixing. The potential adverse effect of temperature and exposure to water on the stability of some drugs may limit the application of wet granulation. In such cases, dry granulation by the older slugging process or the more contemporary roller compaction process can be used to accomplish most of the objectives of granulation, although such dry processes do not inherently provide for the addition of the drug in solution or hydrophilization. Of course, the liquid addition of a low-dose drugs to form an ordered mix also may be accomplished by dissolving the drug, perhaps in a nonaqueous solvent, spraying the solution onto a filler in an appropriate mixing device, and drying.

H. Systematic Formulation Development and Analysis of Critical Variables

More and more, pharmaceutical scientists are adopting systematic approaches to the design, formulation, and optimization of dosage forms. New understandings of biopharmaceutic principles, e.g., the Biopharmaceutical Drug Classification System, coupled with software-driven optimization and decision-making tools, have given pharmaceutical scientists the ability to make logical and deliberate formulation design decisions. Among the tools employed by formulation scientists today are multivariate analysis and response surface methodology [100,140] and artificial intelligence [141–144].

Response Surface Analysis of Piroxicam Capsules

One example of the application of response surface analysis is a study of critical formulation variables for 20 mg piroxicam capsules [100]. Piroxicam is a BCS Class II drug (low solubility and high permeability). This study is particularly informative and useful because it links in vitro outcomes (i.e., dissolution) with in vivo outcomes in human subjects. A resolution V central composite (face-centered) experimental design was implemented in which five formulation (independent) variables were studied at each of three levels. Thirty-two batches of capsules were manufactured in which the variables and their levels were varied. Batch size varied from 5 to 7 kg, depending on the bulk densities of the blends. The five variables studied and their levels appear in Table 5. Note that the effect of piroxicam particle size was evaluated by comparing the piroxicam powder as received, termed "unmilled," with the same lot of piroxicam that was remilled, termed "milled." The capsules were filled using a Zanasi LZ-64 automatic capsule filling machine instrumented to monitor plug compression force. The capsules were filled with a consistent plug compression force. Dissolution profiles (% piroxicam dissolved vs. time) were obtained using methods described in the USP XXIII monograph for piroxicam capsules. Based on the data analysis, the percent lactose, and an interaction between piroxicam particle size and sodium lauryl sulfate level were the most important variables affecting the percent of piroxicam dissolved at 10 minutes. However, the predominant variable affecting the percent dissolved in 45 minutes was the wetting agent, sodium lauryl sulfate, which was followed closely by piroxicam particle size. The apparent reduced significance of the level of lactose at 45 minutes may be due to its complete dissolution. Interestingly, the magnesium stearate level and its blending time were either not significant or among the least significant factors affecting

Table 5 Piroxicam Study Experimental Design

Variable	Level		
	Low	Medium	High
Sodium lauryl sulfate	0%	0.5%	1.0%
Magnesium stearate	0.5%	1.0%	1.5%
Magnesium stearate blending time	2 min	10 min	18 min
Filler: % lactose in binary mixtures with microcrystalline cellulose	0%	50%	100%
% Milled (4.91 M^2/g) piroxicam in binary mixtures with unmilled (1.79 M^2/g) piroxicam	0%	50%	100%

Note: Colloidal silica (glidant) and sodium starch glycolate (disintegrant) were fixed at 0.1% and 5%, respectively, in all batches.
Source: Ref. 100.

piroxicam dissolution. This observation can be largely explained by the ability of sodium lauryl sulfate to overcome the hydrophobicity of magnesium stearate. In addition, the water solubility of lactose and the disintegrant, sodium starch glycolate, also may help overcome any hydrophobic lubricant effects. The plotting of response surfaces permit visualization of the effects of various levels of the independent variables. For example, the response surfaces in Fig. 25 reveal that the ability of sodium lauryl sulfate to enhance the percent dissolved in 10 minutes is most apparent when piroxicam is unmilled. The sodium lauryl sulfate level has comparatively little effect on 10-minute dissolution when the drug is milled and presumably more rapidly dissolving because of a larger specific surface area.

All piroxicam batches were manufactured in compliance with Good Manufacturing Practices, and three formulations having fast, moderate, and slow dissolution were chosen for comparison to a lot of the innovator's product in a human bioavailability study [100]. The resulting pharmacokinetic data provided still another opportunity to examine the effects of formulation variables. To explore the relationship between the in vitro dissolution of piroxicam from these capsules and in vivo absorption, Polli [102] used the following previously described [145] deconvolution-based model:

$$F_a = \frac{1}{f_a}\left(1 - \frac{\alpha}{\alpha - 1}(1 - F_d) + \frac{1}{\alpha - 1}(1 - F_d)^{\alpha}\right) \quad (4)$$

In this equation, F_a is the fraction of the dose of the drug absorbed in time t, and f_a is the fraction of the total amount of drug absorbed at $t = \infty$. α is the ratio of the apparent first-order permeation rate constant, k_p^1, to the first-order dissolution rate constant, k_d. F_d is the fraction of the dose dissolved in time t. The model makes a number of assumptions: apparent first-order permeability, first-order dissolution under sink conditions, drug is stable in the gastrointestinal lumen or at the gastrointestinal wall, in vitro and in vivo dissolution profiles are identical, and the absence of a lag time for permeation or dissolution. Nevertheless, this model does provide some useful and interesting information. Of particular interest is the term α. If $\alpha \gg 1$, the permeation rate constant is much greater than the dissolution rate constant and drug absorption is expected to be dissolution rate limited. If $\alpha \ll 1$, the reverse is true and the rate-limiting step to absorption is intestinal permeation. The values of α for the slow, moderate, and fast formulations and a lot of the innovator product are given in Table 6. These results are consistent with a BCS Class II drug showing dissolution rate–limited absorption. An

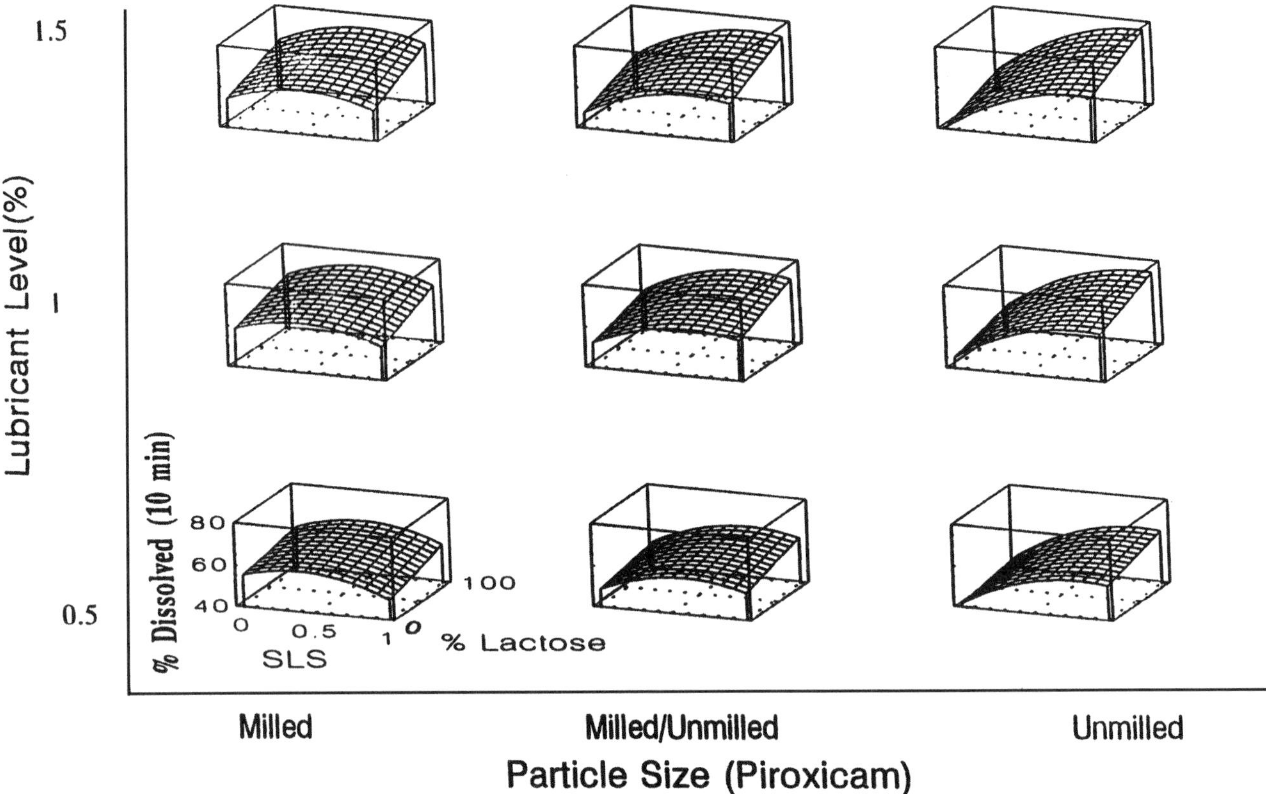

Fig. 25 Response surfaces for the effect of formulation variables on percent of piroxicam dissolving from capsules in 10 minutes. (From Ref. 100.)

examination of Table 6 generally indicates $\alpha \geq 1$ such that piroxicam is generally dissolution rate limited, which is consistent with piroxicam's BCS Class II classification. For the slow formulation, $\alpha = 6.50$, indicating that dissolution was severalfold, dominating over permeability in controlling overall piroxicam absorption. These data also point up the role of formulation. The fast capsule was formulated using the milled piroxicam, 1% sodium lauryl sulfate, and lactose, which promoted dissolution such that $k_d \cong k_p^1$. Indeed, because of formulation design, the fast product is slightly more permeability rate limited than dissolution rate limited, overcoming piroxicam's biopharmaceutic properties.

Table 6 Apparent Permeability and Dissolution Rates for Piroxicam Capsules

Formulation	Apparent permeability rate constant, $k_p^1 \pm$ SE, h^{-1}	First-order dissolution rate constant, $k_d \pm$ SE, h^{-1}	$\alpha = \frac{k_p^1}{k_d} \pm$ SE
Fast (Q45[a] = 95)	7.26 ± 1.12	8.10 ± 0.60	0.896 ± 0.138
Moderate (Q45 = 87)	7.17 ± 1.10	4.66 ± 0.10	1.54 ± 0.24
Innovator (Q45 = 80)	10.7 ± 2.6	3.13 ± 0.20	3.42 ± 0.84
Slow (Q45 = 65)	11.3 ± 3.8	1.75 ± 0.05	6.50 ± 2.17
Mean	9.00 ± 1.14		

SE, Standard error.
[a]% of labeled content dissolving in 45 minutes.
Source: Refs. 100 and 102.

It is interesting that the in vitro dissolution test (USP) was more sensitive to the piroxicam formulation variables than the biodata. The fast, moderate, and slow products were found bioequivalent to each other and to the lot of innovator product studied [100]. It is possible that either the formulation variables studied did not affect in vivo dissolution and/or the differences were not discernible because of the long biological half-life of piroxicam [146].

Expert Systems for Formulation Support

An expert system (ES), is a computer program that attempts to capture the expertise of specialists who have knowledge and experience in a well-defined domain (area). In rule-based systems, the knowledge is often represented as a set of rules that express the relationship between pieces of information in the form of conditional statements that specify actions to be taken or advice to be followed. In principle, the user enters certain information about the properties of the drug (e.g., dose, solubility, particle size, flow properties, BCS classification, etc.) and any specific user requirements (e.g., preferred excipients, method of manufacture, capsule size, etc.), and the expert system returns a suggested formulation. Well-designed expert systems can shorten development time, result in simpler formulations, provide the rationale for the formulation design, serve as a teaching tools for novices, and accumulate and preserve the knowledge and experience of experts who may leave the laboratory through retirement, change of employer, or other reason. However, an ES can only deal with situations that have been anticipated and must, therefore, be designed to handle every contingency. Lai et al. [142] and Bateman et al. [143] have developed expert systems for hard shell capsule powder formulations.

III. SOFT GELATIN CAPSULES [3,147–152]

A. Advantages

Several advantages of soft gelatin capsules derive from the fact that the encapsulation process requires that the drug be a liquid or at least dissolved, solubilized, or suspended in a liquid vehicle. Since the liquid fill is metered into individual capsules via a positive displacement pump, a much higher degree of reproducibility is achieved than is possible with powder or granule feed in the manufacture of tablets and hard gelatin capsule products. Moreover, a higher degree of homogeneity is possible in liquid systems than can be achieved in powder blends. A content uniformity of $\pm 3\%$ has been reported [3] for soft gelatin capsules manufactured in a rotary die process.

Another advantage that derives from the liquid nature of the fill is rapid release of the contents with potential enhanced bioavailability. The proper choice of vehicle may promote rapid dispersion of capsule contents and drug dissolution. Hom and Miskal [151,153] compared the in vitro dissolution rates of 20 drugs from soft gelatin capsules and tablets. The drugs were either dissolved in polyethylene glycol 400 or suspended in polyols or nonionic surfactants. In all cases, more rapid dissolution occurred from the capsules. Several in vivo studies have demonstrated beneficial effects on the bioavailability of drugs administered in soft gelatin capsules [149,152].

For example, single dose studies in humans comparing the sedative temazepam as a powder-filled hard gelatin capsule and as a polyethylene glycol solution in soft gelatin capsules revealed higher and earlier peak plasma levels, although there was no significant difference in their total availabilities [154]. In another example, digoxin dissolved in a vehicle consisting of polyethylene glycol 400, ethanol, propylene glycol, and water and filled in soft gelatin capsules produced higher mean plasma levels in humans during the first 7 hours after administration than either an aqueous solution or commercial tablets [155]. In addition, the areas under the 14-hour plasma concentration curves were also greater for the soft gelatin capsule compared to the solution or tablets.

Soft gelatin capsules are hermetically sealed as a natural consequence of the manufacturing process. Thus, this dosage form is uniquely suited for liquids and volatile drugs. Many drugs subject to atmospheric oxidation may also be formulated satisfactorily in this dosage form. Hom et al. [156] have shown that the soft gelatin shell can be an effective barrier to oxygen.

Soft gelatin capsules are available in a wide variety of sizes and shapes. Specialty packages in tube form (ophthalmics, ointments) or bead form (various cosmetics) are possible [3].

B. Disadvantages

One disadvantage of soft gelatin capsules is that such products often must be contracted out to a limited number of firms having the necessary filling equipment and expertise. Materials must be shipped to the soft gelatin capsule facility, and products must be shipped back to the pharmaceutical manufacturer for final packaging and distribution. Additional quality control measures may be required.

Soft gelatin capsules are not an inexpensive dosage form, particularly when compared to direct compression tablets [3]. There is a more intimate contact between the shell and its liquid contents than exists with dry-filled hard gelatin capsules, which increases the possibility of interactions. For instance, chloral hydrate formulated with an oily vehicle exerts a proteolytic effect on the gelatin shell; however, the effect is greatly reduced when the oily vehicle is replaced with polyethylene glycol [3].

Drugs can migrate from an oily vehicle into the shell, and this has been related to their water solubility and partition coefficient between water and the nonpolar solvent [157]. Studying 4-hydroxybenzoic acid as an encapsulated solution, Armstrong et al. [157] found that most transfer to the shell occurred during drying subsequent to manufacture; however, after completion of drying only a combined 89% of the original amount of solute could be found in the shell and contents. It was thus considered that some of the solute may migrate to the outer shell surface where it can be lost by erosion or washing [157].

The possible migration of a drug into the shell must be considered in the packaging of topical products in soft gelatin tube-like capsules as this could affect drug concentration in the ointment, etc., as applied [3]. For other products such as oral capsules or suppository capsules, both the shell and the contents must be considered in judging drug content when migration occurs. It is interesting that drug in the shell may provide for an initial dissolution of drug prior to shell rupture. When shell migration was negligible, there was a definite lag time in drug dissolution from encapsulated oily solution, indicating that rupture of the shell had to occur before solute release [157]. The larger the proportion of drug in the shell, the more overall drug release was dependent on the dissolution of the shell.

C. Composition of the Shell [3]

Like hard gelatin shells, the basic component of soft gelatin shells is gelatin; however, the shell has been plasticized by the addition of glycerin, sorbitol, or propylene glycol. Other components may include dyes, opacifiers, preservatives, and flavors. The ratio of dry plasticizer to dry gelatin determines the "hardness" of the shell and can vary from 0.3–1.0 for a very hard shell to 1.0–1.8 for a very soft shell. Up to 5% sugar may be included to give a "chewable" quality to the shell. The basic gelatin formulation from which the plasticized films are cast usually consists of one part gelatin, one part water, and 0.4–0.6 part plasticizer. The residual shell moisture content of finished capsules will be in the range of 6–10%.

One physical parameter of finished capsules measured in stability studies is "softness." Whereas this parameter traditionally has been measured subjectively, Vemuri [158] has reported the objective measurement of this property by compression of individual capsules between the platens of a physical testing machine.

D. Formulation of Soft Gelatin Capsules [3,147]

The formulation for soft gelatin capsules involves liquid rather than powder technology. Materials are generally formulated to produce the smallest possible capsule consistent with maximum stability, therapeutic effectiveness, and manufacture efficiency [3].

Soft gelatin capsules contain a single liquid, a combination of miscible liquids, a solution of a drug in a liquid, or a suspension of a drug in a liquid. The liquids are limited to those that do not have an adverse effect on the gelatin walls. The pH of the liquid can be between 2.5 and 7.5. Liquids with more acid pH would tend to cause leakage by hydrolysis of the gelatin. Both liquids with pH > 7.5 and aldehydes decrease shell solubility by tanning the gelatin. Aqueous emulsions cannot be filled because inevitably water will be released, which will affect the shell. Bauer and Dortunc [159] proposed nonaqueous emulsions for both soft and hard gelatin capsules. In general, the emulsions were composed of a hydrophilic liquid such as polyethylene glycol 400 and a triglyceride oil as the lipophilic liquid. Other liquids that cannot be encapsulated include water (>5% of contents) and low molecular weight alcohols such as ethyl alcohol. The types of vehicles used in soft gelatin capsules fall into two main groups:

1. Water-immiscible, volatile, or more likely nonvolatile liquids such as vegetable oils, aromatic and aliphatic hydrocarbons (mineral oil), medium-chain triglycerides, and acetylated glycerides.
2. Water-miscible, nonvolatile liquids such as low molecular weight polyethylene glycol (PEG-400 and PEG-600) have come into use because of their ability to mix with water readily and accelerate dissolution of dissolved or suspended drugs.

All liquids used for filling must flow by gravity at a temperature of 35°C or less. The sealing temperature of gelatin films is 37–40°C.

The limiting particle size for suspensions is that which can be handled by the pump. It is common practice to micronize (colloid mill) all materials during the preparation of the suspension. Typical suspending agents for oily bases and concentration of base are beeswax (5%), paraffin wax (5%), and animal stearates (1–6%). Suspending agents for nonoily bases include PEG 4000 and 6000 (1–5%), solid nonionics (10%), or solid glycol esters (10%). Little work has been published on the physical properties of materials for filling into soft gelatin capsules.

E. Manufacture of Soft Gelatin Capsules [3,148]

Plate Process

The oldest commercial process, this semi-automatic batch process has been supplanted by more modern, continuous processes. Equipment for the plate process is no longer available. In general, the process involved (a) placing the upper half of a plasticized gelatin sheet over a die plate containing numerous die pockets, (b) application of vacuum to draw the sheet into the die pockets, (c) filling the pockets with liquid or paste, (d) folding the lower half of the gelatin sheet back over the filled pockets, and (e) inserting the "sandwich" under a die press where the capsules are formed and cut out.

Rotary Die Process

The first continuous process is the rotary die process, which was invented in 1933 by R. P. Scherer. Aside from its being a continuous process, the rotary die process reduced manufacturing losses to a negligible level and content variation to a ±1–3% range, both major problems with earlier processes. In this process, the die cavities are machined into the outer surfaces of two rollers (i.e., die rolls). The die pockets on the left-hand roller form the left side of the capsule; the die pockets on the right-hand roller form the right side of the die capsule. The die pockets on the two rollers match as the rollers rotate. Two plasticized gelatin ribbons (prepared in the machine) are continuously and simultaneously fed with the liquid or paste fill between the rollers of the rotary die mechanism. The forceful injection of the feed material between the two ribbons causes the gelatin to swell into the left and right-hand die pockets as they converge. As the die rolls rotate, the convergence of the matching die pockets seals and cuts out the filled capsules. The process is illustrated in Fig. 26 and an actual machine is pictured in Fig. 27.

Accogel Process

A continuous process for the manufacture of soft gelatin capsules filled with powders or granules was developed by Lederle Laboratories in 1949. In general, this is another rotary process involving (a) a measuring roll, (b) a die roll, and (c) a sealing roll. The measuring roll rotates directly over the die roll, and the pockets in the two rolls are aligned with each other. The powder or granular fill material is held in the pockets of the measuring roll under vacuum. A plasticized sheet is drawn into the die pockets of the die roll under vacuum. As the measuring roll and die rolls rotate, the measured doses are transferred to the gelatin-lined pockets of the die roll. The continued rotation of the filled die converges with the rotating sealing roll where a second gelatin sheet is applied to form the other half of the capsule. Pressure developed between the die roll and sealing roll seals and cuts out the capsules.

Bubble Method

Truly seamless, one-piece soft gelatin capsules can be made by a "bubble method" [148]. A concentric tube dispenser simultaneously discharges the molten gelatin from the outer annulus and the liquid content from the inner tube. The liquids are discharged into chilled oil as droplets, which consist of a liquid medicament core within a molten gelatin envelope. The droplets assume a spherical shape under surface tension forces, and the gelatin congeals on cooling. The finished capsules then must be degreased and dried.

IV. SOFT/LIQUID-FILLED HARD GELATIN CAPSULES

Perhaps the most important reason soft gelatin capsules became the standard for liquid-filled capsules was the inability to prevent leakage from hard gelatin capsules. The advent of sealing techniques such as banding and of self-locking hard gelatin capsules, together with the development of high-resting-state viscosity fills, has made liquid/semi-solid filled hard gelatin capsules a feasible dosage form today [160]. As of this writing, the only commercial examples in this country are Vancocin[R] HCl (Eli Lilly and Co.) and Gengraf (Abbott/Sangstat).

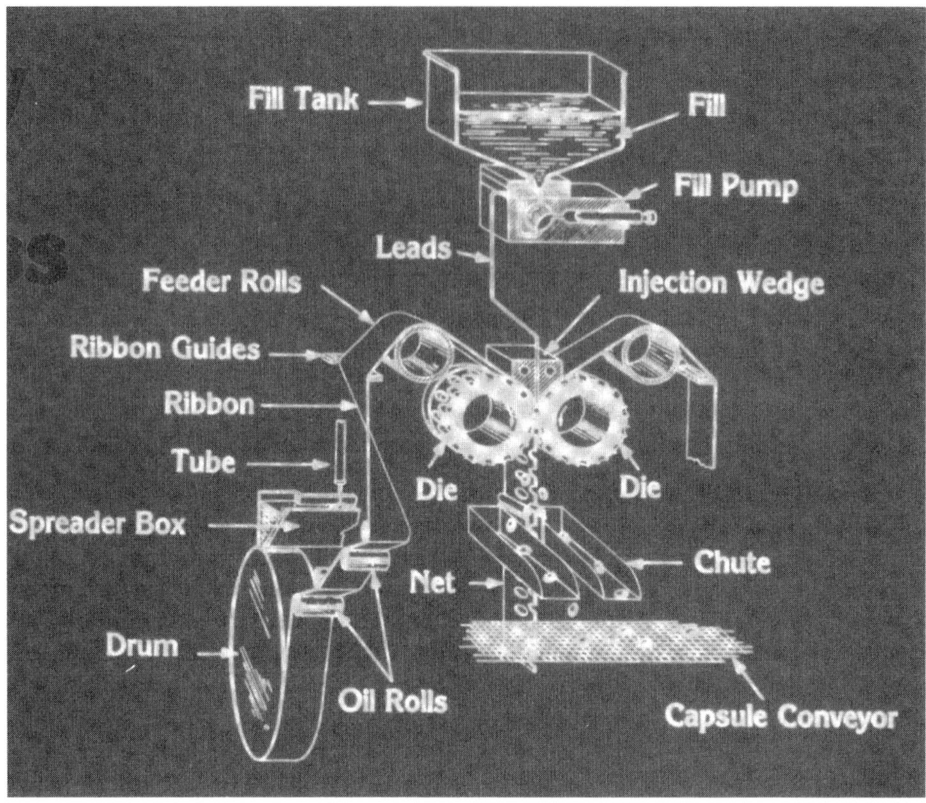

Fig. 26 Illustration of the rotary die process. (Courtesy of R. P. Scherer North America, Clearwater, FL.)

Such a dosage form essentially offers the advantages of soft gelatin capsules. In addition, since most hard shell filling machine manufacturers have developed models capable of filling liquids and semi-solids, this technology can be brought in-house, thus avoiding the necessity of having to contract the work outside to a specialty house [160]. As with soft gelatin capsules, any materials filled into hard capsules must not dissolve, alter, or otherwise adversely affect the integrity of the shell. Generally, the fill material must be pumpable.

Three formulation strategies based on having a high-resting-state viscosity after filling have been described [161,162]:

1. Thixotropic formulations: such systems exhibit shear thinning when agitated and thus are pumpable. Yet, when agitation stops, the system rapidly establishes a gel structure, thereby avoiding leakage.
2. Thermal setting formulations: in this case, excipients are used which are liquid at filling temperatures but which gel or solidify in the capsule to prevent leakage.
3. Mixed thermal/thixotropic systems: improved resistance to leakage may be realized for low or moderate melting point systems. Above its melting point, the liquid can still be immobile because of thixotropy.

A high-resting-state viscosity is not a formulation prerequisite if capsules are banded and the contents have a viscosity of about 100 cps to prevent leakage from the mechanically interlocked capsules prior to banding.

Materials that may be used as carriers for the drug cover a wide range of chemical classes and melting points. These include vegetable oils, hydrogenated vegetable oils, various fats such as carnauba wax and cocoa butter, and polyethylene glycols (molecular weights 200–20,000). For thixotropic systems, the liquid excipient is often thickened with colloidal silicas. In one example [162], the liquid active clofibrate was formulated as a thermal-setting system by adding 30%

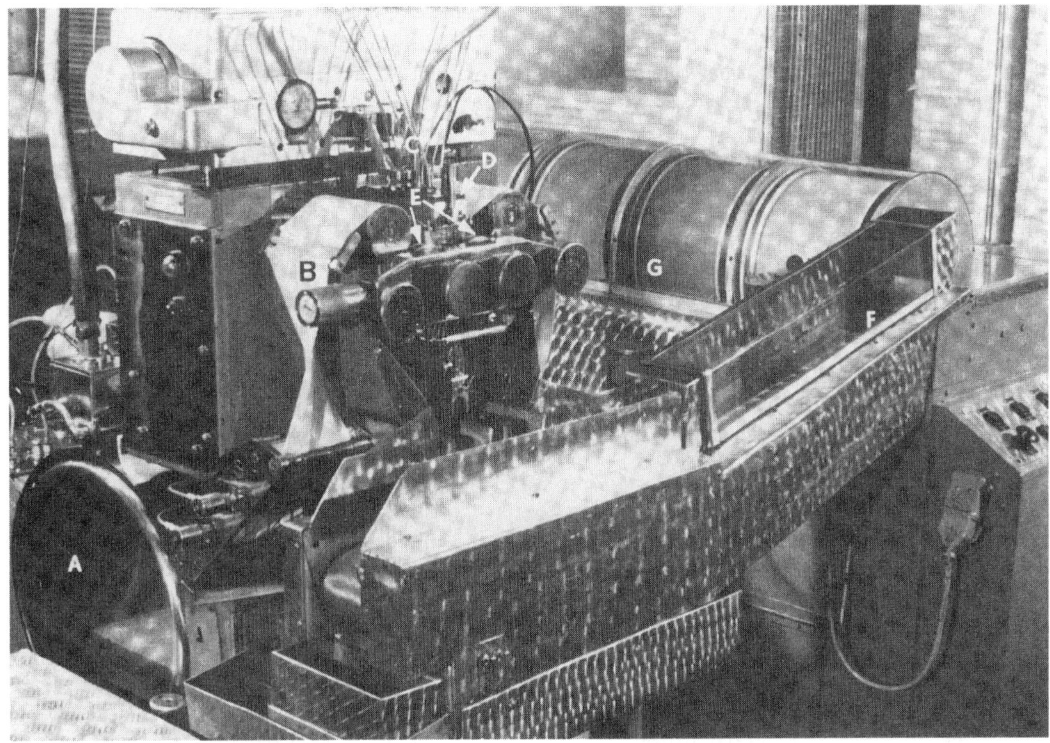

Fig. 27 Rotary die machine. (A) Ribbon casting drum; (B) ribbon; (C) filling leads; (D) injection mechanism; (E) rotary die; (F) capsule wash; (G) infrared dryer. (Courtesy of R. P. Scherer North America, Clearwater, FL.)

(based on total weight) polyethylene glycol 20,000. In another example, [162] vitamin E was filled as a thixotropic system by adding approximately 6% each (based on total weight) beeswax and fumed silicon dioxide. Powdered drugs may be dissolved or suspended in thixotropic or thermal setting systems. In general, the more lipophilic the contents, the slower the release rate. Thus, by selecting excipients with varying hydrophilic/lipophilic balance (HLB), varying release rates may be achieved [162].

GENERAL REFERENCES

V Hostetler, JQ Bellard. Capsules I. Hard capsules. In: L Lachman, H A Lieberman, J L Kanig, eds. The Theory and Practice of Industrial Pharmacy, 2nd ed. Philadelphia: Lea and Febiger, 1976, pp 389–404.

K Ridgeway, Ed. Hard Capsules. Development and Technology. London: The Pharmaceutical Press, 1987.

JP Stanley. Capsules II. Soft gelatin capsules. In: L Lachman, H A Lieberman, J L Kanig, eds. The Theory and Practice of Industrial Pharmacy, 2nd ed, Philadelphia: Lea and Febiger, 1976, pp 404–420.

REFERENCES

1. R Delaney. Surveying consumer preferences. Pharm Executive 2(3):34, 1982.
2. BE Jones, TD Turner. A century of commercial hard gelatin capsules. Pharm J 213:614–617, 1974.
3. JP Stanley. Capsules II. Soft gelatin capsules. In: L Lachman, HA Leiberman, JL Kanig, eds. The Theory and Practice of Industrial Pharmacy, 2nd ed. Philadelphia: Lea & Febiger, 1976, pp 404–420.
4. L Eith, RFT Stepto, F Wittwer, I Tomka. Injection-moulded drug-delivery systems. Manuf Chem 58(1):21, 1987.
5. LM Mortada, FA Ismail, SA Khalil. Correlation of urinary excretion with in vitro dissolution using four dissolution methods for ampicillin capsules. Drug Dev Ind Pharm 11:101–130, 1985.
6. K Arnold, N Gerber, G Levy. Absorption and dissolution studies on sodium diphenylhydantoin capsules. Can J Pharm Sci 5(4):89–92, 1970.
7. AJ Aguiar, LM Wheeler, S Fusari, JE Zelmar. Evaluation of physical and pharmaceutical factors involved in drug release and availability from chloramphenicol capsules. J Pharm Sci 57:1844–1850, 1968.

8. AJ Glazco, AW Kinkel, WC Alegnani, EL Holmes. An evaluation of the absorption characteristics of different chloramphenicol preparations in normal human subjects. Clin Pharmacol Ther 9:472–474, 1968.
9. A study of physician attitudes toward capsules and other pharmaceutical product forms. Elanco Products Co., Div. Eli Lilly & Co., Indianapolis, IN, 1971, El-0004.
10. M Marvola. Adherence of drug products to the oesophagus. Pharmacy Int 3:294–296, 1982.
11. H Hey, F Jorgensen, H Hasselbach, T Wamberg. Oesophageal transit of six commonly used tablets and capsules. Br Med J 285(11):1717–1719, 1982.
12. KS Channer, J Virjee. Effect of posture and drink volume on the swallowing of capsules. Br Med J 285(11):1702, 1982.
13. T Evans, GM Roberts. Where do all the tablets go? Lancet 2 (Oct.-Dec.):1237–1239, 1976.
14. JT Fell. Esophageal transit of tablets and capsules. Am J Hosp Pharm 40:946–948, 1983.
15. GW Martyn, Jr. Production history of hard gelatin capsules from molding through filling, paper presented at Symposium on Modern Capsule Manufacturing, Society of Manufacturing Engineers, Philadelphia, PA, January 31, 1978.
16. LC Lappas. The manufacture of hard gelatin capsules, paper presented to Research and Development Section, The American Drug Manufacturers Association, Atlantic City, NJ, October 8, 1954.
17. GW Martyn, Jr. The people computer interface in a capsule molding operation. Drug Dev Comm l: 39, 1974–5.
18. BE Jones. Hard gelatin capsules and the pharmaceutical formulator. Pharm Technol 9(9):106–108, 110, 112, 1985.
19. LW Buckalew, KE Coffield. An investigation of drug expectancy as a function of capsule color and size and preparation form. J Clin Psychopharmacol 2:245–248, 1982.
20. General worldwide specifications for Capsugel hard gelatin capsules. Revised 11/29/99. Bulletin BAS-203-E. Capsugel, Div. Pfizer, Inc., Greenwood, SC, 1999.
21. Coni-Snap^{R}—the hard gelatin capsule with the advantages that matter. Bulletin BAS-112-E, USA. Capsugel, Div. Pfizer, Inc., Greenwood, SC, 1982.
22. R Shah, LL Augsburger. Oxygen permeation in banded and non-banded hard gelatin capsules (abstr). Pharm Res 6:S–55, 1989.
23. F Wittwer. New developments in hermetic sealing of hard gelatin capsules. Pharm Manuf 2(6):24–29, 1985.
24. D Scott, R Shah, LL Augsburge. A comparative evaluation of the mechanical strength of sealed and unsealed hard gelatin capsules. Int J Pharm 84:49–58, 1992.
25. KS Murthy, I Ghebre-Sellassie. Current perspectives on the dissolution stability of solid oral dosage forms. J Pharm Sci 82:113–126, 1993.
26. K Ito, S-I Kaga, Y Takeya. Studies on hard gelatin capsules I. Water vapor transfer between capsules and powders. Chem Pharm Bull 17:1134–1137, 1969.
27. WA Strickland, Jr., M Moss. Water vapor sorption and diffusion through hard gelatin capsules. J Pharm Sci 51:1002–1005, 1962.
28. Incompatibilities in prescriptions IV. The use of inert powders in capsules to prevent liquefaction due to deliquescence. J Am Pharm Assoc Sci Ed 29:136, 1940.
29. JH Bell, NA Stevenson, JE Taylor. A moisture transfer effect in hard gelatin capsules of sodium cromoglycate. J Pharm Pharmacol 25 (suppl):96P–103P, 1973.
30. MJ Kontny, CA Mulski. Gelatin capsule brittleness as a function of relative humidity at room temperature. Int J Pharm 54:79–85, 1989.
31. G Zografi, GP Grandolfi, MJ Kontny, DW Mendenhall. Prediction of moisture transfer in mixtures of solids: transfer via the vapor phase. Int J Pharm 42:77–88, 1988.
32. JR Schwier, GG Cooke, KJ Hartauer, LYu. Rayon: a source of furfural—a reactive aldehyde capable of insolubilizing gelatin capsules. Pharm Technol 17(5): 78–79, 1993.
33. KS Murthy, NA Enders, MB Fawzi. Dissolution stability of hard-shell products. Part I: the effect of exaggerated storage conditions. Pharm Technol 13(3): 72–86, 1989.
34. KS Murthy, RG Reisch, Jr., MB Fawzi. Dissolution stability of hard-shell capsule products. Part II: the effect of dissolution test conditions on in vitro drug release. Pharm Technol 13(6):53–58, 1989.
35. H Mohamad, R Renoux, S Aiache, J-M Aiache. Etude de la stabilite biopharmaceutique des medicaments application a des gelules de chlorohydrate de tetracycline I. Etude in vitro. STP Pharma 2(17):531–535, 1986.
36. EM Marks, D Tourtellotte, A Andus. The phenomenon of gelatin insolubility. Food Technol 22:1433–1436, 1968.
37. T Dahl, ILT Sue, A Yum. The effect of pancreatin on the dissolution performance of gelatin-coated tablets exposed to high-humidity conditions. Pharm Res 8:412–414, 1991.
38. H Mohamad, J-M Aiche, R Renoux, P Mougin, J-P Kantelip. Etude de la stabilite biopharmaceutique des medicaments application a des gelules de chlorohydrate de tetracycline. IV. Etude complimentaire in vivo. STP Pharma 3(5):407–411, 1986.
39. M Aikman, L Augsburger, I Berry et al. Collaborative development of two-tiered dissolution testing for gelatin capsules and gelatin-coated tablets using enzyme-containing media. Pharmacop Forum 24(5):7045–7050, 1998.
40. G Cole. Capsule filling. Chem Eng (London) 382:473–473, 1982.
41. LL Augsburger, Powdered dosage forms. In: LW Dittert, ed. Sprowl's American Pharmacy, 7th ed. Philadelphia: PA, JB Lippincott, 1974, pp 301–343.
42. H Clement, HG Marquart. The mechanical processing of hard gelatin capsules. News Sheet 3/70, Capsugel, A.G., CH-4000, Basel, Switzerland.

43. K Ridgway, JAB Callow. Capsule-filling machinery. Pharm J 212:281–285, 1973.
44. A look at capsules. Manuf Chem Aerosol News 48(7):26, 1977.
45. V Hostetler, JQ Bellard. Capsules I. Hard capsules. In: L Lachman, HA Lieberman, JL Kanig, eds. The Theory and Practice of Industrial Pharmacy, 2nd ed. Philadelphia: Lea & Febiger, 1976, pp 389–404.
46. K Ito, S-I Kaga, Y Takeya. Studies on hard gelatin capsules II. The capsule filling of powders and effects of glidant by ring filling machine-method. Chem Pharm Bull 17:1138–1145, 1969.
47. G Reier, R Cohn, S Rock, F. Wagenblast. Evaluation of factors affecting the encapsulation of powders in hard gelatin capsules I. Semi-automatic capsule machines. J Pharm Sci 57:660–666, 1968.
48. K Kurihara, I Ichikawa. Effect of powder flowability on capsule filling weight variation. Chem Pharm Bull 26:1250–1256, 1978.
49. Osaka R-180 Brochure, Osaka Automatic Machine. Mfg Co., Osaka 591, Japan.
50. P Heda. A comparative study of the formulation requirements of dosator and dosing disc encapsulators. Simulation of plug formation, and creation of rules for an expert system for formulation design. PhD dissertation, University of Maryland, Baltimore, 1998.
51. GKF, Filling and Sealing Machine for Hard Gelatin Capsules, Hofliger + Karg. Brochure HK/GKF/4/82-2E, Robert Bosch Corp., Packaging Machinery Div., So. Plainfield, NJ.
52. KB Shah, LL Augsburger, LE Small, GP Polli. Instrumentation of a dosing disc automatic capsule filling machine. Pharm Tech 7(4):42–54, 1983.
53. JI Wells. Pharmaceutical Preformulation: The Physicochemical Properties of Drug Substances. Chichester, England: Ellis Horwood LTD, 1988, pp 209–210.
54. LE Small, LL Augsburger. Instrumentation of an automatic capsule filling machine. J Pharm Sci 66:504–509, 1977.
55. LE Stoyle, Jr. Evaluation of the zanasi automatic capsule machine. Proceedings of the Industrial Pharmacy Section, A.Ph.A. 113th Annual Meeting, Dallas, TX, April 1966.
56. Macofar Mod. MT 13-l and 13-2 Brochure, Macofar s.a.s., Bologna, Italy.
57. GM Irwin, GJ Dodson, LJ Ravin. Encapsulation of clomacron phosphate I. Effect of flowability of powder blends, lot-to-lot variability, and concentration of active ingredient on weight variation of capsules filled on an automatic capsule filling machine. J Pharm Sci 59:547–550, 1970.
58. ZT Chowhan, YP Chow. Powder flow studies I. Powder consolidation ratio and its relationship to capsule-filling weight variation. Int J Pharm 4:317, 1980.
59. Y Miyake, A Shimoda, T Jasu, M Furukawa, K Nesuji, K. Hoshi. Packing properties of pharmaceutical powders into hard gelatin capsules. Yakuzaigaku 34:32, 1974.
60. IG Jolliffe, JM Newton, JK Walters. Theoretical considerations of the filling of pharmaceutical hard gelatine capsules. Powder Tech 27:189–195, 1980 .
61. IG Jolliffe, JM Newton. Practical implications of theoretical consideration of capsule filling by the dosator nozzle system. J Pharm Pharmacol 34:293–298, 1982.
62. JB Schwartz. The instrumented tablet press: uses in research and production. Pharm Tech 5(9):102–132, 1981.
63. K Marshall. Instrumentation of tablet and capsule filling machines. Pharm Tech 7(3):68–82, 1983.
64. LL Augsburger. Instrumented capsule filling machines: development and application. Pharm Tech 6(9):111–112, 114, 117–119, 1982.
65. GC Cole, G May. Instrumentation of a hard shell encapsulation machine (abstr). J Pharm Pharmacol 24(suppl):122P, 1972.
66. GC Cole, G. May. The instrumentation of a zanasi LZ/64 capsule filling machine. J Pharm Pharmacol 27:353–358, 1975.
67. LE Small, LL Augsburger. Aspects of the lubrication requirements for an automatic capsule-filling machine. Drug Devel Ind Pharm 4:345–372, 1978.
68. AM Mehta, LL Augsburger. Simultaneous measurement of force and displacement in an automatic capsule filling machine. Int J Pharm 4:347–351, 1980.
69. AM Mehta, LL Augsburger. Quantitative evaluation of force displacement curves in an automatic capsule filling machine. Presented to the IPT Section, A.Ph.A. Academy of Pharmaceutical Sciences, 128th Annual A.Ph.A. Meeting, St. Louis, March-April 1981.
70. R Greenberg. Effects of AZ-60 filling machine dosator settings upon slug hardness and dissolution of capsules. Proceedings of the 88th National Meeting, Am. Inst. Chem. Engrs., Session 11, Philadelphia, PA, June 8–12, 1980 (Fiche 29).
71. JE Botzolakis. Studies on the mechanism of disintegrant action in encapsulated dosage forms. PhD dissertation, University of Maryland, Baltimore, 1985.
72. C Mony, C Sambeat, G Cousin. Interet des measures de pression dans la formulation et le remplissage des gelules. Newsheet 1977. Capsugel A.G., Basel, Switzerland.
73. DJ Rowley, R Hendry, MD Ward, P Timmins. The instrumentation of an automatic capsule filling machine for formulation design studies. paper presented at 3rd International Conference on Powder Technology, Paris, 1983.
74. KB Shah, LL Augsburger, K Marshall. An investigation of some factors influencing plug formation and fill weight in a dosing disk-type automatic capsule-filling machine. J Pharm Sci 75:291–296, 1986.
75. KB Shah, LL Augsburger, K Marshall. Multiple tamping effects on drug dissolution from capsules filled on a dosing-disk type automatic capsule filling machine. J Pharm Sci 76:639–645, 1987.
76. JW Cropp, LL Augsburger, K Marshall. Simultaneous monitoring of tamping force and piston displacement

(F-D) on an Hofliger-Karg capsule filling machine. Int J Pharm 71:127–136, 1991.
77. F Podczeck. The development of an instrumented tamp-filling capsule machine: I. Instrumentation of a Bosch GKF 400S machine. Eur J Pharm Sci 10:267–274, 2000.
78. AM Mehta, LL Augsburger. A preliminary study of the effect of slug hardness on drug dissolution from hard gelatin capsules filled on an automatic capsule filling machine. Int J Pharm 7:327–334, 1981.
79. PK Heda, FX Muller, LL Augsburger. Capsule filling machine simulation I: Low force compression physics relevant to plug formation. Pharm Devel Tech 4(2):209–219, 1999.
80. M Celik, K Marshall. Use of a compaction simulator system in tablet research. Drug Dev Ind Pharm 15:758–800, 1989.
81. AG Stewart, DJW Grant, JM Newton. The release of a model low-dose drug (riboflavine) from hard gelatin capsule formulations. J Pharm Pharmacol 31:1–6, 1979.
82. P Veski, M Marvola. Design and use of equipment for simulation of plug formation in hard gelatin capsule filling machines. Acta Pharm Fennica 100:19–25, 1991.
83. IG Jolliffe, JM Newton, D Cooper. The design and use of an instrumented mG2 capsule filling machine simulator. J Pharm Pharmacol 34:230–235, 1982.
84. IG Jolliffe, JM Newton. An investigation of the relationship between particle size and compression during capsule filling with an Instrumented mG2 simulator. J Pharm Pharmacol 34:415–419, 1982.
85. IG Jolliffe, JM Newton. The effect of dosator nozzle wall texture on capsule filling with the mG2 simulator. J Pharm Pharmacol 35:7–11, 1983.
86. SB Tan, JM Newton. Powder flowability as an indication of capsule filling performance. Int J Pharm 61:145–155, 1990.
87. SB Tan, JM Newton. Influence of capsule dosator wall texture and powder properties on the angle of wall friction and powder-wall adhesion. Int J Pharm 64:227–234, 1990.
88. SB Tan, JM Newton. Capsule filling performance of powders with dosator nozzles of different wall texture. Int J Pharm 66:207–211, 1990.
89. SB Tan, JM Newton. Minimum compression stress requirements for arching and powder retention within a dosator nozzle during capsule filling. Int J Pharm 63:275–280, 1990.
90. SB Tan, JM Newton. Influence of compression setting ratio on capsule fill weight and weight variability. Int J Pharm 66:273–282, 1990.
91. SB Tan, JM Newton. Observed and expected powder plug densities obtained by a capsule dosator nozzle system. Int J Pharm 66:283–288, 1990.
92. JR Britten, MI Barnett. Development and validation of a capsule filling machine simulator. Int J Pharm 71:R5–R8, 1991.
93. JR Britten, MI Barnett, NA Armstrong. Construction of an intermittant-motion capsule filling machine simulator. Pharm Res 12:196–200, 1995.
94. JR Britten, MI Barnett, NA Armstrong. Studies on powder plug formation using a simulated capsule filling machine. J Pharm Pharmacol 48:249–254, 1996.
95. A Ludwig, M Van Ooteghem. Disintegration of hard gelatin capsules. Part 2: disintegration mechanism of hard gelatin capsules investigated with a stereoscopic microscope. Pharm Ind 42:405–406, 1980.
96. A Ludwig, M Van Ooteghem. Disintegration of hard gelatin capsules. Part 5: the influence of the composition of the test solution on disintegration of hard gelatin capsules. Pharm Ind 43:188–190, 1981.
97. GL Amidon, H Lennernas, VP Shah, JR Crison. A theoretical basis for a biopharmaceutic drug classification: the correlation of in vitro drug product dissolution and in vivo bioavailability. Pharm Res 12:413–420, 1995.
98. AS Hussain. Classifying your drug: the BCS guidance. In: GL Amidon, JR Robinson, RL Williams, eds. Scientific Foundations for Regulating Drug Products. Arlington, VA:AAPS Press, 1997, pp 197–204.
99. GS Rekhi, ND Eddington, MJ Fossler, P Schwartz, LJ Lesko, LL Augsburger. Evaluation of in vitro release rate and in vivo absorption characteristics of four metoprolol tartrate immediate release tablet formulations. Pharm Devel Tech 2(1):11–24, 1997.
100. DA Piscitelli, S Bigora, C Propst, S Goskonda, P Schwartz, L Lesko, L Augsburger, D Young. The impact of formulation and process changes on in vitro dissolution and bioequivalence of piroxicam capsules. Pharm Devel Tech 3(4):443–452, 1998.
101. ND Eddington, M Ashraf, LL Augsburger, JL Leslie, MJ Fossler, LJ Lesko, VP Shah, GS Rekhi. Identification of formulation and manufacturing variables that influence in vitro dissolution and in vivo bioavailability of propranolol hydrochloride tablets. Pharm Dev Tech 3(4):535–547, 1998.
102. JE Polli. Analysis of in vitro – in vivo data. In: GL Amidon, JR Robinson, RL Williams, eds. Scientific Foundations for Regulating Drug Products. Arlington, VA: AAPS Press, 1997, pp 335–351.
103. Waiver of in vivo bioavailability and bioequivalence studies for immediate release solid oral dosage forms based on a biopharmaceutics classification system. Center for Drug Evaluation and Research, Food and Drug Administration, issued 8/2000, posted 8/31/2000. http://www.fda.gov/cder/guidance/ index. htm
104. Immediate release solid oral dosage forms; Scale-up and post approval changes: chemistry, manufacturing, and controls; In vitro dissolution testing; In vivo bioequivalence documentation, November, 1995. Center for Drug Evaluation and Research, Food and Drug Administration. http://www.fda.gov/cder/ guidance /index.htm

105. JH Fincher, JG Adams, MH Beal. Effect of particle size on gastrointestinal absorption of sulfisoxazole in dogs. J Pharm Sci 54:704–708, 1963.
106. SM Bastami, MJ Groves. Some factors influencing the in vitro release of phenytoin from formulations. Int J Pharm 1:151–164, 1978.
107. JM Newton, G Rowley. On the release of drug from hard gelatin capsules. J Pharm Pharmacol 22:163 S–168 S, 1970.
108. R Patel, F Podczeck. Investigation of the effect of type and source of microcrystalline cellulose on capsule filling. Int J Pharm 128:123–127, 1996.
109. JM Newton, G Rowley, JFV Tornblom. The effect of additives on the release of drug from hard gelatin capsules. J Pharm Pharmacol 23:452–453, 1971.
110. RJ Withey, CA Mainville. A critical analysis of a capsule dissolution test. J Pharm Sci 58:1120–1126, 1969.
111. JH Tyrer, MJ Eadie, JM Sutherland, WD Hooper. Br Med J 4:271–273, 1970.
112. P York. Studies of the effect of powder moisture content on drug release from hard gelatin capsules. Drug Dev Ind Pharm 6:605–627, 1980.
113. AD Koparkar, LL Augsburger, RF Shangraw. Intrinsic dissolution rates of tablet filler-binders and their influence on the dissolution of drugs from tablet formulation. Pharm Res 7:80–86, 1990.
114. LL Augsburger, RF Shangraw. Effect of glidants in tableting. J Pharm Sci 55:418–423, 1966.
115. P York. Application of powder failure testing equipment in assessing effect of glidants on flowability of cohesive pharmaceutical powders. J Pharm Sci 64:1216–1221, 1975.
116. HM Sadek, JL Olsen, HL Smith, S Onay. A systematic approach to glidant selection. Pharm Tech 6(2):43–62, 1982.
117. RF Shangraw, DA Demarest, Jr. A survey of current industrial practices in the formulation and manufacture of tablets and capsules. Pharm Technol 17:32–44, 1993.
118. B Jones. Two-piece gelatin capsules: excipients for powder products, European practice. Pharm Tech Eur 7(10):25–34, 1995.
119. JM Newton, G Rowley, JFV Tornblom. Further studies on the effect of additives on the release of drug from hard gelatin capsules. J Pharm Pharmacol 23:156S–160S, 1971.
120. JC Samyn, WY Jung. In vitro dissolution from several experimental capsules. J Pharm Sci 59:169–175, 1970.
121. KS Murthy, JC Samyn. Effect of shear mixing on in vitro drug release of capsule formulations containing lubricants. J Pharm Sci 66:1215–1219, 1977.
122. TA Miller, P York. Pharmaceutical tablet lubrication. Int J Pharm 41:1–19, 1988.
123. AC Shah, AR Mlodozeniec. Mechanism of surface lubrication: Influence of duration of lubricant-excipient mixing on processing characteristics of powders and properties of compressed tablets. J Pharm Sci 66:1377–1381, 1977.
124. MR Bolhuis, CF Lerk. Film forming of tablet lubricants during the mixing process of solids. Acta Pharm Technol 23:13–20, 1977.
125. DS Desai, BA Rubitski, SA Varia, AW Newman. Physical interactions of magnesium stearate with starch-derived disintegrants and their effects on capsule and tablet dissolution. Int J Pharm 91:217–226, 1993.
126. I Ullah, GJ Wiley, SN Agharkar. Analysis and simulation of capsule dissolution problem encountered during product scale-up. Drug Dev Ind Pharm 18:895–910, 1992.
127. H Nakagwu. Effects of particle size of rifampicin and addition of magnesium stearate in release of rifampicin from hard gelatin capsules. Yakugaku Zasshi 100:1111–1117, 1980.
128. PT Shah, WE Moore. Dissolution behavior of commercial tablets extemporaneously converted to capsules. J Pharm Sci 59:1034–1036, 1970.
129. FW Goodhart, RH McCoy, FC Ninger. New in vitro disintegration and dissolution test method for tablets and capsules. J Pharm Sci 62:304–310, 1973.
130. RF Shangraw, A Mitrevej, M Shah. A new era of tablet disintegrants. Pharm Tech 4(10):49–57, 1980.
131. RF Shangraw, JW Wallace, FM Bowers. Morphology and functionality of tablet excipients for direct compression: Part II. Pharm Tech 5(10):44, 46, 48, 50, 52, 54, 56, 58, 60, 1981.
132. JE Botzolakis, LE Small, LL Augsburger. Effect of disintegrants on drug dissolution from capsules filled on a dosator-type automatic capsule-filling machine. Int J Pharm 12:341–349, 1982.
133. JE Botzolakis, LL Augsburger. The role of disintegrants in hard-gelatin capsules. J Pharm Pharmacol 37:77–84, 1984.
134. JTH Ong, ZT Chowhan, GJ Samuels. Drug-excipient interactions resulting from powder mixing VI. Role of various surfactants. Int J Pharm 96:231–242, 1993.
135. LH Wang, ZT Chowhan. Drug-excipient interactions resulting from powder mixing V. Role of sodium lauryl sulfate. Int J Pharm 60:61–78, 1990.
136. OI Corrigan, AM Healy. Surfactants in pharmaceutical products and systems. In: J Swarbrick, JC Boylan, eds. Encyclopedia of Pharmaceutical Technology, Vol. 14. New York: Marcel Dekker, 1996, pp 295–331.
137. CF Lerk, M Lagas, JT Fell, P Nauta. Effect of hydrophilization of hydrophobic drugs on release rate from capsules. J Pharm Sci 67:935–939, 1978.
138. CF Lerk, M Lagas, L Lie-A-Huen, P Broersma, K Zuurman. In vitro and in vivo availability of hydrophilized phenytoin from capsules. J Pharm Sci 68:634–637, 1979.
139. M Lagas, HJC de Wit, MG Woldring, DA Piers, CF Lerk. Technetium labelled disintegration of capsules in the human stomach. Pharm Acta Helv 55:114–119, 1980.

140. J Hogan, P-I Shue, F Podczeck, JM Newton. Investigations into the relationship between drug properties, filling, and the release of drugs from hard gelatin capsules using multivariate statistical analysis. Pharm Res 13:944–949, 1996.
141. AS Hussain, X Yu, RD Johnson. Application of neural computing to pharmaceutical product development. Pharm Res 8:1248–1252, 1991.
142. S Lai, F Podczeck, JM Newton, R Daumesnil. An expert system to aid the development of capsule formulations. Pharm Tech Eur 8(Oct.):60–65, 1996.
143. SD Bateman, J Verlin, M Russo, M Guillot, SM Laughlin. The development of a capsule formulation knowledge-based system. Pharm Tech 20(3):174, 178, 180, 182, 184, 1996.
144. RC Rowe, RJ Roberts. Artifical intelligence in pharmaceutical product formulation: neural computing and emerging technologies. PSTT 1(5):200–205, 1998.
145. JE Polli, JR Crison, GL Amidon. Novel approach to the analysis of an in vitro–in vivo relationships. J Pharm Sci 85:753–760, 1996.
146. TA Hicks, B Patel, LL Augsburger, R Shangraw, L Lesko, V Shah, D Young. The effect of relative magnitudes of absorption and elimination half-lives on the decision of Cmax-based bioequivalence (abstr). American Association of Pharmaceutical Scientists, 8th Annual Meeting, Orlando, FL, November 1993.
147. WR Ebert. Soft elastic gelatin capsules: a unique dosage form. Pharm Tech 1(10):44–50, 1977.
148. G Muller. Methods and machines for making gelatin capsules. Manuf Chem 32:63–66, 1961.
149. IR Berry. Improving bioavailability with soft gelatin capsules. Drug Cos Ind 133(3):32, 33, 102, 105–108, 1983.
150. IR Berry. One-piece, soft gelatin capsules for pharmaceutical products. Pharm Eng 5(5):15–19, 1985.
151. FS Hom, JJ Miskel. Enhanced drug dissolution rates for a series of drugs as a function of dosage form design. Lex Sci 8(1):18–26, 1971.
152. H Seager. Soft gelatin capsules: a solution to many tableting problems. Pharm Tech 9(9):84, 86, 88, 90, 92, 94, 96, 98, 100, 102, 104, 1985.
153. FS Hom, JJ Miskel. Oral dosage form design and its influence on dissolution rates for a series of drugs. J Pharm Sci 59:827–830, 1970.
154. LJ Fuccella, G Bolcioni, V Tamassia, L Ferario, G Tognoni. Human pharmacokinetics and bioavailability of temazepam administered in soft gelatin capsules. Eur J Clin Pharmacol 12:383–386, 1977.
155. BF Johnson, C Bye, G Jones, GA Sabey. A completely absorbed oral preparation of digoxin. Clin Pharmacol Ther 19:746–757, 1976.
156. FS Hom, SA Veresh, WR Ebert. Soft gelatin capsules II. Oxygen permeability study of capsule shells. J Pharm Sci 64:851–857, 1975.
157. NA Armstrong, KC James, WKL Pugh. Drug migration into soft gelatin capsule shells and its effect on the in-vitro availability. J Pharm Pharmacol 36:361–365, 1984.
158. S Vemuri. Measurement of soft elastic gelatin capsule firmness with a universal testing machine. Drug Dev Ind Pharm 10:409–424, 1984.
159. KH Bauer, B Dortunc. Non-aqueous emulsions as vehicles for capsule filling. Drug Devel Ind Pharm 10:699–712, 1984.
160. D Francois, BE Jones. Making the hard capsule with the soft center. Manuf Chem Aerosol News 50(3):37, 38, 41, 1979.
161. SE Walker, JA Ganley, K Bedford, T Eaves. The filling of molten and thixotropic formulations into hard gelatin capsules. J Pharm Pharmacol 32:389–393, 1980.
162. The Hard Capsule With the Soft Center, Elanco Products Co., Div. Eli Lilly and Co., Indianapolis, IN.

Chapter 12

Parenteral Products

James C. Boylan

Pharmaceutical Consultant, Gurnee, Illinois

Steven L. Nail

Purdue University, West Lafayette, Indiana

1. INTRODUCTION

The first official injection (morphine) appeared in the *British Pharmacopoeia* (BP) of 1867. It was not until 1898 when cocaine was added to the BP that sterilization was attempted. In this country, the first official injections may be found in the *National Formulary* (NF), published in 1926. Monographs were included for seven sterile glass-sealed ampoules. The NF and the *United States Pharmacopeia* (USP) published chapters on sterilization as early as 1916, but no monographs for ampoules appeared in USP until 1942. The current USP contains monographs for over 500 injectable products [1].

Parenteral administration of drugs by intravenous (IV), intramuscular (IM), or subcutaneous (SC) routes is now an established and essential part of medical practice. Advantages for parenterally administered drugs include the following: rapid onset, predictable effect, predictable and nearly complete bioavailability, and avoidance of the gastrointestinal (GI) tract and, hence, the problems of variable absorption, drug inactivation, and GI distress. In addition, the parenteral route provides reliable drug administration in very ill or comatose patients.

The pharmaceutical industry directs considerable effort toward maximizing the usefulness and reliability of oral dosage forms in an effort to minimize the need for parenteral administration. Factors that contribute to this include certain disadvantages of the parenteral route, including the frequent pain and discomfort of injections, with all the psychological fears associated with "the needle," plus the realization that an incorrect drug or dose is often harder or impossible to counteract when it has been given parenterally (particularly intravenously), rather than orally.

In recent years, parenteral dosage forms, especially IV forms, have enjoyed increased use. The reasons for this growth are many and varied, but they can be summed up as (a) new and better parenteral administration techniques, (b) an increasing number of drugs that can be administered only by a parenteral route, (c) the need for simultaneous administration of multiple drugs in hospitalized patients receiving IV therapy, (d) new forms of nutritional therapy, such as intravenous lipids, amino acids, and trace metals, and (e) the extension of parenteral therapy into the home.

Many important drugs are available only as parenteral dosage forms. Notable among these are numerous biotechnology drugs, insulin, several cephalosporin antibiotic products, and drugs such as heparin, protamine, and glucagon. In addition, other drugs, such as lidocaine hydrochloride and many anticancer products, are used principally as parenterals.

Along with this growth in the use of parenteral medications, the hospital pharmacist has become a very knowledgeable, key individual in most hospitals, having responsibility for hospital-wide IV admixture programs, parenteral unit-dose packaging, and often central surgical supply. By choice, by expertise, and by responsibility, the pharmacist has accumulated the greatest fund of information about parenteral drugs—not only their clinical use, but also their stability, incompatibilities, methods of handling and admixture, and proper packaging. More and more, nurses and physicians are looking to the pharmacist for guidance on parenteral products.

To support the institutional pharmacist in preparing IV admixtures (which typically involves adding one or more drugs to large-volume parenteral fluids), equipment manufacturers have designed laminar flow units, electromechanical compounding units, transfer devices, and filters specifically adaptable to a variety of hospital programs.

The nurse and physician have certainly not been forgotten by manufacturers. A wide spectrum of IV and IM administration devices and aids have been made available in recent years for bedside use. Many innovative practitioners have made suggestions to industry that have resulted in product or technique improvements, particularly in IV therapy. The use of parenteral products is growing at a very significant rate in nonhospital settings, such as outpatient surgical centers and homes. The reduction in costs associated with outpatient and home care therapy, coupled with advances in drugs, dosage forms, and delivery systems, has caused a major change in the administration of parenteral products [2].

II. ROUTES OF PARENTERAL ADMINISTRATION

The major routes of parenteral administration of drugs are subcutaneous, intramuscular, and intravenous. Other more specialized routes are intrathecal, intracisternal, intra-arterial, intraspinal, intraepidural, and intradermal. The intradermal route is not typically used to achieve systemic drug effects. The major routes will be discussed separately. Definitions of the more specialized routes, along with additional information concerning needle sizes, volumes typically administered, formulation constraints, and types of medication administered, are summarized in Table 1.

A. The Subcutaneous Route

Lying immediately under the skin is a layer of fat, the superficial fascia, which lends itself to safe administration of a great variety of drugs, including vaccines, insulin, scopolamine, and epinephrine. Subcutaneous injections are usually administered in volumes up to 2 mL using a 1/2- to 1-in. 23-gauge (or smaller) needle. Care must be taken to ensure that the needle is not in a blood vessel. This is done by lightly pulling back on the syringe plunger (aspiration) before making the injection. If the needle is inadvertently located in a blood vessel, blood will appear in the syringe and the injection should not be made. The injection site may be massaged after injection to facilitate drug absorption. Drugs given by this route will have a slower onset of action than by the IM or IV routes, and total absorption may also be less.

Sometimes dextrose or electrolyte solutions are given subcutaneously in amounts from 250 to 1000 mL. This technique, called hypodermoclysis, is used when veins are unavailable or difficult to use for further medication. Irritation of the tissue is a danger with this technique. Administration of the enzyme hyaluronidase can help by increasing absorption and decreasing tissue distention. Irritating drugs and vasoconstrictors can lead to abscesses, necrosis, or inflammation when given subcutaneously. Body sites suitable for SC administration include most portions of the arms and legs plus the abdomen. When daily or frequent administration is required, the injection site can and should be continuously changed or rotated, especially by diabetic patients self-administering insulin.

B. The Intramuscular Route

The IM route of administration is second only to the IV route in rapidity of onset of systemic action. Injections are made into the striated muscle fibers that lie beneath the subcutaneous layer. The principal sites of injection are the gluteal (buttocks), deltoid (upper arm), and vastus lateralis (lateral thigh) muscles. The usual volumes injected range from 0.5 to 2.0 mL, with volumes up to 4.0 mL sometimes being given (in divided doses) in the gluteal or thigh areas (see Table 1). Again, it is important to aspirate before injecting to ensure that the drug is not administered intravenously. Needles used in administering IM injections range from 1 to 1-1/2 in. and 19 to 22 gauge, the most common being 1-1/2 in. and 22 gauge.

The major clinical problem arising from IM injections is muscle or neuron damage, the injury normally resulting from faulty technique, rather than the medication. Most injectable products can be given intramuscularly, with a normal onset of action from 15

Table 1 Parenteral Routes of Drug Administration

Routes	Usual volume (mL)	Needle commonly used	Formulation constraints	Types of medication administered
Primary parental routes				
Small-volume parenterals				
Subcutaneous	0.5–2	5/8 in., 23 gauge	Need to be isotonic	Insulin, vaccines
Intramuscular	0.5–2	1 1/2 in., 22 gauge	Can be solutions, emulsions, oils, or suspensions, isotonic preferably	Nearly all drug classes
Intravenous	1–1000	Veinpuncture 1 1/2 in., 20–22 gauge	Solutions, emulsions, and liposomes	Nearly all drug classes
Large-volume parenterals	101 and larger (infusion unit)	Venoclysis 1 1/2 in., 18–19 gauge	Solutions and some emulsions	Nearly all drug classes (see precautionary notes in text)
Other parenteral routes				
Intra-arterial: directly into an artery (immediate action sought in peripheral area)	2–20	20–22 gauge	Solutions and some emulsions	Radiopaque media, antineoplastics, antibiotics
Intrathecal (intraspinal; into spinal canal)	1–4	24–28 gauge	Must be isotonic	Local anesthetics, analgesics; neurolytic agents
Intraepidural (into epidural space near spinal column)	6–30	5 in., 16–18 gauge	Must be isotonic	Local anesthetics, narcotics, α_2-agonists, steroids
Intracisternal: directly into caudal region of the brain between the cerebellum and the medula oblongata			Must be isotonic	
Intra-articular: directly into a joint, usually for a local effect there, as for steroid anti-inflammatory action in arthritis	2–20	1.5–2 in., 18–22 gauge	Must be isotonic	Morphine, local anesthetics, steroids, NSAIDs, antibiotics
Intracardial: directly into the heart when life is threatened (epinephrine stimulation in severe heart attack)	0.2–1	5 in., 22 gauge		Cardiotonic drugs, calcium
Intrapleural: directly into the pleural cavity or a lung (also used for fluid withdrawal)	2–30	2–5 in., 16–22 gauge		Local anesthetics, narcotics, chemotherapeutic agents
Diagnostic testing				
Intradermal	0.05	1/2–5/8 in., 25–26 gauge	Should be isotonic	Diagnostic agents

to 30 minutes. As a result, there are numerous dosage forms available for this route of administration: solutions, oil-in-water (o/w) or water in-oil (w/o) emulsions, suspensions (aqueous or oily base), colloidal suspensions, and reconstitutable powders. Those product forms in which the drug is not fully dissolved generally result in slower, more gradual drug absorption, a slower onset of action, and sometimes longer-lasting drug effects.

Intramuscularly administered products typically form a "depot" in the muscle mass from which the drug is slowly absorbed. The peak drug concentration is usually seen within 1–2 hours. Factors affecting the drug-release rate from an IM depot include the compactness of the depot (the less compact and more diffuse, the faster the release), the rheology of the product, concentration and particle size of drug in the vehicle, nature of the solvent or vehicle, volume of the injection, tonicity of the product, and physical form of the product.

Needleless injector systems are sometimes used to administer drugs by either the intramuscular or subcutaneous routes. In needleless injector systems, the drug formulation is propelled by pressure from a cylinder of compressed CO_2 through an orifice, creating a thin stream of liquid that penetrates the skin. The depth of penetration is determined by the size of the orifice used, which in turn determines whether the drug is administered intramuscularly or subcutaneously. Advantages of needleless injector systems include elimination of the "fear of needles," elimination of needle-stick injuries to health care workers, and, in the case of mass immunization programs, lower cost of administration. Limitations of these systems include higher cost for patient-specific drug administration. Also, the incidence of irritation at the site of injection is somewhat higher for needleless injector administration because the formulation is dispersed to a greater extent in the tissue at the site of injection relative to bolus injection via a needle.

C. The Intravenous Route

Intravenous medication is injected directly into a vein either to obtain an extremely rapid and predictable response or to avoid irritation of other tissues. This route of administration also provides maximum availability and assurance in delivering the drug to the site of action. However, a major danger of this route of administration is that the rapidity of absorption makes effective administration of an antidote very difficult, if not impossible, in most instances. Care must often be used to avoid administering a drug too rapidly by the IV route because irritation or an excessive drug concentration at sensitive organs such as the heart and brain (drug shock) can occur. The duration of drug activity is dependent on the initial dose and the distribution, metabolism, and excretion properties (pharmacokinetics) of the drug. For most drugs, the biological half-life is independent of the initial dose because the elimination process is first order. Thus, an intravenous drug with a short half-life would not provide a sustained blood level. The usual method of administration for drugs with short half-lives is to use continuous IV drip (IV infusion). Intravenous injections (venipuncture) normally range from 1 to 1000 mL and are given with either a 19- to 20-gauge 1-in. needle, with an injection rate of 1 mL per 10 seconds for volumes up to 5 mL and 1 mL per 20 seconds for volumes over 5 mL. Only drugs in aqueous solutions, hydroalcoholic solutions, some emulsions, and liposoma formulations are to be given by the IV route.

Large proximal veins, such as those located inside the forearm, are most commonly used for IV administration. Because of the rapid dilution in the circulating blood and the general insensitivity of the venous wall to pain, the IV route may be used to administer drugs that would be too irritating to give by other routes (e.g., nitrogen mustards), provided that proper dosing procedures are employed. The risk of thrombosis is increased when extremities such as the wrist or ankle are used for injection sites or when potentially irritating IV products are used, with the risk further increasing in patients with impaired circulation.

The IV infusion of large volumes of fluids (100–1000 mL) has become increasingly popular. This technique, called *venoclysis*, utilizes products known as large-volume parenterals (LVPs). It is used to supply electrolytes and nutrients, to restore blood volume, and to prevent tissue dehydration. Various parenteral drug solutions can be conveniently added to the LVP solutions as they are being administered, or before administration, to provide continuous and prolonged drug therapy as well as to administer a dilute solution of drugs where either the drug itself or the formulation is too irritating to administer at the concentration used in the formulation provided by the manufacturer. Such drug additions to LVPs have become very common in hospitals. The combination of parenteral dosage forms for administration as a unit product is known as an IV admixture. Pharmacists practicing such IV additive product preparation must be very knowledgeable to avoid physical and chemical incompatibilities in the modified LVP, creation of therapeutic incompatibilities with other drugs, compromising sterility through breaches of aseptic technique, or addition of extraneous particulate matter.

Commonly administered LVPs include such products as Lactated Ringers Injection USP, Sodium Chloride Injection USP (0.9%), which replenish fluids and electrolytes, and Dextrose Injection USP (5%), which provides fluid plus nutrition (calories), or various combinations of dextrose and saline. In addition, numerous other nutrient and ionic solutions are available for clinical use, the most popular of which are solutions of essential amino acids or lipid emulsions. These solutions are modified to be hypertonic, isotonic, or hypotonic to aid in maintaining both fluid, nutritional, and electrolyte balance in a particular patient according to need. Indwelling needles or catheters are required in LVP administration. Care must be taken to avoid local or systemic infections or thrombophlebitis owing to faulty injection or administration technique.

IV infusions can be administered through peripheral veins, typically in the forearm, or through a central line that is surgically implanted in the subclavian vein. Another option for IV infusion that is becoming more popular is the peripherally inserted central cathether (PICC), where the catheter is fed through an incision in a peripheral vein to a large central vein near the heart. Central IV lines are commonly used for administration of very hypertonic formulations that would be excessively irritating to a peripheral vein, and for administration of *vesicants*, or drugs that are damaging to tissue. Introduction of the formulation into an area of high blood flow provides rapid dilution and minimizes irritation.

D. Other Parenteral Routes

Other more specialized parenteral routes are listed and described briefly in Table 1. The intra-arterial route involves injecting a drug directly into an artery. This technique is not simple and may require a surgical procedure to reach the artery. It is important that the artery not be missed, since serious nerve damage can occur to the nerves lying close to arteries. Doses given by this route should be minimal and given gradually, since, once injected, the drug effect cannot be neutralized. As shown in Table 1, the intra-arterial route is used to administer radiopaque contrast media for viewing an organ, such as the heart or kidney, or to perfuse an antineoplastic agent at the highest possible concentration to the target organ.

The intrathecal route is employed to administer a drug directly into the cerebrospinal fluid at any level of the cerebrospinal axis. This route is used when it is not possible to achieve sufficiently high plasma levels to accomplish adequate diffusion and penetration into the cerebrospinal fluid. This is not the same route used to achieve spinal anesthesia, for which the drug is injected within the dural membrane surrounding the spinal cord, or in extradural or epidural anesthesia (caudal or sacral anesthesia), for which the drug is deposited outside the dural membrane and within the body spinal caudal canals. Parenteral products administered by the intrathecal, intraspinal, and intracisternal routes must be formulated at physiological pH, must be isotonic and must not contain antimicrobial preservatives in order to minimize the probability of nerve damage.

Intradermal (ID) administration involves injection into the skin layer. This route is largely limited to injection of materials to detect hypersensitivity reactions for diagnostic purposes. It is important that the product per se be nonirritating. Volumes are normally given at 0.05 mL/dose, and the solutions are isotonic. Intradermal medication is usually administered with a 1/2- or 5/8-in., 25- or 26-gauge needle, inserted at an angle nearly parallel to the skin surface. Absorption is slow and limited from this site since the blood vessels are extremely small, even though the area is highly vascular. The site should not be massaged after the injection of allergy test materials. Skin testing includes not only allergens, such as pollens or dust, but also microorganisms, as in the tuberculin or histoplasmin skin tests.

III. SPECIALIZED LARGE-VOLUME PARENTERAL AND STERILE SOLUTIONS

Large-volume parenterals designed to provide fluid (water), calories (dextrose solutions), electrolytes (saline solutions), or combinations of these materials have been described. Several other specialized LVP and sterile solutions are also used in medicine and will be described here, even though two product classes (peritoneal dialysis and irrigating solutions) are not parenteral products.

A. Hyperalimentation Solutions

Parenteral hyperalimentation involves administration of large amounts of nutrients (e.g., carbohydrates, amino acids, lipids, and vitamins) to maintain a patient who is unable to take food orally for several weeks at caloric intake levels of 4000 kcal/day or more. Earlier methods of parenteral alimentation, which involved IV administration of nutrients through a peripheral vein, were not typically able to maintain patients without a weight loss and gradual deterioration in physical condition because, in order to administer sufficient calories at acceptable volumetric flow rates, the infusion solution must be hypertonic. Development of the technique of subclavian vein cannulation in the early 1950s paved the way for effective parenteral nutrition, since the infused fluid is rapidly diluted by the high blood flow in the subclavian vein. Hyperalimentation formulations commonly consist of mixtures of dextrose, amino acids, and lipids (usually soybean oil, safflower oil, or mixtures of the two) containing added electrolytes, trace metals, and vitamins. The method permits administration of life-saving or life-sustaining nutrients to comatose patients or to patients undergoing treatment for esophageal obstruction, GI diseases (including cancer), ulcerative colitis, and other disease states. As general perioperative support, parenteral nutrition is generally indicated whenever a patient is to take nothing by mouth for periods of 5 days or longer.

B. Cardioplegia Solutions

Cardioplegia solutions are large-volume parenteral solutions used in heart surgery to help prevent ischemic injury to the myocardium during the time the blood supply to the heart is clamped off and during reperfusion, as well as to maintain a bloodless operating field and to make the myocardium flaccid. Cardioplegia solutions are typically electrolyte solutions where the electrolyte composition is intended to maintain diastolic arrest. These solutions are usually admixed by pharmacists in a hospital IV admixture program and are administered cold in order to cool the myocardium and minimize metabolic activity. Cardioplegia solutions are usually slightly alkaline and hypertonic in order to compensate for metabolic acidosis and to minimize reperfusion injury resulting from tissue edema.

C. Peritoneal Dialysis Solutions

The sterile peritoneal dialysis solutions are infused continuously into the abdominal cavity, bathing the peritoneum, and are then continuously withdrawn. The purpose of peritoneal dialysis is to remove toxic substances from the body or to aid and accelerate the excretion function normal to the kidneys. The process is employed to counteract some forms of drug or chemical toxicity as well as to treat acute renal insufficiency. Peritoneal dialysis solutions contain glucose and have an ionic content similar to normal extracellular fluid. Toxins and metabolites diffuse into the circulating dialysis fluid through the peritoneum and are removed. At the same time, excess fluid is removed from the patient if the glucose content renders the dialysis solution hyperosmotic. An antibiotic is often added to these solutions as a prophylactic measure.

D. Irrigating Solutions

Irrigating solutions are intended to irrigate, flush, and aid in cleansing body cavities and wounds. Although certain IV solutions, such as normal saline, may be used as irrigating solutions, solutions designed as irrigating solutions should not be used parenterally. Since irrigating solutions used in treatment of serious wounds infuse into the bloodstream to some degree, they must be sterile, pyrogen-free, and made and handled with the same care as parenteral solutions.

IV. FORMULATION OF PARENTERAL PRODUCTS

A successful therapeutic response following parenteral administration of a drug requires an adequate concentration of drug at the site of action. The intravenous route is characterized by the absence of an absorption step, and a major consideration in formulation of drugs for intravenous administration is assuring adequate solubility of the drug in the solution administered, while minimizing the probability of precipitation of the drug at the site of injection. Intramuscular and subcutaneous administration, however, requires absorption of the drug from the site of injection. This absorption process is determined by physicochemical properties of the drug, the formulation used, and physiological factors such as extent of vascularity at the site of injection, distribution of fat in the tissue, amount of exercise, and condition of the tissue. With an IM suspension, drug dissolution is usually the rate-limiting step in the absorption of the drug at the injection site [3]. The absorption of the drug following IM administration is greatly influenced by the physicochemical properties of the drug.

A. The Active Drug

A thorough evaluation of properties of the active drug or drugs is essential in developing a stable and safe parenteral dosage form. The physical and chemical factors that may significantly affect the development of a parenteral dosage form are discussed in Chapter 7 and by Motola and Agharkar [4]. Important properties include solubility and rate of solution. The most important factor affecting dissolution is the aqueous solubility of the drug itself [5], but other factors that can be important are the physical state of the drug (i.e., crystalline or amorphous), particle size, and perhaps formulation pH.

Crystal Characteristics

Many dry solid parenteral products, such as the cephalosporins, are prepared by sterile crystallization techniques. Control of the crystallization process to obtain a consistent and uniform crystal form, habit, density, and size distribution is particularly critical for drug substances to be utilized in sterile suspensions. For example, when the crystallization process for sterile ceftazidime pentahydrate was modified to increase the density and reduce the volume of the fill dose, the rate of dissolution increased significantly.

To obtain a uniform product from lot to lot, strict adherence to the procedures developed for a particular crystallization must be followed, including control of pH, rates of addition, solvent concentrations and purity, temperature, and mixing rates. Each crystallization procedure has to be designed to ensure sterility and minimize particulate contamination. Changes, such as using absolute ethyl alcohol instead of 95% ethanol during the washing procedure, can destroy the crystalline structure if the material being crystallized is a hydrate structure.

Drugs that associate with water to produce crystalline forms are called hydrates. Water content of the hydrate forms of sodium cefazolin as a function of relative humidity is seen in Fig. 1. As shown in Fig. 1, the sesquihydrate is the most stable structure when exposed to extreme humidity conditions [6]. This figure also shows the importance of choosing the proper combination of hydrate and humidity conditions when designing a manufacturing process or facility.

Chemical Modification of the Drug

Improvement of the properties of a drug may be achieved by the chemical modification of the parent drug. The preparation of an ester, salt, or other modification of the parent structure may be employed with parenteral drugs to increase stability, alter drug solubility, enhance depot action, avoid formulation

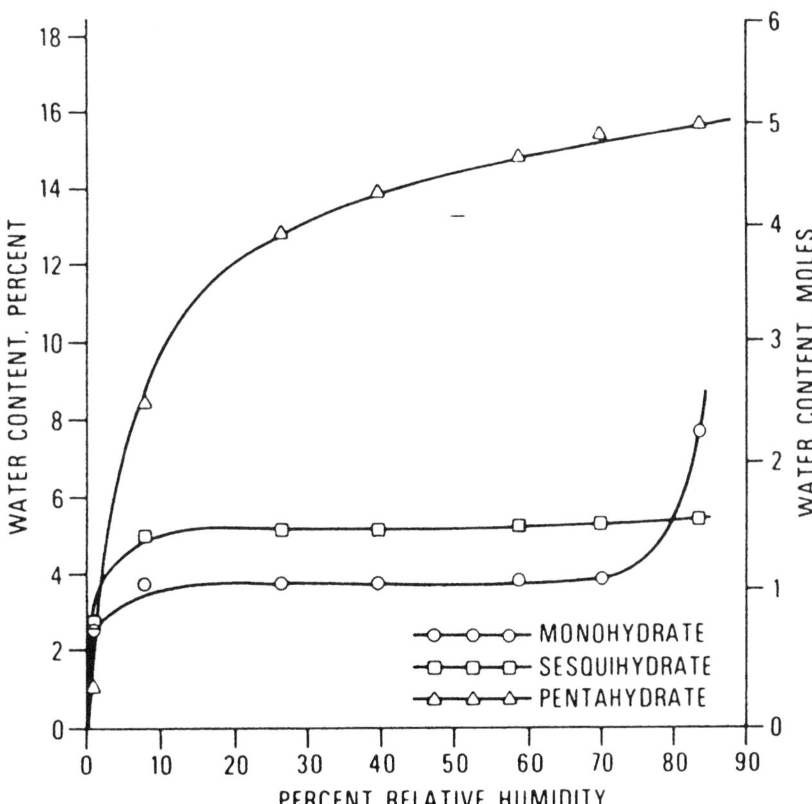

Fig. 1 Water content versus relative humidity for hydrate forms of sodium cefazolin.

difficulties, and, possibly, to decrease pain on injection. The modified drug that converts back to the active parent structure is defined as a prodrug. This conversion usually occurs within the body system or, for some drugs that are formulated as dry powders, occurs on reconstitution. The preparation of prodrugs is becoming a common practice with many types of drugs. Examples of antibiotic prodrugs include benzathine penicillin, procaine penicillin, metronidazole phosphate, and chloramphenicol sodium succinate. Prodrugs are also common for injectable steroids such as methylprednisolone (formulated as methylprednisolone sodium succinate) and hydrocortisone (formulated as hydrocortisone sodium succinate).

The preparation of salts of organic compounds is one of the most important tools available to the formulator. Compounds for both IM and IV solutions may require high solubility in order for the drug to be incorporated into acceptable volumes for bolus administration (see Table 1). Sodium and potassium salts of weak acids and hydrochloride and sulfate salts of weak bases are widely used in parenterals requiring highly soluble compounds, based on their overall safety and history of clinical acceptance.

If the solubility of a drug is to be reduced to enhance stability or to prepare a suspension, the formulator may prepare water-insoluble salts. A classic example is procaine penicillin G, the decreased solubility (7 mg/mL) of which, when compared with the very soluble penicillin G potassium, is utilized to prepare stable parenteral suspensions. Another alternative to preparing an insoluble drug is to use the parent acidic or basic drug and to buffer the pH of the suspension in the range of minimum solubility.

Polymorphism

The literature lists numerous examples of polymorphism; i.e., the existence of several crystal forms of a given chemical that exhibit different physical properties [7]. The conversion of one polymorph to another may cause a significant change in the physical properties of the drug and in critical quality attributes of drug products.

Studies of polymorphs in recent years have pointed out the effects of polymorphism on solubility and, more specifically, on dissolution rates. The aspect of polymorphism that is of particular concern to the parenteral formulator is physical stability of the product [8]. Substances that form polymorphs must be evaluated so that the form used is stable in a particular solvent system. Physical stresses that occur during suspension manufacture may also give rise to changes in crystal form [9].

pH and pK

Profiles of pH versus solubility and pH versus stability are needed for solution and suspension formulations to help assure physical and chemical stability as well as to maximize or minimize solubility. This information is also valuable for predicting the compatibility of drugs with various infusion fluids.

In summary, the physical and chemical data that should be obtained on the drug substance include the following:

Molecular structure and weight
Melting point
Thermal profile
Particle size and shape
Hygroscopicity potential
Ionization constant
Light stability
Optical activity
pH solubility profile
pH stability profile
Polymorphism potential
Solvate formation

B. Added Substances (Excipients) in Parenteral Formulations

To provide efficacious and safe parenteral dosage forms, added substances must frequently be incorporated into the formula to maintain pharmaceutical stability, control product attributes, ensure sterility, or aid in parenteral administration. These substances include antioxidants, antimicrobial agents, buffers, bulking materials, chelating agents, inert gases, solubilizing agents, and protectants. In parenteral product development work, any additive to a formulation must be justified by a clear purpose and function. In addition, every attempt should be made to choose added substances that are accepted by regulatory agencies throughout the world, since most pharmaceutical development is international in scope. Because of the extensive pharmacological and toxicological data required to obtain approval for any new additive, most formulators continue to depend on materials already used in marketed parenteral products.

Some of the most commonly used added substances are listed in Table 2. Pharmacists involved in IV admixture programs must be aware of the types of additives that may be present in the products being combined, since the source of incompatibility between different drugs mixed in solution may be the excipients present. For example, drug formulations containing

Table 2 Classes and Examples of Parenteral Additives

Additive class	Examples	Usual concentration (%)
Antimicrobials	Benzalkonium chloride	0.01
	Benzyl alcohol	1–2
	Chlorobutanol	0.25–0.5
	Metacresol	0.1–0.3
	Butyl *p*-hydroxybenzoate	0.015
	Methyl *p*-hydroxybenzoate	0.1–0.2
	Propyl *p*-hydroxybenzoate	0.2
	Phenol	0.25–0.5
	Thimerosal	0.01
Antioxidants	Ascorbic acid	0.01–0.05
	Cysteine	0.1–0.5
	Monothioglycerol	0.1–1.0
	Sodium bisulfite	0.1–1.0
	Sodium metabisulfite	0.1–1.0
	Tocopherols	0.05–0.5
Buffers	Acetates	1–2
	Citrates	1–5
	Phosphates	0.8–2.0
Bulking Agents	Lactose	1–8
	Mannitol	1–10
	Sorbitol	1–10
	Glycine	1–2
Chelating Agents	Salts of ethylenediaminetetraacetic acid	0.01–0.05
Protectants	Sucrose	2–5
	Glucose	2–5
	Lactose	2–5
	Maltose	2–5
	Trehalose	2–5
	Human serum albumin	0.1–1.0
Solubilizing Agents	Ethyl alcohol	1–50
	Glycerin	1–50
	Polyethylene glycol	1–50
	Propylene glycol	1–50
	Lecithin	0.5–2.0
Surfactants	Polyoxyethylene	0.1–0.5
	Sorbitan monooleate	0.05–0.25
Tonicity-adjusting agents	Dextrose	4–5
	Sodium chloride	0.5–0.9

the preservative benzalkonium chloride, which is positively charged, are commonly incompatible with products containing anionic drugs and excipients.

Antioxidants

Salts of sulfur dioxide, including bisulfite, metasulfite, and sulfite, are the most common antioxidants used in aqueous parenterals. These antioxidants maintain product stability by being preferentially oxidized and gradually consumed over the shelf life of the product. Irrespective of which salt is added to the solution, the antioxidant moiety depends on the final concentration of the thio compound and the final pH of the formulation [10]. While undergoing oxidation reactions, sulfites may be converted to sulfates and other species. Sulfites can also react with certain drug molecules (e.g., epinephrine).

Sulfite levels are determined by the reactivity of the drug, the type of container, single- or multiple-dose use, container headspace, use of inert gas purge, and the expiration dating period to be employed. Upper limits for sulfite levels are specified in most pharmacopeias. Allowances on upper limits are made for concentrated drugs that are diluted extensively before use.

Sulfites have been reported to cause allergic reactions in some asthmatics. If possible, alternative antioxidants should be considered or the product should be manufactured and packaged in a manner such as to eliminate or minimize the concentration of bisulfite required. Deoxygenation of the makeup water, maintaining the solution under a nitrogen atmosphere throughout the manufacturing process, and purging the filled vials with an inert gas may significantly reduce the amount of antioxidant required.

Antimicrobial Agents

A suitable preservative system is required in all multiple-dose parenteral products to inhibit the growth of microorganisms accidentally introduced during withdrawal of individual doses. Preservatives may be added to single-dose parenteral products that are not terminally sterilized as a sterility assurance measure; i.e., to prevent growth of any microorganisms that could be introduced if there were any inadvertent breach of asepsis during filling operations. However, the inclusion of a preservative in single-dose parenteral products must be weighed against the need to develop formulations that are acceptable to regulatory bodies worldwide. Inclusion of a preservative can be a difficult challenge, given the wide range of viewpoints concerning which preservatives are acceptable and when it is appropriate to include them in a formulation. Partly because of this, there is a trend in parenteral product development to eliminate preservatives wherever it is practical to do so. This may require added measures in manufacturing to improve sterility assurance, such as using barrier technology to provide positive separation of personnel from product during aseptic filling and transfer steps.

The formulation scientist must be aware of interactions between preservatives and other components of a formulation that could compromise the efficacy of the preservative. For example, proteins can bind thimerosal, reducing preservative efficacy. Partitioning of preservative into a micellar phase or an oil phase (in an emulsion) can also reduce the effective concentration of preservative available for bactericidal or bacteriostatic action. Preservative efficacy testing should be done on the proposed formulation to assure an effective preservative concentration.

Several investigators have published research on incompatibilities of preservatives with rubber closures and other packaging components, particularly polymeric materials [11]. Again, challenging the product with selected microorganisms to measure bacteriostatic or bactericidal activity is necessary, including evaluation of efficacy as a function of time throughout the anticipated shelf life of the product.

More subtle effects of preservatives on injectable formulations are possible. Formulation of insulin is an illustrative case study. Insulin is usually formulated as a multiple-dose vial, since individual dosage varies among patients. Preservation of zinc insulin with phenol causes physical instability of the suspension, whereas methylparaben does not. However, the presence of phenol is required for obtaining protamine insulin crystals [9].

Buffers

Many drugs require a certain pH range to maintain product stability. As discussed previously, drug solubility may also be strongly dependent on the pH of the solution. An important aid to the formulator is the information contained in a graph of the solubility profile of the drug as a function of pH (Fig. 2). The

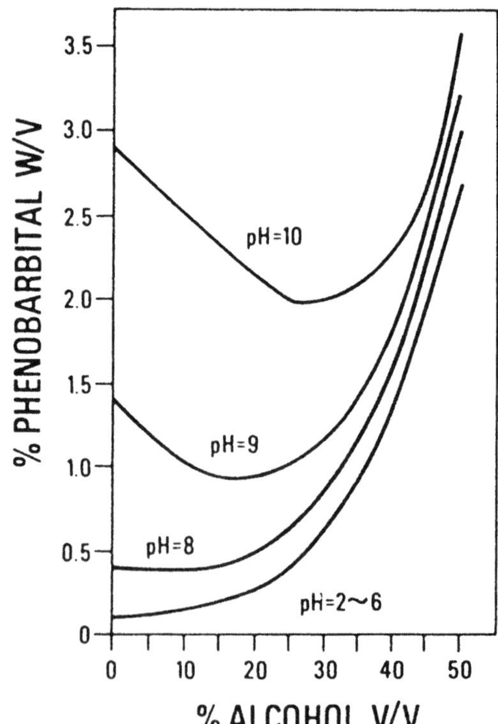

Fig. 2 Solubility of phenobarbital as a function of pH and alcohol concentration. (From Ref. 5).

product can then be buffered to approach maximum or minimum solubility, whichever is desired.

Parenteral products should be formulated to possess sufficient buffer capacity to maintain proper product pH. Factors that influence pH include product degradation, container and stopper effects, diffusion of gases through the closure, and the effect of gases in the product or in the headspace. However, the buffer capacity of a formulation must be readily overcome by the biological fluids; thus, the concentration and ratios of buffer ingredients must be carefully selected.

Buffer systems for parenterals consist of either a weak base and the salt of a weak base or a weak acid and the salt of a weak acid. Buffer systems commonly used for injectable products are acetates, citrates, and phosphates (see Table 2). Amino acids are being increasingly used as buffers, especially for polypeptide injectables.

Chelating Agents

Chelating agents are added to complex and, thereby, inactivate metals such as copper, iron, and zinc that generally catalyze oxidative degradation of drug molecules. Sources of metal contamination include raw material impurities; solvents, such as water, rubber stoppers, and containers; and equipment employed in the manufacturing process [12]. The most widely used chelating agents are edetate disodium derivatives and salts. Citric and tartaric acids are also employed as chelating agents.

Inert Gases

Another means of enhancing the product integrity of oxygen-sensitive medicaments is by displacing the air in the solution with nitrogen or argon. This technique may be made more effective by first purging with nitrogen or boiling the water to reduce dissolved oxygen. The container is also purged with nitrogen or argon before filling and may also be topped off with the gas before sealing.

Glass-seal ampoules provide the most impervious barrier for gas transmission. A butyl rubber stock is used with rubber-stoppered products that are sensitive to oxygen because it provides better resistance to gas permeation than other rubber stocks.

Solubilizing Agents and Surfactants

Drug solubility can be increased by the use of solubilizing agents, such as those listed in Table 2, and by nonaqueous solvents or mixed solvent systems, to be discussed shortly. When using solubilizing agents, the formulator must consider their effect on the safety and stability of the drug.

A surfactant is a surface-active agent that is used to disperse a water-insoluble drug as a colloidal dispersion. Surfactants are used for wetting and to prevent crystal growth in a suspension. Surfactants are used quite extensively in parenteral suspensions for wetting powders and to provide acceptable syringability. They are also used in emulsions and for solubilizing steroids and fat-soluble vitamins.

Tonicity Adjustment Agents

It is important that injectable solutions that are to be given intravenously are isotonic, or nearly so. Because of osmotic pressure changes and the resultant exchange of ionic species across red blood cell membranes, nonisotonic solutions, particularly if given in quantities larger than 100 mL, can cause hemolysis or crenation of red blood cells (owing to hypotonic or hypertonic solutions, respectively). Dextrose, sodium chloride, or potassium chloride is commonly used to achieve isotonicity in a parenteral formula.

Protectants

A protectant is a substance that is added to a formulation to protect against loss of activity caused by some stress that is introduced by the manufacturing process or to prevent loss of active ingredients by adsorption to process equipment or to primary packaging materials. Protectants are used primarily in protein formulations, liposomal formulations, and vaccines. For example, cryoprotectants and lyoprotectants are used to inhibit loss of integrity of the active substance resulting from freezing and drying, respectively. Compounds that provide cryoprotection are not necessarily the same as those that provide lyoprotection. Polyethylene glycol protects lactate dehydrogenase and phosphofructokinase from damage by freezing, but does not protect either protein from damage by freeze-drying. Compounds such as sucrose and trehalose are effective lyoprotectants for both proteins [13]. Effective cryo- and lyoprotectants must be determined on a case-by-case basis, but sugars and polyhydroxy compounds are usually the best candidate compounds. These same types of compounds also tend to markedly improve the stability of proteins against inactivation by thermal denaturation.

Another type of protectant is used to prevent loss of active substance—again, usually a protein and usually present at a very low concentration—by adsorption to materials or equipment in the manufacturing process or to components of the primary package. In manufacturing, particular attention should be given to adsorption of the active entity to filters (especially nylon) and to silicone tubing used for transfer operations. For packaging materials, rubber closures and other polymeric materials should be examined carefully for adsorptive potential. The same consideration applies to infusion equipment, particularly considering that most materials in modern IV infusion therapy—plastic bags, infusion sets, and in-line filters—are polymeric.

Human serum albumin (HSA) may be used as a protectant against adsorptive loss of proteins present at low concentrations. HSA is present at higher concentration than the active substance and is preferentially adsorbed, coating the surface of interest and preventing adsorption of the drug. For example, insulin is subject to adsorptive loss to hydrophobic materials. Addition of 0.1–1.0% HSA has been reported to prevent this adsorptive loss [9].

C. Vehicles

Aqueous Vehicles

Water for injection (WFI) is the most widely used solvent for parenteral preparations. The USP requirements for WFI and purified water have been recently updated to replace the traditional wet and colorimetric analytical methods with the more modern and cost-effective methods of conductivity and total organic carbon. Water for injection must be prepared and stored in a manner to ensure purity and freedom from pyrogens. The most common means of obtaining WFI is by the distillation of deionized water. This is the only method of preparation permitted by the European Pharmacopoeia (EP). In contrast, the USP and the Japanese Pharmacopeias also permit reverse osmosis to be used. The USP has also recently broadened its definition of source water to include not only the U.S. Environmental Protection Agency National Primary Drinking Water Standards, but also comparable regulations of the European Union or Japan.

Microorganisms, dissolved organic and inorganic substances, and foreign particles are the most common contaminants found in water. Inorganic compounds are commonly removed by distillation, reverse osmosis, deionization, or a combination of these processes. Membrane and depth filters are used to remove particulate contaminants, and charcoal beds may be used to remove organic materials. Filtration, chilling or heating, or recirculation of water are used to reduce microbial growth and to prevent pyrogen formation that will occur in a static deionization system. To inhibit microbial growth, WFI must be stored at either 5 or 60–90°C if it is to be held for over 24 hours.

The USP also lists Sterile Water for Injection and Bacteriostatic Water for Injection, which, unlike WFI, must be sterile. Higher levels of solids are allowed in these vehicles because of the possible leaching of glass constituents into the product during high-temperature sterilization and subsequent storage. Bacteriostatic Water for Injection USP must not be placed in containers larger than 30 mL. This is to prevent the administration of large quantities of bacteriostatic agents (such as phenol) that could become toxic if large volumes of solution were administered. Other aqueous vehicles that may be used in place of sterile water for injection or bacteriostatic water for injection for reconstitution or administering drugs include dextrose (5%), sodium chloride (0.9%), and a variety of other electrolyte and nutrient solutions, as noted earlier.

Nonaqueous and Mixed Vehicles

A nonaqueous solvent or a mixed aqueous/nonaqueous solvent system may be necessary to stabilize drugs, such as the barbiturates, that are readily hydrolyzed by water, or to improve solubility (e.g., digitoxin). Nonaqueous solvents must be carefully screened and tested to ensure that they exhibit no pharmacological action, are nontoxic and nonirritating, and are compatible and stable with all ingredients of a formulation.

A major class of nonaqueous solvents is the fixed oils. The USP [1] recognizes the use of fixed oils as parenteral vehicles and lists their requirements. The most commonly used oils are corn oil, cottonseed oil, peanut oil, and sesame oil. Because fixed oils can be quite irritating when injected and may cause sensitivity reactions in some patients, the oil used in the product must be stated on the label.

Sesame oil is the preferred oil for most of the official injections in oil. This is because it is the most stable (except in light) and, thus, will usually meet the official requirements. Fixed oils must never be administered intravenously and are, in fact, restricted to IM use.

The USP usually does not specify an oil, but states that a suitable vegetable oil can be used. The main use of such oils is with the steroids, with which they yield products that produce a sustained-release effect. Sesame oil has also been used to obtain slow release of fluphenazine esters given intramuscularly [14]. Excessive unsaturation of an oil can produce tissue irritation. The use of injections in oil has diminished somewhat in preference to aqueous suspensions, which generally have less irritating and sensitizing properties. Benzyl benzoate may be used to enhance steroid solubility in oils if desired.

Water-miscible solvents are widely used in parenterals to enhance drug solubility and to serve as stabilizers. The more common solvents include glycerin, ethyl alcohol, propylene glycol, and polyethylene glycol 300. Examples of injectable products formulated with nonaqueous solvents are Diazepam Injection USP and Phenytoin Sodium USP. Mixed-solvent systems do not exhibit many of the disadvantages observed with the fixed oils, but may also be irritating or increase toxicity, especially when present in large amounts or in high concentrations. A solution containing a high percentage of ethanol will produce pain on injection.

The formulator should be aware of the potential of nonaqueous solvents in preparing a solubilized or stable product that may not have been otherwise possible. The reader is directed to comprehensive reviews of nonaqueous solvents for additional information [15,16].

D. Parenteral Dosage Forms

Solutions

Most injectable products are solutions. Solutions of drugs suitable for parenteral administration are referred to as *injections*. Although usually aqueous, they may be mixtures of water with glycols, alcohol, or other nonaqueous solvents. Many injectable solutions are manufactured by dissolving the drug and any excipients, adjusting the pH, sterile filtering the resultant solution through a 0.22 μm membrane filter and, when possible, autoclaving the final product. Most solutions have a viscosity and surface tension very similar to water, although streptomycin sulfate injection and ascorbic acid injection, for example, are quite viscous.

Sterile filtration, with subsequent aseptic filling, is common because of the heat sensitivity of many drugs. Those drug solutions that can withstand heat should be terminally autoclave sterilized after filling, since this best assures product sterility.

Large-volume parenterals (LVPs) and small-volume parenterals (SVPs) containing no antimicrobial agent should be terminally sterilized. It is common practice to include an antimicrobial agent in SVPs that cannot be terminally sterilized or are intended for multiple-dose use. The general exceptions are products that pass the USP Antimicrobial Preservative Effectiveness Test [1] because of the antimicrobial activity of the active ingredient, vehicle, pH, or a combination of these. For example, some barbiturate products have a pH of 9–10 and a vehicle that includes propylene glycol and ethanol.

Injections and infusion fluids must be manufactured in a manner that will minimize or eliminate extraneous particulate matter. Parenteral solutions are generally filtered through 0.22 μm membrane filters to achieve sterility and remove particulate matter. Prefiltration through a coarser filter is often necessary to maintain adequate flow rates, or to prevent clogging of the filters during large-scale manufacturing. A talc or carbon filtration aid (or other filter aids) may also be necessary. If talc is used, it should be pretreated with a dilute acid solution to remove surface alkali and metals.

The formulator must be aware of the potential for binding when filtering protein solutions. Because of the cost of most protein materials, a membrane should be used that minimizes protein adsorption to the membrane surface. Typical filter media that minimize this binding include hydrophilic polyvinylidene difluoride and hydroxyl-modified hydrophilic polyamide membranes [17a]. Filter suppliers will evaluate the compatibility of the drug product with their membrane media and also validate bacterial retention of the selected membrane.

The total fluid volume that must be filled into a unit parenteral container is typically greater than the volume that would contain the exact labeled dose. The fill volume is dependent on the viscosity of the solution and the retention of the solution by the container and stopper. The USP provides a procedure for calculating the fill dose that is necessary to ensure the delivery of the stated dose. It also provides a table of excess volumes that are usually sufficient to permit withdrawal and administration of the labeled volume.

Suspensions

One of the most difficult parenteral dosage forms to formulate is a suspension. It requires a delicate balance of variables to formulate a product that is easily resuspended and can be ejected through an 18- to 21-gauge needle through its shelf life. To achieve these properties it is necessary to select and carefully maintain particle size distribution, zeta potential, and rheological properties, as well as the manufacturing steps that control wettability and surface tension. The requirements for, limitations in, and differences between the design of injectable suspensions and other suspensions have been previously summarized [17b, 18,19].

A formula for an injectable suspension might consist of the active ingredient suspended in an aqueous vehicle containing an antimicrobial preservative, a surfactant for wetting, a dispersing or suspending agent, and perhaps a buffer or salt.

Two basic methods are used to prepare parenteral suspensions: (a) sterile vehicle and powder are combined aseptically, or (b) sterile solutions are combined and the crystals formed in situ. Examples of these procedures may be illustrated using Penicillin G Procaine Injectable Suspension USP and Sterile Testosterone Injectable Suspension USP.

In the first example, procaine penicillin, an aqueous vehicle containing the soluble components (such as lecithin, sodium citrate, povidone, and polyoxyethylene sorbitan monooleate) is filtered through a 0.22 μm membrane filter, heat sterilized, and transferred into a presterilized mixing-filling tank. The sterile antibiotic powder, which has previously been produced by freeze-drying, sterile crystallization, or spray-drying, is aseptically added to the sterile solution while mixing. After all tests have been completed on the bulk formulation, it is aseptically filled.

An example of the second method of parenteral suspension preparation is testosterone suspension. Here, the vehicle is prepared and sterile-filtered. The testosterone is dissolved separately in acetone and sterile-filtered. The testosterone-acetone solution is aseptically added to the sterile vehicle, causing the testosterone to crystallize. The resulting suspension is then diluted with sterile vehicle, mixed, the crystals allowed to settle, and the supernatant solution siphoned off. This procedure is repeated several times until all the acetone has been removed. The suspension is then brought to volume and filled in the normal manner.

The critical nature of the flow properties of parenteral suspensions becomes apparent when one remembers that these products are frequently administered through 1-in. or longer needles having internal diameters in the range of only 300–600 μm. In addition, microscopic examination shows a very rough interior needle surface, further hindering flow. The flow properties of parenteral suspensions are usually characterized on the basis of *syringeability* or injectability. The term syringeability refers to the handling characteristics of a suspension while drawing it into and manipulating it in a syringe. Syringeability includes characteristics such as ease of withdrawal from the container into the syringe, clogging and foaming tendencies, and accuracy of dose measurement. The term *injectability* refers to the properties of the suspension during injection; it includes such factors as pressure or force required for injection, evenness of flow, aspiration qualities, and freedom from clogging. The syringeability and injectability characteristics of a suspension are closely related to viscosity and to particle characteristics.

Emulsions

An emulsion is a dispersion of one immiscible liquid in another. This inherently unstable system is made possible through the use of an emulsifying agent, which prevents coalescence of the dispersed droplets. Parenteral emulsions have been used for several purposes, including (a) water-in-oil emulsions of allergenic extracts (given subcutaneously) and (b) oil-in-water sustained-release depot preparations (given intramuscularly). Formulation options are severely restricted through a very limited selection of stabilizers and emulsifiers, primarily owing to the dual constraints of autoclave sterilization and parenteral injection. Additionally, unwanted physiological effects (e.g., pyrogenic reaction and hemolysis) have further limited the use of intravenous emulsions.

An increasingly popular class of intravenous emulsions is lipid emulsions. These preparations have been available in Europe and the United States for over 25 years. Fat is transported in the bloodstream as small droplets called chylomicra. Chylomicra are 0.5 to 1.0 μm spheres consisting of a central core of triglycerides and an outer layer of phospholipids. Intravenous fat emulsions usually contain 10% oil, although they may range up to 20% (Table 3). These emulsions yield triglycerides that provide essential fatty acids and calories during total parenteral nutrition of patients who are unable to absorb nutrients through the gastrointestinal tract. The products commercially available in the United States range from 0.1 to 0.5 μm and have a pH of 5.5–8 (blood plasma has a pH of 7.4). Glycerol is commonly added to make the product isotonic. Intravenous lipid emulsions are usually administered in combination with dextrose and amino acids. Drugs are generally not added to these admixtures, with common exceptions being heparin, insulin, and ranitidine.

Dry Powders

Many drugs are too unstable—either physically or chemically—in an aqueous medium to allow formulation as a solution, suspension, or emulsion. Instead, the drug is formulated as a dry powder

Table 3 Intravenous Fat Emulsions Composition in % (w/v)

Component (g/100 mL)	Intralipid[a]		Liposyn II[b]		Infonutrol[c]		Lipofundin[d]	Liphysan[e]	
	10%	20%	10%	20%	10%	20%	10%	10%	15%
Soybean oil	10	20	5	10					
Safflower oil			5	10					
Cottonseed oil					15		10	10	15
Egg phospholipids	1.2	1.2	1.2	1.2					
Soybean phospholipids					1.2		1.2		
Soybean lecithin								1.5	2
Glycerol	2.25	2.25	2.25	2.25					
Glucose					4				
Sorbitol							5	5	5
Pluronic F-68					0.3				
DL-α-tocopherol								0.05	0.05
Water for injection, q.s.	100 ml		100 ml		100 ml		100 ml	100 ml	

[a]Kabi-Vitrum A.G., Stockolm, Sweden
[b]Abbott Laboratories, North Chicago, IL
[c]Astra-Hewlett, Sodertaye, Sweden
[d]Braun, Melsunger, West Germany
[e]Egic, L' Equilibre Biologique S.A., Loiret, France

that is reconstituted by addition of water before administration. The reconstituted product is usually an aqueous solution; however, occasionally it may be an aqueous suspension (e.g., ampicillin trihydrate and spectinomycin hydrochloride are sterile powders that are reconstituted to form a sterile suspension).

Dry powders for reconstitution as an injectable product may be produced by several methods: filling the product into vials as a liquid and freeze-drying, aseptic crystallization followed by powder filling, and spray-drying followed by powder filling. A brief discussion of each follows.

Freeze-Drying. The most common form of sterile powder is a *freeze-dried*, or *lyophilized*, powder. The advantages of freeze-drying are that (a) water can be removed at low temperature, avoiding damage to heat-sensitive materials; (b) if freeze-drying is done properly, the dried product has a high specific surface area, which facilitates rapid, complete rehydration (or "reconstitution") of the solid; and (c) from an operations point of view, freeze-dried dosage forms allow drug to be filled into vials as a solution. This makes control of the quantity filled into each vial more precise than filling drug into vials as a powder. In addition, since drug is filled as a solution, there is minimal concern with dust containment, cross-contamination, and potential worker exposure to hazardous drugs.

Despite the advantages of freeze-drying, some limitations must be kept in mind.

1. Some drugs, particularly biological systems such as proteins, liposomal systems, and vaccines, are damaged by freezing, freeze-drying, or both. Although the damage can often be minimized by using protective agents in the formulation, the problem is still substantial.
2. Often the stability of a drug in the solid state depends on its physical state (i.e., crystalline or amorphous [8]). If freeze-drying produces an amorphous solid and the amorphous form is not stable, then freeze-drying will not provide an acceptable product.
3. Freeze-drying is a relatively expensive drying operation. Although this is not an issue for many high-cost drug products, it can be an issue for more cost-sensitive products.

In freeze-drying, a solution is filled into vials, a special slotted stopper is partially inserted into the neck of the vial (Fig. 3), and trays of filled vials are transferred to the freeze-dryer. The solution is frozen by circulation of a fluid, such as silicone oil, at a temperature in the range of −35 to about −45°C through internal channels in the shelf assembly. When the product has solidified sufficiently, the pressure in the freeze-dry chamber is reduced to a pressure less that the vapor pressure of ice at the temperature of the product, and heat is applied to the

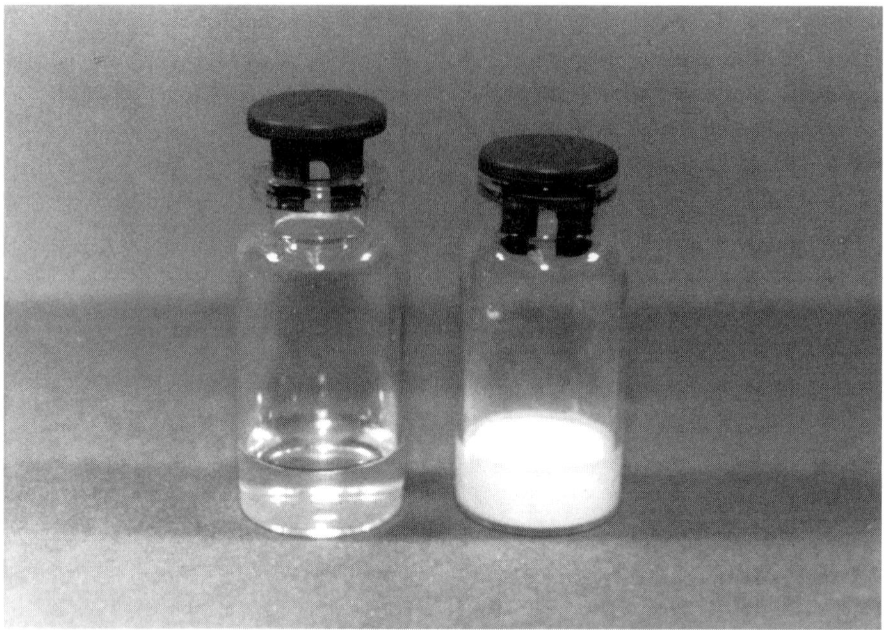

Fig. 3 Vials typically used for lyophilization showing slotted stopper in the open and closed positions.

product by increasing the temperature of the circulating fluid. Under these conditions, water is removed by sublimation of ice, or a phase change from the solid state directly to the vapor state without the appearance of an intermediate liquid phase. The phase diagram in Fig. 4 illustrates the difference between freeze-drying and conventional drying methods, during which drying takes place by a phase change from the liquid state to the vapor state. Freeze-drying takes place below the triple point of water, at which solid, liquid, and vapor all co-exist in equilibrium. As freeze-drying proceeds, a receding boundary can be observed in the vial as the thickness of the frozen layer decreases. This phase is called *primary drying*, during which ice is removed by direct sublimation through open channels created by prior sublimation of ice. After primary drying, additional drying is necessary to remove any water that did not freeze during the freezing process, but instead remained associated with the solute. This is called *secondary drying* and consists of water removal by diffusion and desorption of water from the partially dried solid phase. The phases of a typical freeze-dry cycle-freezing, primary drying, and secondary drying-are illustrated by means of a plot of shelf temperature, chamber pressure, and product temperature in Fig. 5.

The most important objective in developing a freeze-dried product is to assure that critical quality attributes are met initially and throughout the shelf life of the product. Examples of critical quality attributes are recovery of original chemical or biological activity after reconstitution, rapid and complete dissolution,

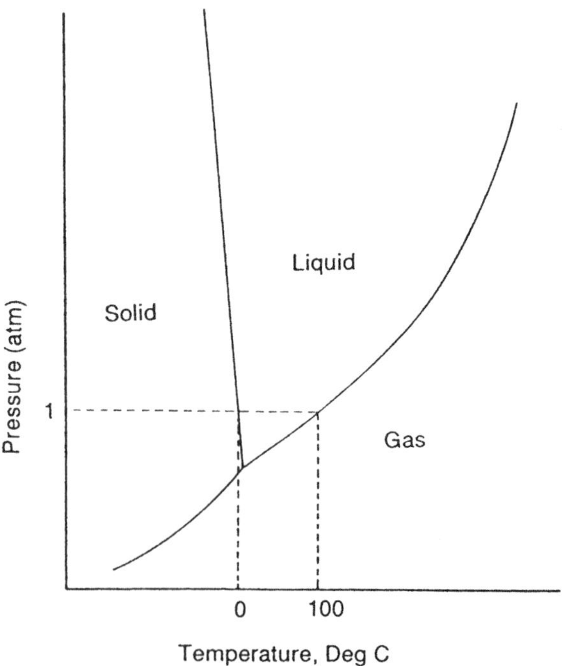

Fig. 4 Phase diagram of water.

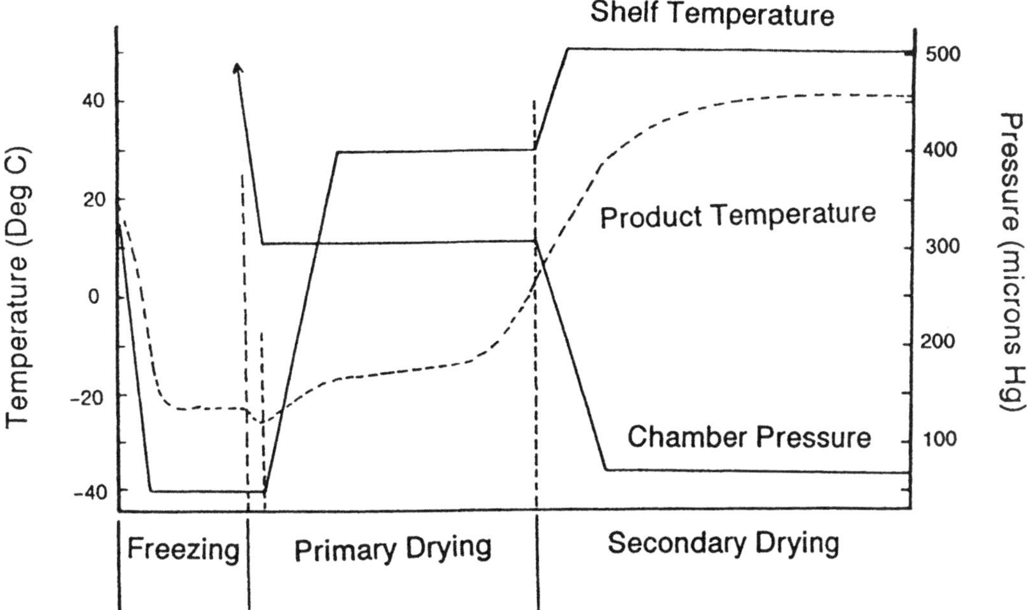

Fig. 5 Process variables during a representative freeze-dry cycle.

appropriate residual moisture level, and acceptable cake appearance. In addition, process conditions should be chosen to maximize process efficiency, i.e. those conditions that minimize drying time without adversely affecting product quality. The driving force for sublimation is the vapor pressure of ice, and the vapor pressure of ice is highly temperature dependent, as shown below:

Temperature (°C)	Vapor pressure (mmHg)
−40	0.096
−30	0.286
−20	0.776
−10	1.950
0	4.579

Therefore, freeze-drying should be carried out at the highest allowable product temperature that maintains the appropriate attributes of a freeze-dried product. This temperature depends on the nature of the formulation. Process development and validation requires characterizing the physical state of the solute, or solutes, that result from the freezing process and identifying a maximum allowable product temperature for the primary drying process [20,21].

The term *eutectic temperature* is often misused in reference to freeze-drying. A eutectic mixture—an intimate mixture of ice and crystals of solute that melts as if it were a single, pure compound—is present only if the solute crystallizes when the solution is frozen. Eutectic melting can often be detected by thermal analysis, such as differential scanning calorimetry (DSC) [22,23]. An example of a eutectic system is neutral glycine in water. The presence of a eutectic mixture is indicated by a melting endotherm in the DSC thermogram of the solution (Fig. 6) in addition to the melting endotherm for ice. In this example, the theoretical maximum allowable product temperature during primary drying is the eutectic melting temperature at −3.5°C. In practice, the product temperature should be maintained a few degrees below this temperature to assure that melting does not occur during the process. Examples of some other common solutes that form eutectics, along with the eutectic temperature, are as follows [23]:

Solute	Eutectic temperature (°C)
Calcium chloride	−51.0
Citric acid	−12.2
Mannitol	−1.0
Potassium chloride	−10.7
Sodium carbonate	−18.0
Sodium chloride	−21.5
Sodium phosphate, dibasic	−0.5

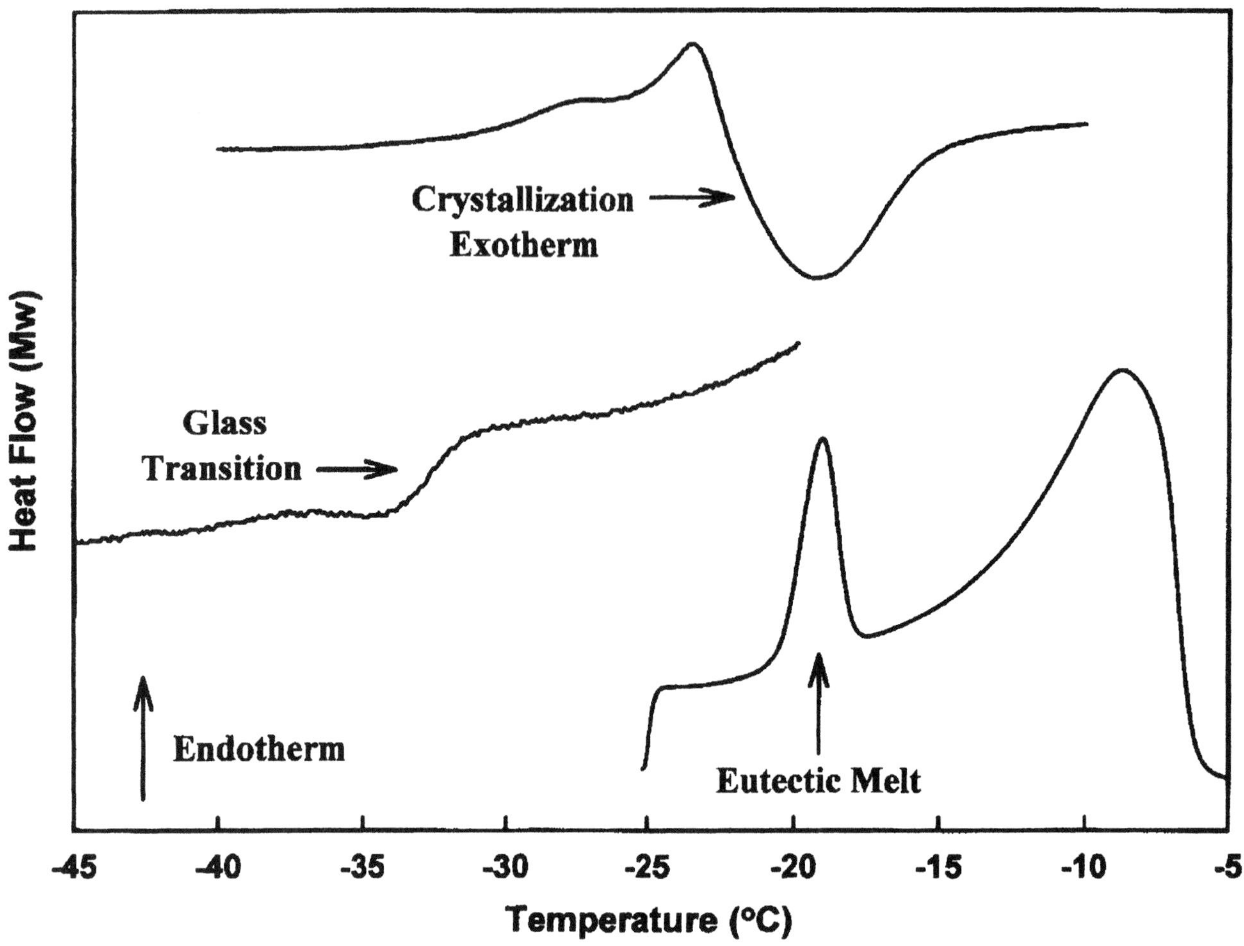

Fig. 6 DSC thermograms showing representative thermal transitions in frozen solutions. The top thermogram is for a mannitol solution and is characteristic of a metastable glass-forming system.

However, many solutes do not crystallize during the freezing process, but instead form a glassy mixture with unfrozen water. Examples include sugars—such as sucrose, lactose, maltose—polymers, and many drugs. In this case, no eutectic mixture is formed. Instead, the freeze concentrate becomes more concentrated and more viscous as the temperature decreases and ice crystals grow. This process continues until a temperature is reached at which the viscosity of the freeze concentrate increases dramatically with only a small change in temperature, and ice crystal growth ceases on a practical time scale. This temperature is a glass transition temperature (called T_g') and is an important characteristic of amorphous systems. Below the glass transition temperature, the freeze concentrate exists as a rigid glass. Above the glass transition temperature, the freeze concentrate behaves as a viscous liquid. The significance of the glass transition temperature of the freeze concentrate is that it is closely related to the *collapse temperature* in freeze-drying. If drying is carried out above the collapse temperature, the freeze concentrate will flow and lose the microstructure established by freezing once the supporting structure of ice crystals is removed. Collapse can be observed in a variety of forms, from a slight shrinkage of the dried cake (where the cake has pulled away from the wall of the vial) to total loss of any cake structure. An example of collapse is shown in Fig. 7.

The glass transition of solutes that remain amorphous during and after the freezing process can often be seen in the DSC thermogram as a shift in the baseline toward higher heat capacity. This is illustrated in the DSC thermogram of sucrose solution in Fig. 6, in which the glass transition is observed at $-34°C$.

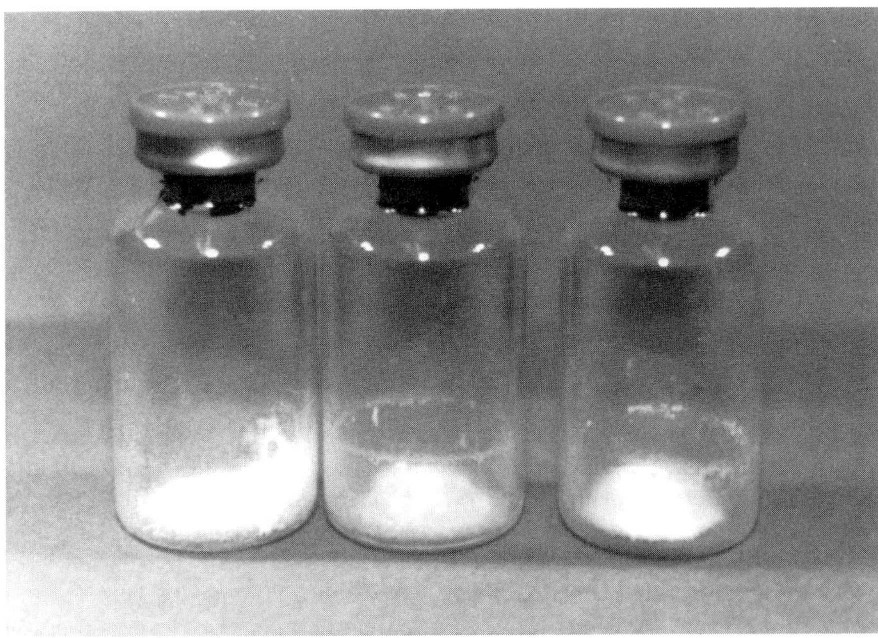

Fig. 7 Collapse is characteristic of amorphous materials, and can occur either during the freeze-dry process or during storage.

Glass transition (Tg') values of some other solutes common to freeze-drying are as follows [24]:

Solute	Glass transition (Tg')
Dextran	−9
Gelatin	−10
Glucose	−43
Lactose	−32
Maltose	−32
Polyvinylpyrrolidone	−24
Sorbitol	−48

Some solutes may form a metastable amorphous phase initially on freezing and then crystallize when the material is heated. Mannitol, a common bulking agent in freeze-dried formulations, is an example of a solute that can, depending on the cooling rate during freezing, form a metastable amorphous system initially, then crystallize from the glass as the system is heated to above the glass transition temperature of the freeze concentrate. The DSC thermogram of a frozen mannitol solution is shown in Fig. 6, where the exotherm indicates crystallization. Crystallization of mannitol during heating is believed to be the underlying cause of vial breakage in mannitol-based formulations [24].

Solutes that form metastable glassy systems upon freezing can sometimes be induced to crystallize by *thermal treatment*, or *annealing*, in the freeze-dry process. The product is first frozen to perhaps −40°C, then heated to a temperature above the glass transition temperature, held for a few hours, and then cooled before starting the drying process. Some cephalosporins have been shown to crystallize during annealing steps [25]. In addition, annealing has been shown to improve both the rate and the vial-to-vial uniformity of primary drying [26].

In general, crystallization of the solute is desirable in terms of freeze-drying properties, as well as quality attributes of the final product, for several reasons. First, when the solute crystallizes, nearly all of the water is present as ice in the frozen matrix, and it is removed by direct sublimation during primary drying. Therefore, there is little water to be removed by secondary drying. This improves process efficiency, since water removed during secondary drying must be removed primarily by the process of diffusion, rather than by bulk flow. Second, eutectic temperatures are usually higher than collapse temperatures, which allows higher product temperatures and more efficient drying. Eutectic temperatures of most organic compounds are in the range of −1 to about −12°C, whereas collapse temperatures commonly are −30°C or lower. Third, the chemical and physical stability of a compound in crystalline form is generally better than that of the same compound in an amorphous form [8,27]. This can be a critical aspect of determining the feasibility of a freeze-dried dosage form.

While crystallinity of a drug is generally desireable for freeze-drying, it is often important for excipients to remain amorphous. In particular, disaccharides (such as sucrose and trehalose) are important as formulation additives to stabilize proteins against damage caused by freezing, freeze-drying, or both. However, in order to be effective stabilizers, it is essential for these compounds to remain amorphous both during freeze-drying and during subsequent storage.

An understanding of the effect of formulation on freeze-drying behavior is important to the pharmaceutical scientist involved in the development of freeze-dried products. Mixtures of components should be expected to behave differently from single-component systems. For example, a compound that crystallizes readily from aqueous solution when it is the only solute present may not crystallize at all when other solutes are present. For solutes that remain amorphous on freezing, the glass transition temperature is affected by the presence of other solutes. Subtle variations in the composition of the formulation, such as changes in ionic strength or pH, may have a significant effect on the physical chemistry of the freezing and freeze-drying processes.

Many drugs are present in a dose too small to form a well-defined freeze-dried cake and must be formulated with a *bulking agent*, the purpose of which is to provide a dried matrix in which the active ingredient is dispersed. Common bulking agents are mannitol, lactose, glycine, and mixtures of these compounds. Buffers are commonly used, such as sodium or potassium phosphate, acetate, citrate, tris-hydroxymethylaminomethane (THAM), or histidine. Formulations of proteins, liposomes, or cells generally require the presence of a *protectant*, or a substance that protects the active compound from damage by freezing, by drying, or both. Disaccharides, such as sucrose and trehalose, are, in general, the most effective protectants [28]. The use of maltose and lactose, also disaccharides, should be approached with caution, since they are both reducing sugars.

In addition to the effects of formulation factors on freeze-drying behavior, it is important for the pharmaceutical scientist to understand basic principles of heat and mass transfer in freeze-drying [29,30]. Because of the high heat input required for sublimation (670 cal/g), transfer of heat from the heated shelf to the sublimation front is often the rate-limiting step in the coupled heat and mass transfer process. There are three basic mechanisms for heat transfer: conduction, convection, and radiation. *Conduction* is the transfer of heat by molecular motion between differential volume elements of a material. *Convection* is the transfer of heat by bulk flow of a fluid, either from density differences (natural convection) or because an external force is applied (forced convection). Because of the relatively low pressures used in freeze-drying, convection is probably not a large contributing factor in heat transfer. Heat transfer by *thermal radiation* arises when a substance, because of thermal excitation, emits radiation in an amount determined by its absolute temperature. Of these mechanisms, heat transfer by conduction is the most important. Heat transfer by conduction takes place through a series of resistances—the bottom of the vial, the frozen layer of product, the metal tray (if used), and the vapor phase caused by lack of good thermal contact between the vial and the shelf. The thermal conductivity of the vapor phase at the pressures used in freeze-drying is dependent on pressure in the chamber. Therefore, to maintain consistent drying conditions from batch to batch, it is as important to control the chamber pressure as it is to control shelf temperature [31]. In addition, changes in the geometry of the system that affect heat transfer will also affect process consistency. Examples include changing from molded to tubing vials, changing the depth of fill in the vials, and changing from trays with metal bottoms to those without bottoms. Thermal radiation is a small, but significant, contributor to the total quantity of heat transferred to the product. This can be a significant issue in scale-up of cycles from pilot dryers to production-scale equipment.

Mass transfer in freeze-drying refers to the transfer of water vapor from the sublimation front through open channels in the partially dried layer, created by prior sublimation of ice, through the headspace of the vial, past the lyostopper, through the chamber, to the condenser.

The reader is referred to basic studies of mass transfer in freeze-drying by Pikal and coworkers for in-depth treatment of the theoretical and practical aspects of mass transfer [29,32]. Briefly, the rate-limiting step in mass transfer is transfer of water vapor through the partially dried matrix of solids. Resistance of the dried layer increases in a more or less continuous fashion as the depth of the dried layer increases, and the resistance also increases with the concentration of solids in the dried layer. Other factors can also affect the resistance of the dried layer, such as the method of freezing; faster freezing tends to create a higher resistance in the dried layer.

Mass transfer of the "unfrozen" water through a glassy phase during secondary drying occurs more slowly than bulk flow of water vapor by direct sublimation, since no open channels are present in the glassy phase. The high resistance of the solid material to mass transfer is why secondary drying can be the most time-consuming phase of the freeze-dry cycle for amorphous solutes containing a large percentage of unfrozen water. According to studies reported by Pikal, shelf temperature is the most critical process variable, affecting the rate of secondary drying and final moisture level [32]. Chamber pressure had no measureable influence on secondary drying kinetics.

The quantity of residual water is frequently a critical product characteristic relative to chemical and physical stability of freeze-dried products, particularly amorphous solids. Water acts as a plasticizer of the solid material, lowering the glass transition temperature. A low glass transition temperature relative to the storage temperature can result in physical instability, such as cake shrinkage or collapse, or accelerated rates of chemical reactions leading to instability. Often a small change in moisture content can result in a large change in the glass transition temperature; therefore, careful consideration of appropriate limits on residual moisture is often an important part of the product development process.

Aseptic Crystallization and Dry Powder Filling. Aseptic crystallization is primarily used for manufacture of sterile aqueous suspensions. However, if the physical form of the drug is critical to quality of the final product, better control over physical form can be attained by aseptic crystallization because a large variety of organic solvents can be used to control the crystallization process. In aseptic crystallization, the drug is dissolved in a suitable solvent and sterile filtered through an appropriate membrane filter. A second solvent—a sterility filtered nonsolvent for the drug—is then added at a controlled rate, causing crystallization and precipitation of the drug. The crystals are collected on a funnel, washed if necessary, and dried by vacuum-drying. After drying, it may be necessary to mill or blend the drug crystals. The powder is then transferred to dry-powder-filling equipment and filled into vials. Although simple in principle, there are obvious drawbacks to this approach. Batch-to-batch variability in crystal habit and crystal size and the resulting variability in physical properties can be troublesome for consistent product quality. Maintenance of asepsis between sterile crystallization and filling of the powder is a challenge during material handling and will usually result in decreased sterility assurance. Also, since the drug is filled into vials as a powder, maintenance of fill weight uniformity is generally more troublesome than when filling with a liquid.

Spray-Drying. A solution of drug is sterile filtered and metered into the drying chamber, where it passes through an atomizer that creates an aerosol of small droplets of liquid (Fig. 8). The aerosol comes into contact with a stream of hot sterile gas—usually air. The solvent evaporates quickly, allowing drug to be collected as a powder in the form of uniform hollow spheres. The powder is then filled into vials using conventional powder-filling equipment. Spray-drying may be more economical than freeze-drying, but challenges in the use of this technique include sterile filtration of very large volumes of air, constructing and maintaining a spray dryer that can be readily sterilized, aseptic transfer of powder from the spray

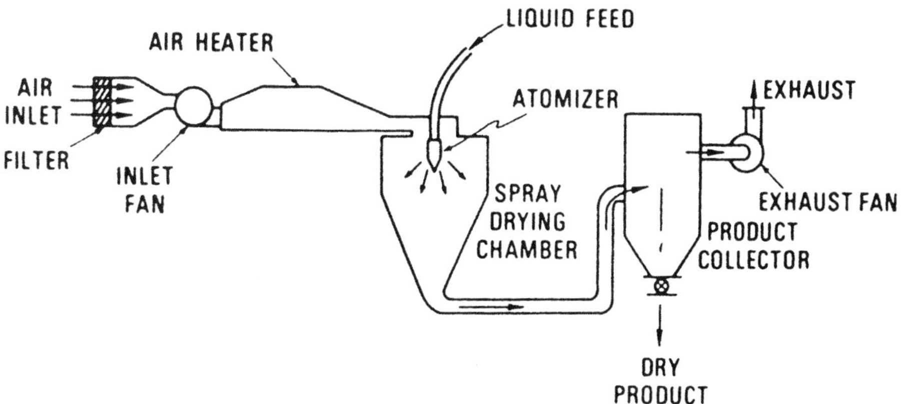

Fig. 8 Schematic drawing of spray dryer.

dryer to the powder-filling line, and precise control of the drying conditions to prevent overheating of the product while providing adequate drying. Probably because of these limitations, the technique is not widely used.

Protein Formulations

The first biotechnology-derived therapeutic agent to be approved by FDA in the United States was human insulin (Humulin, Eli Lilly) in 1982. The number of such products has grown steadily since then, and in 1999 they accounted for well over $10 billion in sales worldwide. This growth is expected to continue during the next decade. Because biotechnology-derived pharmaceuticals are generally proteins and glycoproteins, they require special consideration in formulation and processing.

Special problems with formulation and processing of proteins arise from the hierarchy of structural organization of proteins. In addition to primary structure (the amino acid sequence), proteins have secondary structure (interactions between peptide bonds, resulting in helical or sheetlike structures), tertiary structure (folding of chain segments into a precise three-dimensional arrangement), and, in some, quaternary structure (association of individual protein subunits into a multimeric structure). Disruption of this higher-order structure can lead to loss of the biologically active, or native, conformation, which, in turn, causes physical instability that may accelerate reactions that are characteristic of chemical instability of proteins.

Loss of the native conformation of a protein generally exposes hydrophobic amino acid residues that are normally buried on the inside of the self-associated structure and are shielded from the aqueous environment. This leads to association between the exposed hydrophobic residues of neighboring proteins (aggregation) or between these exposed residues and hydrophobic surfaces that the protein may encounter either in the manufacturing process or in the primary package.

Seemingly subtle aspects of processing may be critical in manufacturing pharmaceutical dosage forms of proteins. For example, vigorous agitation of a protein solution can cause foaming, generating a large air/water interface that is an excellent site for denaturation, aggregation, and perhaps precipitation of protein. Loss of protein by adsorption to surfaces, such as tubing and filters used in manufacturing, can result in subpotent product. Other potentially critical factors in maintenance of the native structure during processing include temperature, pH, the presence of organic solvents, and ionic strength of the formulation.

Disruption of the native structure of a protein can also contribute to chemical instability by accelerating the rates of a variety of degradation routes, including deamidation, hydrolysis, oxidation, disulfide exchange, β-elimination, and racemization.

Formulation strategies for stabilization of proteins commonly include additives such as other proteins (e.g., serum albumin), amino acids, and surfactants to minimize adsorption to surfaces. Modification of protein structure to enhance stability by genetic engineering may also be feasible, as well as chemical modification such as formation of a conjugate with polyethylene glycol.

Most proteins are not sufficiently stable in aqueous solution to allow formulation as a sterile solution. Instead, the protein is freeze-dried and reconstituted before use. Development of a freeze-dried protein formulation often requires special attention to the details of the freezing process (potential pH shifts and ionic strength increase with freezing) as well as to potential loss of activity with drying. Formulation additives, such as sugars and polyhydroxy compounds, are often useful as cryoprotectants and lyoprotectants. Residual moisture may also be critical to the stability of the dried preparation [33].

Novel Formulations

A summary of sustained- and controlled-release parenteral dosage forms is included in Chapter 15. This subject is also covered extensively by Chien [34].

Concepts in drug delivery that have received increasing attention include drug carrier systems, implants, intravenous infusers, and implantable infusion pumps. Carrier systems include microspheres, liposomes, monoclonal antibodies, and emulsions. Drugs are incorporated into these systems to increase the duration of drug action and to provide selective delivery of the drug to a specific target site or organ. Implants are used for the same reason. Unwanted side effects and adverse reactions are usually reduced because of selective delivery, which also results in a lower concentration of drug required to achieve the desired therapeutic effect. Infusion pumps provide a delivery system with uniform, continuous flow. A specific dose of a drug, such as insulin, may be administered to a patient on a continual or intermittent basis.

V. PACKAGING

Container components for parenteral products must be considered an integral part of the product because they can dramatically affect product stability, potency, toxicity, and safety. Parenteral dosage forms, especially solutions, usually require more detailed evaluation of packaging components for product compatability and stability than do other pharmaceutical dosage forms. Common container components in direct contact with the product include various types of glass, rubber, plastic, and stainless steel (needles), all of which may react with the drug. Maintenance of microbiological purity and product stability, adaptability to production operations and inspections, resistance to breakage and leakage, and convenience of clinical use are factors that must be evaluated when selecting the container.

Parenteral packaging includes ampoules, rubber-stoppered vials and bottles, plastic bags and bottles, glass and plastic syringes, and syringe-vial combinations. Glass containers have traditionally achieved widespread acceptability for parenteral products because of their relative inertness. In recent years, hospital preference for unit-dose and clinical convenience has resulted in an increase in products packaged in disposable syringes and the development of polyvinyl chloride, polyester, and polyolefin plastic containers for IV fluids. Package systems, such as dual chamber plastic containers and Add-Vantage, have been developed for combining unstable mixtures of drugs and solutions. Several antibiotics that are unstable in solution are now available as a frozen product in a plastic container. All these systems are designed for convenience and cost efficiency as well as minimizing the potential of contamination when preparing the admixture. Parenteral packaging materials are discussed in Chapter 17.

VI. STABILITY

A formal stability program is needed to assure that all critical attributes of any drug product are maintained throughout the shelf life of the product. A validated stability-indicating assay is essential to measure chemical or biological activity, and acceptance criteria should be established before initiating stability studies. Particular attention should be given to developing a detailed protocol for a stability study before preparing stability samples, including assays to be performed, storage conditions, and sampling intervals.

In general, expiration dating is based on the estimated time required for the active compound to reach 90–95% of labeled potency at the specified storage temperature. However, other considerations may limit the shelf life of the product. For example, the shelf life of products containing a preservative may be determined by adsorption of preservative to a rubber closure or another elastomeric component of the container-closure system. The drug substance itself may be subject to physical instability such as adsorption. The stability program should include placing enough units at the specified storage conditions to allow inspection of a statistically valid number of units to verify acceptable appearance of the product, such as the development of haze or discreet particulate matter in solution products, as well as to check for discoloration or any other physical attribute that would result in unacceptable pharmaceutical elegance. Formulation pH is often a critical attribute that must be monitored during a stability study, since pH may be affected both by chemical reactions in solution or by interactions between the formulation and the container-closure system.

Sterile powders may require special attention to identify which tests are required to assure adequate physical and chemical stability. The stability of many dried products is often sensitive to small differences in the amount of residual water present, requiring monitoring of residual moisture by Karl Fisher titration or loss on drying. This is particularly important for protein formulations. Special efforts may be needed to minimize the residual moisture in rubber stoppers, since water vapor can transfer from the closure to the powder during prolonged storage. Reconstitution time—the amount of time required after addition of diluent until all solids are dissolved—should be measured routinely. For freeze-dried products, cake shrinkage with time is not uncommon. This may be accompanied by discoloration, increased reconstitution time, or crystallization of one or more components of the formulation. The physical state of the drug—crystalline or amorphous—has an important influence on stability, particularly for cephalosporins. Periodic examination of stability samples by x-ray diffraction may be valuable to identify changes in physical state of either drug or excipients that could influence critical quality attributes. For some solid dosage forms subject to oxidative degradation, it is critical to exclude oxygen from the vial headspace. The headspace of selected vials should be analyzed periodically for oxygen. Many freeze-dried powders are stoppered under vacuum or an inert gas. Testing selected vials during the stability study for presence of vacuum in the headspace of the vial is a useful method of verifying container-closure integrity.

Sterile suspensions can be challenging with respect to physical stability, and this should be reflected in the stability protocol. Examples of physical stability issues for suspensions include (a) caking, which causes poor resuspendability; (b) changes in the particle size distribution, particularly growth of large crystals of drug, which can cause poor syringeability; and (c) polymorphic transformations, which can result in changes in dissolution characteristics and, therefore, the bioavailability of the drug.

For parenteral emulsions, the formulation scientist must be particularly aware of changes in particle size distribution of the oil phase. Droplet coalescence results in increased droplet size. As a general rule, average droplet size should be less than 1 μm. Droplet sizes of more than 6 μm can cause blockage of capillaries (capillary emboli).

VII. STERILIZATION METHODS

Five sterilization processes are described in the USP: steam, dry-heat, filtration, gas, and ionizing radiation. All are commonly used for parenteral products, except gas and ionizing radiation, which are widely used for devices and surgical materials. To assist in the selection of the sterilization method, certain basic information and data must be gathered. This includes determining (a) the nature and amount of product bioburden and (b) whether the product and container-closure system will have a predominantly moist or dry environment during sterilization. Both of these factors are of critical importance in determining the conditions (time and temperature) of any sterilization method chosen.

The natural bioburden in a well-maintained pharmaceutical parenteral manufacturing plant is quite low, often to the point that it is difficult to isolate and propagate plant bioburden for sterilization studies. Nevertheless, it is still important to characterize the microbiological bioburden in the process and then monitor it at regular intervals.

For sterilization purposes, microorganisms can be categorized into three general categories: (a) easy to kill with either dry or moist heat, (b) susceptible to moist heat, but resistant to dry heat (e.g., *Bacillus subtilis*), or (c) resistant to moist heat but susceptible to dry heat (e.g., *Clostridium sporogenes*). Organisms such as *B. subtilis* and *C. sporogenes* are often used as biological indicators because they are spore formers of known heat resistance. When used in a known concentration, they will be killed at a reproducible rate. In this manner, when a product has a low bioburden, biological indicator organisms can be used at a concentration of 1×10^3 in kill studies to simulate 10^6 kills of natural (environmental) bioburden. Processing and design of container-closure systems for individual products must be reviewed carefully to ascertain whether moist or dry conditions predominate, particularly in difficult-to-reach inner portions of closures. The use of biological indicators in validating parenteral container-closure systems has been reviewed by Akers and Anderson [35].

The USP also recommends the use of biological indicators, whenever possible, to monitor all sterilization methods except sterile filtration. Biological indicators are generally of two types. If a product to be sterilized is a liquid, microorganisms are added directly to carefully identified representative samples of the product. When this is not practical, as with solids or equipment to be sterilized, the culture is added to strips of filter paper. The organism chosen varies with the method of sterilization.

Sterilization tests are performed to verify that an adequate sterilization process has been carried out. Validation of the sterilization cycle also gives assurance of process integrity. Sterility is not assured simply because a product passes the USP sterility test. As outlined in the USP, the sterility test is described in considerable detail, including procedures for sampling, general conditions of the test, and specific procedures for testing solids and liquids. In addition, guidelines for the design of an aseptic work environment are outlined in some detail. Sample limitations, plus the impossibility of cultivating and testing all viable microorganisms that may be present, affect the reliability of sterility tests. Because of these problems, it is necessary to monitor and test sterilization equipment continuously. The reader is referred to Akers and Anderson for a review of validation of sterile products [35].

A. Sterilization by Steam

When drug solutions and containers can withstand autoclaving conditions, this method is preferred to other sterilization methods because moist heat sterilizes quickly and inexpensively. However, judgment must be exercised and experiments run to ensure that the solution and container are permeable to steam. Oils and tightly closed containers, for example, are not normally sterilizable by steam.

Autoclave steam sterilization is a well-established and widely used procedure. Normally, steam enters through the top of the chamber (Fig. 9). Being lighter than air, it remains at the top of the chamber but steadily and continuously drives the air out of the chamber through the bottom vent throughout the sterilization cycle. The velocity of steam entering the

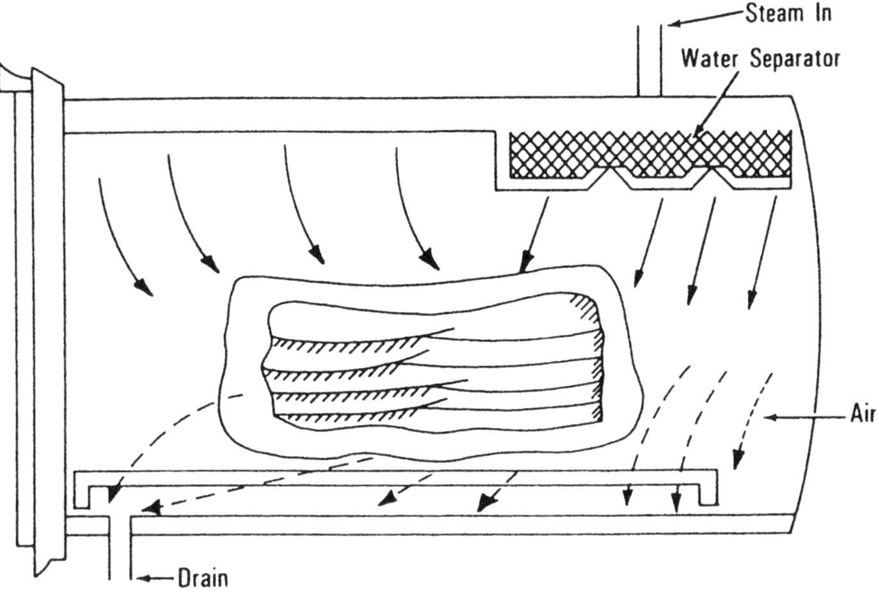

Fig. 9 Gravity displacement steam sterilizer.

autoclave, the efficiency of water separation from incoming steam, the size of the drain, and the amount of vacuum applied are all factors that must be controlled to obtain efficient and reproducible steam sterilization in an autoclave. The reader is referred to a review by Leuthner [36] for a more thorough discussion of the theory and practice of steam sterilization.

With the widespread use of flexible packaging for LVP products, the use of steam sterilization has increased. Compared with the traditional LVP glass bottles closed with rubber stoppers, flexible LVP plastic containers (polyvinyl chloride, polyester, or polyolefin) offer autoclaving advantages. Specifically, (a) a larger surface area is available for heating per unit volume of liquid; (b) if held in a "flattened" position during sterilization, the heat penetration depth required is reduced, resulting in a more uniform thermal mapping of the contents; and (c) shorter heat-up and cool-down periods are required. The net effect is to allow a much shorter sterilization cycle for LVP products packaged in flexible containers, thus exposing the product to less heat, less potential for degradation, and reduced manufacturing costs.

B. Sterilization by Dry Heat

Dry heat is widely used to sterilize glassware and equipment parts in manufacturing areas for parenteral products. It has good penetration power and is not as corrosive as steam. However, heat-up time is slow, necessitating long sterilization periods at high temperatures. It is important to allow sufficient circulation around the materials to be sterilized. Metal cans are often used to contain the parts or containers that are to be sterilized.

The two principal methods of dry-heat sterilization are infrared and convection hot air. Infrared rays will sterilize only surfaces. Sterilization of interior portions must rely on conduction. Convection hot-air sterilizers are normally heated electrically and are of two types: gravity or mechanical. In gravity convection units, a fan is used to promote uniformity of heat distribution throughout the chamber.

Dry-heat processes kill microorganisms primarily through oxidation. The amount of moisture available to assist sterilization in dry-heat units varies considerably at different locations within the chamber and at different time intervals within the cycle. Also, the amount of heat available, its diffusion, and the environment at the spore/air interface all influence the microorganism kill rate. Consequently, cycles tend to be longer and hotter than would be expected from calculations to ensure that varying conditions do not invalidate a run. In general, convection dry-heat sterilization cycles are run above 160°C [37].

C. Sterilization by Ethylene Oxide

Ethylene oxide (ETO), a colorless gas, is widely used as a sterilant in hospitals and industry for items that cannot be sterilized by steam. It is often diluted with carbon dioxide, or sometimes fluorocarbons, to overcome its flammable and explosive nature. The mechanism by which ETO kills microorganisms is by alkylation of various reactive groups in the spore or vegetative cell. One of the more resistant organisms to ETO is *B. subtilis* var. *niger* (*globigii*). It is the USP biological indicator for monitoring the effectiveness of ETO sterilization cycles. Several factors are important in determining whether ETO is effective as a sterilizing gas: gas concentration, temperature, humidity, spore water content, and substrate for the microorganisms. Ethylene oxide should be present at a concentration of about 500 mL/L for maximum effectiveness. Once gas concentration is not a limiting factor, the inactivation rate of spores by ETO doubles for each 10°C rise in temperature. Relative humidity plays an important role in that the sensitivity of spores to ETO largely depends on the water content of the spore.

A "typical" ETO sterilization cycle is shown in Fig. 10. As discussed at the beginning of this section, it is important to determine and monitor the bioburden level of the product entering the sterilizer. Also, the load configuration in the sterilizer is important in achieving uniform and reliable sterilization. Unfortunately, commercially available biological indicators used in ETO sterilization are often unreliable. Hopefully, progress will be made in this field in the years ahead.

Unlike other methods, it is necessary to posttreat the product, either through vacuum purging or by allowing the product to remain at ambient conditions for a time, to allow removal of residual ETO and ethylene chlorhydrin/ethylene glycol by-products before use by the consumer. In addition, in 1984 the U.S. Occupational Safety and Health Agency (OSHA) lowered the maximum permissible operator 8-hour exposure level from 50 to 1 ppm in air (on a time-weighted average) [38].

D. Sterilization by Filtration

It has been only in the past 25 years that filters have become sufficiently reliable to use them on a wide scale to sterilize injectable solutions. Even now it is prudent to use filtration to sterilize only those products that cannot be terminally sterilized.

Filters are of two basic types: depth and membrane. Depth filters rely on a combination of tortuous pathway and adsorption to retain particles or microorganisms. They are made from materials such as diatomaceous earth, inorganic fibers, natural fibers, and porcelain. They carry a nominal rating, i.e., a particle size above which a certain percentage of particles is retained. The major advantage of depth filters is their ability to retain large quantities of particles, including many below the nominal rating of the particular filter. Disadvantages of depth filters include grow-through and reproduction of microorganisms, tendency of the filter components to slough during line surges, and retention of some liquid in the filter. Membrane filters rely on sieving and, to a lesser degree,

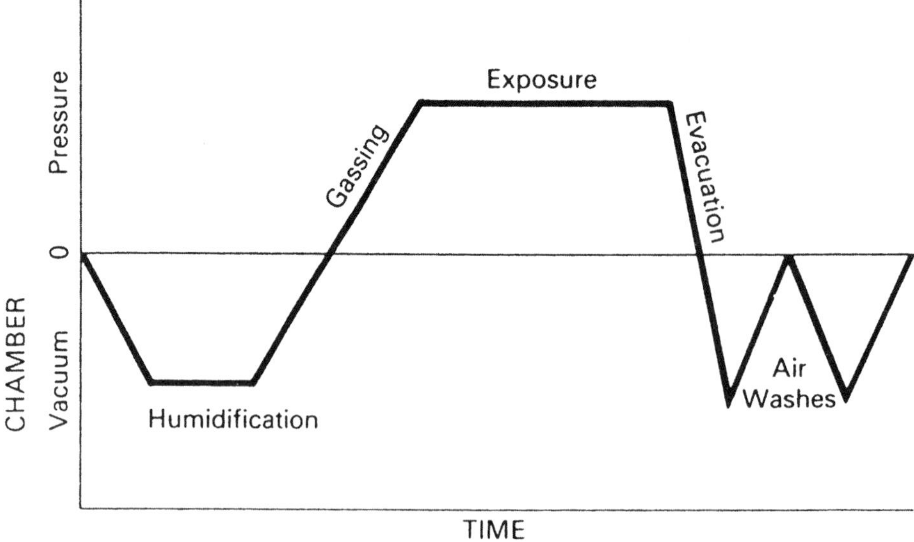

Fig. 10 Ethylene oxide sterilization cycle.

absorption to prevent particles from passing. Although all pores in a membrane filter are not of the same size, nevertheless, the filter can retain all particles larger than the stated size.

Similar to depth filters, membrane filters are made from a variety of materials, although filters made from cellulose ester derivatives are by far the most common. The advantages of membrane filters include no retention of product, no media migration, and efficiency independent of flow-rate pressure differential. The major disadvantages are low capacity before clogging and the need to prewash the filters to remove surfactants. Given the advantages and disadvantages of each type of filter, when large quantities of liquids are to be sterile filtered, such as in industrial applications, it is very common to use a relatively coarse-depth filter (1–5 mm) to remove the great majority of particles and, subsequently, use a membrane filter to remove the remaining particles and microorganisms down to a predetermined size (0.22 μm).

Filter cartridges are used for filtering large volumes of solution or more viscous products because of the large surface area that is available through the pleated design. Hydrophobic filters are also available for sterile filtering of gases and solvents [39].

VIII. CLINICAL CONSIDERATIONS IN PARENTERAL PRODUCT DESIGN

Sterility, freedom from pyrogens, and acceptably low level of extraneous particulate matter are critical quality attributes of all injectable products. Additional critical quality attributes depend on the clinical use of the product. For example, for IV, IM, and SC routes, isotonicity and physiological pH (7.4) are always desirable in order to minimize potential irritation upon injection. Other factors may preclude this, however. If the required dose of drug must be administered in a small volume, it may not be feasible to formulate an isotonic solution. Likewise, solubility or stability considerations may preclude formulation at physiological pH. This explains why formulation pH for injectable drugs varies from about pH 2 to about pH 11.

However, for certain routes of injection, such as intrathecal, intraocular, or into any part of the brain, isotonicity and physiological pH are critical in order to minimize potential nerve damage. Absence of preservatives is also critical for these routes of administration for the same reason.

The effect of isotonicity on reducing pain on injection is somewhat uncertain, although it may at least reduce tissue irritation. Pain on injection may occur during and immediately following the injection, or it may be a delayed or prolonged type of pain that becomes more severe after subsequent injections. The actual cause of the pain is often unknown and varies significantly among patients. In some cases, pain may be reduced by minor formulation changes, such as adjusting tonicity and pH, or by adding an anesthetic agent such as benzyl alcohol or lidocaine hydrochloride. In other cases, pain is attributable to the drug, and pain reduction is more difficult or impossible to resolve. Pain, soreness, and tissue inflammation are often encountered in parenteral suspensions, especially those containing a high concentration of solids.

Thrombophlebitis, an inflammation of the venous walls, may occur during IV infusion and may be related to the drug being infused, pH or tonicity of the formulation, the administration technique, the device being used for the infusion (i.e., a needle or a catheter), the duration of the infusion, and the extent to which the administration device is mechanically stabilized [40]. It is difficult to define the relative importance of each because of the interplay of all these variables. Irritation caused by the drug or the formulation can be minimized by observing published limits on the volumetric rate of infusion. The observance of proper technique should also be emphasized, including selection of the appropriate infusion device, venipuncture technique, stabilization of the catheter, and changing the administration device at appropriate time intervals.

The formulator should be aware of the clinical use of a drug when designing the dosage form. Specific examples are pediatric dosage forms and unit dosage forms, including disposable syringes and special packages for hospital, office, or home administration. Hospital packages can take several forms, depending, for example, on whether the package is to be unit-dose, reconstituted by a nurse, a bulk container for use in the pharmacy, or administered as a secondary "piggyback" IV container.

Drugs that affect tissue properties, particularly blood flow at the absorption site, may be used to control the rate of absorption. Reduced drug absorption may be achieved physiologically with an IM preparation by incorporating epinephrine, which causes a local constriction of blood vessels at the site of injection. Increased muscular activity may enhance drug absorption because of increased drug flow.

When preparing preparations for IV and IM use, the formulator must be aware of the effect of added substances when unusually large doses of the drug are administered. Although the USP limits the use of some added substances (Table 4), these types of problems

Table 4 Maximum Amounts of Added Substances Permitted in USP Injectable Products

Substance	Maximum
Mercury compounds	0.01
Cationic surfactants	0.01
Chlorobutanol	0.5
Cresol	0.5
Phenol	0.5
Sulfur dioxide	0.2
or sodium bisulfite equivalent	0.2
or sodium sulfite equivalent	0.2

cannot always be anticipated. The USP urges special care when administering more than 5 mL [1]. When effects do become apparent, the formulator should consider additional dosage sizes or formulation changes. Sometimes during the life of a drug product, new uses and larger doses make the original formula unsatisfactory. When this happens, a new dosage form should be designed and the appropriate cautionary statements placed on the respective labels. The precautions, problems, hazards, and complications associated with parenteral drug administration are discussed extensively by Duma and Akers [41].

The preparation of a new drug substance or dosage form for evaluation in clinical trials must meet the same regulatory requirements and controls as a marketed product. The cGMP requirements for clinical trial products are outlined by FDA and are discussed in Chapter 20.

A. Toxicity Studies

In toxicity studies, acute toxicity tests are usually carried out in the rat, mouse, cat, and dog. Subacute toxicity studies for IM products are performed by giving SC injections to rats and IM injections to dogs. In IV studies the rat tail vein or a front leg is used. Deliberate overdosing usually "washes out" metabolism differences between species. In dogs it is common to give an IV dose five times that intended for humans. In rats this is increased to 10 times.

Irritation studies are done in rabbits. Each rabbit serves as its own control. The concentration selected for the irritation studies is that intended for humans.

B. Clinical Evaluation

Clinical evaluation of the dosage form is the most expensive and critical phase of product development. All that has been done before this point has been done in an effort to ensure a safe and reliable product for the clinician.

A drug company normally assigns one of its staff physicians as "monitoring" physician for the clinical trial (CT) program. The monitoring physician has the key role in the conduct of the CT program (Fig. 11). He or she coordinates the establishment of clinical protocols, the awarding of grants, the gathering and "in-house" evaluation of clinical data, and preparation of the FDA submission.

The monitoring physician must first establish what the clinical protocol is going to be. With injectable products, this involves both a clinical pharmacology safety test and a dose-ranging study in humans. These studies are normally a single IM injection in several patients. Depending on the drug, clinical studies may proceed eventually to controlled double-blind studies. Care must be exercised to involve a sufficient number of patients to make the studies statistically meaningful. If it is intended that treatment of several clinical conditions is to be claimed for the product, each must be evaluated separately. Throughout the course of the studies, there is a continuing dialogue between FDA and the monitoring physician.

When the clinical program has been approved by a peer review committee and filed with FDA, the monitoring physician requests a sufficient amount of material from the formulator to initiate the clinical program. Before the dosage form is released to the custody of the monitoring physician, the new drug substance and the formulated product must be thoroughly evaluated to ensure proper potency, purity, and safety. Stability studies must also be initiated so that if the product becomes subpotent or physically unstable during the course of the clinical trial, it can be recalled before any harm can result to the patients in the study.

After release of CT material, the monitoring physician supplies it to the clinical investigators with whom the clinical program has previously been discussed. As the clinical investigators use the product, they begin sending reports to the monitoring physician, who evaluates them and sends them to the FDA. Although the concept shown in Fig. 11 is oversimplified, it does convey the principal framework under which the clinical trials are conducted.

IX. QUALITY ASSURANCE

The terms *quality assurance* and *quality control* are sometimes used interchangeably, but there is an important difference. Quality control generally refers to testing of raw materials, packaging components, and

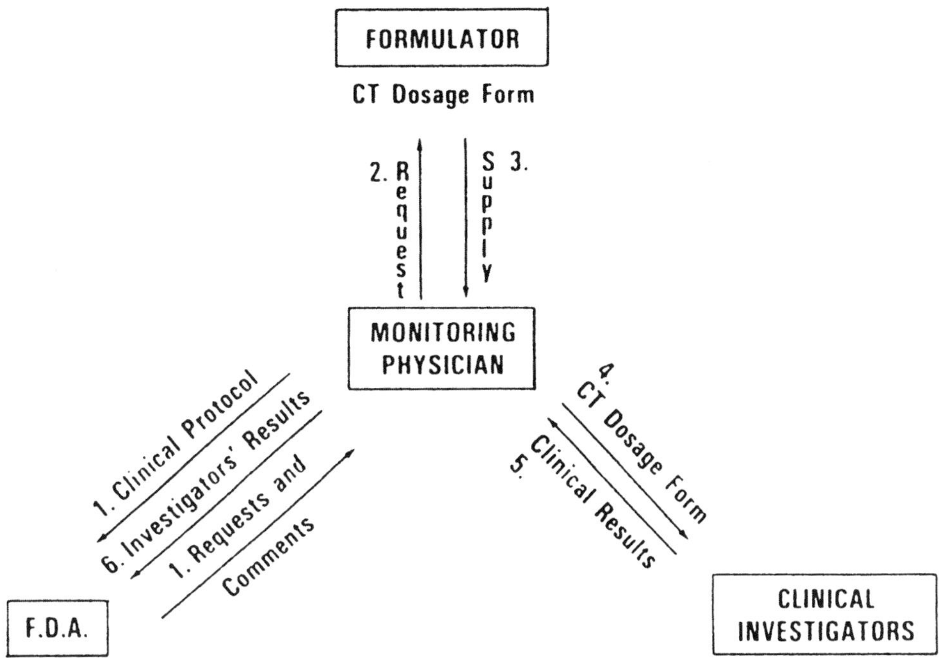

Fig. 11 Clinical trial scheme.

final product for conformance to established requirements. Quality assurance is a term that includes quality control, but has broader meaning to include written operating procedures, personnel training, record keeping, and facility design and monitoring. The philosophy of a quality assurance program is to build quality into the product, rather than to rely only on final product testing to cull out defective product.

Although principles of quality control and quality assurance are important to all pharmaceutical dosage forms, they are especially critical when considering the unique attributes of parenteral dosage forms—sterility, absence of pyrogens, and freedom from extraneous particulate matter. Quality control is generally divided into three areas: raw materials, in-process controls, and product specifications. However, numerous attributes for a product have to be considered throughout all phases of development, evaluation, production, and storage to guarantee good quality.

The factors necessary to achieve quality in a product during the developmental stage have been discussed. The formulator of a new product must consider the manufacturing process to be used for full-scale production of the product. Many new product failures or deficiencies occur because of inability to resolve or foresee production-related problems, rather than to poor product development per se. Therefore, the scientist involved in the development of a product must be involved in development of its manufacturing process and testing. Standards must be carefully established for all raw materials and packaging components used in the product so that the quality of the product will be maintained. Trial production runs should be performed on a new product for stability testing and process evaluation.

A. Regulatory and Compendial Requirements

The manufacture and sale of parenteral products is regulated by federal and state laws, as well as by the USP. Federal drug regulations are discussed in detail in Chapter 20. The USP provides specifications, test procedures, standards, etc. for parenteral products and their packaging components. In addition to individual monographs, the USP limits the use of certain additives (see Table 4), limits the size of multiple-dose containers to 30 mL, and requires a suitable preservative to be added to containers intended for multiple use.

The current Good Manufacturing Practice (cGMP) regulations are guidelines that FDA requires a pharmaceutical manufacturer to meet. Compliance with the cGMPs is a prerequisite for the approval of NDAs, INDs, and antibiotic forms. General areas in which

GMP guidelines must be established and adhered to include:

- Organization and personnel
- Buildings and facilities
- Control of drug components, packaging, and materials
- Production and process control
- Equipment
- Packaging and labeling control
- Holding and distribution
- Laboratory control
- Records and reports

Parenteral formulation and the preparation of parenterals for clinical trial use obviously require adherence to cGMPs. A development group that generates CT materials should have guidelines and written procedures covering such areas as equipment (validation, maintenance, and cleaning), environmental monitoring, instruments (maintenance and calibration), housekeeping, documentation, training, and material handling and storage. Sterilization methods, aseptic processing, and filling techniques and methods must be validated to assure product sterility and quality. *Validation* is the process of proving that a process or equipment does what it is supposed to do within the established limits. All individuals performing an aseptic process must periodically pass a test to verify their aseptic technique.

B. Monitoring Programs

Process Facilities

Continual evaluation of manufacturing processes are necessary to maintain good manufacturing practices. Facilities, buildings, and equipment used in the production of parenteral products must be specially designed for this purpose. Factors to be considered when designing a new plant include environmental conditions, work flow, equipment, choice of materials, personnel, organization, process, documentation, production hygiene, and process controls [42,43]. Thorough planning and engineering of a parenteral facility will not only help maintain the quality of the manufactured products, but will simplify clean-up and maintenance requirements. Contamination of a product is minimized by maintaining a clean facility.

Production Areas

Production areas can be separated into seven general classes: clean-up area, preparation area for packaging materials, preparation area for drug products, sterilization facilities, aseptic filling and processing areas, sorting and product holding areas, and a labeling section.

The exact identity of all packaging components, the bulk and filled product, labels, and so on, must be carefully maintained. The production ticket must be written so that it is easily understood and followed by the appropriate production personnel. All procedures should be clearly outlined and limits established for all operators (e.g., "heat water to 35–45°C" or "autoclave sterilize for 15–20 min at 121–124°C).

All production processes, such as ampoule washing and sterilization, solution filtration, equipment set-up and operation, sorting, and freeze-drier cleaning and operation, should be covered in detail in a procedure manual to ensure that all operations are understood as well as carried out properly and uniformly. Cleaning, sterilization, sterile filtration, filling, and aseptic processing operations must be validated.

Personnel

People are the principal source of contamination in clean room operations. All personnel involved throughout the development and production of a parenteral product must be aware of the factors that influence the overall quality of a product as well as the factors on which they directly impinge. It is of particular importance that production personnel be properly trained so that human error is minimized. They should be made aware of the use of the products with which they are involved and the importance of following all procedures, especially proper aseptic techniques. Procedures must be set up to verify that the product is being manufactured as intended. After manufacture of a batch, production tickets must be carefully checked, sterilization charts examined, and labels verified for correctness and count.

Environmental Monitoring

Control of environmental factors is important to product quality. Air quality and air movement, care and maintenance of the area, and personnel movement and attire are of particular importance.

The air quality in preparation and aseptic areas can be one of the greatest sources of product contamination. However, this problem can be minimized by use of the equipment currently available to provide clean air essentially free from microorganisms and dirt particles. Depth-type filters, electrostatic filters, and dehumidification systems are used to remove the major portion of the airborne contaminants. Air for aseptic areas is then passed through high-efficiency particulate air (HEPA) filters, which remove 99.97% of all particles 0.3 μm or larger. To prevent outside air from entering aseptic areas, a positive pressure is maintained relative to corridors.

A laminar flow enclosure provides a means for environmental control of a confined area for aseptic use. Laminar flow units utilize HEPA filters, with the uniform movement of air along parallel lines. The air movement may be in a horizontal or vertical direction and may involve a confined area, such as a workbench, or an entire room. Laminar flow modules are suspended above filling lines, vial- and stopper-washing equipment, and other processes to provide an aseptic and particulate-free environment.

Regardless of the methods used to obtain a clean air environment, unless the parenteral operator is made completely aware of the limits of laminar flow, uses careful, planned movements, and is wearing proper clothing, he or she can be a source of product contamination. Operator movement within aseptic rooms should be minimized. The rooms must be disinfected regularly and thoroughly before setting up for aseptic operation.

Commonly used environmental monitoring techniques include the following:

Passive Air Sampling: Petri dishes containing microbiological growth media are placed in aseptic areas for specified lengths of time, the "settling plates" are then incubated and colonies are counted and identified. This is a qualitative test, since there is no way of knowing the volume of air represented by a given number of colonies.

Active Air Sampling: Active air sampling provides quantitative data because air at a known flow rate is impacted on a strip of nutrient media, followed by incubation of the nutrient strips and enumeration of colonies. Common active air sampling instruments include the slit-to-agar impact sampler and the centrifugal (Reuter) sampler.

Air-Classification Measurement: Electronic airborne particle–monitoring instruments count and size particulate matter in the sampled air with no consideration of whether the particles are viable or nonviable. Air classification is defined as the number of particles per cubic foot of air that are larger than 0.5 μm in diameter. Climet and HIAC-Royco are common instruments for airborne particulate monitoring).

Surface Monitoring: Contact (or Rodac) plates of growth media are applied to surfaces such as bench tops, walls, and personnel and then incubated. Colony-forming units (cfu) are counted and identified.

Differential Pressure Measurement: Differential manometers are instruments that measure the difference in pressure between two adjacent rooms. Cleaner environments must have a higher pressure than adjacent, less clean environments to prevent flow of relatively dirty air into the cleaner environment. This differential pressure must be monitored and controlled.

C. Product Testing and Evaluation

Quality control testing and evaluation is involved primarily with incoming raw materials, the manufacturing process, and the final product. Testing of incoming raw materials includes routine testing on all drugs, chemicals, and packaging materials.

Process controls include daily testing of water for injection (USP), conformation of fill doses and yields, checking and approving intermediate production tickets, and checking label identity and count. Finished product control includes all the tests necessary to ensure the potency, purity, and identity of the product. Parenteral products require additional tests, which include those for sterility, pyrogens, clarity, and particulate analysis, and for glass-sealed ampoules, leaker testing.

Sterility Testing

The purpose of a sterility test is to determine the probable sterility of a specific batch. The USP lists the procedural details for sterility testing and the sample sizes required [1]. The USP official tests are the direct (or culture tube inoculation) method and the membrane filtration method.

The interpretation of sterility results is divided into two stages by the USP relative to the type of sterility failure if one occurs. If sterility failure of the test samples occurred because of improper aseptic technique or as a fault of the test itself, stage 1 may be repeated with the same sample size. Sample size is doubled in a stage 2 testing, which is performed if microbial growth is observed in stage 1 and there is no reason to believe that the test was invalid. The only absolute method to guarantee the sterility of a batch would be to test every vial or ampoule.

There is a probability of non–product-related contamination in the order of 10^{-3} when performing the sterility test because of the aseptic manipulations necessary to carry out the procedure. This level is comparable with the overall efficiency of an aseptic operation. Confidence in the sterility test is dependent on the fact that the batch has been subjected to a sterilization procedure of proved effectiveness. Records of all sterility tests must be maintained, as well as temperature recordings and records from autoclaves, ovens, or other equipment used during the manufacturing process. All sterilizing equipment must be validated to ensure that the proper temperatures are obtained for the necessary time period. These validations are obtained by the use of thermocouples, chemical and biological indicators, sealed ampoules containing culture medium with a suspension of heat-resistant spores, and detailed sterility testing.

Pyrogen Testing

Pyrogenic substances are primarily lipid polysaccharide products of the metabolism of microorganisms; they may be soluble, insoluble, or colloidal. Pyrogens produced by gram-negative bacilli are generally the most potent. Minute amounts of pyrogens produce a wide variety of reactions in both animals and humans, including fever, leukopenia, and alterations in blood coagulation. Large doses can induce shock and eventually death.

Pyrogens readily contaminate biological materials because of their ability to withstand autoclaving as well as to pass through many filters. Several techniques are used to remove them from injectable products. The ideal situation is one in which no pyrogens are present in the starting materials. This is achieved by strict control of the cleanliness of equipment and containers, distillation of water, and limited processing times. In general, pyrogens may be destroyed by being subjected to prolonged heating. Other pyrogen-removal techniques, which are generally less effective or applicable, include ultrafiltration, absorption or adsorption, chemical (oxidation), aging, or a combination of these.

One pyrogen test is a qualitative biological test based on the fever response of rabbits. If a pyrogenic substance is injected into the vein of a rabbit, a temperature elevation will occur within 3 hours. Many imitative medical agents will also cause a fever.

A preferred method for the detection of pyrogens is the limulus amebocyte lysate (LAL) test. A test sample is incubated with amebocyte lysate from the blood of the horseshoe crab, *Limulus polyphemus*. A pyrogenic substance will cause a gel to form. This is a result of the clottable protein from the amebocyte cells reacting with the endotoxins. This test is more sensitive, more rapid, and easier to perform than the rabbit test.

Leaker Testing and Sealing Verification

Ampoules that have been sealed by fusion must be tested to ensure that a hermetic seal was obtained. The leaker test is performed by immersing the ampoules in a dye solution, such as 1% methylene blue, and applying at least 25 in. (64 cm) of vacuum for a minimum of 15 minutes. The vacuum on the tank is then released as rapidly as possible to put maximum stress on weak seals. Next, the ampoules are washed. Defective ampoules will contain blue solution.

Another means of testing for leakers is a high-frequency spark test system developed by the Nikka Densok Company of Japan, which detects pinholes in ampoules. Some advantages of this system include higher inspection accuracy, higher processing speed, and eliminating the possibility of product contamination [44].

Bottles and vials are not subjected to such a vacuum test because of the flexibility of the rubber closure. However, bottles that are sealed under vacuum may be tested for vacuum by striking the base of the bottle sharply with the heel of the hand to produce a "water hammer" sound. Another test is the spark test, in which a probe is applied outside the bottle. When it reaches the air space of the bottle, a spark discharge occurs if the headspace is evacuated.

The microbiological integrity of various packages, such as vials and stoppers, disposable syringes, and plastic containers, should be determined. A microbiological challenge test is performed by filling the package with a sterile medium and then exposing the sealed container to one of the following tests that is appropriate for the package system: (a) static-aerosol challenge, (b) static-immersion challenge, (c) static-ambient challenge, or (d) dynamic-immersion challenge. The static-immersion challenge test is used commonly with new package combinations. The sealed containers are periodically challenged by immersion into a suspension of challenge organisms. Storing the containers at 5 or 40–50°C, or both, before immersion provides additional stress.

Clarity Testing and Particulate Analysis

Clarity is defined as the state or quality of being clear or transparent to the eye. Clarity is a relative term subject to the visual acuity, training, and experience of the sorter. Clarity specifications are not given in the USP, other than to state that all injections be subjected to visual inspection.

Instruments that measure scattered light, such as the Photo-Nephelometer (Coleman Instruments, Oak Brook, IL), are used to evaluate and set clarity standards for parenteral preparations. It is not possible to establish an overall standard value for all products (e.g., 30 nephelos) because the value itself is relative and influenced by many factors, including concentration, aging, stopper extracts, and the solubility characteristics of the raw materials. Nephelometer readings are insensitive to contamination by large (visible) particulates.

Particulate matter is defined in the USP as extraneous, mobile, undissolved substances, other than gas bubbles, unintentionally present in parenteral solutions. Test methods and limits for particulates are stated in the USP for large-volume injections and small-volume injections.

The development of sorting standards is the responsibility of the manufacturer. Parenteral solutions are sorted for foreign particles, such as glass, fibers, precipitate, and floaters. The sorter also checks for any container deficiency and improper dose volume when feasible. All products containing clear solutions should be inspected against a black and sometimes a white background using a special light source. Although manual visual inspection is the most common means of inspection, electronic particle detection equipment and computer-controlled electro-optic systems are replacing manual inspection and use a light source or camera, or both, positioned behind, above, or below the units being inspected.

The significance of particulate contamination in all parenteral preparations and devices has received much attention. Although it has not been established that particles can cause toxic effects, the pharmaceutical industry, the medical profession, hospital pharmacists, and FDA all realize the importance of reducing particulate levels in all parenteral products and devices.

Sources of particulate matter include the raw materials, processing and filling equipment, the container, and environmental contamination. Several methods have been developed for identifying the source of particulates in a product so that they may be eliminated or reduced. The most effective method is that of collecting the particulates on a membrane filter and identifying and counting them microscopically. However, this method is time-consuming and not adaptable to in-line inspection. Several video image projection methods for in-line detection of particles have been developed that provide potential for mechanizing inspection. Electronic particulate counters have been applied to parenterals because of the rapidity at which they do particulate analysis. Their main disadvantages are the lack of differentiation of various types of particulates including liquids such as silicones and the fact that particle size is measured differently from microscopic analysis. The USP tests for particulate matter in injections utilize both the microscopic and light obscuration methods [1].

Labeling

The package and, in particular, the labeling for parenteral dosage forms are integral and critical parts of the product. The labeling must be legible and clearly identify the drug, its concentration, handling or storage conditions, and any special precautions. The dose or concentration must be prominently displayed when other concentrations of the same drug are marketed. Proper labeling is difficult with the space limitation dictated by small containers used for many parenteral products. Smaller containers have become increasingly popular because of the unit-dose concept.

REFERENCES

1. *The United States Pharmacopeia*, 24th Ed., U. S. Pharmacopeial Convention, Rockville, MD, 2000.
2. S. Turco, *Sterile Dosage Forms*, 4th ed., Lea & Febiger, Philadelphia, 1994.
3. S. Feldman, Physicochemical factors influencing drug absorption from the intramuscular site, Bull. Parenter. Drug. Assoc., 28, 53–63 (1974).
4. S. Motola and S. N. Agharkar, *Preformulation Research of Parenteral Medications*, 2nd Ed., *Pharmaceutical Dosage Forms: Parenteral Medications*, Vol. 1 (K. E. Avis, H. A. Lieberman, and L. Lachman, eds.), Marcel Dekker, New York, 1992, pp. 115–172.
5. K. S. Lin, J. Anschel, and C. J. Swartz, Parenteral formulations IV: solubility considerations in developing a parenteral dosage form, Bull. Parenter. Drug Assoc., 25, 40–50 (1971).
6. G. Engel and R. Pfeiffer, unpublished data, Eli Lilly & Co., Indianapolis, IN.
7. J. K. Haleblian, Characterization of habits and crystalline modification of solids and their pharmaceutical applications, J. Pharm. Sci., 64, 1269–1288 (1975).
8. M. J. Pikal, A. L. Lukes, J. E. Lang, and K. J. Gaines, Quantitative crystallinity determinations for beta-lactam antibiotics by solution calorimetry: correlations with stability, J. Pharm. Sci., 67, 767–773 (1978).
9. L. Brage, *Galenics of Insulin*, Springer-Verlag, New York, 1982, p. 41.
10. L. C. Schroeder, Sulfurous acid salts as pharmaceutical anti-oxidants, J. Pharm. Sci., 50, 891–901 (1961).
11. L. Lachman, P. B. Sheth, and T. Urbanyi, Lined and unlined rubber stoppers for multiple-dose vial solutions, J. Pharm. Sci., 53, 211–218 (1964).

12. S. Motola and C. Clawans, Identification and surface removal of incompatible group II metal ions from butyl stoppers, Bull. Parenter. Drug Assoc., 26, 163–171 (1972).
13. J. F. Carpenter, S. J. Prestrelski, T. J. Anchordoguy, and T. Arakawa, Interactions of stabilizers with proteins during freezing and drying, in *Formulation and Delivery of Peptides and Proteins* (J. L. Cleland and R. Langer, Eds.), ACS Symposium Series 567, Am. Chem. Soc., Washington, DC, 1994, pp. 134–147.
14. J. Freyfuss, J. M. Shaw, and J. J. Ross, Jr., Fluphenazine enanthate and fluphenazine decanoate: intramuscular injection and esterification as requirements for slow-release characteristics in dogs, J. Pharm. Sci., 65, 1310–1315 (1976).
15. A. J. Spiegel and M. M. Noseworthy, Use of nonaqueous solvents in parenteral products, J. Pharm. Sci., 52, 917–927 (1963).
16. S. L. Hem, D. R. Bright, G. S. Banker, and J. P. Pogue, Tissue irritation evaluation of potential parenteral vehicles, Drug. Dev. Commun., 1, 471–477 (1974–75).
17a. A. Pitt, Protein adsorption to microporous filtration membranes, J. Parent. Sci. Tech. 41, 110–114, 1987.
17b. M. J. Akers, A. L. Fites, and R. L. Robison, Formulation design & development of parenteral suspensions, J. Parenter. Sci. Technol., 41, 88–96 (1987).
18. J. C. Boylan, Bull. Parenter. Drug Assoc., 19, 98 (1965).
19. J. C. Boylan and R. L. Robison, Rheological stability of a procaine penicillin G suspension, J. Pharm. Sci., 57, 1796–1797 (1968).
20. A. P. MacKenzie, The physicochemical basis for the freeze-drying process; Dev. Biol. Stand., 36, 51–67 (1977).
21. F. Franks, Freeze drying: from empiricism to predictability, Cryo Lett., 11, 93–110 (1990).
22. S. L. Nail and L. A. Gatlin, in *Pharmaceutical Dosage Forms: Parenteral Medications*, 2nd ed., Vol. 2 (K. Avis, H. Lieberman, and L. Lachman, eds.), Marcel Dekker, New York, 1993.
23. L. M. Her and S. L. Nail, Measurement of glass transitions in frozen solutions by differential scanning calorimetry, Pharm. Res., 11, 54–59 (1994).
24. N. A. Williams, Y. Lee, G. P. Polli, and T. A. Jennings, The effects of cooling rate on solid phase transitions and associated vial breakage occurring in frozen mannitol solutions, J. Parenter. Sci. Technol., 40, 135–141 (1986).
25. L. A. Gatlin and P. P. DeLuca, Kinetics of a phase transition in a frozen solution, J. Parenter. Drug Assoc., 34, 398–408 (1980).
26. J. A. Searles, J. F. Carpenter, and T. W. Randolph, Primary drying rate heterogeneity during pharmaceutical lyophilization, Am. Pharm. Rev., 3, (2000).
27. T. Oguchi, Freezing of drug/additive binary systems II. Relationship between decarboxylation behavior and molecular states of p-aminosalicylic acid, Chem. Pharm. Bull., 37, 3088–3091 (1989).
28. J. Crowe, L. Crowe, and J. Carpenter, Are freezing and dehydration similar stress vectors? A comparison of modes of interaction of biomolecules with stabilizing solutes, Cryobiology, 27, 219–231 (1990).
29. M. J. Pikal, S. Shah, D. Senior, and J. E. Lang, Physical chemistry of freeze drying: measurement of sublimation rates of frozen aqueous solutions by a microbalance technique, J. Pharm. Sci., 72, 635–650 (1983).
30. M. J. Pikal, M. L. Roy, and S. Shah, Mass and heat transfer in vial freeze-drying of pharmaceuticals: role of the vial, J. Pharm. Sci., 73, 1224–1237 (1984).
31. S. L. Nail, The effect of chamber pressure on heat transfer in the freeze drying of parenteral solutions, J. Parenter. Drug Assoc., 34, 358–368 (1980).
32. M. J. Pikal, S. Shah, M. L. Roy, and R. Putman, The secondary drying stage of freeze drying: drying kinetics as a function of shelf temperature and chamber pressure, Int. J. Pharm., 60, 203–217 (1990).
33. T. J. Ahern and M. J. Manning, *Stability of Protein Pharmaceuticals*, Part A, *Chemical and Physical Pathways of Protein Degradation*, Plenum Press, New York, 1992.
34. Y. W. Chien, *Novel Drug Delivery Systems: Fundamentals, Developmental Concepts, Biomedical Assessments*, Marcel Dekker, New York, 1982, pp. 219–292.
35. M. J. Akers and N. R. Anderson, *Pharmaceutical Process Validation* (B. T. Loftus and R. A. Nash, eds.), Marcel Dekker, New York, 1984, pp. 29–97.
36. E. J. Leuthner, *Autoclaves and Autoclaving, Encyclopedia of Pharmaceutical Technology*, Vol. 1 (J. Swarbrick and J. Boylan, eds.), Marcel Dekker, New York, 1988, pp. 393–414.
37. F. M. Groves and M. J. Groves, in *Dry Heat Sterilization and Depyrogenation, Encyclopedia of Pharmaceutical Technology*, Vol. 4 (J. Swarbrick and J. Boylan, eds.), Marcel Dekker, New York, 1991, pp. 447–484.
38. R. R. Reich and D. J. Burgess, in *Ethylene Oxide Sterilization, Encyclopedia of Pharmaceutical Technology*, Vol. 5 (J. Swarbrick, and J. Boylan, eds.), Marcel Dekker, New York, 1992, pp. 315–336.
39. T. H. Meltzer, in *Filters and Filtration, Encyclopedia of Pharmaceutical Technology*, Vol. 6 (J. Swarbrick and J. Boylan, eds.), Marcel Dekker, New York, 1992, pp. 51–91.
40. S. J. Turco, Therapy Hazards Assoc. Parenter. Bull. Parenter. Drug Assoc., 28, 197–204 (1974).
41. R. J. Duma and M. J. Akers, in *Pharmaceutical Dosage Forms: Parenteral Medications*, Vol. I (K. E. Avis, L. Lachman, and H. A. Lieberman, eds.), Marcel Dekker, New York, 1984, p. 35.
42. H. E. Hempel, Large scale manufacture of parenterals, Bull. Parenter. Drug Assoc., 30, 88–95 (1976).
43. R. A. Blackmer, Sterile operations facility, J. Parenter. Sci. Technol., 38, 183–189 (1984).
44. M. J. Akers, in *Parenteral Quality Control: Sterility, Pyrogen, Particulate, and Package Integrity Testing*, Vol. 1 (J. R. Robinson, ed.), Marcel Dekker, New York, 1985, pp. 207–209.

Chapter 13

Design and Evaluation of Ophthalmic Pharmaceutical Products

John C. Lang, Robert E. Roehrs,* Denise P. Rodeheaver, Paul J. Missel, Rajni Jani, and Masood A. Chowhan

Alcon Research Ltd., Fort Worth, Texas

I. INTRODUCTION

Any modern text on the design and evaluation of therapeutic products must place into unique perspective the nature of the eye and requirements of ophthalmic dosage forms. The eye, perhaps better than any other bodily organ, serves as a model structure for the evaluation of drug activity. In no other organ can a practitioner, without surgical or mechanical intervention, so well observe the activity of an administered drug. With such modern instrumentation as the biomicroscope (Fig. 1), the specular microscope (Fig. 2), the confocal microscope capable of viewing the single-layered corneal endothelium, and various devices for measuring intraocular pressure, blood flow, and electroretinal response, the ophthalmologist can readily track changes in ocular structures from the cornea to the retina and monitor their function and physiology. In so doing, the ophthalmologist and diagnostic scientist often detect signs of ocular or systemic disease long before sight-threatening or certain general health-threatening disease states become intractable. With such specialized instrumentation, the practitioner can view the activity of the drug product on the entire eye or, for those products administered to the internal structure of the eye, the activity or effect of the drug product on a cell, a group of cells, or entire tissues.

Ophthalmic pharmaceutical dosage forms serve as delivery vehicles for a wide range of drugs with pharmacological activity in the eye. The most commonly employed ophthalmic dosage forms are solutions, suspensions, and ointments. The characteristics essential for each of these dosage forms have been generally defined in the United States Pharmacopeia (USP) and will be expanded upon in this chapter. Also included are the newest dosage forms for ophthalmic drug delivery—gels, gel-forming solutions, ocular inserts or systems, intravitreal injections, and implants. Common to all ophthalmic dosage forms is the critical requirement for sterility of the finished product as well as appreciation for the sensitivity of ocular tissue to irritation and toxicity and the inherent limitations in topical ocular absorption of most drugs. As will be seen, these are primary factors in the design and evaluation of all ophthalmic pharmaceutical products.

The USP has numerous requirements, e.g., "ophthalmic solutions [need be] essentially free from foreign particles, suitably compounded and packaged for instillation into the eye," or "ophthalmic suspensions [need contain] solid particles dispersed in liquid vehicle intended for application to the eye" [1]. Ophthalmic suspensions are required to be made with the insoluble drug in a micronized form to prevent irritation or scratching of the cornea. A finished ophthalmic ointment must be free from large particles and must meet the requirements for "leakage" and for "metal particles" under "ophthalmic ointments". These and other requirements will be discussed further in subsequent sections.

*Retired.

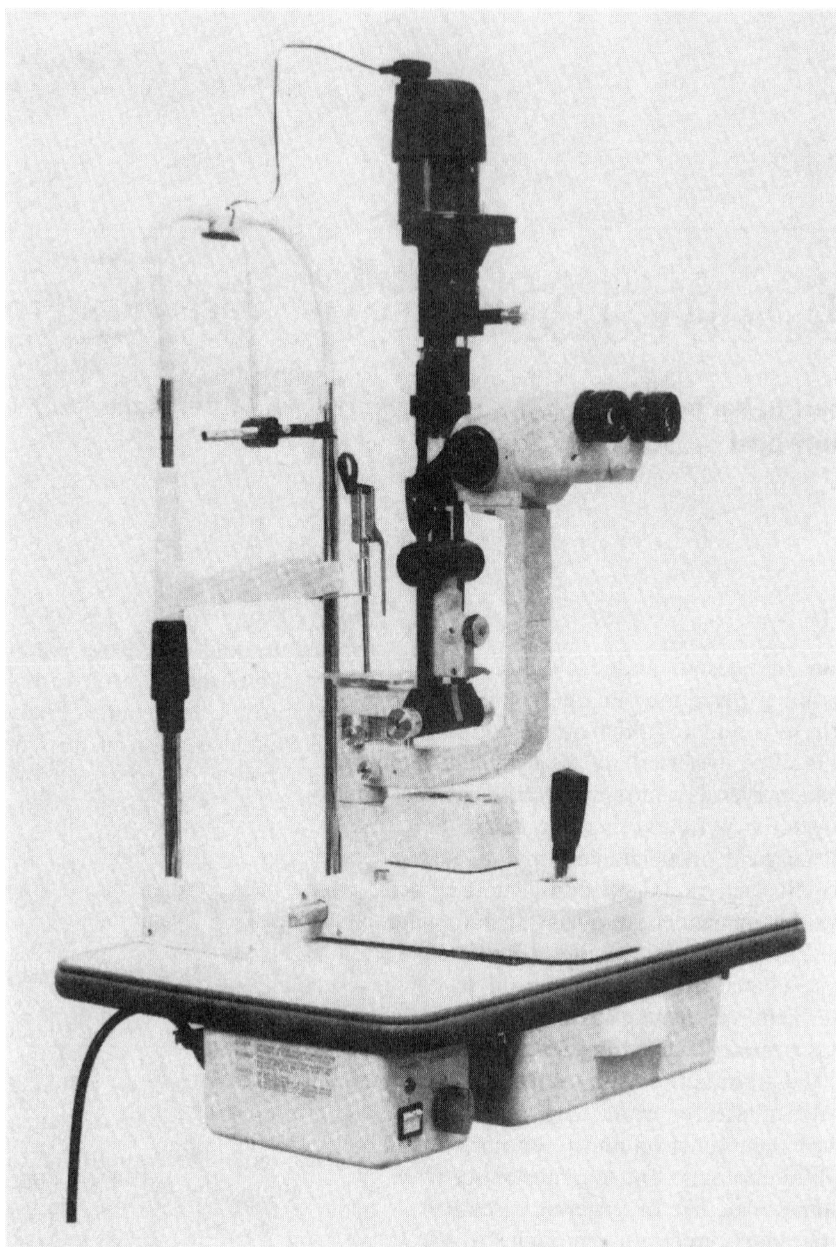

Fig. 1 Topcon slit-lamp biomicroscope.

Behind the relatively straightforward compositional nature of ophthalmic solutions, suspensions, and ointments, however, lie many of the same physicochemical parameters that affect drug stability, safety, and efficacy, as they do for most other drug products. But additionally, specialized dosage forms present the ophthalmic product designer with some extraordinary compositional and manufacturing challenges. These range from concerns for sterility and consistency of parenteral-type ophthalmic solutions for intraocular, subtenon, and retrobulbar use, to resuspendability of such insoluble substances as dexamethasone or fluorometholone, to reconstitution, creating for the patient an apparently conventional solution for compounds such as acetylcholine chloride and epinephrine bitartrate, whose shelf life depends on storage conditions.

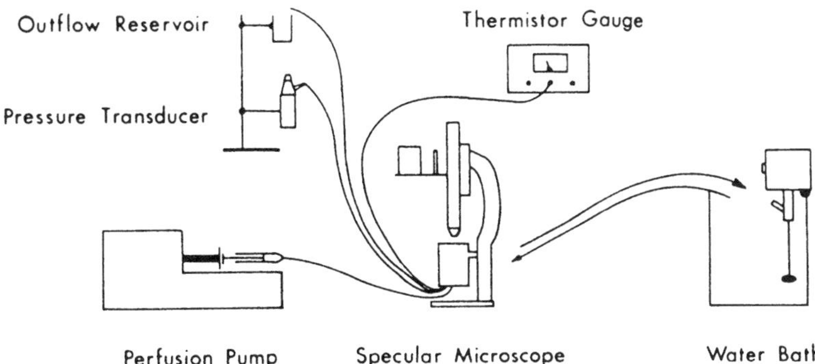

Fig. 2 Specular microscope setup for in vitro evaluation of effect of drugs on ocular tissue.

More recently, the challenge to formulate with consistency highly potent actives present in diminishingly low concentrations raised the bar for formulations another significant notch. Procedures and devices for safe intravitreal implantation of sustained antiviral medication have grown from the advent of new therapies for a life- and eye-threatening new disease, HIV-AIDS.

Like most other products in the medical armamentarium, ophthalmic products are currently undergoing *optimization*. New modes of delivering a drug to the eye are being actively explored, ranging from solid, hydrophobic, or hydrophilic devices that are inserted into the ophthalmic cul-de-sac, to conventionally applied dosage forms that, owing to their formulation characteristics, markedly increase the drug residence time in the fornix of the eye, thereby providing drug for absorption for prolonged periods and reducing the frequency that a given drug product must be administered. Intermediate between these alternatives, in both their physical state and effect on duration, are responsive polymeric systems that undergo transitions from liquid to gel or semisolid [2–7].

In as much as products for the diagnosis and treatment of ocular disease cover the spectrum of practically all dosage forms and, thus, require the same pharmaceutical sciences for their development, in this chapter we discuss the entire scope of considerations involved in the development of ophthalmic products, ranging from regulatory and compendial requirements, through physicochemical, safety, and efficacy considerations, to a discussion of types of dosage forms currently used by the medical practitioner.

The final consideration, but by no means a minor one, is the design and evaluation of contact lens care products, which are regulated by the U.S. Food and Drug Administration (FDA) as medical devices since they are accessory products necessary for the safe and effective use of contact lenses to correct visual acuity. These products include formulations for rinsing, storing, cleaning, and disinfecting contact lenses with specialized compositions for each major type of lens material, i.e., hard, soft hydrophilic, and rigid gas-permeable lenses. Also, lens care products for use in the eye as comfort drops while wearing contact lenses have been developed from similar products using lubricating polymers for treatment of minor eye irritation and tear deficiency (dry eye). The pharmaceutical scientist designing lens care products and improved ophthalmic drug dosage forms have taken advantage of advances in polymer and biomaterial sciences as is evident in the following sections.

II. HISTORICAL BACKGROUND

"If a physician performed a major operation on a seignior [a nobleman] with a bronze lancet and has saved the seignior's life, or he opened the eye socket of seignior with a bronze lancet and has saved the seignior's eye, he shall receive ten shekels of silver." But if the physician in so doing "has caused the seignior's death, or has destroyed the seignior's eye, they shall cut off his hand." The foregoing excerpts are from 2 of 282 laws of King Hammurabi's Code, engraved about 100 B.C. in a block of polished black igneous stone about 2.7 m high, now permanently preserved at the Louvre [8].

Mention is made of the Code of Hammurabi only to place in human history that period when reference to eye medicines or poultices was beginning to appear. The Sumerians, in southern Mesopotamia, are considered to be the first to record their history, beginning about 3100 B.C. The Egyptians used copper compounds, such as malachite and chrysocalla, as green eye makeup with, no doubt, some beneficial effect against infection, owing to the antibacterial properties of copper [9]. The standard wound salve of the Smith Papyrus (approximately 1700 B.C.)—grease, honey and lint—probably served as one of the earliest ointments or ointment bases for the treatment of eye disease or wounds. The Greeks expanded on this basic salve to arrive at a typical enaimon (enheme), a drug for fresh wounds, which might have contained copper, lead, or alum, in addition to myrrh and frankincense [10]. The use of the aromatic substance myrrh in the form of sticks, blocks, or probes has been documented and attributed to the Romans and Greeks. Such sticks were called *collyria* and were dissolved in water, milk, or egg white for use as eyedrops. The Latin word *collyrium* is a derivative of the Greek word, *kollyrien* (in turn derived from *kollyra*, a roll of coarse bread), meaning a glutinous paste made from wheat and water that was rolled into thin cones, rods, or blocks. Often the physician's name was inscribed on these bodies [11]. Pliny the Elder (ca. A.D. 23–79) advocated the use of egg whites to "cool" inflamed eyes, and lycium, one of the most popular of the plant extracts of India, was recommended especially for "eye troubles" [12].

After having placed the origin of at least two dosage forms (solution and ointment) for treating disorders or wounds of the eye between approximately the first and second millennium B.C., we can readily reflect on the progress that the designers of dosage forms for eye products have made down through the ages—until relatively recently, little or none. Over the past two decades, however, we have begun to see new concepts emerging, some receiving the enthusiastic support of the ophthalmologist and optometrist, whereas others, not so fortunate, have been relegated to the status of little-used novelties.

III. ANATOMY OF THE EYE AND ADNEXA

In-depth discussions of the anatomy of the eye and adnexa have been adequately covered elsewhere in the pharmaceutical literature [13–17] and in recent texts on ocular anatomy. Here a brief overview is presented of the critical anatomical features that influence the nature and administration of ophthalmic preparations. In this discussion, consideration will be given primarily to drugs applied topically, that is, onto the cornea or conjunctiva or into the palpebral fornices. Increasingly, drugs are being developed for administration by parenteral-type dosage forms subconjunctivally, into the anterior and posterior chambers, the vitreous chamber, Tenon's capsule, or by retrobulbar injection.

Table 1 Anatomical Structures of the Eye

Conjunctiva	Iris
Inferior conjunctival sac	Uvea
Superior conjunctival sac	Posterior chamber
	Zonules of Zinn
Cornea	Lens
Epithelium	Vitreous humor
Bowman's membrane	
Stroma (substantia propria)	Tenon's capsule
Descemet's membrane	Retina
Endothelium	Ciliary body (zone)
	Meibomian glands
Anterior chamber	
Angle of anterior chamber	Posterior chamber
Schlemm's canal	Vitreous chamber
Spaces of fontana	
Retina	

Because some of the dosage forms described may be considered as adjunctive to ophthalmic surgical procedures, those procedures and the concomitant use of the drug are described in Sec. VIII.D. For orientation, readers are encouraged to familiarize themselves with the anatomical structures of the eye (Table 1), some of which are shown in Fig. 3.

The eye is essentially a globe suspended in the ocular orbit, specialized for sight through an arrangement of multiple tissues that function to focus, transmit, and detect incoming light. There is a central path that light travels to the retina, with all intervening tissues (cornea, aqueous humor, pupil, lens, and vitreous humor) being transparent. All surrounding tissues serve to nourish, support, and protect these essential structures.

The cornea composes only one sixth of the outer surface of the eye, yet it is the first and one of the most important barriers to external materials. The cornea is composed of three layers of varying structural and chemical properties that form barriers based on solubility, polarity and partitioning properties, molecular weight and geometry, and specific binding characteristics. The presence and type of intercellular junctions regulate molecular diffusion around the cells, while the hydrophilic or lipophilic characteristic of each layer controls diffusion across and along the cell membrane. The cornea itself has no blood vessels so it relies on passive diffusion of nutrients from surrounding tissues and aqueous humor.

The outermost layer, the epithelium, is composed of five to seven layers of stratified epithelial cells that makeup only 10% (50 μm) of the total corneal

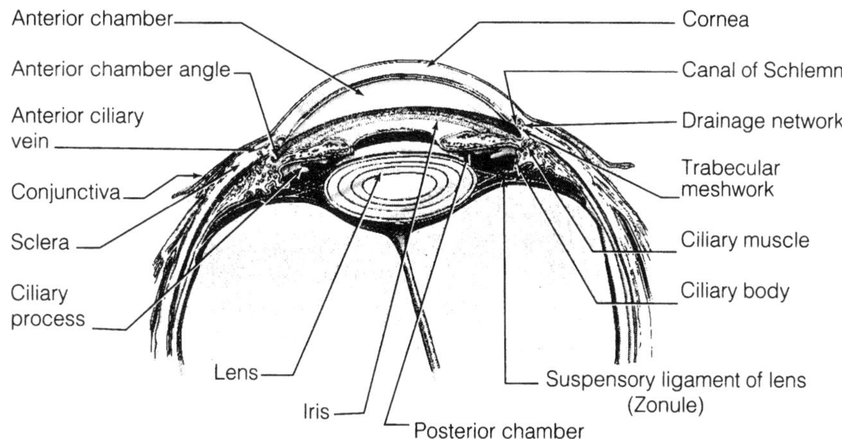

Fig. 3 Anatomical cross section of the human eye.

thickness. Basal cells of the epithelium are mitotically active, providing a regular supply of cells to replenish those lost through normal sloughing or injury. The tight junctions and lipophilic composition of the epithelium combine to form an effective barrier to molecules and foreign substances that are hydrophilic or of high molecular weight. The tears, composed of mucin, aqueous and lipid phases, serve to hydrate the epithelium, prevent adhesion of bacteria and other foreign materials, and influence the distribution and toxicity of foreign materials [18]. Finally, the epithelium is metabolically highly active against xenobiotics; while protective against toxic substances, this activity may also impact drug bioavailability and therapeutic index significantly. Bowman's membrane separates the epithelium from the stroma, the layer that comprises 90% of the cornea.

In contrast to the epithelium, the stroma is 76–80% water and composed mostly of collagen fibrils in a highly organized array with interstices filled with glucosaminoglycan ground substance and a scattering of keratocytes. No junctions are present, yet the hydrophilic composition presents a significant barrier to lipophilic molecules. The stroma is susceptible to swelling, and water content must be actively controlled to prevent opacification. This is a primary function of the endothelium, a single layer of hexagonally arranged cells separated from the stroma by Decemet's membrane. Since the corneal endothelial cells have discontinuous tight junctions, water readily passes from the aqueous humor across to the stroma. To counter this, cellular ion pumps maintain proper hydration of the stroma by active transport of ions out into the aqueous humor with water following the ionic gradient through passive diffusion. These "leaky" junctions may present a constant hazard of overhydration to the stroma and present little or no barrier to drug penetration, but are essential to the diffusion of nutrients from the aqueous humor into the cornea. The endothelium has an overall lipophilic nature that limits diffusion of hydrophilic molecules. It is important to note that the human endothelium has a fixed number of cells that are not mitotically active, instead compensating for cell loss only through migration and hypertrophy of individual cells to cover gaps in the layer. Inability to compensate for cell loss will result in loss of function and corneal opacification. Since endothelial cells are sensitive to chemical and mechanical insult, any ophthalmic preparation that could contact these cells must be carefully evaluated for biocompatibility.

The cornea is connected at the limbus to the opaque sclera, the tough fibroelastic capsule that encloses the eye and provides support and protection for the interior structures. The visible area of the sclera is generally referred to as the conjunctiva. The stroma has loosely packed collagen fibrils with scattered fibrocytes and few blood vessels except in the limbal area. No junctional complexes are present, so the sclera presents only a lipophilic barrier to foreign materials. The limbus is rich in blood vessels, and systemic absorption of topically applied drugs occurs here primarily. Within the interior of the eye, the limbal area contains the trabecular meshwork and canal of Schlemm at the junction of the iris and sclera. These structures drain aqueous humor from the anterior chamber, a function essential to prevent fluid accumulation, increased intraocular pressure, and glaucoma. The iris, a ring of muscular tissue that regulates light entry into the back of the eye through the pupil, is located in front of the lens and physically forms the division between the anterior chamber and the posterior chamber. This structure is rich in blood vessels, which dilate when exposed to severe irritants resulting in iridial hyperemia and edema. The innervation of the iris provides the means by which the practitioner can control pupillary dilation.

The lens is essentially a flattened sphere that is held in place and connected to the ciliary body by fiber-like strands, the zonules of Zinn. Composed of concentric layers of crystalline fibers, the avascular lens has a single layer of epithelial cells on the anterior surface and is surrounded by a thin but tough capsule that conveniently provides the support for an intraocular lens (IOL) once a cataractous lens has been removed. The lens epithelial cells have some mitotic activity, and older cells progressively lose their cellular contents and migrate to form the crystalline fibers. The lens is flexible and changes shape in order to adjust focal length for near objects (accommodation), an ability that is lost with age. It is important to note that there is little exchange of materials in the lens and no loss of cells so that drug accumulation should be investigated for ophthalmic preparations that are absorbed into the eye. The ciliary body has two major functions. The ciliary muscle connects to the zonules of Zinn and controls lens accommodation. The anterior portion of the ciliary body facing the posterior chamber produces the aqueous humor that circulates across and through the pupil to the anterior chamber and out of the eye for a continual turnover of fluid.

Behind the lens is the vitreous chamber that contains vitreous humor, a transparent gelatinous material that has no turnover and is in direct contact with the retina. The retina is a bilayered highly metabolically active tissue that transforms light to an electrical signal, which is processed and transmitted as electronic images to the brain. The tissue is composed of a complex arrangement of photoreceptor cells (rods and cones) overlying the retinal pigmented epithelium (RPE) and is isolated from vascular fluids by the blood-retinal barrier, a combination of endothelial cell tight junctions lining the retinal blood vessels and tight junctions between the RPE cells that restricts diffusion from the systemic circulation. The choroid is a highly vascularized collagenous tissue lying between the retina and the sclera from the ciliary body to the optic nerve. The optic nerve connects to the retina at the optic disk, a highly vascularized area that is susceptible to ocular hypertension and drug effects. Finally, several accessory tissues (adnexa) are essential to proper functioning of the eye. Tenon's capsule, a thin membrane surrounding the sclera, separates the eye from the surrounding socket for freedom of movement. The lacrimal and Meibomian glands provide essential tear and lipid components while the eyelids assist in tear distribution and protect against mechanical injury.

From this discussion, the reader can appreciate the intricacy of the eye and the care required in devising ophthalmic preparations in order to provide safe and effective therapy.

IV. PHARMACOLOGY AND THERAPEUTICS OF OPHTHALMIC MEDICATION

It is not the purpose of this text to present an in-depth review of the pharmacology of ophthalmic drugs. For this purpose the reader is referred to one of the authoritative treatments of this subject [19–21]. However, since this topic is not commonly covered in pharmacy school curricula, a brief treatment is presented here. For the most part, drugs used in the eye fall into one of several categories, including miotics, mydriatics (with or without cycloplegic activity), cycloplegics, anti-inflammatories, anti-infectives (including antibiotics, antivirals, and antibacterials), antiglaucoma drugs, surgical adjuncts, diagnostics, and a category of drugs for miscellaneous uses. The intended ophthalmic use will define more precisely what drug or combination of drugs is to be used, the appropriate dosage form, and route of administration. For example, the practitioner will, with knowledge of certain contraindications, use mydriatic drugs specifically for their pupillary and accommodative effects, both in the process of refraction and in the management of iridocyclitis, iritis, accommodative exotropia, and so on. Atropine, homatropine, scopolamine, tropicamide, and cyclopentolate are examples of parasympathomimetic drugs possessing mydriatic and cycloplegic activity, whereas phenylephrine and epinephrine are examples of sympathomimetic drugs possessing only mydriatic activity.

Drugs that may be chosen for use in the management of glaucoma may be topically applied miotics, such as pilocarpine hydrochloride or nitrate, carbachol, echothiophate iodide, or demecarium bromide; epinephrine prodrugs like dipivefrin hydrochloride, nonselective β-adrenergic blocking agents such as timolol maleate and bunolol hydrochloride, and selective β-adrenergic blocking agents such as racemic- or the more potent *levo*-betaxolol hydrochloride, compounds devoid of pupillary effect; topically administered carbonic anhydrase inhibitors, such as dorzolamide and brinzolamide; prostaglandin analogs of the class $PGF_{2\alpha}$, such as latanoprost and travoprost, capable of lowering intraocular pressure (IOP) significantly with little or no inflammatory or vasodilatory response; or they may be orally administered drugs to present an osmotic effect that will lower intraocular pressure, such as 50% glycerin or 45% isosorbide. Other drugs administered orally to lower intraocular pressure are the carbonic anhydrous inhibitors acetazolamide and methazolamide. Furthermore, the miotic drugs may be chosen to reverse the effect of mydriatics after refraction or during surgical procedures such as cataract removal. There is now available an antimydriatic drug devoid of pupillary activity, dapiprazole hydrochloride, which is gaining importance in the reversal of the effect of mydriatics.

Depending on the location of ocular inflammation, a specific corticosteroid in a specific dosage form may be chosen. For instance, a corticosteroid of high potency, such as prednisolone acetate, fluorometholone, dexamethasone, or rimexolone, may be chosen for deep-seated inflammation of the uveal tract. Further treatment of such inflammation may take the form of subtenon injections or oral (systemic) administration of selected corticosteroids, depending on the indication and the dosage forms available. For inflammation of a more superficial nature, the lower strengths of prednisolone acetate or the lower-potency corticosteroids, such as hydrocortisone or medrysone, will usually be chosen. It is now also possible to treat inflammation with nonsteroidal agents like diclofenac or keterolac, drugs not expected to raise IOP.

Drugs used for the treatment of ocular infection will generally be chosen based on the presumptive diagnosis of the causative agent by the ophthalmologist. Laboratory confirmation by microbial culture and identification is routinely conducted concurrently with the initiation of therapy. This is generally necessary because of the severity and sight-threatening nature of some types of infection. For example, if a patient has a foreign body lodged in the cornea originating from a potentially contaminated environment, the physician may choose to begin treatment of the eye, after foreign body removal, with a single or combination antibiotic, such as gentamicin, tobramycin, chloramphenicol, and a neomycin-polymyxin combination. Recent introduction of quinolone antibiotics like ciprofloxacin, ofloxacin, and norfloxacin have expanded the physician's choice of available products for ocular infections. The application of these agents is considered appropriate, since an infection with *Pseudomonas aeruginosa* can destroy a cornea in 24–48 hours, generally the time it takes to identify an infectious agent. Less fulminating, but no less dangerous, are infections caused by various staphylococcal and streptococcal organisms. For superficial bacterial infections of the conjunctiva and eyelids, sulfonamides, such as sodium sulfacetamide, are usually prescribed, as are yellow mercuric oxide and mild silver protein. Prophylactic therapy for ophthalmia neonaturnum is nearly universally required in the United States, with silver nitrate, penicillin G, or erythromycin being the primary anti-infectives used. Pre- and postsurgical prophylaxis is becoming more commonplace with the popularity of surgically corrected vision, and combinations of anti-infectives with anti-inflammatory agents are frequently used to reduce surgical trauma to the eye.

For fungal and viral infections, there are very few agents that the ophthalmologist can prescribe. These organisms' resistance and similarity to mammalian tissue make it difficult to find effective and safe therapies. For instance, idoxuridine, a selective metabolic inhibitor, has been shown to be useful against herpes simplex virus infection of the cornea. For the trachoma virus and viruses that cause inclusion conjunctivitis [i.e., TRIC (the single largest cause of blindness worldwide)], no specific antiviral agent has demonstrated satisfactory activity, and the secondary bacterial ramifications of this disease are managed by conventional antibiotics, such as tetracycline, chloramphenicol, and erythromycin. The trachoma virus itself seems to be somewhat susceptible to these antibiotics; however, up to 6 weeks of treatment three times per day are required to achieve an 80% cure rate [22,23].

A similar situation exists for the treatment of fungal keratitis. The antifungal antibiotic drugs nystatin and natamycin have been effective to varying degrees in superficial fungal infection, as have copper sulfate and sodium sulfacetamide [24,25]. For both of these drugs iontophoresis of the topically administered drug produces enhanced activities.

Drugs used as surgical adjuncts are primarily irrigating solutions, solutions of proteolytic enzymes, viscoelastics and miotics employed in cataract removal, intraocular lens placement, vitrectomy, and procedures to preserve retinal integrity. These drugs are considered true parenteral dosage forms, the design and evaluation of which are discussed in greater detail elsewhere in this chapter.

Diagnostic drugs, such as sodium fluorescein, are administered topically or intravenously to aid in the diagnosis of such conditions as corneal abrasions or ulceration and various retinopathies. This agent has become the most widely used diagnostic agent in the practice of ophthalmology and optometry. Rose bengal has also been used topically, although to a far lesser degree than sodium fluorescein, which is available as well-preserved alkaline solutions in concentrations ranging from 0.5 to 2.0% [26,27], as fluorescein-impregnated absorbent sterile paper strips [28], or as unpreserved, terminally sterilized intravenous injections in concentrations ranging from 5 to 25% [29].

Several topically applied local anesthetics are routinely used by the eye care specialist in certain routine diagnostic procedures and for various relatively simple surgical procedures such as insertion of punctal plugs and surgical vision correction. The first of these to be used was cocaine, in concentrations ranging from 1 to 4% [30]. More modern local anesthetics, however, such as tetracaine hydrochloride and proparacaine hydrochloride, have replaced cocaine as drugs of choice in these procedures. For surgical procedures of a more complex nature, lidocaine hydrochloride and similar local anesthetics as retrobulbar injections have been used [31].

The foregoing overview has presented the major classes of ophthalmic drugs. One additional class of drugs that merits brief discussion includes drugs used for the treatment of various dry eye syndromes. The most severe of these, *keratoconjunctivitis sicca*, involves diminished secretion of mucins, consisting of glycoproteins and glycosaminoglycans and their complexes. These materials serve to coat the corneal epithelium with a hydrophilic layer that uniformly attracts water molecules, resulting in even hydration of the corneal surface. Diminished secretion of these substances causes dry spots to develop on the cornea, resulting in corneal dehydration, which can lead to ulceration, scarring, or corneal opacities [32]. Modern pharmaceutical products are available (Hypotears, Tears Naturale Forte) that contain mucomimetic high molecular weight polymers that serve to resurface the cornea temporarily, thereby preventing the aforementioned dehydration and affording the dry eye sufferer with a degree of relief previously unavailable [33,34]. These agents are not pharmacologically active, although recent research leads to the promise of drugs that will stimulate tear production for longer-term relief.

V. GENERAL SAFETY CONSIDERATIONS

A. Sterility

Every ophthalmic product must be manufactured under conditions validated to render it sterile in its final container for the shelf life of the product [35,36]. Sterility testing is conducted on each lot of ophthalmic product by suitable procedures, as set forth in the appropriate pharmacopeia and validated in each manufacturer's laboratory. While the majority of ophthalmic preparations contain preservatives for multiple-dose use, sterile preparations in special containers for individual use on a single patient must be made available. This availability is especially critical for every hospital, office, or other installation where accidentally or surgically traumatized eyes are treated, as well as for patients intolerant to preservatives.

The USP recognizes six methods of achieving a sterile product: (a) steam sterilization, (b) dry-heat sterilization, (c) gas sterilization, (d) sterilization by ionizing radiation, (e) sterilization by filtration, and (f) aseptic processing [37]. For ophthalmic products packaged in plastic containers, typical for ophthalmic products, a combination of two or more of these six methods is used routinely. For example, for a sterile ophthalmic suspension, bottles, dropper tips, and caps may be sterilized by ethylene oxide or gamma radiation; the suspended solid may be sterilized by dry heat, gamma radiation, or ethylene oxide; and the aqueous portion of the composition may be sterilized by filtration. The compounding is completed under aseptic conditions.

One can see by the complexity of these types of manufacturing procedures that much care and attention to detail must be maintained by the manufacturer. This sterile manufacturing procedure must then be validated to prove that no more than 3 containers in a lot of 3000 containers (0.1%) are nonsterile. Ultimately, it is the manufacturer's responsibility to ensure the safety and efficacy of the manufacturing process and the absence of any adverse effect on the product, such as the possible formation of substances toxic to the eye, an ever-present possibility with gas sterilization or when using ionizing radiation. For ophthalmic products sterilized by terminal sterilization (sterilization in the final sealed container, e.g., steam under pressure), the sterilization cycle must be validated to ensure sterility at a probability of 10^6 or greater.

Currently, the *British Pharmacopoeia* suggests five methods of sterilization: (a) sterilization by autoclaving, (b) dry-heat sterilization, usually to >60°C, (c) ethylene oxide, (d) ionizing radiation (electron accelerator or gamma radiation), and (e) sterilization by filtration. During the manufacture of an ophthalmic product, sterility may be checked while the finished product is in its bulk form before filling. It is then also tested on a random sampling basis in the finished package. Suggested guidelines for the number of samples are dependent on whether or not sterilization has taken place in the sealed final container. While terminal sterilization (methods a–d) is preferred, sterilization by filtration and aseptic processing have been accepted for preparations that are incompatible with other methods. Class A products are those sterilized in bulk form and filled aseptically into sterile final containers without further sterilization. Class B products are those sterilized in sealed final containers. Class B is further subdivided according to method of sterilization: type 1 comprises those products sterilized by steam under pressure; type 2 comprises those products sterilized by any other means. Class A products require a minimum random sample number of no fewer than 30 items from each filling operation. Class B products require varying sample sizes, generally from 5 to 30 units per lot, depending on whether the sterilization occurs in a chamber or by a continuous process.

B. Ocular Toxicity and Irritation

Assessment of the potential for ocular irritation and toxicity of ophthalmic solutions represents an extremely important step in the development of both over-the-counter (OTC) and prescriptive pharmaceuticals. Excellent reviews of procedures describing these evaluations have been published [38–40,90]. Refinements in procedures, study design, use of objective measures, and standardization of noninvasive methods such as specular microscopy have resulted in greater reliability, detection, and predictability. In addition, the incorporation of structure-activity relationship (SAR) evaluations provides an early assessment of probable toxic effects of the chemical moieties under consideration. The historical evaluation of these procedures can be traced through the literature [41–50], as can an understanding of the mechanisms of ocular response to irritants, based on examination of the conjunctiva [51–54], the cornea [42,55–57], or the iris [42,58,120]. Advances in design and use of ophthalmic drugs and devices have brought ocular toxicity into sharper focus. Many interior structures of the eye adjacent to target tissues, or which are targets of newer therapies themselves, can suffer irreversible damage so safety evaluations must be comprehensive. In general, consideration must also be given to the use of various ophthalmic preparations with other drugs and devices. Testing, therefore, must be based on risk analysis to include both the intended uses of the product as well as reasonably foreseeable misuse.

Albino rabbits have been the primary species used to test ocular toxicity and irritation of ophthalmic formulations. While recent debate has centered on the use of rabbits or other species as predictors for human responses, there is consensus that there is no more reliable model that captures the full complexity of the eye and the ocular response of its intricate biochemical and physiological processes. In addition, the albino rabbit has obvious advantages due to its availability, ease of handling, ease of maintenance, and large prominent unpigmented eye. The ocular structures are easily observed and accessible, including the cornea, bulbar conjunctival iridial vessels, and posterior segment [39]. The primary differences between rabbits and humans in ophthalmic studies relate to decreased tearing in rabbits, decreased blinking rate, presence of lipid from a species-specific gland (Harderian gland), loosely attached eyelids, presence of a nictitating membrane [53,59–61], differences in the structure of Bowman's membrane, slower reepithelialization of the rabbit cornea [42], and regenerative endothelium of the rabbit. The corneal differences result in increased ocular response to irritants in the rabbit. The primate has gained in popularity as an ocular model for the evaluation of drugs and chemicals because it is more similar to human eye [59,60]. However, due to the difficulty and risk inherent in their care and handling, primates are used secondarily and in cases where other species may not provide an accurate assessment. This is especially true for drugs with melanin-binding characteristics that may accumulate in a pigmented iris.

Various governmental agencies have published guidelines for ocular irritancy studies [61,62,77]. These guidelines are directed toward ophthalmic formulations, chemicals, cosmetics, extractables from ophthalmic containers, and other materials that may intentionally or accidentally contact the eye during use. It is the manufacturer's responsibility to determine those studies specifically appropriate for testing the safety of the ophthalmic formulation, yet abiding by general governmental guidelines. The USP presents guidelines for a 72-hour ocular irritation test in rabbits using saline and cottonseed oil extracts of plastic containers used for packaging ophthalmic products. Containers are cleaned and sterilized as in the final packaged product to determine acceptability of the packaging system.

As a part of the Federal Hazardous Substances Act (FHSA), a modified Draize test was adopted [63–65] as the official method for evaluation of acute ocular irritancy [66]. It is a pass/fail determination that remains in effect today. Two refinements have been accepted as alternatives: (a) the test which uses a small volume more consistent with the capacity of the inferior conjunctival sac [67], and (b) assessment of the degree, frequency, and duration of ocular changes using biomicroscopic slit-lamp examination and/or fluorescein staining [39,64,65]. While various in vitro tests have been proposed to replace this in vivo evaluation, none has yet been accepted or validated [68–70].

Current guidelines for toxicity evaluation of ophthalmic formulations involve both single and multiple applications, dependent on the proposed clinical use [39]. The multiple applications may extend over a 9-month period and incorporate evaluations of ocular irritation and toxicity, systemic toxicity, and determinations of systemic exposure (toxicokinetics). In many cases the systemic exposure from an ocular route is less than by parenteral administration, information that will assist in determining whether additional studies may be needed to establish systemic safety of the ophthalmic preparation. U.S. and international guidance documents are available [71,72], and regulations and tests have been summarized for ophthalmic preparations [39,73,74].

As mentioned previously (and discussed in detail in Sec. IX), contact lens products have specific guidelines that focus on compatibility with the contact lens and biocompatibility with the cornea and conjunctiva [75]. These solutions are viewed as new medical devices and require testing with the contact lenses with which they are to be used. Tests include a 21-day ocular study in rabbits and employ the appropriate types of contact lenses with which they are to be used and may include the other solutions that might be used with the lens. Additional tests to evaluate cytotoxicity potential, acute toxicity, sensitization potential (allergenicity), and risks specific to the preparation are also required [75–77]. These tests are sufficient to meet requirements in the majority of countries, though testing requirements for Japan are currently much more extensive.

While systemic exposure is rarely encountered in intraocularly administered drug products, there are safety concerns related to the biocompatibility of these products with ocular tissues. These products have special design and evaluation concerns, since a product instilled into the anterior chamber may contact for up to 2 hours such essential and delicate tissues as the endothelium and trabecular meshwork [78]. For such drug products, it is mandatory to design specific testing that mimics this length of exposure. Methods may include ex vivo models that continuously infuse the specific product composition, both freshly made and aged, into the anterior chamber of excised rabbit eyes for prolonged periods. Judgments for product-tissue compatibility can then be made by observing corneal endothelium with specular microscopy [79] and histopathology. These materials can also be evaluated against specific cell lines in tissue culture, particularly corneal endothelial tissue. As tissue culture technology progresses, cell lines for the other tissues in the anterior segment of the eye are being established and will become useful in tissue compatibility testing as well.

The sensitivity of the intraocular tissues places certain restrictions on intraocular dosage forms. In general, preparations that incorporate fewer ingredients in a properly balanced solution will have less likelihood of tissue incompatibility. This is not to say that a simple solution of drug in water is optimal. Indeed, a simple isotonic solution of sodium chloride is toxic to human corneal epithelial, endothelial, iris, and conjunctival cells, whereas a solution properly balanced with various organic and inorganic ions and nutrients is nontoxic to these cells in vitro and in vivo. In the electron photomicrographs of human corneal endothelium presented in Figs. 4–6, the effect of solution composition on tissue integrity is illustrated. Figure 4 shows human corneal endothelial tissue after corneal perfusion for 3 hours with lactated Ringer's solution, while Fig. 5 illustrates the same tissue perfused for 3 hours with Ringer's solution containing glutathione, adenosine, and bicarbonate. In the former, cell darkening and swelling are in evidence, whereas in the latter, normal cell confluence is retained. Fig. 6 shows the same tissue after a 3-hour perfusion with a solution devoid of ingredients essential for normal cell confluence. The discontinuity of cell structure is quite evident.

Other agents commonly used in topical ocular drugs can be used only sparingly or not at all for intraocular use. The preservative agents commonly used in topical ophthalmic preparations are not compatible with the tissues of the anterior segments of the eye and in several cell lines in tissue culture [80]. The USP recognizes this problem and specifically warns against their use in intraocular solutions [81,82]. Drug stabilizers, such as antioxidants and chelating agents, must be used with care and should be used in absolutely minimal quantities only when necessary. Occasionally, it may seem desirable to solubilize an otherwise sparingly soluble ingredient. Whereas this may be a practical consideration in some injectables, only aqueous solutions should be employed intraocularly. Furthermore, only fairly low concentrations of typical cosolvents such as glycerin and propylene glycol can be employed because of their osmotic effect on the surrounding tissues. Hyperosmotic solutions may elicit some transient desiccation of the anterior chamber tissues, whereas hy-

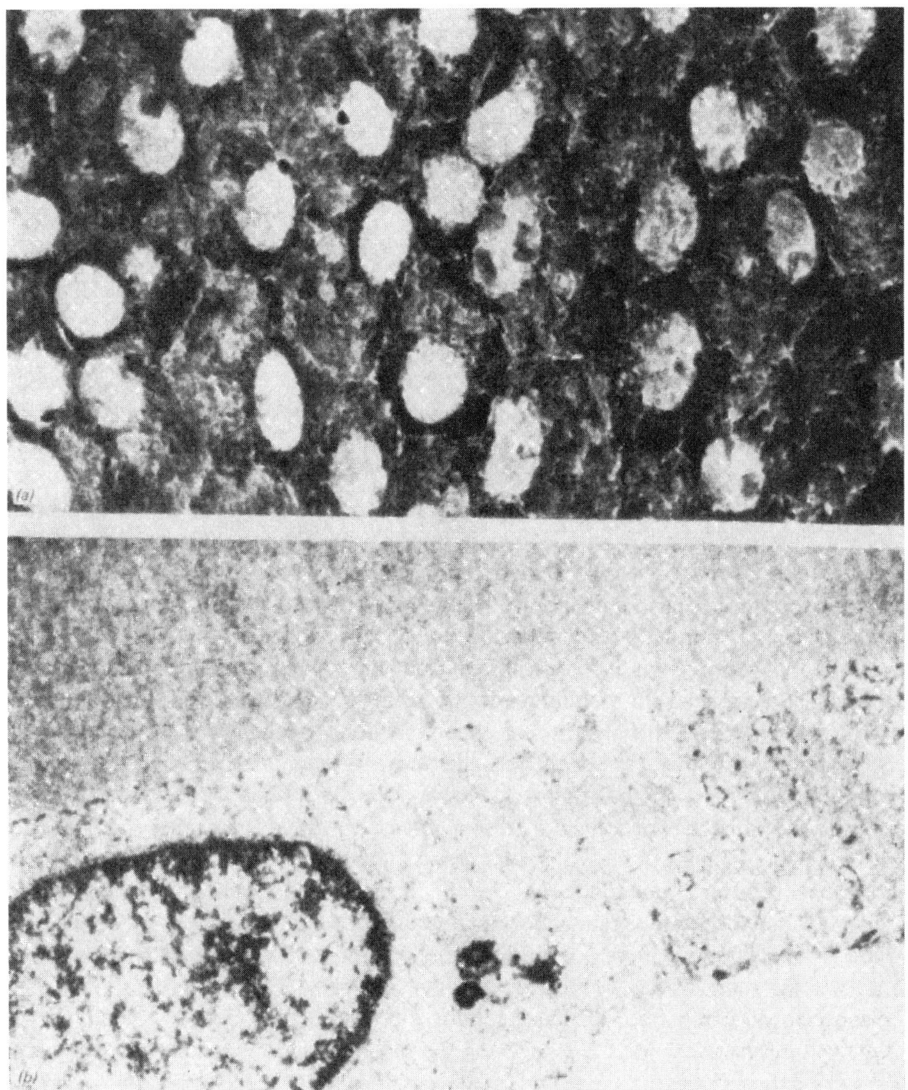

Fig. 4 Human corneal endothelium following 3-hour perfusion with lactated Ringer's solution: (a) scanning electron micrograph (2100 ×); (b) transmission electron micrograph (9100 ×). (Courtesy of H. Edelhauser.)

potonic solutions may cause edema that could lead to corneal clouding. There appears to be little or no experience with these or other common cosolvents in products of this type, and their use should be avoided.

Another formulation variable that must be considered is that of the solution pH and buffer capacity. Since the anterior chamber fluid (aqueous humor) contains essentially the same buffering systems as the blood, products with a pH outside the physiological range of 7.0–7.4 are converted to this range by the buffering capacity of the aqueous humor if a relatively small volume of the solution is introduced. Often, however, aqueous humor is lost in the procedure or the volume of solution is relatively large, therefore, drug products should be formulated as closely as possible to this physiological range although the use of buffering agents should be avoided if possible.

The question of particulate matter is also of great importance. Although the total effect of particulate inclusion in the anterior chamber is not completely known, some possible results have been postulated [82]. Certain amounts of iritis and uveitis might be expected, as well as the production of granulomas similar to the type reported for pulmonary tissue that

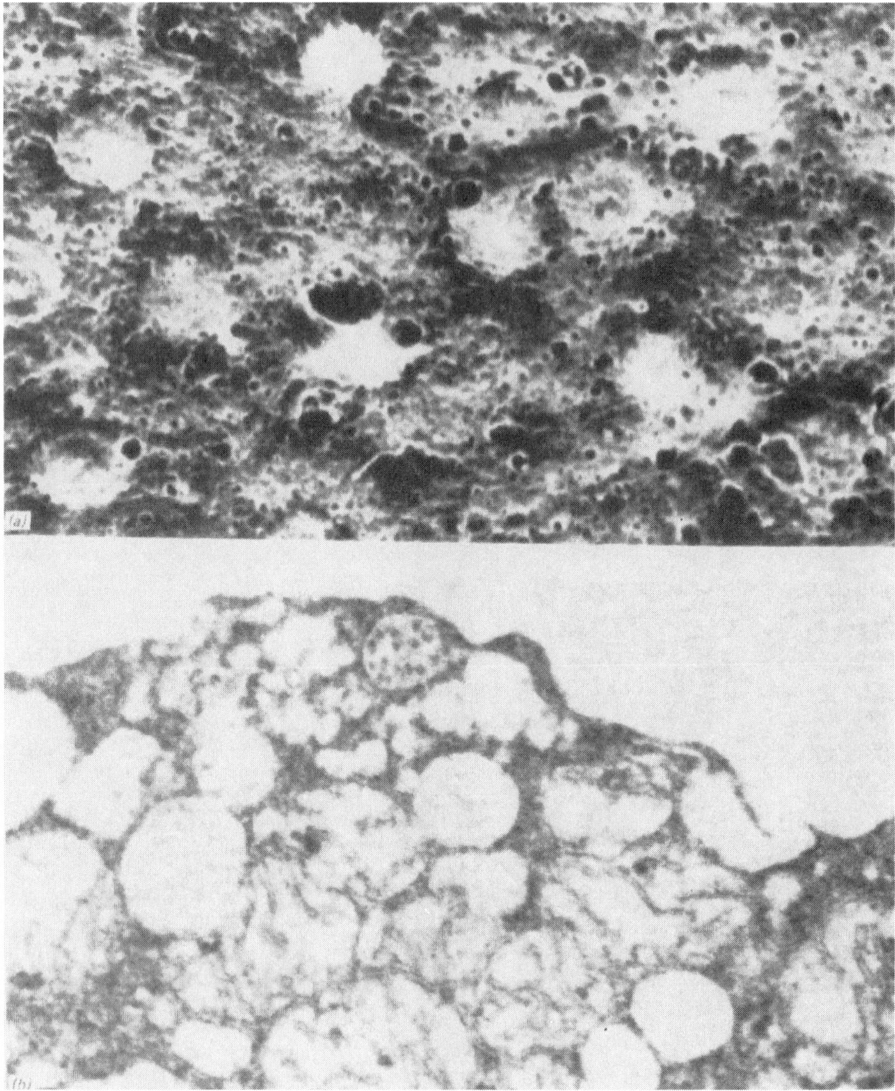

Fig. 5 Human corneal endothelium following 3-hour perfusion with glutathione bicarbonated Ringer's solution: (a) scanning electron micrograph (1950 ×); (b) transmission electron micrograph (8450 ×). (Courtesy of H. Edelhauser.)

results from particulates in large-volume parenterals. At least as important is the possibility that particulate matter can block the canals of Schlemm, which provide the outflow mechanism for the aqueous humor. If this should occur to any great extent, the normal continual production of aqueous humor could lead to a rapid increase in intraocular pressure and the onset of an acute attack of glaucoma. The formulator should be aware that particulates may originate from raw materials as well as glass fragments produced in glass ampoule fracture or elastomeric particles generated during stopper penetration. Very specialized stopper design, cleaning procedures, and lubrication should be considered when the latter type of packaging is used.

To provide a complete assessment of all these variables, the final evaluation of safety must be made in the in vivo model using the preparation under the proposed conditions for use, following tissue compatibility with many of the techniques already discussed. Confocal microscopy is a relatively new noninvasive technique that allows a detailed examination of the endothelium in the live animal, and thus may prove useful in following changes in this delicate tissue over time. As in ex vivo models, the

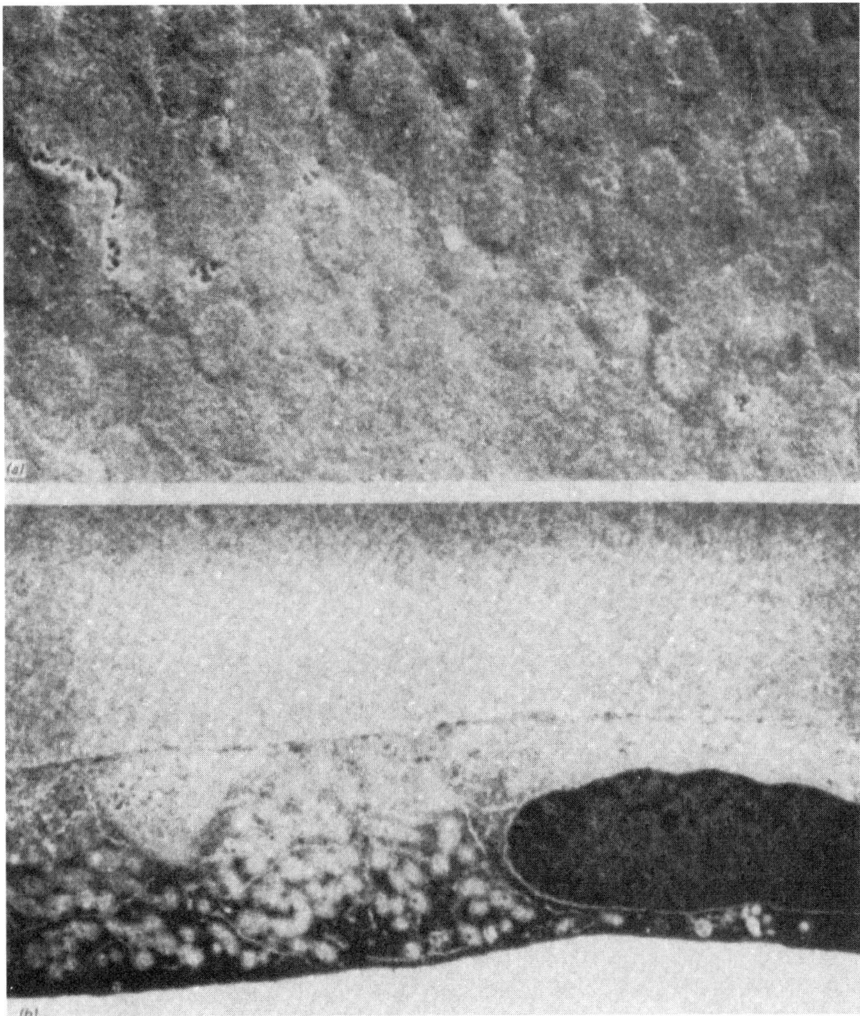

Fig. 6 Human corneal endothelium following 3-hour perfusion with solution devoid of essential nutrients: (a) scanning electron micrograph (2100 ×); (b) transmission electron micrograph (9100 ×). (Courtesy of H. Edelhauser.)

experimental design must address the nature of the intraocular preparation and the type of contact. Irrigating solutions of low viscosity may have limited contact while the gel-like viscoelastic materials that maintain the corneal dome, or the solutions and gases used as vitreous replacements to prevent retinal detachment, may have prolonged contact with delicate ocular tissues or the retina. In vivo studies can thus become quite lengthy even during early phases of development, underscoring the utility of preliminary in vitro or ex vivo evaluations, in which experiments utilize harvested tissues maintained viable for the duration of the evaluation.

A new therapy involves treatment for neovascularization of the retina, a disease in which proliferation of blood vessels can lead to blindness. The treatment combines a systemic chemical that localizes in the new blood vessels followed by laser treatment to destroy the vessels. Such new therapies and new routes of administration require special care in their design and evaluation.

During the application of the various guidelines for ophthalmic, contact lens, and intraocular products, ocular examination and biomicroscopic examination of rabbit eyes are completed with objective reproducible grading for conjunctival congestion, conjunctival swelling, conjunctival discharge, aqueous (humor) flare, iris involvement, severity and area of corneal opacity or cloudiness, pannus, and intensity of fluorescein staining [39,103]. Other available methods measure intraocular pressure, corneal thickness, cells in the aqueous humor, and posterior segment changes.

In addition to in vivo testing of ophthalmic preparations, primarily in rabbit eyes and secondarily in a primate eye, numerous in vitro methods have been developed over the past few years as alternatives to in vivo ocular testing [83–92]. In vivo methods that incorporate new technology and reduced numbers of animals have also been developed. Particular attention has been given recently to evaluation of preservative effects on corneal penetration [93,94], cytotoxicity [95–99], and affects on wound healing [100–102]. These methods have been able so far to mimic only acute dosing regimens, and validation efforts have not substantiated the correlation of any method with rabbit or human responses. However, these methods are useful for comparing relative toxicity under controlled conditions, and several manufacturers currently are using in vitro toxicity tests in the development of ophthalmic solutions.

C. Preservation and Preservatives

In 1953 the FDA imposed the federal requirement that all manufactured ophthalmic solutions be sterile [104]. Preservatives are included as a major component of all multiple-dose eye solutions for the primary purpose of maintaining that sterility in the opened product over its lifetime of use. Packaging ophthalmic solutions in the popular plastic eyedrop container has reduced, but not completely eliminated, the chances of inadvertent contamination. There can be a "suckback" of an unreleased drop when pressure on the bottle is released. If the tip is allowed to touch a nonsterile surface, contamination may be introduced. Therefore, it is important that the pharmacist instruct the patient on the proper method of dispensing from a plastic eyedrop container in order to minimize the hazards of contamination. The hazard is magnified in the busy clinical practice of the eye care professional where a diagnostic solution – there are many, including cycloplegics, mydriatics, and dyes – may be used for many patients from the same container. The cross-contamination hazard can be eliminated by the use of packages containing small volumes designed for single application only (i.e., unit-dose). Since preservatives are not included in solutions packaged in unit-dose containers, and because these single-use packages still contain (as a large-scale manufacturing necessity) an amount in excess of the several drops (0.05–0.20 mL) required, patient and physician alike should be cautioned to avoid exhausting their entire contents in a multi-use application which will increase the hazard of contamination and defeat the purpose of this special packaging.

The USP outlines a test procedure for antimicrobial effectiveness and how to interpret the results. This test is not a mandatory requirement of the USP or FDA [105], but is applied by manufacturers as a guide in developing adequately preserved products. This testing of the antimicrobial characteristics of alternate formulas is carried out as a part of the development sequence. Cultures of *Candida albicans*, *Aspergillus niger*, *Escherichia coli*, *Pseudomonas aeruginosa*, and *Staphylococcus aureus* are used. Standardized inocula with organism counts of 10^5–10^6 per mL for each microorganism are prepared and tested against the preserved formula. The inoculated tubes or containers are incubated at 20 or 25°C for 28 days, with examination at days 7, 14, 21, and 28. The product's preservative is effective if (a) the concentrations of viable bacteria are reduced to no more than 0.1% of the initial concentrations by day 14, (b) the concentrations of viable yeasts and molds remain at or below the initial concentrations during the first 14 days, and (c) the concentration of each test microorganism remains at or below these designated levels during the remainder of the 28-day test period. Importantly, most manufacturers of ophthalmic products apply this as a minimum standard for a preservative and attempt to formulate their products with an even greater margin of safety.

In the ophthalmic literature because of reports of loss of eyes from corneal ulcerations caused by eye solutions contaminated with *P. aeruginosa*, considerable emphasis is placed on the effectiveness of preservatives against *Pseudomonas* species. This organism is not the most prevalent cause of bacterial eye infections, even though it is a common inhabitant of human skin, but it is the most opportunistic and virulent. *Staphylococcus aureus* is responsible for most bacterial infections of the eye. The eye seems to be remarkably resistant to infection when the corneal epithelium is intact due to the barrier properties discussed previously as well as the antimicrobial activity of lysozyme and other enzymes present in tears. When there is a corneal epithelial abrasion, organisms can enter freely and *P. aeruginosa* can grow readily in the cornea, rapidly producing an ulceration and loss of vision. This microorganism has been found as a contaminant in a number of studies on sterility of ophthalmic solutions, particularly in sodium fluorescein solutions used to detect corneal epithelial damage. The chances for serious infections and cross-contamination are greatly enhanced by multiple use of this dye solution—a danger that has led to the practice by the ophthalmologist of using sterile disposable applicator strips of fluorescein. Although infrequent, *P. aeruginosa* has been found on contact lenses.

An additional test procedure employed by one manufacturer is the preservative evaluation "cidal" test. A formulation is tested against 5–14 species of microorganism, including gram-negative and gram-positive bacteria, fungi, and yeasts in a standardized inoculum. Cidal times (no growth) are measured for each organism within 24, 48, and 72 hours of contact.

One area of ophthalmic products for which stricter microbiological guidelines have been imposed recently is in the area of soft (hydrophilic) contact lens accessory products. Specific guidelines have been devised by FDA and international organizations for this area of ophthalmic products and differ primarily in the required kill rate, which depends on the intended use, for a single disinfecting product or in combination with other lens care solutions. The microbiological guidelines, which have evolved during the last decade, are discussed in Sec. IX of this chapter.

In some applications the use of preservatives is not recommended. For example, preservatives should not be used in a corneal storage media for donor corneas; instead, antibiotics such as gentamicin are used. Alternative packaging for multidose nonpreserved preparations [106] and drugs administered in dry form [107] may offer nonpreserved choices for the formulator, but efficacy and compatibility of each drug with these systems must be investigated. Because experimental results reported in the literature have shown a somewhat higher incidence of adverse effects with preserved solutions compared with unpreserved, there is some question of the necessity for preservatives in some applications [108,109]. However, preservatives can enhance drug efficacy, chemically balance a preparation, and enable a dosing form that promotes patient compliance. While some ophthalmic drugs may be formulated in an unpreserved form, many drugs cannot, and it is the challenge of the formulator to provide an acceptable balance of safety and effectiveness.

Although this chapter is directed toward ophthalmic products, it is largely applicable to parenteral and even nonsterile products (solutions, emulsions, and suspensions). The choice of preservative is limited to only a few chemicals that have been found, over the years, to be safe and effective for this purpose. These are benzalkonium chloride, thimerosal, methyl- and propylparaben, phenylethanol, chlorhexidine, polyquaternium-1, and polyaminopropyl biguanide. The chelating agent disodium edetate (EDTA) is sometimes used to increase activity against certain *Pseudomonas* strains, particularly solutions preserved with benzalkonium chloride. Chlorhexidine—as the hydrochloride, acetate, or gluconate salt—is used widely in the United Kingdom and Australia but was not introduced into the United States until 1976, and only then for solutions intended for disinfection of soft contact lenses. This limited choice of preservative agents is further narrowed by the requirements of chemical and physical stability and compatibility with drugs, packaging, and contact lens materials. Many times it is necessary to design the formula to fit the requirements of the chosen preservative system since the buffer system and excipients can alter preservative action significantly. While it is recognized that excipients themselves may produce toxicity and their use needs be controlled, the large variety and number of available excipients prohibits discussion here, and the reader is referred to a recent pharmaceutical text that provides an excellent review [110].

Several guidelines are available in the literature for the pharmacist who must extemporaneously prepare an ophthalmic solution. The USP contains a section on ophthalmic solutions, as do other compendia and several standard textbooks. Since the pharmacist does not have the facilities to test the product, he or she should dispense only small quantities, with an expiration date of no more than 30 days. Refrigeration of the product should also be required as a precautionary measure. To reduce the largest potential source of microbial contamination, only sterile purified water should be used in compounding ophthalmic solutions. Sterile water for injection, USP, from unopened IV bottles or vials is the highest-quality water available to the pharmacist. Prepackaged sterile water with bacteriostatic agents should *not* be used.

Benzalkonium Chloride

The most widely used preservative remains benzalkonium chloride, which often is supplemented with disodium edetate. The benzalkonium chloride defined in the USP monograph is the quaternary ammonium compound alkylbenzyldimethylammonium chloride, in which the alkyl portion is composed of a mixture of chain lengths ranging from C_8 to C_{16}. This compound's popularity is based, despite its compatibility limitations, on its being the most effective and rapid-acting preservative with excellent chemical stability. It is stable over a wide pH range and does not degrade, even under excessively hot storage conditions. It has pronounced surface-active properties, and its activity can be reduced by adsorption. It is cationic, which unfortunately can lead to a number of incompatibilities with large negatively charged molecules with the potential for producing salts of lower solubility and possibly precipitation. For example, it cannot be used with nitrates, salicylate, anionic soaps, and large anionic drugs, such as sodium sulfacetamide and sodium fluorescein. When feasible, it is usually advisable to design the formula to avoid these incompatible anions, rather than to substitute a less effective preservative. There are a number of helpful lists of incompatibilities of benzalkonium chloride in the literature, but they should not be relied upon entirely. Compatibility is determined by the total environment in which the drug molecules exists (i.e., the total product formula). The pharmaceutical manufacturer can sometimes design around what appears to be an incompatibility, whereas the extemporaneous compounder may not have this option or, more importantly, the ability to test the final product for its stability, safety, and efficacy.

The conventional concentration of benzalkonium chloride in eyedrops is 0.01%, with a range of 0.004–0.02% [111]. While uptake of benzalkonium chloride itself into ocular tissues is limited [113], even lower concentrations of benzalkonium chloride have been reported to enhance corneal penetration of other compounds including therapeutic agents [93,112,114]. The differential effect of this preservative on the cornea compared to the conjunctiva can be exploited to target a drug for corneal absorption and delivery to the posterior segment of the eye [115]. Its use has been proposed as a means of delivering systemic doses by an ocular route of administration [116].

Richards [117], Mullen et al. [118], and the American College of Toxicology [119] have summarized the literature of benzalkonium chloride. The conclusion drawn was that benzalkonium chloride, up to 0.02%, has been well substantiated as being suitable for use in topical ophthalmic solutions when the conditions of its use are properly controlled. McDonald [121] found up to 0.02% to be permissible in ophthalmic solutions following extensive testing in rabbits.

Numerous studies comparing benzalkonium chloride with other preservatives have been described in the literature. Many of the articles give conflicting results, not surprising considering the many different test methods, formulas, and criteria used to arrive at these diverse conclusions. However, adequate information is available in the literature to permit the manufacturer to select appropriate tests for nearly any product. Generally, the USP (or similarly validated) test can be employed to decide which preservative system is most compatible with a specific composition. While recent reports show benzalkonium chloride to have a somewhat higher incidence of ocular effects [122–124], this preservative is one of the most effective available and generally assures an adequate level of preservative efficacy.

Some strains of *P. aeruginosa* are resistant to benzalkonium chloride and, in fact, can be grown in solutions concentrated in this agent. This has caused great concern because of the virulent nature of this organism in ocular infections, as discussed previously. Thus, it was an important finding in 1958 that the acquired resistance could be eliminated by the presence of ethylenediaminetetracetic acid (sodium edetate) in the formulation. This action of EDTA has been correlated with its ability to chelate divalent cations, and it is commonly used as a preservative aid [125]. The use of disodium EDTA, where compatible, is recommended in concentrations up to 0.1%.

Other quaternary ammonium germicides, benzethonium chloride and benzalkonium bromide, have been used in several ophthalmic solutions. While these have the advantage of not being a chemical mixture, they do not possess the bactericidal effectiveness of benzalkonium chloride and are subject to the same incompatibility limitations. In addition, the maximum concentration for benzethonium chloride is 0.01%. Several new products that form gels in the eye, like Timolol Gel Forming Solution and Timoptic-XE, employ another quaternary preservative, BDAB, in the formulation.

Organic Mercurials

When benzalkonium chloride could not be used in a particular formulation of a therapeutic agent (e.g., pilocarpine nitrate, serine salicylate, or fluorescein sodium) because of potential anion-cation association, one of three organic mercurials, phenylmercuric nitrate, phenylmercuric acetate, and thimerosal, had until recent years been used. Because of environmental concerns, however, the use of organic mercurials has fallen into disfavor. Although organic mercurials have not been implicated in classical mercurial toxicity, several countries have banned their use entirely, and other countries require its rigorous defense based on the absence of any suitable alternative. In those situations for which the use of an organic mercurial is the only avenue available, the usual range in concentration for the phenylmercuric compounds is 0.002–

0.004% and for thimerosal, 0.02–0.01%. Although they can be used effectively in some products, the mercurials are relatively weak and slow in their antimicrobial activity. The organic mercurials are generally restricted to use in neutral to alkaline solutions; however, they have been used successfully in slightly acid formulations. The phenyl mercuric ion can react with halide ions to form salts of lower solubility, reducing their effectiveness. Thimerosal has a greater solubility and is relatively more stable than the phenylmercuric compounds and has not been shown to deposit in the lens of the eye. The latter phenomenon has been observed with phenylmercury compounds.

Ocular sensitization to thimerosal has been well documented over the years [126–132]. Although thimerosal had at one time been referred to as the preservative of choice for soft contact lens care products [133–135], its use has been supplanted almost completely by the polyquaternium-l and polybiguanide preservatives.

Since the organic mercurials offer an alternative to quaternary ammonium preservatives, and since preservative efficacy of ophthalmic solutions is essential, the choice among these alternatives should be based on a benefit-to-risk analysis as long as a ban is not imposed on the use of these organometallic preservatives.

Chlorobutanol

This aromatic alcohol has been an effective preservative and still is used in several ophthalmic products. Over the years it has proved to be a relatively safe preservative for ophthalmic products [138] and has produced minimal effects in various tests [99,136,139]. In addition to its relatively slower rate of activity, it imposes a number of limitations on the formulation and packaging. It possesses adequate stability when stored at room temperature in an acidic solution, usually about pH 5 or below. If autoclaved for 20–30 minutes at a pH of 5, it will decompose about 30%. The hydrolytic decomposition of chlorobutanol produces hydrochloric acid (HCl), resulting in a decreasing pH as a function of time. As a result, the hydrolysis rate also decreases. Chlorobutanol is generally used at a concentration of 0.5%. Its maximum water solubility is only about 0.7% at room temperature, which may be lowered by active or excipients, and is slow to dissolve. Heat can be used to increase dissolution rate but will also cause some decomposition and loss from sublimation. Concentrations as low as 0.125% have shown antimicrobial activity under the proper conditions.

Methyl- and Propylparaben

These esters of *p*-hydroxybenzoic acid have been used primarily to prevent growth of molds but in higher concentrations possess some weak antibacterial activity. Their effective use is limited by low aqueous solubility and by reports of stinging and burning sensations related to their use in the eye. They bind to a number of nonionic surfactants and polymers, thereby reducing their bioactivity. They are used in combination, with the methyl ester at 0.03–0.1% and the propyl ester at 0.01–0.02%. Parabens have also been shown to promote corneal absorption [140].

Phenylethyl Alcohol

This substituted alcohol has been used at 0.5% concentration, but in addition to its weak activity it has several limitations. It is volatile and will lose activity by permeation through a plastic package. It has limited water solubility, can be "salted out" of solution, and can produce burning and stinging sensations in the eye. It has been recommended primarily for use in combination preservative systems.

Polyquaternium-1 (POLYQUAD®)

This preservative is comparatively new to ophthalmic preparations and is a polymeric quaternary ammonium germicide. Its advantage over other quaternary ammonium seems to be its inability to penetrate ocular tissues, especially the cornea. It has been used at concentrations of 0.001–0.01% in contact lens solutions as well as dry eye products. At clinically effective levels of preservative, POLYQUAD is approximately 10 times less toxic than benzalkonium chloride [87,137]. Various in vitro tests and in vivo evaluations substantiate the safety of this compound [137,141,142]. This preservative has been extremely useful for soft contact lens solutions because it has the least propensity to adsorb onto or absorb into these lenses, and it has a practically nonexistent potential for sensitization. Its adsorption/absorption with high water and high ionic lenses can be resolved by carefully balancing formulation components [143].

Chlorhexidine

Chlorhexidine, a bisbiguanide, has been demonstrated to be somewhat less toxic than benzalkonium chloride and thimerosal at clinically relevant concentrations [87,89,95,144,145]. This work was confirmed in a series of in vitro and in vivo experiments [137,146–148].

Polyaminopropyl Biguanide

This preservative is also comparatively new to ophthalmic formulations and has been used as a disinfectant in contact lens solutions. Polyaminopropyl biguanide (polyhexamethyl biguanide) also is a polymeric compound that has a low toxicity potential at the concentrations generally used in these solutions [141, 149, 150].

Cetrimonium Chloride

This preservative has been used in a dry eye treatment and was shown in a clinical study to have the same biocompatibility as another marketed preparation [152]. Cetrimonium chloride (0.01%) produced the same corneal and conjunctival changes after one-month ocular administration in rats as the effective levels of other major preservatives [153].

VI. OCULAR DRUG TRANSPORT AND DELIVERY

A. Modes of Transport

Passive transport or simple diffusion of molecules is a transport process dependent on water and lipid solubility, size of the molecule, and concentration gradient across the cellular membrane. No energy is expended in the process, and transport will cease when the concentrations of the molecules on both sides of the membrane are equal. Passive transport is not inhibited by metabolic inhibitors (inhibiting ATP production or utilization) or by competitive substrates. In general, hydrophilic molecules pass through proteinaceous pores in the cellular membrane and lipophilic molecules diffuse through the lipid portion of the membrane. Transport through the pores is limited by the pore size that is specific to each tissue. The low lipid solubility of ionized molecules may be increased by altering the degree of ionization with changes in solution pH. Passive transport is important in diffusion of drugs across the cornea and in nutrient uptake across the corneal endothelium.

Active transport is an energy-dependent process requiring ATP, is carrier-mediated, and is capable of transporting substrates against a concentration gradient. Macromolecular carriers are membrane-bound and have varying degrees of substrate specificity. The carrier reversibly binds to the substrate, transports and releases the molecule on the other side of the membrane, and returns to the original state. These characteristics also make active transport subject to metabolic inhibitors, competitive inhibition from other similar substrates, and saturation at high substrate concentrations. Active transport in the corneal endothelium is essential to maintenance of proper stromal hydration.

Facilitated transport combines some properties of both mechanisms discussed above. This type of transport is carrier mediated so that there is substrate specificity, a transport maximum, and competitive inhibition. However, facilitated transport is not energy-dependent and is unable to transport a substrate against a concentration gradient.

B. Biological Barriers and Fundamentals of Passive Transport

Membranes as Barriers

In a very general sense, biological membranes serve an extremely useful function, effectively walling off the body from invasive and destructive pathological microorganisms as well as noxious influences of the environment. They allow tissues to customize their environments. Dosage forms are therefore devised so that either the therapeutic agent is introduced by a physical or chemical means, which penetrates the barrier and introduces the drug behind the impediment, or the drug design or dosage form itself enables the therapeutic agent to penetrate the barrier. If the latter is the preferred means, both the drug and the vehicle need to avoid producing a significant toxic insult to the barrier, lest that barrier be compromised in its ability to prevent intrusion of foreign chemical or biological agents or be rendered sufficiently uncomfortable that the delivery is not effective nor the patient compliant.

The significance of the barrier function of membranes has been the topic of considerable research. The blood-brain barrier and the blood-retinal barrier are well understood, and the microscopic structures imparting and controlling barrier properties have been quite thoroughly investigated and the science reviewed [15, 154–155]. The structures and functions of ocular membranes specific to transport associated with ophthalmic drug administration also have been topics of extensive research [15, 157–158].

The most common means of administering drugs to the eye is by topical administration of agents capable of penetrating the cornea and targeting the appropriate tissue for either physiological or medicinal effect [159,160]. The trilaminar structure of the transparent avascular cornea has been described previously. The corneal epithelium exposes a hydrophobic barrier to hydrophilic therapeutic agents and a hydrophilic corneal stromal barrier to hydrophobic agents. Nonetheless, as the models considered below rationalize, low molecular weight therapeutic agents of modest hydrophobicity and high water solubility are often capable of penetrating the eye, and may be effective ocular therapeutic agents if their potency—or receptor affinity if that is appropriate—can be maintained in the accommodation to these requirements.

More recently alternative routes of drug administration have been sought and utilized. Scientists are developing technologies to circumvent the constraints imposed on molecular weight, water solubility, and modest hydrophobicity by the conventional transcorneal route. Patents exist for ophthalmically acceptable penetration enhancers. More water-soluble therapeutic agents now in use for glaucoma appear to achieve approximately equal access by both scleral-limbal and transcorneal routes of administration [161,162]. Research is ongoing to understand and utilize scleral administration of therapeutic agents; the role of hydrostatic pressure on the transport of both water and drug has been investigated in order to determine the classes of therapeutic agent for which this mode of delivery may be utilized [163–166]. One consequence will be the determination of the diminished transport constraints imposed by a barrier from which the hydrophobic layer is absent. Both academic and industrial investigations have led to technologies for scleral implants and sustained release.

Role of Hydrodynamics

Basic hydrodynamic phenomena govern the duration of exposure of corneal and conjunctival membranes to the therapeutic agents. Rapid clearance provides a temporal barrier to drug delivery.

Drainage of the drop through the nasolacrimal system into the gastrointestinal tract begins immediately on instillation. This takes place when either reflex tearing or the dosage form causes the volume of fluid in the cul-de-sac and precorneal tears to exceed the normal lacrimal volume of 7–10 μL. Reference to Fig. 7 indicates the pathway for this drainage. The excess fluid volume enters the superior and inferior lacrimal puncta, moves down the canaliculi into the lacrimal sac, and continues into the gastrointestinal tract. It is due to this mechanism that significant systemic effects for certain potent ophthalmic medications have been reported [170–172]. This also is the mechanism by which a patient may occasionally sense a bitter or salty taste, typical of therapeutic ammonium salts, following the use of eye drops. The influence of drop size on bioavailability has been investigated thoroughly for conventional formulations and is significant [173,174]. Even for nonconventional viscoelastic formulations, drop volume can be expected to influence efficacy and needs to be optimized [175]. The clinical significance of drainage is so well recognized that manual nasolacrimal occlusion has been recommended as a means of improving the therapeutic index of antiglaucoma medications [176]. Once the dynamics of tear-flow excess have taken their course, steady-state hydrodynamics can be expected.

Loss of drug from a precorneal volume has been investigated both in vivo and in vitro. These studies relate to both design of dosage forms as well as investigations of transport, bioavailability and pharmacokinetics. Simultaneous release profiles of drugs and adjuvant from an artificial in vitro reservoir, designed with its volume to be characteristic of the eye, can be correlated simply with exposure for transmembrane transport [181]. An example of release profiles and the influence of dosage form from one of these models, the CRAS model, is shown in Fig. 8.

Simple hydrodynamic analysis of the in vitro mechanism indicates that the elution concentration, in the absence of absorption, is a linear kinetic process, with a release profile that scales as the ratio of the tear production to the volume of the tear reservoir, $\dot{V}_T/V_T$. Specifically:

$$N_E(t) = N_I\left(1 - \exp\left(\frac{-\dot{V}_T \cdot t}{V_T}\right)\right) \tag{1}$$

where

$N_E(t)$ = time-dependent total amount eluted from volume in time t
V_T = volume of the reservoir
$\dot{V}_T$ = flow rate through reservoir (alternatively, Q_T)
N_I = amount of drug in reservoir at time zero

and where the complementary amount, the amount of drug in the reservoir at time t, is defined as

$$N_T(t) = N_I - N_E(t) \tag{2}$$

characteristic of the stirred-tank chemical reactor models [182–184]. Combining these containment profiles, $N_T(t)$, with diffusional transmembrane transport, yields expected tissue profiles. The time-dependent concentrations are dictated by both containment profile and tissue affinities, and the magnitude is often

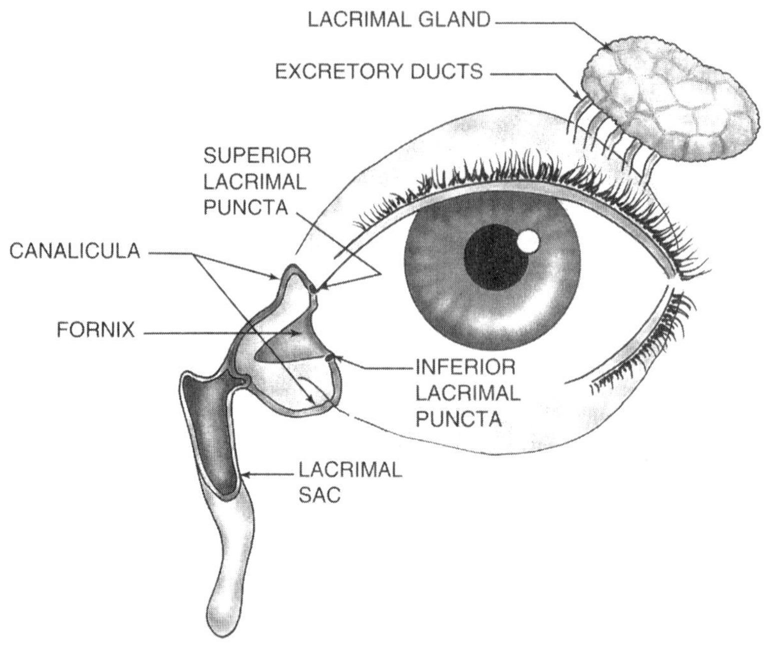

Fig. 7 Anatomical view of the lids and lacrimal systems.

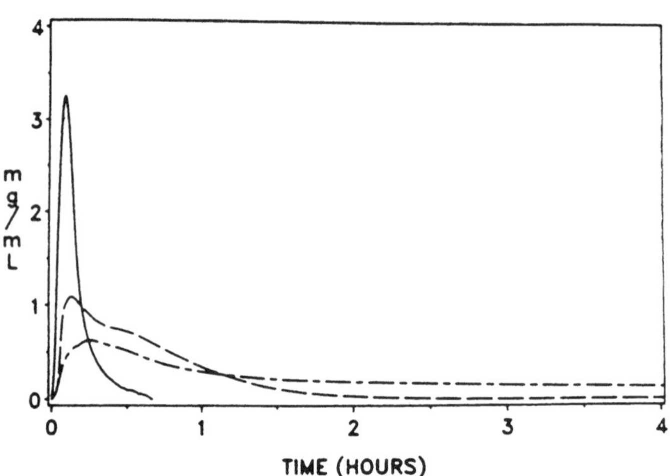

Fig. 8 Comparison of time-release profiles from three different preparations of betaxolol: (—) drug solution representing marketed product; (— —) supension formulation; (- — - —) gel formulation.

dominated by transmembrane flux (below). A pictorial representation of the processes is shown in Fig. 9. Pharmacokinetic modeling with this scheme has been successful in fitting the aqueous humor levels of pilocarpine following topical administration (Fig. 10) [173]. Although this type of data fitting has been quite successful, there has not been a sufficient number of systematic studies to determine the role of every molecular and physiological property influencing each of the various pharmacokinetic parameters. The pharmacokinetic consequences of these competing transport processes have been reviewed [180]. Elaborate analyses of such data using Green's function solutions, for responses to unit impulse, can be integrated as a means of generating responses to more complicated dosage regimens [185,186]. Alternatively,

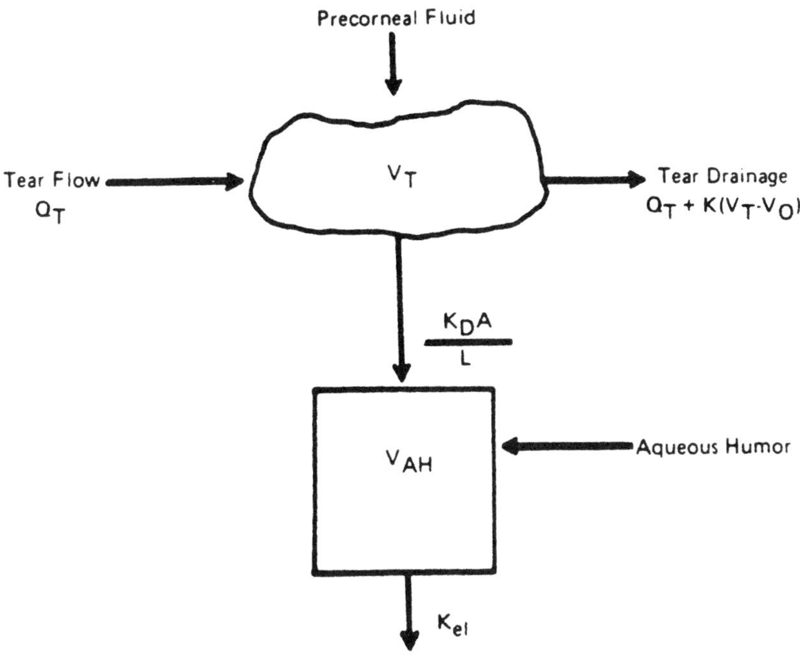

Fig. 9 Pharmacokinetic scheme for ocular absorption, distribution, and elimination.

and more simply, the differential equations representing the coupled effects of instillation, hydrodynamics and drainage, and membrane transport can be readily integrated numerically to provide predictions of the impact of drug and dosage form on bio availability [15].

Mechanisms and Models of Transmembrane Transport

At a physical level the description of the cornea is as a transparent, avascular tissue that, with the adherent precorneal tear film, is the first refracting surface operant in the process of sight. At a morphological and chemical level the description is of a three-layered structure: a multilayered, lipid-rich epithelium, a well-hydrated and lipid-poor stroma, and a lipid-rich endothelium of one-cell-layer thickness. Differential studies of the relative lipid densities for these three corneal layers have shown that the densities of lipid in epithelium and endothelium are approximately 40 times as large as that in the stroma [194], although more recent studies suggest the disparity may be less [195,196]. This can be a primary physiological factor influencing drug penetration through the cornea and into the aqueous humor. For a topically administered drug to traverse an intact cornea and to appear in the aqueous humor, it must possess dual or differential solubility. But as ever more explicit descriptions have been developed by histologists, microscopic anatomists, and electron microscopists, increasingly detailed mechanisms of transport through these tissues have been envisioned and tested.

The multilayered corneal epithelium consists of cells attached by microstructural junctions of well-established morphology and function and separated by water-filled intercellular spaces. Drug transport through such an environment can be imagined to consist of two competing pathways. Predominantly water-soluble compounds presumably pass through the tortuously connected aqueous channels, establishing a path through the maze from epithelial surface to stroma, a paracellular pathway. Predominantly lipid-soluble compounds presumably pass by surface diffusion along the lipid surfaces, passing in a tortuous path from adjacent cell to cell—the transcellular pathway. In either case boundaries of lipid junctions for water-soluble compounds or aqueous channels for lipid-soluble compounds would be more readily surmounted by compounds with shared funtionality. The characteristics of diffusion through and along such well-defined structures is well known, and the statistical mechanics of percolation phenomena governing such random paths has been well investigated.

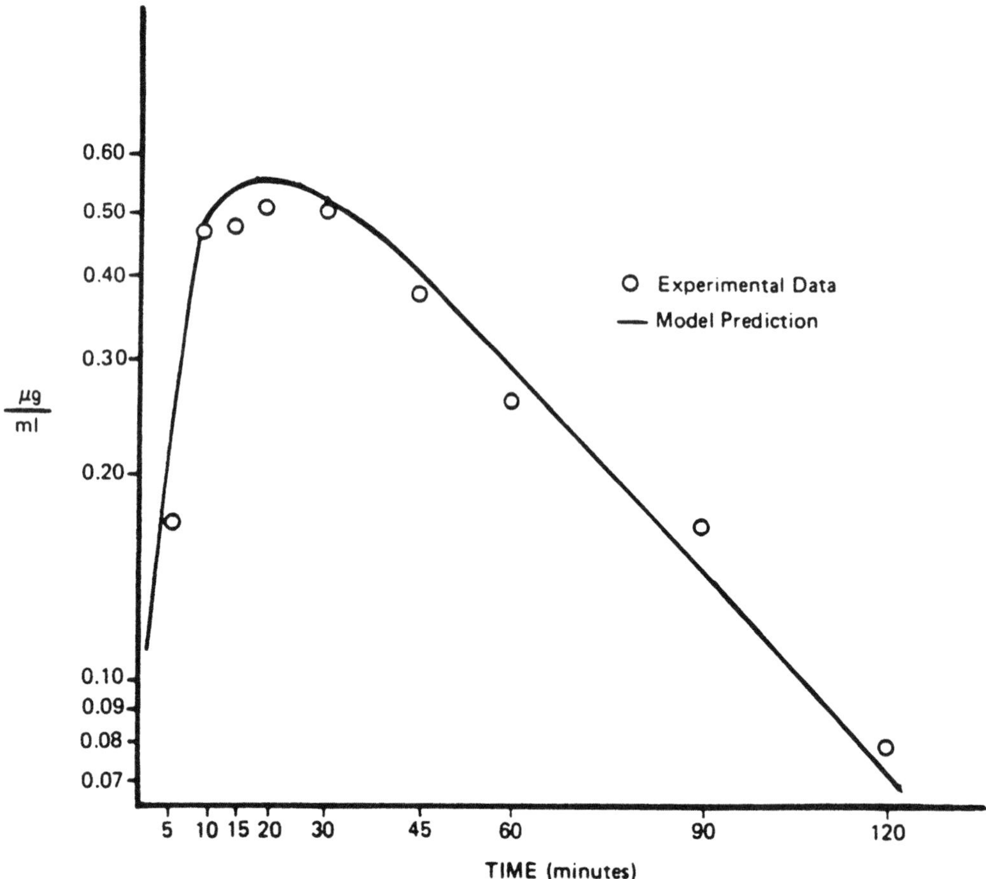

Fig. 10 Comparison of predicted and experimental aqueous humor concentrations following topical administration of pilocarpine.

For example, several recent studies have attempted to provide a molecular basis for the earlier largely empirical observations and essentially macroscopic continuum analyses [197,198]. For the stroma and sclera much is known about their structure and composition. These tissues consist primarily of water, collagen, and glycosaminoglycans wherein the lamellar order is derived primarily from collagen, which has a fivefold organizational hierarchy. The collagen molecule consists of three α-chains of peptides. These α-chains are organized into ordered, relatively stiff collagen fibrils, typically 50 nm in diameter. Many fibrils, along with proteoglycan-rich ground substance, compose collagen fibers, which are about a half micrometer in diameter and in stroma and sclera are organized into nearly lamellar sheets [199–201]. These membranes, over which there will be hydrodynamic pressure gradients, will be barriers to fluid flow, and with the administration of drugs these membranes, over which there will be concentration gradients, will be barriers to molecular diffusional flow. The effects of fibrous obstructions on both fluid flow and solute diffusion have been the topic of intense research in chemical engineering and physics. The flow and diffusional characteristics have been related to the relative dimensions and volume fractions of the fibers and the permeabilities (influenced by the state of hydration) of the different materials to the solvent and solutes, respectively. The diffusional characteristics of solute molecules will be influenced by the relative solubilities of these molecules in the different environments; more water-soluble solutes will diffuse more rapidly through the highly hydrated stroma.

These effects, specialized for the geometries and materials properties of the collagen-rich stroma and sclera, have been calculated in a paper by Edwards and Prausnitz [197]. They also modeled diffusion across the corneal endothelium assuming that the major path was between cells and that this was governed by the most restrictive portion, the diffusion through the tight junctions. The diffusional flow was predicted based on the density and width of these parallel channels. These authors generalized this description for both corneal endothelium and epithelium by allowing there to be a balance between this paracellular pathway and a transcellular pathway. The only difference between the epithelial and endothelial paracellular pathways was the geometry of the junctions and their number, larger for the multilayered epithelium. The transcellular pathway was modeled from the known geometry of the cells, which determined the length of the diffusional pathway, and the partitioning characteristics of the molecules.

The cumulative effects of these barriers and the resistance to flow they produce were computed, and it was demonstrated these macroscopically derived laws applied at molecular dimensions were able to provide semiquantitative agreement with the available data. While further tests of these models will undoubtedly provide refinements to our understanding, the agreement supports our understanding of the basic phenomena regulating transport of therapeutically active substances through these barriers and the role of disease states that impact hydrodynamic pressure on the efficacy of drug delivery.

C. Passive Absorption and Intraocular Delivery

Considerations Influencing Drug Design for Topical Administration

From the perspective of drug design for conventional topical delivery, several requirements need to be satisfied by ophthalmic therapeutic agents. The drug must be (a) both biochemically and pharmacologically potent, (b) nontoxic to both ocular and systemic tissues, (c) sufficiently stable that neither significant loss in potency from diminished availability nor increase in toxicity from by-products of degradation arises, (d) targetable either to tissues and location of primary disease-state etiology or to sites responsible for symptomatic response, and (e) sufficiently compatible with the dosage form, and with the tissues exposed to it, to achieve an effective pharmacokinetic tissue profile.

Often the demand for such a complement of properties requires a hierarchical strategy in which only the broadest possible limits are satisfied by the less demanding design requirements. For example, topical administration assists in limiting toxicity while improving targeting and pharmacokinetic response. On the other hand, the requirements for effective absorption of such topical ophthalmic medications often places significant demands on the physical, chemical, and transport characteristics of the drug, which in most cases was designed primarily to satisfy more stringent biological, physiological and pharmacological criteria. Simple guidelines can be appreciated readily by examining the factors influencing absorption of an antiglaucoma agent administered in the conventional manner as drops into the cul-de-sac, discussed in the next section [167].

Efficacy is also influenced by minimizing those factors that diminish availability. The first factor reducing drug availability is loss of drug from the palpebral fissure. This takes place by spillage of drug from the eye and its removal by the nasolacrimal drainage. The normal volume of tears in the human eye is estimated to be approximately 7 μL, and if blinking occurs the human eye can accommodate a volume of up to 30 μL without spillage from the palpebral fissure. With an estimated drop volume of 50 μL, 70% of the administered volume of two drops can be seen to be expelled from the eye by overflow. If blinking occurs, the residual volume of 10 μL indicates that 90% of the administered volume of two drops will be expelled within the first several minutes [168,169].

Many technologies have been devised, some discussed below, for modifying the dosage form as a means of slowing the escape of drug from the precorneal location from which it can be transported to tissues influencing ocular physiology. In addition, other approaches have been recommended. For example, temporary manual punctal occlusion immediately after instillation of drug transiently prevents drainage of the enriched tears from the puncta. For patients with dry eye, often permanent occlusion, which is implemented either by cautery or by one of several designs of punctal plug, results in a diminished rate of tear clearance. Transient occlusion can be expected to influence drug delivery only modestly and be effective only in rather specific circumstances, when either the molecular weight or the aqueous solubility of the therapeutic agent is high. For those circumstances in which the therapeutic agent is reasonably lipophilic, the kinetics of absorption by transepithelial transport can be quite rapid (see below).

A second factor reducing drug availability is the drainage associated with hydrodynamic flow of tears through the precorneal space and cul-de-sac, discussed above. A third and more difficult problem for delivery by nondirectional technologies and devices is the undesirable adsorption and absorption by nearby noncorneal tissues competing for therapeutic agents.

These include absorption by adjacent palpebral and bulbar conjunctiva, with concomitant rapid removal from ocular-tissues by peripheral blood flow. For example, the extensive vascularity of the uvea underlies the bulbar conjunctiva, a mucous membrane, and the sclera, a white tissue providing a tough outer covering [177]. Binding of drug to either external sites, like the tear polymers such as mucins or lysozyme, or internal tissues like the sclera can be detrimental to efficacy.

To the extent that these competing and detrimental effects can be controlled, delivery can be enhanced. But their control is inconsequential if the molecular properties regulating transmembrane transport are not selected in a manner to facilitate corneal permeation, the topic of the next section. Finally, in competition with the three foregoing forms of therapeutically ineffective drug removal from the palpebral fissure is the transcorneal absorption of drug, often the route most effective in bringing drug to the anterior portion of the eye. Although transport of hydrophilic and macromolecular drugs has been reported to occur by limbal or scleral routes, often this is at rates significantly reduced from those expected for transcorneal transport of conventional, modestly lipophilic agents of low molecular weight [178–180,191–193]. Even here, transmembrane transport is a significant requirement for availability.

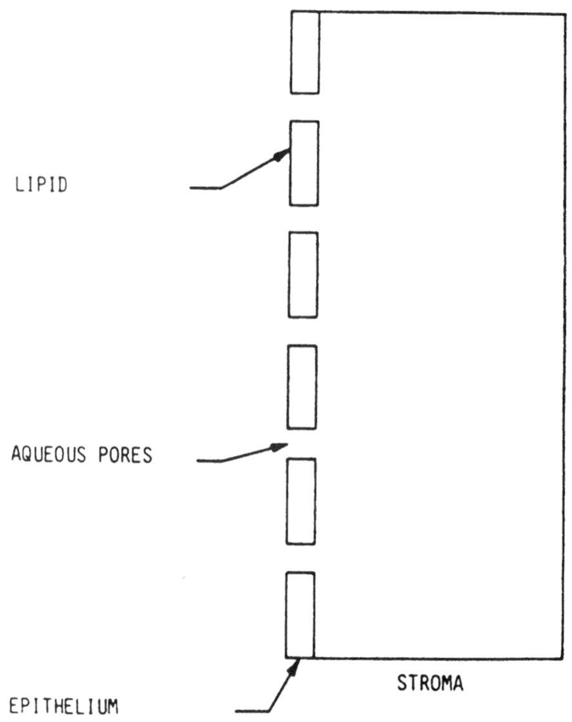

Fig. 11 Schematic diagram of the physical model for transcorneal permeation; features are not to scale.

A Generalized Phenomenological Transport Model and Simple Consequences

One of the key parameters for correlating molecular structure and chemical properties with bioavailability has been transcorneal flux or, alternatively, the corneal permeability coefficient. The epithelium has been modeled as a lipid barrier (possibly with a limited number of aqueous "pores" that, for this physical model, serve as the equivalent of the extracellular space in a more physiological description) and the stroma as an aqueous barrier (Fig. 11). The endothelium is very thin and porous compared with the epithelium [189] and often has been ignored in the analysis, although mathematically it can be included as part of the lipid barrier. Diffusion through bilayer membranes of various structures has been modeled for some time [202] and adapted to ophthalmic applications more recently [203,204]. For a series of molecules of similar size, it was shown that the permeability increases with octanol/water distribution (or partition) coefficient until a plateau is reached. Modeling of this type of data has led to the earlier statement that drugs need to be both oil and water soluble. If pores are not included in the analysis, the steady-state corneal fux, J_s can be approximated by:

$$J_s = \frac{PC_w}{\frac{Pl_s}{D_s} + \frac{l_e}{D_e}} \tag{3}$$

where

C_w = concentration of drug in donor phase
l_s, l_e = stromal and epithelial thickness, respectively
D_s, D_e = corresponding difffusion coefficients
P = distribution coefficient

The permeability coefficient K_{per} is just the flux divided by C_w. It is apparent that the permeability coefficient is linear with P for small distribution coefficients and constant for large P. Thus, for small P the epithelium is the barrier, and for large P the stroma is the barrier. A fit for steroid permeability is shown in Fig. 12, where the regression analysis gave $D_e = 1.4 \times 10^{-9}\,\text{cm}^2/\text{s}$ and $D_s = 2.0 \times 10^{-6}\,\text{cm}^2/\text{s}$ for $l_e = 4 \times 10^{-3}\,\text{cm}$ and $l_s = 3.6 \times 10^{-2}\,\text{cm}$ [205]. These values for the diffusion coefficients are reasonable compared with those of aqueous gels and lipid membranes.

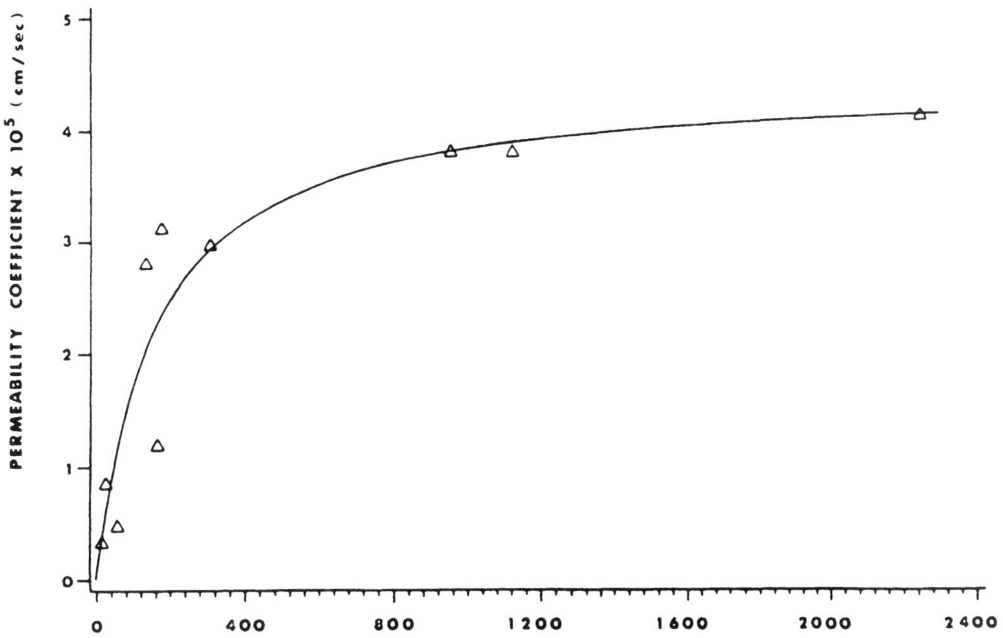

Fig. 12 Predicted versus experimental values for corneal steroid permeability as a function of partition coefficient.

A simple estimate of the diffusion coefficients can be approximated from examining the effects of molecular size on transport through a continuum for which there is an energy cost of displacing solvent. Since the molecular weight dependence of the diffusion coefficients for polymers obeys a power law equation [206], a similar form was chosen for the corneal barriers. That is, the molecular weight (M) dependence of the diffusion coefficients was written as:

$$D_e = D_e^{(0)} M^{\alpha}$$
$$D_s = D_s^{(0)} M^{\delta} \tag{4}$$

Using regression analysis on a data set of about 50 different molecules, it was found that $\alpha = -4.4, \delta = -0.5, D_e^{(0)} = 12\ \text{cm}^2/\text{s}$, and $D_s^{(0)} = 2.5\times\ 10^{-5}\ \text{cm}^2/\text{s}$ [192]. A graphic representation of the effect of relative molecular mass (M_r) and distribution coefficient on corneal permeability is shown in Fig. 13. One observes a rapid reduction in permeability coefficient with decreasing P and increasing M_r. The addition of pores to the model, a mathematical construct, is necessary to account for permeability of polar molecules, such as mannitol and cromolyn. These would also be required for correlating effects of compounds, such as benzalkonium chloride, which may compromise the epithelial barrier by increasing the volume of the extracellular space.

Another perspective provided by this model is the effect of three physiochemical parameters—solubility, distribution coefficient, and molecular mass—on transcoreal flux. All of these properties can be influenced by molecular design. The effects of these properties are illustrated in Fig. 13, in which the logarithm of the flux is plotted as a function of solubility and distribution coefficient for two different M_r. Several features of the model are depicted, and these qualitative, or semi-quantitative, aspects presumably encompass the principles of corneal permeation.

Inferred from this model is the relative independence of the effects of solubility and partitioning. For each property there is a characteristic threshold above which the log of the flux increases more slowly than below it, and the value of the threshold for one variable is not very dependent on the value of the other variable. This tabletop perspective has led to the name *mesa model*. The relative independence signifies that neither property can totally compensate for a deficiency in the other. This is not to say that these properties are independent of one another in a chemical sense—quite the contrary. However, in the hypothetical sense that if one property were varied independently of the other, then the consequences on flux are relatively independent. Clearly dependence

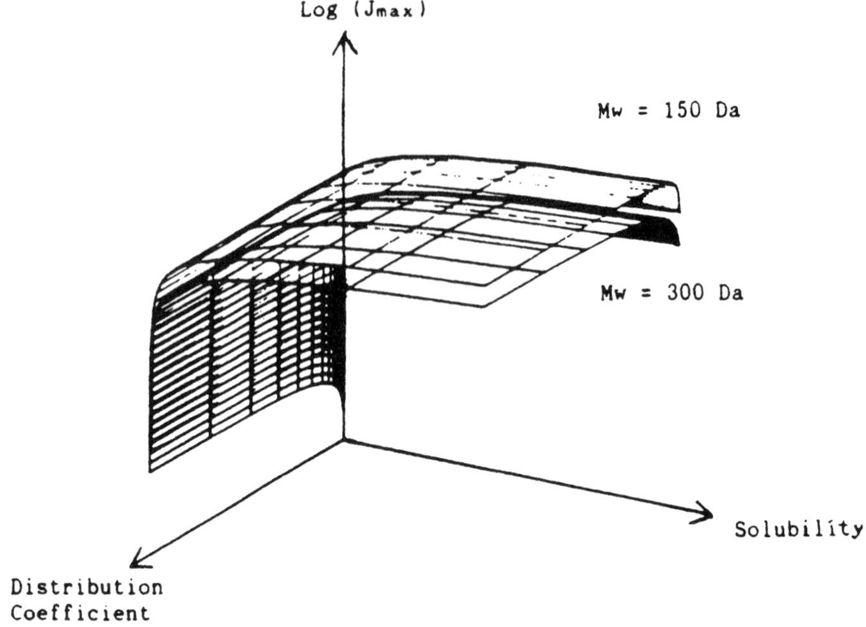

Fig. 13 This figure illustrates the "mesa" response for the diffusion model. Two plateau functions corresponding to different M_r are shown.

on molecular mass, even for relatively low molecular mass agents, can be significant.

Ex vivo studies of transcorneal transport in animal models have been used to establish the characteristics of passive diffusional motion, the conventional means by which drugs reach internal ocular tissues. Although such analysis neglects the complications of tear flow, tear drainage, nonproductive membrane absorption, elimination from the aqueous humor, and so forth, measurements of corneal transport measurements have been important in establishing correlations of model calculations with experimental measurements of transmembrane transport. Modifications [187] of the classical ex vivo experiments of transport across excised, but metabolizing, rabbit corneas [188–191] have provided information both about targeting of similar molecules from the same pharmacological class [192] and confirmation of the balance of different anatomical pathways for accession [193].

The rough brush stroke agreement between model and experiment is illustrated by the results shown in Fig. 14, for which the correspondences of theoretical with experimental permeability coefficients for the compounds listed in Table 2, β-adrenegic blockers studied by Lee et al. [207,208] and Schoenwald and Huang [191], are plotted. The calculated values utilized the physical model with pores [205]. Characteristic of correlations of this type is the slope's value—less than 1. The origin of the smaller calculated values of permeability coefficients is unknown. A reasonable conjecture, however, is that the estimated diffusion coefficients [i.e., the laws presented in Eq. (4) on which the permeability is based] are not quite correct for the drugs in different ocular environments. The predictability of the model is useful both for providing approximate values and for distinguishing departure from simple diffusional transport. Also apparent from a comparison of the last two figures (Figs. 13 and 14) is the significance of solubility, since it is the value of C_w that controls flux by orders of magnitude.

A significant inference from the model is that if, as is the conventional behavior of a family of molecules, the solubility decreases with an increase of distribution coefficient, eventually this effect will profoundly reduce the transcorneal flux. Alternatively and conceptually, for any class of molecules with a desirable physiological response and without significant differences in potency or therapeutic index, the member of that family with the greatest promise for ophthalmic application is the one with the lowest molecular weight, the highest distribution coefficient, and the highest aqueous solubility. However, since the last two requirements are in general inconsistent (the most soluble molecule is generally the one with lowest partition

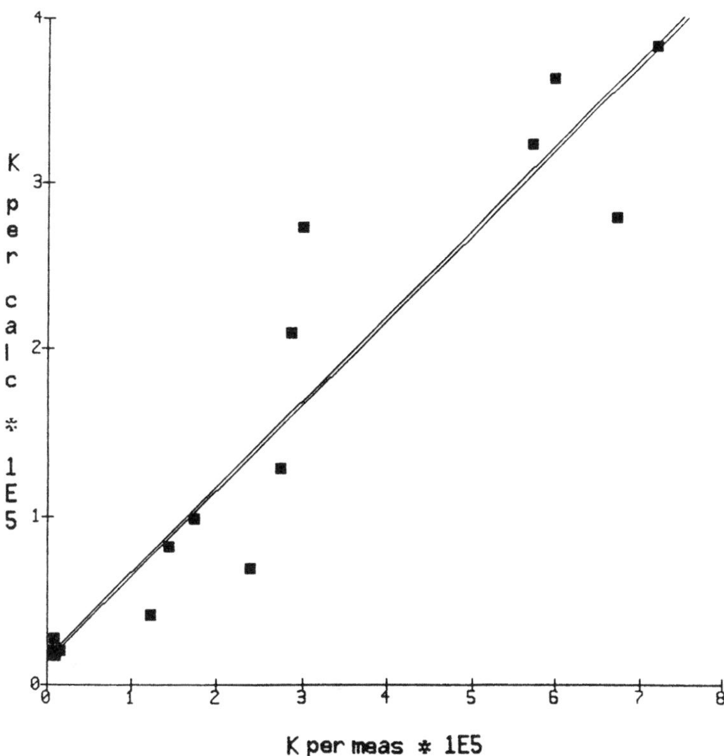

Fig. 14 Plot of data in Table 2: the theoretically computed permeability coefficient versus that measured. The larger influence on flux is often the range of solubility, which can increase the range in flux by several orders of magnitude.

Table 2 Permeability of β-Adrenergic Blockers

Compound	Chemical formula	Molecular weight	Distribution coefficient	K_{per}^{calc} *1E5 cm/s	K_{per}^{meas} *1E5 cm/s
Acebutolol	$C_{18}H_{28}N_2O_4$	336.43	1.58	0.28	0.085
Alprenolol	$C_{15}H_{23}NO_2$	249.34	8.92	2.09	2.86
Atenolol	$C_{14}H_{22}N_2O_3$	266.34	0.03	0.20	0.068
Betaxolol	$C_{18}H_{29}NO_3$	307.44	60.3	2.72	3.02
Bevantolol	$C_{20}H_{27}NO_3$	345.44	154.8	2.78	6.76
Bufuralol	$C_{16}H_3NO_2$	261.36	204.2	3.82	7.24
Labetolol	$C_{19}H_{24}N_2O_3$	328.41	7.77	0.82	1.43
Levobunolol	$C_{17}H_{25}NO_3$	291.39	5.25	0.99	1.74
Metoprolol	$C_{15}H_{25}NO_3$	267.38	1.91	0.69	2.40
Nadolol	$C_{17}H_{27}NO_4$	309.42	0.15	0.17	0.10
Oxprenolol	$C_{15}H_{23}NO_3$	265.34	4.90	1.28	2.75
Penbutolol	$C_{18}H_{29}NO_2$	291.44	338.84	3.62	6.03
Propranolol	$C_{16}H_{21}NO_2$	259.34	41.69	3.22	5.75
Sotalol	$C_{12}H_{20}N_2O_3S$	272.36	0.06	0.20	0.16
Timolol	$C_{13}H_{24}N_4O_3S$	316.42	2.19	0.42	1.23

coefficient), the model helps select the molecular structure for which the flux is greatest.

Perhaps as more is learned about the molecular requirements for binding therapeutic agents to active sites of macromolecules as part of the intention to control physiological function, these simple transport requirements can be incorporated into the molecular design.

Role of Specialized Formulations

Many materials and specialized formulations have been devised with the intention of improving delivery of drugs to intraocular tissues by means of the transcorneal route. Carriers have been used both alone and in conjunction with viscosifying or responsive formulations to control concentration of the active therapeutic compound or sustain delivery. As calculations clearly demonstrate and experiments confirm, the impact on total drug availability for such systems is crucially dependent on the degree to which the vehicle is capable of sustaining residence time of the drug or drug carrier in the eye [15]. The historical and current challenge remains to devise spontaneously responsive systems that are capable of being retained in the eye, sustaining the presence of the carrier without degrading its reservoir and delivery characteristics and without producing such conventional side effects as blurring or undesirable residues.

In recent years a barrage of technologies have been developed for sustaining delivery of drug to the cornea. Corneal collagen shields and contact lenses loaded with drug have been placed directly on the cornea. But undesirable side effects, including blurring, dumping of drug, packaging and storage problems, have prevented these technologies from being successful in the marketplace. Responsive polymeric systems have been more successful to date. Polymers whose solubilities and interactions are dominated by hydrogen bonding can be controlled with temperature, whose solubilities are dominated by coacervation-type interactions can be controlled by the concentration of the complementary polymer, whose solubilities are dominated by weak acid ionization can be controlled by pH, and whose solubilities are dominated by ion pairing condensation can be controlled by ionic strength or even specific ion concentrations. Those systems utilizing mechanisms less influenced by the environment have proven more widely applicable. Polymers like xanthan gum or gelrite, which interact with one or more tear components to form a gel in situ, have been employed in timolol maleate formulations that require dosing only once a day.

D. Active Transport, a Potential Mechanism for Specific Structures

As more is learned about accession of drugs into the eye, it is becoming more obvious that passive diffusion through the cornea is not the only pathway likely to be exploited for future delivery of drugs. Many drugs are known either to bind to, or to be taken up by and accumulated in, epithelial cells. Interesting work is emerging in the areas of facilitated transport in which enhancers are used to diminish diffusional barriers temporarily [209,210] and areas of active transport in which drug carriers can be employed for transport of larger molecules [187].

As ever more potent therapeutic agents are developed, concentrations required diminish and the importance of drug targeting as a means of reducing systemic toxicity increases. For biochemical and therapeutic agents included in specific classes of amino acids, dipeptides, polypeptides with resemblance to specific peptide sequences (e.g., the undecapeptide cyclosporin A), small cationic molecules, or monocarboxylates, and nucleosides, there are known transporters, antiports, co-transporters, etc., in conjunctiva and sometimes in cornea that at low concentrations of a drug may actively contribute to controlling flux into or out of specific tissues [211–216]. Carrier-mediated transport is not restricted to ocular conjunctiva and cornea, of course, but has been identified in other ocular tissues, specifically the retinal pigment epithelium (RPE), as well as in numerous systemic tissues such as gastric, intestinal, hepatic, renal, and cardiac tissues and in some ex vivo cell-culture lines. As a consequence, information concerning structural and geometric specificity, co- or counterion requirements, proton and energy dependence, pump capacity (saturability), total ion flux and current, and directionality of mediated transport have been provided by biochemists, physiologists, and pharmacologists studying a variety of human and mammalian tissues.

For conventional therapeutic agents the presence of active drug transport is either nonexistent or obscured, since while both active and passive transport may occur concurrently at high concentrations, the passive component is the dominating and overwhelming fraction. However, as the concentration decreases, as it will for potent agents for which concentrations in the micromolar range may be adequate, some of these agents will experience facilitated, active, carrier-mediated transport. For example, the flux can be expected to have a complicated concentration dependence:

$$J = \frac{J_{\max}}{\frac{K_m}{[C]} + 1} + K_d[C] \quad (5)$$

where $J_{\max}$ is the maximum saturable flux from the active transport process, K_m is the Michaelis-Menten constant and K_d is the passive diffusive permeation rate [214]. Note both K_m and K_d are temperature-dependent; however, the temperature dependence of K_m is much greater, so that the diagnostic for the presence of active transport is the essentially complete loss of the active component by the time the temperature is reduced to 4°C.

Some measure of the importance of active transport is the diversity of systems where it has been observed. For example, carrier-mediated transport of L-argenine, a substrate for nitric oxide synthase, can impact the concentrations of NO, a neurotransmitter. The same carrier present in the conjunctiva can be inhibited by competitive inhibitors such as nitro-L-argenine. This transporter appears to be coupled to the transport of Na^+ ions and directionally transports the inhibitor preferentially into the tissues from the mucosal exterior surface. The utility of such a path might be to regulate production of NO in vivo and thereby control inflammation, a complication, for example, in Sjögren's syndrome. The potential for delivering a therapeutic agent to the uveal tract is also promising. Nucleoside transport for uridine has also been demonstrated to have similar directionality, preferential flow from mucosal to serosal, or apical to basolateral, sides of the conjunctival cells. Its role is presumably to salvage nucleosides from the tears, and it might be able to be exploited for compounds with antiviral activity.

Not all transporters, however, show the same preferential directions. Lee and coworkers also have discovered a pump glycoprotein in the conjunctiva with preferential flux directed toward the mucosal side of the tissue. This transporter has been shown to restrict conjunctival absorption of therapeutic agents such as cyclosporin A, verapamil, and dexamethasone. In some circumstances, transient inhibition of such xenobiotic transporters might be an effective means of increasing the efficacy of particular classes of therapeutic agents.

E. Delivery to the Vitreous and Posterior Segment

There are a number of drugs that would be of benefit for the treatment of diseases in the interior of the eye, but for which therapeutic levels cannot be achieved by topical administration [217]. Until recently the only method of achieving an effective dose was by direct intravitreal injection, employed first for antibiotics, with animal experiments beginning about the 1940s [218]. A more modern approach has been the use of a sustained-release device for implantation into the vitreous, such as the Vitrasert® (developed by Controlled Delivery Systems), the only such device approved for intraocular implantation [219]. The device contains 4.5 mg of the drug gancyclovir and is used to treat the condition of cytomegaloviral (CMV) retinitis in patients with acquired immunodeficiency syndrome (AIDS). The therapy appears to be effective and well tolerated according to clinical reports and provides sustained therapy over many months [220–222].

Several practical factors must be considered when designing a device intended for intraocular use [223]. For example, the placement of the device should interfere as little as possible with vision. In the case of the Vitrasert, the device is sutured to the sclera in the region of the pars plana (Fig. 15). This region is devoid of retina; the device is also out of the central visual field and is close enough to allow visual inspection to determine when the supply of drug has been exhausted [225]. Drug release is controlled by a rate-controlling membrane.

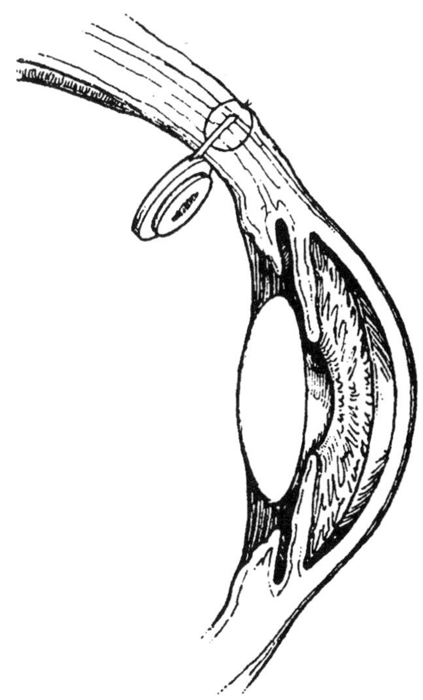

Fig. 15 Drawing showing the optimum placement of an intravitreal sustained-release device in the eye. (From Ref. 224.)

In order to design such an efficient and effective device, one must understand the mechanisms by which drug is transported in the ocular interior. One issue debated in the literature for some time has been the relative importance of transport by passive diffusion versus that facilitated by the flow of fluid in the vitreous (see, e.g., Ref. 226). To predict the geometric distribution even at steady state of drug released from an implant or an intravitreal injection, one must appreciate which of these mechanisms is at work or, as appropriate, their relative balance.

The conclusion that convective flow may provide an important contribution was based upon observations of the distribution of colloidal particles and its evolution following intravitreal injection [227]. Such experiments could have been complicated by the large volumes that were generally injected, which might have created artificial flow channels in the vitreous gel [223], and/or by backflow out through the needle hole [228]. When intravitreal injection is performed through the superior rectus muscle, the latter complication appears to be minimized. When fluorescently labeled polymers are injected intravitreally, the ratio of polymer in the aqueous versus the vitreous cavities is inversely proportional to polymer molecular weight [229]. This suggests that the vitreous cavity is essentially stagnant and that passive diffusion is the major factor determining the flow of any xenobiotic agent.

Elimination from the vitreous occurs by one of two pathways. This can be visualized by injecting fluorescent compounds and examining the concentration distribution in frozen sections obtained after a steady state has been established [230]. If the major route of elimination is by means of the retina/choroid, at steady state the lowest concentration would be in the vicinity of the retina. The contours observed in frozen sections of the rabbit eye obtained after intravitreal injection of fluorescein exhibit this pattern, with the highest concentration immediately behind the lens (Fig. 16A). Compounds not chiefly eliminated through the retina exit the vitreous by passive diffusion and enter the posterior aqueous, where they are eliminated by the natural production and outflow of aqueous humor. In such a situation, the contours would be perpendicular to the retina, with the highest concentration towards the rear of the vitreous cavity. This appears to be the case for fluorescently labeled dextran polymer, whose contours decrease in concentration toward the hyaloid membrane (Fig. 16B).

Various articles have examined the pharmacokinetics of fluorescent compounds in the eye, developing mathematical models for the blood-retinal permeability, mainly in closed form [231–234]. More recently, sophisticated numerical methods have been developed which model the geometrical anatomical and physiological features of the eye more closely. Tojo et al. have applied the method of lines to a cylindrical model of the eye to simulate the biodistribution of several different compounds using extemporaneous Fortran code [235–239]. Begun more recently has been the application of finite element methods, at times harnessing the power of very sophisticated codes traditionally employed in modeling of fluid dynamics and mass transfer [240–245].

The power of these methods for accurately predicting the disposition of drug in the eye is illustrated in Fig. 17, where finite element analysis was used to simulate the experiments of Ref. 230 (FlexPDE was used, www.pdesolutions.com). When the retinal permeability is high, the contours resemble the experimental result for fluorescein, with the highest concentration immediately behind the lens. When the only pathway allowed is through the hyloid membrane, the contours resemble those obtained for the polymer, with the highest concentration at the rear of the vitreous cavity. Other physiological details included in simulations have been the hydrodynamics of the aqueous humor [241], the influence of the directionality of release from an intravitreal device [244], and dynamic partitioning of drug between various ocular tissues [245].

Numerical simulation methods can provide a useful predictive tool for simulating drug release from complex devices [246,247] and can aid in optimizing device design to provide sustained release of drug under idealized conditions. Their proper use will require careful characterization of the important physiological constants that govern the disposition of a particular drug and may indicate the dependency of efficacy on individual-to-individual variation [248,249]. An example of this is demonstrated in Fig. 18. The steady-state drug release profile is predicted for a hypothetical circular intravitreal device, which releases drug from only one side at a fixed rate. In the example, the retinal permeability was taken to be 4.5×10^{-6} cm/s, and the diffusion coefficient was 6×10^{-6} cm^2/s, values appropriate for the drug gancyclovir [244]. The influence of hydrodynamics of the aqueous humor were approximated by applying a permeability boundary condition at the hyloid annulus in which the clearance of drug there was 100 times higher than that for the drug at the retina.

Two issues are suggested by the Fig. 18. First, the drug concentration at the retinal surface varies by

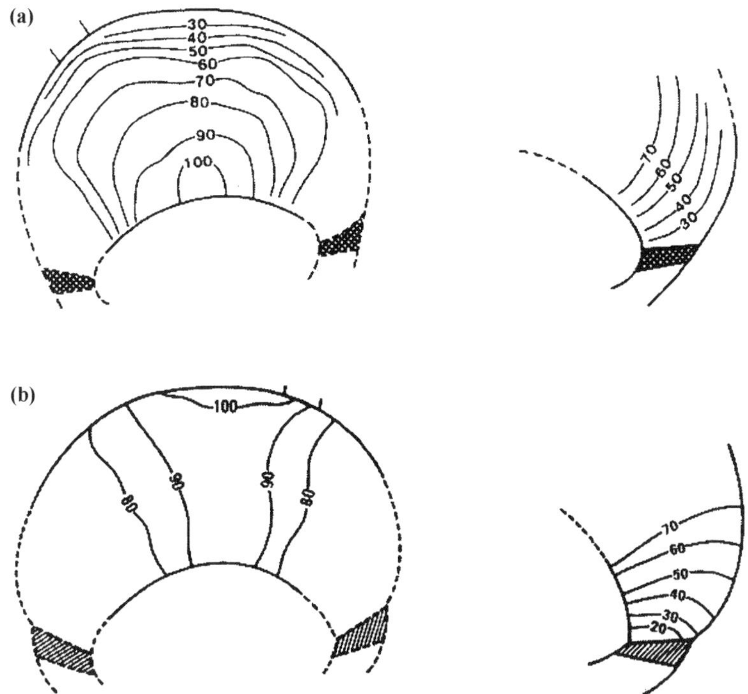

Fig. 16 Contours of fluorescent intensity in frozen sections of the rabbit eye following 15 μL injection of marker solution in the central vitreous cavity; injection was conducted through the superior rectus muscle: 15 hours following injection of 0.2% sodium fluorescein; 14 days following injection of 0.1% FITC-dextran, molecular weight 66,000. (From Ref. 230.)

orders of magnitude depending upon proximity to the implanted device. Depending upon the therapeutic index of the drug, tissues far away from the device may be undertreated, whereas tissues near the device may be overtreated and in danger of toxic exposure. Second, there is a twofold difference in average vitreous drug concentration between the front versus back-facing device, with the higher average concentration resulting from backwards placement. This illustrates the importance of geometric factors when engineering such devices, in that they impact the average and local concentrations and duration of action of therapy.

F. Conclusions

In conclusion, it should be apparent from this discussion of the absorption mechanisms that, although the major features influencing drug absorption are well known, implementation of a coherent delivery strategy is highly specific for any compound, and many variables need to be adjusted for their significant influence on absorption and more importantly, on bioavailability. In addition, from the suggestion of the role of ocular hydrodynamics, delivery strategies will also include consideration of the dosage form and its effect on local systemic and target pharmacokinetics.

Finally, from the available research into the variety of mechanisms for targetting ophthalmic drugs to specific tissues, means for integrating—both figuratively and literally—combinations of effects are now available [15]. Certainly, the combination of hydrodynamics, retention or sustained release, and diffusional or even active transport can be computed, their influence anticipated, and some specific deficiencies addressed. Nonetheless, many unanticipated interactions may often intrude and still leave the field heavily dependent on empirical assessment.

VII. MANUFACTURING CONSIDERATIONS

Because the official compendia require all topically administered ophthalmic medications to be sterile, manufacturers of such medications must weigh numerous alternative approaches as they design manufacturing procedures. Ideally, as preferred by some regulators, especially in Europe, all ophthalmic pro-

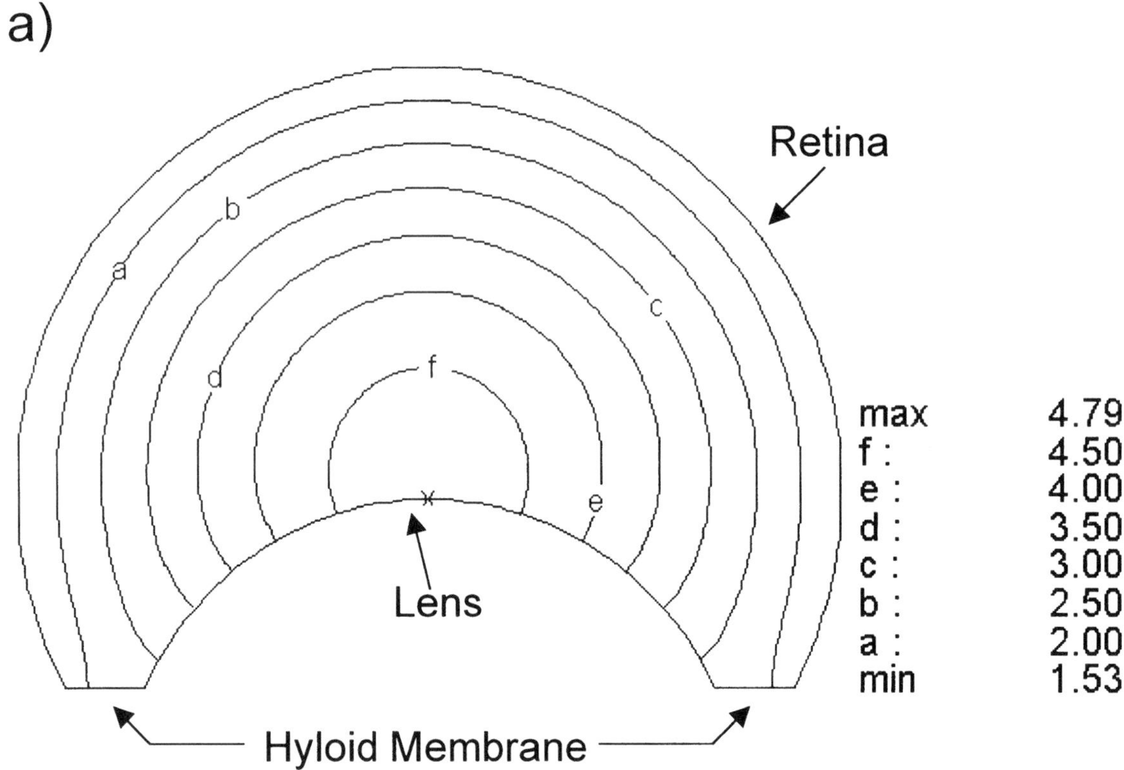

Fig. 17 Finite element modeling of concentration profiles established after central intravitreal bolus injection using FlexPDE v2.17 and a 3-D geometric model for the rabbit eye similar to Ref. 241. Arbitrary concentration units; highest concentration is marked ×. (a) Contours of drug concentration simulated 15 hours after injection, assuming reasonable values[230] for the diffusion coefficient (6×10^{-6} cm^2 s^{-1}) and retinal permeability (2.3×10^{-5} cm s^{-1}) for fluorescein. Permeability across of lens and hyloid membrane is assumed to be negligible. (b) Simulated concentration profile 14 days after injection for FITC-dextran (diffusion coefficient 6×10^{-7} cm^2 s^{-1}), assuming zero retinal permeability, and hyloid permeability 2.3×10^{-5} cm s^{-1}. Finite element mesh used is shown in the inset.

ducts would be terminally sterilized in the final packaging because it offers the best chance of assuring patients of their sterility. In effect, this would rule put any aseptic processing for the manufacture of ophthalmic products; however, the use of sterile filtration and/or aseptic assembly of ophthalmic products has been shown not to constitute a risk to public health.

It is quite rare that the composition or the packaging of an ophthalmic pharmaceutical will lend itself to terminal sterilization, the simplest form of manufacture of sterile products. Only a few ophthalmic drugs formulated in simple aqueous vehicles are stable to normal autoclaving temperatures and times (121°C for 20–30 min). Such heat-resistant drugs may be packaged in glass or other heat-deformation-resistant packaging and thus can be sterilized in this manner. The convenience of plastic dispensing bottles is possible today using modern polyolefins that resist heat deformation with proper sterilization cycles.

Most ophthalmic products, however, cannot be heat sterilized. In general, the active principle is not particularly stable to heat, either physically or chemically. Moreover, to impart viscosity, aqueous products are generally formulated with the inclusion of high molecular weight polymers, which may, similarly, be affected adversely by heat.

Because of these product sensitivities, most ophthalmic pharmaceutical products are aseptically manufactured and filled into previously sterilized containers in aseptic environments using aseptic filling-and-capping techniques. This is the case for ophthalmic solutions, suspensions, and ointments, and specialized technology is involved in their manufacture.

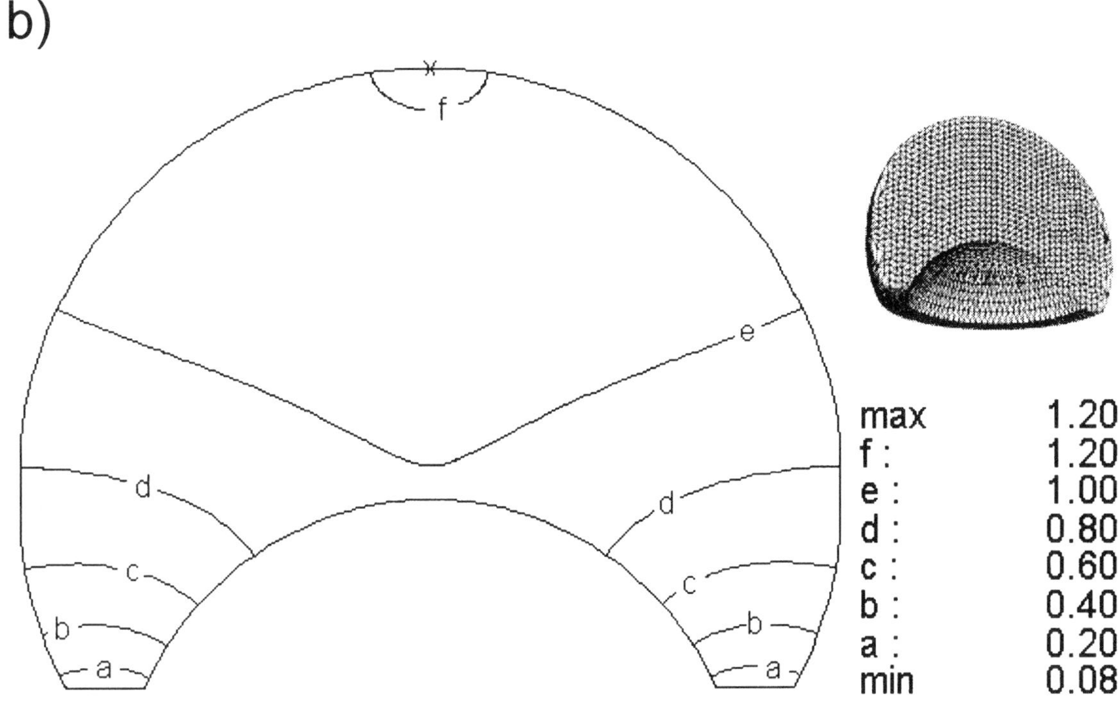

Fig. 17b

All pharmaceutical manufacturers are required to follow Current Good Manufacturing Practice (CGMPs) Part 210—Current Good Manufacturing Practice in Manufacturing, Processing, Packaging, or Holding of Drugs; General Part 211—Current Good Manufacturing Practice for Finished Pharmaceuticals. Readers can access more information from FDA's website at www.fda.gov. These guidelines cover all aspects of manufacture of pharmaceutical products.

A. Manufacturing Environment

Aside from drug safety, stability, efficacy, and shelf-life considerations associated with tonicity, pH, and buffer capacity, the major design criteria of an ophthalmic pharmaceutical product are the additional safety criteria of sterility, preservative efficacy, and freedom from extraneous foreign particulate matter. Current U.S. standards for Good Manufacturing Practices (GMPs) [250] provide for the use of specially designed environmentally controlled areas for the manufacture of sterile large- and small-volume injections for terminal sterilization. These environmentally controlled areas must meet the requirements of class 100,000 space in all areas where open containers and closures are *not* exposed, or where product filling-and-capping operations are *not* taking place. The latter areas must meet the requirements of class 100 space [251]. As defined in Federal Standard 209E, class 100,000 and 100 spaces contain not more than 100,000 or 100 particles, respectively, per cubic foot of air of a diameter of 0.5 μm or larger. The readers are also referred to the British Standard 5295, 1989, for classification of cleanroom environments. Often these design criteria are coupled with laminar airflow concepts [252,253]. This specification deals with total particle counts and does not differentiate between viable and nonviable particles. Federal Standard 209 was promulgated as a "hardware" or mechanical specification for the aerospace industry and has found applications in the pharmaceutical industry as a tool for the design of aseptic and particle-free environments. Class 100,000 conditions can be achieved in the conventionally designed cleanroom, where proper filtration of air supply and adequate turnover rates are provided. Class 100 conditions over open containers can be achieved with properly sized HEPA (high-efficiency particulate air) filtered laminar airflow sources. Depending on the

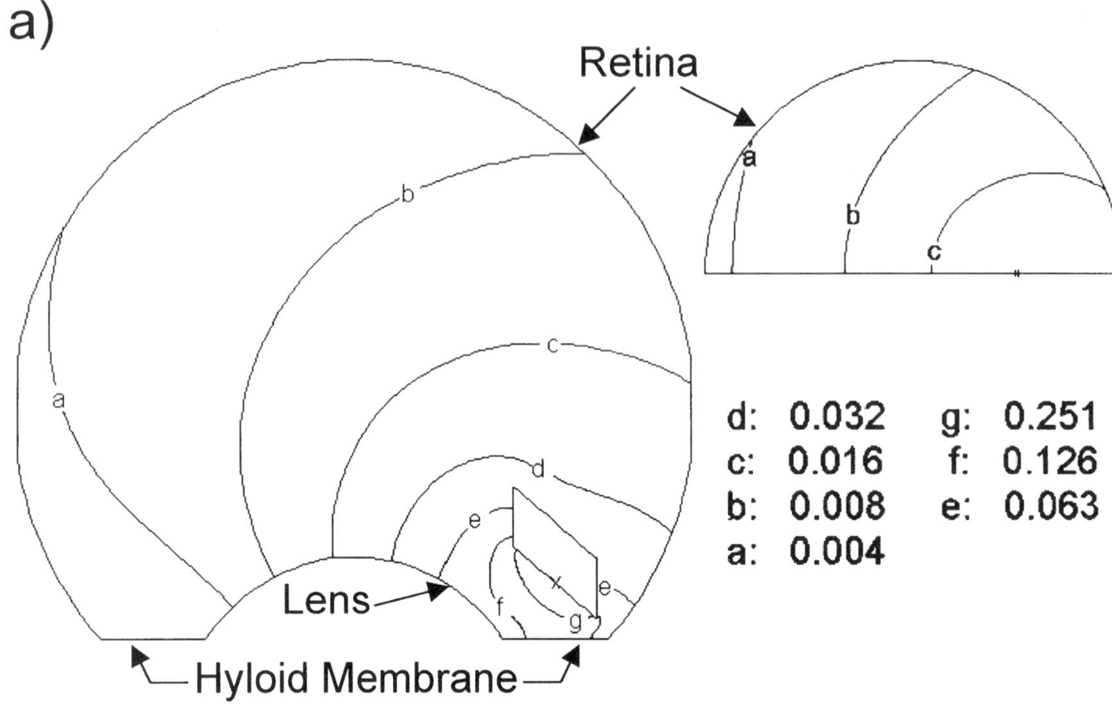

Fig. 18 Finite element modeling of steady-state concentration profiles in the human eye[241] from a hypothetical device that releases from one side only. (a) Device releases towards the front; (b) device releases towards the back. Arbitrary concentration units (scale, inset a); highest concentration marked ×. Contours are shown for x-z plane and for x-y plane through the center. x-z portion of finite element mesh displayed (inset b); device (opaque to diffusion) represented by voided region. (Adapted from Ref. 244.)

product need and funds available, some aseptic pharmaceutical environments have been designed to class 100 laminar-flow specifications throughout the manufacturing area. However, during actual product manufacture the generation of particulate matter by equipment, product, and (most importantly) people may cause these environments to demonstrate particulate matter levels two or more orders of magnitude greater than design. It is for this reason that specialists in the design of pharmaceutical manufacturing and hospital operating room environments are beginning to view these environments not only from the standpoint of total particles per cubic foot of space alone, but also from the standpoint of the types of particles, for example, the ratio of disease-transmitting biocontaminants to inert particulates [254].

Such environmental concepts as mass air transfer may lead to meaningful specifications for the space in which a nonterminally sterilized product can be manufactured with a high level of confidence [255].

When dealing with the environment in which a sterile product is manufactured, the materials used for construction of the facility, as well as personnel attire, training, conduct in the space, the entrance and egress of personnel, equipment, and packaging, and the product, all bear heavily on the assurance of product sterility and minimization of extraneous particulate matter.

The importance of personnel training and behavior cannot be overemphasized in the maintenance of an acceptable environment for the manufacture of sterile ophthalmic products or sterile pharmaceutical agents in general. Personnel must be trained in the proper mode of gowning with sterile, nonshedding garments and in the proper techniques and conduct for aseptic manufacturing. The Parenteral Drug Association can be contacted at their offices in Bethesda, Maryland, for a listing of available training films on this subject. To maximize personnel comfort and to minimize sloughing of epidermal cells and hair, a cool working environment should be maintained, with relative humidities controlled to between 40 and 60%.

Additional guidelines on pharmaceutical cleanroom classifications (which became effective on January 1, 1997, for Europe) are contained in Ref. 263.

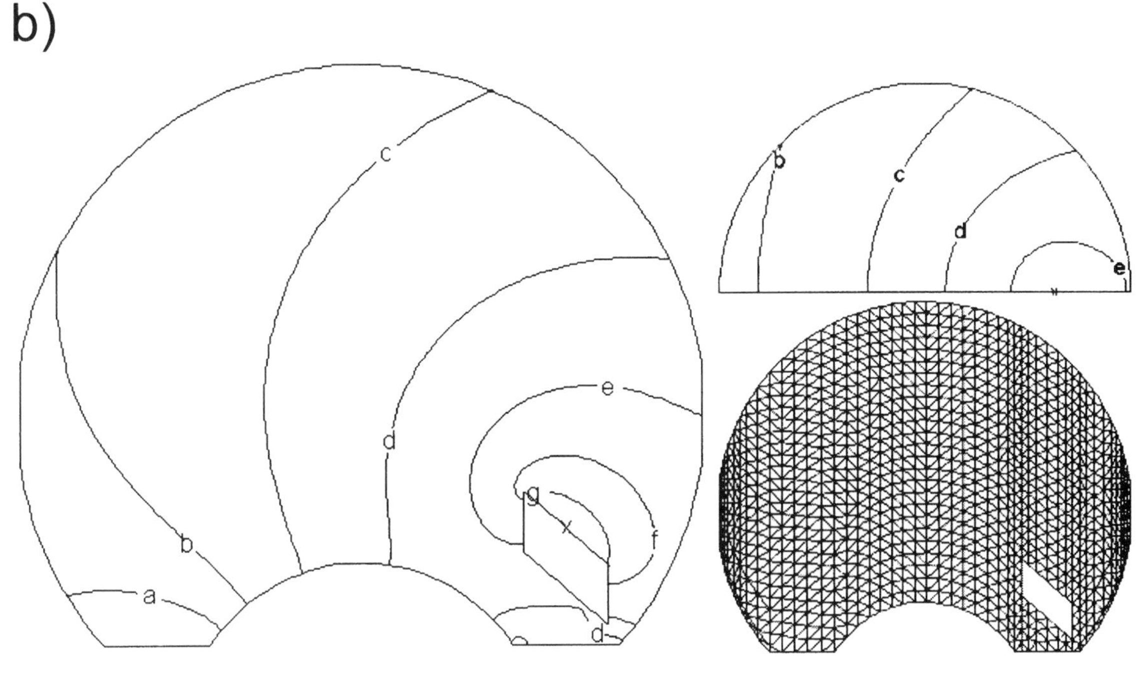

Fig. 18b

B. Manufacturing Techniques

In general, aqueous ophthalmic solutions are manufactured by methods that call for the dissolution of the active ingredient and all or a portion of the excipients into all or a portion of the water and the sterilization of this solution by heat or by sterilizing filtration through sterile depth or membrane filter media into a sterile receptacle. If incomplete at this point, this sterile solution is then mixed with the additional required sterile components, such as previously sterilized solutions of viscosity-imparting agents, preservatives, and so on, and the batch is brought to final volume with additional sterile water.

Aqueous suspensions are prepared in much the same manner, except that before bringing the batch to final volume with additional sterile water, the solid that is to be suspended is previously rendered sterile by heat, by exposure to ethylene oxide or ionizing radiation (gamma or electrons), or by dissolution in an appropriate solvent, sterile filtration, and aseptic crystallization. The sterile solid is then added to the batch, either directly or by first dispersing the solid in a small portion of the batch. After adequate dispersion, the batch is brought to final volume with sterile water. Because the eye is sensitive to particles larger than 25 μm in diameter, proper raw material specifications for particle size of any dispersed solids must be established and verified on each lot of raw material and final product. The control of particle size of the final suspended material is very important, not only for comfort of the product but also for improving physical stability and resuspendability of the suspension throughout the shelf life and the in-use life by patients. Manufacturing of some suspension products [256] may require modified processes in order to control particle size and obtain a sterile product.

When an ophthalmic ointment is manufactured, all raw material components must be rendered sterile before compounding unless the ointment contains an aqueous fraction that can be sterilized by heat, filtration, or ionizing radiation. The ointment base is sterilized by heat and appropriately filtered while molten to remove extraneous foreign particulate matter. It is then placed into a sterile steam-jacketed kettle to maintain the ointment in a molten state under aseptic conditions, and the previously sterilized active ingredient(s) and excipients are added aseptically. While still molten, the entire ointment may be passed through a previously sterilized colloid mill for adequate dispersion of the insoluble components.

After the product is compounded in an aseptic manner, it is filled into previously sterilized containers. Commonly employed methods of sterilization of packaging components include exposure to heat, ethylene oxide gas, and ^{60}Co (gamma) irradiation. When a product is to be used in conjunction with ophthalmic surgical procedures and must enter the aseptic operating area, the exterior of the primary container must be rendered sterile by the manufacturer and maintained sterile with appropriate packaging. This may be accomplished by aseptic packaging or by exposure of the completely packaged product to ethylene oxide gas, ionizing radiation, or heat. Whenever ethylene oxide is used as a sterilant for either the raw material or packaging components, strict processing controls and validated aeration cycles are required to assure lower residual limits permitted by the regulatory agencies.

With the need of, and the preference for, unpreserved formulations of active drug(s) by ophthalmologists and patients, the blow/fill/seal concept, also termed the form/fill/seal method, has gained acceptance for manufacture of unpreserved ophthalmic products, especially for artificial tear products. In this process, the first step is to extrude polyethelene resin at high temperature and pressure and to form the container by blowing the resin into a mold with compressed air. The product is filled as air is vented out, and finally the container is sealed on the top. There are several published articles describing and validating this technology [257–262]. Automatic Liquid Packaging, Incorporated (Woodstock, IL) designs and fabricates Blow/Fill/Seal machines and provides contract manufacture in the United States. Hollopack (BottlePack-6) provides similar equipment in Europe.

C. Raw Materials

All raw materials used in the compounding of ophthalmic pharmaceutical products must be of the highest quality available. Complete raw material specifications for each component must be established and verified for each lot purchased. As many pharmaceutical companies improve efficiency and increase product distribution by qualifying a single plant to provide product globally, it becomes necessary to qualify excipients for global distribution. Excipients used in the product need to be tested for multiple pharmacopeial specifications to meet global requirements (USP, Pharma Europe, Japanese Pharmacopoeia). When raw materials are rendered sterile before compounding, the reactivity of the raw material with the sterilizing medium must be completely evaluated, and the sterilization must be validated to demonstrate its capability to sterilize raw materials contaminated with large numbers (10^5–10^7) of microorganisms that have been demonstrated to be most resistant to the mode of sterilization appropriate for that raw material. As mentioned previously, for raw material components that will enter the eye as a suspension in an appropriate vehicle, particle size must be carefully controlled both before use in the product and as a finished product specification.

As for most sterile (and nonsterile) aqueous pharmaceuticals, the largest portion of the composition is water. At present, USP 24 allows the use of "purified water" as a pharmaceutical aid for all official aqueous products, with the exception of preparations intended for parenteral administration [264]. For preparations intended for parenteral administration, USP 24 requires the use of water for injection (WFI), sterile water injection, or bacteriostatic water for injection as a pharmaceutical aid. Because some pharmaceutical manufacturers produce a line of parenteral ophthalmic drugs and devices (large-volume and small-volume irrigating and "tissue-sparing" solutions) as well as topical ophthalmic drugs, the provision of WFI manufacturing capability is being designed into new and existing facilities to meet this requirement. Some manufacturers have made the decision to compound *all* ophthalmic drugs from WFI, thus employing the highest grade of this raw material economically available to the pharmaceutical industry. In doing so, systems must be designed to meet all the requirements for WFI currently listed in the USP [264] and the guidelines listed for such systems by FDA in its Good Manufacturing Practices guidelines for large- and small-volume parenterals [265]. Briefly, these proposals call for the generation of water by distillation or by reverse osmosis and its storage and circulation at relatively high temperatures of up to 80°C (or, alternatively, its disposal every 24 hours), in all stainless steel equipment of the highest attainable corrosion-resistant quality.

D. Equipment

The design of equipment for use in controlled environment areas follows similar principles, whether for general injectable manufacturing or for the manufacturer of sterile ophthalmic pharmaceuticals. All tanks, valves, pumps, and piping must be of the best available grade of corrosion-resistant stainless steel. In general, stainless steel type 304 or 316 is preferable.

All product-contact surfaces should be finished either mechanically or by electropolishing to provide a surface as free as possible from scratches or defects that could serve as a nidus for the commencement of corrosion [266]. Care should be taken in the design of such equipment to provide adequate means of cleaning and sanitization. For equipment that will reside in aseptic-filling areas, such as filling and capping machines, care should be taken in their design to yield equipment as free as possible from particle-generating mechanisms. Wherever possible, belt- or chain-drive concepts should be avoided in favor of sealed gear or hydraulic mechanisms. Additionally, equipment bulk located directly over open containers should be held to an absolute minimum during filling-and-capping operations in order to minimize introduction of equipment-generated particulate matter or creation of air turbulence. This precaution is particularly important when laminar flow is used to control the immediate environment around the filling-capping operation.

In the design of equipment for the manufacture of sterile ophthalmic (and nonophthalmic) pharmaceuticals, manufacturers and equipment suppliers are turning to the advanced technology in use in the dairy and aerospace industries, where such concepts as CIP (clean-in-place), COP (clean-out-of-place), automatic heliarc welding, and electropolishing have been in use for several years. As a guide here, the reader is referred to the so-called 3A Standards of the dairy industry issued by the U.S. Public Health Service [267].

Some of the newer and more potent drugs, like the prostaglandins, which are produced at very low concentrations in the finished formulation, may require special precautions during compounding and processing in order to prevent loss of actives due to adsorption/absorption to the walls of fill lines and/or storage tanks.

VIII. CLASSES OF OPHTHALMIC PRODUCTS

A. Topical Eyedrops

Administration and Dosage

Although many alternate experimental methods have been tried, the use of eyedrops remains the major method of administration for the topical ocular route. The usual method of self-administration is to place the eyedrop from a dropper or dropper bottle into the lower cul-de-sac by pulling down the eyelid, tilting the head backward, and looking at the ceiling after the tip is pointed close to the sac, and applying a slight pressure to the rubber bulb or plastic bottle to allow a single drop to form and fall into the eye. Most people become quite adept at this method with some practice and may develop their own modifications. However, elderly, arthritic, low-vision, and glaucoma patients often have difficulty in self-administration and may require another person to instill the drops.

The pharmacist should instruct patients to keep in mind the following considerations in administering drops to help improve the accuracy and consistency of dosage and to prevent contamination: be sure that the hands are clean; do not touch the dropper tip to the eye, surrounding tissue, or any surface; prevent squeezing or fluttering of lids which causes blinking; place the drop in the conjunctival sac, not on the globe; close the lids for several moments after instillation. The administration of eyedrops to young children can be a difficult task. A way to simplify the task involves the parent's sitting on the floor or a flat surface and placing the child's head firmly between the parent's thighs and crossing legs over the child's lower truck and legs. The parent's hands are then free to lower the eyelid and administer the drops.

In addition to the proper technique to administer eyedrops, the pharmacist may need to explain to the patient the correct technique for temporary punctal occlusion. Punctal occlusion is usually reserved for use with potent drugs which can have adverse systemic effects from topical ocular administration such as with ocular β-blockers. Tear fluid drains into the nasolacrimal duct via the puncta located on the medial portion of the eyelid and fluid is directed into the puncta by the blinking action of the lids. The nasal meatus is a highly vascular area within the nasal cavity which receives the fluid of the nasolacrimal duct, and drugs contained in tears can be absorbed into the systemic circulation from this area as well as from gastrointestinal absorption. Punctal occlusion can be performed immediately after instillation of an eyedrop by closing the eye and placing a finger between the eyeball and the nose and applying pressure for several minutes.

Eyedrops are one of the few dosage forms not administered by exact volume or weight dosage, yet this seemingly imprecise method of dosing is quite well established and accepted by ophthalmologists. The volume of a drop is dependent on the physiochemical properties of the formulation, particularly surface tension; the design and geometry of the dispensing office; and the angle at which the dispenser is held in relation to the receiving surface. The manufacturer of ophthalmic products controls the tolerances necessary for the dosage form and dispensing container to provide a uniform drop size. How precise does the actual dose have to be? As noted earlier, the normal tear volume is about 7 μL, and with blinking about 10 μL can be retained in the eye. Approximately 1.2 μL of tears is produced per minute, for about a 16% volume replacement per minute. Commercial ophthalmic droppers deliver drops of about 30–50 μL. Therefore, the volumes delivered normally are more than threefold larger than the eye can hold, and the fluid that does remain in the eye is continuously being removed until the normal tear volume is attained. It can be seen, then, that the use of more than 1 drop/dose must take into account the fluid volume and dynamics of the lacrimal system of the eye. If the effect of multiple drops is desired, they should be administered 1 drop at a time with a 3- to 5-minute interval in between dosings. Some doctors may prescribe more than 1 drop/dose to ensure that the patients retains at least 1 drop in the eye.

Dosage Forms

Solutions. The two major physical forms of eyedrops are aqueous solutions and suspensions. Nearly all the major ophthalmic therapeutic agents are water soluble or can be formulated as water-soluble salts. A homogeneous solution offers the assurance of greater uniformity of dosage and bioavailability and simplifies large-scale manufacture. The selection of the appropriate salt form depends on its solubility, therapeutic concentrations required, ocular toxicity, the effect of pH, tonicity, and buffer capacity, its compatibility with the total formulation, and the intensity of any possible stinging or burning sensations (i.e., discomfort reactions). The most common salt forms used are the hydrochloride, sulfate, nitrate, and phosphate. Salicylate, hydrobromide, and bitartrate salts are also used. For drugs that are acidic, such as the sulfonamides, sodium and diethanolamine salts are used. The effect that choice of salt form can have on resulting product properties is exemplified by the epinephrine solutions available, as shown in Table 3. The bitartrate form is a 1:1 salt, and the free carboxyl group acts as a strong buffer, resisting neutralization by the tears, and may cause considerable stinging. The borate form results in a solution with lower buffer capacity, a more nearly physiological pH, and better patient tolerance; however, it is less stable than the other two salts. The hydrochloride salt combines better stability than the borate with acceptable patient tolerance.

Gel-Forming Solutions. One disadvantage of solutions is their relatively short residence time in the eye. This has been overcome to some degree by the development of solutions that are liquid in the container and thus can be instilled as eyedrops but gel on contact with the tear fluid and provide increased contact time with the possibility of improved drug absorption and increased duration of therapeutic effect.

A number of liquid-gel phase transition-dependent delivery systems have been researched and patented. They vary according to the particular polymer(s) employed and their mechanism(s) for triggering the transition to a gel phase in the eye. The mechanisms that make them useful for the eye take advantage of changes in temperature, pH, ion sensitivity, or ionic strength upon contact with tear fluid or due to the presence of proteins such as lysozyme in the tear fluid. Thermally sensitive systems, which are transformed to a gel phase by the change in temperature associated with reaching body temperature, have the disadvantage of possibly gelling in the container when subjected to warmer climatic conditions. The pH-sensitive systems may have limited use for drugs that require a neutral to slightly alkaline environment for stability, solubility, etc.

Gel-forming ophthalmic solutions have been developed and approved by FDA for timolol maleate, which is used to reduce elevated intraocular pressure (IOP) in the management of glaucoma. Timolol maleate ophthalmic solutions, as initially developed, require twice-a-day dosage for most patients. With the gel-forming solutions, IOP-lowering efficacy was extended from 12 to 24 hours and thus required only once-a-day dosing. This extended duration of efficacy was demonstrated for both gel-forming products in controlled clinical

Table 3 Effects of Salt Form on Product Properties

Salt form	Discomfort reaction	pH range	Buffer capacity
Epinephrine hydrochloride	Mild to moderate stinging	2.5–4.5	Medium
Epinephrine bitartrate	Moderate to severe stinging	3–4	High
Epinephrine borate	Only occasional mild stinging	5.5–7.5	Low

trials. The first gel-forming product, Timolol® XE, uses the polysaccharide gellan gum and is reported to gel in situ in response to the higher ionic strength of tear fluid (U.S. Patent 4,861,760). Alternative ion-sensitive gelling systems have been patented [3–5]. The second product, (timolol maleate), uses the polysaccharide xanthan gum as the gelling agent and is reported to gel upon contact with the tear fluid, at least in part due to the presence of tear protein lysozyme (U.S. Patent 6,174,524).

Suspension. If the drug is not sufficiently soluble, it can be formulated as a suspension. A suspension may also be desired to improve stability, bioavailability, or efficacy. The major topical ophthalmic suspensions are the steroid anti-inflammatory agents prednisolone acetate, dexamethasone, fluorometholone, and rimexolone. Water-soluble salts of prednisolone phosphate and dexamethasone phosphate are available; however, they have a lower steroid potency and are poorly absorbed.

An ophthalmic suspension should use the drug in a microfine form; usually 95% or more of the particles have a diameter of 10 μm or less. This is to ensure that the particles do not cause irritation of the sensitive ocular tissues and that a uniform dosage is delivered to the eye. Since a suspension is made up of solid particles, it is at least theoretically possible that they may provide a reservoir in the cul-de-sac for slightly prolonged activity. However, it appears that this is not so, since the drug particles are extremely small, and with the rapid tear turnover rate they are washed out of the eye relatively quickly.

Pharmaceutical scientists have developed improved suspension dosage forms to overcome problems of poor physical stability and patient-perceived discomfort attributed to some active ingredients. An important development aspect of any suspension is the ability to resuspend easily any settled particles prior to instillation in the eye and ensure that a uniform dose is delivered. It would be ideal to formulate a suspension that does not settle since the patient may not always follow the labeled instructions to shake well before using. However, this is usually not feasible or desirable since the viscosity required to retard settling of the insoluble particles completely would likely be excessive for a liquid eyedrop. The opposite extreme, of allowing complete settling between doses, usually leads to a dense layer of agglomerated particles that are difficult to resuspend.

An improved suspension has been developed, which controls the flocculation of the insoluble active ingredient particles, such that they will remain substantially resuspended (95%) for many months and any settled particles can be easily resuspended with only a few seconds of gentle hand shaking. This improved vehicle utilizes a charged water-soluble polymer and oppositely charged electrolyte such as negatively charged carbomer polymer of very high molecular weight and large dimension and a cation such as sodium or potassium. The negatively charged carboxy vinyl polymer is involved in controlling the flocculation of the insoluble particles, such as the steroid rimexolone, and the cation assists in controlling the viscosity of the vehicle such that the settling is substantially retarded, yet can be easily and uniformly resuspended and can be dispensed from a conventional plastic eyedrop container (U.S. Patent 5,461,081).

In some cases it may be advantageous to convert a water-soluble active ingredient to an insoluble form for development as an ophthalmic suspension dosage form. This could be the case when it is beneficial to extend the practical shelf life of the water-soluble form, to improve the compatibility with other necessary compositional ingredients, or to improve its ocular tolerability. Such an example is the β-blocker betaxolol HCL, which is an effective IOP-lowering agent with clinically significant safety advantages for many asthmatic patients. With the ophthalmic solution dosage form some patients experienced discomfort characterized as a transient stinging or burning upon instillation. Although this did not interfere with the safety or efficacy of the product, it was desirable to improve the patient tolerability. Many solution-based formulations were tried but with limited success. It was discovered that an insoluble form of betaxolol (Betoptic®S) could be produced in situ with the use of a combination of a high molecular weight polyanionic polymer such as carbomer and a sulfonic acid cation exchange resin. The resultant optimized suspension increased the ocular bioavailability of betaxolol such that the drug concentration required to achieve equivalent efficacy to the solution dosage form was reduced by one half and the ocular tolerance was improved significantly. It would appear that the sustained release of the active betaxolol occurs through exchange with cations such as sodium and potassium in tear fluid resulting in prolonged tear levels of the drug and substantial increase in ocular bioavailability (U.S. Patent 4,911,920).

Powders for Reconstitution. Drugs that have only limited stability in liquid form are prepared as sterile powders for reconstitution by the pharmacist prior to dispensing to the patient. In ophthalmology, these drugs include α-chymotrypsin, echothiophate iodide

(Phospholine Iodide®), dapiprazole HCl (Rev-Eyes®), and acetylcholine (Miochol®). The sterile powder is usually manufactured by lyophilization in individual glass vials. In powder form these drugs have a much longer shelf life than in solution. Mannitol is usually used as a bulking agent and lyophilization aid and is dissolved in the solution with the drug prior to drying. In the case of echothiophate iodide, it was found that potassium acetate used in place of mannitol as a drying aid produced a more stable product. Apparently the presence of potassium acetate with the drug allows freeze-drying to a lower residual moisture content (U.S. Patent 3,681,495). A stable echothiophate product has also been produced by freeze-drying from an alcoholic solution without a co-drying or bulking agent, but the product is no longer marketed.

A separately packaged sterile diluent and sterile dropper assembly is provided with the sterile powder and requires aseptic technique to reconstitute. The pharmacist should only use the diluent supplied by the manufacturer since it has been developed to maintain the optimum potency and preservation of the reconstituted solution. The storage conditions and expiration dating for the final solution should be emphasized to the patient.

Inactive Ingredients in Topical Drops

The therapeutically inactive ingredients in ophthalmic solution and suspension dosage forms are necessary to perform one or more of the following functions: adjust concentration and tonicity, buffer and adjust pH, stabilize the active ingredients against decomposition, increase solubility, impart viscosity, and act as solvent. The use of unnecessary ingredients is to be avoided, and the use of ingredients solely to impart a color, odor, or flavor is prohibited.

The choice of a particular inactive ingredient and its concentration is based not only on physical and chemical compatibility, but also on biocompatibility with the sensitive and delicate ocular tissues. Because of the latter requirement, the use of inactive ingredients is greatly restricted in ophthalmic dosage forms.

The possibility of systemic effects due to nasolacrimal drainage as previously discussed should also be kept in mind. FDA has catalogued all inactive ingredients in approved drug products and provides this information at www.fda.gov/cder/drug/iig. The listings are alphabetical by inactive ingredient and provide the routes of administration, dosage forms, and quantitative usage ranges.

Tonicity and Tonicity-Adjusting Agents. In the past a great deal of emphasis was placed on teaching the pharmacist to adjust the tonicity of an ophthalmic solution correctly (i.e., exert an osmotic pressure equal to that of tear fluids, generally agreed to be equal to 0.9% NaCl). In compounding an eye solution, it is more important to consider the sterility, stability, and preservative aspects and not jeopardize these aspects to obtain a precisely isotonic solution. A range of 0.5–2.0% NaCl equivalency does not cause a marked pain response, and a range of about 0.7–1.5% should be acceptable to most persons. Manufacturers are in a much better position to make a precise adjustment, and thus their products will be close to isotonic, since they are in a competitive situation and are interested in a high percentage of patient acceptance for their products. In certain instances, the therapeutic concentration of the drug will necessitate using what might otherwise be considered an unacceptable tonicity. This is the case for sodium sulfacetamide, for which the isotonic concentration is about 3.5%, but the drug is used in 10–30% concentrations. Fortunately, the eye seems to tolerate hypertonic solutions better than hypotonic ones. Various textbooks deal with the subject of precise tonicity calculations and determination. Several articles [268] have recommended practical methods of obtaining an acceptable tonicity in extemporaneous compounding. Common tonicity-adjusting ingredients include NaCl, KCl, buffer salts, dextrose, glycerin, propylene glycol, and mannitol.

pH Adjustment and Buffers. The pH and buffering of an ophthalmic solution is probably of equal importance to proper preservation, since the stability of most commonly used ophthalmic drugs is largely controlled by the pH of their environment. Manufacturers place particular emphasis on this aspect, since economics indicate that they produce products with long shelf lives that will retain their labeled potency and product characteristics under the many and varied storage conditions outside the makers' control. The pharmacist and wholesaler must become familiar with labeled storage directions for each product and assure that it is properly stored. Particular attention should be paid to products requiring refrigeration. The stability of nearly all products can be enhanced by refrigeration except for those few in which a decrease in solubility and precipitation might occur. Freezing of ophthalmic products, particularly suspensions, should be avoided. A freeze-thaw cycle can induce particle growth or crystallization of a suspension and increase the chance of ocular irritation and loss of dosage uniformity.

Glass-packaged liquid products may break owing to the volume expansion of the solution when it freezes. It is especially important that the pharmacist fully advise the patient on proper storage and use of ophthalmic products to ensure their integrity and their safe and efficacious use.

In addition to stability effects, pH adjustment can influence comfort, safety, and activity of the product. Comfort can be described as the subjective response of the patient after instillation of the product in the cul-de-sac (i.e., whether it may cause a pain response such as stinging or burning). Eye irritation is normally accompanied by an increase in tear fluid secretion (a defense mechanism) to aid in the restoration of normal physiological conditions. Accordingly in addition to the discomfort encountered, products that produce irritation will tend to be flushed from the eye, and hence a more rapid loss of medication may occur with a probable reduction in the therapeutic response [15].

Ideally, every product would be buffered to a pH of 7.4, considered the normal physiological pH of tear fluid. The argument for this concept is that the product would be comfortable and have optimum therapeutic activity. Various experiments, primarily in rabbits, have shown an enhanced effect when the pH was increased, owing to the solution containing a higher concentration of the nonionized lipid-soluble drug base, the species that can penetrate the corneal epithelial barrier more rapidly. This would not be true if the drug were an acidic moiety. The tears have some buffer capacity of their own, and it is believed that they can neutralize the pH of an instilled solution if the quantity of solutions is not excessive and if the solution does not have a strong resistance to neutralization. Pilocarpine activity is apparently the same whether applied from vehicles with nearly physiological pH values or from more acidic vehicles, provided the latter are not strongly buffered [269]. A pH difference of 6.6 versus 4.2 produced a statistically insignificant difference in pilocarpine miosis [270]. The pH values of ophthalmic solutions are adjusted within a range to provide an acceptable shelf life. When necessary, they are buffered adequately to maintain stability within this range for at least 2 years. If buffers are required, their capacity is controlled to be as low as possible, thus enabling the tears to bring the pH of the eye back to the physiological range. Since the buffer capacity is determined by buffer concentration, the effect of buffers on tonicity must also be taken into account—another reason that ophthalmic products are usually only lightly buffered.

The pH value is not the sole contributing factor to discomfort with use of some ophthalmic solutions. It is possible to have a product with a low pH and little buffer capacity that is more comfortable than a similar product with a higher pH and a stronger buffer capacity. Epinephrine hydrochloride and dipivefrin hydrochloride solutions, used for treatment of glaucoma, have a pH of about 3, yet they have sufficiently acceptable comfort to be used daily for many years. The same pH solution of epinephrine bitartrate has an intrinsically higher buffer capacity and will produce much more discomfort.

The acidic nonsteroidal anti-inflammatory agents produce significant stinging and burning upon topical ocular instillation, and this limits the concentration of drug that can be developed. Caffeine, a xanthine derivative, has been found to improve significantly the comfort of drugs such as suprofen (Profenal®) by forming in situ weak complexes with the NSAID (U.S. Patent 4,559,343).

Stablizers. Stabilizers are ingredients added to a formula to decrease the rate of decomposition of the active ingredients. Antioxidants are the principal stabilizers added to some ophthalmic solutions, primarily those containing epinephrine and other oxidizable drugs. Sodium bisulfite or metabisulfite are used in concentration up to 0.3% in epinephrine hydrochloride and bitartrate solutions. Epinephrine borate solutions have a pH range of 5.5–7.5 and offer a more difficult challenge to formulators who seek to prevent oxidation. Several patented antioxidant systems have been developed specifically for this compound. These consist of ascorbic acid and acetylcysteine, and sodium bisulfite and 8-hydroxyquinoline. Isoascorbic acid is also an effective antioxidant for this drug. Sodium thiosulfate is used with sodium sulfacetamide solutions.

Surfactants. The use of surfactants is greatly restricted in formulating ophthalmic solutions. The order of surfactant toxicity is anionic > cationic >> nonionic. Several nonionic surfactants are used in relatively low concentrations to aid in dispersing steroids in suspensions and to achieve or to improve solution clarity. Those principally used are the sorbitan ether esters of oleic acid (Polysorbate or Tween 20 and 80), polymers of oxyethylated octyl phenol (Tyloxapol), and polyoxyl 40 stearate. The lowest concentration possible is used to perform the desired function. Their effect on preservative efficacy and their possible binding by macromolecules must be taken into account, as well as their effect on ocular irritation. The use of surfactants as cosolvents for an ophthalmic solution of chloramphenicol has been described [271]. This composition includes polyoxyl 40 stearate and polyethylene glycol to solubilize 0.5% chloramphenicol. These surfactants-cosolvents provide a clear aqueous solution of chloramphenicol and a stabilization of the antibiotic in aqueous solution. Polyethoxylated ethers of castor oil are used reportedly for solubilization in Voltaren® (diclofenac sodium) ophthalmic solution (U.S. Patent 4,960,799).

Viscosity-Imparting Agents. Polyvinyl alcohol, methylcellulose, hydroxypropyl methylcellulose, hydroxyethylcellulose, and one of the several high molecular weight cross-linked polymers of acrylic acid, known as Carbomers [270], are commonly used to increase the viscosity of ophthalmic solutions and suspensions. Although they reduce surface tension significantly, their primary benefit is to increase the ocular contact time, thereby decreasing the drainage rate and increasing drug bioavailability. A secondary benefit of the polymer solutions is a lubricating effect that is largely subjective, but noticeable to many patients. One disadvantage to the use of the polymers is their tendency to dry to a film on the eyelids and eyelashes; however, this can be easily removed by wiping with a damp tissue.

Numerous studies have shown that increasing the viscosity of ophthalmic products increases contact time and pharmacological effect, but a plateau is reached after which further increases in viscosity produce only slight or no increase in effect. The location of the plateau is drug- and formulation-dependent. Blaugh and Canada [271] using methylcellulose solutions found increased contact time in rabbits up to 25 cP (centipoise) and a leveling off at 55 cP. Linn and Jones [272] studied the rate of lacrimal excretion in humans using a dye solution in methylcellulose concentration from 0.25 to 2.5%, corresponding to viscosities of 6–30,000 cP, the latter being a thick gel. The results are shown in Table 4.

Chrai and Robinson [273] conducted studies in rabbits and found that, over a range of 1.0–12.5 cP viscosity, there is a threefold decrease in the drainage rate constant and a further threefold decrease over the viscosity range of 12.5–100 cP. This decrease in drainage rate increased the concentration of drug in the precorneal tear film at zero time and subsequent time periods, which resulted in a higher aqueous humor drug concentration. The magnitude of the increase in drug concentration in the aqueous humor was smaller than the increase in viscosity, about 1.7 times, for the range 1.0–12.5 cP, and only a further 1.2-fold increase at 100 cP. Since direct determination of ophthalmic bioavailability in humans is not possible without endangering the eye, investigators have used fluorescein to study factors affecting bioavailability in the eye, because its penetration can be quantified in humans through the use of slit-lamp fluorophotometer. Adler et al. [274], using this technology, found only small increases in dye penetration over a wide range of viscosities. The use of fluorescein data to extrapolate vehicle effects to ophthalmic drugs in general would be questionable owing to the large differences in chemical structure, properties, and permeability existing between fluorescein and most ophthalmic drugs.

Table 4 Effect of Viscosity on Product Contact Time

Methylcellulose concentration (%)	Time to dye appearance through nasolacrymal duct (s)
0.0	60
0.25	90
0.50	140
1.00	210
2.50	255

The major commercial viscous vehicles are hydroxypropyl methylcellulose (Isopto®) and polyvinyl alcohol (Liquifilm®). Isopto products most often use 0.5% of the cellulosic and range from 10 to 30 cP in viscosity. Liquiflm products have viscosities of about 4–6 cP and use 1.4% polymer.

Although usually considered to be inactive ingredients in ophthalmic formulations added because they impart viscosity, many of these polymers function as ocular lubricants. They are marketed as the active ingredients in OTC ocular lubricants used to provide relief from dry eye conditions. The regulatory requirements for these OTC products are found in the FDA Code of Federal Regulations (21CFR349.12), and their formulations are presented in the Twelfth Edition of the *APhA Handbook of Nonprescription Drugs*.

In summary, there are numerous variables to be adjusted and many choices of excipients required when tailoring a formulation of a particular therapeutic agent for ophthalmic application. But ultimately the choice rests on finding an economically viable formulation that clinically enhances the therapeutic index for that drug.

Vehicles. Ophthalmic drops are, with few exceptions, aqueous fluids using purified water USP as the solvent. Water for injection is not required as it is in parenterals. Purified water meeting USP standards may be obtained by distillation, deionization, or reverse osmosis. All ophthalmic drops must be rendered sterile.

Oils have been used as vehicles for several topical eyedrop products that are extremely sensitive to moisture. Tetracycline HCl is an antibiotic that is stable for only a few days in aqueous solution. It is supplied as a 1% sterile suspension with Plastibase 50W and light liquid petrolatum. White petrolatum and its combination with liquid petrolatum to obtain a proper consistency is routinely used as the vehicle for ophthalmic ointments.

When oils are used as vehicles in ophthalmic fluids, they must be of the highest purity. Vegetable oils such as olive oil, castor oil, and sesame oil have been used for extemporaneous compounding. These oils are subject to rancidity and, therefore, must be used carefully. Some commercial oils, such as peanut oil, contain stabilizers that could be irritating. The purest grade of oil, such as that used for parenteral products, would be advisable for ophthalmics.

Packaging

Eyedrops have been packaged almost entirely in plastic dropper bottles since the introduction of the Drop-Tainer® plastic dispenser in the 1950s. A few products still remain in glass dropper bottles because of special stability considerations. The main advantage of the Drop-Trainer and similarly designed plastic dropper bottles are convenience of use by the patient, decreased contamination potential, lower weight, and lower cost. The plastic bottle has the dispensing tip as an integral part of the package. The patient simply removes the cap and turns the bottle upside down and squeezes gently to form a single drop that falls into the eye. The dispensing tip will deliver only one drop or a stream of fluid for irrigation, depending on the tip design and pressure applied. When used properly, the solution remaining in the bottle is only minimally exposed to airborne contaminants during administration; thus, it will maintain very low to nonexistent microbial content as compared with the old-style glass bottle with its separate dropper assembly.

The plastic bottle and dispensing tip is made of low-density polyethylene (LDPE) resin, which provides the necessary flexibility and inertness. Because these components are in contact with the product during its shelf life, they must be carefully chosen and tested for their suitability for ophthalmic use. In addition to stability studies on the product in the container over a range of normal and accelerated temperatures, the plastic resins must pass the USP biological and chemical tests for suitability. The LDPE resins used are compatible with a very wide range of drugs and formulation components. Their one disadvantage is their sorption and permeability characteristics. Volatile ingredients such as the preservatives chlorobutanol and phenylethyl alcohol can migrate into the plastic and eventually permeate through the walls of the container. The sorption and permeation can be detected by stability studies if they are significant. If the permeating component is a preservative, a repeat test of the preservative effectiveness with time will determine if the loss is significant. If necessary, a safe and reasonable excess of the permeable component may be added to balance the loss during the product's shelf life. Another means of overcoming permeation effects is to employ a secondary package, such as a peel-apart blister or pouch composed of nonpermeable materials (e.g., aluminum foil or vinyl). The plastic dropper bottles are also permeable to water, but weight loss by water vapor transmission has a decreasing significance as the size of the bottle increases. The consequences of water vapor transmission must be taken into consideration when assessing the stability of a product.

The LDPE resins are translucent, and if the drug is light-sensitive, additional package protection may be required. This can be achieved by using a resin containing an opacifying agent such as titanium dioxide, by placing an opaque sleeve over the exterior of the container, or by placing the bottle in a cardboard carton. Extremely light-sensitive drugs, such as epinephrine and proparacaine, may require a combination of these protective measures. Colorants, other than titanium dioxide, are rarely used in plastic containers; however, the use of colorants is common for the cap. Red has historically been used for mydriatics such as atropine and green for miotics such as pilocarpine. FDA and the ophthalmic industry have extended the cap color scheme to differentiate different classes of newer prescription drugs for the benefit of the patient who may be using more than one product. The intent is to help prevent errors in medication and improve patient compliance. It is important for the pharmacist to explain this color coding to the patient and/or caregiver since it can be defeated if the cap is not returned to the proper container after each use. Colors used for certain medications are as follows:

β-Blockers: Yellow or blue
Nonsteroids: Grey
Anti-infectives: Brown, Tan
Carbonic anhydrous inhibitors: Orange

The pharmacist should dispense the sterile, ophthalmic product only in the original unopened container. A tamper-evident feature such as a cellulosic or metal band around the cap and bottleneck is provided by the manufacturer, and the container should not be dispensed if these are missing or there is evidence of prior removal and reapplication. The LDPE resin used for the bottle and the dispensing tip cannot be autoclaved, and they are sterilized either by ^{60}Co gamma irradiation or ethylene oxide. The cap is designed such that when it is screwed tightly onto the bottle, it mates with the dispensing tip and forms a seal. The cap is usually made of a harder resin than the bottle, such as polystyrene or polypropylene, and is also sterilized by gamma radiation or ethylene oxide gas exposure. A plastic ophthalmic package has been introduced that uses a special grade of polypropylene that is resistant to deformation at autoclave temperatures. With this specialized packaging, the bottle can be filled, the dispensing tip and cap applied, and the entire product sterilized by steam under pressure at 121°C.

The glass dropper bottle is still used for products that are extremely sensitive to oxygen or contain permeable components that are not sufficiently stable in plastic. Powders for reconstitution also use glass containers, owing to their heat-transfer characteristics, which are necessary during the freeze-drying process. The glass used should be USP type I for maximum compatiblity with the sterilization process and the product. The glass container is made sterile by dry heat or steam autoclave sterilization. Amber glass is used for light resistance and is superior to green glass. A sterile dropper assembly is usually supplied separately. It is usually gas-sterilized in a blister composed of vinyl and Tyvek, a fused, porous polypropylene material. The dropper assembly is made of a glass or LDPE plastic pipette and a rubber dropper bulb. The manufacturer carefully tests the appropriate plastic and rubber materials suitable for use with the product; therefore, they should be dispensed with the product. The pharmacist should place the dropper assembly aseptically into the product before dispensing and instruct the patient on precautions to be used to prevent contamination.

Multidose Packaging of Unpreserved Topical Drops. In some cases it may be desirable to provide a product without an antimicrobial preservative for patients who exhibit sensitivity to various preservatives. This can be accomplished with the use of unit dose containers, but these usually contain more than that needed for a single use, so if the patient ignores the labeling and makes multiple use of the contents there is increased risk for contamination.

FDA regulations for ophthalmic liquids allow the use of unpreserved multidose packaging if the product is packaged and labeled in such a manner as to afford adequate protection and minimize the hazards resulting from contamination during use (21CFR 200.50). Thus, the same unit dose containers can be modified to use a resealable cap, the labeling modified to limit the usage to a minimum number of doses such as to discard after 12 hours from initial use and limit the content volume to the expected number of doses with only a small overfill if necessary. It may be necessary to use a secondary package to retard moisture vapor transmission significantly, depending on the surface-to-volume ratio of the primary package.

B. Semisolid Dosage Forms: Ophthalmic Ointments and Gels

Formulation

The principle semisolid dosage form used in ophthalmology is an anhydrous ointment with a petrolatum base. The ointment vehicle is usually a mixture of mineral oil and white petrolatum. The mineral oil is added to reduce the melting point and modify the consistency. The principal advantages of the petrolatum-based ointments are their blandness and their anhydrous and inert nature, which make them suitable vehicles for moisture-sensitive drugs. Ophthalmic ointments containing antibiotics are used quite frequently following operative procedures, and their safety is supported by the experience of a noted eye surgeon [275], who, in over 20,000 postsurgical patients, saw no side effects secondary to ointment use. No impediment to epithelial or stromal wound healing was exhibited by currently used ophthalmic ointments tested by Hanna et al. [276]. The same investigators reported that, even if these ointments were entrapped in the anterior chamber and did not exceed 5% of the volume, little or no reaction was caused [277]. Granulomatous reactions requiring surgical excision have been reported secondary to therapeutic injection of ointment into the lacrimal sac [278].

The chief disadvantages of the use of ophthalmic ointments are their greasy nature and the blurring of vision produced. They are most often used as adjunctive nighttime therapy, with eyedrops administered during the day. The nighttime use obviates the difficulties produced by blurring of vision and is stated to prolong ocular retention when compared with drops. Ointments are used almost exclusively as vehicles for antibiotics, sulfonamides, antifungals, and anti-inflammatories. The petrolatum vehicle is also used as an ocular lubricant following surgery or to treat various dry eye syndromes. Anesthesiologists may prescribe the ointment vehicle for the non-ophthalmic surgical patients to prevent severe and painful dry eye conditions that could develop during prolonged surgeries. A petrolatum ointment is recognized as a safe and effective OTC emollient (21CFR 349.14), and marketed OTC emollient products are discussed in the twelfth edition of the *APhA Handbook of Nonprescription Drugs*.

The anhydrous petrolatum base may be made more miscible with water through the use of an anhydrous liquid lanolin derivative. Drugs can be incorporated into such a base in aqueous solution if desired. Polyoxyl 40 stearate and polyethylene glycol 300 are used in an anti-infective ointment to solubilize the active principle in the base so that the ointment can be sterilized by aseptic filtration. The cosmetic-type bases, such as the oil-in-water (o/w) emulsion bases popular in dermatology, should not be used in the eye, nor should liquid emulsions, owing to the ocular irritation produced by the soaps and surfactants used to form the emulsion.

In an attempt to formulate an anhydrous, but water-soluble, semisolid base for potential ophthalmic use, five bases were studied [279]. The nonaqueous portion of the base was either glycerin or polyethylene glycols in high concentrations. The matrix used to form the phases included silica, Gantrez® AN-139, and Carbopol® 940. Eye irritation results were not reported, but the authors studied representative bases from that research report and found them to be quite irritating in rabbit eyes. The irritation is believed to be primarily due to the high concentration of the polyols used as vehicles.

An aqueous semisolid gel base has been developed that provides significantly longer residence time in the cul-de-sac and increases drug bioavailability and, thereby, may prolong the therapeutic level in the eye. The gel contains a high molecular weight cross-linked polymer to provide the high viscosity and optimum rheological properties for prolonged ocular retention. Only a relatively low concentration of polymer is required, so that the gel base is more than 95% water.

Schoenwald et al. [280] demonstrated the unique ocular retention of this polymeric gel base in rabbits, in which the miotic effect of pilocarpine was significantly prolonged. The use of other polymers, such as cellulosic gums, polyvinyl alcohol, and polyacrylamides at comparable apparent viscosities, did not provide a significantly prolonged effect. The prolonged effect of pilocarpine has also been demonstrated in human clinical trials, in which a single application of 4% pilocarpine HCl–containing carbomer gel at bedtime, provided a 24-hour duration of reduced intraocular pressure (IOP), compared with the usually required q.i.d. dosing for pilocarpine solution [281]. As a result, some glaucoma patients can now use pilocarpine in this aqueous gel base (Pilopine® HS Gel), dosing only once a day at bedtime to control their IOP without the significant vision disturbance experienced during the day for the use of conventional pilocarpine eyedrops. The gel is applied in a small strip in the lower conjunctival sac from an ophthalmic ointment tube.

The carbomer polymeric gel base itself has been used successfully to treat moderate to severe cases of dry eye (*keratoconjunctivitis sicca*) [282]. The dry eye syndrome is usually characterized by deficiency of tear production and, therefore, requires frequent instillation of aqueous artificial tear eyedrops to keep the corneal epithelium moist. The gel base applied in a small amount provides a prolonged lubrication to the external ocular tissues, and some patients have reduced the frequency of dosing to control their symptoms to three times a day or fewer.

Sterility and Preservation

Since October 1973, FDA regulations require that all U.S. ophthalmic ointments be sterile. This legal requirement was a result of several surveys on microbial contamination of ophthalmic ointments, and followed reports in Sweden and the United Kingdom of severe eye infections resulting from use of nonsterile ointments. In its survey published in 1973, FDA found that of 82 batches of ophthalmic ointments tested from 27 manufacturers, 16 batches were contaminated, including 8 antibiotic-containing ointments. The contamination levels were low and were principally molds and yeasts [283]. The time lag in imposition of a legal requirement for sterility of ointments compared with solutions and suspensions was due to the absence of a reliable sterility test for the petrolatum-based ointments until isopropyl myristate was employed to dissolve these ointments and allow improved recovery of viable microorganisms by membrane filtration. Manufacturers found that, in fact, many of their ointments were sterile, but they revised their manufacturing procedures to increase the assurance of sterility.

A suitable substance or mixture of substances to prevent growth of, or destroy, microorganisms accidentally introduced during use must be added to ophthalmic ointments that are packaged in multiuse containers, regardless of the method of sterilization employed, unless otherwise directed in the individual monograph, or unless the formula itself is bacteriostatic (USP 24). Schwartz [284] commented that a sterile ointment cannot become excessively contaminated by ordinary use because of its consistency and the fact that in a nonaqueous medium microogranisms merely survive but do not multiply. Antimicrobial preservative effectiveness is evaluated by use of the USP 24 testing methodology and criteria for ointments with aqueous bases (Category 1) or nonaqueous bases (Category 2). The test criteria for an anhydrous petrolatum ointment are met if there is no increase in the initial concentration of viable bacteria, yeast, or molds at 14 and 28 days of the test.

Packaging

Ophthalmic ointments are packaged in small collapsible tin tubes, usually holding 3.5 g of product. The pure tin tube is compatible with a wide range of drugs in petrolatum-based ointments. Aluminum tubes have been considered and may eventually be used because of their lower cost and as an alternative should the supply of tin become a problem. Until internal coating technology for these tubes advances, the aluminum tube will be a secondary packaging choice. Plastic tubes made from flexible LDPE resins have also been considered as an alternative material, but they do not collapse and tend to suck back the ointment. Plastic tubes recently introduced as containers for toothpaste have been investigated and may offer the best alternative to tin. These tubes are laminates of plastic and various materials, such as paper or foil. A tube can be designed by selection of the laminate materials and their arrangement and thickness to provide the necessary compatibility, stability, and barrier properties. The various types of metal tubes are sealed using an adhesive coating covering only the inner edges of the bottom of the open tube to form the crimp, which does not contact the product. Laminated tubes are usually heat-sealed. The crimp usually contains the lot code and expiration date. Filled tubes may be tested for leakers by storing them in a horizontal position in an oven at 60°C for at least 8 hours. No leakage should be evidenced except for a minute quantity that could only come from within the crimp of the tube or the end of the cap. The screw cap is made of polyethylene or polypropylene. Polypropylene must be used for autoclave sterilization, but either material may be used when the tubes are gas sterilized. A tamper-evident feature is required for sterile ophthalmic ointments and may be accomplished by sealing the tube or the carton holding the tube such that the contents cannot be used without providing visible evidence of destruction of the seal. The Teledyne Wirz tube used by most manufacturers has a flange on the cap that is visible only after the tube has been opened the first time.

The tube can be a source of metal particles and must be cleaned carefully before sterilization. The USP contains a test procedure and limits the level of metal particles in ophthalmic ointments. The total number of metal particles detected under $30\times$ magnification that are 50 µm or larger in any dimension is counted. The requirements are met if the total number of such particles counted in 10 tubes is not more than 50 and if not more than one tube is found to contain more than 8 such particles.

C. Solid Dosage Forms: Ocular Inserts

In earlier times lamellae or disks of glycerinated gelatin were used to supply drugs to the eye by insertion beneath the eyelid. The aqueous tear fluids dissolved the lamella and released the drug for absorption. The medical literature also describes a sterile paper strip impregnated with drug for insertion in the eye. These appear to have been the first attempts at designing a sustained-release ocular dosage form.

Nonerodible Ocular Inserts

In 1975, the first controlled-release *topical* dosage form was marketed in the United States by the Alza Corporation. Zaffaroni [285] describes the Alza therapeutic system as a drug-containing device or dosage form that administers a drug or drugs at programmed rates, at a specific body Site, for a prescribed time period to provide continuous control of drug therapy and to maintain this control over extended periods. Therapeutic systems for uterine delivery of progesterone, transdermal delivery of scopolamine, and oral delivery of systemic drugs have also been developed.

The Ocusert® Pilo-20 and Pilo-40 Ocular Therapeutic System is an elliptical membrane that is soft and flexible and designed to be placed in the inferior cul-de-sac between the sclera and the eyelid and to release pilocarpine continuously at a steady rate for 7 days. The design of the dosage form is described by Alza in terms of an open-looped therapeutic system, having three major components: (a) the drug, (b) a drug-delivery module, and (c) a platform. In the Ocusert Pilo-20 and Pilo-40 systems, the drug-delivery module consists of (a) a drug reservoir, pilocarpine (free base), and a carrier material, alginic acid; (b) a rate controller, ethylene vinyl acetate (EVA) copolymer membrane; (c) an energy source, the concentration of pilocarpine in the reservoir; and (d) a delivery portal, the copolymer membrane. The platform component for the pilocarpine Ocusert consists of the EVA copolymer membranes, which serve as the housing, and an annular ring of the membrane impregnated with titanium dioxide that forms a white border for visibility. The laminate structure of the Ocusert is seen in Fig. 19. The free-base form of pilocarpine is used, since it exhibits both hydrophilic and lipophilic characteristics. Use of the extremely water-soluble salts of pilocarpine would have necessitated the use of a hydrophilic membrane, which, if it osmotically imbibed an excessive amount of water, would cause a significant decline in the release rate with time. Use of the free base allowed a choice of more hydrophobic membranes that are relatively impermeable to water; accordingly the release rate is independent of the environment in which it is placed. EVA, the hydrophobic copolymer chosen, was found to be very compatible with the sensitive ocular tissues [286], an important feature.

The pilocarpine Ocusert is seen by Alza to offer a number of theoretical advantages over drop therapy for the glaucoma patient. The Ocusert exposes a patient to only one-fourth to one-eighth the amount of pilocarpine, compared with drop therapy. This could lead to reduced local side effects and toxicity. It provides continuous around-the-clock control of IOP, whereas drops used four times a day can permit periods where the IOP might rise. Additionally, the Ocusert provides for more patient convenience and improved compliance, as the dose needs to be administered only once per week. However, clinical experience seems to indicate that the Ocusert has a compliance problem of its own (i.e., retention in the eye for the full 7 days). The patient must check periodically to see that the unit is still in place, particularly in the morning on arising. Replacement of a contaminated unit with a fresh one can increase the price differential of the already expensive Ocusert therapy compared with the inexpensive drop or once-a-day gel therapy. In addition, some patients find positioning the Ocusert in the eye to be challenging.

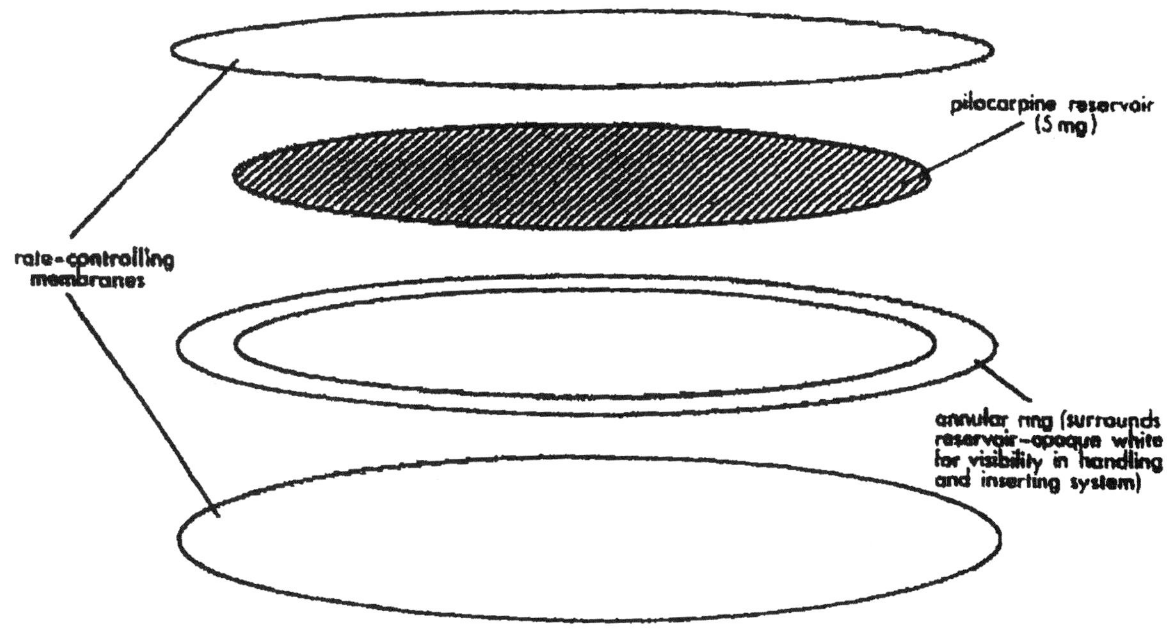

Fig. 19 Elements and dimensions of pilocarpine Ocusert system.

Soft contact lenses, made of the same hydrophilic plastic materials used for vision correction, are also used as corneal bandages to protect the cornea during the healing process following surgery. They can be fitted to the eye and inserted and removed by the ophthalmologist. They are usually used without correction (plano lens) and removed by the ophthalmologist. Since they are used in a compromised cornea, great care must be taken to prevent microbial contamination.

Erodible Ocular Inserts

Since polymers have been added to solutions to increase viscosity and ocular retention, it is not surprising that similar solutions have been dried to form films of the polymer-drug system. These films inserted into the lower cul-de-sac of the eye have been reported to increase retention time, increase drug bioavailability, and prolong therapeutic effect. Ocular inserts made with water-soluble polymers imbibe the tear fluid and slowly dissolve and erode, releasing their drug content. The erodible inserts have the potential advantages of not having to be removed at the end of their useful dosing interval, providing a more precise dosage to the eye from a unit dosage form, and requiring no preservative, thus reducing the risk of inducing sensitivity. Also, it may be possible to reduce the applied dose compared to conventional eyedrops and reduce the risk of local or systemic adverse effects. Potential disadvantages include the difficulty of achieving constant zero-order drug delivery as the matrix is eroding, and in some cases they may be squeezed out of the eye due to movement of the eyelids before their delivery cycle is complete. They may require terminal sterilization, and this may adversely affect stability and could produce unwanted degradation products. Considerable drug-delivery research has been conducted and reported for various erodible ocular inserts [287–291].

An erodible insert developed as a potential ocular drug-delivery system is marketed as a prescription drug for the lubricant properties of the polymer base. Lacrisert® is a sterile ophthalmic insert used in the treatment of moderate to severe dry eye syndrome and is usually recommended for patients unable to obtain symptomatic relief with artificial tear solutions. The insert is composed of 5 mg of hydroxypropylcellulose in a rod-shaped form about 1.27 mm diameter by about 3.5 mm long. No preservative is used, since it is essentially anhydrous. The quite rigid cellulose rod is placed in the lower conjunctival sac and first imbibes water from the tears and after several hours forms a gel-like mass, which gradually erodes as the polymer dissolves. This action thickens the tear film and provides increased lubrication, which can provide symptomatic relief for dry eye states. It is usually used once or twice daily.

Corneal shields are medical devices used as bandages for protection of the cornea and to allow healing following surgery. Initially, hydrophilic soft contact lenses used for vision correction were employed as corneal shields. Collagen was then introduced as a substitute for the plastic noneroding bandage lens. They are widely used today as temporary protective devices for healing corneas. In addition to their approved use of corneal bandages, they have been investigated as drug-delivery vehicles to provide sustained delivery of drugs to the cornea by the ophthalmologist [292].

Collagen is widely used for biomedical applications. It accounts for about 25% of the total body protein in mammals and is the major protein of connective tissue, cartilage, and bone. Importantly, the secondary and tertiary structures of human, porcine, and bovine collagen are very similar, making it possible to use animal-sourced collagen in the human body. Collagen shields are designed to be sterile, disposable, temporary bandage lenses that conform to the shape of the eye and protect the cornea. They are not optically clear and reduce visual acuity to the 20/80–20/200 range. They differ mainly in the source of collagen, usually bovine or porcine, and their dissolution time on the cornea, ranging from 12 to 72 hours. The dissolution time is controlled during manufacture by varying the degree of cross-linking usually by exposure to ultraviolet light.

D. Intraocular Dosage Forms

Opthalmic products, which are introduced into the interior structures of the eye primarily during ocular surgery, are a special class that require the application of technology from parenteral dosage forms in their design, packaging, and manufacture. The development of cytomegalovirus (CMV) retinitis as a common opportunistic infection in patients with AIDS has resulted in expansion of this class of ocular product to include solid inserts and injections of antiviral agents administered directly to the vitreous cavity. As discussed previously, topical and systemic administration often fails to achieve therapeutic concentrations in the vitreous cavity.

Ophthalmic surgery has rapidly advanced in the last three decades, particularly with the ability of the surgeon to operate in the posterior segment. The ophthalmologist can perform vitreoretinal surgery and restore significant visual function in patients with diabetic complications, endophthalmitis, and retinal tears and detachments. Also, significant advances have been made in anterior segment surgery, especially for cataract surgery, where replacement of a cloudy or opaque natural crystalline lens with a plastic or silicone intraocular lens can restore visual acuity and allow the patient to achieve a significant improvement in his or her quality of life. These technological advances have placed greater emphasis on the development of products specifically formulated and packaged for intraocular use. This has led to the development of improved irrigating solutions, intraocular injections, viscoelastics, vitreous inserts, and intravitreal injections.

Intraocular Irrigating Solutions

An essential component of ocular surgery is the use of a simulated physiological solution to moisten and irrigate ocular tissue on the external surface as well as intraocular anterior and posterior segments of the eye. Externally, the solution maintains a moist surface preventing cellular desiccation, which can inhibit the surgeon's ability to see inside the eye. The solution also acts as a substitute for the natural aqueous intraocular fluid and aids in the removal of blood and cellular debris. Normal saline and lactated Ringer's solution were used initially since they were available in parenteral dosage form, but they lacked key components of ocular fluids. In the 1960s a balanced salt solution was developed specifically for ocular surgical use and became widely used. It contains the five essential ions: sodium, potassium, calcium, magnesium, and chloride. It also contains citrate and acetate ions, which provide some buffer capacity and a potential source of bicarbonate. It is formulated to be isoosmotic with aqueous humor (about 305 mOsm) and has a neutral to slightly alkaline physiological pH [293–295].

Balanced salt solution (BSS®) provided an improved ocular irrigating solution; however, as the surgical techniques for cataract surgery evolved and new vitreoretinal surgical procedures were introduced, larger volumes of irrigating solutions were used, and surgical operating times for the very delicate vitreoretinal procedures can now exceed several hours. This has placed additional physiological demands on the irrigating solution, and an enriched balanced salt solution (BSS® Plus) was developed. The enriched product contains the essential electrolyte components of BSS with the addition of glutathione (oxidized) and dextrose as energy sources, bicarbonate as a physiological buffer, and a phosphate buffer system to maintain the products storage pH in the physiological range [296,297].

The enriched BSS formulation presented chemical and physical stability issues not present in the original BSS product. It was necessary to use a two-part formulation in order to develop a commercially viable product with several years of storage stability; the two parts are aseptically combined just prior to surgery. The two-part formulation consists of a large volume part containing sodium, potassium, chloride, phosphate, and bicarbonate components at physiological pH and osmolality. The second part contains the calcium and magnesium divalent ions and the oxidized glutathione and dextrose in an acidic environment for long-term storage stability. The smaller-volume second part has a minimal buffer capacity and, when added to the larger-volume first part, does not significantly change the final product's physiological pH. Once aseptically combined, it is stable for at least 24 hours, although it is labeled to be used within 6 hours as a sterility precaution.

Providing the product as a two-part system was necessary to overcome the physical and chemical incompatibilities inherent in the final composition. Bicarbonate is stable only in an alkaline environment, while glutathione and dextrose are stable in a pH range of about 3–5. Consideration was also given to which of the two parts should be the larger volume in the irrigation bottle, since inadvertent failure to mix the two parts prior to use could occur. The large-volume component contains a bicarbonate saline solution at physiological pH and osmolality and thus would be more tissue compatible than irrigating with a hypo-osmotic acidic pH solution.

The large-volume part is packaged in Type 1 glass IV bottle and as such can be autoclaved sterilized. The quality of the glass is important to prevent leaching of silicates, which can increase pH during autoclaving and storage. IV parenteral grade rubber stoppers must be used to minimize coring and extraction. Type 1 glass is also used for the additive part vial with a parenteral grade rubber stopper. The smaller-volume part is added aseptically to the larger-volume container via a sterile transfer needle.

Intraocular irrigating solutions are required to be preservative-free to prevent toxicity to the internal tissues of the eye, particularly the corneal endothelium, lens, and retina [298,299]. These products are intended for single use only to prevent intraocular infections, which can be difficult to treat and seriously threaten sight. In addition to being sterile, they must be non-pyrogenic, therefore requiring sterile water for injection (WFI) as the vehicle.

These irrigating solutions have been developed and are labeled to be used without the addition of any drugs, i.e., not as a delivery vehicle. However, some drugs such as epinephrine are added to the irrigating solution prior to surgery and used extensively by cataract surgeons to achieve and maintain pupillary dilation, facilitating removal of the natural lens and insertion of the prosthetic intraocular lens. Use of some commercial epinephrine injections that contain sodium bisulfite in addition to their acidic pH as the source for the epinephrine additive have been reported to be the cause of intraocular toxicity, even though it is diluted as much as 500-fold before irrigation [300].

FDA has approved a generic version of the enriched BSS product. The generic product is equivalent only in the final composition after mixing the two parts. To avoid the originator's patents, the generic uses different compositions in the two-part formulations. The larger volume part is an acidic solution, and the second part is a lyophilized product for stability of the dextrose and glutathione components. If the larger volume part is used without the addition of the second part, the eye will be irrigated with an acidic nonphysiological solution.

Intraocular Injections

Very few injectable dosage forms have been specifically developed and approved by FDA for intraocular use. However, the ophthalmologist uses available parenteral dosage forms to deliver antiinfectives, corticosterioids, and anesthetic products to achieve higher therapeutic concentrations intraocularly than can ordinarily be achieved by topical or systemic administration. These unapproved or off-label uses have developed over time as part of the physician's practice of medicine. However, these drugs are usually administered by subconjunctival or retrobulbar injection and rarely are they injected directly in the eye [301].

FDA approved intraocular injections include miotics, viscoelastics, and viscoadherents and an antiviral agent for intravitreal injection. The approved intraocular miotics, carbachol (Miostat®) and acetylcholine (Miochol®), are injected into the anterior chamber at the end of cataract surgery to constrict the pupil and allow the iris to cover the implanted intraocular lens. Carbachol is formulated in a BSS vehicle in sterile water for injection at a physiological pH and packaged in a rubber-stoppered glass vial. Acetylcholine has very limited stability and so is lyophilized with mannitol in a two-chambered vial with a modified BSS vehicle in sterile water for injection in the upper chamber. The product is reconstituted just prior to use. Both products are introduced into the sterile surgical field, and therefore the primary package vial must have a sterile exterior. This is accomplished by ethylene oxide sterilization of the vial in a special secondary package that is permeable to the sterilant gas but protective to contamination of the vial prior to use.

Viscoelastics

Highly purified fractions of sodium hyaluronate have become an important ocular surgical adjunct because of their lubricant and viscoelastic properties. They are injected into the anterior segment of the eye during surgery for removal of cataracts and implantation of an IOL, trabeculectomy, and corneal transplantation. They are also used as a surgical aid in the vitreous cavity during retinal surgery. Their viscoelasticity provides a mechanical barrier between tissues and allows the surgeon more space for manipulation with less trauma to surrounding tissues, particularly the corneal endothelium. It is also used to coat the IOL prior to insertion and lessen the potential for tissue damage upon implantation. In posterior segment surgery, it is used to separate tissue away from the retina and as a tamponade to maneuver tissue, such as a detached retina, back into place for reattachment. The viscoelastic material is usually removed at the end of the surgery since it may take several days to be cleared from the eye and has the potential to elevate IOP.

Sodium hyaluronate is a high molecular weight polysaccharide which is widely distributed throughout the tissues of the body of animals and humans. The viscoelastic materials used as ocular surgical aids are specific fractions from animal tissue, which are highly purified to remove foreign proteins and are tested to be nonantigenic and noninflammatory in the eye. The purified fraction is formulated to yield a high viscoelasticity determined by the interplay of molecular weight and concentration. The solution is packaged in disposable glass syringes, which are terminally sterilized and aseptically packaged so that they can be used in the sterile surgical field (Healon®, ProVisc®, Amvisc®).

Chondroitin sulfate (Viscoat®, DuoVisc®) is also used in combination with sodium hyaluronate as a viscoelastic surgical aid to provide higher viscosities, which may provide additional tissue protection during the irrigation and aspiration accompanying phacoemulsification, a common means of removing the cloudy crystalline lens prior to IOL implantation.

Nonpyrogenic solutions of sterile hydroxypropyl methylcellulose are also used as ocular surgical aids similar to the viscoelastics in cataract surgery (OcuCoat®). These lubricants are sometimes classified as viscoadherents because they are used to coat the IOL prior to implantation and the tips of surgical instruments prior to deployment inside the eye. This is the same cellulosic material but in a highly purified form, serving as a viscosifying agent in topical eyedrops and as an OTC ocular lubricant. Since it is not a natural product, it does not have the antigenic potential of the other viscoelastics. It can be stored at room temperature, whereas the sodium hyaluronate solutions must be stored in the refrigerator.

Intravitreal Injection and Implant

Antivirals are used to treat the ocular sequelae of AIDS such as CMV retinitis. They are treated with systemic administration, but with the need for higher localized ocular therapeutic concentrations, products have been developed and approved for direct administration into the vitreous cavity.

An intravitreal implant containing ganciclovir was the first such ophthalmic product developed and approved for CMV retinitis (Vitrasert®, cf. Section 6 and Fig. 15). The sterile implant is a tablet of ganciclovir with magnesium stearate and is coated to retard drug release with polyvinyl alcohol and ethylene vinyl acetate polymers such that the device when surgically implanted in the vitreous cavity releases drug over a 5- to 8-month period. When the implant is visually observed to be depleted, and based on clinical observation of the progression of the disease, it is surgically removed and replaced with a new implant. The implant is provided in a sterile Tyvek package and contains a suture tab for handling prior to and during implantation so that the polymer release rate controlling coating is not damaged. Also, precautions for handling and disposal of antineoplastic agents should be observed.

A new antiviral agent, developed for treatment of CMV retinitis, can be administered by intravitreal injection. Formivirsen sodium is a phosphorothioate oligonucleotide that inhibits CMV replication through an antisense mechanism. It is formulated as a sterile and preservative-free solution and supplied in single-use vials (Vitravene®). The product is administered directly into the vitreous cavity posterior to the limbus through a 30-gauge needle. This procedure can be performed on an outpatient basis—an advantage over an intravitreal device, which must be surgically implanted and removed. The frequency of injection, based on the clinical progression of the disease, is every 2–4 weeks.

IX. CONTACT LENS CARE PRODUCTS

Contact lenses are optical devices that are either fabricated from preformed polymers or polymerized during lens manufacture. The main purpose of contact lenses is to correct defective vision. For this application, they are called *cosmetic lenses*. Contact lenses used medically for the treatment of certain corneal diseases are called *bandage lenses*.

A. Evolution of Contact Lenses

In 1508 Leonardo da Vinci conceived the concept of the contact lens. It was not until 1887 that scleral contact lenses were fabricated by Dr. A. E. Fick, a physician in Zurich; F. A. Mueller, a maker of prosthetic eyes in Germany; and Dr. E. Kalt, a physician in France. Muller, Obrig, and Gyorry fabricated contact lenses made from polymethyl methacrylate (PMMA) in the late 1930s. K. Tuohy filed the patent for contact lens design in 1948; the lenses were made of PMMA material [302]. Although they were safe and effective, these lenses were uniformly uncomfortable, thus suppressing their potential use for contact lens wear. Lenses made from polyhydroxyethyl methacrylate (HEMA), so-called soft lenses or hydrophilic lenses, were introduced in 1970. Since then, significant technological advances have been made in lens materials, lens fabrication, and lens designs [303]. Consequently, a phenomenal growth in lens wearers necessitated the need for, and development of, lens care products. Today, rigid lenses made from materials polymerized with PMMA and in combination with various siloxanes and fluorocarbons are available to meet the broadest needs of lens wearers.

B. Composition of Contact Lenses

Contact lenses are broadly classified as PMMA, rigid gas-permeable (RGP), and soft hydrogel (HEMA) lenses. Dyes may be added during polymerization or after fabrication to improve lens handling or to change the color of the lens wearer's eyes. Lenses made from numerous polymers are available today [304]. In soft hydrogel lenses, HEMA is a commonly used monomer. However, to avoid infringement of existing patents, many comonomers, e.g., methyl methacrylic acid or a blend of comonomers, are used. Comonomers produce changes in the water content or ionic nature of lenses that is significantly different from HEMA lenses. For example, addition of acrylic acid in HEMA increases the water content and ionic nature of lenses. Some lenses are made from *n*-vinylpyrrolidone and have high water contents. Such lenses have pore sizes that are much larger than low water content lenses. Cross-linkers, such as ethyleneglycol dimethacrylate, and initiators such as benzyl peroxide in appropriate amounts are added for polymerization and to achieve desirable physical and chemical properties. Recently, contact lenses made from HEMA and silicone were made available. These lenses combine the properties of hydrogel and gas-permeable polymers [305]. Table 5 gives a list of monomers, comonomers, and cross-linkers along with their effects on polymer properties. In 1985, FDA published a classification for soft hydrophilic lenses based on their water content and ionic nature. Groupings for soft lenses and their generic names are listed in Table 6. Adequate levels of oxygen are necessary to maintain normal corneal metabolism [306]. Lenses that are poorly designed and worn overnight deprive the cornea of oxygen, causing edema [307].

Generally, oxygen permeability for soft lenses is acceptable when worn on a daily basis. Hypoxia related side effects such as corneal swelling, epithelial microcysts, limbal redness, neovascularization, epithelial polymegathism and blebs are well known and mainly observed with extended contact lens wear. Recent development of hydrophilic silicone hydrogel materials combines the high oxygen permeability of silicone with the good water and ion permeability of hydrogels resulting in acceptable extended wear lenses. The oxygen (gas) transmissibilty of these lenses is greater than all other available lenses.

Contact lenses made from PMMA materials are virtually impermeable to gases [308]. The PMMA lenses are also inflexible, causing discomfort in a large percentage of individuals while the lens is worn. During the 1980s, lenses were made from either cellulose acetate butyrate (CAB) or silicone elastomer. Although comfortable and flexible, such lenses accumulated lipids, were nonwettable, and adhered to the cornea. Several reports detailing difficulty in removing CAB and silicone lenses appeared in the published literature [309]. Lenses made from fluorocarbons and in various combinations of fluorocarbon, silicone, methyl methacylate, and acrylic acid are currently available. Desirable properties of these lenses include flexibility, wettability, and gas transmissibility. Grouping for rigid gas-permeable lenses was published by FDA in 1989. The generic names and oxygen permeabilities of rigid gas-permeable (RGP) lens materials are provided in Table 7 [310].

C. Complications of Contact Lens Wear and the Need for Care Products

Lens design, user compliance with manufacturer's instructions, hygiene, environmental conditions, poor fit, lens materials, and tear chemistry are the major causes of lens wear complications. Complications owing to lens design, compliance, hygiene, environmental conditions, and poor fit are beyond the scope of this chapter and are not critical to an understanding of the concepts required for the development of care products. However, knowledge of tear chemistry is important in understanding the complex chemical interactions between tear components and contact lenses. The tear film can be broadly divided into three distinct layers: lipids, aqueous, and mucin [311]. Each layer of the tear film performs a specific function. The mucin layer spreads and coats the hydrophobic corneal cells and extends into the aqueous layer. The aqueous layer contains 98% water and 2% solids. Dissolved solids in this layer are predominately the electrolytes (Na^+, K^+, C^{2+}, Mg^{2+}, Cl^-, and HCO_3^-), nonelectrolytes (urea and glucose), and proteins. Major proteins in the tear film are presented in Table 8.

The lipid layer, which consists of cholesterol esters, phospholipids, and triglycerides, prevents and regulates aqueous evaporation from the tear film.

Components of the tear attach to contact lenses by electrostatic and van der Waals forces and build up to form deposits. Deposits on the surface and in the lens matrix may result in reduced visual acuity, irritation, and in some instances serious ocular complications. The composition of deposits vary because of the complexity of an individual's ocular physiology-pathology. Lysozyme is a major component of soft lens deposits, especially found on high-water-content ionic lenses [312]. Calcium [313] and lipids [314] are infrequent components of deposits, occurring as inorganic salts, organic salts, or as an element of mixed deposits, or as a combination thereof [315,316].

Lenses are exposed to a broad spectrum of microbes during normal wear and handling and become contaminated relatively quickly. Failure to remove microorganisms effectively from lenses can cause ocular infections. Ocular infections, particularly those caused by pathogenic microbes, such as *P. aeruginosa*, can lead to the loss of the infected eye if left untreated.

Table 5 Commonly Used Monomers, Comonomers, and Cross-Linkers in Contact Lens Polymers

Name	Abbreviation	Lens properties
Acrylic acid	AA	Flexibility Hydrophilicity pH sensitivity —acidic Reactivity—ionically interacts with positively charged tear components Wettability
Butyl methacrylate	BMA	Softness Flexibility Hydrophobicity—attracts lipids Wettability Gas transmissibility
Cellulose acetate butyrate	CAB	Clarity Wettability Gas transmissibility Physical stability
Dimethyl siloxane	DMS	Hydrophobicity Wettability Gas transmissibility Physical stability
Diphenyl siloxane	DPS	Hydrophobicity Wettability Gas transmissibility Physical stability
Ethonylethyl methacrylate	EOEMA	Flexibility Softness Hydrophobicity Wettability Gas transmissibility
Ethylene glycol dimethacrylate	EGDMA	Hydrophobicity Wettability
Glyceryl methacrylate	GMA	Wettability Gas transmissibility Hydrophilicity Machineability
Hydroxyethyl methacrylate	HEMA	Flexibility Wettability Gas transmissibility Softness Machineability
Methacrylic acid	MA	Hardness Machineability Wettability Gas transmissibility Hydrophobicity
Methyl methacrylate	MMA	Hardness Machineability Wettability Gas transmissibility Hydrophobicity
Methylphenyl siloxane	MPS	Hydrophobicity Gas transmissibility
Methyl vinyl siloxane	MVS	Hydrophobicity

Table 5 (Continued)

Name	Abbreviation	Lens properties
N-Vinyl pyrrolidone	NVP	Gas transmissibility Hydrophilicity Wettability Machineability
Siloxanyl methacrylate	SMA	Color, clarity Hardness Wettability Gas transmissibility

Table 6 FDA Grouping for Soft Hydrophilic Lenses and Generic Names

Group 1 Low water (< 50%H_2O) nonionic polymers	Group 2 High water (> 7.50%H_2O) nonionic polymers	Group 3 Low water (< 50%H_2O ionic polymers	Group 4 High water (> 50%H_2O) ionic polymers
Tefilcon (38%)	Lidofilcon (70%)	Etafilcon (43%)	Bufilcon A (55%)
	Lidofilcon B (79%)		
Tetrafilcon A (43%)	Surfilcon (74%)	Bufilcon A (45%)	Perfilcon (71%)
Grofilcon (39%)	Vilifilcon A (55%)	Deltafilcon A (43%)	Etafilcon A (58%)
Dimefilcon A (38%)	Scafilcon A (71%)	Dronifilcon A (47%)	Ocufilcon C (55%)
Hefilcon A (43%)	Xylofilcon A (67%)	Phenifilcon A (38%)	Phenfilcon A (55%)
		Ocufilcon (44%)	Tetrafilcon B (58%)
Hefilcon B (43%)		Mafilcon (33%)	Methafilcon (55%)
Phenifilcon A (30%)			Vifilcon A (55%)
Isofilcon (36%)			
Polymacon (38%)			
Mafilcon (33%)			

D. Types of Lens Care Products

Contact lens care products can be divided into three categories: cleaners, disinfectants, and lubricants. Improperly cleaned lenses can cause discomfort, irritation, decrease in visual acuity, and giant papillary conjunctivitis (GPC). This latter condition often requires discontinuation of lens wear, at least until the symptoms clear. Deposits can also accumulate preservatives from lens care products and produce toxicity and can act as a matrix for microorganism attachment to the lens [317]. Thus, cleaning with the removal of surface debris, tear components, and contaminating microorganisms is one of the most important steps contributing to the safety and efficacy of successful lens wear [318].

Daily cleaners and weekly cleaners are employed to clean deposits that accumulate on lenses during normal wear. A list of cleaning agents commonly used in daily cleaners is provided in Table 9. Single cleaning agents or combinations of cleaning agents may be used in a cleaner. Surfactant(s), surface-active polymer(s), solvent(s), and complexing agent(s) chosen for cleaner formulations must be capable of solubilizing lens deposits and must have low irritation potential. They must be rinsed easily, leaving very low or nondetectable residue levels on the lens. Many problems that contact lens wearers experience with their lenses are the results of incomplete removal of deposit(s) [319]. Nonionic and amphoteric surfactants are commonly used in daily cleaner products. Because of their toxicity to the cornea and binding to the lenses, anionic and cationic surfactants are avoided. Solvents capable of solubilizing lens deposits without altering the lens polymer properties should be selected carefully. Complexing agents, such as citrates, are included in daily cleaner formulations [320]. They retard the binding of positively charged proteins to the lenses and by ion pairing or salt formation render the proteins more soluble in the media.

Table 7 FDA Grouping of Hydrophobic Hard and Rigid Gas-Permeable Lenses

Lens materials	Generic name	D_k
Cellulose acetate butyrate	Cabufocon A	> 150
	Powfocon A	> 150
	Powfocon B	> 150
t-Butylstyrene	Aufocon A	> 150
Silicone	Elastofilcon A	> 150
	Dimofocon	> 150
	Dilafilcon A	> 150
t-Butylstyrene-silicon acrylate	Pentasilcon P	120
Fluoracrylate	Fluorofocon A	100
Fluoro silicone acrylate	Itafluorofocon A	60
	Porflufocon A	30–92
Silicone acrylate	Pasifocon A	14
	Pasifocon B	16
	Pasifocon C	45
	Itafocon A	14
	Itafocon B	26
	Nefocon A	20
	Telefocon A	15–45
	Amefocon A	40

Table 8 Major Proteins of the Tear Film

Name	Total protein (%)	Function
Lysozyme	30–40	Antimicrobial, collagenase regulator
Lactoferin	2–3	Bacteriostatic, anti-inflammatory
Albumin	30–40	Anti-inflammatory
Immunoglobins	0.1	Immunological, anti-inflammatory

Mechanical force is a key aspect in the cleaning process. For daily cleaning, mechanical force is generally provided through the rubbing action of the fingers over the lens during the actual cleaning process. Rubbing typically removes 1.7 ± 0.5 log of microorganisms, rinsing the lens removes 1.9 ± 0.5 log of microorganisms, and cleaning and rinsing the lens removes 3.7 ± 0.5 log of microorganisms of a typical challenge by 10^6 colony-forming units (cfu)/mL [320]. Abrasive particles are included in products to enhance the mechanical force applied to the lens during the cleaning process [321]. The abrasive properties are evaluated by testing the hardness of the included abrasive particles. Typically particles that have Rockwell hardness lower than the hardness of the lens polymers are used. If the hardness of abrasive particles is higher than the hardness of the lens polymer, it is possible that the lens would be damaged. Some contact lenses are reported to require special treatment. Abrasive particles may alter surface treatment effects even when their hardness is lower than that of the lens polymer. Development of potent preservative systems and the use of complexing agents like citrates have led to the availability of multi-purpose solutions. These single-solution products are carefully designed to meet the cleaning and microbiological requirements without a lens rubbing step.

Enzymatic cleaners contain enzymes derived from animals, plants, or microorganisms. Plant and microorganism-derived enzymes may cause sensitization in many lens wearers [322]. A list of commonly used enzymes is provided in Table 10. All of these enzymes are effective in removing deposits from the contact lens surface [323]. They are biochemical catalysts that are specific for catalyzing certain chemical reactions. Those

Table 9 Cleaning Agents Commonly Used in Daily Cleaners

Class	Trade name	Chemical name
Abrasive particles	Nylon 11	11-Aminoundecanoic acid
	Silica	Silicon dioxide
Complexing agents	Citric acid	2-Hydroxy-1,2,3-propane tri-carboxylic acid
Solvents	Isopropyl alcohol	2-Propanol
	Propylene glycol	1,2-Propanediol
	Hexamethylene glycol	1,6-Hexanediol
Surfactants (nonionic)	Tween 21	Polysorbate 21
	Tween 80	Polysorbate 80
	Tyloxapol	4-(1,3,3-Tetramethylbutyl)-phenol polymer with formaldehyde and oxirane
	Pluronic	Poloxamer
	Tetronic	Poloxamine
Surfactants (ionic)	Miracare	Cocoamphocarboxy-glycinate

Table 10 Enzymes Commonly Used in Weekly Cleaners

Name	Origin	Active against	Active at pH
Pancreatin	Animal (Porcine)		
Proteases		Proteins	7.0
Lipase		Lipids	8.0
Amylase		Carbohydrates	6.7–7.2
Papain	Plant (papaya)	Proteins	5.0
Subtilisin A	Microorganisms	Proteins	8–10
Subtilisin B	Microorganisms	Proteins	8–10

that aid in removing debris from contact lenses are protease (protein-specific enzyme), lipase (lipid-specific enzyme), and amylase (polysaccharide-specific enzyme). Such enzymes catalyze breakdown of substrate molecules—protein, lipid, and mucin—into smaller molecular units. This process yields fragments that are readily removed by mechanical force and rinsing.

In the past, only tablet dosage forms of enzymatic cleaners were available. They required soaking lenses in solutions prepared from a tablet for a period of 15 minutes to more than 2 hours before disinfecting the lenses. Although this process provided sufficient time for cleaning, it was a cumbersome process and required multiple steps. Complicated or cumbersome processes inevitably lead to poor user compliance. Enzymes in aqueous liquid compositions are inherently unstable. New technological advances have led to the stabilization of enzymes in liquid vehicles which are compatible with soft and RGP contact lenses [324]. The newer products are either in a tablet or a solution product form. Simultaneous cleaning and disinfection can be achieved, which reduces care time and the need for multiple steps [325].

Contact lenses are contaminated with microorganisms during lens handling and lens wear. They must be disinfected to prevent ocular infections, especially from pathogenic microorganisms. The two disinfection methods used are thermal and chemical. In thermal disinfection systems, lenses are placed in preserved or unpreserved solution in a lens case and then heated sufficiently by a device to kill the microorganisms. The current FDA requirement for thermal disinfection requires heating at a minimum of 80°C for 10 minutes. The unpreserved salines are either packaged in a unit-dose or an aerosol container, and they do have some antimicrobial activity [326]. Preservatives must be used in salines packaged in nonaerosol multidose containers. The types and names of preservatives and antimicrobial disinfectants commonly used in lens care products are listed in Table 11. Thimerosal and sorbic acid are commonly used preservatives in these products; however, concerns of sensitization potential and discoloration of lenses have led to the introduction of new

Table 11 Antimicrobial Agents Commonly Used in Lens Care Products

Class	Generic	Molecular weight	Used in lens type: Soft	Used in lens type: RGP, PMMA
Acids	Benzoic acid	122	No	Yes
	Boric acid	62	Yes	Yes
	Sorbic acid	112	Yes	Yes
Alcohols	Benzyl alcohol	108	No	Yes
	Phenyl ethyl alcohol	122	No	Yes
Biguanides	Chlorhexidine	505	Yes	Yes
	Polyaminopropyl biguanide	~1200	Yes	Yes
Mercurial	Thimerosal	404	Yes	Yes
	Phenylmercuric nitrate	634	Yes	Yes
Oxidizing	Hydrogen peroxide	34	Yes	No
	Sodium dichloroisocyanurate	220	Yes	No
Quaternary	Tris(2-hydroxyethyl) tallow ammonium chloride	≈424	Yes	No
	Benzalkonium chloride	≈363	No	Yes
	Benzethonium chloride	448	No	Yes
	Polyquaternium-1	≈6000	Yes	Yes

and safer molecules like Polyquad (a polymeric quaternary ammonium compound) and Dymed. Specifically, Polyquad is resistant to absorption into the lenses; thus, there is little to diffuse out of the lens into the eye, leading to corneal toxicity, an inherent problem associated with nonpolymeric quaternary ammonium compounds. FDA and the USP have specific standards for preservative effectiveness that these products must meet. The FDA standards detailing the method were published in 1985 [327]. Oxidizing agents and nonoxidizing chemical disinfectants that are nontoxic at product concentrations are used to disinfect lenses chemically. Hydrogen peroxide is used primarily as an oxidizing agent [328]. It is used in concentrations of 0.6–3.0%. Peroxides are very toxic to the cornea of the eye. After the disinfection cycle, and before placing the lens in the eye, hydrogen peroxide must be completely neutralized by reducing agents, catalase, or transition metals, such as platinum.

An ideal chemical-disinfecting agent would have the following properties: (a) it should be nonirritating, nonsensitizing, and nontoxic in tests for cytotoxicity; (b) it should have an adequate antimicrobial spectrum and be able to kill ocular pathogens during a short lens-soaking period; (c) it should not bind to the lens surface; and (d) it should be compatible with the lens and not cause lens discoloration or alter the tint of colored contact lenses. Polyquad and Dymed have most of these characteristics. They have been introduced recently into the marketplace and are performing to expectations [329,330].

Contact lens wearers may experience increasing awareness of their lenses during the day owing to ocular dryness [331]. With some lens materials, this increase in awareness may arise from a decrease in the wettability of the lens surface. Dehydration of the lens or accumulation of debris on the lens surface can cause similar symptoms [332]. The lens wearer may achieve relief from these symptoms with periodic administration of lubricating rewetting drops [333]. These solutions contain polymers or surfactants that enhance the wettability of the surface, facilitate the spreading of tears, and improve the stability of the tear film. They may also provide cushioning and lubrication actions, thereby reducing the frictional force between the eyelids and the lens. Some products are specifically designed to rehydrate the lens. These products are unpreserved and packaged in a unit-dose. However, a preservative is required for a multidose product.

The emphasis that patients place on convenience has led to the development of single-bottle care products referred to as "multi-purpose solutions." Such products do not require a separate cleaner and in some instances can be used as a rewetting drop. However, they require rubbing and rinsing lenses in order to achieve adequate cleaning. Recent advances in technology along with careful selection of formulation components have resulted in a product that does not require a rubbing step [334]. This product has met all the microbiological and cleaning efficacy requirements, including those proposed in the ISO Guidelines.

Table 12 Types of Tests and Requirements Proposed by FDA for Product Development

I. Chemistry/manufacturing
- A. Solution/container descriptions
- B. Solution stability testing
- C. Lens group selection for solution testing

II. Toxicology
- A. Solution testing
  1. Acute oral toxicity assessment
  2. Acute systemic toxicity assessment
  3. Acute ocular irritation and cytotoxicity assessment
  4. Sensitization/allergic response assessment
     - a. Preservative uptake and release test
     - b. Guinea pig maximization testing
- B. Container/accessory testing
  1. In vitro testing
  2. Systemic toxicity testing
  3. Primary ocular irritation testing

III. Microbiology
- A. Sterilization of the solution by the manufacturer
  1. Validation of the sterilization cycle
  2. USP sterility tests
  3. USP type preservative effectiveness test
  4. USP microbial limits test
- B. Shelf life testing requirements
  1. Shelf life sterility
  2. Shelf life preservative effectiveness
  3. Extension of shelf life protocol
- C. Disinfection of the lens
  1. Chemical disinfection systems
     - a. Contribution of elements test
     - b. D-value determinations
     - c. Multi-item microbial challenge test

IV. Clinical
- A. Patient characteristics
- B. Number of eyes duration and number of investigators
- C. Initial patient visit parameters

D. Summary

Generally, contact lens products are sterile solutions or suspensions. Formulators for these products must have training in technologies practiced during development of sterile pharmaceutical products, such as injectable and large-volume intravenous fluids. The products must be effective and compatible with a wide range of lens materials. Components of the formulations should not accumulate in the lens or change the lens properties. They must be preserved adequately and be well tolerated by the sensitive ocular tissues. The products should also be simple to use in order to assure good compliance on the part of lens wearers. Additionally, they should be developed following the guidelines enumerated in Table 12.

ACKNOWLEDGMENT

The authors thank Ms. Cathy Hughes for her assistance in preparing the manuscript.

REFERENCES

1. *The United States Pharmacopeia 24* (USP)/*The National Formulary 1*, U.S. Pharmacopeial Convention, Rockville, MD, 1999, pp. 2113–2114.
2. C. Mazuel and M.-C. Friteyre, U.S. Patent 4,861,760 (1989).
3. J. C. Lang, J. C. Keister, P. J. T. Missel, and D. J. Stancioff, U.S. Patent 5,403,841 (1995).
4. P. J. T. Missel, J. C. Lang, and R. Jani, U.S. Patent 5,212,162 (1993).
5. R. Bawa, G. D. Cagle, R. Hall, B. Kabra, K. Markwardt, M. Shah, and J. Teague, PCT Application, WO 99/51273.
6. A. Rozier, C. Mazuel, J. Grove, and B. Plazonnet, Int. J. Pharm., 153, 191 (1997).
7. G. Meseguer, R. Gurny, P. Buri, A. Rozier and B. Plazonnet, Int. J. Pharm., 95, 229 (1993).
8. G. Majno, *The Healing Hand—Man and Wound in the Ancient World*, Harvard University Press, Cambridge, MA, 1975, pp. 43–45.
9. G. Majno, *The Healing Hand—Man and Wound in the Ancient World*, Harvard University Press, Cambride, MA, 1975, pp. 112–114.
10. G. Majno, *The Healing Hand—Man and Wound in the Ancient World*, Harvard University Press, Cambridge, MA, 1975, pp. 154.
11. G. Majno, *The Healing Hand—Man and Wound in the Ancient World*, Harvard University Press, Cambridge, MA, 1975, pp. 216, 359.
12. G. Majno, *The Healing Hand—Man and Wound in the Ancient World*, Harvard University Press, Cambridge, MA, 1975, pp. 348, 377.
13. D. L. Deardorf, *Remington's Pharmaceutical Sciences*, 14th ed., Mack Publishing, Easton, PA, 1970, pp. 1545–1548.
14. S. Riegleman and D. L. Sorby, *Dispensing of Medication*, 7th ed., Mack Publishing, Easton, PA, 1971, pp. 880–884.
15. J. C. Lang and M. M. Stiemke, Biological barriers to ocular delivery in *Ocular Therapeutics and Drug Delivery, A Multidisciplinary Approach* (I. K. Reddy, ed.), Technomic Publishing Company, 1996, pp. 51–132.
16. G. C. Y. Chiou, Toxicol. Methods, 2, 139 (1992).
17. S. J. Tuft and D. J. Costner, Eye, 4, 389 (1990).
18. J. W. Cheng, S. S. Matsumoto and C. B. Anger, J. Toxicol Cutaneous Ocul. Toxicol. 14, 287 (1995).
19. W. H. Havener, *Ocular Pharmacology*, 2nd ed., C. V. Mosby, St. Louis, MO, 1970.
20. B. Smith, *Handbook of Ocular Pharmacology*, Publication Sciences Group, Action, MA, 1974.
21. P. Ellis and D. L. Smith, *Ocular Therapeutics and Pharmacology*, 3rd ed., C. V. Mosby, St. Louis, MO, 1969.
22. J. T. Grayston, S. P. Wang, R. L. Woolridge, and P. B. Johnson, JAMA, 172, 602 (1962).
23. J. D. Bartlett and S. D. Jaanus, *Clinical Ocular Pharmacology*, Butterworth-Heinemann, 1995, p. 275.
24. J. L. Byers, M. G. Holland, and J. H. Allen, Am. J. Ophthalmol., 49, 267 (1960).
25. W. D. Gingrich, JAMA, 179, 602 (1962).
26. S. Mishima and D. M. Maurice, Invest. Ophthalmol., 1, 794 (1962).
27. D. M. Maurice, Invest. Ophthalmol., 6, 464 (1967).
28. S. J. Kimura, Am. J. Ophthalmol., 34, 446 (1951).
29. A. Wessing, *Fluorescein Angiography of the Retina* (trans. by G. K. von Noorden), C. V. Mosby, St. Louis, MO, 1969.
30. K. Koller, Arch. Ophthalmol., 13, 404 (1884).
31. Council on Drugs, New drugs and developments in therapeutics, JAMA, 183, 178 (1963).
32. M. A. Lemp, C. H. Dohlman, and F. J. Holly, Ann. Ophthalmol., 2, 258 (1970).
33. M. A. Lemp and E. S. Szymanski, Arch. Ophthalmol., 93, 134 (1975).
34. M. A. Lemp, Scientific Exhibit, American Academy of Ophthalmology and Otolaryngology, Dallas, Sept. 1975.
35. *USP 24*, U.S. Pharmacopeal Convention, Rockville, MD, 1999, <71>, p. 1818.
36. *British Pharmacopoeia 2000*, Department of Health. The Stationery Office, London, 2000, Appendix 307.
37. *USP 24*, U.S. Pharmacopeal Convention, Rockville, MD, 1999, <1211>, p. 2144.
38. F. N. Marzulli and M. E. Simon, Am. J. Optom., 48, 61 (1971).
39. R. B. Hackett and T. O. McDonald, Eye irritation, in *Dermatoxicology*, 5th ed. (F. N. Marzulli and H. L. Maibach, eds.), Hemisphere Publishing, Washington, DC, 1996, pp. 299–305, 557–566.

40. P. K. Basu, J. Toxicol, Cutan. Ocul. Toxicol., 2, 205 (1984).
41. J. S. Friedenwald, W. F. Hughes, Jr., and H. Hermann, Arch. Ophthalmol., 31, 379 (1944).
42. C. Carpenter and H. Symth, Am. J. Ophthalmol., 29, 1363 (1946).
43. L. W. Hazelton, Proc. Sci. Sect. Toilet Goods Assoc., 17, 490 (1973).
44. L. M. Carter, G. Duncan, and G. K. Rennie, Exp. Eye Res., 17, 5 (1952).
45. J. H. Kay and J. C. Calandra, J. Soc., Cosmet. Chem., 13, 281 (1962).
46. K. L. Russell and S. G. Hoch, Pro. Sci. Sect. Toilet Goods Assoc., 37, 27 (1962).
47. I. Gaunt and K. H. Harper, J. Soc. Cosmet. Shem., 15, 290 (1964).
48. S. P. Battista and E. S. McSweeney, J. Soc. Cosmet. Chem., 16, 119 (1965).
49. J. H. Becklet, Am. Perum. Cosmet., 80, 51 (1965).
50. C. T. Bonfield and R. A. Scala, Proc. Sci. Sect. Toilet Goods Assoc., 43, 34 (1965).
51. E. V. Buehler and E. A. Newmann, Toxicol. Appl. Pharmacol., 6, 701 (1964).
52. C. H. Dohlman, Invest. Ophthalmol., 10, 376 (1971).
53. M. J. Hogan and L. E. Zimmerman, in *Ophthalmic Pathology: An Atlas and Textbook*, 2nd ed., W. B. Saunders, Philadelphia, 1962.
54. R. R. Phister, Invest. Ophthalmol., 12, 654 (1973).
55. D. M. Maurice, *The Eye*, Vol. 1 (H. Davson, ed.), Academic Press, New York, 1969, pp. 489–600.
56. J. H. Prince, C. D. Diesen, I. Eglitis, and G. L. Ruskell, *Anatomy and Histology of the Eye and Orbit in Domestic Animals*, Charles C Thomas, Springfield, IL, 1960.
57. H. Davson, in *The Eye*, Vol. 1 (H. Davson, ed.), Academic Press, New York, 1969, pp. 217–218.
58. B. S. Fine and M. Yanoff, *Ocular Histology: A Text and Atlas*, Harper & Row, New York, 1972.
59. W. R. Green, J. B. Sullivan, R. M. Hehir, L. G. Scharpf, and A. W. Dickinson, *A Systemic Comparison of Chemically Induced Eye Injury in the Albino Rabbit and Rhesus Monkey*, Soap and Detergent Association, New York, 1978, pp. 405–415.
60. B. S. Fine and M. Yanoff, *Ocular Histology: A Text and Atlas*, Harper & Row, New York, 1972.
61. Committee for the Revision of NAS Publication 1138, National Research Council, *Principles and Procedures for Evaluating the Toxicity of Household Substances*, National Academy of Sciences, Washington, DC, 1977, pp. 41–56.
62. Interagency Regulatory Liaison Group, Testing Standards and Guidelines Work Group, *Recommended Guidelines for Acute Eye Irritation Testing*, Jan. 1981.
63. J. H. Draize, Food Drug Cosmet. Law J., 10, 722 (1955).
64. J. H. Draize and E. A. Kelley, Proc. Sci. Sect. Toilet Goods Assoc., 17, 1 (1959).
65. J. H. Draize, J. Pharmacol. Exp. Ther., 82, 377 (1944).
66. Food Drug Cosmet. Law Rep., 233, 8311; 440, 8313; 476, 8310.
67. L. H. Bruner, R. D. Parker and R. D. Bruce, Fund. Appl. Toxicol., 19, 330 (1992).
68. M. York and W. Steiling, J. Appl. Toxicol., 18, 233 (1998).
69. R. B. Nussenblatt, A. Bron, W. Chambers, J. P. McCulley, M. Pericoi, J. L. Ubels, and H. F. Edelhauser, J. Toxicol. Cut. Ocular Toxicol., 17, 103 (1998).
70. M. Balls, P. A. Botham, L. H. Bruner and H. Spielmann, Toxic. In Vitro 9, 871 (1995).
71. Guidance on Nonclinical Safety Studies for the Conduct of Human Clinical trials for Pharmaceuticals. FDA Docket No 97D-0147. Fed. Reg. 62(227), 62,922 (1997).
72. Timing of Non-Clinical Safety Studies for the Conduct of Human Clinical trials for Pharmaceuticals. Fourth International Conference on Harmonization. International Conference on Harmonization, Brussels, 1997.
73. R. B. Hackett, Lens Eye Toxic. Res. 7, 181 (1990).
74. A. W. Hayes, *Principles and Methods of Toxicology*, 3rd ed., Raven Press, New York, 1994.
75. Guidance for Industry: Premarket Notification (510(k)) Guidance Document for Contact Lens Care Products. Center for Devices and Radiologic Health, FDA, Rockville, MD, 1997.
76. Biological evaluation of medical devices—Part 5: Tests for cytotoxicity: in vitro methods. ISO 10993-5:1992(E). International Standards Organization, 1992.
77. Biological evaluation of medical devices—Part 10: Tests for irritation and sensitization. ISO 10993-10:1992. International Standards Organization, 1992.
78. J. W. Shell and R. W. Baker, Ann. Ophthalmol., 7, 1637 (1975).
79. W. M. Grant, *Toxicology of the Eye*, Charles C Thomas, Springfield, IL, 1974, p. 259.
80. H. F. Edelhauser, D. L. Van Horn, R. W. Scholtz, and R. A. Hyndiuk, Am. J. Ophthalmol., 81, 473 (1976).
81. S. E. Herrell and D. Heilman, Am. J. Med. Sci., 206, 221 (1943).
82. *USP 24*, U. S. Pharmacopeial Convention, Rockville, MD, 1999, <771>, p. 1965.
83. C. Shopsis, E. Borenfreund, J. Walberg, and D. M. Stark, *Alternative Methods in Toxicology*, Vol. 2 (A. M. Goldberg, ed.), Mary Ann Liebert, New York, 1984, pp. 103–114.
84. E. Borenfreund and O. Borrero, Cell Biol. Toxicol., 1, 55 (1984).
85. C. Shopsis and S. Sathe, Toxicology, 29, 195 (1984).
86. R. Neville, P. Dennis, D. Sens, and R. Crouch, Curr. Eye Res., 5, 367 (1986).
87. M. E. Stern, H. F. Edelhauser, and J. W. Hiddemen, Methods of Evaluation of Corneal Epithelial and Endothelial Toxicity of Soft Contact Lens Preservatives. Presented at Contact Lens International Congress, Las Vegas, Nevada, March 1985.

88. H. F. Edelhauser, M. E. Antione, H. J. Pederson, J. W. Hiddemen, and R. G. Harris, J. Toxicol. Cutan. Ocul. Toxicol., 2(1), 7 (1983).
89. S. J. Krebs, M. E. Stern, J. W. Hiddemen, and H. F. Edelhauser, CLAO J., 10(1), 35 (1984).
90. H. E. Seifried, J. Toxicol. Cutan. Ocul. Toxicol., 5, 89 (1986).
91. D. M. Stark, C. Shopsis, E. Borenfreund, and J. Walberg, *Alternative Methods of Toxicology*, Vol. 1, *Product Safety Evaluation*, Mary Ann Liebert, New York, 1983, pp. 127–204.
92. J. M. Frazier, *Dermatotoxicology*, 4th ed. (F. N. Marzulli and H. L. Maibach, eds.), Hemisphere Publishing, Washington, DC, 1991.
93. N. L. Burstein, Invest. Ophthalmol. Vis. Sci., 25, 1453 (1984).
94. D. Maurice and T. Singh, A permeability test for acute corneal toxicity, Toxicol. Lett., 31, 125 (1986).
95. N. L. Burstein, Invest. Ophthalmol. Vis. Sci., 7, 308 (1980).
96. R. R. Pfister and N. Burstein, Invest. Ophthalmol. Vis. Sci., 15, 246 (1976).
97. A. M. Tonjum, Acta Ophthalmol., 53, 358 (1975).
98. H. Ichijima, W. M. Petroll, J. V. Jester, and H. D. Cavanagh, Cornea, 11, 221 (1992).
99. P. S. Imperia, H. M. Lazarus, R. E. Botti, Jr., and J. H. Lass, J. Toxicol. Cutan. Ocul. Toxicol., 5, 309 (1986).
100. H. B. Collins and B. E. Grabsch, Am. J. Optom. Physiol. Opt., 59, 215 (1982).
101. J. Ubels, J. Toxicol. Cutan. Ocul. Toxicol., 1, 133 (1982).
102. B. J. Tripathi and R. C. Tripathi, Lens Eye Toxicol. Res., 6, 395 (1987).
103. H. A. Baldwin, T. O. McDonald, and C. H. Beasley, J. Soc. Cosmet. Chem., 25, 181 (1973).
104. Fed. Reg., 18, 351 (1953).
105. C. W. Bruch, Drug Cosmet. Ind., 118(6), 51 (1976).
106. C. Teping and B. Wiedemann, Klin. Monatsbl. Augenheilkd., 205, 10 (1994).
107. M. Diestelhorst, S. Grunthal, and R. Suverkrup, Graefe's Arch. Clin. Exp. Ophthalmol., 237, 394 (1999).
108. F. Levrat, P. J. Pisella and C. Baudouin, J. Fr. Ophtalmol., 22, 186 (1999).
109. F. Becquet, M. Goldschild, M. S. Moldovan, M. Ettaiche, P. Gastaud, and C. Baudouin, Curr. Eye Res. 17, 419 (1998).
110. M. L. Weiner and L. A. Kotkoskie, eds., *Excipient Toxicity and Safety*, Marcel Dekker, New York, 2000.
111. K. Green and J. M. Chapman, J. Toxicol. Cutan. Ocul. Toxicol., 5, 133 (1986).
112. C. Thode and H. Kilp, Fortschr. Ophthalmol., 79, 125 (1982).
113. K. Green, J. Chapman, L. Cheeks, and R. Clayton, Conc. Toxicol., 4, 126 (1987).
114. A. R. Gassett, Y. Ishii, H. E. Kaufman, and T. Miller, Am. J. Ophthalmol., 78, 98 (1975).
115. H. Sasaki, T. Nagano, K. Yamamura, K. Nishida, and J. Nakamura, J. Pharm. Pharmacol., 47, 703 (1995).
116. H. Sasaki, C. Tei, K. Yamamura, K. Nishida, and J. Nakamura, J. Pharm. Pharmacol., 46:871 (1994).
117. R. M. E. Richards, Aust. J. Pharm. Sci., 55, S86, S96 (1967).
118. W. Mullen, W. Shephard, and J. Labovitz, Surv. Ophthalmol., 17, 469 (1973).
119. W. Johnson, J. Am. Coll. Toxicol., 8, 589 (1989).
120. W. H. Havener, *Ocular Pharmacology*, C. V. Mosby, St. Louis, MO, 1966.
121. T. O. McDonald, Technical Report, Alcon Laboratories Inc., August 1975.
122. C. Baudouin, P. J. Pisella, K. Fillacier, M. Goldschild, F. Becquet, M. De Saint-Jean, and A. Bechetoille, Ophthalmology, 106, 556 (1999).
123. M. De-Saint-Jean, F. Brignole, A. F. Bringuier, A. Bauchet, G. Feldmann, and C. Baudouin, Invest. Ophthalmol. Vis. Sci., 40, 619 (1999).
124. C. Debbasch, M. De-Saint-Jean, P. J. Pisella, P. Rat, J. M. Warnet, and C. Baudouin, J. Toxicol. Cutaneous Ocul. Toxicol., 19, 79 (2000).
125. M. J. Miller, in *Handbook of Disinfectants and Antiseptics*, (J. M. Ascenzi, ed.), Marcel Dekker, New York, 1996, pp. 83–110.
126. P. S. Binder, D. Rasmussen, and M. Gordon, Arch. Ophthalmol., 99, 87 (1981).
127. A. Tosti and G. Tosti, Contact Dermatitis, 18, 268 (1988).
128. E. Shaw, Contact Intraocul. Lens Med. J., 6, 273 (1980).
129. J. Molinari, R. Nash, and D. Badham, Int. Contact Lens Clin., 9, 323 (1982).
130. E. L. Gual, J. Invest. Dermatol., 31, 91 (1958).
131. F. A. Ellis and H. M. Robinson, Arch., Fermatol. Syphilol., 46, 425 (1941).
132. R. E. Reisman, J. Allergy, 43, 245 (1969).
133. D. Mackeen, Contact Lens J., 7, 14 (1978).
134. R. C. Meyer and L. B. Cohn, J. Pharm. Sci., 67, 1636 (1978).
135. W. R. Baily, Contact Lens Soc. Am. J., 6, 33 (1972).
136. E. M. Salonen, A. Vaheri, T. Tervo, and R. Beuerman, J. Toxicol. Cutan. Ocul. Toxicol., 10, 157 (1991).
137. B. J. Tripathi, R. C. Tripathi, and P. K. Susmitha, Lens Eye Toxicol. Res., 9, 361 (1992).
138. W. M. Grant, *Toxicology of the Eye*, 4th ed., Charles C Thomas, Springfield, IL, 1993, p. 365.
139. M. J. Doughty, Optom. Vis. Sci., 71, 562 (1994).
140. H. Sasaki, C. Tei, K. Yamamura, K. Nishida, and J. Nakamura, J. Pharm. Pharmacol., 46, 871 (1994).
141. D. E. Rudnick, H. F. Edelhauser, C. L. Hendrix, D. P. Rodeheaver, and R. B. Hackett, ARVO, 1997.
142. J. H. Chang, H. Ren, W. M. Petroll, H. D. Cavanagh, and J. V. Jester, Curr. Eye Res., 19, 171 (1999).

143. M. A. Chowhan, D. O. Helton, R. G. Harris, and C. L. Luthy (to Alcon Laboratories, Inc), U.S. Patent 5,037,647.
144. N. L. Burstein, Invest. Ophthalmol., 53, 358 (1975).
145. A. M. Tonjum, Acta Ophthalmol., Vis. Sci., 19, 308 (1980).
146. J. A. Dormans and J. J. Van Logten, Toxicol. Appl. Pharmacol., 62, 251 (1982).
147. A. R. Gassett and Y. Ishii, Can. J. Ophthalmol., 10, 98 (1975).
148. K. Green, V. Livingston, K. Bowman, and D. S. Hull, Arch. Ophthalmol., 19, 1273 (1980).
149. C. G. Begley, P. J. Waggoner, G. S. Hafner, T. Tokarski, R. E. Meetz, and W. H. Wheeler, Opt. Vis. Sci., 68, 189 (1991).
150. K. Green, R. E. Johnson, J. M. Chapman, E. Nelson, and L. Cheeks, Lens Eye Toxicol. Res., 6, 37 (1989).
151. Reference deleted.
152. A. J. Bron, P. Daubas, R. Siou-Mermet, and C. Trinquand, Eye 12, 839 (1998).
153. F. Becquet, M. Goldschild, M. S. Moldovan, M. Ettaiche, P. Gastaud, and C. Baudouin, Curr. Eye Res., 17, 419 (1998).
154. E. A. Neuwelt, ed., *Implications of the Blood-Brain Barrier and Its Manipulation*, Vol. 1, *Basic Science Aspects*, Plenum Medical Book Company, New York, 1989.
155. M. B. Segal, ed., *Barriers and Fluids of the Eye and Brain*, CRC Press, Cleveland, OH, 1992.
156. Reference deleted.
157. H. E. Kaufman, B. A. Barron, M. B. McDonald, and S. R. Waltman, eds., *The Cornea*, Churchill Livingstone, New York, 1988.
158. A. K. Mitra, ed., *Ocular Drug Delivery Systems*, Marcel Dekker, New York, 1993.
159. B. S. Fine and M. Yanoff, *Ocular Histology*, Harper & Row, NY, 1979.
160. J. R. Robinson, ed., *Ophthalmic Drug Delivery Systems*, Academy of Pharmaceutical Sciences, American Pharmaceutical Association, Washington, DC, 1980.
161. C. W. Conroy and T. H. Maren, J. Ocul. Pharm. Ther., 15, 179 (1999).
162. C. W. Conroy and T. H. Maren, J. Ocul. Pharm. Ther., 4, 565 (1998).
163. T. W. Olsen, H. F. Edelhauser, J. I. Lim, and D. H. Geroski, Invest. Ophthal. Vis. Sci., 36, 1893 (1995).
164. T. W. Olsen, S. Y. Aaberg, D. H. Geroski, and H. F. Edelhauser, Am. J. Ophth., 125, 237 (1998).
165. D. H. Geroski and H. F. Edelhauser, Invest. Ophthal. Vis. Sci., 41, 961 (2000).
166. D. E. Rudnick, J. S. Noonan, D. H. Geroski, M. Prausnitz, and H. F. Edelhauser, Invest. Ophthal. Vis. Sci., 40, 3054 (1999).
167. J. D. Mullins and G. Hecht, Ophthalmic preparations, in *Remington's Pharmaceutical Sciences*, Vol. 18 (A. R. Genaro, Ed.), Mack Publishing, Easton, PA, 1990, pp. 1581–1595.
168. R. A. Moses, *Adler's Physiology of the Eye*, 5th ed., C. V. Mosby, St. Louis, MO, 1970, p. 49.
169. S. S. Chrai, M. C. Makoid, S. P. Eriksen, and J. R. Robinson, J. Pharm. Sci., 63, 333 (1974).
170. D. I. Weiss and R. D. Schaffer, Arch. Ophthalmol., 68, 727 (1962).
171. F. T. Fraunfelder and S. M. Meyer, *Drug-Induced Ocular Side Effects and Drug Interactions*, Lea & Febiger, Philadelphia, 1989, pp. 442–487.
172. B. C. P. Polak, Drugs used in ocular treatment, in *Meyler's Side Effects of Drugs* (M. N. G. Dukes, ed.), Elsevier, New York, 1988, pp. 988–998.
173. T. F. Patton, in *Ophthalmic Drug Delivery Systems* (J. R. Robison, ed.), Academy of Pharmaceutical Sciences, American Pharmaceutical Association, Washington, DC, 1980, pp. 23–54.
174. J. C. Keister, B. R. Cooper, P. J. Missel, J. C. Lang, and D. F. Hager, J. Pharm. Sci., 80, 50 (1991).
175. A. Rozier, C. Mazuel, J. Grove, and B. Plazonnet, Int. J. Pharm., 57, 163 (1989).
176. T. J. Zimmerman, M. Sharir, G. F. Nardin, and M. Fuqua, Am. J. Ophthalmol., 114, 1 (1992).
177. A. Durward, The skin and the sensory organs, in *Cunningham's Testbook of Anatomy* (G. J. Romanes, ed.), Oxford University Press, London, 1964, p. 796.
178. O. A. Candia, Invest. Ophthalmol. Vis. Sci., 33, 2575 (1992).
179. A. J. Huang, S. C. Tseng, and K. R. Kenyon, Invest. Ophthalmol. Vis. Sci., 30, 684 (1989).
180. N. Narawane, Oxidative and hormonal control of horseradish peroxidase transytosis across the pigmented rabbit conjunctiva, Ph.D. thesis, University of Southern California, 1993.
181. L. E. Stevens, P. J. Missel, and J. C. Lang, Anal. Chem., 64, 715 (1992).
182. R. H. Perry and C. H. Chilton, *Chemical Engineer's Handbook*, 5th ed., McGraw-Hill, New York, 1973, Sec. 4.
183. J. M. Smith, *Chemical Engineering Kinetics*, 3rd ed., McGraw-Hill, New York, 1981, Chap. 3.
184. C. G. Hill, *An Introduction to Chemical Engineering Kinetics and Reactor Design*, John Wiley & Sons, New York, 1977.
185. P. Veng-Pedersen and W. R. Gillespie, S. Pharm. Sci., 77, 39 (1988).
186. W. R. Gillespie, P. Veng-Pedersen, E. J. Antal, and J. P. Phillips, J. Pharm. Sci., 77, 48 (1988).
187. E. Hayakawa, D.-S. Chien, K. Ingagaki, A. Yamamoto, W. Wang, and V. H. L. Lee, Pharm. Res., 9, 769 (1992).
188. H. F. Edelhauser, J. R. Hoffert, and P. O. Fromm, Invest. Ophth., 4, 290 (1965).
189. D. M. Maurice and S. Mishima, *Ocular Pharmackinetics* (M. L. Sears, ed.), Springer-Verlag, Berlin, 1984, pp. 19–116.

190. R. D. Schoenwald and R. L. Ward, J. Pharm. Sci., 67, 786 (1978).
191. R. D. Schoenwald and H. S. Huang, J. Pharm. Sci., 72, 1266 (1983).
192. R. D. Schoenwald, Clin. Pharmacokinet, 18, 255 (1990).
193. D.-S. Chien, J. J. Homsy, C. Gluchowaski, D. D.-S. Tang-Liu, Curr. Eye Res., 9, 1051 (1990).
194. D. M. Maurice and M. V. Riley, The cornea, in *Biochemistry of the Eye* (C. N. Graymore, ed.), Academic Press, New York, 1970, Chap. 1.
195. E. R. Berman, *Biochemistry of the Eye*, Plenum Press, New York, 1991.
196. H. E. P. Bazan, private communications.
197. A. Edwards and M. R. Prausnitz, AICHE J., 44, 214 (1998).
198. A. Edwards and M. R. Prausnitz, to be published.
199. B. Alberts, D. Bray, J. Lewis, M. Raff, K. Roberts and J. D. Watson, *Molecular Biology, of the Cell*, Garland Publishing, Inc., New York, 1983.
200. L. Stryer, *Biochemistry*, W. H. Freeman and Company, 1981.
201. H. Lodish, D. Baltimore, A. Berk, S. L. Zipursky, P. Matsudaira, J. Darnell, *Molecular Cell Biology*, W. H. Freeman and Company, 1995.
202. G. L. Flynn, S. H. Yalkowsky, and T. J. Roseman, J. Pharm. Sci., 63, 479 (1974).
203. E. R. Cooper and G. Kasting, J. Controlled Release, 6, 23 (1987).
204. G. Hecht, R. E. Roehrs, E. R. Cooper, J. W. Hiddemen, F. F. Van Duzee, in *Modern Pharmaceutics*, 2nd Ed. (G. S. Banker and C. T. Rhodes, eds.), Marcel Dekker, New York, 1990, Chap. 14.
205. E. R. Cooper, *Optimization of Transport and Biological Response with Epithelial Barriers in Biological and Synthetic Membranes*, Alan R. Liss, New York, 1989, pp. 249–260.
206. R. W. Baker and H. K. Lonsdale, *Controlled Release: Mechanisms and Rates* (A. C. Tanquary and R. E. Lacy, eds.), Plenum Press, New York, 1974, pp. 15–71.
207. W. Wang, H. Sasaki, D.-S. Chien, and V. H. Lee, Curr. Eye Res., 10, 57 (1991).
208. P. Ashton, S. K. Podder, and V. H. Lee, Pharm. Res., 8, 1166 (1991).
209. J. Liaw and J. R. Robinson, Ocular penetration enchancers, in *Ocular Drug Delivery Systems* (A. K. Mitra, ed.), Marcel Dekker, 1993, pp. 369–381.
210. Y. Rojanaskul, J. Liaw, and J. R. Robinson, Int. J. Pharm., 66, 133 (1990).
211. K.-I. Hosoya, Y. Horibe, K.-J. Kim, and V. H. L. Lee, J. Pharm. Exp. Therap., 285, 223 (1998).
212. K.-I. Hosoya, Y. Horibe, K.-S. Kim, and V. H. L. Lee, Inv. Ophth. Vis. Sci., 39, 372 (1998).
213. P. Saha, J. J. Yang, and V. H. L. Lee, Inv. Ophth. Vis. Sci., 39, 1221 (1998).
214. K.-I. Hosoya, Y. Horibe, K.-J. Kim, and V. H. L. Lee, Inv. Ophth. Vis. Sci., 39, 1436 (1998).
215. S. K. Basu, I. S. Haworth, M. B. Bolger, and V. H. L. Lee, Inv. Ophth. Vis. Sci., 39, 2365 (1998).
216. H. Ueda, Y. Horibe, K.-J. Kim, and V. H. L. Lee, Inv. Ophth. Vis. Sci., 41, 870 (2000).
217. D. M. Maurice, *Symposium on Ocular Therapy*, Vol. 9, John Wiley & Sons, New York, 1976.
218. I. H. Leopold and H. G. Scheie, Arch. Ophthalmol., 29, 811 (1943).
219. *Physician's Desk Reference for Ophthalmology*, 28th Ed., 2000, Section 9.
220. D. F. Martin, F. L. Ferris, D. J. Parks, R. C. Walton, S. D. Mellow, D. Gibbs, N. A. Remaley, P. Ashton, M. D. Davis, C. C. Chan, and R. B. Nussenblatt, Arch. Ophthalmol., 115, 1389 (1997).
221. M. P. Hatton, J. S. Duker, E. Reichel, M. G. Morley and C. A. Puliafito, Retina, 18, 50 (1998).
222. B. Dhillon, A. Kamal, and C. Leen, Int. J. STD AIDS, 9, 227 (1998).
223. D. M. Maurice, private communication.
224. T. J. Smith, P. A. Pearson, D. L. Blandford, J. D. Brown, K. A. Goins, J. L. Hollins, E. T. Schmeisser, P. Glavinos, L. B. Baldwin, and P. Ashton, Arch. Ophthalmol., 110, 255 (1992).
225. G. E. Sanborn, R. Anand, R. E. Torti, S. D. Nightingale, S. X. Cal, B. Yates, P. Ashton, and T. Smith, Arch. Ophthalmol., 110, 188 (1992).
226. J. Xu, J. Heys, V. H. Barocas, and T. W. Randolph, Pharm. Res., 17, 664 (2000).
227. S. S. Hayreh, Exp. Eye Res., 5, 123 (1966).
228. M. Maurice, Am. J. Physiol., 252, F104 (1987).
229. S. Johnson and D. M. Maurice, Exp. Eye Res., 39, 791 (1984).
230. M. Araie and D. M. Maurice, Exp. Eye Res., 52, 27 (1991).
231. A. G. Palestine and R. F. Brubaker, Invest. Ophthalmol. Vis. Sci., 21, 544 (1981).
232. H. Lund-Andersen, B. Krogasaa, M. La Cour, and J. Larsen, Invest. Ophthalmol. Vis. Sci., 26, 698 (1985).
233. A. Hosaka, Acta Ophtallmol. Suppl., 185, 95 (1988).
234. A. Yoshida, S. Ishiko, and M. Kojima, Graefe's Arch. Clin. Exp. Ophthalmol., 230, 78 (1992).
235. K. J. Tojo and A. Ohtori, Proceed. Int. Symp. Control. Rel. Bioact. Mater., 20, 45 (1993).
236. A. Ohtori and K. Tojo, Biol. Pharm. Bull., 17, 283 (1994).
237. K. Tojo and A. Ohtori, Math. Biosci., 123, 59 (1994).
238. K. Uno, K. Nakagawa, A. Ohtori, and K. Tojo, Drug Deliv. Systems (Jpn), 11, 133 (1998).
239. K. Tojo and A. Ohtori, Eur. J. Pharm. Biopharm., 47, 99 (1999).
240. P. M. Pinsky, D. M. Maurice and D. V. Datye, Invest. Ophthalmol. Vis. Sci. Suppl., 37, S700 (1996).
241. S. Friedrich, Y. L. Cheng, and B. Saville, Ann. Biomed. Eng., 25, 303 (1997).

242. S. Friedrich, Y. L. Cheng, and B. Saville, Curr. Eye Res., 16, 663 (1997).
243. S. Friedrich, B. Saville, and Y. L. Cheng, J. Ocular Pharm. Ther., 13, 445 (1997).
244. S. Friedrich, thesis, University of Toronto, Department of Chemical Engineering and Applied Chemistry, 1996.
245. P. J. Missel, Ann. Biomed. Eng., 28, 1307 (2000).
246. Y. Zhou and X. Y. Wu, J. Controlled Rel., 49, 277 (1997).
247. X. Y. Wu and Y. Zhou, J. Controlled Rel., 51, 57 (1998).
248. K. Tojo, Y. Morita, and A. Ohtori, Proceed. Int. Symp. Control. Rel. Bioact. Mater., 18, 293 (1991).
249. K. Uno, A. Ohtori, and K. Tojo, Atarashii Ganka (J. Eye, Japan) 11, 607 (1994).
250. Code of Federal Regulations, 21, § 210–211.
251. Clean Room and Work Station Requirements, Controlled Environment, Sec. 1–5 Federal Standard 209, Office of Technical Services, U.S. Department of Commerce, Washington, DC, Dec. 16, 1963.
252. P. R. Austin and S. W. Timmerman, *Design and Operation of Clean Rooms*, Business News Publishers, Detroit, MI, 1965.
253. P. R. Austin, *Clean Rooms of the World*. Ann Arbor Science Publishers, Ann Arbor, MI, 1967.
254. K. R. Goddard, Air filtration of microbial particles, Publication 953, U.S. Public Health Service, Washington, DC, 1967.
255. K. R. Goddard, Bull. Parente, Drug Assoc., 23, 699 (1969).
256. U.S. Patent 6,071,904, issued June 6, 2000 to Alcon Laboratories, Inc.
257. D. Jones, PDA J., 49(5), 226 (1995).
258. J. R. Sharp, Pharm. J., 239, 106 (1987).
259. J. R. Sharp, Manufact. Chem., Feb., 22, 55 (1988).
260. F. Leo, *Blow/Fill/Seal Aseptic Packaging Technology in Aseptic Pharmaceutical Technology for the 1990's*, Interpharm Press, Prairie View, IL. 1989, pp. 195–218.
261. J. R. Sharp, J. Parenter. Sci. Technol., 44(5) (1990).
262. A. Bradely, S. P. Probert, C. S. Sinclaire, and A. Tallentire, J. Parenter. Sci. Technol., 45(4), 187.
263. *The Rules Governing Medicinal Products in the European Union*, Vol. 4, Good Manufacturing Practices—Medicinal Products for Human and Vetrinary Use, Annex I Manufacture of Sterile Medicinal Products, Commission Directive 91/356/EEC of 13 June 1991.
264. *USP 24*, U.S. Pharcacopeial Convention, Rockville, MD, 1999, pp. 1752–1753.
265. Fed. Reg., 41, 106, June 1, 1976.
266. T. L. Grimes, D. E. Fonner, J. C. Griffin, and L. R. Rathburn, Bull. Parenter. Drug Assoc., 29, 64 (1975).
267. E-3A Accepted Practices for Permanently Installed Sanitary Product Pipeline and Cleaning Systems, Serial E-60500, U.S. Public Health Service, Washington, DC.
268. D. E. Cadwallader, Am. J. Hosp. Pharm., 24, 33 (1967).
269. F. G. Kronfeld and J. E. McDonald, J. Am. Pharm. Assoc. (Sci. Ed.), 42, 333 (1951).
270. S. Riegelman and D. G. Vaughn, J. Am. Pharm. Assoc. (Pract. Pharm. Ed.), 19, 474 (1958).
271. S. M. Blaugh and A. T. Canada, Am. J. Hosp. Pharm., 22, 662 (1965).
272. M. L. Linn and L. T. Jones, Am. J. Ophthalmol., 65, 76 (1968).
273. S. S. Chrai and J. R. Robinson, J. Pharm. Sci., 63, 1218 (1974).
274. C. A. Adler, D. M. Maurice, and M. E. Patterson, Exp. Eye Res., 11, 34 (1971).
275. R. Castroviejo, Arch. Ophthalmol., 74, 143 (1965).
276. C. Hanna, F. T. Fraunfelder, M. Cable, and R. E. Hardberger, Am. J. Ophthalmol., 76, 193 (1973).
277. F. T. Fraunfelder, C. Hanna, M. Cable, and R. E. Hardberger, Am. J. Ophthalmol., 76, 475 (1973).
278. R. Mouly, Ann. Chir. Plast., 17, 61 (1972).
279. D. W. Newton, C. H. Becker, and G. Torosian, J. Pharm. Sci., 62, 1538 (1973).
280. R. L. Schoenwald, R. L. Ward, L. M. DeSantis, and R. E. Roehrs, J. Pharm. Sci., 67, 1280 (1978).
281. W. F. March, R. M. Stewart, A. I. Mandell, and L. Bruce, Arch. Ophthalmol., 100, 1270 (1982).
282. H. M. Liebowitz, R. K. Chang, and A. I. Mandell, Ophthalmology, 91, 1199 (1984).
283. F. W. Bowman, E. W. Knoll, M. White, and P. Mislivic, J. Pharm. Sci., 61, 532 (1972).
284. T. W. Schwartz, Am. Perum. Cosmet., 86, 39 (1971).
285. A. Zaffaroni, *Proc. 31st International Congress on Pharmaceutical Science*, Washington, DC, 1971.
286. J. W. Shell and R. W. Baker, Ann. Ophthalmol., 7, 1037 (1975).
287. S. Lerman and B. Reininger, Can. J. Ophthalmol., 6, 14 (1971).
288. Y. F. Maichuk, Invest. Ophthalmol., 14, 87 (1975).
289. S. P. Loucas and H. M. Haddad, J. Pharm. Sci., 61, 985 (1972).
290. J. Hiller and R. W. Baker, (to Alza Corporation), U.S. Patent 3,811,444 (1974).
291. A. Michaels (to Alza Corporation), U.S. Patent 3,867,519 (1975).
292. N. Keller, A. M. Longwell, and S. A. Biros, Arch. Ophthalmol., 94, 644 (1976).
293. H. F. Edelhauser, Arch. Ophthalmol., 93, 649 (1975).
294. W. H. Havener, *Ocular Pharmacology*, 2nd ed., C. V. Mosby, St. Louis, MO, 1970, p. 27.
295. J. W. Shell and R. W. Baker, Ann. Ophthalmol., 7, 1637 (1975).
296. W. M. Grant, *Toxicology of the Eye*, Charles C Thomas, Springfield, IL, 1974, p. 259.
297. B. E. McCarey, H. F. Edelhauser, and D. L. Van Horn, Invest. Ophthalmol., 12, 410 (1973).

298. D. L. Merrill, T. C. Fleming, and L. J. Girard, Am. J. Ophthalmol., 49, 895 (1960).
299. L. J. Girard, *Proceedings International Congress on Ophthalmology*, Brussels, Sept. 1958.
300. H. F. Edelhauser, D. L. Van Horn, R. W. Scholtz, and R. A. Hyndiuk, Am. J. Ophthalmol., 81, 473 (1976).
301. S. E. Herrell and D. Heilman, Am. J. Med. Sci., 206, 221 (1943).
302. N. S. Jaffee, Bull. Parenter. Drug Assoc., 24, 218 (1970).
303. N. J. Baily, Contact Lens Spectrum, 2(7), 6 (1987).
304. K. J. Randeri, R. P. Quintana, and M. A. Chowhan, Lens care products, in *Encyclopedia of Pharmaceutical Technology*, Vol. 8 (J. Swarbrick and J. C. Boylan, eds.), Marcel Dekker, New York, 1993, pp. 361–402.
305. J. Tan, L. Keay, and D. Sweeney, Contact Lens Spectrum, July, 42 (2000).
306. P. R. Kastl, M. J. Refojo, and O. H. Dabezies, Jr., Review of polymerization for the contact lens fitter, in *Contact Lenses: The CLAO Guide to Basic Science and Clinical Practice*, 2nd ed., Vol. 1 (O. H. Dabezies, Jr., ed.), Little, Brown & Co., Boston, 1989, pp. 6.21–6.24.
307. K. A. Polse and R. B. Mandell, Arch. Ophthalmol., 84, 505 (1970).
308. P. S. Binder, Ophthalmology, 86, 1093 (1978).
309. I. Fatt and R. M. Hill, Am. J. Optom. Arch. Am. Acad. Optom., 47, 50 (1970).
310. I. Fatt, Contacto, 23(1), 6 (1978).
311. Food and Drug Administration, *Guidance Document for Class III Contact Lenses*, U.S. Food and Drug Administration, Silver Springs, MD, 1989.
312. N. J. Van Haeringen, Surv. Opthalmol., 26(2), 84 (1981).
313. E. J. Castillo, J. L. Koenintg, and J. M. Anderson, Biomaterials, 7, 89 (1986).
314. M. Ruben, Br. J. Ophthalmol., 59, 141 (1975).
315. D. E. Hart, Int. Contact Lens Clin., 11, 358 (1984).
316. C. G. Begley and P. J. Waggoner, J. Am. Optom. Assoc., 62, 208 (1991).
317. R. C. Tripathi, B. J. Tripathi, and C. B. Millard, CLAO J., 14, 23 (1988).
318. M. J. Miller, L. A., Wilson, and D. G. Ahrean, J. Clin. Microbiol., 16, 513 (1988).
319. M. Chowhan, T. Bilbault, R. P. Quintana, and R. A. Rosenthal, Contactologia, 15, 190 (1993).
320. R. Jacob, Int. Contact Lens Clin., 15, 317 (1988).
321. D. Holsky, J. Am. Optom. Assoc., 55, 205 (1993).
322. M. M. Hom and M. Pickford, Int. Eyecare, 2, 325 (1986).
323. R. L. Davis, Int. Contact Lens Clin., 10, 277 (1983).
324. M. A. Chowhan, R. P. Quintana, B. S. Hong, T. Bilbault, and R. A. Rosenthal (to Alcon Laboratories, Inc.) U.S. Patent 5,948,738.
325. C. G. Begley, S. Paraguia, and C. Sporm, J. Am. Optom. Assoc., 61, 190 (1990).
326. N. Tarrantino, R. C. Courtney, L. A. Lesswell, D. Keno, and I. Frank, Int. Contact Lens Clin., 15, 25 (1988).
327. R. D. Houlsby, M. Ghajar, and G. Chavez, J. Am. Optom. Assoc., 59, 184 (1988).
328. C. B. Anger, K. Ambrus, J. Stocker, S. Kapadia, and L. Thomas, Spectrum, 9, 46 (1990).
329. M. Chowhan, T. Bilbault, R. P. Quintana (to Alcon Laboratories, Inc.), U.S. Patent 5,370,744.
330. M. Chowhan, D. Keith, H. Chen, R. Stone, Poster at Annual Meeting, CLAO, Las Vegas, 1998.
331. Food and Drug Administration, *Draft Testing Guidelines for Class III Soft (Hydrophilic) Contact Lens Solutions*, U.S. Food and Drug Administration, Silver Springs, MD, 1985.
332. N. A. Brennan and N. Efron, Optom. Vis. Sci., 66, 834 (1989).
333. N. Efron, T. R. Goldwig, and N. A. Brennan, CLAO J., 17, 114 (1991).
334. M. Chowhan, H. Chen, R. Stone, R. A. Rosenthal, D. Keith, and J. Stein, Alcon Laboratories, Inc., Technical Report.

Chapter 14

Delivery of Drugs by the Pulmonary Route

Anthony J. Hickey

University of North Carolina, Chapel Hill, North Carolina

I. INTRODUCTION

A. Background and Historical Perspective

Inhaled therapies have existed for at least 5000 years [1]. Modern drug therapy can be traced to the propellant-driven metered-dose inhaler (pMDI) of the 1950s [2]. The surge in interest that has arisen in the last decade relates to the chlorofluorocarbon (CFC) propellant ban and the development of biotechnology products. The observation that CFC propellants play a significant role in ozone depletion in the upper atmosphere [3], which in turn results in greater surface ultraviolet (UV) radiation and impact on public health, particularly the incidence of skin cancer, led to regulation in the late 1980s [4]. In addition, the burgeoning biotechnology industry of the late 1980s and early 1990s actively sought alternative methods of delivering macromolecular drugs, which were difficult to deliver in therapeutic doses by the oral or parenteral route [5]. The urgent need for alternative methods explains the diversity of devices that have been described in the patent literature, many of which are currently under development.

The factors governing lung deposition may be divided into those related to the physicochemical properties of the droplets or particles being delivered, the mechanical aspects of aerosol dispersion usually associated with the delivery device, and the physiological and anatomical considerations associated with the biology of the lungs.

B. Physicochemical Factors Governing Lung Deposition

A number of physicochemical properties are associated with aerosol droplets of particles, which impact upon their characteristics as aerosols. The most important of these may be related to the aerodynamic properties of aerosols [6].

The size of any particle may be related to a characteristic dimension [7]. As examples, visual examination allows determination of projected area diameter, surface area measurement allows determination of equivalent surface diameter, and volume displacement allows determination of equivalent volume diameter. A full discussion of particle size measurement is beyond the scope of this commentary. It is sufficient to acknowledge that the method of describing particle size most relevant to describing aerosol particles is based on the aerodynamic behavior of the particle being studied. The size may then be described in terms of the equivalent diameter of a unit density sphere with the same terminal settling velocity as the particle being studied. The terms of an expression relating different particle diameters in terms of terminal settling velocity take the following form [8]:

$$V_T = \frac{\rho_p g D_e^2 C(D_e)}{\kappa_p 18\eta} = \frac{\rho_0 g D_{ae}^2 C(D_{ae})}{\kappa_0 18\eta} \tag{1}$$

where κ_p and κ_0 are the shape factors for the particle (>1) and an equivalent sphere (1), ρ_p and ρ_0 are the densities of the particle and a unit density (1 g cm^{-3}) sphere, $C(D_e)$ and $C(D_{ae})$ are the slip correction factors for an equivalent volume and an aerodynamically equivalent sphere, D_e and D_{ae} are the equivalent volume diameter

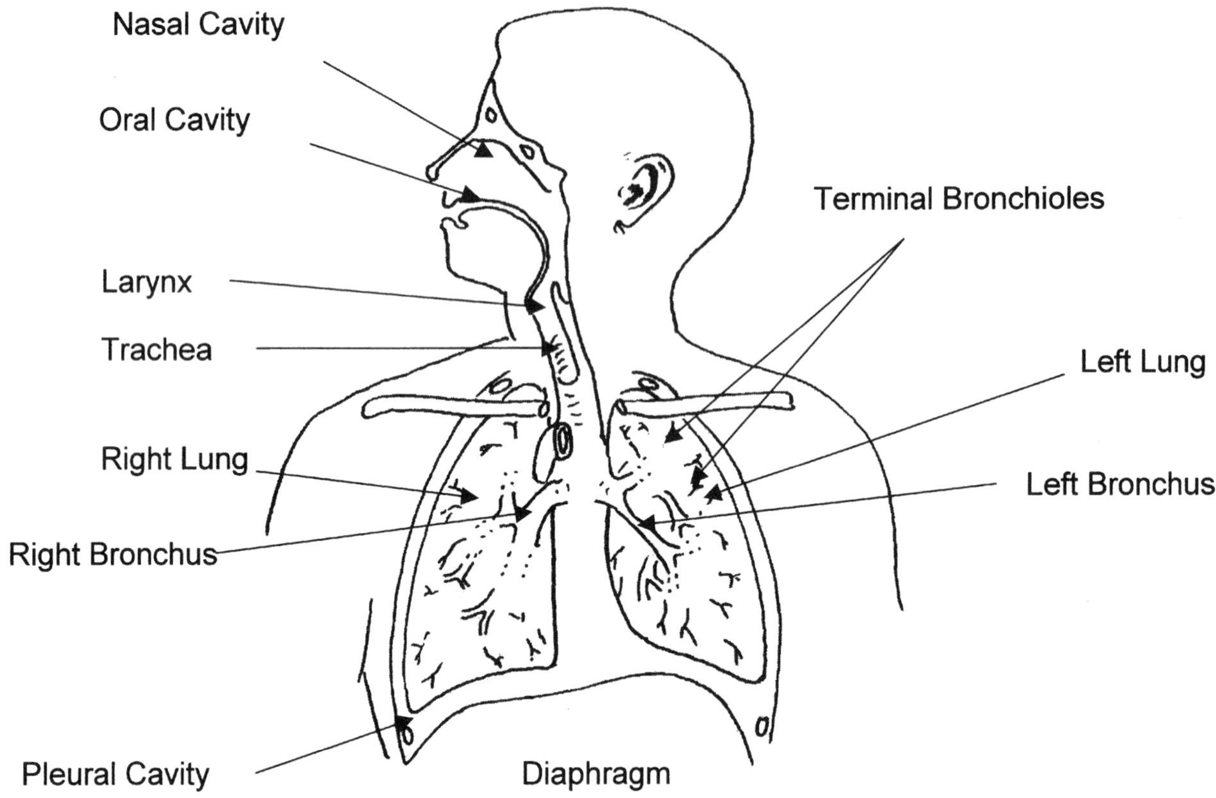

Fig. 1 The anatomy of the lungs showing the major airway subdivisions.

and aerodynamically equivalent (aerodynamic) diameter, and g is the acceleration due to gravity.

Equation (1) points to a number of important particle properties. Clearly the particle diameter, by any definition, plays a role in the behavior of the particle. Two other particle properties, density and shape, are of significance. The shape becomes important if particles deviate significantly from sphericity. The majority of pharmaceutical aerosol particles exhibit a high level of rotational symmetry and consequently do not deviate substantially from spherical behavior. The notable exception is that of elongated particles, fibers, or needles, which exhibit shape factors, κ_p, substantially greater than 1. Density will frequently deviate from unity and must be considered in comparing aerodynamic and equivalent volume diameters.

The slip correction factors are important for particles smaller than 1 μm in diameter, which is rarely the case for pharmaceutical aerosols. Slip correction is required for the Stokes' equation to remain predictive of particle behavior for these small particles. Therefore, assuming the absence of shape effects for particles in the Stokes' regime of flow, Eq. (1) collapses into the following expression:

$$D_{ae} = (\rho_p)^{0.5} D_e \tag{2}$$

The capacity for aerosols to take on moisture by hygroscopicity gives rise to a kinetic phenomenon of change in particle size as a function of residence time at a particular ambient relative humidity. This phenomenon can best be described in terms of the relationship between saturation ratio and particle size according to the following expression [9]:

$$p/p_s = [1 + (6imM_w/M_s\rho\pi d_p^3)]^{-1} \exp(4\gamma M_w/(RTd_p) \tag{3}$$

where p and p_s are the partial and saturation vapor pressure of water in the atmosphere, M_s and M_w are the molecular weights of the solute and water, ρ and γ are the density and surface tension of the solution, respectively, i is the number of ions into which the solute dissociates, and d_p is the particle diameter. This phenomenon is of significance, since a change in size of particles in transit through the high-humidity environment of the lungs (99.5% RH at 37°C) will give rise to altered deposition characteristics [10,11].

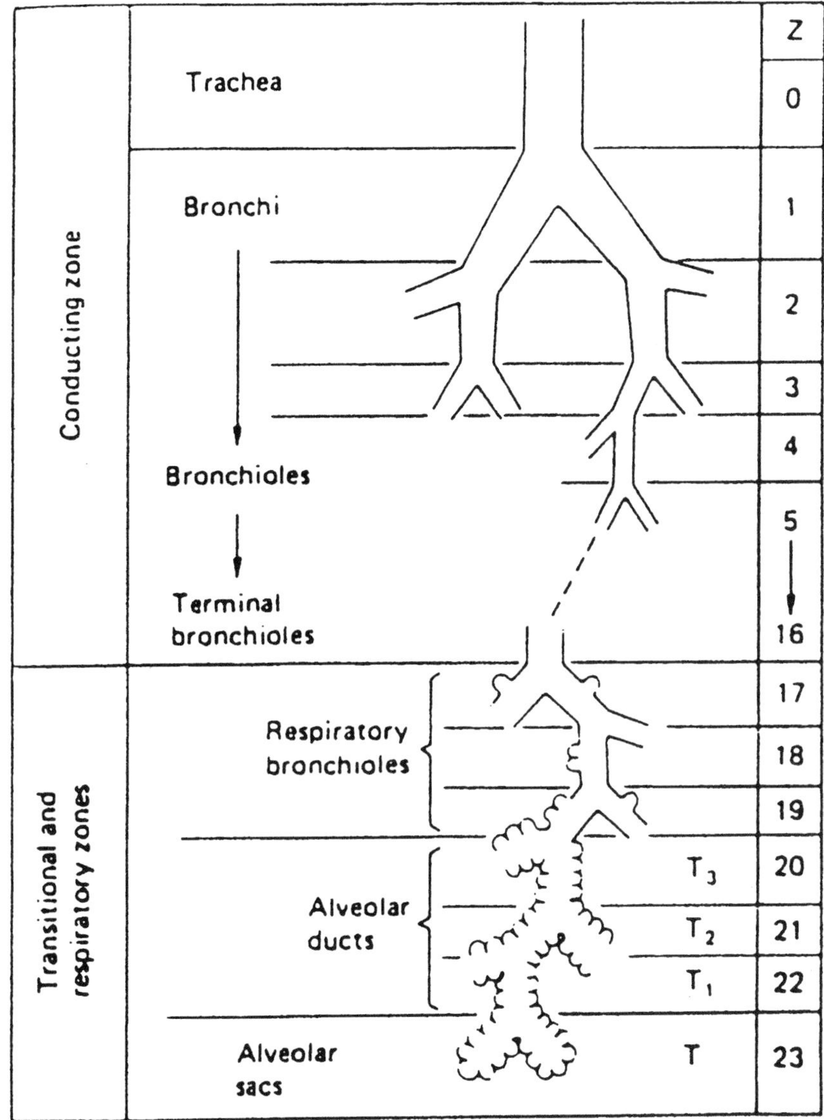

Fig. 2 The Weibel symmetrical branching model of the lung. (From Ref. 12.)

C. Physiological and Anatomical Features Governing Lung Deposition

Anatomically the lung is a series of bifurcating tubes, which begin at the trachea, divide into the main bronchii, the conducting bronchioles, and conclude in the terminal bronchioles and the alveoli, as shown in Fig. 1. Casts of the upper airways have been constructed in an attempt to predict aerosol deposition in the lungs. From these casts a number of anatomical models have been constructed, the most notable assuming symmetrical [12] and asymmetrical [13] branching. Figure 2 illustrates the Weibel symmetrical branching model of the lung. The average lengths, cross-sectional areas, and linear velocities achieved at various locations in the lungs were estimated early in the last century [14], and some examples are shown in Table 1.

Most lung deposition models are based on the influence of particle size on aerosol deposition. Breathing parameters, such as breathing frequency and tidal volume, play a key role in lung deposition [15]. Table 2 shows the breathing parameters for healthy male volunteers subjected to various levels of exercise on a bicycle ergometer [16]. There are known differences in these parameters based on gender, age, and disease

Table 1 Estimates of the Length, Cross-Sectional Areas, and Linear Velocities of Airways Indicating the Geometry and Dynamics of Discrete Regions of the Lungs

Lung region	Length (cm)	Cross-sectional area (cm^2)	Linear velocity (cm/s)
Trachea	11.0	1.3	150
Main bronchi	6.5	1.1	180
Second-order bronchi	1.5	3.1	65
Terminal bronchiole	0.3	150	1.3
Alveolar duct	0.02	8200	0.025

Table 2 Respiratory Rates,[a] Tidal, [b] and Minute[a] Volumes for Healthy Young Men at Rest and Under Two Levels (Light, 622 kg-m min^{-1}; and Heavy, 1660 kg-m min^{-1})

Degree of exertion	Respiratory rate (breaths/min)	Tidal volume (L)	Minute volume (L)
Sedentary	14.6	0.705	10.3
Light	23.0	1.622	37.3
Heavy	47.6	2.391	113.8

[a]Measured.
[b]Calculated.

Table 3 Resting Respiratory Rates, Tidal and Minute Volumes in Laboratory Animals[a]

Species	Respiratory rate (breaths/min)	Tidal volume (mL)	Minute volume (L)
Dog	18	320.0	5.2
Cat	25	12.4	0.32
Rat	85	1.5	0.1
Mouse	163	0.15	0.023
Guinea pig	90	1.8	0.16
Rabbit	46	21.0	1.07

[a]Measured.
Source: Modified from Ref. 17.

state, all of which should be considered in evaluating aerosol therapies.

A variety of species of laboratory animal are employed to study aerosol deposition for both efficacy and toxicity. It is important to recognize that the breathing parameters [17], not to mention the anatomy [18], of these animals differ substantially from humans. Table 3 shows a range of breathing parameters for several species of laboratory animal. Clearly there is a matter of scale involved in that small animals cannot generate the same airflow volumes as humans and to some extent compensate by increasing their respiratory rate.

The physicochemical properties of particles influence their behavior in transit through the airways of the lungs according to three mechanisms: impaction, sedimentation, and diffusion.

The principle of inertial impaction is employed to sample aerosols aerodynamically for characterization of particle size and will be dealt with theoretically later in this chapter.

Sedimentation of particles follows the principle outlined above [Eq. (1)] in which particles in the Stokes' regime of flow have attained terminal settling velocity. In the airways this phenomenon occurs under the influence of gravity. The angle of inclination, ψ, of the tube of radius R, on which particles might impact, must be considered in any theoretical assessment of sedimentation [14,19]. Landahl's expression for the probability, S, of deposition by sedimentation took the form:

$$S = 1 - \exp[-(0.8V_T \cdot t \cdot \cos\psi)/R] \tag{4}$$

where $V_T \cdot t \cdot \cos\psi/R$ has been designated the deposition parameter.

From Eq. 1, V_T includes a term for the particle size and gravitational acceleration. Landahl's expression adds terms describing the geometry of the tube and the residence time of the particle to allow a probability of deposition to be derived. As an example of the manner in which this expression is applied, assuming a deposition parameter of one and a probability of deposition of 55% for 2 μm particles, then 1 and 0.5 μm particles would be expected to deposit with 29% and 10% efficiency, respectively. The probabilities of particle deposition, by the U. S. Atomic Energy Commission and American Conference of Governmental and Industrial Hygienists, have been used to designate the fraction of an aerosol that is respirable as shown in Table 4. This considers deposition in all of the airways of the lungs. Thorough descriptions of theoretical and experimental studies of lung deposition have been collated and may be found in the literature [20].

Particulate diffusion does not play a significant role in the deposition of pharmaceutical aerosols. However, it is worth noting the mechanism by which diffusion of particles occurs in the lungs. The principle of Brownian motion is responsible for particle deposition under the influence of impaction with gas molecules in the airways. The amplitude of particle displacement is given by the following equation:

$$\Lambda = [(RT/N)(Ct/3\pi\eta d)]^{0.5} \tag{5}$$

Table 4 Respirable Fractions as Designated by the American Conference of Governmental and Industrial Hygienist and the U.S. Atomic Energy Commission

Aerodynamic diameter (μm)	Respirable fraction[a] (%)	Respirable fraction[b] (%)
10	1	0
8	5	–
5	30	25
4	50	–
2	91	100
1	97	–

[a]ACGIH (1997).
[b]USAEC (1961).

where R is the gas constant, T is absolute temperature (Kelvin), N is Avogadro's number, C is the slip correction factor, t is time, η is the air viscosity and d is the particle diameter.

Diffusion plays an important role in one of the most efficient aerosol-delivery devices, the cigarette. It is conceivable that the next generation of inhalers may take greater advantage of this mechanism of delivery. However, the major limitation to this approach is that an aerosol with a significant submicrometer fraction tends to be exhaled without depositing. The closer the particle size approaches the mean free path of the conducting gas, the more likely that deposition will not occur within usual lung residence times.

D. Mechanism of Drug Clearance and Pharmacokinetics of Disposition

The first purified and characterized drug substances were administered as aerosols as a topical treatment for asthma approximately 50 years ago. More recently, drugs have been evaluated for systemic delivery. For each category of drug the mechanism of clearance from the airways must be considered. These mechanisms may be listed as mucociliary transport, absorption, and cell-mediated translocation. The composition and residence time of the particle will influence the mechanism of clearance.

The importance of clearance mechanisms from the lungs relates to the action of the drug. For drugs, that act in the lungs, such as bronchodilators or anti-inflammatories, an extended residence time in the lungs might be beneficial. For drugs intended to act systemically, such as ergotamine alkaloids for migraine or insulin for the treatment of *diabetes mellitus*, rapid absorption may be desirable. This is not to imply that all systemically acting agents must be delivered rapidly, but this allows a contrast in rates of delivery.

The nature of the mechanisms involved and the interaction with the aerosol particles complicate the pharmacokinetics of drug clearance from the lungs. Figure 3 illustrates the sites of deposition in the lungs, the nasal and oropharyngeal, tracheobronchial, and pulmonary regions. Also shown in this figure are the routes for clearance by absorption into the blood circulation, by mucociliary transport to the gastrointestinal tract, and cell-mediated transport to the lymphatics and from there to the blood circulation.

Mucociliary transport in the conducting airways takes approximately 24 hours from the lung periphery to the epiglottis. Absorption takes place at a rate dictated by the physicochemical properties of the drug (hydrophobic, hydrophilic, strong or weak electrolyte, molecular weight). These properties impact upon the paracellular and transcellular mechanisms of transport across the alveolar or bronchiolar epithelium. Studies of fluorescent dextrans of a range of molecular weights have shown that paracellular transport occurs more rapidly for small molecular weight molecules than for large ones [21]. A plot of log clearance (min^{-1}) against log molecular weight (D) appears to be linear in the range of clearances of 10^{-1}–10^{-4}, for molecular weights of 10^2–10^5 D, respectively [21]. The data were collected for a number of different species (rat, rabbit, dog, sheep, lamb, dog, and human).

Particles, that exhibit long residence times in the periphery of the lungs, beyond the mucociliary escalator, are subject to uptake by alveolar macrophages, phagocytic cells responsible for clearing debris from the pulmonary region of the lungs. These cells are also the primary immunological defense, presenting the initial response to antigenic materials, usually foreign material of biological origin including infectious microorganisms (bacteria, viruses, and fungi). Cellular clearance may take weeks or months depending upon the nature of the particles.

Mathematical models for drug disposition have been proposed [22] and elaborated upon [23]. The latter model proposed dividing the airways into tracheobronchial and two pulmonary regions, long and short residence time regions, also considering the availability of drug that enters the gastrointestinal tract. A series of equations were derived for fraction remaining in each of the regions under steady-state conditions. These models examine thoroughly the influence of the physicochemical properties on drug disposition from the lungs. More subtle models have

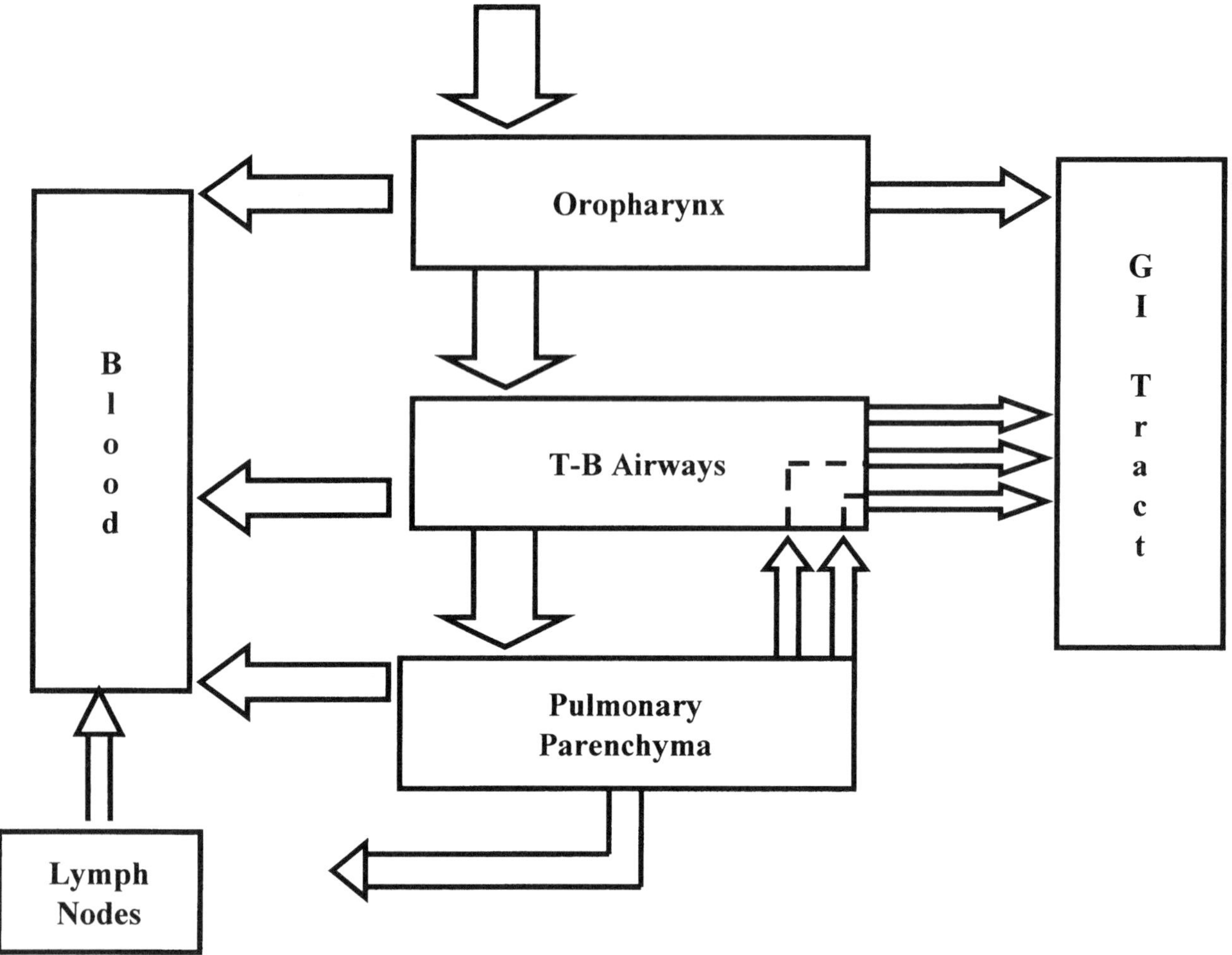

Fig. 3 Sites of deposition in the lungs, the oropharynx, tracheobronchial, and pulmonary regions.

also been evaluated based on receptor occupancy of glucocorticoids [24].

II. CATEGORIES OF AEROSOL-DELIVERY DEVICE

Before discussing the three categories of delivery device, the nature of the emitted aerosol will be considered. Droplet formation may be characterized in terms of the nature of the propulsive force and the liquid being dispersed, and this topic is dealt with for specific situations in the following sections. However, dry particles, which are delivered from suspension in pMDIs or from DPIs alone or from a blend, must be prepared in respirable sizes. The production of respirable aerosol particles has traditionally been achieved by micronization of the drug [25]. This involves the introduction of bulk particles on a gas stream into the path of an opposing gas stream under high pressure. Particles impact on each other and are thereby ground into small particles, which ultimately pass through a cyclone separator and are collected in a vessel or a bag filter. These particles can be produced in size ranges less than 5 μm, which is suitable for lung deposition. In recent years, spray-drying has been employed as an alternative method of production [26]. This method has the advantage that particles produced are frequently spherical. In addition, it may be the case that the particles are not subject to such high energy input as the jet milling, and consequently this may be more suitable for thermolabile materials. As more sophisticated techniques are being developed for the production of particles, they are finding applications in the production of aerosol particles. One of the more successful of these approaches is the supercritical fluid method of manufacture, which involves controlled crystallization of drugs from dispersion in supercritical fluids, notably carbon dioxide [27].

A. Propellant-Driven Metered Dose Inhalers

The formulation for a pMDI consists of several key components: propellant(s), drug, cosolvents, and surfactants.

Propellants may be of a number of different types: CFCs, hydrofluoroalkanes (HFAs), or alkanes. The composition impacts upon performance. A numerical system is employed to identify fluorinated propellants. The rules governing this numbering system allow the molecular structure to be derived from the numerical descriptor. The rules may be listed as follows:

The digit on the extreme right, e.g., propellant 114, represents the number of chlorine atoms.

The second digit from the right, e.g., propellant 114, represents one more than the number of hydrogen atoms.

The third digit from the right, e.g., propellant 114, represents one less than the number of carbon atoms.

A subscripted lowercase letter represents the symmetry of the molecule: the earlier in the alphabet, the more symmetrical the molecule being described, e.g., propellant 134a.

Two additional rules have not been required for pharmaceutical purposes but may be included for completeness:

A fourth number from the right indicates the number of double bonds in the molecule.

A prefixed lowercase c indicates that the molecule is cyclic.

The vapor pressure and density of propellants are employed to assist in formulation. The vapor pressure dictates the force of emission of the droplets from the metering valve of the inhaler. The force of emission is derived from the difference between the product vapor pressure and atmospheric pressure. The density of the propellant may be matched to the drug particles to assist in the suspension formulation stability. Table 5 shows characteristic physicochemical properties of the common propellants.

Hydrocarbons have also been considered as potential propellants for pharmaceutical aerosols. To date concerns regarding flammability seem to have precluded significant developments with propane, isobutane, butane, and mixtures of these alkanes [28].

A cosolvent, typically ethanol, may be used to bring drug into solution. A small number of surfactants (sorbitan trioleate, oleic acid, and lecithin) may be dispersed in propellant systems and can aid in suspension stability and in valve lubrication.

The significance of a propellant is its ability to generate high-velocity emission as it vaporizes upon equilibrium with atmospheric pressure. Raoult's and Dalton's laws may be applied to estimate the vapor pressure of propellant blends.

Raoult's law states that the partial pressure (P') is equal to the product of the pure vapor pressure (P^0) and the mole fraction (X) of the component being considered as follows [29]:

$$P' = P^0 X \tag{6}$$

where for a two-component system (a and b):

$$X_a = n_a/(n_a + n_b)$$

and

$$X_b = n_b/(n_a + n_b)$$

where n_a and n_b are the number of moles of components a and b, respectively, present in the product.

Dalton's law states that the total vapor pressure (P_T) over a solution is equal to the sum of partial vapor pressures attributable to each component $(a, b, \ldots n)$.

Table 5 Physicochemical Properties of Chlorofluorocarbon and Alternative Hydrofluorcarbon Propellants

Propellant (structure)	Molecular wt. (g/mol)	Vapor press. (psia at 25°C)	Boiling pt. (°C at 1 atm)	Density (gcm^{-3}@25°C)
011 (CCl_3F)	137.4	13.4	23.8	1.48
012 (CCl_2F_2)	120.9	94.5	− 29.8	1.31
114 ($C_2Cl_2F_4$)	170.9	27.6	3.8	1.46
134a(CH_2FCF_3)	102.0	96.0	− 26.5	1.20
227($CHF_2C_2F_5$)	170.0	72.6	− 17.3	1.42

$$P_T = P'_a + P'_b + \cdots + P'_n \qquad (7)$$

An empirical relationship between median droplet diameter and atomizer conditions has been demonstrated [30]. The relationship is described in the following expression.

$$D_i = \frac{C_s}{Q_e^m[(P_e - P_A)/P_A]^n} \qquad (8)$$

where

C_s = a constant, relating pressure and quality to droplet size
Q_e = mass fraction of vapor phase in the expansion chamber
m = a constant relating quality of flow to droplet size
n = a constant relating pressure to droplet size
P_e and P_A = are the pressure downstream of discharge orifice and atmospheric pressure, respectively

A theoretical approach has also been taken to predicting the droplet formation from a pMDI, and this was followed by experimental validation studies [31,32].

The container components include a canister, valve, and actuator. Each of these components should be considered in the preparation of a pMDI product. The majority of products marketed are in either plastic-coated glass or aluminum containers of various sizes. Figure 4A shows the assembled components of a pMDI in operation. The therapeutic usefulness of this device stems from the accurate metering of small doses of drug, which is achieved by a small but complex metering valve. The components of a metering valve are shown in Fig. 4B.

The performance should be evaluated in terms of drug and component physical and chemical compatibilities. Particle size and emitted dose determinations are required. Through-life performance should be evaluated as this is a multidosing reservoir system. The influence of temperature and humidity on stability and performance of the product should also be considered.

Filling may be conducted at low temperature or high pressure and requires specialized equipment. Low-temperature filling is carried out at a temperature substantially lower than the boiling point of the propellant to allow manipulation at room temperature in an open vessel. Pressure filling is conducted in a sealed system from which the propellant is dispensed at its equilibrium vapor pressure at room temperature through the valve of the container [33].

B. Dry Powder Inhalers

The forces of interaction between particles present barriers to their flow and dispersion. The major forces of interaction are van der Waals, electrostatic, and capillary forces [34].

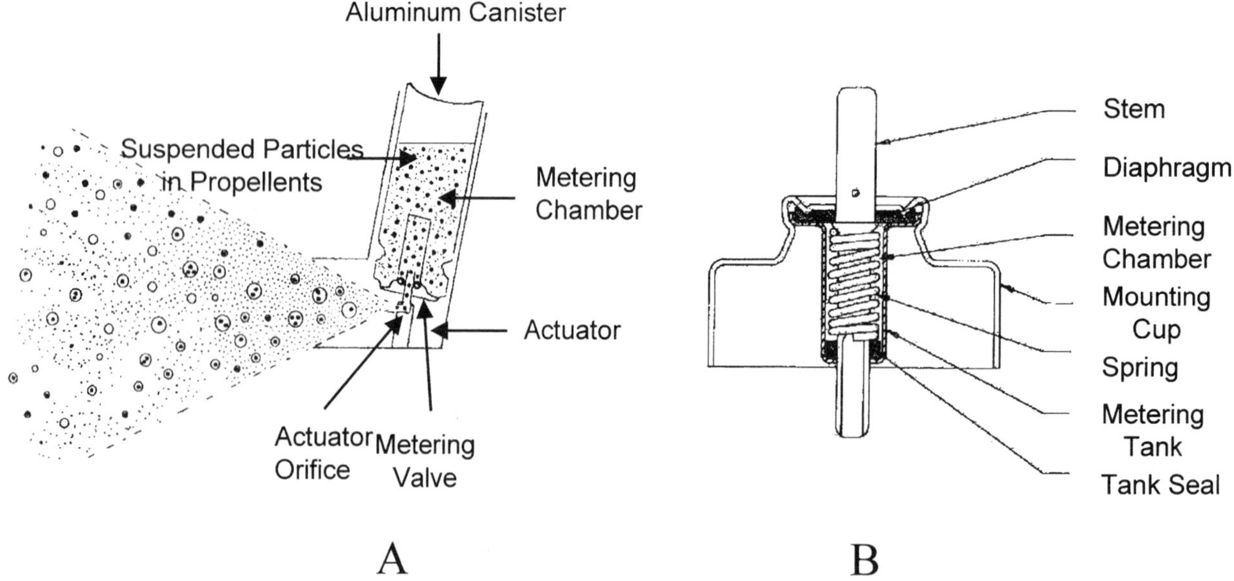

Fig. 4 (A) Propellant-driven metered dose inhaler. (B) Metering valve.

Van der Waals forces are derived from the energy of interaction between two molecules, V_{ss}. These can be derived from London's theory as follows:

$$V_{ss} = -\frac{3}{4} h\nu_0 \frac{\alpha^2}{\alpha^6} \tag{9}$$

where α is the polarizability, h is Planck's constant, and ν_0 the characteristic frequency. Because γ_0 is found in the ultraviolet region of the absorption spectra and plays a key role in optical dispersion, the intermolecular London–van der Waals forces are also called dispersion forces. These forces operate at short ranges but when integrated over all molecules give rise to large interparticulate forces.

The dipole-induced dipole interactions are summed over all atoms and expressed as the Hamaker constant (A). The total molecular potential, U_m, for two perfectly spherical particles with diameters d_1 and d_2 is:

$$U_m = \frac{A d_1 d_2}{12z(d_1 + d_2)} \tag{10}$$

where z is the shortest interparticle distance.

The Hamaker constant is given by:

$$A = \pi^2 n_2 n_2 C_{ss} \tag{11}$$

where n_1 and n_2 are molecular densities and C_{ss} is the London–van der Waals constant.

Two dissimilar materials, with Hamaker constants, A_{11} and A_{22}, interact as follows:

$$A_{12} = (A_{11} \cdot A_{22})^{0.5} \tag{12}$$

Equation (10) may be applied when $z \ll D = d_1 d_2/(d_1 + d_2)$. This is not a practical limitation, but an applicable equation can be obtained by differentiating Eq. (10) with respect to z:

$$F = \frac{\delta}{\delta z}(U_m) = \frac{AD}{12z^2} \tag{13}$$

The attractive force (F) is dependent on the Hamaker constant and the shortest distance between the particles, z. F may be decreased by decreasing A or increasing z. Theoretically, the Hamaker constant can be decreased by decreasing the densities of the two interacting particles. Since the separation distance plays a significant role in van der Waals attraction, any means to increase this distance will reduce the attractive force and increase the ease of dispersion. Surface roughening and the use of spacer particulates can increase interparticulate separation with the improved particle dispersion.

Electrostatic forces are smaller than van der Waals forces for conducting particles, but most pharmaceutical products are poor conductors. Therefore, electrostatic charge must be considered. Two adjacent solid surfaces give rise to a contact potential and in turn electrostatic attractive forces that increase powder aggregation. Particle collisions and surface contacts give rise to contact charging and additional electrostatic interactions. Tribo-electric charging, a potential difference between two interacting particles having different work functions, further contributes to electrostatic interactions. The potential difference causes electrons to migrate from the body that has a smaller work function to that with the larger until equilibrium is achieved. A reduction in charge does not always occur on contact with another particle whether the latter is charged or uncharged. A persistent charge will induce an equal and opposite charge on neighboring particles or surfaces. This induced electrical force on a particle may be expressed as follows:

$$F_1 = \frac{\varepsilon q^2}{h^2} \tag{14}$$

where q is the charge on the particle and h is the separation distance between the adhering particles in a dielectric medium, ε.

The Coulomb equation describes tribo-electric charging (F_c) between spherical particle and an adjacent uncharged particle:

$$F_c = q^2\left(1 - \frac{h}{(R^2 + h^2)^{0.5}}\right) \times \frac{1}{16\pi\varepsilon_0 h^2} \tag{15}$$

where R is the particle radius, q the charge, h the separation distance, and ε_0 the permittivity of vacuum. This Coulomb attraction reduces to zero in a humid environment because of decharging of the system, but attractive forces then become complicated by capillary forces of interaction.

In the presence of a potential difference particles of different work functions are brought into contact by a force of attraction defined as follows:

$$F_W = \pi\varepsilon_0 \frac{R(\Delta U)^2}{h} \tag{16}$$

Capillary forces increase in relationship to the relative humidity (RH) of the ambient air. At greater than 65% RH, fluid condenses in the space between adjacent particles. This leads to liquid bridges causing attractive forces due to the surface tension of the water.

For smooth, spherical particles the force experienced is:

$$F_H = 2\pi\gamma R \tag{17}$$

where γ is the surface tension completely wetting the surface of particles of radius, R.

Liquid between the surface of two solid bodies gives rise to boundary forces. A pressure difference arises and is known as the capillary pressure (P_c). This can be calculated from Laplace's equation.

$$P_c = \gamma(1/R_1 + 1/R_2) \tag{18}$$

where γ is the surface tension at the liquid/gas interface, R_1 and R_2 are the principal radii of curvature of the interface.

It should also be remembered that surface asperities might increase the potential for mechanical interlocking of particles, which will influence the aggregation state and ease of dispersion of particles.

The formulation of dry powder inhalers is dependent upon the nature of particles employed in the formulation. The delivery of dry powder products is dependent upon effective dispersion of particles in respirable size ranges. This has been brought about by blending with carrier particles, most notably lactose [35]. Other approaches include developing particles to overcome the forces of interaction, which include van der Waals forces, capillary forces, electrostatic forces, and mechanical interlocking. Porous particles have been produced that exhibit unique properties of dispersion and aerodynamic behavior. These particles disperse readily since their van der Waals forces are smaller and since they also have fewer points of contact for electrostatic and capillary forces to develop. Once airborne, these particles, which may be geometrically large, behave as aerodynamically small particles, following Eq. (2).

The metering of dry powder inhalers is closely linked to the device itself and may be divided into three common systems: capsules, multidosing blister packs, and reservoir systems. The consideration that goes into these metering systems include convenience to the patients, stability on storage, compatibility with product, and ease of filling.

The components of a DPI are the formulation, themetering system, and the device. The device may involve various dispersion mechanisms, pressure drops.

The performance of a dry powder inhaler involves evaluation of component compatibility and influence on device performance. The performance of commercial passive inhaler devices is influenced by the pressure drop generated by a patient during an inspiratory flow cycle [36]. Recently, it has been suggested that particle size and emitted dose determinations should be conducted as a function of pressure drop. For reservoir powder devices, such as the Turbuhaler [37], evaluation throughout the life of the device is required as part of a stability program. For unit dose systems such as the Spinhaler [38], barrier integrity must be evaluated for the unit dose packaging.

Figure 5 shows examples of two dry powder inhalers, the Turbuhaler and the Diskus, currently marketed in the United States for the delivery of the steroids, budesonide and fluticosone, respectively. Table 6 shows the major elements of a number of passive dry powder inhalers. In addition to the commercially available passive inhalation products, a number of active dispersion systems are under development; the key characteristics of selected devices are shown in Table 7.

C. Nebulizers

Nebulizer formulation conforms to sterile product preparation, which means that drug stability in solution in the presence of additives must be evaluated. Historically, it was sufficient to use antimicrobial agents in the formulation, notably benzalkonium chloride. Adding antimicrobials is not now considered an acceptable approach to the formulation of nebulizer solutions. The solubility of the drug is important since it may impact upon the performance of the solution in a selected nebulizer. Additives may form complexes with the drug.

Components include an energy source (gas, electrical), a site of energy input to solution (capillary tubes, piezoelectric plate), a means of removing large droplets (baffle plate), and tubing and a face mask to deliver aerosol.

The mechanisms of delivery are either air-blast or air-jet and ultrasonic systems. The theory for each of these mechanisms has been elucidated to the same degree.

Droplet delivery from an airblast nebulizer is governed by the surface tension, density and viscosity of the fluid, and the applied pressure, which can be passive or forced. Droplet breakup is illustrated in Fig. 6. Droplets form during this breakup at a critical Weber number (We):

$$We_{\text{crit}} = 8/C_D \tag{19}$$

where C_D is the coefficient of discharge, and

$$We = \rho_A \frac{U_R^2}{\eta} D \tag{20}$$

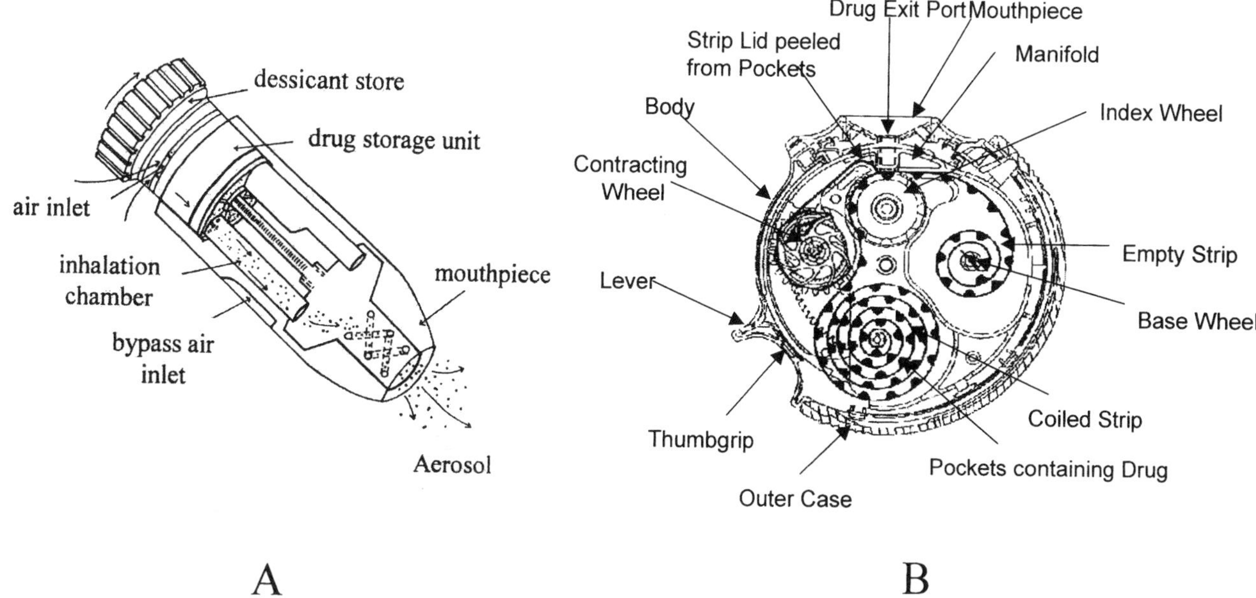

Fig. 5 Examples of two dry powder inhalers: (A) the Turbuhaler™; (B) the Discus™.

Table 6 Characteristics for Selected Passive Dry Powder Inhalers

Inhaler	Carrier	Dose	Powder supply	Passive fluidization	Dispersion
Inhalator Ingelheim™	Glucose	6	Capsules	Capillary	Shear force
Diskhaler™	Lactose	4, 8	Blister	Shear force	Turbulence
Diskus™	Lactose	60	Blister	Shear force	Turbulence
Turbuhaler™	–	200	Reservoir	Shear force, capillary	Shear Force
Easyhaler™	Lactose	200	Reservoir	Shear force	Turbulence
MAGhaler™	Lactose	200–500	Tablet	Mechanical	Mechanical

Source: Modified from Ref. 35.

Table 7 Characteristics for Selected Active Dispersion Dry Powder Inhalers

Inhaler	Carrier	Doses	Powder supply	Active fluidization	Dispersion
Spiros™	n/a	1, 16, or 30	Unit dose blister or casette	Mechanical	Turbulence, impaction, shear force
Prohaler™	Mannitol			Gas assist	Turbulence, shear force
Dynamic Powder Disperser™	Lactose	12	Cartridge	Gas assist	Turbulence, shear force
Inhale Device™	Lactose	1	Blister	Gas assist	Turbulence, shear force

n/a, Information not available.
Source: Modified from Ref. 35.

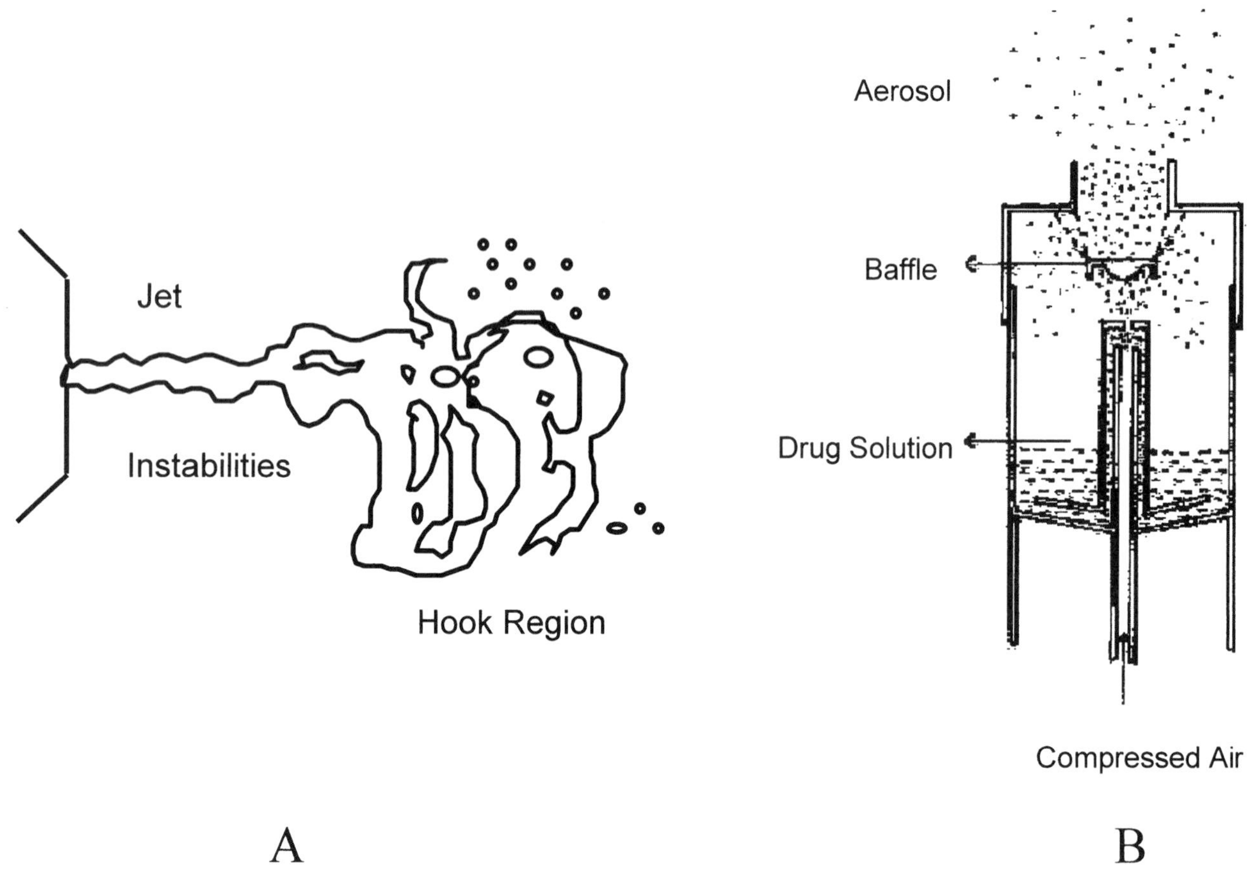

Fig. 6 (A) Droplet formation. (B) Droplet delivery from an airblast nebulizer.

where:

ρ_A = the air density
U_R = the velocity
D = the diameter of the nozzle
η = the liquid viscosity

Droplets are dispersed from nebulizer nozzles by one of five basic mechanisms based on Bernoulli (Venturi) effect.

There are two categories of arrangement of liquid feed supply with respect to the driving gas supply: separate liquid and air feed nozzles and coaxial nozzles. The latter coaxial arrangement has four potential orientations: central gas with internal mixing, central gas with external mixing, central liquid with internal mixing, and central liquid with external mixing. The high-pressure airstream passes over or around the liquid feed nozzle, inducing a low-pressure region, which draws solution through a capillary. The liquid is subsequently dispersed in the air.

Performance of nebulizers is not measured in the same manner as pMDIs and DPIs. Since the drug solution is not supplied with the device, the time scale of compatibility is much smaller. Droplet size and distribution and dose delivery are, however, very important.

The manifestation of through-life evaluation, which is important to these devices, is the delivery of a single dose. The emitted dose and droplet size may vary from the beginning to the end of the delivery period.

III. CHARACTERIZATION OF PHARMACEUTICAL AEROSOLS

A. Emitted Dose

The therapeutic effect of aerosols is dependent upon their delivery to the lungs. Clearly, the first measure of the potential to deliver drug to the lungs is the dose delivered from the device. A number of methods have been suggested for this purpose. Two unit dose samplers are popular and are shown in Fig. 7. A sampler consisting of a tube and absolute filter, through which air is drawn, enables the collection of bolus aerosols delivered by MDIs and DPIs, as shown in Fig. 7A. These airborne particulates are sampled at a fixed flow rate of 60 L/min. Nebulizer output is more difficult to collect as it is delivered over an extended period of time and often saturates filters, compromising their collection efficiency. These devices may more easily be evaluated by passing them through an immersed sintered glass or steel frit, as shown in Fig. 7B.

B. Particle Size Characterization

In Vitro Characterization

Inertial impaction is the method of choice for evaluating particle or droplet size delivery from pharmaceutical aerosol systems. This method lends itself readily to theoretical analysis. It has been evaluated in general terms [39] and for specific impactors [40]. Inertial impaction employs Stokes' law to determine aerodynamic diameter of particles being evaluated. This has the advantage of incorporating shape and density effects into a single term.

The collection efficiency of particles at a stage of an impactor is based on curvilinear motion and assumes Reynolds' numbers for flow greater than 500 but less than 3000. Figure 8A illustrates the principle of inertial sampling in which particles with high momentum travel in the initial direction of flow of an airstream impacting on an obstructing surface and those with low momentum adjust to the new direction of flow and pass around the obstruction. The efficiency of this phenomenon can be described as follows:

$$d_{50}[C(D)]^{0.5} = \left(\frac{9(D_j(Stk_{50}))}{\rho_p U}\right)^{0.5} \tag{21}$$

where d_{50} is the 50% collection efficiency cut-off diameter for the stage, D_j and U are the jet diameter and linear velocity, respectively, Stk_{50} is the Stokes' number for 50% efficiency, which by definition for circular orifices is 0.22, and ρ_p is the particle density usually taken as unity (1 g cm^{-3}) for aerodynamic purposes.

The linear velocity can be derived from the ratio of the volumetric flow rate through the impactor divided by the cross-sectional area of the orifice(s).

Theoretical approximations of deposition on impactor collection plates can be validated by calibration

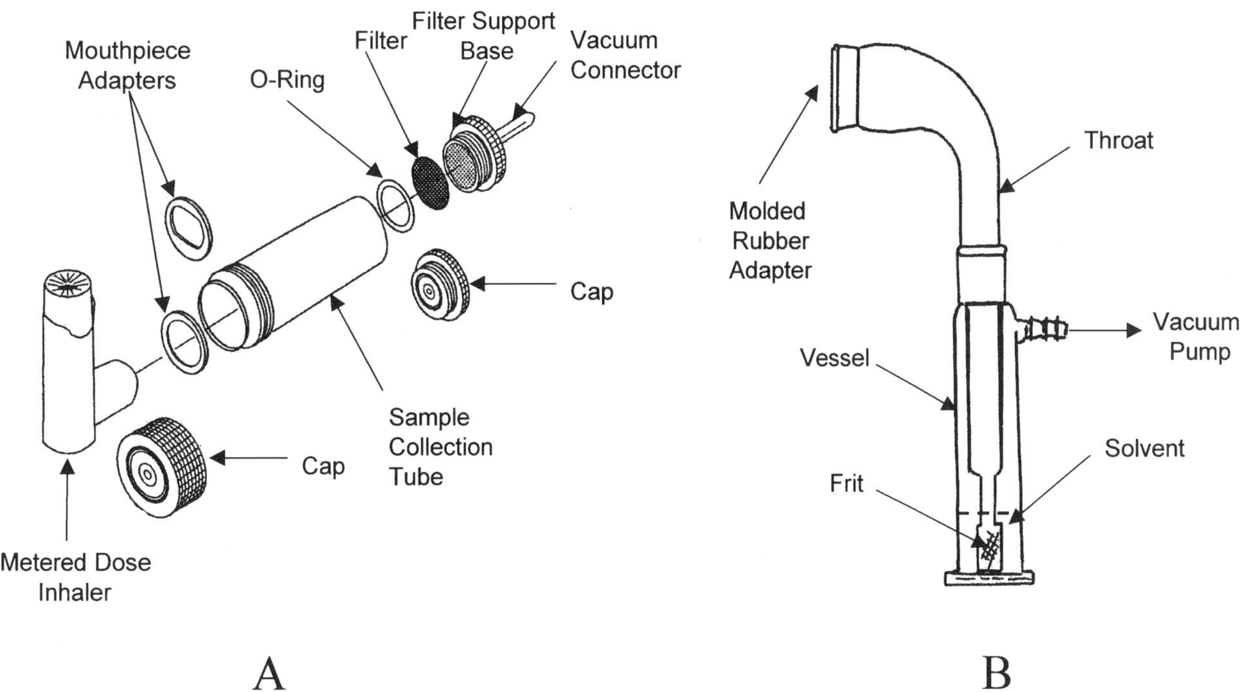

Fig. 7 Unit dose collection: (A) teflon tube; (B) glass samplers.

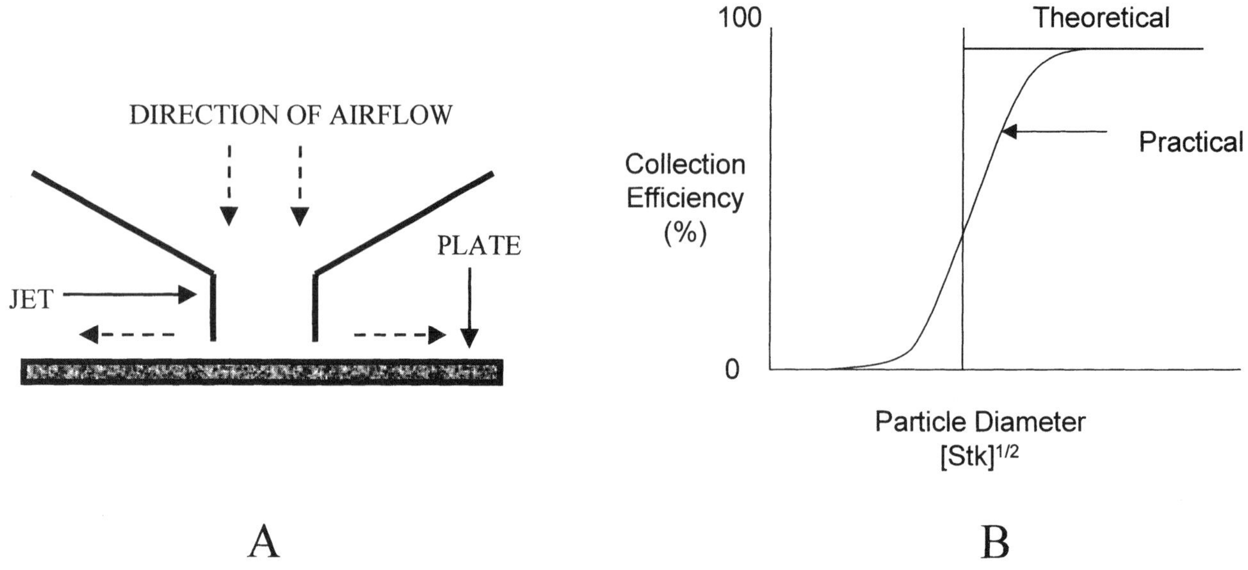

Fig. 8 (A) General principle of inertial sampling through a jet onto a collection plate. (B) Generalized collection efficiency curve.

of the instrument using monodisperse aerosol particles. A number of methods exist for the preparation of monodisperse aerosols, including vibrating orifice aerosol generation [41] and spinning disc aerosol generation [42]. Schematic diagrams of the key elements of these devices are shown in Fig. 9. Each of these methods lends itself to theoretical prediction of particle size output, which is important to the calibration process.

The droplet size delivered from a vibrating orifice monodisperse aerosol generator can be derived from the following expressions:

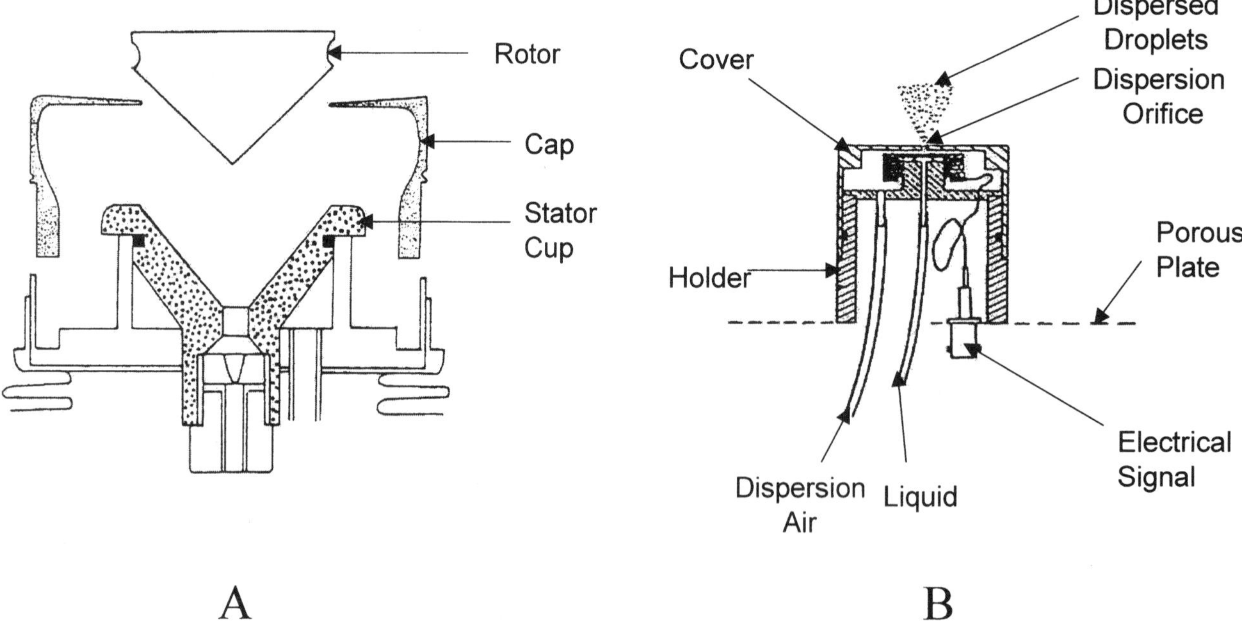

Fig. 9 (A) Exploded diagram of spinning disc aerosol generator. (B) Vibrating orifice aerosol generator.

$$d_d = ((6Q)/(\pi f)^{0.33} \quad (22)$$

where Q is the volumetric flow rate and f is the frequency of the piezoelectric ceramic.

When a nonvolatile solute is incorporated in a volatile solvent droplet, the dry particle diameter can be derived from the following expression:

$$d_p = C^{0.33}\, d_d \quad (23)$$

where C is the volumetric concentration of the nonvolatile solute.

The droplet size delivered from a spinning disc monodisperse aerosol generator can be derived from the following expressions:

$$d = (k/\omega)[\gamma/(D\rho_l)]^{0.5} \quad (24)$$

where:

ω = the angular disk velocity
γ = the surface tension
D = the disc diameter
ρ_l = the liquid density

when the liquid fed to the disk contains solids in a concentration, C, and the droplets are dried slowly in air, the diameter of the resultant spherical particles, d_p, is given by:

$$d_p = [C/\rho]^{0.33} d \quad (25)$$

An alternative method of calibration involves the dispersion of monodisperse polystyrene microparticles. This has recently been made an efficient process by the incorporation of these particles in pMDI suspension to allow for metering of small well-dispersed boluses sufficient for use as aerosol calibration standards [43].

Figure 8B shows the characteristic theoretical and practical collection efficiency curve. The x-axis may be plotted as particle diameter, in which case a series of curves at ever-decreasing sizes representing different stages of the impactor would exist. Converting the data to the square root of Stokes' number overlays each of the particle size curves. The characteristic Stokes' number for circular jets is 0.22.

Figure 10A depicts a stacked Andersen eight-stage impactor with calibrated cut-off diameters of 9.0, 5.8, 4.7, 3.3, 2.1, 1.1, 0.7, and 0.4 μm and a lower absolute filter (0.22 μm) when operated at 28.3 L/min. Figure 10B depicts a four-stage liquid impinger with

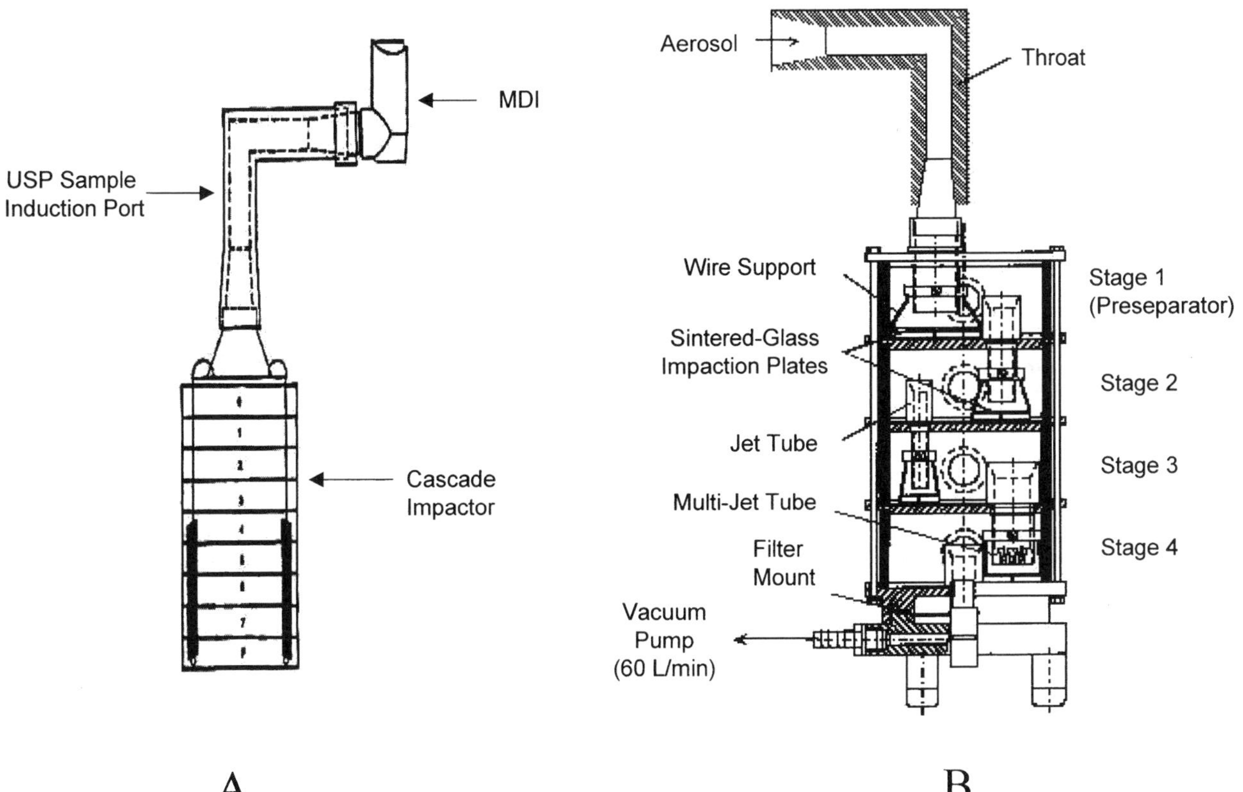

Fig. 10 (A) Andersen eight-stage nonviable inertial sampler. (B) Four-stage liquid impinger.

calibrated cut-off diameters of 13.3, 6.7, 3.2, and 1.7 μm at 60 L/min.

Inertial impactors are calibrated at designated flow rates. This may vary depending on the instrument [35]. The range of flow rates selected for early impactors was based on passive inhalation of environmental and occupational particulates. Thus, the Delron, Batelle Type, six-stage impactor operates at 12.5 L/min and the Andersen eight-stage nonviable impactor operates at 28.3 L/min (1 ACFM). The sampling of pharmaceutical aerosols has proven more difficult than ambient particulates. After a period of debate regarding suitable inlets for the device, the USP adopted a right-angled tube as the standard for sampling pMDI output [44]. When used with the Andersen impactor, the inlet is arranged immediately above the first stage of the impactor.

Dry powder aerosols are more complicated to sample as the commercially available devices disperse the aerosol on the patient's inspiratory flow. In order to challenge the efficiency of these devices, it is important to sample at multiple flow rates. The standard flow rate has become 60 L/min. Additional flow rates of 30 (28.3) and 90 L/min have also been employed. Each impactor must be calibrated at the different flow rates employed. In recent compendial specifications the duration of sampling (4 s) and pressure drop across the device (4 kPa) has also been suggested. This corrects for the effort on the part of a patient in a single breath.

There have been attempts to conduct in vitro experiments in a manner that gives more meaningful data with regard to lung deposition. These methods, which are loosely based on inertial impaction, utilize inspiratory flow cycles rather than fixed flow rates for sampling the aerosol. These "electronic lung" approaches give interesting results, which may prove useful in the development of aerosol products. Their suitability as quality control tools is influenced by the effect of variable flow rates on impactor calibration.

General Sizing Methods

A number of alternative sizing methods are available, and these are described in Table 8. The American Association of Pharmaceutical Scientists, Inhalation Focus Group conducted a comprehensive review of available methods, which was published in a series of articles identified in the last column of the table. All of the methods described either have been or are currently employed in the development of aerosol products. However, at this time only the inertial samplers, cascade impactors and impingers appear in compendial standards and in regulatory guidelines [44–46]. Other methods such as thermal imaging are also under development and may give complementary size information to the current methods.

In Vivo Characterization

The use of animals to evaluate aerosol performance has certain limitations. Toxicological studies have been conducted utilizing whole body or nose-only exposure chambers [47]. However, since pharmaceutical aerosols are not administered as standing clouds, dose estimation by this method would be difficult. Certain species are good pharmacological or immunological models for humans. Only large animals are capable of inhaling or receiving a propelled bolus dose equivalent to

Table 8 General Sizing Methods

Sizing technique	Description	Size range (μm)	Limitations	Ref.
Microscopy with image analysis	Light SEM	1–300 0.2–300	Sampling shape effects	49
Inertial sampling methods	Impactors impingers	0.2–20 0.2–20	Number of data points to construct distribution, re-entrainment	50, 51
Right angle light scattering	Population measure	0.5–40	Sampling refractive Index	52
Phase doppler anemometry	Cumulative with time	>0.5[a]	Limited to droplets, sampling	53
Laser diffraction	Population measure	0.1–800	Obscuration, sampling	54
Time-of-flight	Cumulative with time	0.4–100	Co-incidence errors, sampling	55
Holography	Population measure	3–1000	Obscuration, co-incidence, sampling	56
Direct imaging	Photography	5–1000	Obscuration, coincidence, sampling	57

[a]Depends on optical configuration [58].

a human. Consequently, instillation and insufflation have been employed to deliver drugs to the lungs of various rodent species. Figure 11 shows an insufflator (PennCentury, Philadelphia, PA) and illustrates the dimensions of the device, which is suitable for delivery of powders to rats or guinea pigs [48]. Similar devices are available for delivery of drugs to mice and for the delivery of aqueous solutions. Solution volumes are limited to several hundred microliters.

The field of aerosol science is somewhat behind other areas in terms of in vivo/in vitro correlations. Gamma scintigraphic and single positron emission computer-aided tomography imaging methods have been used to evaluate the site of deposition of drugs administered as aerosols. Gamma scintigraphy has become a routine method for the comparison of the performance of various products [59,60]. It has been proposed that comparison of lung deposition might be employed as a surrogate bioequivalence measure for drugs that act in the lung. This seems a reasonable proposition as the receptors being targeted are located in the airways. It is not quite as clear that site of deposition translates into bioequivalence for systemically acting agents.

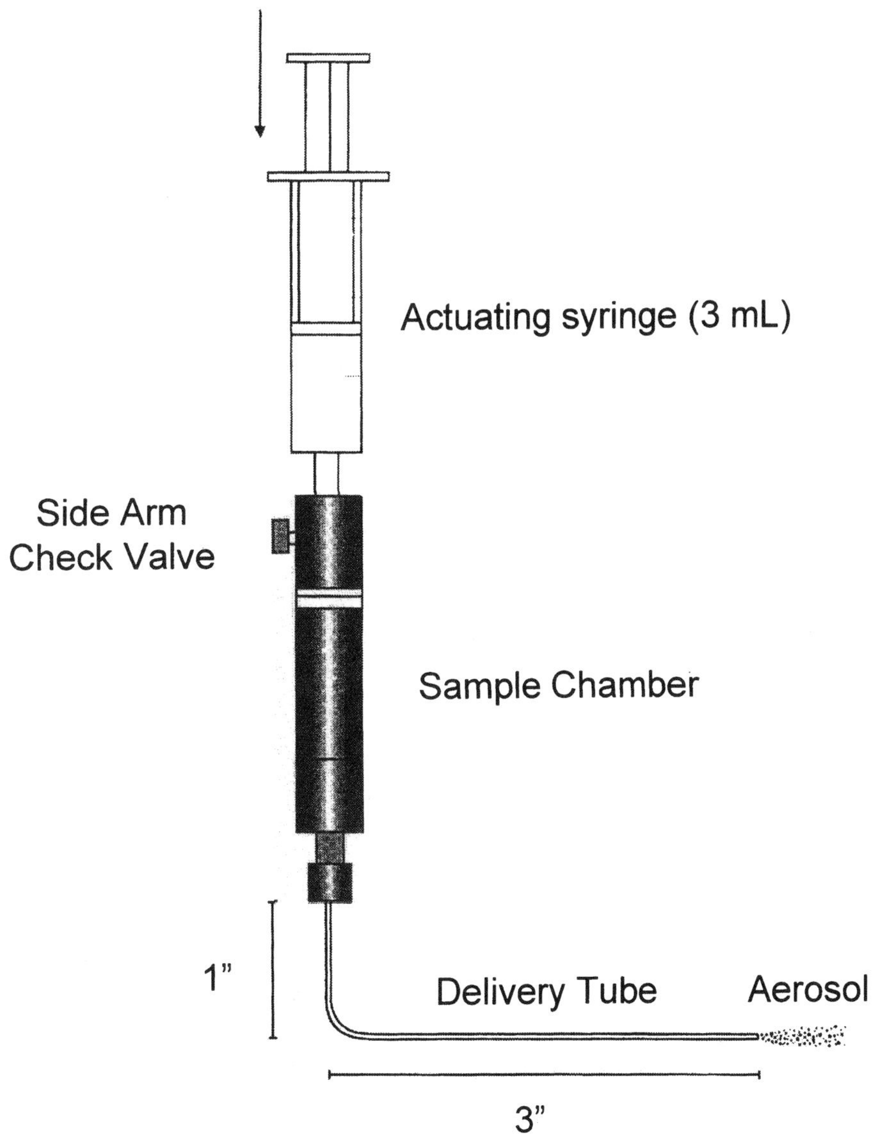

Fig. 11 PennCentury powder insufflator.

Table 9 Examples of Polypeptides and Their Residence Times in the Lungs

Polypeptide	Molecular Weight	*t*max (h)
Leuteinizing hormone–releasing hormone	1,067	1
1-Deamino-8-D-arginine vasopressin	1,209	0.5
Calcitonin	3,418	0.25
Parathyroid hormone	4,109	0.25
Insulin	5,700	0.25
Granulocyte colony–stimulating factor	18,600	1.5
Interferon-α	19,000	6
Human growth hormone	22,000	0.75
Alpha-1-anti	45,000	12
Albumin	68,000	20
Immunoglobulin G	150,000	16

Source: Ref. 64.

C. Efficacy

In the years since the first pMDI asthma therapy was introduced, a host of new products have been developed. The major therapeutic categories are β_2-adrenergic agonists, anticholinergics, glucocorticosteroids, and other anti-inflammatory agents (cromolyn, nedocromil) [61]. The β_2-adrenergic agonists and anticholinergics act on the parasympathetic and sympathetic nervous system to induce bronchodilatation, which relieves bronchoconstriction, a symptom of asthma. Since the underlying cause of asthma is small airways inflammation, glucocorticoids act as anti-inflammatories. Cromolyn blocks the production of histamine, an inflammatory mediator, by stabilizing mast cells, among other actions, which are not fully understood.

Long-acting agents such as salmeterol and formoterol have superseded short-duration bronchodilators such as albuterol and fenoterol. In addition, more potent, site-specific, rapid-onset glucocorticoids, such as fluticosone and budesonide, have superseded the delayed onset of action of less specific molecules such as budesonide.

As greater control of the disease state is achieved with aerosol therapy, manufacturers are considering combining some of their most successful products to achieve bronchodilation and anti-inflammatory effect in a single dose. These combinations may increase interest in the use of anticholinergics in addition to β_2-adrenergic agonists.

The systemic delivery of drugs was pioneered with a pMDI product, leuprolide acetate, for the treatment of prostate cancer. A considerable amount of work was conducted to demonstrate feasibility of delivery of this nonapeptide [62]. Insulin aerosol development has followed closely behind leuprolide, with a number of companies now looking at various formulations of insulin [63] from pMDI, DPI, and aqueous delivery systems. A range of polypeptide molecules have been studied for their potential, as shown in Table 9. It is now accepted that as a general guide the window of opportunity for acceptable rates of delivery of such molecules ranges from 5 to 20 kDa [64].

IV. CONCLUSION

Drug delivery to the respiratory tract has been characterized in the past decade by an increase in knowledge of drug droplet or particle manufacture, behavior, aerosol dispersion, lung deposition and clearance. The number of diseases for which aerosol therapy may be applicable has increased dramatically. The pharmaceutical scientist is no longer limited to pulmonary diseases as therapeutic targets. Substantial progress has been made in every area of pharmaceutical aerosol science, and it is anticipated that this will ultimately lead to many new therapies.

BIBLIOGRAPHY

A. L. Adjei and P. K. Gupta, *Inhalation Delivery of Therapeutic Peptides and Proteins*, Marcel Dekker, New York, 1997.

P. R. Byron, *Respiratory Drug Delivery*, CRC, Boca Raton, FL, 1990.

H. Derendorf and G. Hochhaus, *Handbook of Pharmacokinetic/Pharmacodynamic Correlation*, CRC Press, Boca Raton, FL, 1995.

P. Gehr and J. Heyder, *Particle-Lung Interactions*, Marcel Dekker, New York, 2000.

N. A. Fuchs, *Mechanics of Aerosols*, Dover Press, Minneola, NY, 1964.

D. Ganderton and T. Jones, *Drug Delivery to the Respiratory Tract*, VCH/Ellis Horwood, New York, 1987.

A. J. Hickey, *Pharmaceutical Inhalation Aerosol Technology*, Marcel Dekker, New York, 1992.

A. J. Hickey, *Inhalation Aerosols*, Marcel Dekker, New York, 1996.

W. C. Hinds, *Aerosol Technology*, 2nd ed., John Wiley and Sons, New York, 1999.

M. A. Kaliner, P. J. Barnes, and C. G. A. Persson, *Asthma, Its Pathology and Treatment*, Marcel Dekker, New York, 1991.

A. H. Lefebvre, *Atomization and Sprays*, Hemisphere Publishing Corporation, New York, 1989.

S. P. Newman, *Deposition and Effects of Inhalation Aerosols*, AB DRACO (subsidiary to ASTRA), Lund, Sweden, 1983.

T. S. Purewal and D. J. W. Grant, *Metered Dose Inhaler Technology*, Interpharm Press, Inc., Buffalo Grove, IL, 1998.

P. Reist, *Aerosol Science and Technology*, 2nd Ed., 1993.

REFERENCES

1. JJ Sciarra. Pharmaceutical aerosols. In: L Lachman, HA Lieberman, JL Kanig, eds. The Theory and Practice of Industrial Pharmacy. Philadelphia: Lea and Febiger, 1970, pp. 605–638.
2. CG Thiel. From Susie's question to CFC free: an inventor's perspective on forty years of MDI development and regulation. Phoenix, Arizona: Respiratory Drug Delivery, V, 1996, pp. 115–123.
3. MJ Molina, FS Rowland. Stratospheric sink for chlorofluoromethanes: chlorine atom catalyzed destruction of ozone. Nature 249:1810, 1974.
4. Montreal Protocol on Substances That Deplete the Ozone Layer, 26 1LM 1541, 1987.
5. AJ Hickey, CA Dunbar. A new millenium for inhaler technology. Pharm Technol 21:116–125, 1997.
6. I Gonda. Targeting by Deposition. In: AJ Hickey, ed. Pharmaceutical Inhalation Aerosol Technology. New York: Marcel Dekker, Inc., 1992, pp. 61–82.
7. T Allen. Particle Size Measurement. 4 ed. London: Chapman and Hall, 1993.
8. OG Raabe. Aerosol aerodynamic size conventions for inertial sampler calibration. J Air Pollution Control Assoc 26:856–860, 1976.
9. WC Hinds. Aerosol Technology. 2nd ed. New York: John Wiley and Sons, Inc., 1999.
10. GA Ferron, G Oberdorster, R Henneberg. Estimation of the deposition of aerosolized drugs in the human respiratory tract due to hygroscopic growth. J Aerosol Med 2:271–283, 1989.
11. AJ Hickey, TB Martonen. Behavior of hygroscopic pharmaceutical aerosols and the influence of hydrophobic additives. Pharm Res 10:1–7, 1993.
12. ER Weibel. Morphometry of the Human Lung. Berlin: Springer Verlag, 1963.
13. K Horsfield, MJ Woldenberg. Branching ratio and growth of tree-like structures. Respir Physiol 63:97–107, 1986.
14. W Findeisen. Über das Absetzen kleiner, in der Luft suspendierten Teilchen in der menschlichen Lunge bei der Atmung. Arch Ges Physiol 236:367, 1935.
15. TB Martonen, I Katz, K Fults, AJ Hickey. Use of analytically defined estimates of aerosol respirable fraction to predict lower lung deposition. Pharm Res 9:1634–1639, 1992.
16. TF Hatch, P Gross. Physical factors in respiratory deposition of aerosols. In: Pulmonary Deposition and Retention of Inhaled Aerosols. New York: Academic Press, 1964, pp. 27–43.
17. VW Chaffee. Surgery of laboratory animals. In: EC Melby, NH Altman, eds. Handbook of Laboratory Animal Science. Cleveland: CRC Press, Inc., 1974, pp. 233–273.
18. RF Phalen, MJ Oldham. Tracheobronchial airway structure as revealed by casting techniques. Am Rev Respir Dis 128:S1–S4, 1983.
19. HD Landahl. On the removal of air-borne droplets by the human respiratory tract. I. The lung Bull Math Biophys 12:43, 1950.
20. ICRP, Publication 66. Human respiratory tract model for radiological protection. Ann ICRP 24:1–3, 1994.
21. RM Effros, GR Mason. Measurements of pulmonary epithelial permeability in vivo. Am Rev Respir Dis 125:S59–S65, 1983.
22. PR Byron. Prediction of drug residence times in regions of the human respiratory tract following aerosol inhalation. J Pharm Sci 75:433–438, 1986.
23. I Gonda. Drugs Administered Directly into the Respiratory Tract: Modeling of the Duration of Effective Drug Levels. J Pharm Sci 77:340–346, 1988.
24. G Hochhaus, S Suarez, RJ Gonzalez-Rothi, H Schreier. Pulmonary Targeting of Inhaled Glucocorticoids: How Is It Influenced by Formulation? Respiratory Drug Delivery VI, Hilton Head, SC, 1998, pp. 45–52.
25. AJ Hickey. Lung deposition and clearance of pharmaceutical aerosols: What can be learned from inhalation toxicology and industrial hygiene? Aerosol Sci Technol 18:290–304, 1993.
26. MT Vidgren, PA Vidgren, TP Paronen. Comparison of physical and inhalation properties of spray-dried and mechanically micronized disodium cromoglycate. Int J Pharm 35:139–144, 1987.
27. M Sacchetti, MM Van Oort. Spray-drying and supercritical fluid particle generation techniques. Inhalation Aerosols: Physical and Biological Basis for Therapy 1996:337–384.

28. RN Dalby. Halohydrocarbons, pharmaceutical uses. In: J Swarbrick, JC Boylan, eds. Encyclopedia of Pharmaceutical Technology. New York: Marcel Dekker, Inc., 1993, pp. 161–180.
29. A Martin, J Swarbrick, A Cammarata. Physical Pharmacy. 3rd ed. Philadelphia: Lea & Febiger, 1983.
30. AR Clark. Metered Atomisation for Respiratory Drug Delivery. PhD thesis, Loughborough University of Technology, UK, 1991.
31. CA Dunbar, AP Watkins, JF Miller. An experimental investigation of the spray issued from a pMDI using laser diagnostic techniques. J Aerosol Med 10:351–368, 1997.
32. CA Dunbar, AP Watkins, JF Miller. A theoretical investigation of the spray issued from a pMDI. Atomiz Sprays 7:417–436, 1997.
33. C Sirand, J-P Varlet, AJ Hickey. Aerosol-filling equipment for the preparation of pressurized pack pharmaceutical formulations. In: AJ Hickey, ed. Pharmaceutical Inhalation Aerosol Technology. New York: Marcel Dekker, Inc., 1992, pp. 187–217.
34. AJ Hickey, NM Concessio, MM Van Oort, RM Platz. Factors influencing the dispersion of dry powders as aerosols. Pharm Tech 18:58–64, 82, 1994.
35. CA Dunbar, AJ Hickey, P Holzner. Dispersion and characterization of pharmaceutical dry powder aerosols. KONA 16:7–44, 1998.
36. AR Clark, AM Hollingworth. The relationship between powder inhaler resistance and peak inspiratory conditions in healthy volunteers—implications for in vitro testing. J Aerosol Med 6:99–110, 1993.
37. KIL Wetterlin. Turbuhaler: a new powder inhaler for administration of drugs to the airways. Pharm Res 5:506–508, 1988.
38. Intal-Cromolyn—A Monograph. Bedford, MA: Fisons Corporation, 1973.
39. VA Marple. Simulation of respirable penetration characteristics by inertial impaction. J Aerosol Sci 9:125–134, 1978.
40. NP Vaughan. The Andersen Impactor: calibration, wall losses and numerical simulation. J Aerosol Sci 20:67–90, 1989.
41. RN Berglund, BYH Liu. Generation of monodisperse aerosol standards. Environ Sci Technol 7:147–152, 1973.
42. PR Byron, AJ Hickey. Spinning-disk generation and drying of monodisperse solid aerosols with output concentrations sufficient for single-breath inhalation studies. J Pharm Sci 76:60–64, 1987.
43. C Vervaet, PR Byron. Polystyrene microsphere spray standards based on CFC-free inhaler technology. J Aerosol Med 13:105–115, 2000.
44. USP24. <601> Aerosols, Metered Dose Inhalers, and Dry Powder Inhalers. The United States Pharmacopoeia and National Formulary 1895–1912, 2000.
45. Draft Guidance for Industry—Nasal Spray and Inhalation Solution, Suspension and Spray Drug Products Chemistry, Manufacturing, and Controls, May 26, 1999.
46. Draft Guidance for Industry-Metered Dose Inhaler (MDI) and Dry Powder Inhaler (DPI) Drug Products Chemistry, Manufacturing, and Controls Documentation, Nov. 13, 1998.
47. BKJ Leong, ed. Inhalation Toxicology and Technology. Ann Arbor, MI: Ann Arbor Science, 1981.
48. NM Concessio, MM Van Oort, M Knowles, AJ Hickey. Pharmaceutical dry powder aerosols: correlation of powder properties with dose delivery and implications for pharmacodynamic effect. Pharm Res 16:833–839, 1999.
49. R Evans. Determination of drug particle size and morphology using optical microscopy. Pharm Technol 17:146–152, 1993.
50. SM Milosovich. Particle-size determination via cascade impaction. Pharm Technol 16:82–86, 1992.
51. PJ Atkins. Aerodynamic particle-size testing—impinger methods. Pharm Technol 16:26–32, 1993.
52. PD Jager, GA DeStefano, DP McNamara. Particle-size measurement using right-angle light scattering. Pharm Technol 17:102–120, 1993.
53. JA Ranucci, FC Chen. Phase doppler anemometry: a technique for determining aerosol plume-particle size and velocity. Pharm Technol 17:62–74, 1993.
54. J Ranucci. Dynamic plume-particle size analysis using laser diffraction. Pharm Technol 16:109–114, 1992.
55. RW Niven. Aerodynamic particle size testing using a time-of-flight aerosol beam spectrometer. Pharm Technol 17:72–78, 1993.
56. WG Gorman, FA Carroll. Aerosol particle-size determination using laser holography. Pharm Technol 17:34–37, 1993.
57. AJ Hickey, RM Evans. Aerosol generation from propellent-driven metered dose inhalers. In: AJ Hickey, ed. Inhalation Aerosols. New York: Marcel Dekker, Inc., 1996, pp. 417–439.
58. CA Dunbar, AJ Hickey. Selected parameters affecting characterization of nebulized aqueous solutions by inertial impaction and comparison with phase-doppler analysis. Eur J Pharm Biopharm 48:171–177, 1999.
59. M Dolovich. Lung dose, distribution, and clinical response to therapeutic aerosols. Aerosol Sci Technol 18:230–240, 1993.
60. M Vidgren, J Arppe, P Vidgren, P Vainio, M Silvasti, H Tukiainen. Pulmonary deposition of 99mTc-labelled salbutamol particles in healthy volunteers after inhalation from a metered-dose inhaler and from a novel multiple-dose powder inhaler. S.T.P. Pharm Sci 4:29–32, 1994.
61. MA Kaliner, PJ Barnes, CGA Persson. Asthma, Its Pathology and Treatment. New York, Marcel Dekker, 1991.
62. A Adjei, J Garren. Pulmonary delivery of peptide drugs: effect of particle size on bioavailability of

leuprolide acetate in healthy male volunteers. Pharm Res 7:565–569, 1990.

63. JS Patton, J Bukar, S Nagarajan. Inhaled insulin. Advanced Drug Deliv Rev 35:235–247, 1999.

64. PR Byron, JS Patton. Drug delivery via the respiratory tract. J Aerosol Med 7:49–75, 1994.

Chapter 15

Sustained- and Controlled-Release Drug-Delivery Systems

Gwen M. Jantzen and Joseph R. Robinson

School of Pharmacy, University of Wisconsin, Madison, Wisconsin

I. INTRODUCTION

Over the past 30 years, as the expense and complications involved in marketing new drug entities have increased, with concomitant recognition of the therapeutic advantages of controlled drug-delivery, greater attention has been focused on development of sustained- or controlled-release drug-delivery systems. There are several reasons for the attractiveness of these dosage forms. It is generally recognized that for many disease states, a substantial number of therapeutically effective compounds already exist. The effectiveness of these drugs, however, is often limited by side effects or the necessity to administer the compound in a clinical setting. The goal in designing sustained- or controlled-delivery systems is to reduce the frequency of dosing or to increase effectiveness of the drug by localization at the site of action, reducing the dose required, or providing uniform drug delivery.

If one were to imagine the ideal drug-delivery system, two prerequisites would be required. First, it would be a single dose for the duration of treatment, whether it be for days or weeks, as with infection, or for the lifetime of the patient, as in hypertension or diabetes. Second, it should deliver the active entity directly to the site of action, thereby minimizing or eliminating side effects. This may necessitate delivery to specific receptors, or to localization to cells or to specific areas of the body.

It is obvious that this imaginary delivery system will have changing requirements for different disease states and different drugs. Thus, we wish to deliver the therapeutic agent to a specific site, for a specific time. In other words, the objective is to achieve both spatial and temporal placement of drug. Currently, it is possible to only partially achieve both of these goals with most drug-delivery systems.

In this chapter we present the theory involved in developing sustained- and controlled-release delivery systems and applications of these systems as therapeutic devices. Although suspensions, emulsions, and compressed tablets may demonstrate sustaining effects within the body compared with solution forms of the drug, they are not considered to be sustaining and are not discussed in this chapter. These systems classically release drug for a relatively short period, and their release rates are strongly influenced by environmental conditions.

II. TERMINOLOGY

In the past, many of the terms used to refer to therapeutic systems of controlled and sustained release have been used in an inconsistent and confusing manner. Although descriptive terms such as "timed release" and "prolonged release" give excellent manufacturer identification, they can be confusing to health care practitioners. For the purposes of this chapter, sustained release and controlled release will represent separate delivery processes. *Sustained release* constitutes any dosage form that provides medication over an extended time. *Controlled release*, however, denotes that the system is able to provide some actual therapeutic control, whether this be of a temporal nature, spatial nature, or both. In other words, the system attempts to control drug concentrations in the target issue. This correctly suggests that there are sustained-release systems that cannot be considered controlled-release systems.

In general, the goal of a sustained-release dosage form is to maintain therapeutic blood or tissue levels of the drug for an extended period. This is usually accomplished by attempting to obtain *zero-order* release from the dosage form. Zero-order release constitutes drug release from the dosage form that is independent of the amount of drug in the delivery system (i.e., a constant release rate). Sustained-release systems generally do not attain this type of release and usually try to mimic zero-order release by providing drug in a slow first-order fashion (i.e., concentration-dependent). Systems that are designated as prolonged release can also be considered as attempts at achieving sustained-release delivery. Repeat-action tablets are an alternative method of sustained release in which multiple doses of a drug are contained within a dosage form, and each dose is released at a periodic interval. Delayed-release systems, in contrast, may not be sustaining, since often the function of these dosage forms is to maintain the drug within the dosage form for some time before release. Commonly, the release rate of drug is not altered and does not result in sustained delivery once drug release has begun. Enteric-coated tablets are an example of this type of dosage form.

Controlled release, although resulting in a zero-order delivery system, may also incorporate methods to promote localization of the drug at an active site. In some cases, a controlled-release system will not be sustaining, but will be concerned strictly with localization of the drug. *Site-specific* systems and *targeted-delivery* systems are the descriptive terms used to denote this type of delivery control.

The ideal of providing an exact amount of drug at the site of action for a precise time period is usually approximated by most systems. This approximation is achieved by creating a constant concentration in the body or an organ over an extended time; in other words, the amount of drug entering the system is equivalent to the amount removed from the system. All forms of metabolism and excretion are included in the removal process: urinary excretion, enterohepatic recycling, sweat, fecal, and so on. Since for most drugs these elimination processes are first-order, it can be said that at a certain blood level, the drug will have a specific rate of elimination. The idea is to deliver drug at this exact rate for an extended period. This is represented mathematically as

$$\text{Rate in} = \text{rate out} = k_{\text{elim}} \times C_d \times V_d$$

where C_d is the desired drug level, V_d is the volume of distribution, and k_{elim} is the rate constant for drug elimination from the body. Often such exacting delivery rates prove to be difficult to achieve by administration routes other than intravenous infusion. Noninvasive routes (e.g., oral) are obviously preferred.

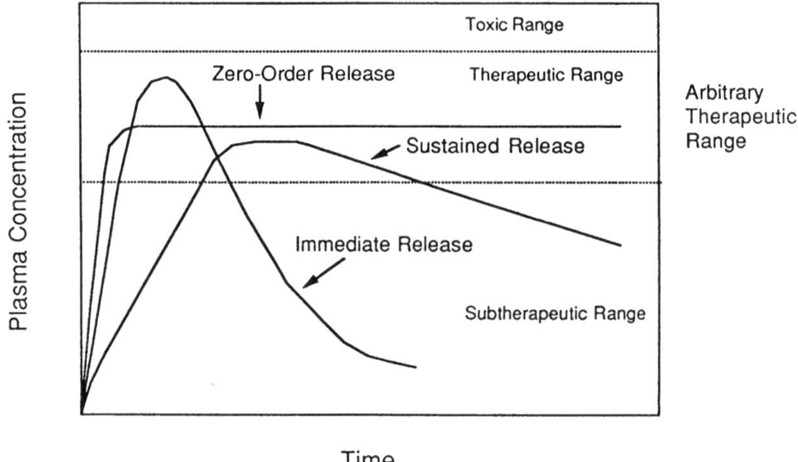

Fig. 1 Drug level versus time profile showing differences between zero-order controlled release, slow first-order sustained release, and release from a conventional tablet or capsule.

Figure 1 shows comparative blood level profiles obtained from administration of conventional, controlled-, and sustained-release dosage forms. The conventional tablet or capsule provides only a single and transient burst of drug. A pharmacological effect is seen as long as the amount of drug is within the therapeutic range. Problems occur when the peak concentration is above or below this range, especially for drugs with narrow therapeutic windows. The slow first-order release obtained by a sustained-release preparation is generally achieved by slowing the release of drug from a dosage form. In some cases this is accomplished by a continuous release process; however, systems that release small bursts of drug over a prolonged period can mimic the continuous-release system.

Before treating the various classes of sustained- and controlled-release drug-delivery systems in this chapter, it is appropriate to note that drug delivery may be incorporated in other chapters where the various classes of drug products and routes of administration are discussed. In addition, the reader is referred to Chapter 14 on target-oriented drug-delivery systems.

III. ORAL SYSTEMS

Historically, the oral route of administration has been used the most for both conventional and novel drug-delivery systems. There are many obvious reasons for this, not the least of which would include acceptance by the patient and ease of administration. The types of sustained- and controlled-release systems employed for oral administration include virtually every currently known theoretical mechanism for such application. This is because there is more flexibility in dosage design, since constraints, such as sterility and potential damage at the site of administration, axe minimized. Because of this, it is convenient to discuss the different types of dosage forms by using those developed for oral administration as initial examples.

With most orally administered drugs, targeting is not a primary concern, and it is usually intended for drugs to permeate to the general circulation and perfuse to other body tissues (the obvious exception being medications intended for local gastrointestinal tissue treatment). For this reason, most systems employed are of the sustained-release variety. It is assumed that increasing concentration at the absorption site will increase the rate of absorption and, therefore, increase circulating blood levels, which in turn, promotes greater concentrations of drug at the site of action. If toxicity is not an issue, therapeutic levels can thus be extended. In essence, 'drug delivery by these systems usually depends on release from some type of dosage form, permeation through the biological milieu, and absorption through an epithelial membrane to the blood. There are a variety of both physicochemical and biological factors that come into play in the design of such systems.

A. Biological Factors Influencing Oral Sustained-Release Dosage Form Design

Biological Half-life

The usual goal of an oral sustained-release product is to maintain therapeutic blood levels over an extended period. To achieve this, drug must enter the circulation at approximately the same rate at which it is eliminated. The elimination rate is quantitatively described by the half-life ($t_{1/2}$). Each drug has its own characteristic elimination rate, which is the sum of all elimination processes, including metabolism, urinary excretion, and all other processes that permanently remove drug from the bloodstream.

Therapeutic compounds with short half-lives are excellent candidates for sustained-release preparations, since this can reduce dosing frequency. However, this is limited, in that drugs with very short half-lives may require excessively large amounts of drug in each dosage unit to maintain sustained effects, forcing the dosage form itself to become limitingly large. In general, drugs with hall-lives shorter than 2 hours, such as furosemide or levodopa [1], are poor candidates for sustained-release preparations. Compounds with long half-lives, more than 8 hours are also generally not used in sustaining forms, since their effect is already sustained. Digoxin, warfarin, and phenytoin are some examples [1]. Furthermore, the transit time of most dosage forms in the gastrointestinal (GI) tract (i.e., mouth to ileocecal junction) is 8–12 hours making it difficult to increase the absorptive phase of administration beyond this time frame. Occasionally, absorption from the colon may allow continued drug delivery for up to 24 hours.

Absorption

The characteristics of absorption of a drug can greatly affect its suitability as a sustained-release product. Since the purpose of forming a sustained-release product is to place control on the delivery system, it is necessary that the rate of release is much slower than the rate of absorption. If we assume that the transit time of most drugs and devices in the absorptive areas of the GI tract is about 8–12 hours, the maximum half-life for absorption should be approximately 3–4 hours; otherwise, the device will pass out of the potential absorptive regions before drug release is complete. This corresponds to a minimum apparent absorption rate constant of 0.17–0.23 h^{-1} to give 80–95% over this time period [3]. The absorption rate constant is an apparent rate constant and should, in actuality, be the release rate constant of the drug from the dosage form. Compounds that demonstrate true lower absorption rate constants will probably be poor candidates for sustaining systems.

The foregoing calculations assume that absorption of the therapeutic agent occurs at a relatively uniform rate over the entire length of the small intestine. For many compounds this is not true. If a drug is absorbed by active transport or transport is limited to a specific region of the intestine, sustained-release preparations may be disadvantageous to absorption. Absorption of ferrous sulfate, for example, is maximal in the upper jejunum and duodenum, and sustained-release mechanisms that do not release drug before passing out of this region are not beneficial [5].

One method to provide sustaining mechanisms of delivery for compounds such as these has been to try to maintain them within the stomach. This allows slow release of the drug, which then travels to the absorptive site. These methods have been developed as a consequence of the observation that coadministration of food results in a sustaining effect [6]. Although administration of food can create highly variable effects, there have been methods devised to circumvent this problem. One such attempt is to formulate low-density pellets, capsules [7] or tablets [8]. These float on top of the gastric juice, delaying their transfer out of the stomach [9]. The increase in gastric retention results in higher blood levels for *p*-aminobenzoic acid, a drug with a limited GI absorption range [10], but drugs that have widespread absorption in the intestinal system would likely not benefit from an increase in emptying time [11].

Another approach is that of bioadhesive materials. The principle is to administer a device with adhesive polymers having an affinity for the gastric surface, most probably the mucin coat [12]. Bioadhesives have demonstrated utility in the mouth, eye, and vagina, with a number of commercially available products. To date, use of bioadhesives in oral drug delivery is a theoretical possibility, but no promising leads have been published.

An alternative to GI retention for drugs with poor absorption characteristics is to use chemical penetration enhancers. Membrane modification through chemical enhancers has been very well demonstrated for a variety of tissues in the body, including the gastrointestinal tract. Concern about this approach is the potential toxicity that may arise when protective membranes are altered. Although there are numerous safety studies for oral products containing surfactants, which are known penetration enhancers, there has not been a definitive safety study in humans using an agent that is specifically present in the formulations as a penetration enhancer.

Metabolism

Drugs that are significantly metabolized before absorption, either in the lumen or the tissue of the intestine, can show decreased bioavailability from slower-releasing dosage forms. Most intestinal wall enzyme systems are saturable. As the drug is released at a slower rate to these regions, less total. drug is presented to the enzymatic process during a specific period, allowing more complete conversion of the drug to its metabolite. For example, aloprenolol was more extensively metabolized in the intestinal wall when given as a sustained-release preparation [13]. High concentrations of dopa-decarboxylase in the intestinal wall will result in a similar effect for levodopa [14]. If levodopa is formulated in a dosage form with a drug compound that can inhibit the dopa-decarboxylase enzyme, the amount of levodopa available for absorption increases and can sustain its therapeutic effects. Formulation of these enzymatically susceptible compounds as prodrugs is another viable solution.

B. Physicochemical Factors Influencing Oral Sustained-Release Dosage Form Design

Dose Size

For orally administered systems, there is an upper limit to the bulk size of the dose to be administered. In general, a single dose of 0.5–1.0 g is considered maximal for a conventional dosage form [15]. This also holds for sustained-release dosage forms. Those compounds that require a large dosing size can sometimes be given in multiple amounts or formulated into liquid systems. Another consideration is the margin of safety involved in administration of large amounts of a drug with a narrow therapeutic range.

Ionization, pK_a, and Aqueous Solubility

Most drugs are weak acids or bases. Since the unchanged form of a drug preferentially permeates across lipid membranes, it is important to note the relationship between the pK_a of the compound and the absorptive environment. It would seem, intuitively, that presenting the drug in an uncharged form is advantageous for drug permeation. Unfortunately, the situation is made more complex by the fact that the drug's aqueous solubility will generally be decreased by conversion to an uncharged form. Delivery systems that are dependent on diffusion or dissolution will likewise be dependent on the solubility of drug in the aqueous media. Considering that these dosage forms must function in an environment of changing pH, the stomach being acidic and the small intestine more neutral, the effect of pH on the release processes must be defined. For many compounds, the site of maximum absorption will also be the area in which the drug is the least soluble. As an example, consider a drug for which the highest solubility is in the stomach and is uncharged in the intestine. For conventional dosage forms, the drug can generally fully dissolve in the stomach and then be absorbed in the alkaline pH of the intestine. For dissolution- or diffusion-sustaining forms, much of the drug will arrive in the small intestine in solid form, meaning that the solubility of the drug may change several orders of magnitude during its release.

Compounds with very low solubility (<0.01 mg/mL) are inherently sustained, since their release over the time course of a dosage form in the GI tract will be limited by dissolution of the drug. Examples of drugs that are limited in absorption by theft dissolution rate are digoxin [16], griseofulvin [17], and salicylamide [18]. The lower limit for the solubility of a drug to be formulated in a sustained-release system has been reported to be 0.1 mg/mL [19], so it is obvious that the solubility of the compound will limit the choice of mechanism to be employed in a sustained-delivery system. Diffusional systems will be poor choices for slightly soluble drugs, since the driving force for diffusion, which is the drug's concentration in solution, will be low.

Partition Coefficient

When a drug is administered to the GI tract, it must cross a variety of biological membranes to produce a therapeutic effect in another area of the body. It is common to consider that these membranes are lipidic; therefore, the partition coefficient of oil-soluble drugs becomes important in determining the effectiveness of membrane barrier penetration. *Partition coefficient* is generally defined as the ratio of the fraction of drug in an oil phase to that of an adjacent aqueous phase. Accordingly, compounds with a relatively high partition coefficient are predominantly lipid-soluble and, consequently, have very low aqueous solubility. Furthermore, these compounds can usually persist in the body for long periods, because they can localize in the lipid membranes of cells. Phenothiazines are representative of this type of compound [20]. Compounds with very low partition coefficients will have difficulty penetrating membranes, resulting in poor bioavailabiity. Furthermore, partitioning effects apply equally to diffusion through polymer membranes. The choice of diffusion-limiting membranes must largely depend on the partitioning characteristics of the drug.

Stability

Orally administered drugs can be subject to both acid-base hydrolysis and enzymatic degradation. Degradation will proceed at a reduced rate for drugs in the solid state; therefore, this is the preferred composition of delivery for problem cases. For drugs that are unstable in the stomach, systems that prolong delivery over the entire course of transit in the GI tract are beneficial; this is also true for systems that delay release until the dosage form reaches the small intestine. Compounds that are unstable in the small intestine may demonstrate decreased bioavailability when administered from a sustaining dosage form. This is because more drug is delivered in the small intestine and, hence, is subject to degradation. Propantheline [21] and probanthine [22] are representative examples of such drugs.

C. Oral Sustained- and Controlled-Release Products

Because of their relative ease of production and cost compared with other methods of sustained or controlled delivery, dissolution and diffusion-controlled systems have classically been of primary importance in oral delivery of medication. Dissolution systems have been some of the oldest and most successful oral systems in early attempts to market sustaining products.

D. Dissolution-Controlled Systems

It seems inherently obvious that a drug with a slow dissolution rate will demonstrate sustaining properties, since the release of drug will be limited by the rate of dissolution. This being true, sustained-release preparations of drugs could be made by decreasing their rate of dissolution. The approaches to achieve this include preparing appropriate salts or derivatives, coating the drug with a slowly dissolving material, or

Table 1 Encapsulated Dissolution Products

Product	Active ingredient(s)	Manufacturer
Ornade Spansules	Phenylpropanolamine hydrochloride, chlorpheniramine maleate	SmithKline Beecham
Thorazine Spansules	Chlorpromazine hydrochloride	SmithKline Beecham
Contac 12-hour capsules	Phenylpropanolamine hydrochloride, chlorpheniramine maleate, atropine sulfate, scopolamine hydrobromide, hyoscyamine sulfate	SmithKline Consumer Products
Artane Sequels	Trihexyphenidyl hydrochloride	Lederle
Diamox Sequels	Acetazolamide	Lederle
Nicobid Temples	Nicotinic acid	Rorer
Pentritol Temples	Pentaerythritol tetranitrate	Rorer
Chlor-Trimeton Repetabs	Chlorpheniramine maleate	Schering
Demazin Repetabs	Chlorpheniramine maleate, phenylephrine hydrochloride	Schering
Polaramine Repetabs	Dexchlorpheniramine maleate	Schering

incorporating it into a tablet with a slowly dissolving carrier. Representative products using dissolution-controlled systems are listed in Tables 1 and 2.

Dissolution-controlled systems can be made to be sustaining in several different ways. By alternating layers of drug with rate-controlling coats, as shown in Fig. 2, a pulsed delivery can be achieved, If the outer layer is a quickly releasing bolus of drug, initial levels of drug in the body can be quickly established with pulsed intervals following. Although this is not a true controlled-release system, the biological effects can be similar. An alternative method is to administer the drug as a group of beads that have coatings of different thicknesses (Fig. 3). Since the beads have different coating thicknesses, their release will occur in a progressive manner, Those with the thinnest layers will provide the initial dose. The maintenance of drug levels at later times will be achieved from those with thicker coatings. This is the principle of the Spansule capsule marketed by SmithKline Beecham.

This dissolution process can be considered to be diffusion-layer controlled. This is best explained by considering the rate of diffusion from the solid surface to the bulk solution through an unstirred liquid film as the rate-determining step. This dissolution process at steady state is described by the Noyes-Whitney equation:

Table 2 Matrix Dissolution Products

Product (tablets)	Active ingredient(s)	Manufacturer
Dimetane Extentabs	Brompheniramine maleate	Robins
Dimetapp Extentabs	Brompheniramine maleate, phenylephrine hydrochloride, phenylpropanolamine hydrochloride	Robins
Donnatal Extentabs	Phenobarbital, hyoscyamine sulfate, atropine sulfate, scopolamine hydrobromide	Robins
Quinidex Extentabs	Quinidine sulfate	Robins
Mestinon Timespans	Pyridostigmine bromide	ICN
Tenuate Dospan	Diethylpropion hydrochloride	Merrel
Disophrol Chronotabs	Dexbrompheniramine maleate, pseudoepherine sulfate	Schering

$$\frac{dC}{dt} = k_D A(C_s - C) = \frac{D}{h} A(C_s - C) \quad (1)$$

where

dC/dt = dissolution rate
k_D = dissolution rate constant
D = diffusion coefficient
C_s = saturation solubility of the solid
C = concentration of solute in the bulk solution

It can be seen that the dissolution rate constant k_D is equivalent to the diffusion coefficient divided by the thickness of the diffusion layer (D/h).

Equation (1) predicts that the rate of release can be constant only if the following parameters are constant: (a) surface area, (b) diffusion coefficient, (c) diffusion layer thickness, and (d) concentration difference. These parameters, however, are not easily maintained constant, especially surface area. For spherical particles, the change in surface area can be related to the weight of the particle; that is, under the assumption of sink conditions, Eq. (1) can be rewritten as the cube-root dissolution equation:

$$W_0^{1/3} - W^{1/3} = k_D t \quad (2)$$

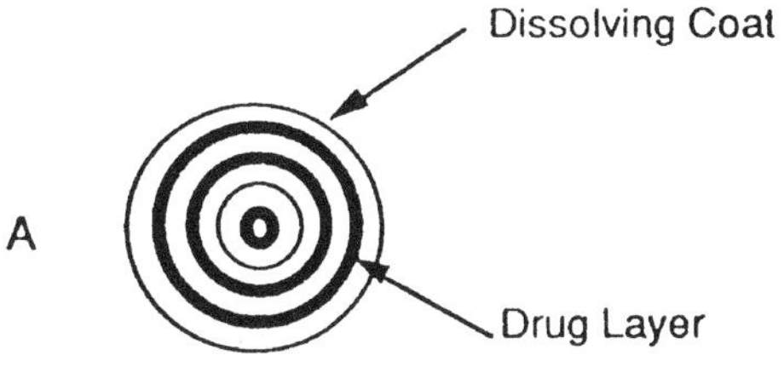

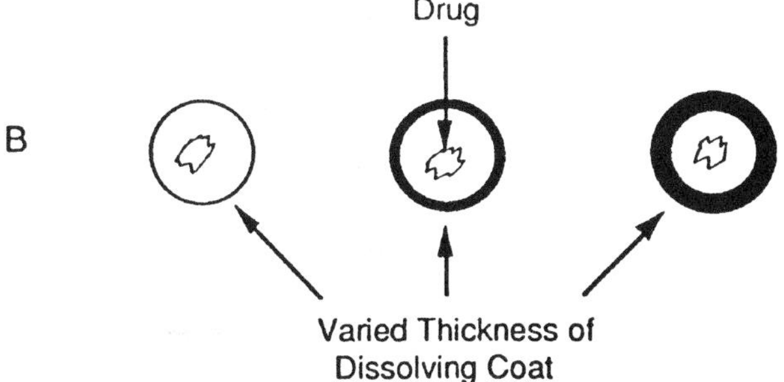

Fig. 2 Two types of dissolution-controlled, pulsed delivery systems: (A) single bead-type device with alternating drug and rate-controlling layers; (B) beads containing drug with differing thickness of dissolving coats.

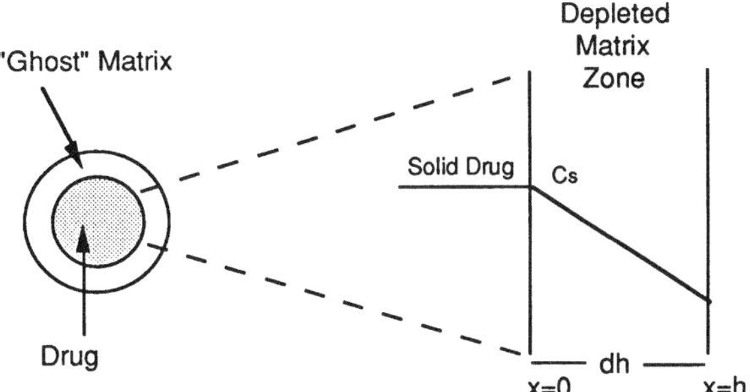

Fig. 3 Schematic representation of a matrix release system. C_s is the saturation concentration of drug controlling the concentration gradient over the distance, h, of the remaining ghost matrix.

where k_D is the cube-root dissolution rate constant and W_0 and W are the initial weight and the weight of the amount remaining at time t, respectively.

E. Diffusional Systems

Diffusion systems are characterized by the release rate of a drug being dependent on its diffusion through an inert membrane barrier. Usually this barrier is an insoluble polymer. In general, two types or subclasses of diffusional systems are recognized: reservoir devices and matrix devices. These will be considered separately.

Reservoir Devices

Reservoir devices, as the name implies, are characterized by a core of drug, the reservoir, surrounded by a polymeric membrane. The nature of the membrane determines the rate of release of drug from the system. A schematic description of this process is given in Fig. 4, and characteristics of the system are listed in Table 3.

The process of diffusion is generally described by a series of equations that were first detailed by Fick [23]. The first of these states that the amount of drug passing across a unit area is proportional to the concentration difference across that plane. The equation is given as

$$J = -D\frac{dC}{dX} \quad (3)$$

where the flux J, given in units of amount/area – time, D, is the diffusion coefficient of the drug in the membrane in units of area/time. This is a reflection of the drug molecule's ability to diffuse through the solvent

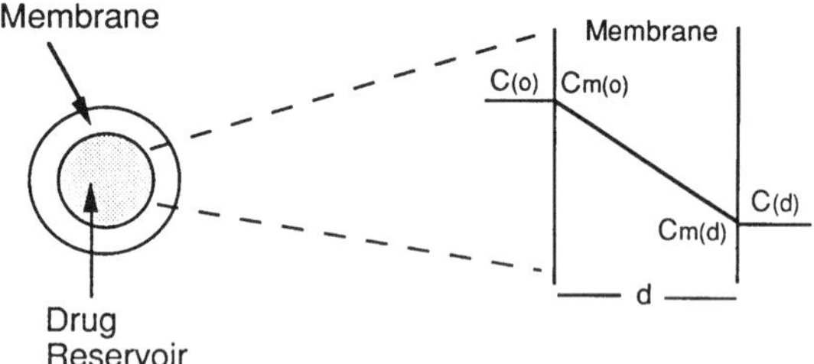

Fig. 4 Schematic representation of a reservoir diffusional device. $C_{m(0)}$ and $C_{m(d)}$ represent concentrations of drug at inside surfaces of the membrane, and $C_{(0)}$ and $C_{(d)}$ represent concentrations in the adjacent regions. (From Ref. 29.)

and is dependent on such factors as molecular size and charge.

This coefficient may be dependent on concentration [24]; hence, its designation as a coefficient and not a constant, although for the purpose of designing a pharmaceutical system it is usually considered a constant [25]. dC/dX represents the rate of change in concentration C relative to a distance X in the membrane.

It is useful to make the assumption that a drug on either side of the membrane is in equilibrium with its respective membrane surface. There is, then, an equilibrium between the membrane surfaces and their bathing solutions, as shown in Fig. 4. This being so, the concentration just inside the membrane surface can be related to the concentration in the adjacent region by the following expressions:

$$K = \frac{C_{m(0)}}{C_{(d)}} \quad \text{at } x = 0 \tag{4}$$

$$K = \frac{C_{m(d)}}{C_{(d)}} \quad \text{at } x = d \tag{5}$$

where K is the partition coefficient. This coefficient denotes the ratio of drug concentration in the membrane to that in the bathing medium at equilibrium. In general, a hydrophilic molecule will partition favorably to the medium, whereas a hydrophobic compound will preferentially partition to the polymer. C_m is the concentration of drug on the inside surface of the membrane, $C_{m(d)}$ the concentration on the outside surface, and d the thickness of the diffusion layer, the diffusional path length.

Assuming that D and K are constant, Eq. (3) can be integrated and simplified to give

$$J = \frac{DK\,\Delta C}{d} \tag{6}$$

where ΔC is the concentration difference across the membrane. The other variables are as defined previously. Drug release will vary, depending on the geometry of the system. The simplest system to consider is that of a slab, where drug release is from only one surface, as shown in Fig. 5. In this case, Eq. (6) can be written as

$$\frac{dM_t}{dt} = \frac{ADK\,\Delta C}{d} \tag{7}$$

where M_t is the mass of drug released after time t, dM_t/dt the steady-state release rate at time t, and A the surface area of the device. Equations of a similar form can be written for other geometries, such as spheres or cylinders [26].

Since the left side of Eq. (7) represents the release rat of the system, a true controlled-release system with a zero-order release rate can be possible only if all of the variables on the right side of Eq. (7) remain constant. A constant effective area of diffusion, diffusional path length, concentration difference, and diffusion coefficient are required to obtain a release rate that is constant. These systems often fail to deliver at a constant rate, since it is especially difficult to maintain all these

Table 3 Characteristics of Reservoir Diffusional Systems

Description	Drug core surrounded by polymer membrane that controls release rate
Advantages	Zero-order delivery is possible
	Release rate variable with polymer type
Disadvantages	System must be physically removed from implant sites
	Difficult to deliver high molecular weight compounds
	Generally increased cost per dosage unit
	Potential toxicity if system fails

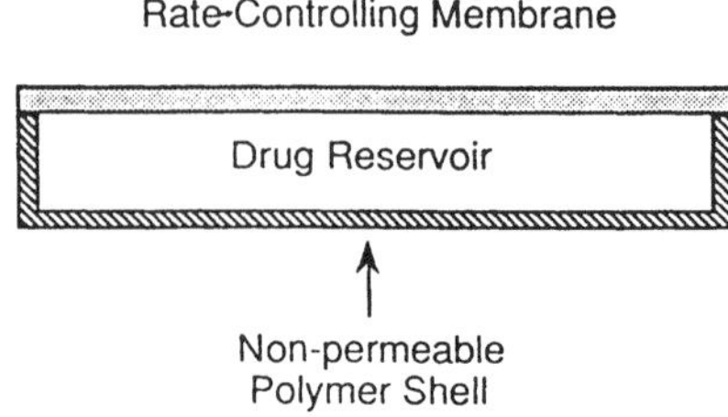

Fig. 5 Diagrammatic representation of the slab configuration of a reservoir diffusional system.

parameters constant. The use of a solid drug core reservoir results in a constant effective concentration, that of the solubility of the drug. Often, however, the polymer may be affected by the bathing medium. Swelling or contraction of the polymer membrane causes a change in the diffusional path length of the diffusion coefficient of the drug through the barrier. For example, if the polymer swells, the diffusion path length will increase. The ability of the drug to diffuse through the membrane, however, will increase. This is because the diffusion coefficient of the drug in the bathing medium, which has perfused the polymer during swelling, will be greater than in the unswelled polymer.

Although the partition coefficient is expected to remain constant, its magnitude is important. Since this coefficient represents the concentration of drug in the membrane relative to that in the core, an excessively high partition coefficient will allow quick depletion of the core and an ineffective delivery system. For effective diffusional systems, the partition coefficient should be less than unity. If the value of this coefficient is greater than 1, the surrounding polymer does not represent a barrier, and drug release becomes first-order.

Although diffusional systems can provide constant release at steady state, they will demonstrate Initial release rates, which may be faster or slower. This depends on the device [27]. For reservoir devices, a system that is used relatively soon after construction will demonstrate a large time in release, since it will take time for the drug to diffuse from the reservoir to the membrane surface. On the other hand, systems that are stored will demonstrate a burst effect, since, on standing, the membrane becomes saturated with available drug. The magnitude of these effects is dependent on the diffusing distance (i.e., the membrane thickness). Figure 6 gives examples of this phenomenon. This plot shows the approach to steady-state release for a typical reservoir device that has been stored (burst effect) and for a device that has been freshly made (time lag).

Reservoir diffusional systems have several advantages over conventional dosage forms. They can offer zero-order release of drug, the kinetics of which can be controlled by changing the characteristics of the polymer to meet the particular drug and therapy conditions. The inherent disadvantages are that, unless the polymer used is soluble, the system must somehow be removed from the body after the drug has been released. This is an important dosage form consideration with implantable systems. A silicone elastomer reservoir has been used to orally deliver iodine through

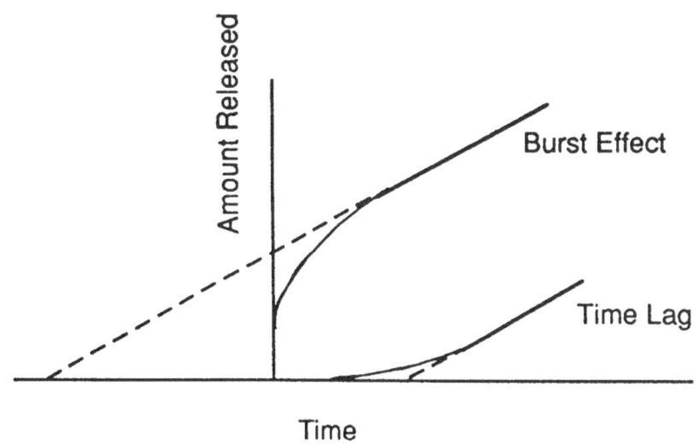

Fig. 6 Plot showing the approach to steady state for a reservoir device that has been stored for an extended period (the burst effect curve) and for a device that has been freshly made (the lag time curve). (From Ref. 29.)

the water supply to large populations suffering from deficiency [28]. For a system such as this, the nonerodible device poses no significant problem; however, the appearance of the drug-depleted matrix in the stool can often alarm a naive patient.

Another important point to consider is that, in general, the amount of drug contained in the reservoir is far greater than the usual dose needed, since the dosage form is designed to sustain delivery over many dosing intervals. Any error in production or any accidental damage to the dosage form that would directly expose the reservoir core could expose the patient to a potentially toxic dose of drug. This becomes important when designing these dosage forms for drugs with narrow therapeutic ranges or high toxicity. Table 4 gives a representative listing of available products employing reservoir diffusion systems.

Matrix Devices

A matrix device, as the name implies, consists of drug dispersed homogeneously throughout a polymer matrix as represented in Fig. 7. In the model, drug in the outside layer exposed to the bathing solution is dissolved first and then diffuses out of the matrix. This process continues with the interface between the bathing solution and the solid drug moving toward the interior. Obviously, for this system to be diffusion-controlled, the rate of dissolution of drug particles within the matrix must be much faster that the diffusion rate of dissolved drug leaving the matrix. Derivation of the mathematical model to describe this system involves the following assumptions [29,30]: (a) a pseudo-steady state is maintained during drug release, (b) the diameter of the drug particles is less than the

Table 4 Reservoir Diffusional Products

Product	Active ingredient(s)	Manufacturer
Duotrate	Pentaerythritol tetranitrate	Jones
Nico-400	Nicotinic acid	Jones
Nitro-Bid	Nitroglycerin	Marion
Cerespan	Papaverine hydrochloride	Rhône-Poulenc Rorer
Nitrospan	Nitroglycerin	Rorer
Measurin	Acetylsalicylic acid	Sterling Winthrop

average distance of drug diffusion through the matrix, (c) the bathing solution provides sink conditions at all times, (d) the diffusion coefficient of drug in the matrix remains constant (i.e., no change occurs in the characteristics of the polymer matrix).

The next equations, which describe the rate of release of drugs dispersed in an inert matrix system, have been derived by Higuchi [29]. The following equation can be written based on Fig. 3:

$$\frac{dM}{dh} = C_0 dh - \frac{C_s}{2} \tag{8}$$

where

dM = change in the amount of drug released per unit area
dh = change in the thickness of the zone of matrix that has been depleted of drug

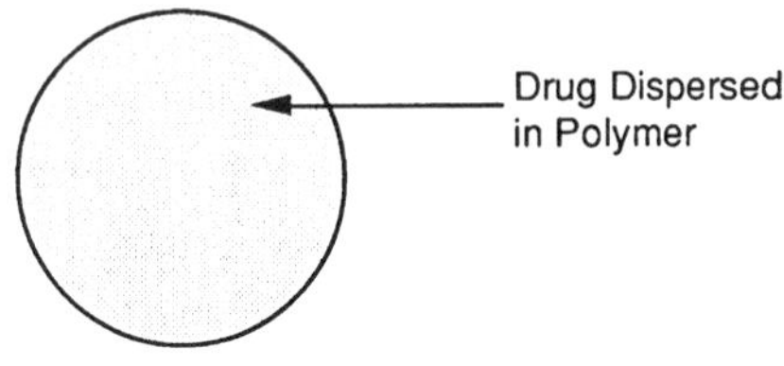

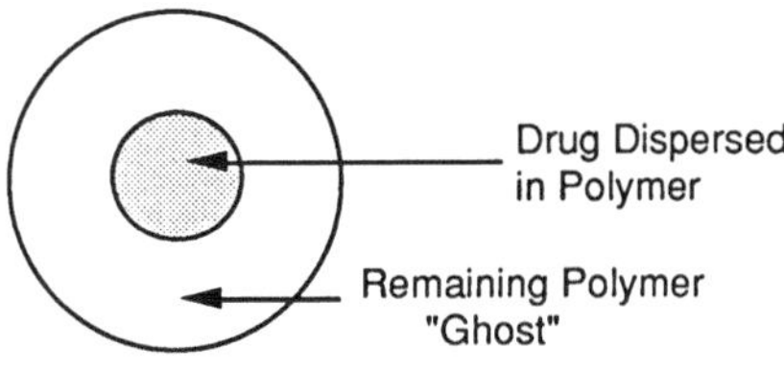

Fig. 7 Matrix diffusional system before drug release (time = 0) and after partial drug release (time = t).

C_0 = total amount of drug in a unit volume of the matrix
C_s = saturated concentration of the drug within the matrix

From diffusion theory,

$$dM = \frac{D_m C_s}{h} dt \tag{9}$$

where D_m is the diffusion coefficient in the matrix. Equating Eqs. (8) and (9), integrating, and solving for h gives:

$$M = [C_s D_m (2C_0 - C_s)t]^{1/2} \tag{10}$$

When the amount of drug is in excess of the saturation concentration, that is, $C_0 \gg C_s$,

$$M = (2C_s D_m C_0 t)^{1/2} \tag{11}$$

which indicates that the amount of drug released is a function of the square root of time. In a similar manner, the drug release from a porous or granular matrix can be described by

$$M = \left[D_s C_a \frac{p}{T}(2C_0 - pC_a)t\right]^{1/2} \tag{12}$$

where

p = porosity of the matrix
T = tortuosity
C_a = solubility of the drug in the release medium
D_s = diffusion coefficient in the release medium

This system is slightly different from the previous matrix system in that the drug is able to pass out of the matrix through fluid-filled channels and does not pass through the polymer directly.

For purposes of data treatment, Eq. (11) or (12) can be reduce to

$$M = kt^{1/2} \tag{13}$$

where k is a constant, so that a plot of amount of drug released versus the square root of time will be linear, if

Table 5 Characteristics of Matrix Diffusion Systems

Description	Homogeneous dispersion of solid drug in a polymer mix
Advantages	Easier to produce than reservoir devices
	Can deliver high molecular weight compounds
Disadvantages	Cannot obtain zero-order release
	Removal of remaining matrix is necessary for implanted systems

the release of drug from the matrix is diffusion-controlled. If this is the case, then, by the Higuchi model, one may control the release of drug from a homogeneous matrix system by varying the following parameters [31–35]: (a) initial concentration of drug in the matrix, (b) porosity, (c) tortuosity, (d) polymer system forming the matrix, and (e) solubility of the drug.

Matrix systems offer several advantages. They are, in general, easy to make and can be made to release high molecular weight compounds. Since the drug is dispersed in the matrix system, accidental leakage of the total drug component is less likely to occur, although, occasionally, cracking of the matrix material can cause unwanted release. The primary disadvantages of this system are that the remaining matrix "ghost" must be removed after the drug has been released. Also, the release rates generated are not zero-order, since the rate varies with the square root of time. A substantial sustained effect, however, can be produced through the use of very slow release rates, which in many applications are indistinguishable from zero-order. The characteristics of the system are summarized in Table 5, and a representative listing of available products is given in Table 6.

F. Bioerodible and Combination Diffusion and Dissolution Systems

Strictly speaking, therapeutic systems will never be dependent on dissolution only or diffusion only. However, in the foregoing systems, the predominant mechanism allows easy mathematical description. In practice, the dominant mechanism for release will overshadow other processes enough to allow classification as either dissolution rate–limited or diffusion-controlled. Bioerodible devices, however, constitute a group of systems for which mathematical descriptions of release characteristics can be quite complex. Characteristics of this type of system are listed in Table 7. A typical system is shown in Fig. 8. The mechanism of release from simple erodible slabs, cylinders, and spheres has been described [36]. A simple expression describing release from all three of these erodible devices is

$$\frac{M_t}{M} = 1 - \left(1 - \frac{k_0 t}{C_0 a}\right)^n \tag{14}$$

where $n = 3$ for a sphere, $n = 2$ for a cylinder, and $n = 1$ for a slab. The radius of a sphere, or cylinder, or the half-height of a slab is represented by a. M_t is the mass of a drug release at time t, and M is the mass released at infinite time. As a further complication, these systems can combine diffusion and dissolution of both the matrix material and the drug. Not only can drug diffuse out of the dosage form, as with some previously described matrix systems, but the matrix itself undergoes a dissolution process. The complexity of the system arises from the fact that, as the polymer dissolves, the diffusional path length for the drug may change. This usually results in a moving-boundary diffusion system. Zero-order release can occur only if surface erosion occurs and surface area does not change with time. The inherent advantage of such a system is that the bioerodible property of the matrix does not result in a ghost matrix. The disadvantages of these matrix systems are that release kinetics are often hard to control, since many factors affecting both the drug and the polymer must be considered.

Another method for the preparation of bioerodible systems is to attach the drug directly to the polymer by

Table 6 Matrix Diffusional Products

Product (tablets)	Active ingredient(s)	Manufacturer
Desoxyn-Gradumet	Methamphetamine hydrochloride	Abbott
Fero-Gradumet	Ferrous sulfate	Abbott
Tral Filmtab	Hexocyclium methylsulfate	Abbott
PBZ-SR	Tripelennamine	Geigy
Procan SR	Procainamide hydrochloride	Parke-Davis
Choledyl SA	Oxtriphylline	Parke-Davis

Table 7 Characteristics of Bioerodible Matrix Systems

Description	A homogeneous dispersion of drug in an erodible matrix
Advantages	All the advantages of matrix dissolution system
	Removal from implant sites not necessary
Disadvantages	Difficult to control kinetics owing to multiple processes of release
	Potential toxicity of degraded polymer must be considered

a chemical bond [37]. Generally, the drug is released from the polymer by hydrolysis or enzymatic reaction. This makes control of the rate of release somewhat easier. Another advantage of the system is the ability to achieve very high drug loading, since the amount of drug placed in the system is limited only by the available sites on the carrier.

A third type, which in this case utilizes a combination of diffusion and dissolution, is that of a swelling-controlled matrix [38]. Here the drug is dissolved in the polymer, but instead of an insoluble or eroding polymer, as in previous systems, swelling of the polymer occurs. This allows entrance of water, which causes dissolution of the drug and diffusion out of the swollen matrix. In these systems the release rate is highly dependent on the polymer-swelling rate, drug solubility, and the amount of soluble fraction in the matrix [39]. This system usually minimizes burst effects, since polymer swelling must occur before drug release.

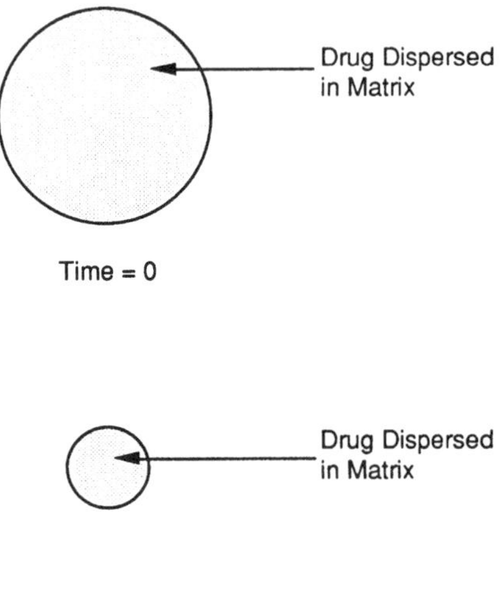

Fig. 8 Representation of a bioerodible matrix system. Drug is dispersed in the matrix before release at time = 0. At time = t, partial release by drug diffusion or matrix erosion has occurred.

G. Osmotically Controlled Systems

In these systems, osmotic pressure provides the driving force to generate controlled release of drug. Consider a semipermeable membrane that is permeable to water, but not to drug. A tablet containing a core of drug surrounded by such a membrane is shown in Fig. 9. When this device is exposed to water or any body fluid, water will flow into the tablet owing to the osmotic pressure difference. The rate of flow, dV/dt, of water into the device can be represented as

$$\frac{dV}{dt} = \frac{Ak}{h(\Delta\Pi - \Delta P)} \tag{15}$$

where

k = membrane permeability
A = area of the membrane

Type A

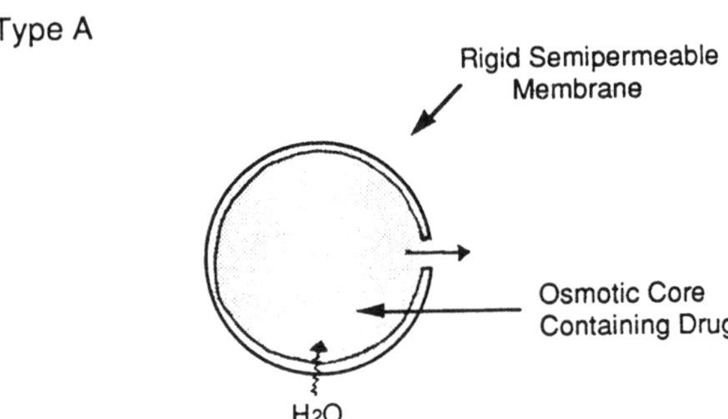

Type B

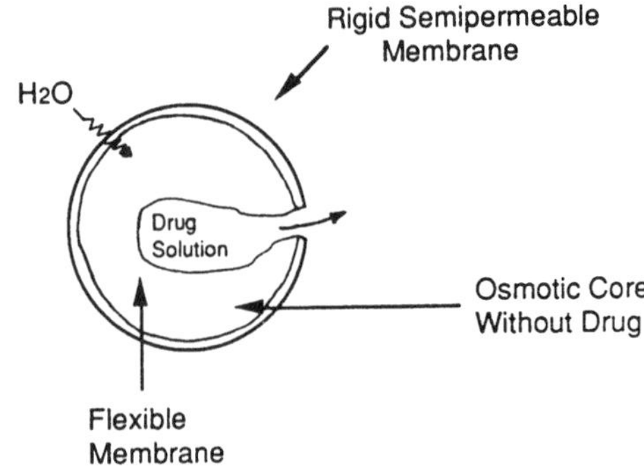

Fig. 9 Diagrammatic representation of two types of osmotically controlled systems. Type A contains an osmotic core with drug. Type B contains the drug solution in a flexible bag, with the osmotic core surrounding.

h = membrane thickness
$\Delta\Pi$ = osmotic pressure difference
ΔP = hydrostatic pressure difference

These systems generally appear in two different forms, as depicted in Fig. 9. The first contains the drug as a solid core together with electrolyte, which is dissolved by the incoming water. The electrolyte provides the high osmotic pressure difference. The second system contains the drug in solution in an impermeable membrane within the device. The electrolyte surrounds the bag. Both systems have single or multiple holes bored through the membrane to allow drug release. In the first example, high osmotic pressure can be relieved only by pumping solution, containing drug, out of the hole. Similarly, in the second example, the high osmotic pressure causes compression of the inner membrane, and drug is pumped out through the hole.

In the system with the bag, or if the hole is large enough in either system, the hydrostatic difference becomes negligible, and Eq. (15) becomes

$$\frac{dV}{dt} = \frac{Ak}{h(\Delta\Pi)} \tag{16}$$

indicating that the flow rate of water into the tablet is governed by permeability, area, and thickness of the membrane. The rate of drug leaving the orifice, dM/dt, is equivalent to the flow rate of incoming water multiplied by the solution concentration of drug, C_s, within the device:

$$\frac{dM}{dt} = \frac{dV}{dt} C_s \tag{17}$$

Osmotic systems have application in pharmacological studies, implantation therapies, and oral drug delivery.

In systems with solid drug dispersed with electrolyte, the size or number of bored hole(s) are the rate-limiting factors for release of drug. Quality control of the manufacture of these systems must be exceptional, since any variation in boring of the hole, accomplished with a laser drill, can have a substantial effect on release characteristics. Most of the orally administered osmotic systems are of this variety. A variation on this theme is an osmotic system of similar design without a hole. The building osmotic pressure causes the tablet to burst, causing all the drug to be rapidly released [40]. This design is useful for drugs that are difficult to formulate in tablet or capsule form.

These osmotic systems are advantageous in that they can deliver large volumes, and some are refillable. Most important, the release of drug is in theory independent of the drug's properties [41,42]. This allows one dosage form design to be used for almost any drug. Disadvantages are that the systems are relatively expensive and, for certain applications, require implantation. For drugs that are unstable in solution, these systems may be inappropriate because the drug remains in solution form for extended periods before release. System characteristics are summarized in Table 8.

Table 8 Characteristics of Osmotically Controlled Devices

Description	Drug surrounded by semipermeable membrane and release governed by osmotic pressure
Advantages	Zero-order release obtainable
	Reformulation not required for different drugs
	Release of drug independent of the environment of the system
Disadvantages	Systems can be much more expensive than conventional counterparts
	Quality control more extensive than most conventional tablets

H. Ion-Exchange Systems

Ion-exchange systems generally use resins composed of water-insoluble cross-linked polymers. These polymers contain salt-forming functional groups in repeating positions on the polymer chain. The drug is bound to the resin and released by exchanging with appropriately charged ions in contact with the ion-exchange groups.

$$\text{Resin}^+ - \text{drug}^- + \text{X}^- \rightarrow \text{resin}^+ - \text{X}^- + \text{drug}^-$$

conversely,

$$\text{Resin}^- - \text{drug}^+ + \text{Y}^+ \rightarrow \text{resin}^- - \text{Y}^+ + \text{drug}^+$$

where X^- and Y^+ are ions in the GI tract. The free drug then diffuses out of the resin. The drug–resin complex is prepared either by repeated exposure of the resin to the drug in a chromatography column or by prolonged contact in solution.

The rate of drug diffusing out of the resin is controlled by the area of diffusion, diffusional path length, and rigidity of the resin, which is a function of the amount of cross-linking agent used to prepare the resin.

This system is advantageous for drugs that are highly susceptible to degradation by enzymatic processes, since it offers a protective mechanism by temporarily altering the substrate. This approach to

Table 9 Ion-Exchange Products

Product	Active ingredient(s)	Manufacturer
Biphetamine capsules	Amphetamine, dextroamphetamine	Fisons
Tussionex suspension	Hydrocodone, chlorpheniramine	Fisons
Ionamin capsules	Phenteramine	Pennwalt
Delsym solution	Dextromethorphan hydrobromide	McNeil

sustained release, however, has the limitation that the release rate is proportional to the concentration of the ions present in the area of administration. Although the ionic concentration of the GI tract remains rather constant with limits [15], the release rate of drug can be affected by variability in diet, water intake, and individual intestinal content. A representative listing of ion-exchange products is given in Table 9.

An improvement in this system is to coat the ion-exchange resin with a hydrophobic rate-limiting polymer, such as ethylcellulose or wax [43]. These systems rely on the polymer coat to govern the rate of drug availability.

IV. TARGETED DELIVERY SYSTEMS

Targeted systems represent the next level in state-of-the-art controlled drug-delivery systems. These systems address the problem of spatial placement of therapeutic compounds. Since the site of drug action is the target of these systems, oral administration is generally not used as a method of delivery. Targeted drug-delivery systems have received much attention for cancer chemotherapy. A very extensive review on this subject and on novel drugs describes the enormous potential for the discovery of innovative cancer treatments with improved efficacy and selectivity for the third millennium [44]. The review focuses on new technologies and on mechanism-based agents and systems directed to molecular pathways and targets that are casually involved in cancer formation and progression.

A. Liposomes

Liposomes have been, and continue to be, of considerable interest in drug-delivery systems. A schematic diagram of their production is shown in Fig. 10. Liposomes are normally composed of phospholipids that spontaneously form multilamellar, concentric, bilayer vesicles, with layers of aqueous media separating the lipid layers. These systems, commonly referred to as multilamellar vesicles (MLVs), have diameters in the range of 1–5 μm. Sonication of MLVs results in the production of small unilamellar vesicles (SUVs), with diameters in the range 0.02–0.08 μm. These vesicles are a single, lipid outer layer, with an aqueous inner core. Large unilamellar vesicles (LUVs) can also be made by evaporation under reduced pressure, resulting in liposomes with a diameter of 0.1–l μm. Further extrusion of LUVs through a membrane filter will also result in SUVs.

To use liposomes as delivery systems, drug is added during the formation process. Hydrophilic compounds usually reside in the aqueous portion of the vesicle, whereas hydrophobic species tend to remain in the lipid proteins. The physical characteristics and stability of lipsomal preparations depend on pH, ionic strength, the presence of divalent cations, and the nature of the phospholipids and additives used [45–47].

In general, these vesicle systems demonstrate low permeability to ionic and polar substances, but this varies greatly with liposome composition. Those made with positively charged phospholipids are impermeable to cations, whereas negatively charged liposomes are permeable to cations, and both types are readily permeated by anions [48]. The degree of saturation or the length of the phospholipid fatty acid chain will also greatly affect the solute permeability of the liposomes [49]. An increase in temperature can also alter permeability [50] by causing the lipids to undergo a phase transition to a less-ordered, more fluid configuration. Again, the transition is characteristic for differing types of lipids. This has been employed in a unique targeting approach by creating an environment of local hypothermia; the liposomes are encouraged to release their encapsulated cargo in that specified area, for example, a capillary bed [51,52].

Some proteins, such as those found in serum, are able to deform, penetrate the bilayer, or remove lipid components, resulting in changes in liposome permeability [53]. Many additives, such as cholesterol, are able to inhibit this effect, stabilizing the membrane structure of the vesicle and limiting cargo leakage [54]. This is achieved by allowing closer lipid packing [55]. The fact that impurities, such as cholesterol or free

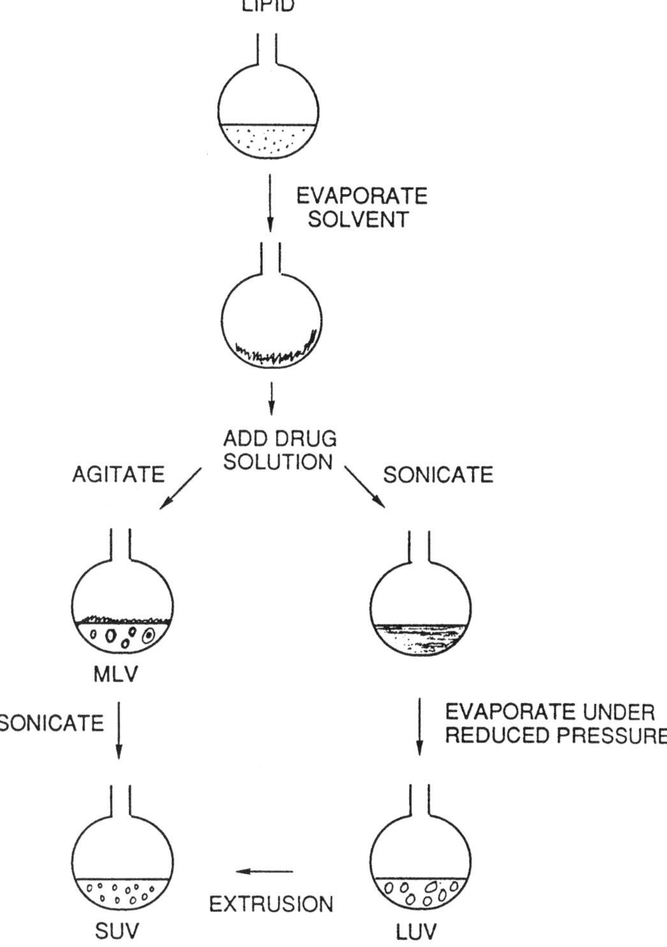

Fig. 10 Schematic representation of a procedure for the production of liposomes.

fatty acids [56], can dramatically change the permeability and surface charge of liposomes points to the necessity for strict controls on the quality and purity of lipids used in liposomal preparation.

Liposomes that remain impermeable to their contents cannot release these compounds without interaction with cells. This cellular interaction occurs by three different mechanisms (Fig. 11) [57]. Of these, fusion and adsorption usually involve drug leakage, whereas effective drug delivery results from endocytosis.

1. *Fusion of the liposome with the cell membrane.* For this, the lipid portion of the vesicle becomes part of the cell wall.
2. *Adsorption to the cell wall.* For this, transfer of liposome content must be by diffusion through the lipids of the liposome and the cell membrane.
3. *Endocytosis of the vesicle by the cell.* The entire liposomal contents are made available to the cell.

The advantageous effects of liposomal carrier systems include protection of compounds from metabolism or degradation, as well as enhanced cellular uptake. Liposome-mediated delivery of cytotoxic drugs to cells in culture has resulted in improved potency [58,59]. Prolonged release of encapsulated cargo has also been demonstrated [60,61]. More recently, liposomes with extended circulation half-lives and dose-independent pharmacokinetics (Stealth liposomes) [62] have shown promise in delivery of drugs that are normally very rapidly degraded.

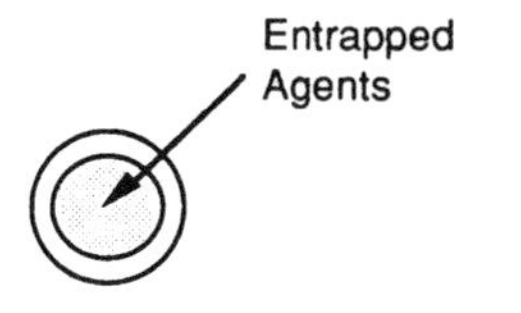

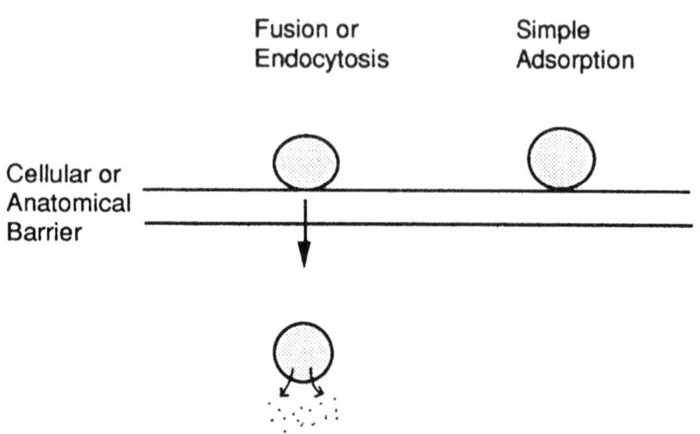

Fig. 11 Schematic representation of liposome interactions at a membrane surface.

Liposomes, however, also have inherent disadvantages in the areas of stability and uniformity of production. Once a system has demonstrated merit for treatment of a particular disease state, the following must be determined before a formulation is acceptable for marketing and human use: (a) lipid purity and stability; (b) drug stability and leakage from the vesicles; (c) lipid-drug cargo interaction; and (d) control of vesicle size and drug-loading efficiency for large-batch production.

The potential of liposomes in oral drug delivery has been largely disappointing. However, the use of polymer-coated, polymerized, and microencapsulated liposomes have all increased their potential for oral use [63], and it predicted that a greater understanding of their cellular processing will ultimately lead to effective therapies for oral liposomes.

Progress in employing liposomes and nanoparticles for the targeted delivery of antibiotics over the past 20 years was recently summarized. These systems may provide stealthy strategies to avoid drug uptake by mononuclear phagocytes following IV injection, allowing extended systemic presence of the drug and increased drug concentrations at infected sites while reducing drug toxicity [64].

Advances in liposome technology that have resulted in the development of ligand-targeted liposomes capable of selectively increasing the efficacy of carried agents against receptor-bearing tumor cells have been extensively reviewed [65]. Receptors for vitamins and growth factors are attractive targets for ligand-directed liposomal therapies due to their high expression levels on various forms of cancer.

External stimuli have also been used to further target liposomes. In one such study magnetite particles were incorporated in radiolabeled liposomes and a magnet positioned over the right kidney of a test animal. The liposomes were selectively targeted to that kidney in concentrations that were viewed as significantly high for relevant clinical applications [66].

Mention should also be made in this section of niosomes, which are nonionic surfactant vesicles that have shown promise as inexpensive and chemically stable alternatives to liposomes [67].

A challenge in designing liposome systems is the assessment of drug release from such systems in vitro. Use of agarose gel matrices has been reported as one approach to evaluate the release kinetics of liposome-encapsulated materials in the presence of biological components [68].

B. Prodrugs

A *prodrug* is a compound resulting from chemical modification of a biologically active compound that will liberate the active form in vivo by enzymatic or hydrolytic cleavage. The primary purpose in forming a prodrug is to modify the physicochemical properties of the drug, usually to alter the membrane permeability of the parent compound. This change in physicochemical properties of the drug influences the ultimate localization of the drug. There are various reasons for formulating a prodrug system. If the parent compound is insoluble, this can be modified [69]. If it is easily degraded, modification can protect the parent compound from enzymatic of hydrolytic attack. Modifications can also reduce side effects, such as GI irritation [70]. Several drugs are now marketed in the form of a prodrug; for example, sulindac, a nonsteroidal anti-inflammatory agent, and numerous angiotension-converting enzyme (ACE) inhibitors. The necessary conversion of prodrug to parent can occur by a variety of reactions, the most common being hydrolytic cleavage [71]. The prodrug ester forms of a hydroxyl or carboxyl group of the parent compound can be readily cleaved by blood esterase. Other activation processes may include biochemical reduction or oxidation.

However the conversion occurs, to achieve sustained drug action the rate of conversion from prodrug to active compound should not be too high [72]. Site-specific, controlled delivery is achieved by the antiviral prodrug acyclovir, which is converted to active form by a virus-specific enzyme [73]. Sustained release of steroid prodrugs, especially progestagens and progestagen-estrogen combinations, have seen a substantial amount of clinical experience, both as a means of birth control and as symptomatic menopausal treatment [74].

The concept of the double prodrug (proprodrugs) may allow more controlled delivery of various prodrug compounds [75]. For example, if a prodrug shows site-specific activation but has poor transport properties or stability problems, it could be converted to a proprodrug that transported better or is more stable (Fig. 12). Prodrug systems have been taken even further by including as prodrugs polymer prodrugs, in which a drug is covalently linked to a polymer backbone. This type of system could encompass a staggering number of possibilities. Encouraging results have been shown with mitomycin [76,77], for example. A model, the Ringsdorf model, has been developed to depict the ideal drug-delivery system for polymeric prodrugs, which has all the desired physicochemical properties to deliver the drug at the desired tissue or intracellular region [78].

The most serious disadvantage of the prodrug approach to controlled sustained delivery is that extensive development must be undertaken to find the correct chemical modification for a specific drug. Additionally, once a prodrug is formed, it is a new drug entity and, therefore, requires extensive and costly studies to determine safety and efficacy.

C. Nanoparticles

Nanoparticles are solid colloidal particles ranging in size from 10 to 1000 nm. They can be used as drug carriers, with the drug encapsulated, dissolved, adsorbed, or covalently attached [79,80]. The small size of the nanoparticles permits administration by intravenous injection and also permits their passage through capillaries that remove larger particles. They are usually taken up by the liver, spleen, and lungs [81,82].

Preparation of nanoparticles can be by a variety of different ways. The most important and frequently used is emulsion polymerization; others include interfacial polymerization, solvent evaporation, and desolvation of natural proteins. The materials used to prepare nanoparticles are also numerous, but most commonly they are polymers such as polyalklcyanoacrylate, polymethylmethacrylate, polybutylcyanoacrylate, or are albumin or gelatin. Distribution patterns of the particles in the body can vary depending on their size, composition, and surface charge [83–85]. In particular, nanoparticles of polycyanoacrylate have been found to accumulate in certain tumors [86,87].

There are several possible ways that the drug cargo can be incorporated into nanoparticles. They may be bound by polymerization of the nanoparticles in the presence of drug solution or by absorption of the drug onto prepolymerized nanoparticles. The drug will be dispersed in the particle's polymer matrix [88] or adsorbed to the surface, depending on its affinity to the polymer. Drugs used for nanoparticle delivery have been, for the most part, cytotoxic agents such as dactinomycin (actinomycin D) [89], 5-fluorouracil [90,91], doxorubicin [92,93], and methotrexate [94], but have also included delivery of bioactive peptides and proteins, for example, growth hormone–releasing factor [95,96].

Nanoparticles show great promise as devices for the controlled release of drugs, provided that the choice of material for nanoparticle formation is made with the appropriate considerations of the drug cargo, administration route, and the desired site of action. The use of nano- and microparticles as controlled drug-delivery devices has recently been extensively reviewed [97].

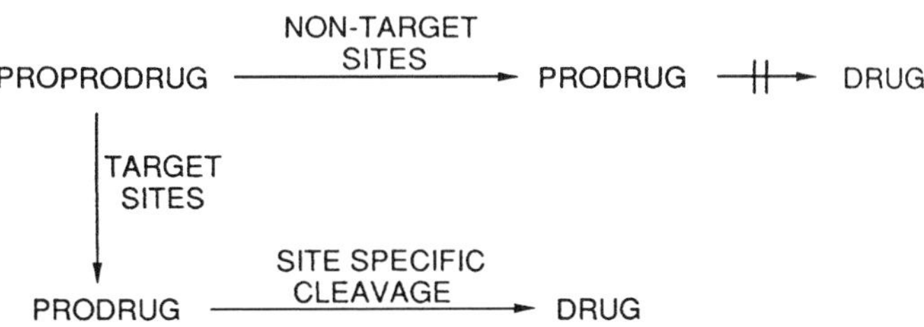

Fig. 12 Illustration of prodrug and proprodrug concept.

In addition, biodegradable nanoparticles for sustained release formulations to improve site-specific drug delivery has also been reviewed [98].

D. Resealed Erythrocytes

When red blood cells are placed in hypotonic media, they swell, which causes rupturing of the membrane and formation of pores. These pores allow free exchange of intra- and extra-cellular components. Readjustment of the solution tonicity to isotonic allows resealing of the membrane. This technique usually allows encapsulation of up to 25% of the drug or enzyme in solution [99]. In addition to this method, called the preswell dilution technique, there are other ways to form drug-loaded erythrocytes. In the dialysis technique, the red blood cells are placed in dialysis tubes that are immersed in a hypotonic medium. This results in retention of cytoplasmic components when the cells are resealed. Another method involves subjecting the cells to an intense electric field, causing pores to form, which again can be resealed after drug uptake.

The potential advantages of loaded red blood cells as delivery systems are as follows [100]:

1. They are biodegradable and nonimmunogenic.
2. They can be modified to change their resident circulation time, depending on their surface (cells with little membrane damage can circulate for prolonged periods).
3. Entrapped drug is shielded from immunological detection and external enzymatic degradation.
4. The system is relatively independent of the physicochemical properties of the drug (i.e., it does not require chemical modifications).

In general, normally aging erythrocytes and slightly damaged cells are sequestered in the spleen, whereas those heavily damaged or modified are removed from circulation by the liver [101]. This along with a short storage life of about 2 weeks [102], constitutes the major drawback of using resealed erythrocytes as drug carriers.

Before treating the various classes of sustained- and controlled-release drug-delivery systems in this chapter, it is appropriate to note that drug delivery may be incorporated in other chapters where the various classes of drug products and routes of administration are discussed. In addition the reader is referred to Chapter 16 on target-oriented drug-delivery systems.

E. Antibody-Targeted Systems

An alternative drug-delivery system makes use of macromolecular attachment for delivery using immunoglobulins as the macromolecule. The obvious advantage of this system is that it can be targeted to the site of the antibody specificity. Although this usually does not provide much of a sustaining mechanism, the problem of spatial placement is addressed. The advantage in this is that far less drug is used, and side effects can be reduced substantially.

Drugs are linked, covalently or noncovalently, to the antibody [103] or placed in vesicles such as liposomes or microspheres, and the antibody used to target the liposome [104,105] (Fig. 13). Covalent attachment is generally not very efficient and also diminishes the antigen-binding capacity [106,107]. There are only a few functional groups available per antibody that can be used for chemical coupling without affecting the antibody's binding activity. If conjugation is done through an immediate carrier molecule, one can increase the drug/antibody ratio [108,109]. Such intermediates have included dextran or poly-L-glutamic acid [110–112].

Many drugs have been conjugated to antibodies or their fragments, including daunomycin [113], cyclosporine [114], platinum [115], chlorambucil [116], and vindesine [117]. When choosing a drug for this type of

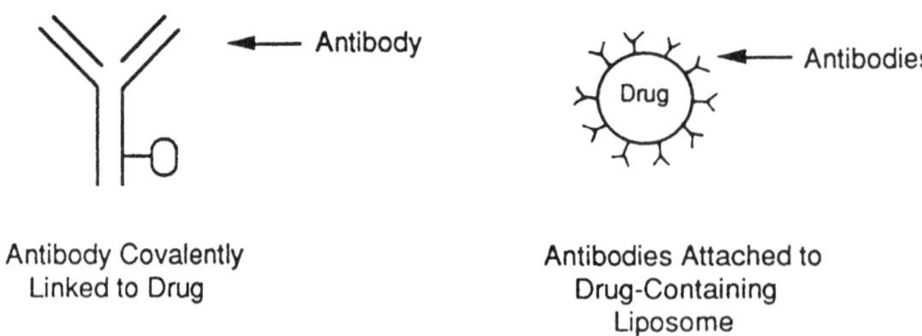

Fig. 13 Diagrammatic representation of two types of antibody-targeted systems. Drug is either covalently linked directly to the antibody or is contained in liposomes that are targeted by attached antibodies.

delivery, one must consider many facts [118], such as whether the drug is active extra- or intracellularly, if it must be cleaved from the antibody to be active, and the strength and method of coupling.

Immunoliposomes—liposomes loaded with drug cargo that have been surface-conjugated to antibodies or antibody fragments—have also been investigated by a number of researchers. Linkage of antibody to a liposome can be covalent or noncovalent. Spacers are used for covalent binding, or the antibody is modified by attaching an "anchor group [119] for noncovalent coupling. The anchor group, which is hydrophobic, inserts into the bilayer of the liposome, "anchoring" the antibody to the vesicle. Numerous antibody–liposome combinations have been looked at, delivering both drugs [120–122] and genetic material [123–125].

The obvious advantage to antibody-targeted systems is that through the use of monoclonal antibodies, which recognize only the tumor antigen, side effects of cytotoxic chemicals on the rest of the body could be greatly reduced [126,127]. These systems represent a novel and currently high-interest research area of drug delivery. Their potential value in the delivery of compounds to directed targets has generated considerable interest.

V. DENTAL SYSTEMS

Controlled and sustained drug delivery has recently begun to make an impression in the area of treatment of dental diseases. Many researchers have demonstrated that controlled delivery of antimicrobial agents, such as chlorhexidine [128–130], ofloxacin [131–133], and metronidazole [134], can effectively treat and prevent periodontitis. The incidence of dental caries and formation of plaque can also be reduced by controlled delivery of fluoride [135,136]. Delivery systems used are film-forming solutions [129,130], polymeric inserts [132], implants, and patches. Since dental disease is usually chronic, sustained release of therapeutic agents in the oral cavity would obviously be desirable.

VI. OCULAR SYSTEMS

The eye is unique in its therapeutic challenges. An efficient mechanism, that of tears and tear drainage, which quickly eliminates drug solution, makes topical delivery to the eye somewhat different from most other areas of the body [137]. Usually less than 10% of a topically applied dose is absorbed into the eye, leaving the rest of the dose to potentially absorb into the bloodstream [138], resulting in unwanted side effects. The goal of most controlled-delivery systems is to maintain the drug in the precorneal area and allow its diffusion across the cornea. Suspensions and ointments, although able to provide some sustaining effect, do not offer the amount of control desired [139,140]. Polymeric matrices can often significantly reduce drainage [141], but other newer methods of controlled drug delivery can also be used.

The application of ocular therapy generally includes glaucoma, artificial tears, and anticancer drugs for intraocular malignancies. The sustained release of artificial tears has been achieved by a hydroxypropylcellulose polymer insert [142]. However; the best-known application of diffusional therapy in the eye, Ocusert-Pilo, the device shown in Fig. 14, is a relatively simple structure with two rate-controlling membranes surrounding the drug reservoir containing pilocarpine. Thus, a thin, flexible lamellar ellipse is created and serves as a model reservoir device. The unit is placed in the eye and resides in the lower cul-de-sac, just below the cornea. Since the device itself remains in the eye, the drug is released into the tear film.

The advantages of such a device are that it can control intraocular pressure for up to a week [143]. Control is achieved with less drug and fewer side effects, since the release of drug is zero-order. The system is more convenient, since application is weekly, as opposed to the four times a day dosing for pilocarpine solutions. This greatly improves patient compliance and assures round-the-clock medication, which is of great importance for glaucoma treatment. The main disadvantage of the system is that it is often difficult to retain in the eye and can cause some discomfort.

Another method of delivery of drug to the anterior segment of the eye that has proved successful is prodrug administration [144]. Since the corneal surface presents an effective lipoidal barrier, especially to hydrophilic compounds, it seems reasonable that a prodrug that is more lipophilic than the parent drug will be more successful in penetrating this barrier.

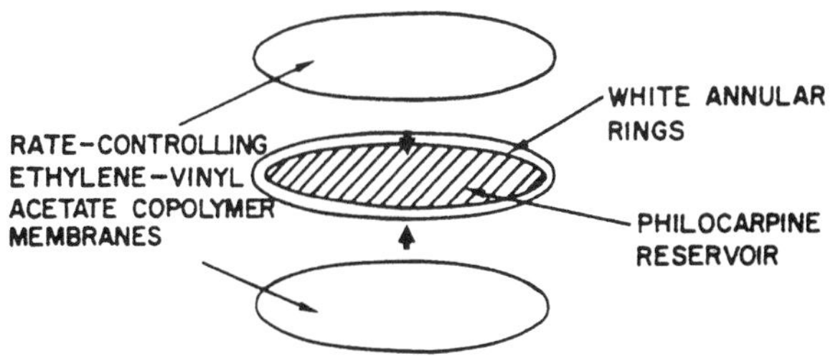

Fig. 14 Schematic diagram of the Ocusert intraocular device for release of pilocarpine.

One drug that has been formulated in this manner is dipivalyl epinephrine (Dividephrine), a dipivalyl ester of epinephrine. Epinephrine itself is poorly absorbed owing to its polar characteristics and is highly metabolized. The prodrug form is approximately 10 times as effective at crossing the cornea and produces substantially higher aqueous humor levels [144,145]. For another prodrug, phenylephrine pivalate, there is some possibility that the prodrug itself is therapeutically active [146,147]. Many other drugs have been derivatized for prodrug ocular delivery: timolol [148,149], nadolol [150], pilocarpine [151,152], prostaglandin $F_{2\alpha}$ [153,154], terbutaline [155], acyclovir [156], vidarabine [157], and idoxuridine [158,159].

New sustained-release technologies are gaining in ocular delivery, as in other routes. Liposomes as drug carriers have achieved enhanced ocular delivery of certain drugs [160], antibiotics [161–163], and peptides [164]. Biodegradable matrix drug delivery to the anterior segment has also been studied [165,166]. Prolonged delivery of pilocarpine can be achieved with a polymeric dispersion [167] or submicrometer emulsions [168]. Implantation of polymers containing endotoxin for neovascularization [169], gancyclovir [170], 5-flurouracil [171], and injections of doxorubicin (adriamycin) [172] have also resulted in sustained delivery. However, topical ocular delivery is much preferred over implants and injections.

VII. TRANSDERMAL SYSTEMS

The transdermal route of drug administration offers several advantages over other methods of delivery. For some cases, oral delivery may be contraindicated, or the drug may be poorly absorbed. This would also include situations for which the drug undergoes a substantial first-pass effect [173] and systemic therapy is desired.

The skin, although presenting a barrier to most drug absorption, provides a very large surface area for diffusion. Below the barrier of the stratum corneum is an extensive network of capillaries. Since the venous return from these capillary beds does not flow directly to the liver, compounds are not exposed to these enzymes during absorption [173]. A most notable example of such a drug is nitroglycerin, which has been administered both sublingually and transdermally to avoid first-pass metabolism. Other drugs that have seen success in controlled transdermal delivery are testosterone [174], fentanyl [175,176], bupranolol [177], and clonidine.

Transdermal controlled-release systems can be used to deliver drugs with short biological half-lives and can maintain plasma levels of very potent drugs within a narrow therapeutic range for prolonged periods. Should problems occur with the system or a change in the status of the patient require modification of therapy, the system is readily accessible and easily removed.

One of the primary disadvantages to this method of delivery is that drugs requiring high blood levels to achieve an effect are difficult to load into a transdermal system owing to the large amount of material required. These systems would naturally be contraindicated if the drug or vehicle caused irritation to the skin. Also, various factors affecting the skin, such as age, physical condition, and device location, can change the reliability of the system's ability to deliver medication in a controlled manner. In other words, both the drug and the nature of the skin can affect the system design.

Current controlled transdermal-release systems can be classified into four types, as follows, with a representative product and manufacturer:

1. Membrane permeation-controlled system in which the drug permeation is controlled by a polymeric membrane: Transderm-Scop (scopolamine; Ciba-Geigy).
2. Adhesive dispersion-type system, which is similar to the foregoing but lacks the polymer membrane; instead the drug is dispersed into an adhesive polymer: Deponit (nitroglycerin; Wyeth).
3. Matrix diffusion-controlled system in which the drug is homogeneously dispersed in a hydrophilic polymer; diffusion from the matrix controls release rate: Nitrodur (nitroglycerin; key).
4. Microreservoir dissolution-controlled system in which microscopic spheres of drug reservoir are dispersed in a polymer matrix: Nitrodisc (nitroglycerin; Searle).

Most marketed systems are of the polymeric membrane-controlled type; representative of these is Transderm-Scop. This product, shown in Fig. 15, is designed to deliver scopolamine over a period of days without the side effects commonly encountered when the drug is administered orally [178]. The system consists of a reservoir containing the drug dispersed in a separate phase within a highly permeable matrix. This is laminated between the rate-controlling microporous membrane and an external backing that is impermeable to drug and moisture. The pores of the rate-con-

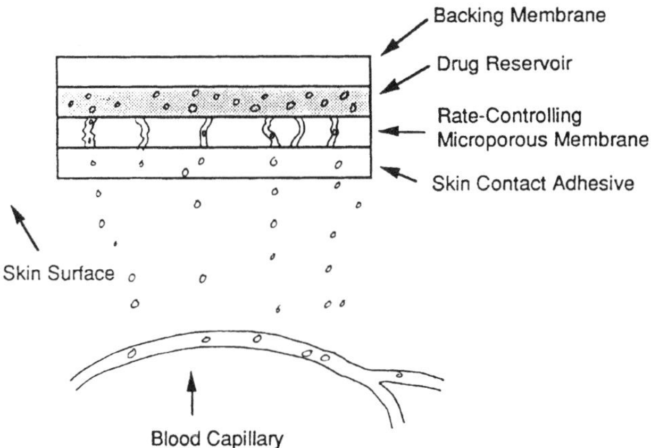

Fig. 15 Schematic diagram of a transdermal device for the delivery of scopolamine.

trolling membrane are filled with a fluid that is highly permeable to scopolamine. This allows delivery of the drug to be controlled by diffusion through the device and skin. Control is achieved because at equilibrium the membrane is rate-limiting for drug permeation. To initiate an immediate effect, a priming dose is contained in a gel on the membrane side of the device.

Another drug that is popular for controlled transdermal release is nitroglycerin. Conventionally, this drug is administered sublingually, although the duration of action by this route is quite short. This is acceptable for acute anginal attacks, but not for prophylactic treatment. Oral administration has the disadvantage that large fractions of the dose are lost to first-pass metabolism in the liver. Topical ointments have long been used for prophylactic treatment of angina, but their duration is only 4–8 hour and, in addition, they are not aesthetically acceptable. The transdermal nitroglycerin devices employ a variety of systems to provide 24-hour delivery.

An electrochemical method to provide pulsed delivery of nitroglycerin, on demand, by the transdermal route has been described [179]. Transdermal iontophoresis is another technique to provide noninvasive, continuous, pulsatile, or preprogrammed dosing that, as disclosed in a review, is showing good promise for many drugs including some peptides and proteins [180]. Another promising new approach in transdermal and transmucosal drug delivery is the use of high-velocity powder injection. This approach, which uses a helium gas jet to accelerate fine drug particles (20–100 μm diameter) into skin or mucosal sites, has also recently been reviewed [181]. Yet another new transdermal system has been developed to deliver nitric oxide (NO) which is a mediator of a number of biological processes, including vasodilation, wound healing, and antimicrobial activity. A chemical generator of NO is placed on one side of a selective permeable membrane (to NO but not to the generator chemicals), with the skin on the other side [182].

VIII. VAGINAL AND UTERINE SYSTEMS

Sustained- and controlled-release devices for drug delivery in the vaginal and uterine areas are most often for the delivery of contraceptive steroid hormones. The advantages in administration by this route—prolonged release, minimal systemic side effects, and an increase in bioavailability—allow for less total drug than with an oral dose. First-pass metabolism that inactivates many steroid hormones can be avoided [183,184].

One such application is the medicated vaginal ring [185]. Therapeutic levels of medroxyprogesterone have been achieved at a total dose that was one-sixth the required oral dose [186]. Ring delivery devices have several problems that have limited their use—vaginal wall erosion and ring expulsion, to name a few. Microcapsules have also recently been useful for vaginal and cervical delivery [187]. Local progesterone release from this dosage form can alter cervical mucus to interfere with sperm migration [188]. Other steroids have also attained sustained delivery by an intracervical system [189]. The sustained release of progesterone from various polymers given vaginally have also been found useful in cervical ripening and the induction of labor [190–192]. A possible new use of the vaginal route is for long-term delivery of antibodies. When various antibodies, including monoclonal IgG and IgM, were administered from polymer vaginal rings in test animals, antibody concentrations remained high over 30 days in vaginal secretions and detectable in blood and tissues, suggesting the route as a reasonable approach to achieve sustained mucosal and systemic antibody levels [193].

A more common contraceptive device is the intrauterine device (IUD). The first type of intrauterine device used was undedicated. These have received increased attention since the use of polyethylene plastics and silicone rubbers [194–196]. These materials had the ability to resume their shape following distortion. Because they are unmedicated, these IUDs cannot be classifieds as sustained-release products. It is believed that their mechanism of action is due to local endometrial responses, both cellular and cytosecretory

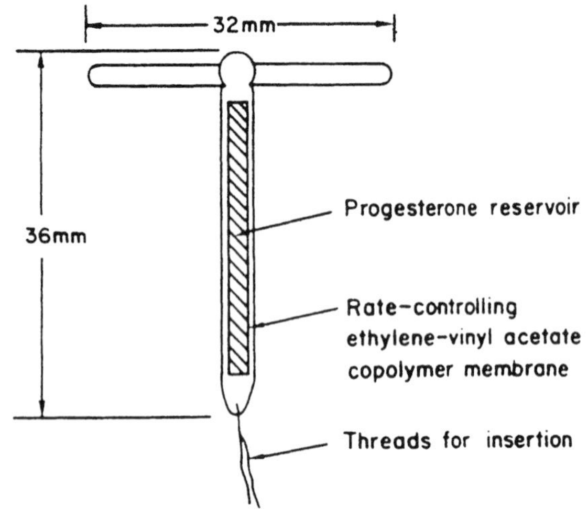

Fig. 16 Schematic diagram of the Progestasert intrauterine device for the release of progesterone.

[197]. Initial investigations of these devices led to the conclusion that the larger the device, the more effective it was in preventing pregnancy. Large devices, however, increased the possibility of uterine cramps, bleeding, and expulsion of the device.

Efforts to improve IUDs have led to the use of medicated devices. Two types of agents are generally used—contraceptive metals and steroid hormones. The metal device is exemplified by the CU-7, a polypropylene plastic device in the shape of the number 7. Copper is released by a combination of ionization and chelation from a copper wire wrapped around the vertical limb. This system is effective for up to 40 months.

The hormone-releasing devices have a closer resemblance to standard methods of sustained release because they involve the release of a steroid compound by diffusion [198,199]. The Progestasert, a reservoir system, is shown in Fig. 16. Progesterone, the active ingredient, is dispersed in the inner reservoir, surrounded by an ethylene/vinyl acetate copolymer membrane. The release of progesterone from this system is maintained almost constant for 1 year. The effects of release are local, with none of the systematic side effects observed with orally administered contraceptives [200–207].

IX. INJECTIONS AND IMPLANTS

One of the most obvious ways to provide sustained-release medication is to place the drug in a delivery system and inject or implant the system into the body tissue. The concept of such delivery methods is not new, but the technology applied is contemporary. Administration of these systems often requires surgical implantation or specialized injection devices. The fact that these systems are in constant contact with exposed tissue components places certain requirements on the systems and their polymer composition.

In general, the materials used must be biocompatible, that is, the polymers themselves must not cause irritation at the implantation site or promote infectien or sterile abscess. The most common polymers used are hydrogels, silicones, and biodegradable materials [208]. Hydrogels have the advantageous property of being able to retain large amounts of water within their structure without dissolving [209]. This high aqueous content makes them very compatible with living tissues but unfortunately allows low molecular weight substances to diffuse out quickly. Cross-linking agents can be used to reduce this diffusional loss and to provide structural rigidity, but this can increase the frictional irritation of the hydrogel with its surrounding tissue.

Subcutaneous implantation is currently one of the most utilized routes to investigate the potential of sustained-delivery systems. This is because favorable absorption sites are available and removal of the device can be accomplished at any time. Surgery is often required and in itself can be considered a disadvantage, as is the fact that once implanted, the delivery rate of the drug is usually fixed until the device is removed. The development of implants has a long history, starting initially with investigations on implanted silicone devices. The most notable new implantable product is Norplant, a contraceptive device releasing levonorgestrel for up to 5 years [210]. This product is implanted subdermally and requires only a local anesthetic. A variety of other drugs have also been used, including thyroid hormones, steroids, cardiovascular agents [211–213], insulin [215], and nerve growth factor [216].

Sustained-release injections, subcutaneous and intramuscular, have been investigated in a variety of different formulations [217,218]. Injections of degradable microspheres have efficiently prolonged delivery of numerous drugs [219–222], even antigenic substances and vaccines to produce immunity [223,224].

Some implantation devices have extended well beyond the classic diffusional systems and have included not only bioerodible devices, but also implantable therapeutic systems that can be activated. There are devices activated by change in osmotic pressure to deliver insulin [225], morphine release trigger by vapor pressure [226], and pellets activated by magnetism to release their encapsulated drug load [227]. Such external control of an embedded device would eliminate many of the disadvantages of most implanted delivery systems.

In the delivery of therapeutic proteins, although recent advances in transdermal and oral delivery have been significant, logarithmic increases in the bioavailability of these drugs must be achieved to make them candidates for commercialization by these routes. Therefore, in the years immediately ahead, protein delivery for commercial products will likely be limited to injection forms, depot systems, and pulmonary administration [228]. As a result a great deal of research is now directed to such areas as increasing the functionalization of polymer carrier material surfaces to meet the demands of the biological host system [229]. Included in this general approach are adherent bilayer hydrogels carrying proteins for intraarterial delivery [230]. Another approach involves the chemical modification of proteins to facilitate their formulation into or conjugation with the parenteral polymeric carriers [231].

X. OTHER TARGETED SITES

Sites along the small intestine and in the colon are increasingly becoming specific locations for drug delivery. A wide variety of transporters are found in the intestine and are involved in the transport of dietary nutrients. These transporters, located in the brush border membrane and basolateral membrane, exhibit unique substrate specificities. The development of prodrugs that target intestinal transporters has been successful in some cases, and the intestinal peptide transporter is used to increase the bioavailability of several peptidomimetic drugs. Recent advances in gene cloning and molecular biology techniques are making it possible to study the characteristics and distribution of transporters at a molecular level. This field and the promise for targeting specific intestinal transporters in drug delivery has recently been comprehensively reviewed [232].

The colon represents an important and challenging target site in the gastrointestinal tract to provide more effective treatments for ulcerative colitis, Crohn's disease, and colorectal cancer. In addition, colonic delivery of vermicides and diagnostic agents is enhanced. Special "superenteric" polymer coatings continue to be investigated; these transit not only to the stomach, but also to the small intestine before releasing all or most of their "encapsulated" drug [233,244]. Several very comprehensive reviews on colonic drug targeting have been published [235,236]. Various prodrug conjugates of 5-aminosalicylic acid have also been used to deliver that drug to the colon for site-specific release [237].

Another very important site for drug delivery is the central nervous system (CNS). The blood-brain barrier presents a formidable barrier to the effective delivery of most agents to the brain. Interesting work is now advancing in such areas as direct convective delivery of macromolecules (and presumably in the future macromolecular drug carriers) to the spinal cord [238] and even to peripheral nerves [239]. For the interested reader, the delivery of therapeutic molecules into the CNS has also been recently comprehensively reviewed [240].

Polymers have historically been the key to the great majority of drug-delivery systems. It is expected that this will be the case in the foreseeable future. A class of polymers growing in importance in this regard are phase-transition polymers. These materials undergo physical changes, which may, for example, trigger drug release in response to external stimuli (pH, temperature including microwave response, light sources, chemicals including metabolites, electric current, magnetic field, etc.). The significance of these polymers is that they may not only dictate where a drug is delivered, but when and at what time intervals it is released. A paper has summarized these polymers and their applications to modulated drug delivery [241].

XI. CONCLUSIONS

The space limitations of a text such as this do not permit a complete discourse on all of the sustained and controlled mechanisms available for possible drug delivery. Instead an attempt has been made to cover as completed as possible the major and currently marketed types, of drug delivery while also providing some insights into likely future advances. Sustained and controlled drug-delivery systems are becoming more the norm rather than the exception in modem pharmaceutical development, to enhance and even optimize drug product effectiveness, reliability, and safety. Current research in this area involves numerous new and novel systems, many of which have strong therapeutic potential. Furthermore, many if not most of the drugs that will derive from the biotechnology scientific revolution in the years and decades ahead will require the application of effective and innovative drug-delivery technology. The future of this area is limited only by the imagination of those who choose to become involved in the field.

REFERENCES

1. V. H. Lee and J. R. Robinson, in *Sustained and Controlled Release Drug Delivery Systems* (J. R. Robinson, ed.), Marcel Dekker, New York, 1978, p. 71.
2. M. E. Jacobson, Postgrad. Med., 49, 181 (1971).
3. B. Beerman, K. Helstrom, and A. Rosen, Clin. Pharmacol. Ther., 13, 212 (1972).
4. A. B. Morrison, C. B. Perusse, and J. A. Campbell, N. Engl. J. Med., 263, 115 (1960).
5. E. J. Middleton, E. Nagy, and A. B. Morrison, N. Engl. J. Med., 274, 136 (1966).
6. P. G. Welling and R. H. Barbhaiya, J. Pharm. Sci., 71, 32 (1982).
7. B. C. Thanoo, M. C. Sunny, and A. Jayakrishnan, J. Pharm. Pharmacol., 45, 21 (1993).
8. W. L. Xu, X. D. Tu, and Z. D. Lu, Acta Pharm. Sin., 26, 541 (1991).
9. S. Watanabe, M. Kayano, Y. Ishino, and K. Miyao, U.S. Patent 3, 976,764 (1976).
10. S. Watanabe, M. Ichikawa, and Y. Miyake, J. Pharm. Sci., 80, 1062 (1991).
11. S. Watanabe, M. Ichikawa, T. Kato, M. Kawahara, and M. Kayano, J. Pharm. Sci., 80, 1153 (1991).
12. S. S. Leung and J. R. Robinson, J. Controlled Release, 5, 223 (1988).
13. R. Johansson, C. G. Regardh, and S. Sjogren, Acta Pharm. Suec., 8, 59 (1971).
14. A. C. Woods, G. A. Glaubiger, and T. N. Chase, Lancet, 1, 1391 (1973).
15. S. Eriksen, in *The Theory and Practice of Industrial Pharmacy* (L. Lachman, H. A. Lieberman, and J. L. Kanig, eds.), Lea & Febiger, Philadelphia, 1970, p. 408.
16. V. Manninen, K. Ojala, and P. Reisell, Lancet, 2, 922 (1972).
17. J. G. Wagner, P. G. Welling, K. O. Lee, and J. E. Walker, J. Pharm. Sci., 69, 666 (1971).
18. T. R. Bates, D. A. Lambert, and W. H. Jones, J. Pharm. Sci., 58, 1488 (1969).
19. J. H. Fincher, J. Pharm. Sci., 57, 1825 (1968).
20. N. P. Salzman and B. B. Brodie, J. Pharmacol. Exp. Ther., 118, 46 (1956).
21. B. Beerman, K. Helstrom, and A. Rosen, Clin. Pharmacol. Ther., 13, 212 (1972).
22. W. H. Bachrach, Am. J. Dig. Dis., 3, 743 (1958).
23. A. Fick, Poggendorffs Ann., 94, 59 (1885).
24. R. M. Barrier, Discuss. Faraday Soc., 21, 138 (1956).
25. G. L. Flynn, S. H. Yalkowsky, and T. J. Roseman, J. Pharm. Sci., 63, 479 (1974).
26. J. Crank, *The Mathematics of Diffusion*, Oxford University Press, Oxford, 1956.
27. R. W. Baker and H. K. Lonsdale, in *Controlled Release of Biologically Active Agents* (A. C. Tanquary and R. E. Lacey, eds.), Plenum Press, New York, 1974, p. 15.
28. A. Fisch, E. Pichard, T. Prazuck, R. Sebbag, G. Torres, G. Gernez and M. Gentilini, Am. J. Public Health, 83, 540 (1993).
29. T. Higuchi, J. Pharm. Sci., 50, 874 (1961).
30. G. L. Flynn, S. H. Yalkowsky, and T. J. Roseman, J. Pharm. Sci., 63, 479 (1974).
31. S. J. Desai, P. Singh, A. P. Simonelli, and W. I. Higuchi, J. Pharm. Sci., 55, 1224 (1966).
32. S. J. Desai, A. P. Simonelli, and W. I. Higuchi, J. Pharm. Sci., 54, 1459 (1965).
33. S. J. Desai, P. Singh, A. P. Simonelli, and W. I. Higuchi, J. Pharm. Sci., 55, 1230 (1966).
34. S. J. Desai, P. Singh, A. P. Simonelli, and W. I. Higuchi, J. Pharm. Sci., 55, 1235 (1966).
35. H. Lapidus and N. G. Lordi, J. Pharm. Sci., 55, 840 (1966).
36. H. B. Hopfenberg, in *Controlled Release Polymeric Formulations* (D. R. Paul and F. W. Harris, eds.), American Chemical Society, Washington, DC, 1976, p. 26.
37. E. Goldberg, in *Polymeric Delivery Systems, Midland Macromolecular Symposium* (R. J. Kostelnek, ed.), Gordon and Breach, New York, 1978, p. 227.
38. H. B. Hopfenberg and K. C. Hsu, Polym. Eng. Sci., 18, 1186 (1978).
39. H. Nakagami and M. Nada, Drug Design Discovery, 8, 103 (1991).
40. R. W. Baker, U.S. Patent 3,952,741 (1976).
41. W. Bayne, V. Place, F. Theeuwes, J. D. Rogers, R. B. Lee, R. O. Davies, and K. C. Kwan, J. Clin. Pharmacol. Ther., 32, 270 (1982).
42. R. Theeuwes, J. Pharm. Sci., 64, 1987 (1975).
43. S. Motycka and J. G. Naira, J. Pharm. Sci., 67, 500 (1978).
44. M. D. Garrett and P. Workman, Eur. J. Cancer, 35(14), 2010 (1999).
45. G. Gregoriadis, in *Drug Carriers in Biology and Medicine* (G. Gregoriadis, ed.), Academic Press, London, 1979.
46. H. K. Kimelberg and G. G. Meyhem, CRC Crit. Rev. Toxicol., Dec., 25 (1978).
47. G. Gregoriadis, C. Kirby, P. Large, A. Meehan, and J. Senior, in *Targeting of Drugs* (G. Gregoriadis, J. Senior, and A. Trouet, eds.), Plenum Press, New York, 1982, p. 155.
48. D. Chapman in *Liposome Technology*, Vol. 1 (G. Gregoriadis, ed.), CRC Press, Boca Raton, FL, 1984.
49. J. de Gien, J. G. Mandersloot, and L. L. M. van Deenen, Biochim. Biophys. Acta, 150, 166 (1968).
50. B. D. Ladbrooke and D. Chapman, Chem. Phys. Lipid, 3, 304 (1969).
51. R. L. Magin and J. N. Weinstein, in *Liposome Technology*, Vol. 3, (G. Gregoriadis, ed.), CRC Press, Boca Raton, FL, 1984.
52. J. N. Weinstein, R. L. Mahin, R. L. Cysyk, and D. S. Zaharko, Cancer Res., 40, 1388 (1980).

53. J. D. Morrissett, R. L. Jackson, and A. M. Gotto, Biochim. Biophys. Acta, 472, 93 (1977).
54. F. Szoka and D. Papahadjopoulos, Annu. Rev. Biophys. Bioeng., 9, 467 (1980).
55. R. A. Damel, S. C. Kinsky, C. B. Kinsky, and L. L. M. Van Deenen, Biochim Biophys. Acta, 150, 655 (1968).
56. H. L. Kantor and J. H. Prestegard, Biochemistry, 14, 1790 (1975).
57. R. E. Pagano and J. N. Weinstein, Annu. Rev. Biophys. Bioeng., 7, 435 (1978).
58. T. D. Heath, N. G. Lopez, J. R. Piper, J. A. Montgomery, W. H. Stern, and D. Papahadjopoulos, Biochim. Biophys. Acta, 862, 72 (1986).
59. T. D. Heath and C. S. Brown, J. Liposome Res., 1, 303 (1989).
60. J. Vaage and E. Mayhew, Int. J. Cancer, 47, 582 (1991).
61. H. A. Titulaer, W. M. Eling, D. J. Crommelin, P. A. Peeters, and J. Zuiderma, J. Pharm. Pharrnacol. 42, 529 (1990).
62. T. M. Allen, T. Mehra, C. Hansen, and Y. C. Chin, Cancer Res. 52, 2431 (1992).
63. J. A. Rogers and K. E. Anderson, Crit. Rev. Ther. Drug Carrier Syst. 15(5), 421 (1998).
64. H. Pinto-Alphandary, A. Andremont, and P. Couveur, Int. J. Antimicrob. Agents, 13(3), 155 (2000).
65. D. C. Drummond, K. Hong, J. W. Park, C. C. Benz, and D. B. Kirpotin, Vitam. Horm., 60, 285 (2000).
66. M. Babincova et a1., Zeitschr. Naturforsch. J. Biosci., 5 (3–4), 278 (2000).
67. A. Namideo and N. K. Jain, J. Microencap, 16(6), 731 (1999).
68. R. Peschka, C. Dennehy, and F. C. Szoka Jr., J. Contr. Rel., 56(l–3), 41 (1998).
69. G. L. Amidon, G. D. Leesman, and R. L. Elliot, J. Pharm. Sci., 69, 1363 (1980).
70. G. W. Carter, P. R. Young, L. R. Swett, and G. Y. Paris, Agents Actions, 10, 240 (1980).
71. J. Bungaard, in *Bioreversible Carriers in Drug Design, Theory and Application* (E. B. Roche, ed.). Pergammon Press, New York, 1987.
72. H. Bungaard, in *Design of Prodrugs* (H. Bungaard, ed.), Elsevier, Amsterdam, 1985.
73. G. B. Elion, J. A. Fyfe, L. Beauchamp, P. A. Furman, P. De Miranda, and H. J. Schaeffer, Proc. Natl. Acad. Sci. USA, 74, 5716 (1977).
74. A. A. Sinkula, in *Design of Prodrugs* (Bungaard, ed.), Elsevier, Amsterdam, 1985.
75. A. Bundgaard, Adv. Drug Deliv. Rev., 3, 39 (1989).
76. T. Kojima, M. Hashida, S. Muranishi, and H. Sezaki, J. Pharm. and Pharmacol., 32, 30 (1980).
77. A. Kato, Y. Takakura, M. Hashida, T. Kimura, and H. Sezaki, Chem. Pharm. Bull. 30, 2951 (1982).
78. H. N. Joshi, Pharm. Tech., June, 118 (1988).
79. J. Kreuter and W. Liehl, J. Pharm. Sci., 70, 367 (1981).
80. J. Kreuter, Pharm. Acta Helv., 58, 196 (1983).
81. R. C. Oppenhem, in *Drug Delivery Systems* (R. L. Juliano, ed.), Oxford University Press, New York, l982, p. 182.
82. J. Kreuter, Pharm. Acta Helv., 58, 217 (1983).
83. L. Illum and S. S. Davis, FEBS Lett., 167, 79 (1984).
84. D. Leu, B. Manthey, J. Kreuter, P. Speiser, and P. P. DeLuca, J. Pharm. Sci., 73, 1433 (1984).
85. S. D. Troster, U. Mueller, and J. Kreuter, Int. J. Pharm., 61, 85 (1991).
86. L. Grislain, P. Couvreur, V. Lenaerts, M. Roland, D. Deprez-Decampeneere, and P. Speiser, Int. J. Pharm., 15, 335 (1983).
87. E. M. Gipps, R. Arshady, J. Kreuter, P. Groscurth, and P. P. Speiser, J. Pharm. Sci., 75, 256 (1986).
88. T. Harmia, P. Speiser, and J. Kreuter, J. Microencapsul., 3, 3 (1986).
89. F. Brasseur, P. Couvreur, B. Kante, L. Deckers-Passau, M. Roland, C. Deckers, and P. Speiser, Eur. J. Cancer, 16, 1441 (1980).
90. J. Kreuter and H. R. Hartmann, Oncology, 40, 363 (1983).
91. K. Sugibayashi, M. Akimoto, Y. Morimoto, T. Nadai, and Y. Kato, J. Pharmicobiodyn., 2, 350 (1979).
92. P. Couvreur, B. Kante, L. Grislain, M. Roland, and P. Speiser, J. Pharm. Sci., 71, 790 (1982).
93. Y. Morimoto, K. Sugibayashi, and Y. Kato, Chem. Pharm. Bull., 29, 1433 (1981).
94. J. Kreuter, in *Drug Targeting* (P. Buri and A. Gumma, eds.), Elsevier, Amsterdam, 1985.
95. J. L. Grangier, M. Puygrenier, J. V. Hautier, and P. Couvreur, J. Controlled Deliv., 15, 3 (1991).
96. J. C. Gautier, J. L. Grangier, A. Barbier, P. Dupont, D. Dussossoy, G. Pastor, and P. Couvreur, J. Controlled Release, 20, 67 (1992).
97. N. V. Majeti and R. Kumar, J. Pharm. Pharmaceut. Sci., 3(2), 234 (2000).
98. J. C. Levoux, E. Allermann, F. DeJaeghere, E. Doelker, and R. Gurny, J. Contr. Rel., 39, 339 (1996).
99. E. Pitt, C. M. Johnson, D. A. Lewix, D. A. Jenner, and R. B. Offord, Biochem. Pharmacol., 32, 3359 (1983).
100. G. Ihler, in *Drug Carriers in Biology and Medicine* (G. Gregoriadis, ed.), Academic Press, London, 1979, p. 287.
101. R. A. Cooper, in *Hematology*, 2nd ed. (W. J. Williams, E. Beutler, A. J. Erslev, and R. W. Rundles, eds.), McGraw-Hill, New York, 1977, p. 216.
102. D. A. Lewis and H. O. Alpar, Int. J. Pharm., 22, 137 (1984).
103. C. A. Scheinberg and M. Strand, Cancer Res., 42, 44 (1982).
104. G. Gregoriadis, Drugs, 24, 261 (1982).
105. L. D. Lesserman, J. Barbet, F. Kourilsky, and J. N. Weinstein, Nature, 288, 602 (1980).
106. P. N. Kulkarni, P. H. Blair, and T. Ghose, Fed. Proc., 40, 642 (1982).

107. G. F. Rowland, R. G. Simmons, J. R. F. Corvalan, R. W. Baldwin, J. P. Browns, M. J. Embelton, C. H. J. Ford, K. E. Hillstorm, I. Hellstrom, J. T. Kemshead, C. E. Newmans, and X. S. Woodhouse, in *Proteins of the Biological Fluids*, Proceedings Colloquim 30 (H. Peters, ed.), Pergammon Press, New York, 1983.
108. J. M. Whitely, Ann. NY Acad. Sci., 79, 621 (1982).
109. M. Muirhead, P. J. Martin, B. Torok-Storb, J. W. Uhr, and S. Vitelia, Blood, 62, 327 (1983).
110. G. F. Rowland, in *Targeted Drugs* (E. P. Goldberg, ed.), Wiley-Interscience, New York, 1983.
111. M. B. Primm, J. A. Jones, M. R. Price, J. G. Middle, M. J. Embleton, and R. W. Baldwin, Cancer Immunol. Immunother., 12, 125 (1982).
112. Z. Brich, S. Ravel, T. Kissel, J. Fritsch, and A. Schoffmann, J. Controlled Release, 19, 245 (1992).
113. I. Tsukada, W. K. Bishop, N. Hibe, H. Hirai, B. Hurwitz, and M. Sela, Proc. Natl. Acad. Sci. USA, 79, 621 (1982).
114. B. Rihoua, A. Jegorov, J. Strohalm, W. Matha, P. Rossmann, L. Fornusek, and K. Ulbrich, J. Controlled Release, 19, 25 (1992).
115. F. Hurwitz, R. Kashi, and M. Wilcheck, J. Natl. Cancer Inst., 69, 47 (1982).
116. L.G. Bernier, M. Page, R. C. Gaudreault, and L. P. Joly, Br. J. Cancer, 49, 245 (1984).
117. M. J. Embleton, G. F. Rowland, R. S. Simmonds, E. Jacobs, C. H. Marsden, and R. W. Baldwin, Br. J. Cancer, 47, 43 (1983).
118. J. B. Cannon and H. W. Hui, in *Targeted Therapeutic Systems* (P. Tyle and B. P. Ram, eds.), Marcel Dekker, NY, 1990.
119. S. Wright and L. Huang, Adv. Drug Deliv. Rev., 3, 343 (1989).
120. M. Udayachander, A. Meenakshi, R. Muthiah, and M. Sivanandham, Int. J. Radiol. Oncol. Biol. Phys., 13, 1713 (1987).
121. A. K. Agrawal, A. Singhal, and C. M. Gupta, Biochim. Biophys. Res. Commun., 148, 357 (1987).
122. T. Tadakuma, in *Medical Applications of Liposomes* (K. Yagi, ed.), Japan Scientific Society Press, Tokyo, 1986.
123. C. Y. Wang and L. Huang, Proc. Natl. Acad. Sci. USA, 84, 7851 (1987).
124. P. Machy and L. D. Lesernman, Biochim. Biophys. Acta, 730, 313 (1983).
125. K. K. Matthay, T. D. Heath, and D. Papahadjopoulos, Cancer Res., 44, 1850 (1984).
126. D. Paphadjopoulous, T. Heath, F. Martin, F. Fraley, and R. Straubinger, in *Targeting of Drugs* (G. Gregoriadis, J. Senior, and A. Trouet, eds.), Plenum Press, New York, 1982.
127. W. Magee, H. Croneberger, and D. E. Thor, Cancer Res., 38, 1173 (1978).
128. F. Cervone, L. Tronstad, and B. Hammond, Endodont. Dent. Traumatol., 6, 33 (1990).
129. D. Steinberg, N. Friedman, A. Soskolne, and M. N. Sela, J. Periodontol., 61, 393 (1990).
130. A. Kozlorsky, A. Sintor, Y. Zubery, and H. Tal, J. Dent Res., 71, 1577 (1992).
131. K. Higashi, K. Morisaki, S. Hayashi, M. Kitamura, N. Fujimoto, S. Kimura, S. Ebisu, and H. Okada, J. Periodont. Res., 25, 1 (1990).
132. H. Yamagami, A. Takomori, T. Sakamotok, and H. Okada, J. Periodontol., 63, 2 (1992).
133. S. Kimura, H. Toda, Y. Shimabukuro, M. Kitamura, N. Fujimoto, Y. Miki, and H. Okada, J. Periodont. Res., 26, 33 (1991).
134. J. P. Fiorellini and D. W. Paguette, Curr. Opin. Dent., 2, 63 (1992).
135. K. S. Aithal, A. R. Moor, Y. B. Pathak, and J. Uchil, Indian J. Dent. Res., 2, 174 (1990).
136. S. Tamburic, G. Vuleta, M. Gajic, R. Stevanovic, Slomatoloski Glasnik Srbije, 37, 307 (1990).
137. M. C. Makoid and J. R. Robinson, J. Pharm. Sci., 68, 435 (1978).
138. H. Benson, Arch. Ophthalmol., 91, 313 (1974).
139. J. W. Seig and J. R. Robinson, J. Pharm. Sci., 68, 724 (1979).
140. R. D. Schoenwald and P. Stewart, J. Pharm. Sci., 69, 391 (1980).
141. J. W. Shell, Surv. Ophthalmol., 26, 207 (1982).
142. D. W. Lamberts, D. P. Langston, and W. Chu, Ophthalmology, 85, 794 (1978).
143. J. W. Shell and R. W. Baker, Ann. Ophthalmol., 6, 1037 (1974).
144. J. A. Anderson, W. L. Davis, and C. Wei, Invest. Ophthalmol. Visual Sci., 19, 817 (1980).
145. A. I. Mandell, F. Stentz, and A. E. Kitabchi, Ophthalmology, 85, 268 (1978).
146. J. S. Mindel, S. T. Shaikewite, and S. M. Podos, Arch. Ophthalmol., 98, 2220 (1980).
147. D. S. Chien and R. D. Schoenwald, Pharm. Res., 7, 476 (1990).
148. D. S. Chien, H. Bundgaard, A. Buur, and V. H. L. Lee, J. Ocular Pharmacol., 4, 137 (1988).
149. H. Bundgaard, A. Buur, S. C. Chang, and V. H. L. Lee, Int. J. Pharm., 33, 15 (1986).
150. E. Duzman, C. C. Chen, J. Anderson, M. Blumenthal, and L. Twizer, Arch. Ophthalmol., 100, 1916 (1982).
151. H. Bundgaard, E. Falch, C. Larsen, and T. J. Mikkelson, J. Pharm. Sci., 75, 775 (1986).
152. G. L. Mosher, H. Bundgaard, E. Falch, C. Larsen, and T. J. Mikkelson, Int. J. Pharm., 39, 113 (1986).
153. L. Z. Bito and R. A. Baroody, Exp. Eye Res., 44, 217 (1984).
154. O. Camber, P. Edman, and L. I. Olsson, Int. J. Pharm. 37, 27 (1987).
155. T. L. Phipps, D. B. Potter, and J. M. Rowland, J. Ocular Pharmacol., 2, 109 (1986).
156. P. C. Maudgal, K. D. Clercq, J. Descamps, and L. Missotten, Ardh. Ophthalmol. 102, 140 (1984).

157. D. Pavan-Langston, R. D. North, P. A. Geary, and A. Kinkel, Arch. Ophthalmol., 94, 1585 (1976).
158. M. M. Narurkar and A. K. Mitra, Pharm. Res., 6, 887 (1989).
159. M. M. Narurkar and A. K. Mitra, Pharm. Res., 5, 734 (1988).
160. V. H. L. Lee, P. T. Ureaa, R. B. Smith, and D. J. Schanzlin, Surv. Ophthalmol., 29, 335 (1985).
161. M. W. Fountain, A. S. Janoff, M. J. Ostro, M. C. Popescu, and A. L. Weiner, 10th Int. Symp. Contr. Rel. Bioactive Mat., 1983.
162. K. Singh and M. Mezei, Int. J. Pharm., 19, 263 (1984).
163. A. G. Palestine, R. B. Nussenblatt, M. V. W. Bergamini, I. E. Bolcsak, and W. T. Robinson, Invest. Ophthalmol. Vis. Sci., 27 (3 suppl.), 112 (1986).
164. M. Barza, J. Baum, and F. Szoka, Invest. Ophthalmol. Vis. Sci., 25, 486 (1984).
165. G. M. Grass, J. C. Cob, and M. C. Makoid, J. Pharm. Sci., 75, 618 (1984).
166. J. W. Shell, Sur. Ophthalmol. 29, 117 (1984)
167. S. P. Vyas, S. Ramchandraiah, C. P. Jain, S. K. Jain, J. Microencapsul., 9, 347 (1992).
168. M. Sznitowska et al., J. Microencapsul., 18(2). 173 (2001).
169. W. W. Li, G. Grayson, J. Folkman, and P. A. D'Amore, Invest. Ophthalmol. Vis. Sci., 32, 2906 (1991).
170. R. Anand, S. D. Nightingale, R. H. Fish, T. J. Smith, and P. Ashtor, Arch. Ophthalmol., 111, 223 (1993).
171. D. L. Blondford, T. J. Smith, J. D. Brown, P. A. Pearson, and P. Ashtor, Invest. Ophthalmol. Vis. Sci., 32, 2906 (1991).
172. J. Kimura, Y. Ogura, T. Moritera, Y. Honda, R. Wada, and S. H. Hyon, Invest. Ophthalmol. Vis. Sci., 33, 3436 (1992).
173. S. K. Chandrasekaran, W. Bayne, and J. E. Shaw, J. Pharm. Sci., 67, 1370 (1978).
174. M. Bals-Pratsch, Y. D. Yoon, U. A. Knuth, and E. Nieschlag, Lancet, 2, 943 (1986).
175. D. J. R. Duthie, D. J. Rowbotham, R. Wyld, P. D. Henderson, and W. S. Nimmo, Br. J. Anaesth., 60, 614 (1988).
176. F. O. Holley and C. van Steenis, Br. J. Anaesth., 60, 608 (1988).
177. A. Wellstein, H. Kuppers, H. F. Pitscher, and D. Palm., Eur. J. Clin. Pharmacol., 31, 419 (1986).
178. S. K. Chandrasekaran, H. Benson, and J. Urquhart, in *Sustained and Controlled Release Delivery Systems* (J. R. Robinson, ed.), Marcel Dekker, New York, 1978, p. 578.
179. R. Groning and U. Kuhland, Internat. J. Pharmaceut., 193(1), 57 (1999).
180. O. Pillai, V. Nair, R. Poduri, and R. Panchagnula, Methods Findings Exp. Clin. Pharmacol., 21(3), 229 (1999).
181. T. L. Burkoth et al., Crit. Rev. Ther. Drug Carrier Systems, 16(4), 331 (1999).
182. J. B. Hardiwick, A. T. Tucker, M. Wilks, A. Johnson, and N. Benjamin, Clin. Sci., 100(4), 395 (2001).
183. D. P. Benziger and J. Edelson, Drug Metab. Rev., 14, 137 (1983).
184. D. J. Back, A. Breckenridge, M. E. Orme, and M. A. Shaw, Lancet, 1(8369), 171 (1984).
185. E. Diczfalusy and B. M. Landgren, in *Long-Acting Contraceptive Delivery Systems* (G. I. Zatuchni, A. J. Sobero, J. J. Speidel, and J. J. Sciarra, eds.), Harper & Row, New York, 1984.
186. Y. W. Chien, in *Drug Delivery Systems* (R. L. Juliano, ed.), Oxford University Press, New York, 1982, p. 42.
187. G. A. Digenis, M. Jay, R. M. Beihn, T. R. Rice, and L. R. Beck, in *Long-Acting Contraceptive Delivery Systems* (G. I. Zatuchni, A. J. Sobero, J. J. Speidell, and J. J. Sciarra, eds.). Harper & Row, New York, 1984.
188. N. S. Mason, D. V. S. Gupta, D. W. Liller, R. S. Youngquist, and R. S. Sparks, in *Biomedical Applications of Microencapsulation* (R. Lim, ed.), CRC Press. Boca Raton, FL, 1984.
189. P. Lahteenmaki, H. Kurunmaki, T. Luukkainer, P. O. A. Lahteenmaki, K. Ratsula, and J. Toivonen, in *Biomedical Applications of Microencapsulation* (R. Lim, ed.), CRC Press, Boca Raton, FL, 1984.
190. T. A. Johnson, I. A. Green, R. W. Killy, and A. A. Calder, Brit. J. Ob. Gyn., 99, 877 (1992).
191. F. R. Witter, L. E. Rocco, and T. R. Johnson, Am. J. Obstet. Gynecol., 99, 877 (1992).
192. A. V. Taylor, J. Boland, and I. Z. MacKenzie, Prostaglandins, 40, 89 (1990).
193. W. M. Saltzman, J. K. Sherwood, D. R. Adams, and P. Haller, Biotechnol. Bioeng., 67(3), 253 (2000).
194. W. Oppenheimer, Am. J. Obstet. Gyncecol., 78, 446 (1959).
195. A. Ishihama, Yokahama Med. Bull., 20, 89 (1959).
196. A. Ishihama, T. Kagabu, T. Iamai, and M. Shimal, Acta Cytol., 14, 35 (1970).
197. M. Rowland, *Response to Contraception*, W. B. Saunders, Philadelphia, 1973, p. 111.
198. Alza Corporation, Palo Alto, CA.
199. V. A. Place and B. B. Pharriss, J. Reprod. Med., 13, 66 (1974).
200. R. Aznar-Ramos, B. B. Pharriss, and J. Martinez-Mamautou, Fertil. Steril., 25, 308 (1974).
201. B. D. Kulkarni, T. D. Avila, B. B. Pharriss, and A. Scommegna, Contraception, 8, 299 (1973).
202. U. Leone, Int. J. Fertil., 19, 17 (1974).
203. A. Scommegna, Obstet, Gynecol., 43, 769 (1974).
204. A. Zaffaroni, Acta Endocrinol., 75 (Suppl. 185), 423 (1974).
205. V. A. Place and B. B. Pharriss, J. Reprod. Med., 13, 66 (1974).

206. A. Rosado, J. J. Hicks, R. Aznar, and E. Mercado, Contraception, 9, 39 (1974).
207. B. Seohadri, Y. Gibor, and A. Scommegna, Am. J. Obset. Gynecol., 109, 536 (1971).
208. R. Langer, Chem. Eng. Commun., 6, 1(1980).
209. T. Tanaka, Sci. Am., 224, (1) 124, 138 (1981).
210. C. M. Klaisle and S. Wysocke, Clin. Issues Perinat. Wom. Health, 3, 267 (1992).
211. H. M. Creque, R. L. Langer, and T. Folkham, Diabetes, 29, 39 (1980).
212. Y. W. Chien and E. P. K. Lau, J. Pharm. Sci., 65, 488 (1976).
213. A. S. Lifichez, Fertil. Steril., 21, 426 (1970).
214. A. Cuadros, A. Brinson, and K. Sundaram, Contraception, 2, 29 (1970).
215. P. Y. Wans, Biomaterials, 12, 57 (1991).
216. E. M. Powell, M. R. Sobarzo, and W. M. Saltzman, Brain Res., 515, 309 (1990).
217. J. Skarda, J. Slaba, P. Krejci, and I. Mikular, Physiol. Res., 41, 151 (1992).
218. F. M. Kahan and J. D. Rogers, Chemotherapy, 2, 21 (1991).
219. S. Li, M. Lepage, Y. Merand, A. Belanger, F. Labrie, Breast Cancer Res. Treat., 24, 127 (1993).
220. T. Hashimoto, T. Wada, N. Fukuda, and A. Nagoaka, J. Pharm. Pharmacol., 45, 94 (1993).
221. R. A. Burns, K. Vitale, and L. M. Sanders, J. Microencapsul., 7, 397 (1990).
222. N. S. Jones, M. G. Glenn, L.A. Orloff, and M. R. Mayberg, Arch. Otolaryngol., 116, 779 (1990).
223. D. T. O'Hagan, D. Ragman, J. P. McGee, H. Jeffrey, M. C. Davies, P. Williams, S. S. Davis, and S. J. Challacombe, Immunology, 73, 239 (1991).
224. D. T. O'Hagan, H. Jeffrey, M. J. Roberts, J. P. McGee, and S. S. Davis, Vaccine, 9, 768 (1991).
225. Y. W. Chein, in *Novel Drug Delivery Systems* (T. J. Roseman and S. Z. Mansdorf, eds.), Marcel Dekker, New York, 1982.
226. Implantable pump for morphine, Am. Pharm., NS24, 9, 20 (1984).
227. D. S. T. Hsieh and R. Langer, in *Controlled Release Delivery Systems* (T. J. Roseman and S. Z. Mansdorf, eds.), Marcel Dekker, New York, 1983.
228. J. L. Cleland, A. Daugherty and R. Mrsny, Curr. Opin. Biotechnol. 12(2), 212 (2001).
229. B. Kasemo and J. Gold, Adv. Dental Res., 13, 8 (1999).
230. Y. An and J. A. Hubbell, J. Contr. Rel., 64(1–3), 205 (2000).
231. T. K. Kim and D. J. Burgess, J. Pharm. Pharmacol., 53(1), 23 (2001).
232. D. M. Oh., H. K. Han and G. L. Amidon, Pharmac. Biotech. 12, 59–88 (1999).
233. E. Fukui, N. Miyamura, K. Uemura and M. Kobayashi, Int. J. Pharm. 204 (1–2): 7–15 (2000).
234. V. Carelli, G. DiColo, E. Nannipieri, B. Poli and M.F. Serafina, Int. J. Pharm. 202 (1–2): 103–112 (2000).
235. R. Kinget, W. Kalala, L. Vervoort, and G. van den Mooteer, J. Drug Targeting 6 (2): 129–149 (1998).
236. E. Schacht et al., J. Contr. Rel. 39, 327–339 (1996).
237. Y. J. Jung, S. L. Jeoung and M. K. Young, J. Pharm. Sci. 89 (5), 594–556 (2000).
238. R. R. Lonser, N. Gogate, P. F. Morrison, J. D. Wood and E. H. Oldfield, J. Neurosurg. 89 (4): 616–622 (1998).
239. R. R. Lonser, R. J. Weil, P. F. Morrison, L. S. Governale and E. H. Oldfield, J. Neurosurg. 89 (4): 610–615 (1998).
240. M. E. Emborg and J. H. Kordower, Prog. Brain Res. 128, 323–332 (2000).
241. S. H. Yuk and Y. H. Bae, Crit. Revs. in Ther. Drug Carrier Systems 16 (4): 385–423 (1999).

Chapter 16

Target-Oriented Drug-Delivery Systems

Vijay Kumar and Gilbert S. Banker

University of Iowa, Iowa City, Iowa

I. INTRODUCTION

The idea of drug targeting to a specific site in the body, was first introduced almost a century ago by Ehrlich [1]. However only in recent years has the field emerged as an important area of research. This long silence in the field through most of the twentieth century can be attributed to an inadequate understanding of various diseases; a lack of a detailed description, at the cellular-molecular level, of how drugs are processed; and difficulties in identifying and producing carrier molecules specific to the targeted organs, cells, or tissues. The recent advent of recombinant DNA technology and progress in biochemical pharmacology and molecular biology have not only provided a clearer elucidation of pathogenesis of many diseases and identification of various types of surface cell receptors, but also enabled the production of several new classes of highly potent protein and peptide drugs (e.g., homo- and heterologous peptidergic mediators and sequence-specific oilgonucleotides) [2]. For these new drugs, and for some conventional drugs (e.g., antineoplastic agents) that have narrow therapeutic windows and require localization to a particular site in the body, it is essential that they be delivered to their target sites intact, in adequate concentrations, and in an efficient, safe, convenient, and cost-effective manner. Most drug therapies currently available provide little, if any, target specificity. The selective delivery of drugs to their pharmacological receptors should not only increase the therapeutic effectiveness, but also limit side effects and increase safety.

In this chapter, various target-specific drug-delivery systems will be described, and biological events and processes that influence drug targeting will be discussed. In addition, many of the drugs that have been incorporated in target-specific delivery systems and the therapeutic impact of this technology on disease state management are comprehensively treated, with the goal of providing the reader with an insight into the rapid developments and likely future of this growing field.

II. RATIONALE FOR TARGETED DRUG DELIVERY

Most drugs, after administration in a conventional immediate- or controlled-release dosage form, freely distribute throughout the body, typically leading to uptake by cells, tissues, or organs other than where their pharmacological receptors are located. Figure 1 illustrates the distribution, metabolism, and elimination of drugs that may occur by natural pathways. The lack of target specificity, illustrated in Fig. 1, for the most part can be attributed to the formidable barriers that the body presents to a drug. For example, a drug taken orally (most drugs are administered by this route, if possible) must withstand large fluctuations in pH as it travels along the gastrointestinal (GI) tract, as well as resist the onslaught of the enzymes that digest food and metabolism by microflora that live there. To be systemically active, the drug must then be absorbed from the GI tract into the blood before it passes its region of absorption in the tract. Once in the blood, it

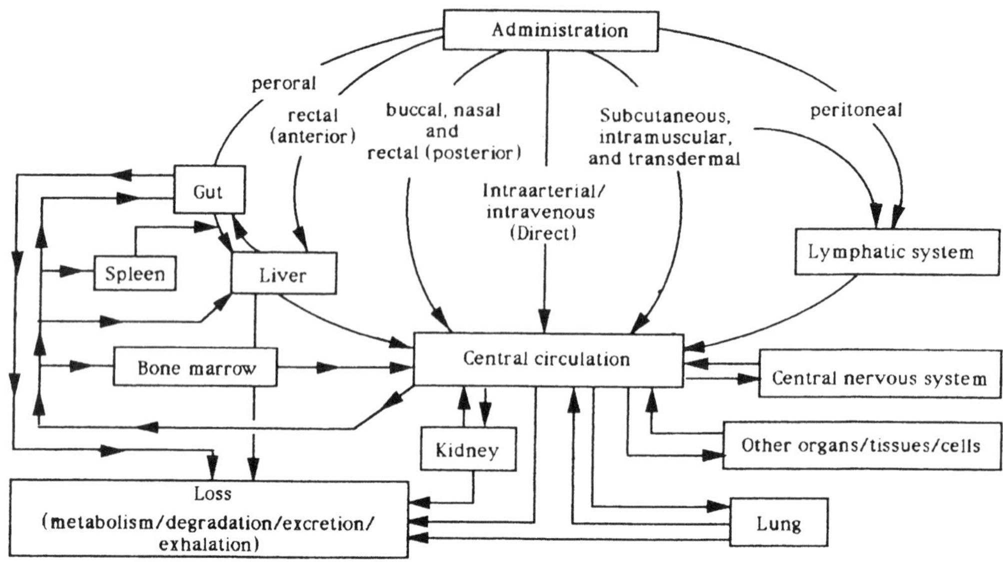

Fig. 1 A schematic representation of drug disposition in the body.

needs to survive inactivation by metabolism and extraction (first-pass effects). To produce its therapeutic effect(s), the drug must then selectively access and interact with its pharmacological receptor(s). The concentration of drug at the active site must also be adequate. Administration of drugs by parenteral routes avoids GI-associated problems, but deactivation and metabolism of the drug and dose-related toxicity are frequently observed. Furthermore, it cannot be assured that, of all the paths the drug may take following administration, one of them will lead the drug to its desired destination in adequate concentrations. There are many diseases for which accessibility is poor. These include rheumatoid arthritis, diseases of the central nervous system, some cancers, and intractable bacterial, fungal, and parasitic infections. The treatment of these diseases often requires high doses and frequent administration of drugs, which can lead to toxic manifestations, inappropriate pharmacodisposition, untoward metabolism, and other deleterious effects.

Reasons enumerating why it is preferable to direct drugs to their sites of action are listed in Table 1 [3]. Thus, a target-oriented drug-delivery system may best supply drug selectively to its site(s) of action(s) in a manner that provides maximum therapeutic activity (through controlled and predetermined drug-release kinetics), preventing degradation or inactivation during transit to the target sites, and protecting the body from adverse reactions because of inappropriate disposition. For drugs that have a low therapeutic index (ratio of toxic dose to therapeutic dose), targeted drug delivery may provide an effective treatment at a relatively low drug concentration. Other requirements for target-oriented drug delivery include that (a) the delivery system should be biochemically inert (nontoxic), nonimmunogenic, and physically and chemically stable in vivo and in vitro; (b) the carrier must be biodegradable, or readily eliminated without problems; and (c) the preparation of the delivery system must be reproducible, cost-effective, and reasonably simple.

Table 1 Reasons for Site-Specific Delivery of Drugs

Pharmaceutical
Drug instability as delivered from conventional formulation
Solubility
Biopharmaceutical
Low absorption
High membrane binding
Biological instability
Pharmacokinetic and pharmacodynamic
Short half-life
Large volume of distribution
Low specificity
Clinical
Low therapeutic index
Anatomical or cellular barriers
Commercial
Drug presentation

Source: Ref. 3.

III. BIOLOGICAL PROCESSES AND EVENTS INVOLVED IN DRUG TARGETING

Drug targeting has been classified into three types: (a) first-order targeting—this describes delivery to a discrete organ or tissue; (b) second-order targeting—this represents targeting to a specific cell type(s) within a tissue or organ (e.g., tumor cells versus normal cells and hepatocytic cells versus Kupffer cells); and (c) third-order targeting—this implies delivery to a specific intracellular compartment in the target cells (e.g., lysosomes) [4]. Basically, there are three approaches for drug targeting. The first approach involves the use of biologically active agents that are both potent and selective to a particular site in the body (magic bullet approach of Ehrlich). The second approach involves the preparation of pharmacologically inert forms of active drugs, which upon reaching the active sites become activated by a chemical or enzymatic reaction (prodrug approach). The third approach utilizes a biologically inert macromolecular carrier system that directs a drug to a specific site in the body where it is accumulated and effects its response (magic gun or missile approach). Regardless of the approach, the therapeutic efficacy of targeted drug-delivery systems depends on the timely availability of the drug in active form at the target site(s) and its intrinsic pharmacological activity. The intrinsic pharmacokinetic properties of the free drug should be the same, irrespective of whether or not it is introduced into the body attached to a carrier. Figure 2 shows a schematic representation of possible anatomical and physiological pathways that a drug may follow to reach its target site(s) [5]. As shown in this figure, a drug can selectively access to, and interact with, its pharmacological receptors, either passively or by active processes. Passive processes rely on the normal distribution pattern of a drug–drug-carrier system, whereas the active routes use cell receptor–recognizing ligand(s) or antibodies ("homing" or "vector" devices) to access specific cells, tissues, or organs in the body. Various biological processes and events that govern drug targeting are discussed in the following sections.

A. Cellular Uptake and Processing

Following administration, a drug frequently passes through various cells, membranes, and organs to reach its target site(s). Various passive and active processes or mechanisms by which the drug can achieve this are shown in Fig. 2 [5]. These pathways offer opportunities for cell selection and access by targeted drug delivery.

Low molecular weight drugs can enter into, or pass through, various cells by simple diffusion processes. Targeted drug-delivery systems often comprise macromolecular assemblies and are unable to enter into cells by such simple processes. Instead, they are captured by a process called endocytosis. Endocytosis is defined as a phenomenon that involves internalization of the plasma membrane, with concomitant engulfment of the extracellular material (particulate or fluid). This process can be constitutive or nonconstitutive. Other methods of gaining access to cells include passive diffusion, membrane fusion, and binding to either specific or nonspecific regions of the cell.

Endocytosis is divided into two types: phagocytosis and pinocytosis (Fig. 3). The former refers to the capture of particulate matter, whereas the latter represents engulfment of fluids. Phagocytosis is carried out by specialized cells of the mononuclear phagocyte system (MPS), called phagocytes. It is mediated by the adsorption of specific blood components [e.g. immunoglobulin (Ig) G, complement C3b, and fibronectin], called opsonins, and relevant receptors located on macrophages. The extent to which a drug is opsonized, and by what plasma protein, depends on the size and surface characteristics of the particles. This, in turn, determines the engulfment mechanism. For example, red blood cells treated with glutaraldehyde are opsonized by IgG and rapidly phagocytosed by the Fc receptor. In contrast, cells treated with *n*-ethylmaleimide are opsonized by C3b factor and are engulfed with a minimal membrane-receptor contact. Changes in the glycoprotein levels of patients may lead to variations in the opsonization of administered particles and, consequently, their ultimate distribution in the body [6]. Particles with higher hydrophilic surface characteristics tend to undergo opsonization to a lesser extent and, as a result, exhibit decreased phagocytic uptake [7–10]. This has direct implications in targeting microparticulate drugs to cells other than those of the reticuloendothelial system (RES), because the longer the drug stays in the central circulation, the greater the chances of uptake by other cells. Nonspecific phagocytic uptake of particles, triggered by particle size and hydrophilic coatings [11] and mediated by membrane components [12], has also been reported.

Following ingestion, the phagocytic vacuole (or phagosome) fuses with one or more lysosomes to form phagolysosomes (or secondary lysosomes) (see Fig. 3A). It is here that the digestion of particles by lysosomal acid hydrolases (e.g., proteinases, glycosidases, nucleases, phospholipases, phosphatases, and sulfatases) occurs, making the drug available to exert

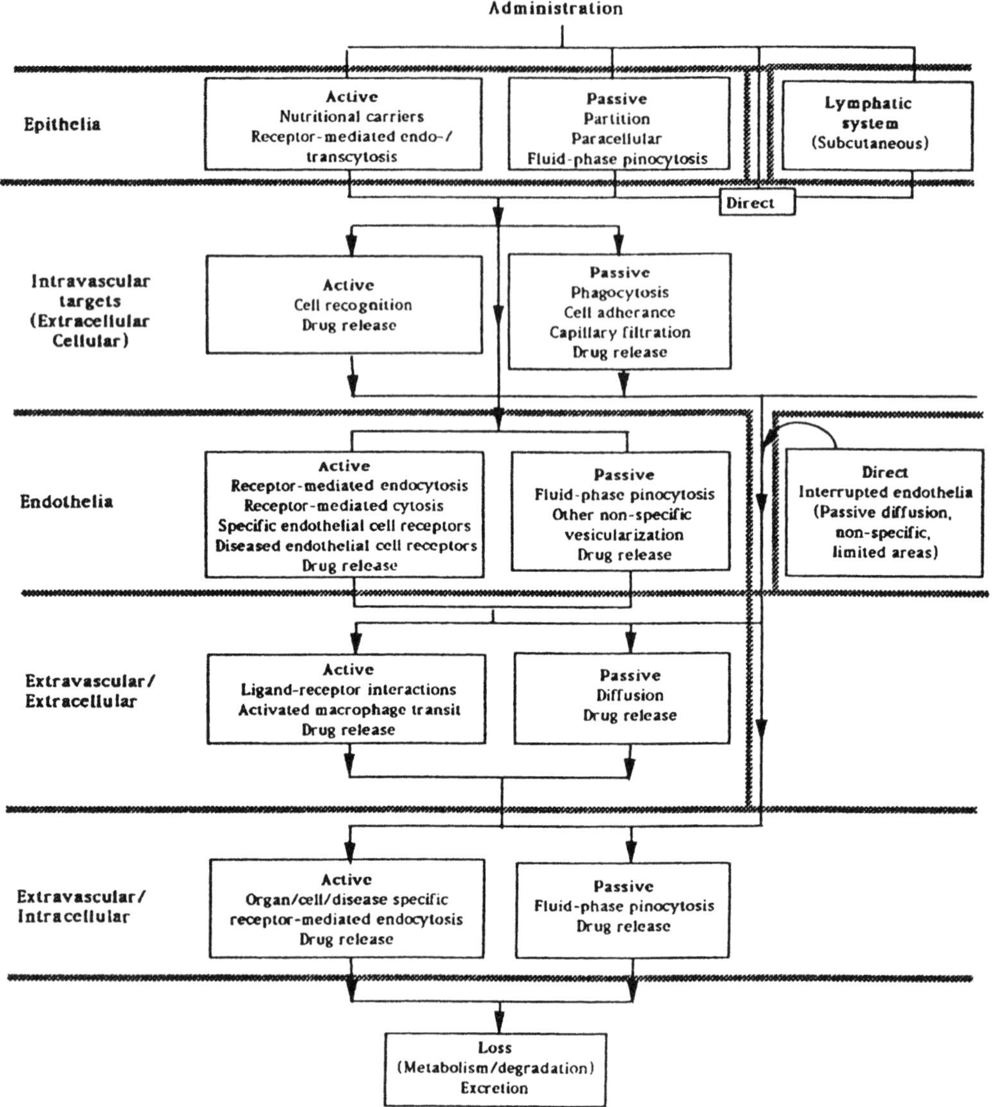

Fig. 2 Anatomical and physiological pathways for site-specific delivery. (From Ref. 5.)

its therapeutic effect. The internal pH of lysosomes is between 4.5 and 5.5.

Compared with phagocytosis, pinocytosis appears to be a universal phenomenon in all cells, including phagocytes. Unlike phagocytosis, which is mediated by the serum opsonin, pinocytosis does not require any external stimulus. Pinocytosis is divided into two types: fluid-phase pinocytosis and adsorptive pinocytosis (see Fig. 3B). Fluid-phase pinocytosis is a nonspecific, continuous process, and it is believed to be useful as a general process for transporting macromolecular constructs through epithelia, some endothelia, and into various blood cells. Adsorptive pinocytosis, in contrast, refers to internalization of macromolecules that bind to the cell surface membrane. If the macromolecule adheres to a general cell surface site, then uptake is referred to as simply nonspecific pinocytosis. However, if it binds to a specific cell receptor site, then the process is called receptor-mediated pinocytosis. Before membrane internalization, the pinocytic substrate often patches into domains or areas of the membrane called coated pits. Coated pits have a cytoplasmic coat consisting of clathrin and other proteins. Once internalized, the pinocytic vesicles can interact among themselves or with vesicles of other intracellular origins, such as endosomes and

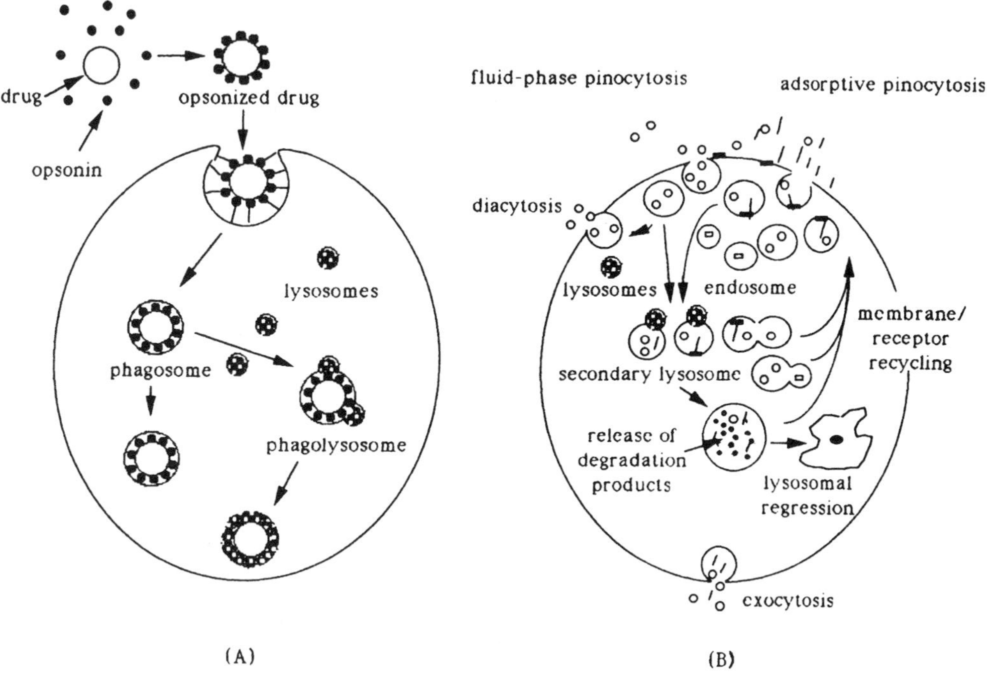

Fig. 3 (A) Phagocytic and (B) pinocytic uptake of drugs.

lysosomes. Endosomes are rich in pinocytic receptors and contain an active ATP-powered proton pump (not identical with that present in lysosomes) that maintains the internal pH between 5.0 and 5.5. The mild internal acidic pH condition induces dissociation of the receptor–drug carrier complex, freeing the receptor for recycling. Endosomes also serve as a sorting station to route internalized substrates to their appropriate intracellular locations. Internalized substrates that remain intact in the endosome are usually then transferred to the lysosome (transcellular transfer), where their digestion by acid hydrolases continues. In some cells (e.g., endothelial cells) the endosomes, instead of transferring their contents to the lysosome, release them outside the cell. This process is termed diacytosis or retroendocytosis and can achieve a vectorial translocation of substances through an otherwise impenetrable barrier of cells [13]. In cells such as secretory polymeric IgG in the neonatal gut, polymeric IgA in hepatocytes, and low-density lipoprotein (LDL) in endothelia, the secondary lysosome transports its contents to the other side of the membrane by a process called transcytosis. The secondary lysosome can also regress to form residual bodies that continue to retain nondegraded macromolecules.

Nonspecific pinocytic uptake appears to be dependent on the size (molecular weight and configuration), charge, and hydrophobicity of the pinocytic substrates. Polycation macromolecules have increased pinocytic uptake in rat yolk sacs and rat peritoneal macrophages cultured in vitro, compared to neutral and anionic macromolecules [14–16]. The rate of pinocytic uptake in different cells also increases with an increase in the size and hydrophobicity of the substrates. The molecular size of the pinocytic substrate is detrimental to the movement of macromolecules from one compartment to another.

The receptor-mediated form of endocytic uptake has been identified for a wide variety of physiological ligands, such as metabolites, hormones, immunoglobulins, and pathogens (e.g., virus and bacterial and plant toxins). Several endosomotropic receptors identified in cells are listed in Table 2.

Compared with phagocytosis, fluid-phase pinocytic capture of molecules is relatively slower, being directly proportional to the concentration of macromolecules in the extracellular fluid. It is also dependent on the size (molecular weight) of macromolecules; lower molecular weight fractions are captured faster than the higher molecular weight fractions. The magnitude of the rate of capture by adsorptive pinocytosis is higher than fluid-phase pinocytosis and relates to the nature of substrate-membrane interactions.

Table 2 Distributions of Some Endosomotropic Receptors (Various Species)

Cell	Receptor for
Hepatocytes	Galactose, low-density lipoprotein, polymeric IgA
Macrophages	Galactose (particles), mannose-fucose, acetylated LDL, alpha$_2$-macroglobulin–Protease complex (AMPC)
Leukocytes	Chemotactic peptide, complement C3b, IgA
Basophils, mast cells	IgE
Cardiac, lung, diaphragm endothelia	Albumin
Fibroblasts	Transferrin, epidermal growth factor, LDL, mannose-6-phosphate, transcobalamine II, AMPC, mannose
Mammary acinar	Growth factor
Enterocytes	Maternal IgG, dimeric IgA, transcobalamine–B_{12}/intrinsic factor
Blood-brain endothelia	Transferrin, insulin

Source: Ref. 5.

B. Transport Across the Epithetial Barrier

The oral, buccal, nasal, vaginal, and rectal cavities are all internally lined with one or more layers of epithelial cells. Depending on the position and function in the body, epithelial cells can be of varied forms, ranging from simple columnar, to cuboidal, to squamous types. Irrespective of their morphological differences, these cells are extremely cohesive. The lateral membrane of these cells exhibits several specialized features that form intercellular junctions (tight junction, zonula adherens, and gap junction), which serve not only as sites for adhesion, but also as seals to prevent flow of materials through the intercellular spaces (paracellular pathway) and to provide a mechanism for intercellular communication. The strong intercellular cohesion is partly due to the binding action of the glycoproteins, which are an integral part of the plasma membrane and of a small amount of the intercellular proteoglycan. Calcium ions also play a role in maintaining this cohesion. Below the epithelial cells is a layer of connective tissue called the lamina propria, which is bound to epithelium by the basal lamina. The latter also connects epithelium to other neighboring structures. The luminal side of the epithelium is covered with a more or less coherent, sticky layer of mucus. This is the layer that first interacts with foreign materials (e.g., food, drugs, bacterial organisms, and chemicals). Mucus contains the glycoproteins (mucins), water, electrolytes, sloughed epithelial cells, enzymes, bacteria and bacterial products, and various other materials, depending on the source and location of the mucus. Mucin, which is synthesized by goblet cells or by special exocrine cells, acini, constitutes about 5% of the total weight of mucus. The structure of mucin consists of a polypeptide backbone with oligosaccharide side chains. Each oligosaccharide chain contains 8–10 monosaccharide residues of a molecular weight of 320–4500 and has sialic acid or L-fucose as the terminal group. The oligosaccharide side chains are covalently linked to hydroxyamino acids, serine, and threonine residues along the polypeptide backbone.

The absorption of low molecular weight drugs from oral, buccal, nasal, vaginal, and rectal cavities is well known and established. Various transport processes used by drugs to cross the epithelial barrier lining these cavities include passive diffusion, carrier-mediated transfer systems, and selective and nonselective endocytosis. Additionally, polar materials also can diffuse through the tight junctions of epithelial cells (the paracellular route). However, there is now evidence to suggest that macromolecules (particulate and soluble), including peptides and proteins, can also reach the systemic circulation, albeit in small amounts, following administration by these routes. This may have far-reaching consequences in certain therapies, such as immune reactions and hormone-replacement treatment. Both passive and active transport path ways are energy-dependent processes, and they may occur simultaneously. Passive transport is usually higher in damaged mucosa, whereas active transport depends on the structural integrity of epithelial cells.

Harris [17] reported that nasal administration of biopharmaceuticals (polypeptides) resulted, in bioavailabilities of the order 1–20% of administered dose, depending on the molecular weight and physiochemical properties of the drug. It is widely accepted that (macro)molecules with a molecular weight of less than 10,000 can be absorbed from the nasal epithelium into the systemic circulation in sufficient amounts without the need for added materials. except for bioadhesives [18]. Larger molecules, such as proteins [e.g., interferon, granulocyte colony-stimulating factor (G-CSF), human growth hormone], however, require both a penetration enhancer (e.g., bile salts and surfactants) and bioadhesives. Since the entire dose passes through one tissue, these flux enhancers may cause deleterious effects to the nasal mucosa and muciliary function. Thus, caution must be exercised in using them. Recently, cyclodextrin [19] and phospholipids [20] have been reported to significantly increase the absorption of macromolecules, without causing any damage to the nasal mucosal membrane. The phospholipid approach is particularly attractive, in that phospholipids are biocompatible and bioresorbable and, thus, pose no threat of toxicity.

The transport of macromolecules across intestinal epithelium may occur by cellular vesicular processes involving either fluid-phase pinocytosis or specialized (receptor-mediated) endocytic processes [21]. Matsuno et al. [22] reported that spheres of 20 nm diameter, when given orally to suckling mice, pass through the epithelial layer and become localized in the momentum, the Kupffer cells of the lumen, the mesenteric lymph nodes, and even the thymic cortex. Recent studies with polyalkylcyanoacrylate nanocapsules smaller than 300 nm in size suggest that particles can also pass intact through the intestinal barrier by the paracellular route [23]. The M cells found in Peyer's patches have also been suggested to transport paticles that exist within the epithelium membrane. These are specialized absorptive cells known to absorb and transport indigenous bacteria (i.e. *Vibrio cholerea*); macromolecules, such as ferritin ad horseradish peroxidase; viruses; and carbon particles, from the lumen of the intestine to submucosal lymphoid tissue [21,24]. Further transport of absorbed materials to the systemic circulation through lymph fluid and by lymphocytes has been suggested as possible. An increase in the lymph flow or a decrease in the blood supply could make lymphatic uptake of particle important [24]. Since Peyer's patches are more prevalent and larger in young individuals and drastically decrease with increasing age, the transport by this route may only be of significance in younger individuals [25].

Various factor influencing the absorption of drugs, including peptides, from the GI tract have recently been reviewed [26,27]. Table 3 lists some of the parameter discussed in these reviews, including important physiological and biochemical variables affecting drug absorption, such as pH, enzymes, surface area, segment length, microflora, and transit time. A variety of penetration enhancers have been used to improve intestinal absorption of peptides and other macromolecular drugs. These include chelators (e.g., ethylenediaminetetraacetic acid, citric acid, salicylates, *N*-acetyl derivatives of collagen, and enamines); natural, semisynthetic, and synthetic surfactants (e.g., bile salts, derivatives of fusidic acid, sodium lauryl sulfate, polyoxyethylene-9-laurylether, and polyoxyethylene-20-cetylether); fatty acids and their derivatives (e.g., sodium caprate, sodium laurate, oleic acid, monoolein, and acrylcarntines); and a variety of mixed micelle solutions [28,29]. The different regions of the GI tract show different sensitivity to penetration enhancers. The following order of sensitivity is suggested: rectum > colon > small intestine > stomach. Present evidence, however, suggests that oral

Table 3 Factors Influencing the Absorption of Drugs

Location	Average length/diameter (cm)	Average surface area (m^2)	Average pH (range)	Enzymes and others	Mean transit times	Microflora per gram content
Mouth cavity	15–20/10	0.07	6.4 (5.8–7.1)	Ptyalin, maltose, mucin	At will	
Esophagus	25/2.5	0.02	5.6		9–15 s	
Stomach	20/15	0.11	1.5 (1.0–3.5)	Pepsin, lipase, rennin, HCl	0.5–4.5 h	
Duodenum	25/5	0.09	6.9 (6.5–7.6)	Bile, trypsin, chymotrypsin, amylase, maltase, lipase, nuclease, peptidases		$< 10^3$
Jejunum	300/5	60	6.9 (6.3–7.3)	Erepsin, amylase, maltase, lactase, sucrase, peptidases	1–4 h	
Ileum	300/5	60	7.6 (6.9–7.9)	Lipase, nuclease, enterokinase, nucleotidase, peptidases		10^5–10^7
Cecum	10–30/7	0.05	7.7 (7.5–8.0)		4–16 h	
Colon	150/5	0.25	7.95 (7.9–8.0)			10^{10}–10^{13}
Rectum	15–19/2.5	0.015	7.7 (7.5–8.0)		2–8 h	

Source: Ref. 27.

administration of peptides and proteins results in less than 1% bioavailability [30].

There is very little evidence to suggest that soluble or particulate macromolecules can be transported across the buccal mucosa [31]. More work is needed to determine whether this route could be of any benefit in drug targeting.

The absorption of drugs from the rectal [32] cavity has been studied in some detail. Muranishi et al. [34] have shown that a significant increase in the absorption and lymphatic uptake of soluble and colloidal macromolecules can be achieved by pretreating the rectal mucosal membrane with lipid–nonionic surfactant mixed micelles. They found no evidence of serious damage of the mucosal membrane. Davis [30] suggested that the vaginal cavity could be an effective delivery site for certain pharmaceuticals, such as calcitonin, used for the treatment of postmenopausal osteoporosis.

C. Extravasation

Many diseases result from the dysfunction of cells located outside the cardiovascular system. Thus, for a drug to exert its therapeutic effects, it must egress from the central circulation and interact with its extravascular-extracellular or extravascular-intracellular target(s). This process of transvascular exchange is called extravasation, and it is governed by the permeability of blood capillary walls. The main biological features that control permeability of capillaries include the structure of the capillary wall, under normal and (patho)physiological conditions, and the rate of blood and lymph supply. Physicochemical factors of compounds that are of profound importance in extravasation are molecular size, shape, charge, and hydrophilic-lipophilic balance (HLB) characteristics.

The structure of the blood capillary wall is complex and varies in different organs and tissues. It consists of a single layer of endothelial cells joined together by intercellular junctions. Each endothelial cell, on an average, is 20–40 μm long, 10–15 μm wide, and 0.1–0.5 μm thick, and contains 10,000–15,000 uniform, spherical vesicles called plasmalemmal vesicles. These vesicles range in size between 60 and 80 nm in diameter. About 70% of these vesicles open on the luminal side of the endothelial surface, and the remaining open within the cytoplasm. Plasmalemmal vesicles are believed to be involved in the pinocytic transport of substances across the endothelium. The transition time of pinocytic vesicles across the cell is about 1 second. Fusion of plasmalemmal vesicles leads to the formation of transendothelial channels. The endothelial cells are covered, on the luminal side, with a thick (10–20 nm) layer of a glycosaminoglycan coating. This layer continues into the plasmalemmal vesicles and into trans-endothelial channels and is believed to be involved in cell adhesion, the stabilization of receptors, cellular protection, and the regulation of extravasation. It also provides many microdomains of differing charge or charge density on the endothelial cell surface. On the external side, the endothelium is supported by a 5- to 8-nm-thick membrane called the basal lamina. Below the basal lamina a layer of connective tissues is present, called adventitia. The connective tissues surround the basal lamina as well as blending externally with the surrounding fibroaerolar tissues.

Depending on the morphology and continuity of the endothelial layer and the basement membrane, blood capillaries are divided into three types: continuous, fenestrated, and sinusoidal. The distribution of these capillaries in the body and their characteristics are presented in Table 4, and a schematic representation of the differences in their structures is shown in Fig. 4 [35]. Continuous capillaries are common and widely distributed in the body. They exhibit tight interendothelial junctions and an uninterrupted basement membrane. Fenestrated capillaries show interendothelium gaps of 20–80 nm at irregular intervals. These gaps have a thin membrane, which is believed to be derived from the basal membrane. Sinusoidal capillaries show interendothelial gaps of up to 150 nm. Depending on the tissue or organ, the basal membrane in sinusoidal capillaries is either absent (e.g., in liver) or present as a discontinuous membrane (e.g., in spleen and bone marrow). Sinusoidal capillaries are also wider in diameter, have an irregular lumen, and their wall is very thin. Furthermore, they have hardly any connecting tissues between the endothelial cells and the cells in which they are located. This area is occupied by a variety of cells, including highly active phagocytic cells.

There are also numerous important variations in the microvasculature bed (i.e., arterioles, capillaries, and venules) that affect permeability. For example, venular portions of the capillaries have thin endothelial cells (170 nm), with frequent interendothelial discontinuities. About 30% of venular junctions are believed to have gaps of about 6 nm. Arterioles, in contrast, have endothelial cells that are linked by the tight junctions and communicating junctions, whereas the capillary endothelium contains

Table 4 Distribution and Characteristics of Endothelium in Various Tissues

Tissue	Characteristics
Continuous endothelium	
Connective tissue, muscle (skeletal and smooth), heart, pancreas, brain, lung, gonads, mesentery	Tight junctions (up to 2 nm) with continuous basement membrane; extravasation mainly by vesicular trafficking
Discontinuous endothelium	
Fenestrated	
Kidney glomeruli, GI tract mucosa, exocrine and endocrine glands, certain tumors, pertibular capillaries, choroid plexus, pancreas, intestinal wall	Interruptions (20–80 nm) between cell junctions; membrane thickness 4–6 nm; basement membrane continuous
Sinusoidal	
Liver, spleen, red bone marrow, suprarenal and parathyroid glands, certain tumors, carotid and coccygeal bodies	Junctions up to 150 nm, basement membrane absent in liver and discontinuous in spleen and bone marrow

only occluding junctions. Communicating gaps are small and rare in muscular venules and are absent in capillaries and pericytic venules. Endothelial cells in capillaries have more vesicles than those in arterioles ($1000/\mu m^3$ VS. $190/\mu m^3$).The intercellular sealing is strong in arterioles, well developed in capillaries, and particularly loose in venules. Furthermore, capillaries and venules have more transendothelial channels.

The transport of macromolecules across endothelium has been reviewed [36,37]. Macromolecules can traverse the normal endothelium by passive processes, such as nonspecific fluid-phase transcapillary pinocytosis and passage through interendothelial junctions, gaps, or fenestrae, or by receptor-mediated transport systems. Passive extravasation is affected by regional differences in capillary structure, the disease state of the tissue or organ, the number and size of the microvascular surface area, and the physicochemical characteristics of the macromolecules. In general, the transfer of macromolecules across endothelium decreases progressively with an increase in molecular size. It is widely recognized that low molecular weight solutes and a large number of macromolecules, up to 30 nm in diameter, can cross the endothelium under certain normal and pathophysiological conditions [24].

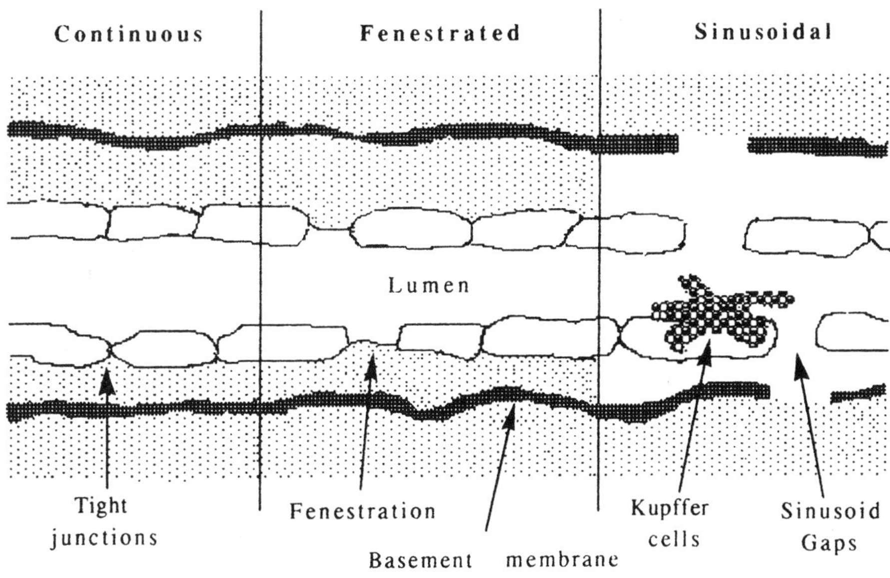

Fig. 4 The endothelial barrier. (From Ref. 35.)

For proteins, the threshold restricting free passage through the glomerular endothelium is at a molecular weight of 60,000 and 70,000. Molecules with a molecular weight larger than 70,000 are predominantly retained in the blood until they are degraded and excreted. Certain hydrophilic polymers, such as polyvinylpyrrolidone (PVP), dextran, polyethylene glycol (PEG), and *N*-(2-hydroxypropyl)methacrylamide (HPMA), exhibit much greater hydrodynamic radii, compared with proteins of the same molecular weight, and consequently, the threshold molecular weight restricting glomerular filtration is lower than for proteins (25,000 for PVP; 50,000 for dextran; and 45,000 for HPMA) [38].

Because of the presence of anionic sites on the endothelium and on the glycocalyx layer, anionic macromolecules show a significantly slower rate of extravasation compared with neutral and cationic macromolecules. Kern and Swanson [39] found a threefold increase in the permeability of the pulmonary vascular system to cationic albumin, compared with native albumin of the same molecular weight and hydrodynamic radius.

Regional differences in the capillary structure and the number and size of the microvascular surface area determine the flux of macromolecules in the interstitium [24]. For example, organs such as the lung with very large surface areas will have a proportionately large total permeability and, consequently, a high extravasation. Renal endothelium has a thick basement membrane, which contains anionic groups and heparin sulfate proteoglycan. Thus, extravasation through this membrane will largely depend on the molecular charge, shape, size, and lipophilic-drophilic balance characteristics of the macromolecules. Intestinal endothelium, although fenestrated, is highly restrictive to passage of macromolecules. The absolute rate of extravasation varies considerably from one region to another within the alimentary canal. There is a large difference in permeation of solute macromolecules with a radius of less than 6 nm and no decrease in the permeation for molecules with a radius between 6 and 13.5 nm [40]. The lung endothelium, which is nonfenestrated and has vesicles with a size of 50–100 nm, is more selective to the passage of macromolecules; the lymph/plasma ratio was decreased from 0.7 to 0.25 when the molecular radius of the macromolecule increased from 3.7 to 11.0 nm [41]. Skeletal muscle, adipose tissue, liver, and myocardial endothelia all show extravasation as a function of macromolecular size. The endothelium of the brain is the tightest of all endothelia in the body. It is formed by continuous, nonfenestrated endothelial cells and shows virtually no pinocytic activity. There are, however, certain regions of the brain (e.g., choroid plexus) that have fenestrated endothelium. Macromolecules such as horseradish peroxidase reach the cerebrospinal fluid by this route. Also, certain pathophysiological conditions, such as osmotic shocks, thermal injury, arterial hypertension, air or fat embolism, hypovolemia, and traumatic injury, cause transcapillary leakage and onset of pinocytic activity. This may have some implications in extravasation of macromolecules across the blood-brain barrier.

The changes in the permeability of capillaries as a result of inflammation are believed to be due to the effect of histamine, bradykinin, and a variety of other mediators [36]. The latter act directly on the capillary venule and endothelial vessel wall, effecting a rapid interaction between venular endothelial cells and circulating neutrophils. Damaged capillaries, in general, show increased openings (ranging in size between 80 and 140 nm) in the endothelium and, hence, increased transport activity. Macromolecules of up to 300,000 are capable of extravasation from blood vessels within experimental solid tumor, whereas molecules between 70,000 and 150,000 extravasate mainly from the vascular plexus induced around solid tumors. It has been suggested that inflamed tissues also show changes in the glycocalyx layer, which causes increased vesicular trafficking and, consequently, increased extravasation of bloodborne materials. The metabolic changes, which are mediated through a reduced oxygen concentration, an increased carbon dioxide concentration, and a local increase in pH owing to accumulation of various metabolites, also affect extravasation.

Soluble macromolecules permeate the endothelial barrier more readily than particulate macromolecules. The rate of movement of fluid across the endothelium appears to be directly related to the difference between the hydrostatic and osmotic forces.

Receptor-mediated transport systems include both the fluid phase and constitutive and nonconstitutive endocytosis or transcytosis. It appears that particles smaller than 40 nm in diameter are able to enter these pathways. Ghitescu et al. [42], using 5 nm gold-albumin particles, showed that particles are first adsorbed onto specific binding sites of the endothelia examined (i.e., in lung, heart, and diaphragm), and are then transported in transcytotic vesicles across the endothelium by receptor-mediated transcytosis and, to a lesser extent, by fluid-phase processes. Low-density lipoproteins pass through sinusoids, enter the space of Disse, and then are processed into the liver hepatocytes after interaction with the apolipoprotein ligands on the surface of the hepatocytes. Studies indicate that particles can be directed to other cells in the liver by altering the surface with ligands specific for the plasma membrane of those cells. Table 2 lists various receptors and the cells that have them.

D. Lymphatic Uptake

Following extravasation, drug molecules can either reabsorb into the bloodstream directly by the enlarged postcapillary interendothelial cell pores found in most tissues [43] or enter into the lymphatic system and then return with the lymph (a constituent of the interstitial fluid) to the blood circulation (Fig. 5). Also, drugs administered by subcutaneous, intramuscular, transdermal, and peritoneal routes can reach the systemic circulation by the lymphatic system (see Fig. 1). A schematic representation of the integration of lymph and blood circulation is shown in Fig. 6 [44]. As shown in Fig. 6, the lymphatic system originates in tissues as a network of fine capillaries. These capillaries coalesce regionally to form large vessels (referred to as afferent vessels), which extend centrally to one or more lymph nodes. The (efferent) ducts from the centrally located lymph nodes unite and form the major lymph trunks (e.g., intestinal, cervical, and thoracic ducts), which finally coalesce with the venous supply at the root of the neck.

Similar to blood capillaries, the lymphatic capillaries consist of a single layer of endothelial cells joined together by intercellular junctions. The diameter of small pores is 12 nm, whereas large pores range between 50 and 70 nm. The rate of formation of lymph depends on the hydrostatic pressure of blood and the permeability of the capillary wall. As blood enters the arterial end of the capillary, the hydrostatic pressure increases and, consequently, extravasation of water, electrolytes, and other bloodborne substances (e.g., proteins) occurs. By the time blood reaches the venular end of the capillary, the hydrostatic pressure drops, and some water and other low molecular weight (10,000) substances are reabsorbed. However, there is a net excess of extravasation over reabsorption, which results in accumulation of excess lymph in the tissues. This accumulation of excess fluid causes an increase in the interstitial pressure, which forces the lymph to enter the lymphatic system. The larger lymphatic vessels contain bicuspid valves, which prevent the retrograde flow of the lymph, while a coat of circular smooth muscle propels the lymph to flow centrally at a rate proportion to its rate of formation [45]. Following absorption in the peripheral capillary bed, the lymph is transported (by large lymph capillaries) to the regional lymph node where lymphocytes are added. The lymph is then taken to the next node up the chain and, finally, into the great vein.

Factors known to influence the clearance of drugs from interstitial sites, following extravasation or parenteral interstitial or transepithelial administration, include size and surface characteristics of particles, formulation medium, the composition and pH of the interstitial fluid, and disease within the interstitium. Studies indicate that soluble macromolecules smaller than 30 nm can enter the lymphatic system, whereas particulate materials larger than 50 nm are retained in the interstitial sites and serve as a sustained-release depot. The use of lipids or an oil in a formulation and the presence of a negative surface charge all appear to

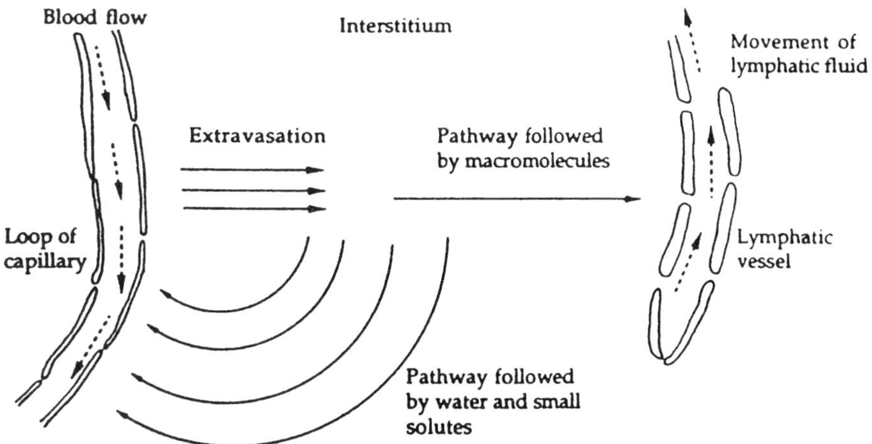

Fig. 5 Schematic representation of extravasation and lymphatic drainage. (From Ref. 38.)

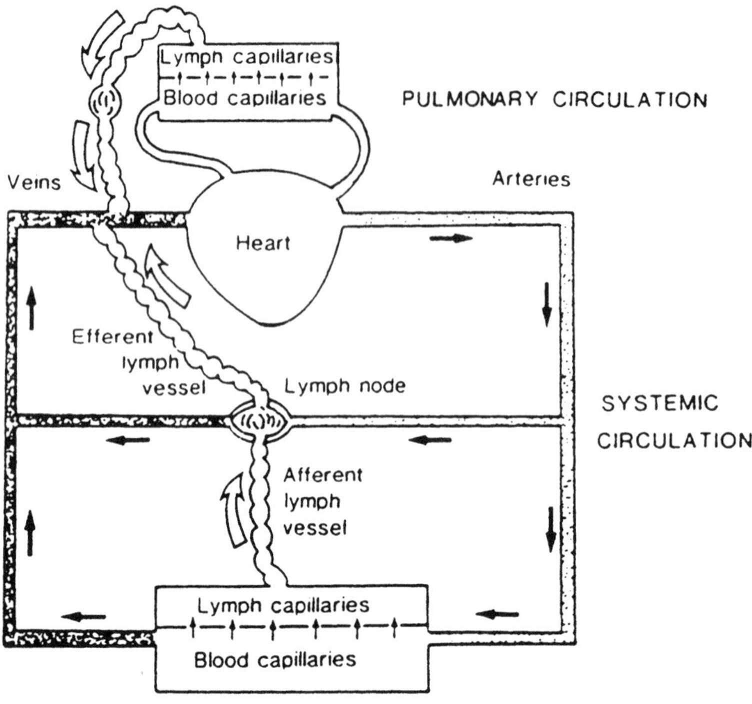

Fig. 6 Schematic representation of lymphatic and blood vasular systems. (From Ref. 44.)

facilitate the absorption of particles into the lymphatic system.

Solid tumors, in general, lack lymphatic drainage; therefore, macromolecular drugs that enter tumor interstitium, by extravasation remain there. This mechanism is commonly referred to as the tumor enhanced permeability and retention (EPR) effect. The trapped drug in the tumor interstitium may then be released, either intra- or extracellularly, by tumor-associated proteolytic enzymes. The released drug is then able to penetrate readily through cell membranes and reach its intracellular targets. Possible exploitation of this phenomenon in selective tumor therapy has been discussed in detail by Seymour [38]. The direct delivery of drugs into lymphatics has also been proposed as a potential approach to kill malignant lymphoid cells located in lymph nodes.

IV. PHARMACOKINETIC AND PHARMACODYNAMIC CONSIDERATIONS

The human body can be considered to be made up of a series of anatomically discrete compartments connected to each other through the circulatory system and by physiological and biochemical links. When a drug is administered, it is readily distributed to various compartments by blood. The relative amounts of drug available at the target (response compartment) and nontarget (toxicity compartment) sites determine the therapeutic effect and toxicities relative to that effect. In conventional therapy, the natural distribution characteristics of the drug determine the ratio of therapeutic response to the toxic effects.

Targeted drug-delivery systems are designed to maximize therapeutic response by delivering drug selectively to its pharmacological site(s). Several factors determine the availability of drug at the target site [46,47]. These include the rates of (a) input of targeted drug into the body plasma, (b) distribution of targeted drug to the active site, (c) release of active drug from the targeted drug at the site of action, (d) removal (elimination) of targeted drug and free drug from the target site, (e) diffusion or transport of targeted drug and free drug from the active site to nontarget sites, and (f) blood and lymph flow to and from the target site. A three-compartment pharmacokinetic model used by Boddy et al. [46] to describe these processes is schematically shown in Fig. 7. The release of free drug from the targeted drug-delivery system may occur either passively or by an active mechanism mediated by an internal or external stimulus (e.g., pH, temperature,

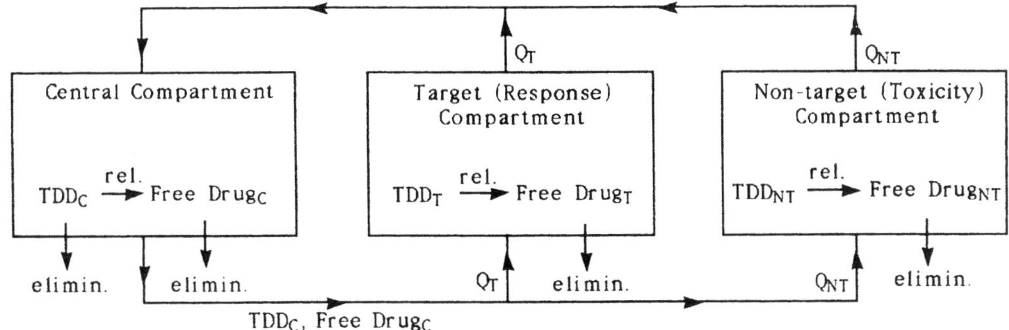

Fig. 7 A three-compartment pharmacokinetic model describing targeted drug delivery. (From Ref. 46.)

and enzymes). Thus, the rate of release of drug varies, depending on the mechanism involved. In enzyme-mediated reactions, the rate of release of free drug depends on the activity and concentration of the enzyme involved, whereas in reactions that are selective but nonspecific to the local chemical characteristics of the active site, the rate of release of free drug depends on the concentration of the targeted drug available at that site.

Thus, if the rate of distribution of targeted drug delivery to active site(s) is slow, or if the rate of elimination of targeted drug from the active site is faster than the rate of delivery to this site, then a sufficient amount of drug may not be available at the target site to produce the desired pharmacological effect [46]. The rate of distribution of targeted drug delivery to the target site depends on the rate of blood flow, whereas the removal of targeted delivery and free drug from the active site depends on the permeability of the endothelial barrier, on the rates of flow of blood and lymph to and from the target site, and on the rate of release of free drug. The upper limit of distribution of targeted drug or free drug to a specific tissue or organ in the body is provided by the product of blood flow and the concentration of the species in the blood. The inability of macromolecules or charged species to cross membrane barriers can limit their access to, and removal from, the target sites. The binding of the targeted drug-delivery system or drug within the target site reduces the concentration available for removal. For drugs that are active only in the free form, the binding may also reduce the effective amount required to produce the desired therapeutic effect. Levy [48], on the basis of the assumption that the targeted drug-delivery product will be transported from the target site to the rest of the body (which acts at least initially as an infinite sink), by diffusion, convection, or transport processes, concluded that (a) drug elimination from the target site will frequently be much more rapid than drug elimination from the body as a whole; (b) the duration of action of a targeted bolus dose will often be much shorter than the duration of action of a conventionally administered bolus dose and, consequently, the rate of drug administration to maintain a constant pharmacological effect will need to be much higher for targeted drug than for conventionally administered drug; and (c) changes in the biotransformation and excretion kinetics or of other processes (e.g., the liver perfusion rate) that determine the systemic clearance of a drug by the body will have no effect on the kinetics of elimination of targeted drug from the site of action.

According to Levy [48], if there is a large difference between the rates of drug elimination from the active site and from the body, if the ratio of the effective dose at the active site and in body plasma is small, and if elimination at the target site does not represent biotransformation, then the amount of drug in the body will gradually accumulate if the targeted drug-delivery system is continuously administered. As a result, the pharmacological effect will gradually increase. However, this will also lead to the loss of drug-targeting selectivity because the amount of drug in the body plasma will continue to rise. Thus, to maintain the selectivity of drug targeting, the delivery system must be designed to require a very low continuous input relative to the rate of elimination of drug from the body [48].

In conventional delivery, the pharmacological response to a drug is assumed to be linearly related to the drug concentration in the plasma. This relationship between concentration and effect is much more complex in targeted drug delivery. It can vary in different organs or tissues, depending on access, retention (maintenance of adequate levels of targeted delivery and free drug at the active site), and timing of release of drug within that site.

The various approaches used to quantitate targeted drug-delivery systems have been reviewed by Gupta and Hung [49]. These authors suggested that the overall drug-targeting efficiency (T_e^*), which represents selectivity of a delivery system for the target tissue (T), compared with n nontarget (NT) tissues, can be reliably calculated according to the following expression:

$$\%T_e^* = \frac{(AQU_0^\infty)_T \times 100}{\sum_{i=1}^{n}(AQU_e^\infty)_{NT}}$$

where (AQU_0^∞) is the area under the amount of drug (Q) in a tissue versus time curve. Q can be obtained, at any time t, by the relationship $Q = CV$ (or W), where C is the concentration of drug at time t and V and W are the volume and weight, respectively, of that tissue.

V. TARGETED DRUG-DELIVERY SYSTEMS

As noted in Sec. III, three strategies have been used to achieve drug targeting. These include use of site-specific, pharmacologically active molecules (magic bullet approach); preparation of pharmacologically inert agents that are activated only at the active site (prodrugs); and use of biologically inert carrier systems that selectively direct drugs to a specific site in the body (magic gun/missile, or drug-carrier approach). In this section, prodrugs and drug-carrier–delivery systems are discussed in detail.

A. Prodrugs

A prodrug is a pharmacologically inert form of an active drug that must undergo transformation to the parent compound in vivo by either a chemical or an enzymatic reaction to exert its therapeutic effects. The theory and practice of prodrugs have been reviewed by Notari [50]. Stella and Himmelstein [51,52] have critically reviewed the use of prodrugs in site-specific delivery. For a prodrug to be useful in site-specific delivery, it must exhibit adequate access to its pharmacological receptor(s). Also, the enzyme or chemical agent responsible for reactivating the prodrug should show major activity only at the target site. Furthermore, the enzyme should be in adequate supply to produce the required level of drug to manifest its pharmacological effect. Finally, the active drug produced in situ must remain at the target site and not leak out into the systemic circulation, which could lead to adverse effects. Thus, prodrugs are designed to alter the absorption, distribution, and metabolism of the parent compound and, thereby, to increase its beneficial effects and decrease its toxicity. Prodrugs are also used to overcome formulation problems and to avoid an unpleasant taste or odor of the parent compounds.

Table 5 lists some commonly used types of prodrugs and their methods of regeneration [53]. Many of these prodrugs are simple esters and can be reactivated in vivo by an esterase enzyme. Prodrugs containing an amide bond can be regenerated by peptidases, but their use in vivo has had varying degrees of success. The chemically reconvertible prodrugs frequently lack selectivity of activation at the target sites and, thus, offer little opportunity for drug targeting (a detailed discussion of prodrugs listed in Table 5 can be found in Refs. 54 and 55).

Numerous reports of prodrugs in the literature show improved drug effects. Prodrugs that have shown some measure of success for site-specific delivery include L-3,4-dihydroxyphenylalanine (L-dopa) to the brain [56], dipivaloyl derivative of epinephrine to the eye [57], γ-glutamyl-L-dopa to the kidney [58], β-D-glucoside dexamethasone and prednisolone derivatives to the colon [59], thiamine-tetrahydrofuryldisulfide to red blood cells, and various amino acid derivatives of antitumor agents such as daunorubicin [61,62], acivicin [63], doxorubicin [63], and phenylenediamine [63] to tumor cells.

The selective delivery of drugs to the brain has been, and continues to be, one of the greatest challenges. Only highly lipid-soluble drugs can cross the blood-brain barrier. Prodrugs with high lipid solubility can be used, but they may show increased partitioning to other tissues and, thereby, cause adverse reactions. For example, L-dopa, the precursor of dopamine, when administered orally, readily partitions throughout the body, including the brain. Its conversion to dopamine in the corpus striatum produces the therapeutic response, whereas its conversion in the peripheral tissues results in many undesirable side effects. Although many of these side effects can be overcome by additional administration of an inhibitor of aromatic amino acid decarboxylase, such as carbidopa (this does not penetrate into the brain and thereby permits the conversion of L-dopa to dopamine in the brain, but prevents its transformation in the peripheral tissues), the direct delivery of dopamine to the brain constitutes an attractive alternative. One approach that has been used is a prodrug carrier system developed by Bodor and

Table 5 Prodrug Modifications and Method of Regeneration

Drug	Prodrug	Regeneration method
R-OH (alcohols and phenols)	Alkyl esters and half esters	Enzyme
	Phosphate and sulfate esters	Enzyme
	Sulfoacetyl, dialkyl aminoacyl	Enzyme
	Acyloxyalkyl ethers and thioethers	Enzyme
	Carbamates	Enzyme
R-COOH	Alkyl and glyceryl esters	Enzyme
	Acyloxyalkyl and lactonyl esters	Enzyme
	Alkoxycarbonyloxyalkyl esters	Enzyme
	(2-Oxo-1,3-dioxolenyl)alkyl esters	Enzyme
	Amides and amino acid derivatives	Enzyme
RNH_2, R_2NH, and R_3N	Enamines, Schiff bases, Mannich bases, and oxalzolidines	Chemical
	Amides and peptides	Enzyme
	Hydroxymethyl derivatives	Chemical
	Hydroxymethyl esters	Enzyme
	Soft quaternary ammonium slats	Enzyme
	Carbamates	Enzyme
R-CHO and >C=O	Enol esters	Enzyme
	Thiazolidines and oxazolidines	Chemical
R-C(O)-NH_2 and imides	Hydroxymethyl derivatives	Chemical
	Hydroxymethyl esters such as acetate and phosphates	Enzyme
	Mannich bases	Chemical

Source: Ref. 53.

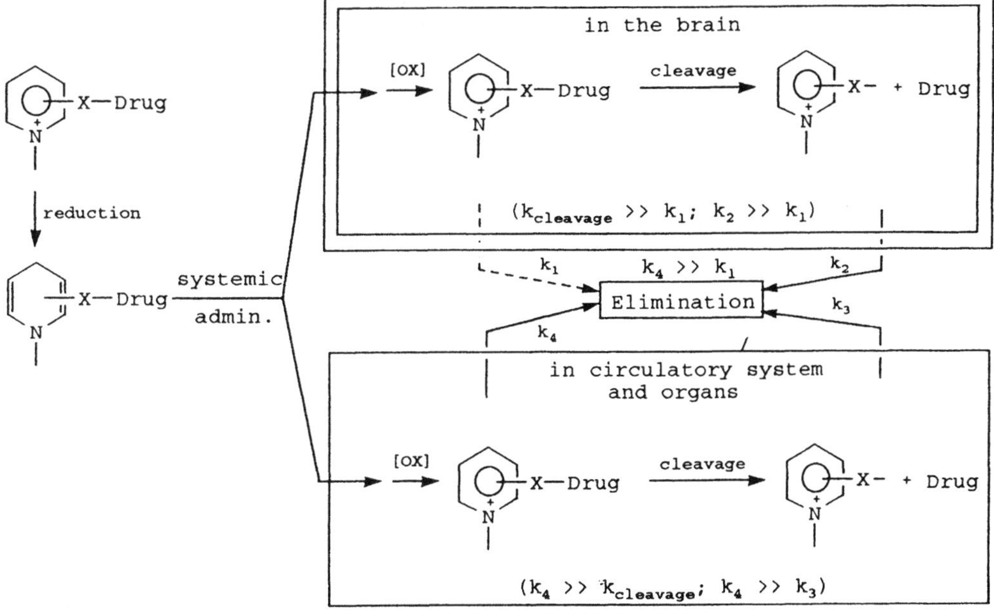

Fig. 8 Schematic representation of dihydropyridine-pyridinium redox delivery system. (From Ref. 66)

Simpkins (Fig. 8) [64]. This approach is based on the observation that certain dihydropyridines fairly readily enter the brain, where they are oxidized to the corresponding quaternary salts. The latter, owing to difficulty in crossing the blood-brain barrier, remain in the brain. The formation of quaternary salts in the peripheral tissues, on the other hand, rapidly accelerates their removal by renal or biliary mechanisms. This results in a significant buildup of the quaternary salt concentration in the brain and a significant reduction in systemic toxicity. Chemical or enzymatic hydrolysis of the quaternary salt (in the brain) then slowly releases the drug in the cerebrospinal fluid, allowing the therapeutic concentration to be maintained over some period. Examples of drugs that have been investigated using this approach include pralidoxime iodide (2-pyridine aldoxime methyl iodide) [65], phenylethylamine [66], dopamine [67], 3′-azido-2′,3′-dideoxyuridine (Azddu) [68], 3′-azido-3′-deoxythymidine (AZT; zidovudine) [68–70], and sex hormones.

B. Drug-Carrier–Delivery Systems

Drug-carrier–delivery systems employ biologically inert macromolecules to direct a drug to its target site in the body. These are divided into two types: particulate and soluble macromolecular. Depending on the carrier system, the drug can be either molecularly entrapped within the carrier matrix or covalently linked to the carrier molecules. The major advantage of drug-carrier–delivery systems is that the distribution of drugs in the body depends on the physicochemical properties of the carrier, not those of drugs. This implies that targeting can be manipulated by choosing an appropriate carrier, or by alterations in the physicochemical properties of the carrier. There are, however, several other factors that must be considered in the pharmaceutical development and clinical use of both soluble macromolecular and particulate biotechnical and synthetic site-specific systems. These are listed in Table 6.

Targeting with drug-carrier systems can be divided into three types: passive, active, and physical [38,72,73]. Passive targeting relies on the natural distribution pattern of the drug–drug-carrier system. For example, particles with a diameter of 5 μm or smaller are readily removed from the blood by macrophages of the RES when administered systemically. This natural defense mechanism of the RES thus provides an opportunity to target drugs to macrophages if they are encapsulated in or conjugated with an appropriate carrier system. Mechanical filtration of particulate carriers larger than 5–7 μm by capillary blockage can also be exploited to target drugs to the lungs by the venous supply and to other organs through the appropriate arterial supply. By controlling the rate of drug release, one can achieve the desired therapeutic action in the targeted organ. Passive targeting also includes delivery of drug-carrier systems directly to a discrete region in the body (e.g., different regions of the GI tract, eye, nose, knee joints, lungs, vagina, rectum, respiratory tract, or other). This offers the opportunity for the treatment of diseases that require a persistent and sustained presentation of drug at that site.

Active targeting employs a deliberately modified drug–drug-carrier molecule capable of recognizing and interacting with a specific cell, tissue, or organ in the body. Modifications of the carrier system may include a change in the molecular size, alteration of the surface properties, incorporation of antigen-specific antibodies, or attachment of cell receptor-specific ligands [73].

Physical targeting refers to delivery systems that release a drug only when exposed to a specific microenvironment, such as a change in pH or temperature, or the use of an external magnetic field [73].

A detailed discussion of particulate and soluble macromolecular delivery systems is presented in the following sections.

Particulate Drug-Delivery Systems

The concept of using particles to deliver drugs to selected sites in the body originated from their use as radiodiagnostic agents in medicine in the investigation of the RES (liver, spleen, and bone marrow), and lymph nodes, gastrointestinal examinations, and so on. Particles ranging in sizes from 20 to 300 μm have been proposed for drug targeting. Because of the small size of the particles, particulate drug–delivery systems can be introduced directly into the central circulation by intra-articular or intravenous injection or delivered to a given body compartment, for example, by injection into a joint or by administration by an aerosol to the lungs and nose. Subcutaneous and intraperitoneal administration routes have also been used to deliver drugs to the lymphatic system and regional lymph nodes. Some suggested uses of particulate drug-delivery systems in drug targeting are presented in Table 7 [24].

Particulate drug-delivery systems can be monolithic (i.e., containing an intimate mixture of drug and the core material), capsular (in which the drug is surrounded by the carrier material), or emulsion (in which the drug is dispersed in a suspension of the carrier material) types. The biofate (passive targeting) of particulate drug-delivery systems depends on the size, shape, charge, and surface hydrophobicity of the particles. A relation between particle size and biological targeting, after intravascular injection, is schematically

Table 6 Considerations in the Pharmaceutical Development and Clinical Use of Both Soluble Macromolecular and Particulate Biotechnical and Site-Specific Drug-Delivery Systems

Specification/activity

- I. Pharmaceutical development
  - A. Production
    - 1. Purity
    - 2. Evaluation of novel production safety hazard (e.g., sparkling with particulate)
  - B. Characterization
    - 1. Identity
    - 2. Conformation
    - 3. Size
    - 4. Size distribution
    - 5. Charge, aggregation
    - 6. Density
    - 7. Surface configuration, homogeneity of attachment moieties:
      - Polymers
      - Ligands
      - Spacers
  - C. In vitro functionality
    - 1. Drug loading efficiency
    - 2. Drug release
    - 3. Retention of recognition characteristics
  - D. Stability
    - 1. Characteristics of the breakdown products
      - In storage formulation
      - In biological fluids
    - 2. Parameters to be assessed on storage:
      - Chemical stability
      - Character
      - In vitro functionality
      - Sterility and functionality
      - Colloidal character (e.g., aggregation, size, charge)
      - Surface properties (including conformation and epitopic character)
- II. Safety pharmacology (nonhuman)
  - A. General considerations
    - 1. General safety
    - 2. Sterility and pyrogenicity
      - Major organ function tests
      - Acute and subacute toxicity studies
  - B. Potential novel toxicities
    - 1. MPS uptake
    - 2. Uptake in specialized immune
    - 3. Depression/exhaustion of MPS
      - Bone marrow
      - Bacterial and viral infections
      - Immunological depression
      - Hemorrhagic and endotoxin shock
      - Altered drug response

Table 6 (continued)

Specification/activity

- 4. Low level activation of MPS
  - Interleukin-I
  - Amyloidosis
  - Hyperplastic liver foci
  - Altered stem cell kinetics
  - Altered drug metabolism
  - Altered response to drugs
- C Biotechnics: For biotechnics (and specifically monoclonal antibodies), factors affecting safety include
  - 1. Hybridoma background:
    - Murine-murine
    - Human-human
    - Interspecies (chimerics)
  - 2. Contaminants
    - General safety
    - Pyrogens
    - Sterile
    - Free of hazardous viruses
    - Free of detectable DNA
  - Interaction with the host
    - Immunogenicity
    - Cross-reactivity
    - Hypersensitivity to foreign epitopes
    - Anti-idiotypic response to normal cells
    - Immune complex disease
    - Potential MPS toxicity
- D. Specific specificity
  - 1. Issues include altered drug disposition/metabolism, and the need for a tier assessment of safety to include knowledge on
    - Pathology of lymphoid tissues
    - Antibody and cell-mediated immunity
    - Host cell resistance
    - Phagocytic cell function
    - Immune/immunotoxicity reaction
    - Testing
    - Antigen specificity
    - Complement binding
- III. Metabolism: Issues here include species-specific metabolism (related to novel pattern of drug release at receptor sites), and possible use of novel paracrine- and endocrine-like peptidergic mediators. These could manifest themselves in novel:
  - Dose response
  - Absorption sites/rates
  - Bioavailabilities (at receptor)
  - Organ, tissue, cell disposition
  - Disease-dependent release
  - Excretion routes/rates

Table 6 (continued)

Specification/activity
IV. Efficacy: Major considerations in the clinical development of a site-specific system, relating to effect, utility, and efficacy could include:
Novel pharmacokinetic and disposition
Novel modalities of cell/tissue/receptor exposure
Utilization of novel cellular transport processes
Species-specific drugs and delivery modalities
Novel drug interactions
Novel drug metabolism
Local versus general distribution
Biphasic drug action
Chronopharmacology
New routes of administration: transmucosal; specific regional uptake in gastrointestinal tract
New pattern of drug release: bolus/flrst order/pulsatile; feedback control; disease-related release of drug
(Analytical techniques will need to encompass the identification of very low levels of site-specific systems and their degradation and metabolic products.)
V. Extended nonclinical development: these parallel activities will include
Reproductive toxicology
Chronic toxicology
Selection of market formulation
Definition of marketed specifications
Development of implementation of market-related scale-up
Confirmation of specification following scale-up

Source: Ref. 24.

depicted in Fig. 9 [73]. After intravenous administration, particles larger than 7 μm are normally mechanically filtered by the smallest capillaries of the lungs (particles of 15 μm have been homogeneously distributed throughout the lung, whereas particles of 137 μm exhibited a more peripheral distribution [74]), and particles smaller than 7 μm in diameter (between 2 and 7 μm) may pass the smallest lung capillary beds and be entrapped in the capillary network of the liver and spleen. Larger particles can also be injected intra-arterially. Here, particles will be retained in the first capillary bed encountered (first-order targeting). For example, administration into the mesenteric, portal, or renal artery leads to complete entrapment of particles in gut, liver, or kidneys, respectively. For organs that bear solid tumors, this approach may lead to localization in the tumor cells. Particles between 0.05 and 2 μm in size are rapidly cleared from the bloodstream by macrophages (primarily by the Kupffer cells of the liver) of the RES after intravenous, intra-arterial, or intraperitoneal administration. Extraction of particles by macrophages of the RES can be 90% or greater, with a half-life of less than 1 minute. This natural targeting to the liver offers opportunities for the treatment of tropical diseases (leishmaniasis) and fungal infections (candidiasis). Because of the dominant role of Kupffer cells, other cells of the RES play a small role in removing particles from the blood. Since the fenestrae of the liver endothelium have a diameter of 0.1 μm, particles smaller than 0.1 μm can pass through the sieve plates of the sinusoid and become localized in the spleen and bone marrow.

Negatively charged particles are more rapidly cleared from the blood than are neutral and positive ones [75]. The clearance rate of particles by the reticuloendothelial system is inversely related to the load of the particles; that is, the rate of clearance of a larger dose of microparticulate is slower than for a smaller dose [76].

The targeting of drugs to sites in the body other than the RES (e.g., parenchymal cells or tumor cells of the liver or monocytes in the blood) has been extensively studied. In vitro studies show that this can be achieved by linking particles to monoclonal antibodies [77–80] or to cell-specific ligands (e.g., desialyated fetuin [81], glycoproteins [82], native immunoglobins [83], or heat-aggregated immunoglobins [84]) or by alterations of the particles' surface characteristics (e.g., by using bioadhesives [85] or nonionic surfactants [7]), so that they are not recognized by the RES as being foreign (active targeting) [73]. Changes in the surface properties can prevent particles from adhering to the macrophages and, consequently, their endocytosis. For example, coating particles with high molecular weight copolymers, consisting of a long hydrophobic chain (e.g., poloxmers), to anchor the polymers on the surface of the particles, and two or more hydrophilic chains that prevent endocytosis by steric stabilization, has significantly reduced uptake by the RES, and as a result the particles are distributed to other parts of the body where they do not normally localize (Table 8) [7].

Other approaches used to avoid RES uptake of particles include incorporation of ferromagnetic materials, such as carboxyl-iron powder and Fe_3O_4 [86]; formulation of particles in oils [87]; and the use of an appropriate carrier (e.g, phospholipids) capable of degrading and releasing the drug into the surrounding tissues with slight changes in temperature [88] or in pH [89] conditions. The approach involving magnetic materials has been successfully used in humans in the therapy of carcinoma of the prostate and bladder [90].

Table 7 Some Uses for Particulate Drug-Delivery Systems

Target site/purpose (Particle size)	Disease/therapy
Direct administration to discrete compartments (0.05–100 μm)	
Eye	Infection
Lung	Allergy
Joints	Arthritis
Gastrointestinal tract	Crohn's disease. immunization
Intralesional	Tumor
Bladder	Infection
Cerebral ventricles	Infection
Interstitial administration (0.005–100 μm)	
Subcutaneous	Lymph node targeting (e.g., some cancers)
Intramuscular	Depot for anesthetics, proteins
Intravascular targets	
Diseased macrophages (0.1–1.0 μm)	Parasitic, fungal, viral, enzyme storage disease; autoimmune diseases; gene therapy
Other blood cells (0.1–1.0 μm)	Cancerous; platelets; gene therapy (bone marrow erythroblasts); immune cells (vaccination/adjuvant); antivirals
Circulating depot (0.1–1.0 μm)	Anti-infectives; antileukemics: antithrombotics; antivirals; release of polypeptides and protein drugs
Capillary filtration (> 1.0 μm)	Cancer; emphysema; thrombi: drug acting on local endothelia
Extravascular targets	
Macrophages activation (0.1–1.0 μm)	Abnormal cells (e.g., cancerous and virally infected)
Discontinuous endothelia (<0.15 μm)	
Basement membrane	Spleen
Parenchymal cells	Liver
Diseased endothelia (< 0.5 ? μm)	Rheumatoid arthritis, malignant hypertension, myocardial infarct, transluminal angioplasty
Ex vivo (> 0.5–50 μm)	
Cells	Cell targeting (e.g., for gene therapy)

Source: Ref. 24.

It allows maneuvering of the delivery system with external magnetic fields. The particle-in-oil approach has been used by Sezaki et al. [87] in the treatment of VXZ carcinoma in rabbits and cystic hygroma in pediatric patients. They reported a significant increase in the survival rate of the rabbits and the management of 22 cases of pediatric cystic hygroma when treated with a bleomycin–gelatin microsphere–oil emulsion. Cystic hygroma are benign tumors that are difficult to remove completely by surgery. Free bleomycin had no effect on these tumors.

The various particulate drug-carrier systems that have been investigated can be grouped into the following classes:

Microparticles and Nanoparticles. Colloidal particles ranging in size between 10 and 1000 nm (1 μm) are known as nanoparticles, whereas particles larger than 1 μm but small enough not to sediment when suspended in water (but large enough to scatter incoming light) are called microparticles. A partial list of various natural and synthetic materials used in the preparation of microparticles and nanoparticles is presented in Table 9 [3]. Also included in the list are the sizes of particles investigated, the names of the active agents entrapped or proposed for entrapment, and the intended or suggested use in drug targeting.

The most commonly practiced methods to prepare microparticles and nanoparticles are emulsion, micelle, and interfacial polymerization, and coacervation. The emulsion polymerization method involves heating a mixture of monomer and active agent(s) in an aqueous or nonaqueous phase that contains an initiator, a surfactant (employed usually in excess of its critical micelle concentration), and a stabilizer. Vigorous agitation is employed during the emulsion formation to produce particles smaller than 100 μm, usually less than 1 μm. The smaller particle size assures good tissue tolerance, uptake, and transfer, and causes no foreign body reaction. Examples of carrier systems prepared by the emulsion polymerization approach include poly(methyl methacrylate) nanoparticles, which exhibit excellent adjuvant properties for vaccines [91], and polyalkylcyanoacrylate nanoparticles [92], which are biodegradable. The main advantage of emulsion polymerization is that higher molecular weight polymers are usually formed at a faster rate and a lower temperature. A major disadvantage, however, is that the product cannot be readily freed from the residual monomers. Micellar polymerization differs from emulsion polymerization only in that the monomers and active agent(s) are contained within the micelles

Table 8 Uptake of Polystyrene Microsphere (60 nm diameter) in Rat Organs Following IV Injection

System	Liver	Spleen	Blood[a]	Femurs
Uncoated control	47.4[b] + 2.6 (7)	1.05 + 0.65 (4)	3.7 + 0.28 (7)	0.059 + 0.002 (3)
Coated with poloxamer 338	3.5 + 1.1 (2)	0.39 + 0.015 (2)	39.2 + 5.4 (2)	0.142 + 0.037 (2)
Coated/uncoated ratio	0.073	0.36	10.6	2.4

[a]Blood volume taken as 6.5 ml/100 g body weight.
[b]Percentage uptake at 1 h.
Source: Ref. 7.

formed by a suitable concentration of a surfactant before the polymerization is commenced. This allows very little, if any, increase in particle size as polymerization proceeds.

In interfacial polymerization, monomers react at the interface of two immiscible liquid phases to produce a film that encapsulates the dispersed phase. The process involves an initial emulsification step in which an aqueous phase, containing a reactive monomer and a core material, is dispersed in a nonaqueous continuous phase. This is then followed by the addition of a second monomer to the continuous phase. Monomers in the two phases then diffuse and polymerize at the interface to form a thin film. The degree of polymerization depends on the concentration of monomers, the temperature of the system, and the composition of the liquid phases.

The coacervation approach uses heating or chemical denaturation and desolvation of natural proteins or carbohydrates. As much as 85% of water-soluble drugs can be entrapped within a protein matrix by freeze-drying the emulsion prepared in this manner. For water-insoluble drugs, a microsuspension-emulsion procedure has been suggested as a method of choice to achieve high drug payloads.

Most products investigated to date are designed as sterile, freeze-dried, free-flowing powders, usually containing 0.1% w/w of a nonionic surfactant to assist redispersion in saline. These can be administered either systemically or by an intramuscular route. As is obvious from Table 7, the major use of microspheres and nanospheres, including magnetic microspheres, has been in tumor therapy. Microsphere-in-oil emulsions have been used as lysosomotropic systems. After subcutaneous administration, the oily product is readily taken up by the lymphatic system, not by the cardiovascular system [87]. Recently, biodegradable polymeric nanospheres, with potential applications in medical imaging, gene therapy, and drug targeting to specific cells or tissues, have been developed [93]. These nanospheres have a polymer core in which a drug is dispersed. The core is, in turn, covalently linked to a polyethylene glycol coating that prevents rapid clearance of the particles from the body. The drug releases by diffusion through the coating or as the nanospheres break down. The nanospheres can carry high doses of drug or agent (up to 45% of particle weight), with an entrapment efficiency of over 95%. Antibodies or other protein ligands can also be attached to nanospheres.

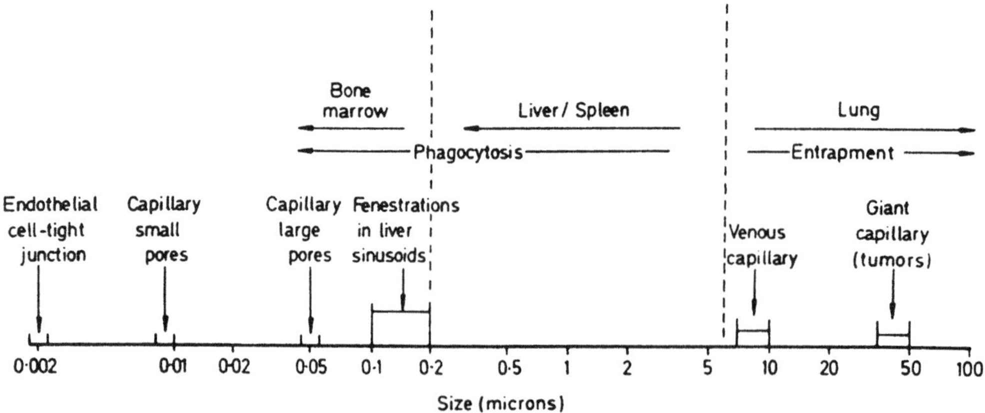

Fig. 9 The vascular bed and passive targeting. (From Ref. 73.)

Table 9 Particulate Drug-Delivery Systems

Matrix material	Diameter (μm)	Intended or suggested use	Actual or suggested active molecules
Chylomicron	0.1–0.5		Factor VIII
Low-density lipoprotein	0.017–0.025	Delivery to neoplastic cells	Methotrexate, anticancer agents
High-density lipoprotein	0.007–0.012	Delivery to adrenals and ovaries after intravenous injection	Gram-negative lipopolysaccharide
Polyalkylcyanoacrylate	0.2	Lysosomtropic after intravenous injection	Antimitotics (e.g., daunorubicin, actinomycin D, doxorubicin)
	0.213	Blood glucose regulators after intra-articular injection	Insulin, triamcinolone diacetate
Ferromagnetic			
Poly(isobutylcyanoacrylate)	0.22	Biodegradable TDS with extracorporeal guidance	[^{3}H]Dactinomycin
Poly(methylmethacrylate)	0.1–1.0	Vaccine therapy	Vaccines
Polyamide	60–120	Oral for saccharose tolerance	L-Invertase
Polyacrylamide	0.3, 18, 36	Intraperitonial, intravenous for acute leukemia	L-Asparaginase
	0.25–3	Intramuscular/subcutaneous for reduction in enzyme antibody effects	L-Asparaginase
	0.7	Lysosomotropic after intravenous injection to treat enzyme deficiencies (e.g., adult Gaucher's disease)	Enzymes
Polyacryldextran		Biodegradable TDS for protein delivery	Proteins (e.g., L-asparaginase)
DL-polylactic acid	25–75	Subcutaneous delivery of local anesthetics	Dibucaine; tetracaine
	125	Subdermal antimalarial implant	Quinazoline analogs
Sulfonic ion-exchange resin	38–297	Oral, anthelminitic	Levamisole
Carnauba	30–800	Chemoembolism TDS for intra-arterial delivery of cytostatics	5-Fluorouracil, CCNU, methotrexate
Ethylcellulose	225 (mean)	Arterial cheamoembolism for delivery of cytostatics to kidney and liver	Mitomycin
Ferromagnetic ethylcellulose	307	Extracorporeal guidance to tumors	Mitomycin
Modified cellulose	40–160	Nondegradable (model) parenteral TDS for delivery to lungs	Methotrexate
Gelatin	0.301	Intra-articular injection	Triamcinolone diacctate
	1.6, 1.9	Intralymphatic delivery (lymphotropic), as microspheres-in-oil emulsion for delivery of cytostatics	5-Fluorouracil
	0.28	Delivery to liver and spleen after intravenous injection	Bleomycin, water-soluble drugs
Gelatin core with dextran conjugate of drug	15	Lung, after intravenous injection	Mitomycin-dextran conjugate

Table 9 (continued)

Matrix material	Diameter (μm)	Intended or suggested use	Actual or suggested active molecules
Dextran cross-linked functionalized by carboxymethylation	10–30	Intratumor direct delivery	Doxorubicin; mitomycin
Self-forming microspheres polymercaptol	0.8	Oral and hemoperfusion for treatment of heavy metal poisioning	Mercaptol
Insulin	0.2	Oral and intramuscular delivery for treatment of diabetes	Insulin
Hemoglobin	5–60	Oxygen transport function	Hemoglobin
Polystyrene	3–25	Percorneal retention studies	
Agarose		Injection into tumor tissue	Mitomycin
Starch (Spherex)	40	Intra-arterial administration of cytostatics	5-Fluorouracil, hepatic BCNU, renal actinomycin D
Ferromagnetic starch	1–50	Extracorporeal maneuvering to tumor tissue after IV injection	Ethanolamine and albumin as model compounds
Albumin	0.1–1	IV immunosuppressives delivery: infestation of the RES (e.g., histoplasmosis, typhoid)	[^{14}C]Mercaptopurine-8-hydrate
	0.169	Intra-articular injection	Triamcinolone diacetate
	0.66	Intravenous delivery to liver (RES)	[^{3}H]5-Fluorouracil
	10–30	Intrarenal delivery to tumors	Doxorubicin, bleomycine, 5-fluorouracil, methotrexate
	10	Intravenous delivery to lungs of antiallergic compounds	Sodium cromoglicate (Cromolyn sodium)
	7, 15	Treatment of emphysema (IV)	Leukocyte elastase inhibitor
	10–200	Intramuscular or subcutaneous depot	Norgestrone, progesterone
	All sizes	Variously: intra-arterial, intravenous	Antiasthmatics, analgesics, bronchodialators; narcotics; mucolytics; antibacterials; antituberculars; hypoglycemics; steroids; antitumor agents; amino acids
	10–40	Supplementation of drug therapy using internal radiation by intra-arterial delivery of radiolabeled microspheres	Yttrium 90
Ferromagnetic albumin	1–2	Delivery to tumors by extracorporeal guidance	Doxorubicin
	1–2; 2–4; 3–7	Intravenous delivery to lung; renal artery delivery	Doxorubicin
	1	Probe for neurological function	Mylein basic protein
	7	Immunoglobulin incorporation using staphylococcal protein A	

Source: Ref. 2.

Solid lipid nanoparticles have been reported which substantially increase permeation of glucocorticoids through human epidermis [94]. Polyethylene glyco–coated polycyanoacrylate nanoparticles have been described that reduce hepatic uptake, thereby facilitating a greatly increased that reduced hepatic uptake, thereby facilitating a greatly increased uptake in the spleen, providing an interesting perspective for the targeting of drugs to tissues other than the liver [95]. Solid lipid nonoparticles have also shown promise to facilitate targeting of antineoplastic agents to the brain [96]. The use of a variety of nonoparticles that have the critical size (2–200 nm) and surface characteristics (neutral to weekly negative) to target solid tumors has been reviewed [97]. The nanospheres can be freeze-dried and reconstituted.

Various factors that influence the release of drugs from particulate carriers are listed in Table 10. Drugs can be released by diffusion or by surface erosion, disintegration, hydration, or breakdown (by a chemical or an enzymatic reaction) of the particles. The release of drugs from microspheres follows a biphasic pattern; that is, an initial fast release followed by a slower first-order release (Fig. 10) [98]. The higher the solubility of a drug in water, the greater will be the release rate from the microspheres. Yapel [99] reported that, for epinephrine, the release from (albumin) microspheres becomes monophasic when the drug load exceeds 30%, by weight. The release (of drug) is also dependent on the degree of cross-linking (or heat denaturation) of the polymer and on the size of the particles. At least over some initial range, the higher the cross-linking, the greater the water uptake characteristics of the polymer and, consequently, the slower the release rates. This suggests that the release of a drug from albumin microspheres with extended cross-linking is primarily due to the hydration of the polymer, rather than degradation. Figure 10 also shows the effect of microsphere size on the release rate. It is obvious that the release rate decreases as the size of microspheres decreases, suggesting that the release of cromolyn sodium (sodium cromoglycate) from albumin microspheres is a diffusion-controlled process. Sezaki et al. [87] reported that incorporation of a gelatin-mitomycin drug conjugate, instead of free mitomycin into gelatin microspheres, leads to a monophasic drug release, similar to the rate of hydrolytic cleavage of the conjugate linkage. In magnetic microspheres, the release rate of drug apparently depends on the strength of the magnetic field, the frequency of oscillation [100], the shape of the embedded magnet [101], and the composition of the polymer [102,104]. Nano- and microparticles have been extensively reviewed by Kumar [105].

Table 10 Factors Affecting the Release of Drugs from Particulate Carriers

Drug
Position in the particle
Molecular weight
Physicochemical properties
Concentration
Drug-carrier interaction
Diffusion; desorption from surface; ion exchange
Particles
Type and amount of matric material
Size and density of the particle
Capsular or monolithic
Extent and nature of any cross-linking; denaturation of polymerization
Presence of adjuvants
Surface erosion; particle diffusion and leaching
Total disintegration of particles
Environment
Hydrogen ion concentration
Polarity
Ionic strength
Presence of enzymes
Temperature
Microwave
Magnetism
Light

Source: Ref. 3.

Liposomes. Liposomes are versatile, efficient, and probably the most extensively studied class of carrier systems. They have been used experimentally in many areas of medicine. A comprehensive review of the preparation, analysis, drug entrapment, and interactions with the biological milieu, including drug targeting, can be found in a compendium entitled *Liposome Technology*, edited by Gregoriadis [106,107]. There are several books [108–111], book chapters [112–116], and review articles [117–124] that cover various aspects of liposome technology. A general discussion of liposomes as a dispersed system, including preparation, characterization, and uses in pharmacy, is presented in Chapter 9 of this book.

The important attributes of liposomes as a drug carrier are: (a) they are biologically inert and completely biodegradable; (b) they pose no concerns of toxicity, antigenicity, or pyrogenicity, because phospholipids are natural components of all cell membranes; (c) they can be prepared in various sizes, compositions, surface charges, and so forth, depending on the requirements of

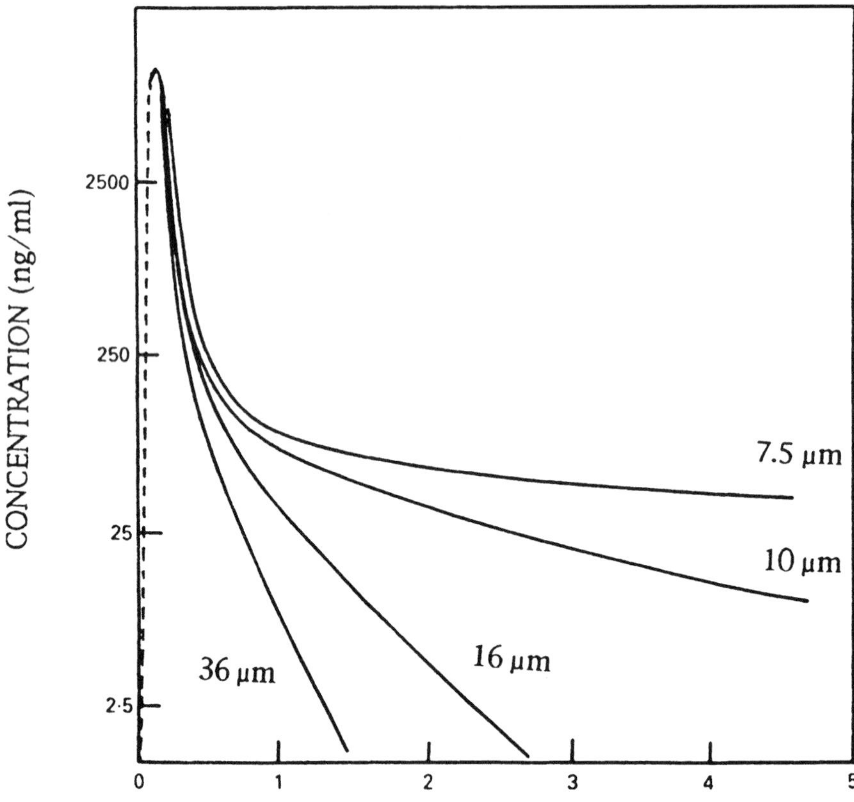

Fig. 10 Release of cromolyn sodium (sodium cromoglycate) from human serum albumin microspheres prepared using a water–oil emulsion technique with 5% glutaraldehyde as cross-linking agent. Dissolution medium: pH 7 phosphate buffer. (From Ref. 98.)

a given application; (d) they can be used to entrap or encapsulate a wide variety of hydrophilic and lipophilic drugs, including enzymes, hormones, vitamins, antibiotics, and cytostatic agents; (e) drugs entrapped in liposomes are physically separated from the environment and, thus, are less susceptible to degradation or deactivation by the action of external media (e.g., enzymes or inhibitors); and (f) liposome-entrapped drugs offer new possibilities for drug targeting, since entrapped drugs follow the fate of liposomes and are released only at the site of liposome destruction.

The drug-loading capacities of liposomes depend on the properties of the drug, the phospholipids, and other additives used. Typically, hydrophobic drugs are solubilized with lipid(s) in an organic solvent that is then dried and subsequently hydrated to yield lipospmal drug formulations. The loading of hydrophilic drugs is limited by their aqueous solubility and is dependent on the entrapment efficiency of the formulation method. By submitting the liposome-drug solution to several freeze-thaw cycles, the entrapment efficiency of water-soluble drugs can be increased from 1–5% to 50–80%. However, this is possible only at high lipid concentrations [125]. The loading of cationic (or anionic) drugs can be significantly improved by using liposomes containing negatively (or positively) charged lipids. Gabizon [126] reported that the entrapment efficiency can be increased from 10% for neutral liposomes to 60% for charged liposomes. Another approach to increase entrapment efficiency is the use of transmembrane pH gradients. For example, liposomes with low internal pH will accommodate a higher loading of cationic drugs, whereas a high intraliposomal pH will enable increased entrapment of negatively charged (anionic drugs) and amphiphilic drugs [127]. Recently, a new dehydration-rehydration approach has been developed that allows entrapment of drugs in a concentration range of 50–85%. This method is easy to scale up, and the liposome vesicles containing drug, including protein, can be freeze-dried and reconstituted with saline solution without affecting the entrapped drug [118]. Proteins, sugar residues, and antibodies can also be incorporated into liposomes. The various approaches used include physical adsorption, incorporation during liposomal preparation, and covalent binding (direct or through a spacer) to the active drug or an inert additive (e.g., polymer), incorporated into the liposomal membrane [124,128,129].

After intravenous administration, liposomes are rapidly removed from blood, primarily by cells of the RES, and foremost by the liver (Kupffer cells). The half-lives of liposomes in the blood stream may range from a few minutes to many hours, depending on the nature and compositions of the lipids, surface properties, and size of the liposomal vesicles. In general, smaller unilamellar vesicles (SUVs) show much longer half-lives in the blood than multilamellar vesicles (MLVs) and large unilamellar vesicles (LUVs). Negatively charged liposomes are cleared more rapidly from the circulation than corresponding neutral or positively charged liposomes. Also, the uptake by the spleen is greater for negatively charged liposomes than for positive or neutral liposomes. The SUVs can penetrate 0.1 μm fenestrations located in the endothelium of discontinuous (sinusoidal) capillaries lining the liver, spleen, and bone marrow [130] and reach the underlying parenchymal cells. The endothelium of the hepatic sinusoid contains openings larger than 0.1 μm in diameter, and this may allow penetration of MLVs and LUVs. An increase in the liposome dose causes a relative decrease in liver uptake and, consequently, an increase in blood levels and, to some extent, in spleen and bone marrow uptake [130]. Prolongation of the blood clearance times of the liposomes by blocking the RES uptake may increase the likelihood of liposomes to interact with vascular endothelial cells and circulating blood cells.

Irrespective of size, liposomes, when injected intraperitoneally, partially accumulate in the liver and spleen. It has been suggested that transport of liposomes from the peritoneal cavity to the systemic circulation, and eventually to tissues, occurs by lymphatic pathways. Local injection of larger liposomes leads to quantitative accumulation at the site of injection. The slow disintegration of the carrier than releases the drug, which diffuses into the blood circulation. Smaller liposomes, on the other hand, enter the lymph nodes and blood circulation and eventually accumulate in the liver and spleen.

Since the RES is the natural target, liposomes have been extensively investigated as carriers for the treatment of liver and RES organ diseases (passive targeting) Belchetz et al. [131] reported that liposome-entrapped glucocerebroside, when administered intravenously in patients suffering with Gaucher's disease, reduced liver size significantly. The effect is attributed to the penetration ability of the liposomal drug into the cells. The native enzyme gave no effects because of its inability to penetrate the cells. A similar finding was reported in patients suffering with glycogenesis type II disease following administration of amyloglycosidase entrapped in liposomes [132]. Encapsulation of antimonial drugs within liposomes has increased the efficacy by 800- to 1000-fold, compared with the free drug, against experimental visceral and cutaneous leishmaniasis in rats [133–135]. Bakker-Woudenberg et al. [136] found about a 90-fold increase in the therapeutic efficacy following administration of liposome-encapsulated ampicillin, compared with free ampicilin, against *Listeria monocytogenes* infection.

Liposomes have also been used for delivering immunomodulating agents to macrophages. Macrophages are immunologically competent, extravascular cells that contribute to host defense mechanisms. Activated macrophages are capable of selectively killing tumor cells, thereby leaving normal cells unharmed. Fidler et al. [137] have shown that lymphokines (macrophage-activating factor, interferon), muramyl dipeptide, and a lipophilic derivative of muramyl tripeptide, encapsulated within liposomes are highly effective in activating antitumor functions in rodent and human macrophages in vitro, and in the mouse and the rat in vivo. Dose-response measurements show that liposome-encapsulated preparations of these agents induce maximum levels of macrophage activation at a significantly lower dose than needed for equivalent activation by the nonencapsulated preparation [138–140]. Roerdnik et al. [113] reported a 50–60% increase in the tumoricidal activity of muramyl dipeptide when encapsulated within liposomes, compared with free drug, against B-16 melanoma cells in vitro. The free drug gave a maximum activity of 30% cytotoxicity versus a 250- to 1000-fold increase in potentiation of muramyl-induced cytotoxicity as a result of encapsulation within liposomes. Fidler et al. [141,142] and Sone et al. [143] have found that encapsulation of more than one agent within the same liposome produces synergistic activation of macrophages in vitro and in vivo. The activation of macrophages, in general, requires phagocytosis of the liposome, followed by a lag period of 4–8 hours before tumoricidal activity is expressed [139]. No participation of macrophage surface receptors is required. This suggests that tumoricidal activity of macrophages results from the interaction of immunomodulating agents with intracellular targets [144].

Liposomes also serve as carriers for a variety of antineoplastic drugs. Mayhew and Rustum [145] demonstrated that liposomes containing doxorubicin

(Adriamycin) are 100 times more effective, compared with free drug, against the liver metastasis of the M5076 tumor. Liposomal encapsulation of amphotericin B, a potent, but extremely toxic, antifungal drug, also resulted in much reduced toxicity, while it maintained potency [146]. Rosenberg et al. [147] and Burkhanov et al. [148] have reported that liposomes prepared using autologous phospholipids obtained from tumor cells are taken up by the tumor cells two to six times better than a control egg lecithin liposome.

Liposomes containing specific targeting molecules, such as tumor-specific antibodies or cell receptor–specific ligands (e.g., glycolipids, lipoproteins, and amino sugars), have been prepared to provide liposomes with increased direct transport properties [124]. These cell-specific targeting molecules can be either adsorted on or covalently attached, directly or by a spacer, to the outer surface of the liposomal membrane. The use of spacers enables binding of considerable quantities of targeting molecules, without affecting its specific binding properties or the integrity of the liposomes.

Temperature- and pH-sensitive liposomes have been investigated for targeting drugs to primary tumors and metastases or sites of infection and inflammation [72]. The basis for the temperature-sensitive drug delivery is that at elevated temperatures, above the gel to liquid-crystalline phase transition temperature (T_c), the permeability of liposomes markedly increases, causing the release of the entrapped drug. The release rate depends on the temperature and the action of the serum components, principally the lipoproteins. Weinstein et al. [149] investigated the effect of heating on incorporation of [^{3}H]methotrexate, administered in the free form and encapsulated in 7:3 (w/w) dipalmitoyl and distearoyl phosphatidylcholine liposomal vesicles, in L1210 tumors implanted in the hind feet of mice. They found about a 14% increase in [^{3}H]methotrexate incorporation from the liposomal form, compared with the free drug, after heating. This approach has been extended to a bladder transitional cell carcinoma, implanted in the hind legs of C^3H/Bi mice [150], and for delivery of cisplatin (*cis*-diamminedichloroplatinum) selectively to tumors [151].

The pH-sensitive liposomes consist of mixtures of several saturated egg phosphatidylcholines and several *N*-acylamino acids. The release of drug is suggested to be a function of acid-base equilibrium effected by the interaction between ionizable amino acids and *N*-acylamino acid headgroups of the liposomes. There appears to be a close relation between T_c and pH effect [72].

Liposomes also offer potential for use as carriers to transfer genetic materials to cells. Nicolau et al. [152] reported that a recombinant plasmid containing the rat preproinsulin I gene, encapsulated in large liposomes, when injected intravenously, resulted in the transient expression of this gene in the liver and spleen of the recipient animals. A significant fraction of the expressed hormone was in physiologically active form. Recently, liposomes have also been used to block the initial binding of human immunodeficiency virus (HIV) to host cells [113]. This binding takes place between a glycoprotein (gp 120) on the virus coat and the CD4 receptor on the surface of T-helper lymphocytes and other cells. Antiviral drugs, such as zalcitabine (2′,3′-dideoxycytidine)-5′-triphosphate [153] and zidovudine (AZT) [154], have also been incorporated into liposomes and studied for their antiviral activities.

The incorporation of magnetic particles in liposomes, combined with an externally applied magnetic field, has recently demonstrated in vivo the ability to slectively target a specific organ, i.e., one kidney over the other [155].

The use of nanoparticles and liposomes to target and increase the bioavailability of antibiotics has been a research activity over the last 20 years and has been recently reviewed [156]. Ocular drug targeting by liposomes is another important area of research [157]. Oral liposome drug delivery has been the subject of considerable cynicism. However, polymerized micro-encapsulated and polymer-coated liposomes have increased the potential for liposomes via the oral route as well as a greater understanding of their cellular processing, as extensively reviewed by Rogers and Anderson [158].

Niosomes. Niosomes are globular submicroscopic vesicles composed of nonionic surfactants. They can be formed by techniques analogous to those used to prepare liposomes [159]. To predict whether the surfactant being used will produce micelles or bilayer niosome vesicles, an arbitrary critical packing parameter (CPP) can be used, i.e., $v/a \cdot l$, where v and l are specific volume and length of the hydrophilic portion of the surfactant, and a is the area of the hydrophobic segment of the surfactant [160]. A CPP value of 0.5 or less favors the formation of micelles, whereas a value between 0.5 and 1.0 favors the formation of vesicles. The various types of nonionic surfactants used to prepare niosomes include polyglycerol alkylethers [161], glucosyl dialkylethers [162], crown ethers [163], and polyoxyethylene alkylethers [163]. Similar to liposomes, niosome vesicles can be unilamellar, oligolamellar, or multilamellar. A variety of lipid additives, such as cholesterol, can be incorporated in the niosome bilayer. Incorporation of cholesterol in the niosome bilayer enhances the stability of niosomes against destabilizing effects of plasma and serum proteins and decreases the permeability of the vesicle to entrapped solute [164]. Niosomes are osmotically active and require no special conditions for handling and storage.

Niosomes have been investigated as drug carriers in experimental cancer chemotherapy and in murine visceral leishmaniasis [164]. The structures of nonionic surfactants (polyglycerol-based) employed to prepare niosomes used in these studies are shown in Fig. 11 Surfactants I and II contain an ether linkage, whereas surfactant III has an ester linkage. The latter can be degraded in vivo by esterase enzymes. When compared with free drug, niosomal forms of methotrexate, prepared using nonionic surfactant I, cholesterol, and dicetylphosphate, after intravenous administration by the tail vein in mice, exhibited prolonged lifetimes in the plasma and produced increased methotrexate levels in the liver and the brain. In addition, encapsulation within niosomes caused a reduction in the metabolism and urinary and fecal excretion of methotrexate [165,166]. Polysorbate 80, a nonionic surfactant that does not form niosomes, when coadministered with free methotrexate, provided reduced efficacy, compared with methotrexate encapsulated in niosomes [166]. This suggests that it is essential for surfactants to have a vesicular structure to effect enhanced targeting of drugs. Niosomal delivery has also been reported for 5-fluorouracil [167].

The delivery of doxorubicin to the S180 sarcoma (tumor) in mice, using niosomes as a carrier, has been studied by Rogerson [168]. Much higher tumor drug levels were reported with niosomes prepared using the nonionic surfactant I and 50% cholesterol than with free drug or drug encapsulated in cholesterol-free niosomes. The initial serum drug concentrations were higher following administration of free drug, but between 2 and 6 hours after administration the concentrations dropped and were lower than those observed using niosomal drugs, suggesting a rapid metabolism or distribution of free drug from the vascular system.

Niosomes (prepared using surfactant I and surfactant I, II, or III and 30% cholesterol) containing stibogluconate have been as effective as the corresponding liposomal drugs in the visceral leishmaniasis model. Free drug showed reduced efficacy [169].

Lipoproteins. A lipoprotein is an endogenous macromolecule consisting of an inner apolar core of cholesteryl esters and triglycerides surrounded by a monolayer of phospholipid embedded with cholesterol and apoproteins. The functions of lipoproteins are to transport lipids and to mediate lipid metabolism. There are four main types of lipoproteins (classified based on their flotation rates in salt solutions): chylomicrons, very-low-density lipoprotein (VLDL), low-density lipoprotein (LDL), and high-density lipoprotein (HDL). These differ in size, molecular weight, and density and have different lipid, protein, and apoprotein compositions (Table 11). The apoproteins are important determinants in the metabolism of lipoproteins—they serve as ligands for lipoprotein receptors and as mediators in lipoproteins interconversion by enzymes.

A schematic representation of the metabolism of lipoproteins is shown in Fig. 12 [170]. Chylomicrons are synthesized and secreted by the small intestine. They are hydrolyzed in blood by the enzyme lipoprotein lipase

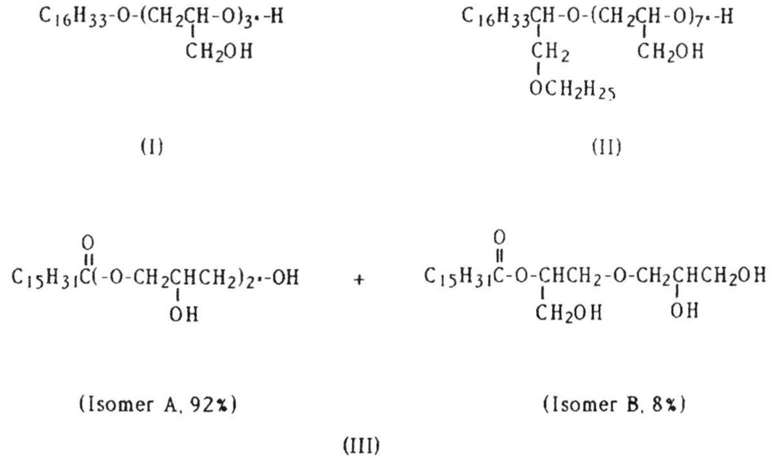

$C_{16}H_{33}\text{-}O\text{-}(CH_2\underset{|}{C}H\text{-}O)_{3^*}\text{-}H$ with CH_2OH on the CH

(I)

$C_{16}H_{33}CH\text{-}O\text{-}(CH_2CH\text{-}O)_{7^*}\text{-}H$ with CH_2–OCH_2H_{25} on the first CH and CH_2OH on the second CH

(II)

$C_{15}H_{31}C(=O)(\text{-}O\text{-}CH_2CH(OH)CH_2)_{2^*}\text{-}OH$ + $C_{15}H_{31}C(=O)\text{-}O\text{-}CH(CH_2OH)CH_2\text{-}O\text{-}CH_2CH(OH)CH_2OH$

(Isomer A, 92%) (Isomer B, 8%)

(III)

Fig. 11 Structures of three polyglycerol-based nonionic surfactants used in the preparation of nionsomes (* represents an average number value of glycerol units).

Table 11 Physicochemical Properties and Composition of Human Lipoproteins

Lipoproteins	Chylomicrons	VLDL	LDL	HDL
Density (g/ml)	< 0.950	< 1.006	1.019–1.063	1.063–1.210
Size (nm)	80–1000	30–90	20–25	8–12
Molecular weight, *M*	10^9	10×10^6	2.3×10^6	300,000
Composition (%)				
Phospholipids	3–6	15–20	18–24	26–32
Cholesterol	1–3	4–8	6–8	3–5
Cholesterol esters	2–4	16–22	45–50	15–20
Triglycerides	80–95	45–65	4–8	2–7
Protein	1–2	6–10	18–22	45–55
Apoproteins[a]				
Major	A-I, A-IV, B-48, C-I, C-II, C-III	B-100, C-I, C-II, C-III, E	B-100	A-I, A-II, E
Minor	A-II, E	A-I, A-II, Ed	C-I, C-II, C-III	C-I, C-II, C-II, D, E

[a] Designations A, B, and C represent heterogeneous groups of apoproteins, each containing more than one polypeptide.
Source: Refs. 170, 252.

(LPL; found on the endothelial surfaces of the blood capillaries) to produce chylomicron remnants, which are then removed from the circulation by specific remnant receptors located on parenchymal liver cells. VLDLs are secreted by the liver. Following their secretion in blood, VLDLs undergo metabolism in a way analogous to chylomicron. The resulting VLDL remnants are either removed by the hepatic remnant receptors or further metabolized to LDL, the major cholesterol-carrying lipoprotein in humans. LDLs are removed from the circulation mainly by the liver and, to some extent, by peripheral cells. The HDL

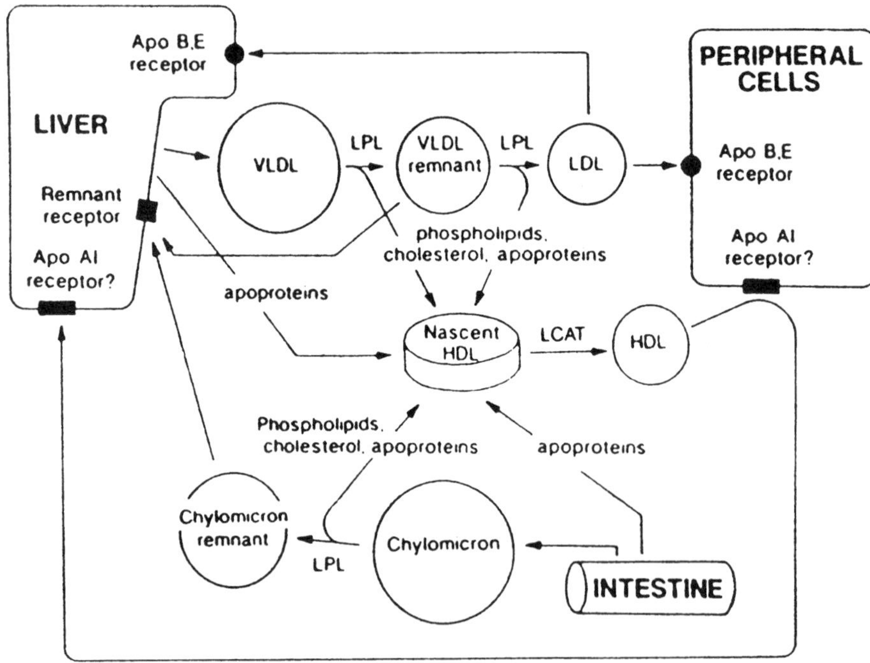

Fig. 12 Schematic representation of lipoprotein metabolism. (From Ref. 170).

apoproteins are synthesized and secreted by the liver and the intestine. These apoproteins combine with the phospholipids, cholesterol, and protein components, produced as side products during in vivo conversion of chylomicrons and VLDL to the corresponding remnants by the lipoprotein lipase enzyme, and form the nascent HDL intermediate. The later is then converted to HDL by the enzyme lecithin cholesterylacyltransferase (LCAT). Depending on the types of apoproteins present, HDL can be removed from the circulation by LDL-specific receptors, remnant receptors, or by specific high-affinity HDL-binding sites present on adipocytes, adrenocortical cells, and various liver cells. The function of HDL is to transport cholesterol from peripheral tissues to the liver. It also serves as the site of plasma cholesterol esterification [171].

Lipoproteins have been suggested as potential drug carriers because (a) they are natural macromolecules and thus pose no threats of any anti-immunogenic response; (b) unlike other particulate carriers, lipoproteins are not rapidly cleared from the circulation by the reticuloendothelial system; (c) the cellular uptake of lipoproteins is by high-affinity receptors; (d) the inner core of a lipoprotein, which comprises triglycerides and cholesterol, provides an ideal domain for transporting highly lipophilic drugs, whereas amphiphilic drugs can be incorporated in the outer phospholipid coat of the core; (e) drugs incorporated in the core are protected from the environment during transport, and the environment is protected from the drug; and (f) drugs located in the core do not affect the specificity of the ligand(s) present on the surface of the particle for binding to various cells.

Several methods are known to entrap or incorporate drugs into lipoproteins. The three most commonly practiced procedures include [170]: (a) direct addition of an aqueous solution of a drug to the lipoprotein; (b) transfer of a drug from a solid surface (e.g., the wall of a glass tube, glass beads, or small siliceous earth crystals) to the lipoprotein; and (c) delipidation of lipoprotein with sodium desoxycholate or an organic solvent, followed by reconstitution with drug-phospholipid microemulsion or drug alone.

The use of LDL and other lipoproteins in drug targeting has been reviewed [170,172]. Damle et al. [173] have shown that radiopharmaceuticals, such as iopanoic acid, a cholecystographic agent, could be incorporated in chylomicron remnants by esterification with cholesterol and used for liver imaging. About 87% of the chylomicron remnant–loaded iopanoic acid accumulated in the liver within 0.5 hour after administration, compared with 31% accumulated using a saline solution containing the same amount of the drug. The LDLs have been used as a carrier to selectively deliver chemotherapeutic agents to neoplastic cells. The rationale is that tumor cells, compared with normal cells, express higher amounts of LDL receptors and, thus, can be selectively targeted with LDL. Thus, Samadi-Baboli et al. [174] have shown that LDL loaded with 9-methoxyellipticin incorporated in an emulsion containing dimyristoylphosphatidylcholine and cholesteryl oleate exhibited much higher activity than free drug against L1210 and P388 murine leukemia cells in vitro. The eradication of the L1210 cells by the drug-LDL complex occurred exclusively by an LDL receptor mechanism. The LDL-drug complex showed higher cytotoxicity against cells preincubated with lipoprotein-deficient serum than those incubated in fetal serum, confirming that higher LDL expression on the cells leads to a higher uptake of LDL. Another study [175] indicated that acrylophenon antineoplastic molecules when incorporated within LDL can be delivered selectively to cancer cells without being entrapped in other blood proteins and cleared by the reticuloendothelial cells.

Kempen et al. [176] synthesized a water-soluble cholesteryl-containing trigalactoside, Tris-Gal-Chol (**I**), which when incorporated in lipoproteins allows the utilization of active receptors for galactose-terminated macromolecules as a trigger for the uptake of lipoproteins. The effect of increasing concentrations of Tris-Gal-Chol on the removal of LDL and HDL from serum and their quantitative recovery in the liver is shown in Fig. 13. These data show that lipoproteins containing Tris-Gal-Chol can be used as a liver-specific drug-carrier system.

LDL and HDL have also been chemically modified to provide new recognition markers so that they can be selectively targeted to various types of cells in the liver [170,172]. Lactosylated LDL and HDL, which contain D-galactose residues as a ligand, can be prepared by incubating the corresponding protein with lactose (D-galactosyl-D-glucose) and sodium cyanoborohydride. Incubation of LDL with acetic anhydride produces the acetylated LDL. When injected intravenously in rats, both lactosylated LDL and HDL and acetylated LDL are rapidly cleared from the circulation by the liver (Table 12). Lactosylated LDL is specifically taken up by the Kupffer cells, whereas lactosylated HDL is mainly cleared by the parenchymal cells. Acetylated LDL shows a higher accumulation in endothelial and parenchymal cells than in Kupffer cells. Thus, lactosylated HDL can be used to deliver antiviral drugs to parenchymal cells, whereas lactosylated LDL may serve as a carrier for immunomodulators, antivirals, and antiparasitic drugs

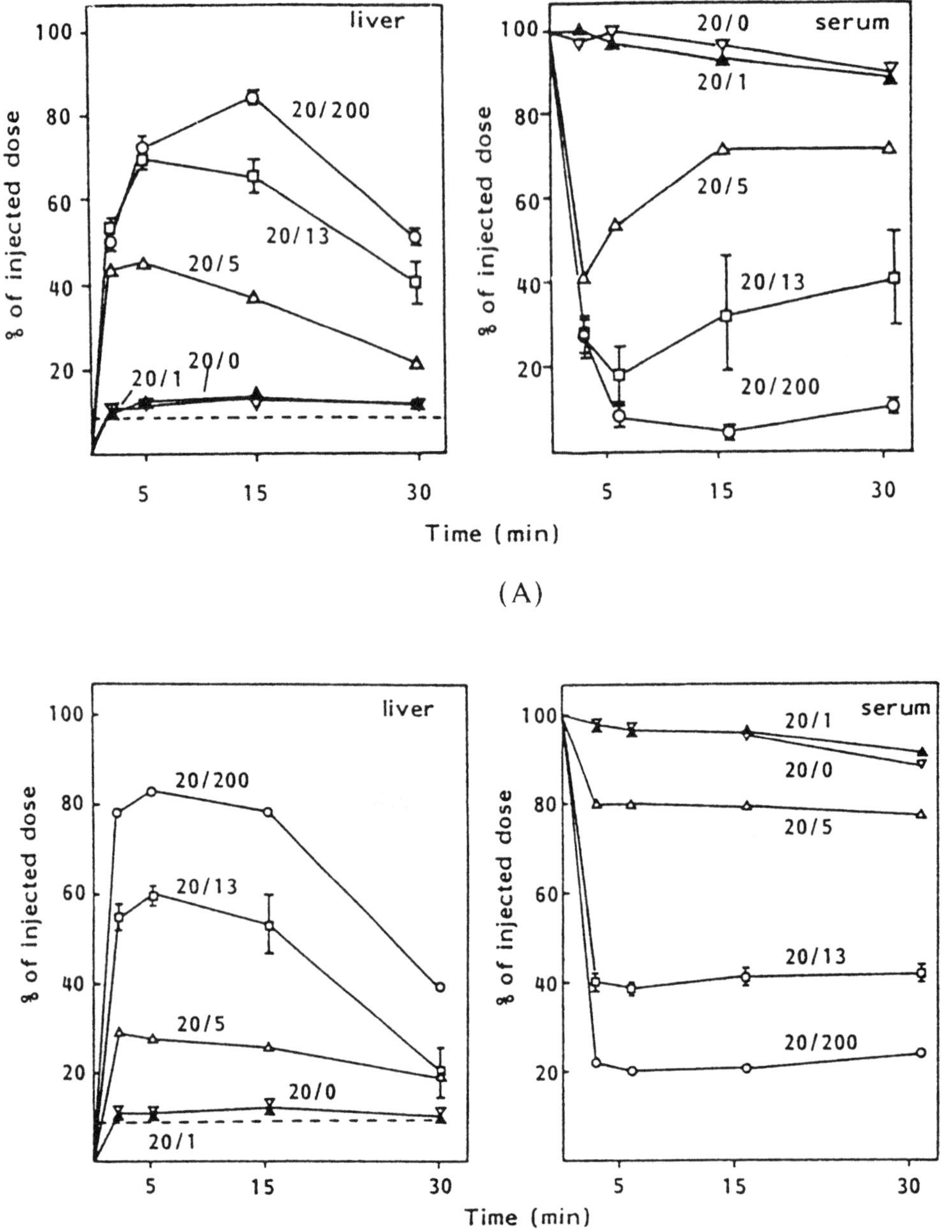

Fig. 13 The effect of Tris-Gal-Chol concentration (A) (0, 5, 13, and 200 μg) on the liver association and serum decay of ^{125}I-LDL and (B) ^{125}I-HDL (20 μg). The dotted line represents the maximal contribution of the serum value to the liver uptake. (From Ref. 170.)

to Kupffer and parenchymal cells. Acetylated LDL, on the other hand, is suitable for targeting anti-infective drugs to parenchymal and endothelial liver cells. Both Kupffer and endothelial cells have been implicated in HIV infections [177].

Activated Carbon (Charcoal). Activated carbon is commonly used as an adsorbent. It has a microporous structure and possesses a large surface area for adsorption. Drugs or chemicals adsorbed on activated carbon particles exist in dynamic equilibrium with nonadsorbed drugs. The aqueous suspension forms of activated carbon, available commercially under the trade name Actidose with Sorbitol and Actidose-Aqua (208 mg/mL), have been accepted for oral use in humans to remove toxic substances.

Table 12 Distribution of Acetylated LDL, Lactosylated LDL, and Lactosylated HDL Over Liver Cell Types

	Percentage of total liver uptake ($n = 3$)		
	Acetylated LDL	Lactosylated LDL	Lactosylated HDL
Parenchymal cells	38.8 ± 5.8	31.8 ± 4.9	98.1 ± 0.6
Kupffer cells	7.4 ± 1.7	57.1 ± 1.9	1.0 ± 0.5
Endothelial cells	53.8 ± 5.7	11.1 ± 3.2	0.9 ± 0.2

Source: Ref 170.

Activated carbon, when injected into tissues, is taken into the lymphotic capillaries and becomes localized in the regional nodes. When administered into a cancerous pleural or abdominal cavity, activated carbon was adsorbed onto cancer and serosal surfaces. Takahashi [178] reported that mitomycin binds reversibly to activated carbon with desorption rates of 90 ± 4.8% and 107.2 ± 7.3% in saline and Ringer's solutions, respectively. Activated carbon adsorbs 20–500 times more mitomycin than considered to be effective for cancer cells. The acute toxicity, evaluated in vivo in non–tumor-bearing and tumor-bearing humans and animals, showed an increase in the median lethal dose (LD_{50}) value with an increase in the amount of activated carbon. When administered peritoneally in non–tumor-bearing rats, activated carbon–mitomycin particles (equalivalent to 5.0 mg of mitomycin) deposited in the omentum and peritoneum cavities and were odserved in to the lymphatic system. In tumor-bearing rats, particles were observed in lymph nodes of the omentum, paar aorta, perirenal, and thoracic angle 10 minutes after administration. There were no particles in the lymph nodes displaced by tumor tissues at a terminal stage, suggesting that the administered activated charcoal–mitomycin particles are delivered to distant lymph nodes with metastasis through the lymph vessels. A graphic presentation of the mitomycin concentration of ascites in Donryu male rats bearing ascites hepatoma AH130, following intraperitoneal administration of mitomycin–activated charcoal and free mitomycin in saline solutions, is shown in Fig. 14. Table 13 lists the concentration of mitomycin in tumors and body organs. In rabbits, mitomycin was delivered only to the lymphatic system [178].

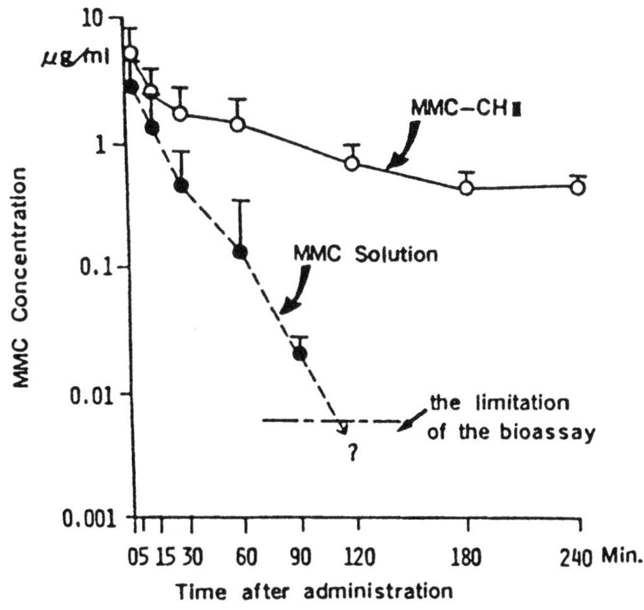

Fig. 14 Mitomycin concentration of ascites in rates bearing AH-130 after intraperitoneal administration (dose: 2 mg/kg in saline solution; open circles, mitomycin adsorbed on activated carbon; solid circles, free mitomycin; $n = 5$). (From Ref. 178.)

Table 13 Mitomycin Concentration (mg/g) in Tumors and Organs After Intraperitoneal Administration of Mitomycin–Activated Carbon and Mitomycin in Saline Solutions (dose: 2 mg/kg)

	Mitomycin solution					Mitomycin–activated carbon				
Time after injection (min)	5	30	60	120	240	5	30	60	120	240
Tumor of greater omentum						0.95	0.55	0.09	0.13	0.013
Tumor of mesentrium						0.06	0.35	0.014	0.082	0.37
Tumor of epidermis		[a]				0.20	0.61	0.08	0.036	0.046
Spleen						0.01	0.029	0.10	0.14	0.082
Retroperitoneum						0.15	0.89	0.67	0.066	0.096
Lung	0.09	[a]								
Heart	[a]									

[a]Below the limitation of the bioassay (<0.005 mg/g).
Source: Ref. 178.

Studies in dogs indicated that mitomycin-activated carbon, when injected into the canine gastric wall, is taken up primarily by the lymphatic system and transported rapidly to the regional lymph nodes, with drug activity being retained [178]. A similar observation was made by Ito et al. [179] following an administration of activated charcoal–mitomycin suspension into the sub-serosal space. In both studies, compared with a mitomycin solution, a significant inhibition of lymph node metastasis was noted with mitomycin-activated charcoal. In humans, both early stomach cancers and advanced cancers of Borrmann I type either decreased by more than 50% in size or completely disappeared following the local injection of mitomycin–activated charcoal. No significant effect was noted in advanced cancers with Borrmann II, III, and IV types. High drug activity was demonstrated in regional lymph nodes for a prolonged period. The drug in the peripheral blood was scarce. Patients tolerated about a five times larger dose of the anticancer agent when presented in the activated charcoal adsorbed form than in free form [178].

It appears that activated carbon might be a potential carrier for lymphatic delivery, or to peritoneal or pleural cavities, the most common sites in cancer metastasis. Minimal side effects are expected, since constant low concentrations of drug are maintained in the general circulation.

Cellular Carriers. Erythrocytes, leukocytes, platelets, islets, hepatocytes, and fibroblasts have all been suggested as potential carriers for drugs and biological substances. They can be used to provide slow release of entrapped drugs in the circulatory system, to deliver drugs to a specific site in the body, as cellular transplants to provide missing enzymes and hormones (in enzyme–hormone replacement therapy), or as endogenous cells to synthesize and secret molecules that affect the metabolism and function of other cells. Because these carriers are actual endogenous cells, they produce little or no antigenic response, and when old or damaged, they, like normal cells, are removed from the circulation by macrophages. Another important feature of these carriers is that, once loaded with drug, they can be stored at 4°C for several hours to several days, depending on the storage medium and the entrapment method used.

Since erythrocytes, platelets, and leukocytes have received the greatest attention, the discussion that follows will be limited to these carriers. Fibroblasts [180] and hepatocytes [181] have been specifically used as viable sources to deliver missing enzymes in the management of enzyme-deficiency diseases, whereas islets are useful as a cellular transplant to produce insulin [182,183].

ERYTHROCYTES. Erythrocytes are biconcave disk-shaped, blood cells (with pits or depressions in the center on both sides), the primary function of which is to transport hemoglobin, the oxygen-carrying protein. The biconcave shape of the erythrocyte provides a large surface volume ratio and thereby facilitates exchange of oxygen. The average diameter of erythrocytes is 7.5 μm, and thickness at the rim is 2.6 μm and in the center about 0.8 μm. The normal concentration of erythrocytes in blood is approximately 3.9–5.5 million cells per μL in women and 4.1–6 million cells per μL in men. The total life span of erythrocytes in blood is 120 days.

The erythrocyte cell is surrounded by a membrane called the plasmalemma, which consists of equal weights of lipid (major components: phospholipids, cholesterol, and glycolipids) and protein (glycophorin. ankyrin, and protein 4.1) components. The lipid portion of the membrane exists as a bilayer. The preponderant phospholipid constituents of the lipid bilayer membrane include phosphatidylcholine, phosphatidylethanolamine, phosphatidylserine, phosphatidylinositol, and sphingomylein. The polar headgroups of the outer lipid layer face out to the extra-cellular fluid, whereas those of the inner lipid layer face inward to the cells. The hydrocarbon portions of the lipid lie adjacent to each other in the middle. Glycolipids are present only as a minor component. About half of the protein present in the plasmalemma spans the lipid bilayer. Erythrocytes show a net negative surface charge (owing to the presence of carboxylic groups of sialic acids), which prevents erythrocytes from agglutinating in the presence of IgG. In addition to lipids and proteins, some membranes contain carbohydrates, which are responsible for some of their surface antigenic properties.

Erythrocytes have been suggested as potential carriers for a number of biologically active substances, including drugs, nucleic acids, and enzymes [184–186]. They can be used as storage depots for sustained-drug release or potentially be modified to permit targeting to specific cell types in the blood (e.g., direct targeting to cells in leukemia [187]. Although constrained to move within blood vessels, erythrocytes can exit from blood vessels into tissues [188], potentiating their use as carriers in treating inflammations. Examples of drugs used for entrapment within erythrocytes and their suggested action against disease or their site specificity in the body is presented in Table 14. A number of enzymes such as β-glucuronidase, β-fructofuranosidase, β-galactosidase, glutaminase, urease, hexosaminidase B, uricase, neuraminidase, thymidine

Table 14 Examples of Erythrocyte-Targeted Drug-Delivery Systems

Agents	Entrapment method	Suggested action against target/disease
As circulating carriers		
l-Asparaginase	a	Leukemia
Indolyl-3-alkane-α-hydroxylase	a	Sarcomas/carcinomas
Arginase	a, b	Hyperargininemia
δ-Aminolevulinate dehydratase	a	Porphyrias
Factor IX hemophilia	b	Hemophilia B
Desferroxamine	a	Excess body iron storage
Ara-C and phosphorylated Ara-C	a, b	Histiocytic medullary reticulosis/leukemia
Primaguine phosphate	c	Casual prophylaxis and radical cure of malaria
Insulin	b	Diabetes mallitus
Dideoxycytidine-5′-phosphate		AJDS
As targeted drug carriers		
Carboplatin		Liver
Rubomycin		Tumor P388
Daunomycin	a, d	Leukemia
Actinomycin D-DNA	a	Tumor
Doxorubicin		Liver tumor
Adriamycin	b	Liver and lung tumors
Methotrexate	a, b, e	Liver tumor
Daunorubicin	f	Leukemia
Bleomycin	a	RES
Genlamicin	b	RES
Antibodies	b	Diphtheria toxin; T cells
Diflubenzuron	b	Blood-sucking flies
Soybean trypsin inhib.	b	Blood-sucking flies
Imidocarb	b	Babesiasis
β-Glucoceribrosidase	a, b	Gaucher's disease
Meglumine antimoniate	g	Leishmaniasis
Pentamidine		Leishmaniasis
Heparin	b	Thromboembolism

a, Dilution; b, dialysis; c, endocytosis; d, amphotericin B; e, dielectric breakdown; f, coupling reaction; g, preswell.

kinase, and hypoxanthine-guanine phosphoribosyltransferase have also been entrapped within erythrocyte and used for treating enzyme deficiency [185]. Erythrocytes are removed from the circulation by the RES, especially by cells located in the spleen and the liver.

Several methods have been used to incorporate exogenous substances within erythrocytes [185]. These include hypotonic hemolysis, dielectric breakdown, endocytosis, and entrapment without hemolysis, using amphotericin B. Of these, hypotonic hemolysis is most commonly used. It involves placing the cell in a hypotonic solution containing the drug or chemical substance to be incorporated. As a result the cell swells. When the internal (osmotic) pressure exceeds a critical value, the cell ruptures and releases its content in the external medium. Substances present in the external medium enter into the cell at this time and become entrapped after the erythrocyte membrane is resealed. Resealing of the erythrocyte membrane can be achieved by incubating the entrapped cells at 37°C under isotonic conditions. This is the fastest and simplest method of drug incorporation, and works efficiently for encapsulation of low molecular weight (< 130,000) substances. The major disadvantages of the method, however, are: (a) it requires a relatively large amount of the starting material (owing to the large extracellular volume compared with the small intercellular volume); (b) a substantial percentage of the cellular content of erythrocyte enzymes and hemoglobin is lost during lysis; (c) a small change in ionic strength of the external medium may cause a significant alteration in the structure of the cell membrane (owing to the loss of membrane polypeptides) and, consequently, a decrease in the life span of the erythrocytes.

Several modifications in the foregoing method (hypotonic hemolysis) have been made to circumvent the disadvantages just noted. For example, the loss of enzymes and hemoglobin during lysis can be reduced by using hypotonic solution and resealing hemolysates prepared by the lysis and dialysis of other erythrocytes, or by preswelling the erythrocytes in 0.6% NaCl solution before subjecting them to hypotonic hemolysis. The morphological and structural integrity of the resealed erythrocytes can be preserved by hemolyzing and resealing erythrocyte cells in a dialysis tube. The dialysis approach allows a slow and gradual decrease in the ionic strengths and, consequently, preserves the elasticity of the erythrocyte membrane. Other advantages of the dialysis method are: (a) entrapped materials do not leak out to an appreciable extent; (b) the use of a high hematocrit during dialysis allows more efficient encapsulation; and (c) erythrocytes with appreciably higher drug percentages can be prepared. Several factors can influence the optimal encapsulation of the drug and the integrity of the erythrocytes and need to be properly optimized, including the composition of the buffer solution, centrifugation speed, osmolarity of the hypotonic buffers, the hematocrit, the temperature during hemolysis and resealing, the time of resealing, and the nature of the lysis procedure.

The dielectric breakdown method involves application of an electric pulse to a suspension of erythrocytes in isotonic or slightly hypotonic solution. Hemolysis is typically achieved at 0–4°C for 1/2–1 hour. It occurs as a result of dielectric breakdown of the cell membrane, which, in turn, causes a reversible change in the permeability of the membrane. An increase in the temperature to 37°C intitiates the resealing process, and the original membrane resistance and impermeability of the erythrocytes are restored within minutes at this temperature. A major advantage of this method is that the size of the pore during lysis and, hence, the permeability of the membrane can be controlled by appropriate manipulations of the electric pulse intensity, pulse duration, or the ionic strength of the pulsation medium. The electric breakdown technique has also been used to prepare "magnetic" erythrocytes [189]

The loading of drugs in erythrocytes by endocytosis typically involves incubating the intact or resealed erythrocytes with the substance to be entrapped for 30 min at 37°C in the presence of varying amounts of membrane-active agents, such as primaquine or chlorpromazine, in a buffer solution. Drugs can also be loaded in erythrocytes without lysing them first [190]. This can be achieved by first incubating the erythrocytes with amphotericin B in an isotonic medium for 30 min at 37°C and then with the material to be encapsulated for another 30 min at 37°C. This method causes no observable structural changes in the erythrocyte cell membrane. Other methods that have been used include chemical-induced isotonic lysis of cells [191] and the use of anesthetic agents, such as halothane [192]. The latter method avoids the use of both isotonic and hypotonic solutions. Recently a method of convalently linking drug pharmacophores to red cell surfaces has been reported [193].

PLATELETS. Platelets are nonnucleated discoid or elliptical cells that originate from the fragmentation of giant polyploid megakaryocytes located in the bone marrow. The average diameter of the platelet is 1.5 μm. Each platelet is surrounded by a trilaminar membrane, and its cytoplasm contains a dense body (delta granule), a surface-connected canalicular system, microchondrion, alpha granules, a lysosome, peroxisomes, glycogen, and a dense tubular system. The normal platelet count ranges from 1.5 to 4.0 $\times$ 10^{10}/dL of blood. Once they enter the blood, platelets have a total life span of about 10 days. Although the primary role of platelets is in controlling hemorrhage, they are also involved in immune reactions, inflammation, maintenance of vascular wall integrity, and the evolution of vascular diseases (e.g., vasculitis and atherosclerosis) [194,195].

Platelets have been used as a carrier for several biological substances and drugs useful in the management of various hematological diseases [194]. Platelets can accumulate drugs by selective active transport. Certain drugs, such as angiotensin, hydrocortisone, imipramines, vinca alkaloids (vinblastine and vincristine), and many others, are known to bind platelets. The first clinical trial of platelet-loaded vinca alkaloids in the treatment of idiopathic thrombocytopenic purpura, an autoimmune disorder characterized by decreased platelets counts, was reported by Ahn et al. [196]. The platelets were loaded with vinblastine and vincristine, separately, by incubation at 37°C in the dark for an hour. Following removal of the unbound drug, the platelets were resuspended in the donor's plasma and then infused to the patients over a period of 30 minutes. They found that patients treated with platelet-loaded alkaloids, compared with free drugs, required fewer treatments to provide a long-lasting remission from the disorder, without any form of maintenance therapy. Despite its success, the technique has several limitations, such as the tedious preparation and high cost for platelet-drug production and, thus, is restricted to those patients refractory of readily available therapies. The use of vinca-loaded platelets has also been reported in the management of autoimmune hemolytic anemia [197], an autoimmune disease of red cells in which they become sensitized with autoantibodies of IgG and are cleared by macrophages, and of various malignant disorders of the mononuclear phagocyte system (e.g., malignant histiocytosis, Rosai Dorfman syndrome, hairy cell leukemia, monocytic leukemia, familial erythrophagocytic lymphohistiocytosis, and other platelet phagocytosing tumors) [198–200].

LEUKOCYTES. Leukocytes are white blood cells involved in the cellular and humoral defense of the organism against foreign materials. They are grouped into two classes: polymorphonuclear leukocytes, which comprise neutrophils, eosinophils, and basophils, and mononuclear leukocytes that include lymphocytes and monocytes. Of these, neutrophils and lymphocytes have been suggested as potential cellular carriers.

Neutrophils constitute about 60–80% of the total blood leukocyte level. They are spherical, with a diameter ranging between 12 and 15 μm. Their total life span is about 6–7 hours. They are known to carry a wide range of digestive enzymes and carrier proteins. Unlike erythrocytes, which are constrained to move within blood vessels, neutrophils can leave the capillaries and accumulate in large numbers at localized areas of disease. This property, their ready availability (the average production per day in adults is 1 $\times$ 10^{11}), and their highly pure form make them very attractive as a natural drug carrier. Segal and coworkers [201] reported that neutrophils containing ^{111}In-oxinate complex as a radiolabel marker, when administered intravenously in patients with abscesses and inflammation, preferentially accumulated at the diseased sites. Gainey and McDougall [202] successfully used this approach for the detection of acute inflammation in children and adolescents. Neutrophils could also be used as carriers for drugs that are effective in the treatment of pyrogenic infections, including diseases such as ulcerative colitis, acute arthritis, and other infections.

Sioux and Teissie [203] loaded propidium iodide in 70% leukocytes in whole blood using the dielectric breakdown method. The entrapped drug showed a half-life of longer than 4 hours at 4 and 37°C. When compared with the nonpulsed cells, leukocytes loaded with the drug showed 10 times more accumulation in the inflammation area than in control areas.

Lymphocytes are of two sizes: smaller lymphocytes, with a diameter of 6–8 μm, and larger lymphocytes, with a diameter up to 18 μm. They are found not only in blood, but in lymph and in every tissue of the body. Larger lymphocytes are believed to be cells that differentiate into T and B lymphocytes when activated by specific antigens. The life span of lymphocytes may vary from a few days to many years. Lymphocytes have been suggested as potential carriers for transporting macromolecules, particularly DNA, to other cells. Low molecular weight exogenous substances can be introduced into lymphocytes by electrical breakdown methods.

Soluble Macromolecular and Other Drug-Delivery Systems

Soluble macromolecules of both natural and synthetic origin have been used as drug carriers. When compared with the particulate carriers, soluble macromolecules (a) encounter fewer barriers to their movement around the body and can enter into many organs by transport across capillary endothelium or in the liver by passage through the fenestration connecting the sinusoidal lumen to the space of Disse; (b) penetrate the cells by pinocytosis, which is a phenomenon universal to all cells and that, unlike phagocytosis. does not require an external stimulus; and (c) can be found in the blood many hours after their introduction (particulate carriers, in contrast, are rapidly cleared from the blood by the RES). The fate of soluble macromolecules in animals and humans, with special reference to the transfer of polymers from one body compartment to another, has been reviewed by Drobnik and Rypacek [43].

Macromolecular drugs, in general, can be divided into four types: (a) polymeric drugs—these represent macromolecules that themselves display pharmacological activity, and polymers that contain therapeutically active groups as an integral part of the main chain; (b) macromolecule-drug analogs—these are derivatives of drugs that require no separation from the macromolecule to fulfill their therapeutic actions; (c) macromolecular prodrugs (or macromolecule-drug conjugates)—these represent drugs that must be detached from the macromolecule at the target site(s) to exert their therapeutic effects; and (d) noncovalently linked macromolecule–drug complexes. In this section, only macromolecule–drug conjugates are discussed.

A general configuration of an ideal macromolecula-drug conjugate is shown in Fig. 15 [206]. The drug can be attached to the macromolecule (or polymer chain) either directly or by a spacer and may present as pendant groups or as a terminal (not shown in Fig. 15) group. The macromolecule-drug conjugate may also contain a homing or vector device (e.g., antibodies or receptor-specific ligands) to achieve selective access to, and interaction with, the target cell, and a moiety for controlling physical and chemical properties of the conjugate. The use of a spacer arm to attach a drug to a macromolecule enhances both configuration and drug-receptor interaction efficiencies.

Depending on the chemical functional groups present on the drug and on the macromolecule, a variety of methods can be used to prepare covalently linked macromolecule-drug conjugates. The most commonly used coupling reactions are shown in Fig. 16. Proteinaceous compounds can be conjugated using the free thiol groups of cysteine, whereas the coupling between carboxylic acid-containing macromolecules and amine drugs, or vice versa, is achieved by the carbodiimide method. Polysaccharides can be attached to amine drugs by an dialdehyde intermediate, prepared using periodates. The covalently linked antibody-toxin conjugates are typically prepared by using the *N*-succinimidyl-3-(2-pyridyldithio)propionate (SDPD) reagent. It is important that the coupling reaction being used does not adversely affect the therapeutic activity of the drug.

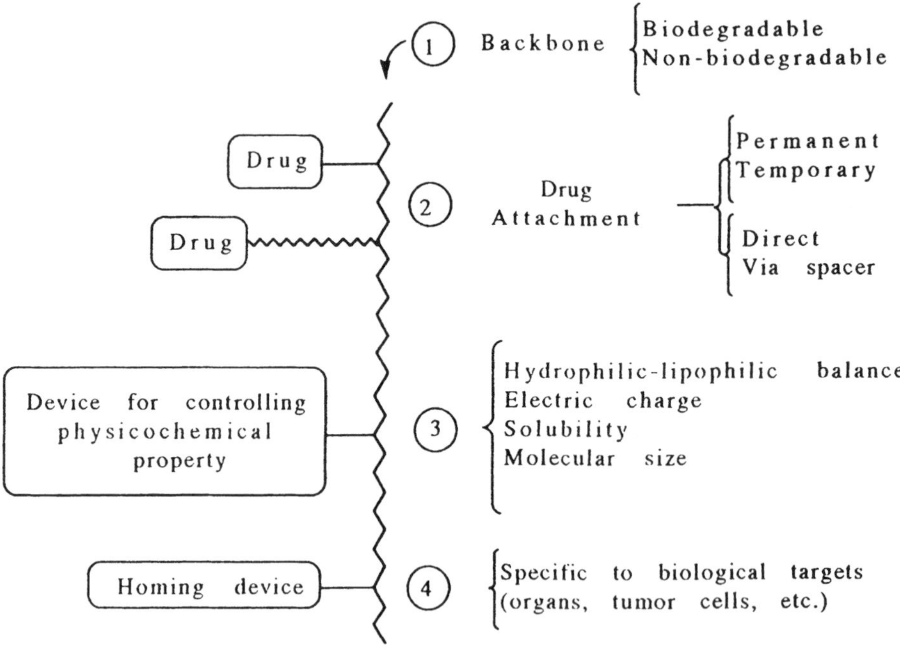

Fig. 15 A schematic representation of an ideal macromolecule-drug conjugate. (From Ref. 206.)

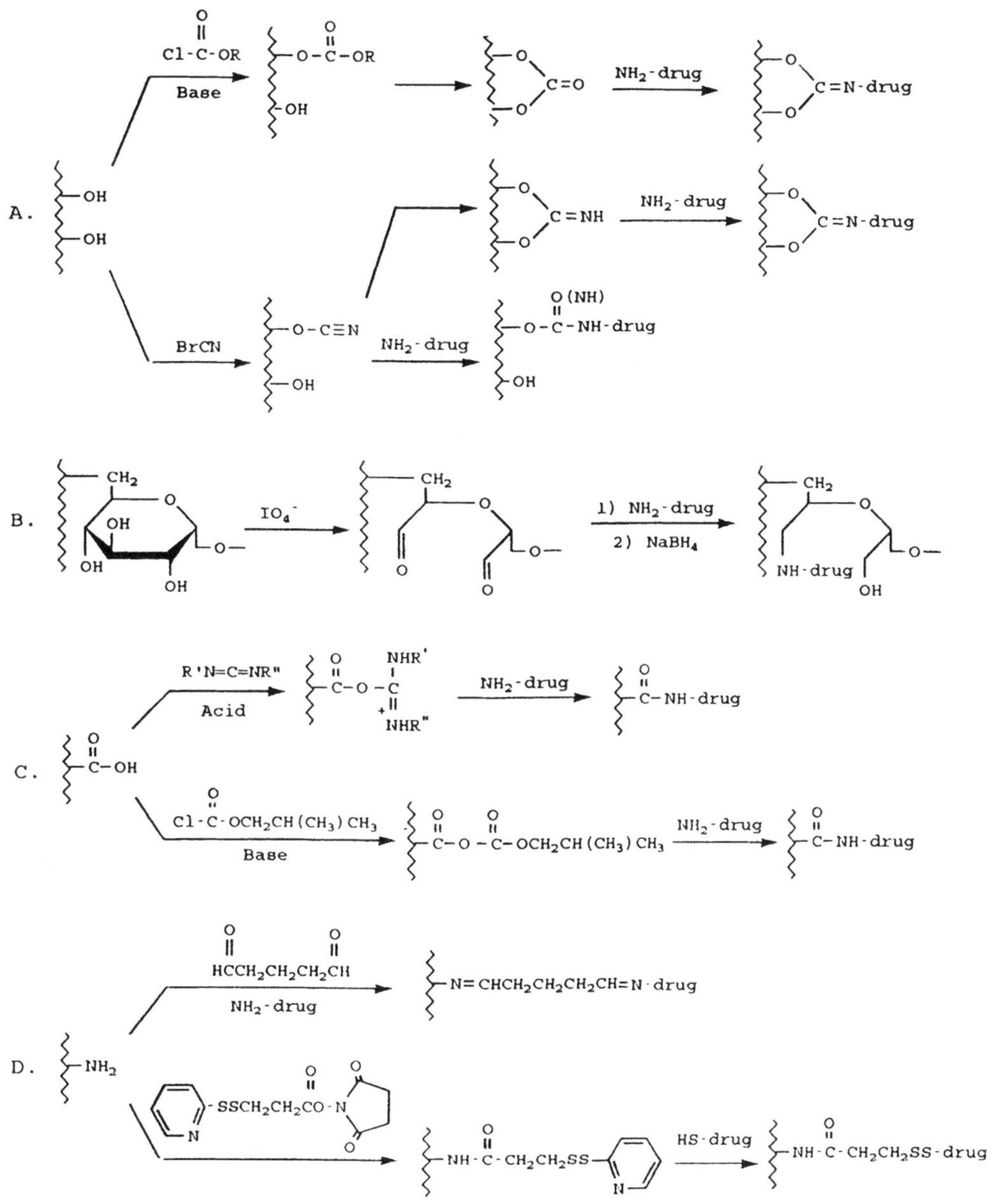

Fig. 16 Commonly used coupling methods for the preparation of macromolecule-drug conjugates. Functional groups of the drug and macromolecule are interchangeable with each other.

The fate of macromolecular drug conjugates in vivo depends on their distribution and elimination properties. In general, the plasma half-life of a macromolecule-drug conjugate depends on its molecular weight, ionic nature, configuration, and interaction tendencies in the physiological milieu. Although the RES is the natural target, other organs in the body can be targeted as well. Because many tumors possess vasculature that is hyperpermeable to macromolecules, soluble macromolecules also serve as potential drug carriers in the treatment of cancers. Present evidence suggests that the greatest levels of tumors accumulation are achieved using macromolecules that carry a negative charge. Several excellent reviews that describe the distribution of soluble macromolecules in biological systems have been published [24,36,38,43,207].

The choice of a macromolecular carrier depends on the intended clinical objectives and the nature of the therapeutic agents being used. In general, the properties of an ideal soluble carrier system include the following

[206,208]: (a) The carrier and its degradation products must be biodegradable (or at least, should not show accumulation in the body), the carrier must be nontoxic and nonantigenic and not alter the antigenicity of the therapeutic agents being transported. (b) The carrier must have an adequate drug-loading capacity; that is, the carrier must have functional groups for chemical fixation of the therapeutic agent. (c) The carrier must remain soluble in water when loaded with drug. (d) The molecular weight of the carrier should be large enough to permit glomerular filtration, but small enough to reach all cell types. (e) The carrier-drug conjugate must retain the specificity of the original carrier and must maintain the original activity of the therapeutic agent until it reaches the targeted site(s). (f) The carrier-drug conjugate must be stable in body fluids, but should slowly degrade in extracellular compartments or in lysosomes. (g) For lysosomotropic drug delivery, the macromolecule should not interfere with pinosome formation at the cell surface and subsequent intracellular fusion events. Furthermore, the macromolecule-drug linkage must be sensitive to acid hydrolysis or degradation by specific lysosomal enzymes.

Various natural and synthetic soluble macromolecules that have been investigated together with their uses are listed in Table 15. Natural polymers are monodisperse (i.e., same chain lengths), have rigid structures, and are generally more biodegradable. The rigid structures may facilitate interactions between the determinant groups on the natural polymer and the binding region of immunoglobulin. Synthetic polymers, by contrast, are less immunogenic and can be better tailor-made to predetermined specifications (i.e., molecular size, charge, hydrophobicity, and their capacity for drug-loading can be optimized). Synthetic polymers are also easier and cheaper to produce in large quantity and high purity, and the chemistry to load drugs is much less laborious. In addition, they are more robust and, thus, are more stable during manipulation and storage. Another interesting field that is developing is the design of polymers that mimic biopolymers. These synthetic polymers have properties similar to those of proteins and RNA, and are teaching us how to design new novel structures with desirable functions including drug therapy. This field has recently been reviewed [209]. A detailed discussion of some natural and synthetic soluble carrier systems follows.

Antibodies. Antibodies are circulating plasma proteins of the globulin group. They are produced by plasma cells that arise as a result of differentiation and proliferation of B lymphocytes. Antibodies interact specifically with antigenic determinants (molecular domains of the antigens) that elicit their formation. In humans, there are five main types of antibodies, commonly designated as IgG, IgA, IgM, IgE, and IgD. Of these, IgG is the most abundant. It constitutes 75% of the serum immunoglobulins and is the only immunoglobulin that crosses the placental barrier and is incorporated in the circulatory systems of the fetus, thereby protecting newborn from infection. The basic structure of the immunoglobulin molecule consists of

Table 15 Suggested Soluble Macromolecular Drug–Delivery Systems and Their Uses

Carrier	Targets/diseases/therapy
Proteins	
Antibodies; antibody fragments (e.g., collagen-specific drug-toxin conjugates)	Injured sites of blood vessels walls; tumor cells
Albumin-drug conjugates; glycoproteins	Hepatocyte-specific agents (infections disease especially viruses)
Lipoproteins	Liver; cancers of ovaries and gonads
Lectins	General carrier/recognition ligands
Hormones (toxin-drug-hormone conjugates)	Tumors
Dextrans (e.g., enzyme-drug-dextran conjugates)	Tumors
Deoxyribonucleic acid (lysosomotropic carrier)	Cancer cells
Synthetic polymers	
Poly-L-lysine and polyglutamic acid	Carrier for targeting to cancer
Poly-L-aspartic acid	Hydrolyzable targeting carrier for cancer
Polypeptide-mustard conjugates	Lung targeting; tumor targeting
HPMA	Lysosomotropic carrier for cytotoxics
Pyran copolymers	Lysosomotropic carrier for cytotoxics

Source: Ref 24.

two identical heavy (long) chains, each with a molecular weight of 50,000, and two light (short) chains with a molecular weight of 23,000 (Fig. 17). These chains are held together by noncovalent forces as well as by disulfide linkages. Each chain also contains interchain disulfide linkages. In addition, each chain contains a region of a constant amino acid sequence and a region of variable amino acid sequence. Antibodies belonging to the same class share the constant region in their heavy chains and may have kappa- or lambda-type light chains. The ends of the constant region (carboxyl ends) of the heavy chains form the Fc region, which is responsible for binding to Fc receptors present on many cells. The specificity of a particular antibody is determined by amino acid sequences of the variable region that are similar in the light and heavy chains. The ends of the variable region, referred to as amino (NH_2) terminals, serve as the binding sites for antigens.

The use of antibodies for active targeting of drugs to specific cell types in vivo has long been recognized [210–214]. They have been extensively explored as carriers in cancer diagnosis and in targeting drugs, toxins, and other therapeutic agents to tumor cells. Monoclonal antibodies of defined class and antigen specificity can be obtained in a highly purified form, and in virtually unlimited amounts, by immunizing mice with human tumor cells, followed by hybridizing their spleen cells with myeloma cells and, subsequently, screening the hybridoma cells for the formation of antibodies that bind only to immunizing tumor cells. The clinical usefulness of a given antibody in drug targeting, however, depends on its degree of cross-reaction with normal tissues and its affinity to target antigens. The presence of free antigens in the general circulation is also an important determinant in drug targeting, because an anti-body specific to these antigens would combine with it prematurely, thereby lowering site specificity. To improve specificity of action and to aid penetration into the target site (e.g., tumor cells), antibodies have been broken enzymatically to Fab′ fragments (see Fig. 17) and used in drug-targeting.

The various cytotoxic drugs that have been investigated using antibodies as a carrier include alkylating agents (e.g., chlorambucil [215], trenimon [216], and *p*-phenylenediamine mustard [217]; antimetabolites (e.g., methotrexate [218,219]); antitumor drugs (e.g., daunomycin [220,221]); and toxic proteins (e.g., A-chains of diphtheria toxin and ricin). Depending on the nature of the drug, the antibody-drug conjugates can be prepared by a carbodiimide [221], mixed anhydride, periodate, or glutaraldehyde [222]-mediated coupling reaction (see Fig. 16). Diphtheria toxin has been linked to antibodies using either a homobifunctional (e.g., glutaraldehyde) or heterobifunctional (e.g., toluene diisocyanate) agent, or through disutfide groups by using the SPDP reagent. Antibodies, in general, are fairly robust molecules and are little affected by chemical manipulations during conjugate synthesis. However, a method that works well with one monoclonal antibody may not necessarily produce the same (intended) conjugated product

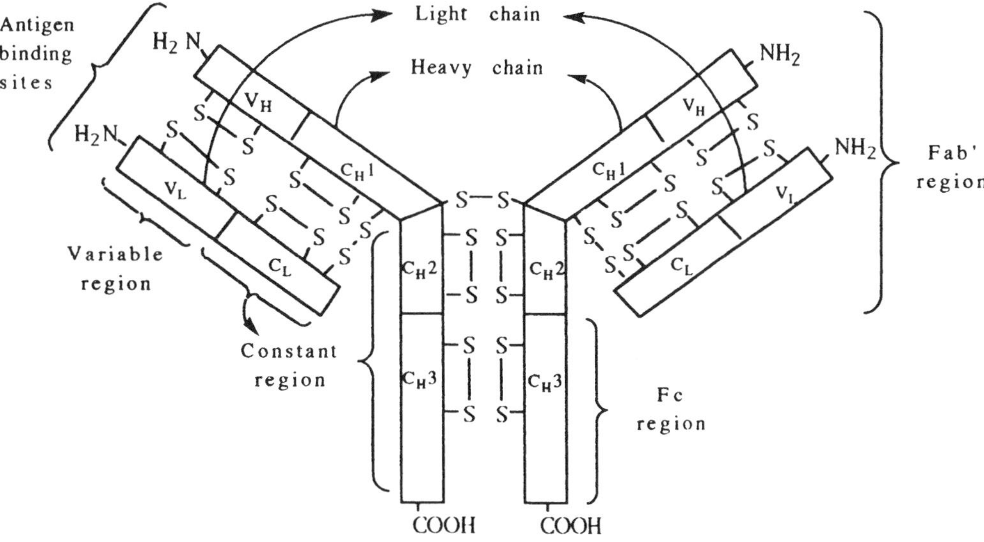

Fig. 17 Schematic representation of structure of an antibody.

with another monoclonal antibody. Rowland et al. [223] found that four monoclonals, recognizing different human tumor-associated antigens, when conjugated using an active azide derivative of a vinca alkaloid, produced vindsine–monoclonal antibody conjugates with a drug/antibody conjugation ratio varying from 3:1 to 10:1, depending on the antibody used. The percentage activity of the vindsine–monoclonal conjugate coupled at 6:1 was 98%, whereas the conjugate with a drug/antibody ratio of 4:1 showed only 2% activity.

Samokhin et al. [224] demonstrated that biotinated red blood cells complexed with biotin–antihuman collagen antibodies (by an avidin cross-linking molecule) bind efficiently and specifically to collagen-coated surfaces, and thus can be used to deliver drugs to injured sites of blood vessel walls. Biotinylated antibodies specific to tumor-associated ganglio-*N*-triosylceramide (GalNAcβ1→4GalNAcβ1→4Glcβ1→ceramide) have been prepared and found very effective in killing tumor cells that express ganglio-*N*-triosylceramide [225].

Antibodies have also been adsorbed or covalently linked to a variety of other carrier systems, such as liposomes [124], erythrocytes [226,227], and microcapsules and nanospheres, to selectively target them to a specific site in the body.

Deoxyribonucleic Acid. Deoxyribonucleic acid (DNA) has been suggested as a potential carrier for drugs that show a strong affinity for DNA and that can be released from DNA by a simple equilibrium process, or after digestion of DNA by extra- or intracellular enzymes. This approach has been extensively investigated in chemotherapy for a number of malignant disorders, because (a) DNA complexed with drugs acts as a lysosomotropic drug system (b) DNA itself is a potent inducer of pinocytosis and is easily degraded by lysosomal hydrolases; and (c) compared with normal cells, tumor cells exhibit higher endocytic activity. To avoid clearance by the RES, DNA-drug complexes are usually administered intraperitoneally [228].

The DNA forms stable complexes with doxorubicin (Adriamycin, ADR) and daunorubicin (DNR). Doxorubicin and DNR, although structurally similar, show distinctly different properties: ADR is more toxic and active than DNR in the treatment of various human solid tumors; the apparent binding affinity of ADR to DNA is about 1.8 times higher than that of DNR to DNA. Trouet et al. [229] found the ADR-DNA complex to be more active than ADR, DNR, or DNR-DNA in subcutaneously inoculated leukemic mice, whereas the DNR-DNA complex showed the highest activity against intravenously inoculated leukemic cells. Similar results have been reported in other tumor models. A recent pharmacokinetics study in patients revealed an enhanced uptake into leukemic cells and a reduction in distribution volume, cardiotoxicity, and rates of plasma clearance following administration of DNA conjugates compared to the free drug [230].

DNA has also been tested as a carrier for ethidium bromide, a drug used in the treatment of protozoal diseases. When compared with free drug, the DNA-bound drug showed decreased toxicity and higher therapeutic efficacy in mice infected with *Trypanosoma cruzi* [231].

A major advantage of DNA as a carrier is that no chemical synthesis or manipulations are needed to obtain DNA-drug complex. The efficacy of the DNA-drug complex depends on stability in the bloodstream, endocytic behavior of normal and tumor cells, presence of extra-cellular deoxyribonuclease activity in the tumor tissues, and capillary barriers that separate normal and tumor cells from the bloodstream.

Low Molecular Weight Proteins. Low molecular weight proteins, such as lysozyme, have been recently suggested as a potential carrier for targeting drugs to the kidney [232]. The rationale is that these endogenous proteins, when administered intravenously, rapidly and extensively, accumulate in the proximal tubule cells of the kidney [233]. Following glomerular filtration, the proteins are endocytosed into the cells and are taken to lysosomes, where their hydrolysis into amino acids occurs by the lysosomal enzymes, causing the release of free drug. The released drug can act either locally or be transferred into the tubular lumen of the kidney. This approach showed effective specific delivery of captopril to the kidney in a recent study [234].

Glycoproteins. Glycoproteins are endogenous substances consisting of a polypeptide backbone, with oligosaccharides as side chains. Each oligosaccharide chain contains monosaccharide residues and has sialic acid as the terminal group. The exact sequence of carbohydrate groups varies in different glycoproteins. The sialic acid groups from the terminal carbohydrate residues can be removed by treatment with the enzyme neuraminidase. When the sialic acid groups are removed, the resulting asialoglycoproteins are readily recognized and cleared by certain cells of the liver, depending on the sugar residues exposed. Hepatocytes recognize and internalize mainly galactose- and *N*-acetylgalactosamine–terminated glycoproteins, whereas Kupffer cells and endothelial cells recognize fucose-, mannose-, or *N*-acetylglucosamine–terminated glycoproteins. Kupffer cells also endocytose particulate material to which galactose groups are attached. Thus, asialoglycoproteins covalently linked to drug, protein, or diagnostic agent can be used as hepatocyte-specific carriers [235].

Recently, a variety of glycoconjugates (also known as neoglycoproteins), such as mannosylated albumin, lactosylated albumin, galactosylated poly(L-lysine), and Ficoll (a polycarbohydrate), and galactosylated poly(hydroxymethylacrylamide) [235–237] have been prepared. These, like glycoproteins, are readily recognized by various liver cell types. A partial list of drug substrates used to target various liver cell types with glycoproteins and glycoconjugates as carriers is presented in Table 16. The rationale for using asialoglycoproteins as a carrier for antiviral drugs is that the sugar residues (e.g., mannose, fucose, and galactose) on the carrier are capable of recognizing lectin receptors on the T lymphocytes and, thus, enhance targeting of antiviral drugs.

Albumin. Albumin is available in highly pure and uniform form, and exhibits low toxicity and good biological stability. It has been used as a carrier for methotrexate and a variety of antiviral drugs [amantadine, fioxuridine (5-fluorodeoxyuridine), and cytarabine (cytosinc arabinoside)] to treat macrophage tumors and infections caused by DNA viruses growing in macrophages. Heavily modified albumins are known to be readily endocytosed by cells of the macrophage system. After penetration into the cell, albumin is digested by lysosomal enzymes, causing the release of free drug. Albumin (bovine and murine)–methotrexate conjugates as well as galactosylated albumin-methotrexate systems exhibit improved liver targeting, or higher and more prolonged serum levels and decreased excretion rates than the free drug. When administered intraperitoneally into L1210 tumor-bearing mice, the methotrexate-albumin conjugate produced increased localization of methotrexate in the ascitic fluid and elevated intracellular methotrcxate levels [238,239]. It was also more effective, compared with free drug, in reducing the number of metastases in female (C57BL/6 × DBA/2)F mice bearing subcuataneously implanted Lewis lung carcinoma [240]. Whiteley et al. [241] examined the mechanism of the therapeutic activity of the conjugate using the methotrexate transport–resistant strain of Reuber hepatoma H35 cells. They found no suppression of the tumor growth, suggesting that the observed increased therapeutic activity of the conjugate occurs either through the transport of free drug following its extracellular release from the albumin, or the conjugate invokes a specific transport system to penetrate the cell. Fibrosis of the liver results from extracellular matrix deposition caused by activation of hepatic stellate cells (HSCs), making this cell type an important target. However,

Table 16 Targeting of Drugs to the Liver with Glycoproteins and Glycoconjugates

Drug/substrate	Glycoprotein carrier-glycoconjugates	Species
Antiviral agents		
Ara-Amp, acyclovir	Lactosaminated HSA	Woodchuck [292], rat [293]
Ara-Amp	Galactosylated poly-L-lysine	Mouse [294]
PMEA	Mannosylated poly-L-lysine	Mouse [295]
Ara C	Galactose-mannose carboxymethyldextran	Mouse
N-Acetylmuramyl peptide	Mannosylated BSA	Mouse [296]
Antiparasitic agents		
Alloprinol riboside	Mannosylated poly-L-lysine	Mouse [297]
Antineoplastic agents		
Mitomycin	Asialofetuin	Rat [298]
Agents affecting lipid metabolism		
LDL	Lactosaminated antiapolipoprotein B antibodies	Rat [299]
HDL	tris-Galactosyl cholesterol	Rat [299]
Antitoxicants/cytoprotective agents		
Uridine monophosphate	Polylysine asialofetuin	Rat in vivo [300]
Naproxen	Galactosyl-mannosyl HSA	Rat [301]
Superoxide dismutase	Mannosylated form	Rat [293]

Source: Courtesy of Professor D. K. F. Meijer, University Center of Pharmacy, University of Groningen, Groningen, The Netherlands. Other examples of drug targeting with glycoproteins and neoglycoproteins can be found in Ref. 235.

antifibratic drugs are not effectively taken up by HSCs. The recent finding that albumin modified with mannose-6-phosphate does selectively target these cells in animals may offer promise to much more efficiently treat fibrosis of the liver [242].

The conjugates of antiviral drugs have been investigated to treat *ectromelia*, a virus known to infect Kupffer cells of the liver [243]. Albumins containing a variety of carbohydrate residues (e.g., lactosyl, galactosyl, and mannosyl) as terminal groups have also been chemically prepared and used as carriers to selectively deliver antitumor and antiviral drugs to the liver cells [235,237]. The homing of negatively charged albumins to the lymphatic system has recently been proposed as a method of facilitating the distribution of anti-HIV-1 agents [244].

Hormones. Hormones, such as human placental lactogen, human chroionic gonadotropin, epidermal growth factor, and melanotropin, have been suggested as carriers to deliver toxins (e.g., ricin and diphtheria toxin) and antineoplastic agents (e.g., daunomycin) to cancer cells. The rationale is that cancer cells frequently possess receptors for hormones; thus, drugs covalently linked to hormones can be selectively targeted to these cells. Other reasons include: (a) hormones are easy to obtain in a chemically pure form; (b) they are not bound by Fc receptors on macrophages; and (c) they cause no allergic reactions since hormones from different species are structurally similar [245].

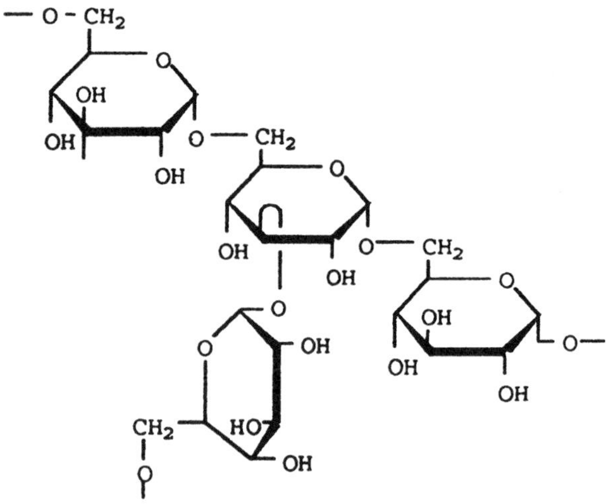

Fig. 18 Structure of dextran.

Dextran and Other Polysaccharides. Dextrans (Fig. 18) are colloidal, hydrophilic, and water-soluble substances produced from sugar by microorganisms of the Lactobacillaceae family or by cell-free systems containing dextran sucrase. Pharmaceutical and commercial dextrans of different molecular weights are produced by controlled hydrolysis and repeated fractionation of native dextran. Dextrans are inert in biological fluids, and do not affect cell viability. Colloidal dextrans of 40,000, 70,000, and 110,000 molecular weight can be used in the prevention of thromboembolic diseases in high-risk surgical patients [246]. The immunogenicity of dextran increases with increasing molecular weight and branching. Dextrans of molecular weight equal to or smaller than 45,000 are completely excreted in the urine within 48 hours following intravenous administration, whereas those with a molecular weight higher than 45,000 remain in the blood for a long period. However, they are eventually cleared by the RES cells. Dextrans are slowly hydrolyzed in vivo into soluble sugars (the major products being isomaltose and isomaltotriose) by dextranase, an enzyme found in the intestinal mucosa and in RES cells [247]. Despite their removal, administration of large doses of dextran can cause a storage problem.

Dextrans have been used as carriers for a variety of drugs and enzymes, including antimicrobial agents (e.g., ampicillin, kanamycin, and tetracycline), cytostatic agents [e.g., mitomycin, methotrexate, bleomycin, daunorubicin, daunomycin, and cytarabine (cytosine-1-β-D-arabinoside)], cardiac drugs (e.g., alprenolol and procainamide), peptides and proteins (e.g., asparaginase, carboxypeptidase α- and β-amylase, and insulin), enzyme inhibitors (e.g., pancreatic trypsin inhibitor), [248] and antineoplastic agents [249]. Drugs or enzymes can be coupled to dextrans either directly, or through a spacer (e.g., γ-aminobutyric acid, ε-aminocaproic acid, and ω-caprylic acid), via activated intermediates produced from reactions with alkali metal periodates, cyanogen bromide, carbodiimide, or chloroformate (see Fig. 16), depending on the nature of the drug and carrier molecules. The direct esterification reaction can be used to link organic acids to dextrans. Drugs coupled to dextran by hydrolyzable covalent linkages are more efficacious than free drugs or drug-dextran conjugates containing nonhydrolyzable covalent linkages. Studies have also revealed that direct substitution of drugs to antibody (4–6 moles of a drug per mole of antibody) causes a significant loss of antibody activity, whereas antibody-dextran conjugates of drugs, with and without a spacer, show increased stability, longer duration of activity, reduced toxicity, and enhanced cell selection activity (drug targeting). The antitumor activity of dextran-mitomycin conjugates against B16 melanoma has been shown to be molecular weight dependent [250]. Modifications of dextran-drug conjugates by an appropriate choice of linkage has permitted the synthesis of a variety of cationic and anionic forms. In vivo studies in mice bearing subcutaneous sarcoma 180 showed that cationic forms clear much more quickly from the bloodstream than anionic forms, accumulating primarily in liver and spleen, with little uptake into tumor tissues. Anionic conjugates with molecular weight ranging between 10,000 and 50,000, on the contrary, show greater tumor accumulation (following intravenous administration) and, thereby, are more effective in the treatment of a subcutaneous tumor. This probably occurs as a result of prolonged residence time of anionic conjugates in the bloodstream. β-Cyclodextrin has also been reported to produce site-directed inclusion complexes with several cytotoxic drugs [251].

Other polysaccharides that have been suggested as potential carriers in drug targeting are chondroitin sulfate, heparin sulfate, dermatin sulfate, hyaluronic acid, and keratin sulfate. All are highly water-soluble, linear polyanions composed of 1:1 mixture of uronic acid and hexosamine (Fig. 19). These are commonly called glycosaminoglycans (GAGs) and are generally biocompatible, nonimmunogenic, and biodegradable. They contain carboxylic and sulfate groups, in addition to primary and secondary hydroxyl groups, and thus provide additional sites for drug attachment. Since polyanions interact with cell membranes, it is proposed that the use of GAGs may facilitate transport to drugs into the interior of cells [252]. *O*-Palmitoylamylopectin, another polysaccharide, has been used to coat liposomes to alter their distribution in vivo.

Synthetic Polymers. Synthetic polymers are versatile and offer promise for both targeting and extracellular-intracellular drug delivery. Of the many soluble synthetic polymers known, the poly(amino acids) [poly(L-lysine), poly(L-aspartic acid), and poly(glutamic acid)], poly(hydroxypropylmethacrylamide) copolymers (polyHPMA), and maleic anhydride copolymers have been investigated extensively, particularly in the treatment of cancers. A brief discussion of these materials is presented.

POLY(AMINO ACIDS). Both anionic [e.g., poly(L-aspartic acid) and poly(glutamic acid)] and cationic [e.g., poly[L-lysine)] poly(amino acids) have been suggested as potential drug carriers. Poly(L-lysine) is a homopolymer cosisting of repeating units of L-lysine. It exhibits some affinity for cancer cells and possesses antimicrobial and antiviral properties. It also shows some activity against murine tumors. The covalently linked methotrexate conjugate of poly(L-lysine), prepared by the carbodiimide method, penetrated Chinese hamster ovary cells faster, and was more effective, than free durg [253]. A poly(D-lysine)–methotrexate conjugate, by contrast, had no effect, because it is resistant to degradation by intracellular enzymes. In vitro growth inhibition studies revealed that the poly(L-lysine)–methotrexate conjugate was more effective against five cell lines of human solid tumors than five cell lines of lymphocytes [254].

Poly(amino acids) can be covalently linked to daunorubicin by a nucleophilic susbstitution reaction of the 14-bromo derivative of the drug [255]. This method avoids alteration or modification of the amino sugar moiety of the drug. When compared with free drug, the poly(L-asparitic acid)–daunorubicin conjugate prepared by this method was less toxic to HeLa cells in vitro, but more effective against P388 leukemia, Gross leukemia, and MS-2 sarcoma in vivo. The corresponding conjugate of poly(L-lysine) showed markedly reduced activity overall. This was attributed to the more stable amide linkage in the poly(L-lysine) conjugate compared with that of the poly(L-aspartic acid) conjugate [255].

Hurwitz et al. [256] used a hydrazide derivative of poly(glutamic acid) as a carrier for daunamycin. This was less toxic than free drug against mouse lymphoma in vitro, but it was as effective, or more effective, against the same lymphoma in vivo.

Poly(L-lysine) has also been suggested as a carrier for pepstatin, a specific inhibitor of the lysosomal proteinase cathepsin D, responsible for causing muscle-wasting diseases, such as muscular dystrophy [257].

POLY(HYDROXYPROPYLMETHACRYLAMIDE) COPOLYMER. Poly(hydroxypropylmethacrylamide) copolymer (polyHPMA) (Fig. 20A) is a nonbiodegradable, nonimmunogenic, biocompatible polymer. It has been extensively investigated as a plasma expander and as a carrier for a variety of anthracycline antibiotic–antitumor agents (e.g., doxorubicin and daunorubicin), alkylating agents (e.g., sarcolysin and melphalan), chlorin e_6 (phytochlorin), and mesalamine (5-aminosalicylic acid) [258]. It is cleared from the circulation, depending on the molecular weight. The molecular weight threshold permitting renal excretion was 45,000. In general, the lower the molecular weight, the faster the clearance rate. Larger polymers are more susceptible to capture by RES cells and have little chance of passing the basement membrane and other natural barriers.

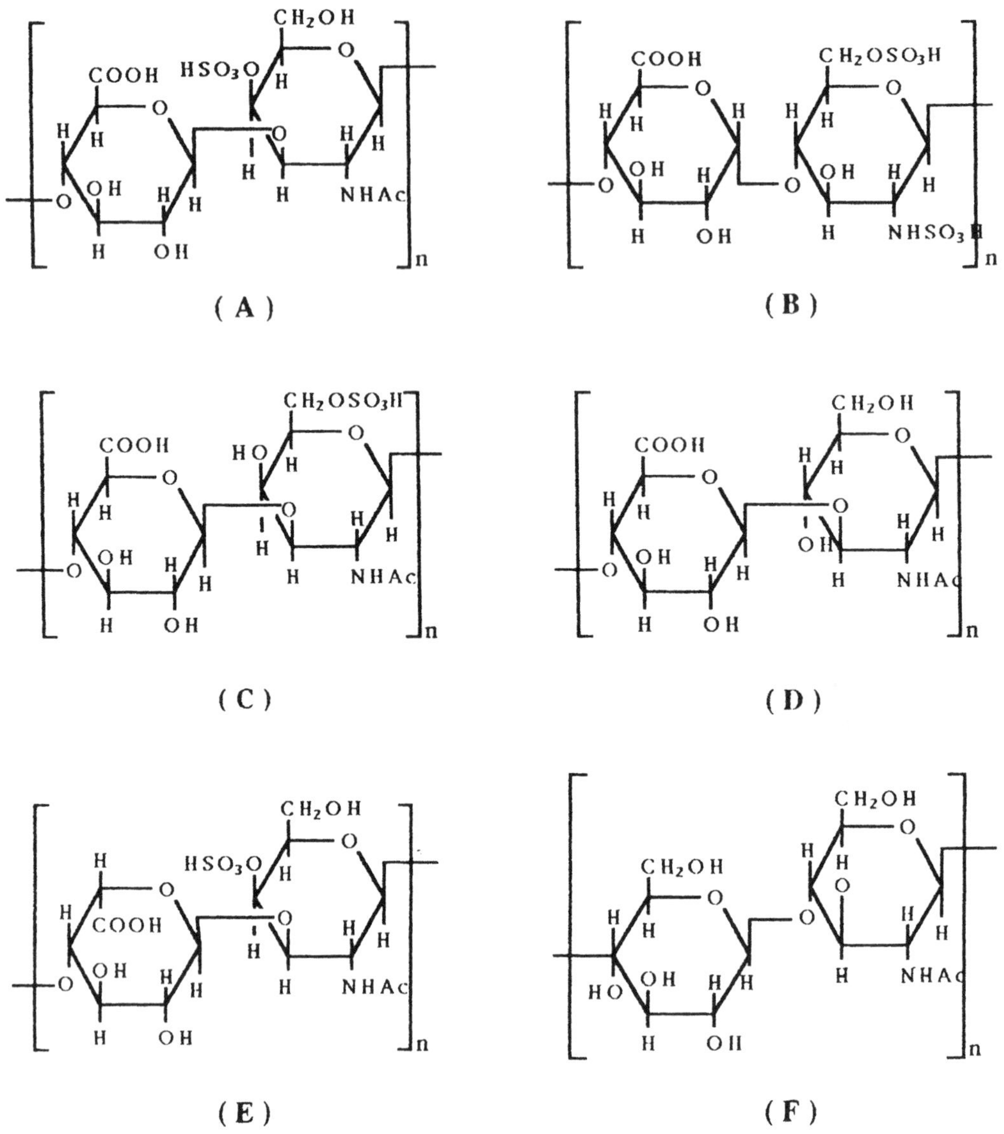

Fig. 19 Structures of glycosaminoglycans: (A) chondroitin-4-sulfate; (B) heparin sulfate; (C) dermatin sulfate; (D) hyaluronic acid; (E) chondroitin-6-sulfate; (F) keratin sulfate.

PolyHPMA has been linked to drugs by oligopeptidyl linkages (e.g., Gly-Phe-Leu-Gly) [207]. These degrade under the influence of lysosomal enzymes, causing the release of free drug. The digestibility of oligopeptides by lysosomal enzymes depends on the length and detailed structure of the oligopeptide sequence and follows the order: tetrapeptide > tripeptide > dipeptide. It is important that the oligopeptide linkage used to attach a drug to the polymer not be susceptible to degradation during transit in the bloodstream. The Gly-Phe-Leu-Gly tetrapeptide sequence fulfills this and the intralysosomal digestibility criteria.

Targeting to a specific cell has been accomplished by attaching appropriate cell receptor–specific ligands to polyHPMA. Thus, polyHPMA derivatized with glycylglycylgalactosamine (Gly-Gly-GalNH$_2$), when injected into the bloodstream of rats, was very efficiently removed by the liver parenchmal cells and taken into the lysosomes. Only 5–10% hydroxypropyl residues need to be substituted to achieve maximal targeting [208]. Studies have shown that the presence of low levels of side chains decreases the pinocytic uptake, which, in turn, causes targeting residues to achieve maximum targeting. More complex targeting

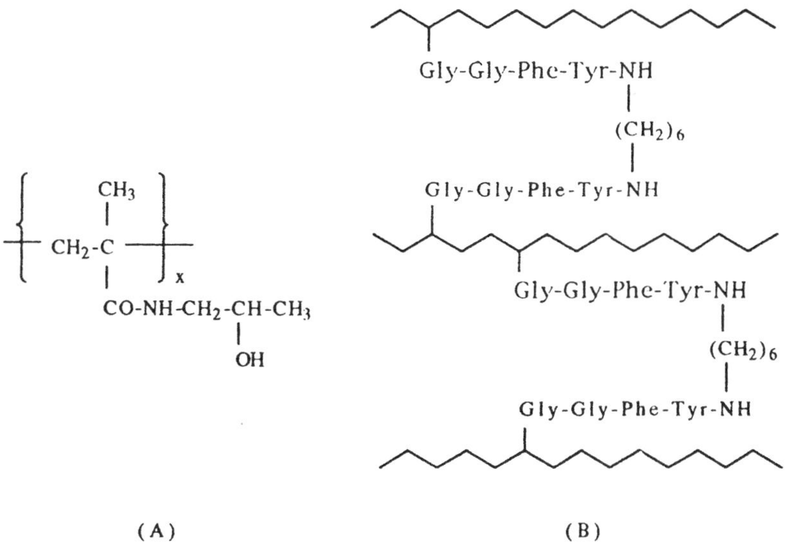

(A) (B)

Fig. 20 (A) Structure of polyHMPA copolymer and (B) schematic representation of cross-linked polyHMPA copolymer.

systems, such as the use of melanocyte-stimulating hormone [259] and antibodies [80], have also been investigated.

To obviate the accumulation of polyHPMA in the body (polyHPMA copolymers are not biodegradable), low molecular weight fractions (small enough to pass through the glomerular filtrate) of polyHPMA have been cross-linked by diamine-containing oligopeptidyl sequences and used as drug carriers (see Fig. 20B) [207]. Similar to non–cross-linked polyHPMA, these are also cleared from the circulation in a molecular weight–dependent fashion. In vivo studies in rats revealed the appearance of lower molecular weight polymer chains in the urine 8–24 hours after intravenous administration.

Recently, polyHPMA copolymers containing galactosamine–chlorin e_6 (phytochlorin) and anti-Thy 1.2 antibody–chlorin e_6 have been developed as targetable polymeric photoactivable drugs [260]. When compared with polyHPMA–chlorine e_6, the polyHPMA–galactosamine–chlorin e_6 conjugate was more active against human hepatoma cell line (PLC/PRF/5; Alexander cells) in vitro. The polyHPMA–anti-Thy 1.2 antibody–chlorin e_6 conjugate was prepared in two ways—one was linked by N^{ϵ}-amino groups of lysine residues, and the other by oxidized carbohydrate. Both showed higher activity toward mouse splenocytes than the nontargeted conjugate. The polyHPMA–anti-Thy 1.2 antibody–chlorin e_6 conjugate linked by oxidized carbohydrate was the most active in its photodynamic effect on the viability of splenocytes and the suppression of the primary antibody response of mouse splenocytes toward sheep red blood cells in vitro.

MALEIC ANHYDRIDE COPOLYMERS. Examples of this class of drug carriers include styrene–maleic anhydride (SMA) and divinyl ether–maleic anhydride (DIVEMA) copolymers (Fig. 21). Both SMA and DIVEMA have been suggested as potential carriers for neocarzinostatin (NCS), a naturally occurring antitumor antibiotic, and other antitumor agents. NCS is more potent than many conventional antitumor drugs (e.g., mitomycin and doxorubicin). It is composed of a protein (molecular weight 12,000) and a low molecular weight cytotoxic chromophore. Following release from the protein, the chromophore enters neighboring cells and interacts with the DNA and, eventually, kills the cells. Despite its higher antitumor activity, NCS cannot be used clinically because (a) it is nonspecific in its action, and (b) it is rapidly cleared ($t_{1/2} = 1.8$ min) by urinary excretion following intravenous administration.

Maeda et al. [261] synthesized styrene–maleic anhydride conjugates of NCS by reacting the two amino groups (one belonging to Ala-1 and the other to Lys-20 residues) on NCS, with the anhydride group of SMA at a pH of 8.5 for 10–12 hours. Compared with free NCS, the SMA-NCS conjugate was retained longer in the blood circulation ($t_{1/2} = 18$ min in mice) and, consequently, promoted accumulation of NCS in peripheral tumor tissues (by up to eightfold in a solid

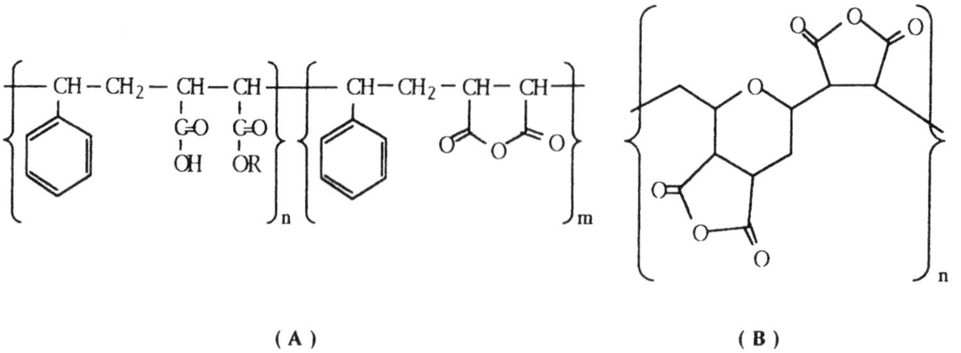

(A) (B)

Fig. 21 Structures of (A) SMA-NCS and (B) DIVEMA.

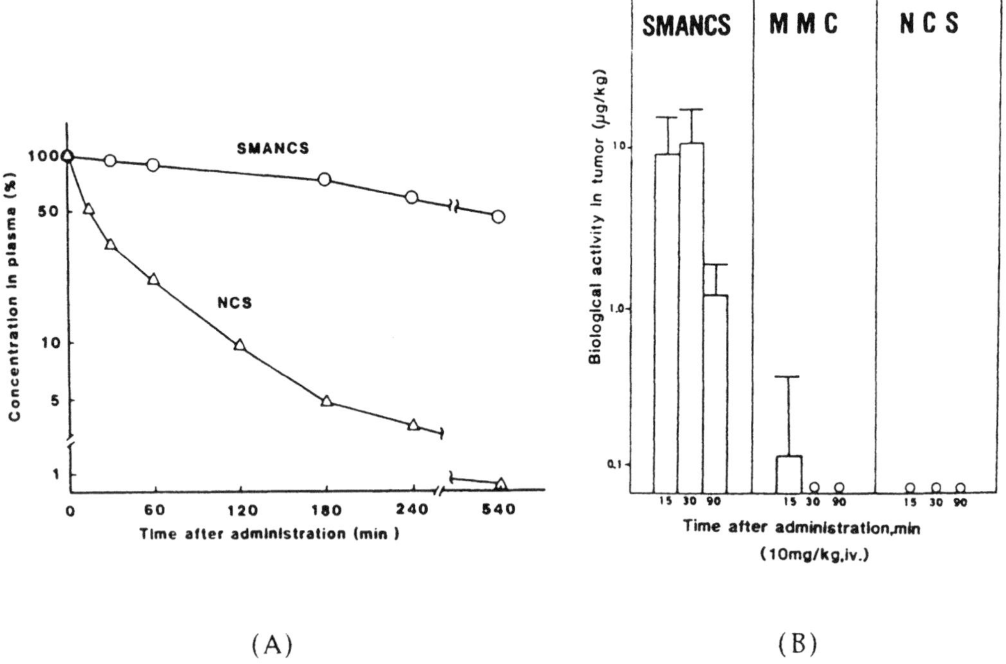

Fig. 22 (A) Plasma concentration of SMA-NCS and NCS in human after an intravenous bolus injection. (B) Intratumor concentration of SMA-NCS, NCS, and mitomycin (MMC). SMA-NCS exhibits a much higher and more prolonged tumor concentration than MMC and NCS. All drugs were given as an intravenous bolus at 10 mg/kg to rabbits bearing VX-2 tumor in the liver (assayed by antibacterial activity). (From Ref. 265.)

sarcoma 180) (Fig. 22). The SMA-NCS conjugate was also effective against lymphatic metastases [261]. Various vasoactive agents can be used to modulate the rates of extravasation and, consequently, penetration of SMA-NCS in tumor tissue [262]. A multi-instutional Phase II clinical trial of SMA-NCS, formulated in an oily lipid contrast medium, Lipiodol (an ethyl ester of iodinated poppyseed oil, 37% w/w in iodine content, used clinically as a lymphographic agent) was completed in Japan in 1990. The tumor/blood ratio was greater than 2500 following intra-arterial administration of this formulation. The results of the first pilot study (total number of patients 44) revealed detectable tumor shrinkage in 95% of the cases [263]. Of 21 patients, 9 showed a 40–99% reduction in tumor mass within 1–5 months, and extensive necrosis was seen in biopsy specimens. Mean survival rate was greater than 18 months for the treated patients, compared with 3.7 months for the controls. In a parallel study, 24 patients with tumors other than hepatoma were included, and SMA-NCS was administered by various arterial routes [264]. The results showed a regression of the tumors in 6 of 9 patients, with metastatic liver cancer, 4 of 4 with adenocarcinoma of the lung, and 1 of 3 patients with unresectable gallbladder tumors.

SMA-NCS can also be used to activate macrophages, natural cells, and T cells and to induce interferon-gamma production [265].

A DIVEMA-NCS conjugate, on the contrary, exhibited cytotoxic activity (on a molar basis) in vitro against eight cell lines and bone marrow cells similar to that observed with free NCS [266]. In vivo toxicity data indicated about a 1.7-fold higher LD_{50} value for the conjugate than for NCS. Studies also revealed a lower distribution of the conjugate than that for NCS in bone marrow and spleen cells and, to some extent, in other organs. The biological activity of DIVEMA-NCS in plasma was about 2.2 times higher than that of NCS. Because of reduced acute toxicity, DIVEMA-NCS showed a 10 times higher antitumor activity than NCS (after 5 mm of injection) at a high dose. At lower doses, there was no difference in the antitumor activities of DIVEMA-NCS and free NCS. The relatively low antitumor activity of DIVEMA-NCS, compared with SMA-NCS, has been attributed to its rapid clearance from the circulation [266].

The DIVEMA copolymer has also been covalently linked to methotrexate [267]. This polymer spontaneously released methotrexate from the polymer backbone by hydrolysis. The DIVEMA-methotrexate conjugate (molecular weight 22,000) was more effective against L1210 leukemia and Lewis lung carcinoma at optimal equivalent doses than either DIVEMA or NCS alone or the combination of DIVEMA and NCS. As such, DIVEMA also shows various biological properties. It is a well-known interferon inducer and shows activity against several solid tumors and virus. It also possesses antibacterial, antifungal, anticoagulant, and anti-inflammatory properties and is capable of stimulating macrophage activation. Biological studies have revealed that the toxicity of DIVEMA increases with an increase in its molecular weight. Low molecular weight pyrans stimulate phagocytosis, whereas high molecular weight copolymers decrease the rate of uptake. The inhibition of polymer metabolism also increases with an increase in the molecular weight [268].

VI. TARGETING IN THE GASTROINTESTINAL TRACT AND TO OTHER MUCOSAL SURFACES

The alimentary canal has been, and continues to be, the preferred route for drug administration for systemic drug action. Thus, there is a growing interest in developing oral dosage forms that can be targeted in the GI tract to either (a) exert a therapeutic effect at a specific site in the GI tract (see Ref. 26 for diseases of the GI tract) or (b) allow systemic absorption of drugs or prodrugs utilizing a specific region of the alimentary canal, without being affected by the GI fluid, pH fluctuations, enzymes, and microflora, while traveling along the GI tract. The various anatomical, physiological, physicochemical, and biochemical features of various regions of the alimentary canal including intestinal transporters that influence drug targeting, and possible formulation approaches that can be used, have been reviewed by Ritschel [27] and Oh et al. [269].

Depending on the site in the GI tract where drug release is sought, a variety of approaches can be used. Bioadhesive polymers are used to prepare adhesive tablets and films for use in the buccal cavity and other regions of the alimentary canal [270]. These polymers adhere to biological tissue for an extended period, thereby providing increased local therapeutic effect or prolonged maintenance of therapeutic amounts of drug in the blood. Examples of bioadhesive polymers commonly used include hydroxypropylcellulose, polyacrylic acid (Carbopol), and sodium carboxymethylcellulose. Enteric polymers (e.g., cellulose acetate phthalate, hydroxypropylcellulose acetate phthalate, polyvinyl acetate phthalate, methacrylate–methacrylic acid copolymers, styrol maleic acid copolymers, and others), which remain insoluble in the stomach, but dissolve at higher pH of the intestine, are used to deliver drugs to the small intestine. Enteric coating also prevents drugs from degradation by gastric fluid and enzymes and protects the gastric mucosa from irritating properties of certain drugs. Recently, Klokkers-Bethke and Fisher [271] developed a multiple-unit drug-delivery system to target the lower parts of the intestine, one formulation releasing the drug in the lower part of the small bowel and the second targeting release in the colon. Drug delivery to the stomach can be achieved using hydrodynamically balanced (floating) dosage forms. Because of lower bulk density, such dosage forms stay buoyant in the stomach, thereby resisting gastric emptying. Drug-delivery systems that contain inflatable chambers (these become gas-filled at body temperature) or solids (e.g., carbonates and bicarbonates) that form gas when in contact with gastric fluid also stay buoyant and are used to target drugs for release in the stomach. A variety of techniques have been advocated for drug targeting to the small intestine, including the use of polysaccharide swellable hydrogels [272].

The successful delivery of drugs to the colon, either for local treatment, such as ulcerative colitis and irritable bowel syndrome, or for the systemic absorption of drugs that are not well absorbed from the other regions of the GI tract, can be achieved either by entrapment within or by coating drugs with azopolymers [273–275]. These polymers form a network or an impermeable film that is resistant to proteolytic digestion in the stomach and small intestine. In the colon, the azopolymer reduces into its corresponding amines by the indigenous microflora; consequently, the film breaks, causing the release of free drug. Targeting in the colon may be of significance to polypeptide delivery, because there are no digestive enzymes in the colon, and the duration of residence is longer in the colon than in other regions of the GI tract (see Table 3). Targeting in the colon is also feasible by time-pulsatile systems. Rectal delivery, depending on the position of the dosage form in the rectum, can be used to target either the systemic circulation or the liver. For systemic targeting, the dosage form should be placed and located directly behind the internal rectal sphincter, whereas targeting to the liver requires the dosage form to be placed in the ampulla recti (about 12–15 cm up the rectum).

Targeting to esophageal mucosa and other regions of the GI tract can also be achieved using bioadhesive magnetic granules [276]. The various parameters that influence targeting to a specific site using bioadhesive magnetic granules include the composition of the formulation, the amount of the magnetic material in the granules, and the magnitude of the magnetic field. This approach can be used for local chemotherapy of esophageal cancer and for other diseases in the alimentary canal [276].

Although most drugs are absorbed from the intestine by the blood capillary network in the villi, they can also be taken up by the lymphatic system (an integral and necessary part of the vascular system, the function of which is to collect extra tissue fluid and return it to the vascular compartment), particularly by M cells that reside in the Peyer's patch regions of the intestine. Peyer's patches have also been implicated in the regulation of the secretory immune response. Wachsmann et al. [277] reported that an antigenic material encapsulated within a liposome, when administered perorally, is taken up by these M cells and exhibited better saliva and serum IgA (primary and secondary) immune response than from a simple solution of antigen (Fig. 23). In an attempt to demonstrate the use of microparticles as potential oral immunological adjuvants, O'Hagan et al. entrapped ovalbumin, a model, but poor, immunogen, into polyacrylamide (2.55 μm diameter) [278] poly(butyl-2-cyanoacrylate)(3 μm and 100 nm) [279], and poly(D, L-lactide-co-glycolide [280–282] particles, and found significantly elevated secretory IgA and systemic lgG antibody responses in rats, compared with soluble antigen, following oral administration. Woodley recently reviewed the use of lectins (naturally occurring proteins) as drug carriers that selectively bind to the surfaces of cells in the intestinal tract [283]. Although additional work is needed, these

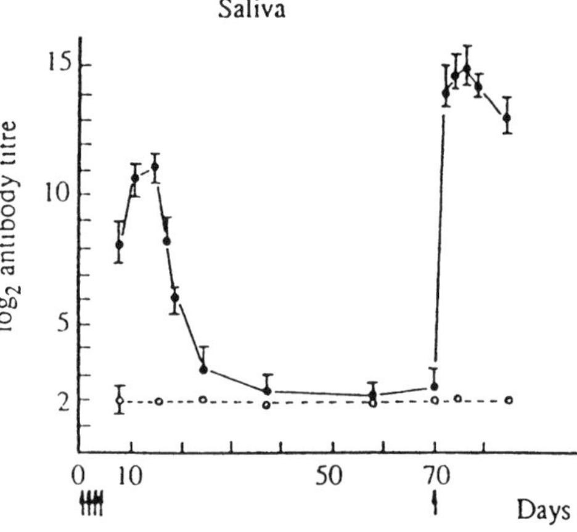

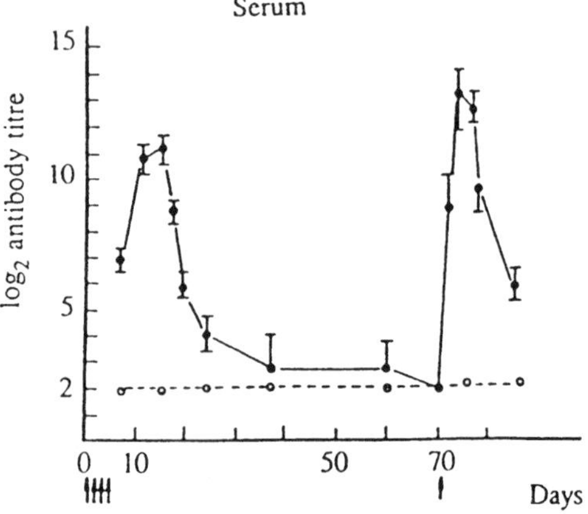

Fig. 23 Saliva and serum IgA (primary and secondary) response following orally administered soluble antigen *Streptococcus mutans* cell wall extract (open circles, soluble antigen; solid circles, liposome-encapsulated material) (phosphatidylcholine, phosphatidic acid, cholesterol). (From Ref. 277).

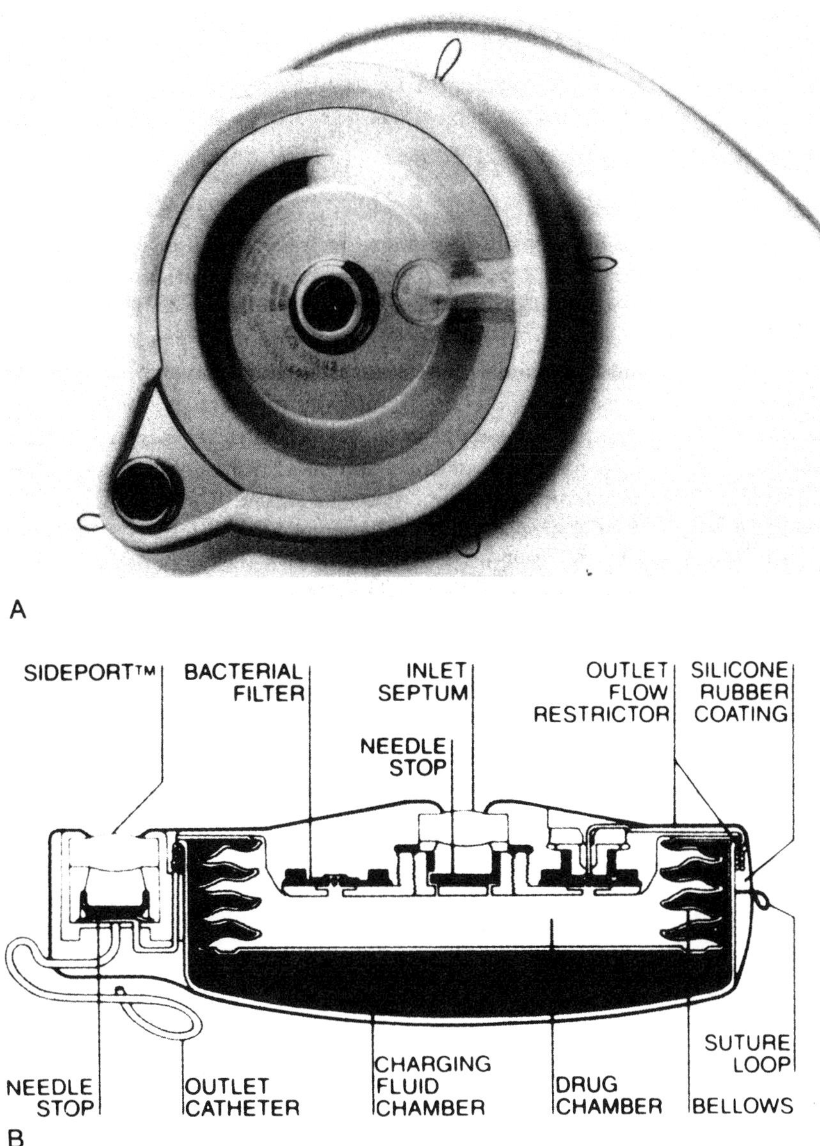

Fig. 24 (A) top view and (B) a cross-sectional illustration of the INFUSAID Model 400 implantable pump. (Courtesy of Infusaid Inc., Norwood, MA.)

studies show that microparticles can be used as potential oral adjuvants for the induction of long-term immune responses.

VII. MECHANICAL PUMPS

The mechanical pump approach employs miniature mechanical devices, such as implantable and portable infusion pumps and percutaneous infusion catheters, to deliver drugs into appro priate blood vessels or to a discrete site in the body. When compared with the conventional drug therapy, these devices offer several advantages: (a) the rate of the drug infusion can be better controlled; (b) a relatively large volume of relatively dilute drug solutions can be administered; (c) the drug dose can be readily changed, stopped, or alternated with other drugs, or a placebo, when required; and (d) the drug can be directed into a vascular site or body cavity using the drug-delivery cannula (e.g., hepatic arterial chemotherapy, intrathecal morphine infusion for pain control, intraventricular and intra-articular treatment of central nervous system tumors, intravenous infusions of heparin in thrombotic disorders, and intravenous infusions of insulin in type II diabetes). Several excellent review articles describing design and applications of infusion and implantable pumps in drug therapy, particularly insulin therapy, have been published [284–290]. A diagram of the INFUSAID Model 400 implantable Pump produced by infusaid Inc (Norwood, MA) is shown in Fig. 24. Drugs such as floxuridine, (5-fluorodexyuridine) [291] and zidovudine (3′-azido-2′3′-dideoxythymidine, AZT) [291] have also been delivered using an implantable pump.

VIII. SUMMARY

The field of targeted drug delivery has grown rapidly in the last three decades. Several delivery systems based on passive, active, and physical targeting strategies have been explored. the two approaches that have received the most attention include prodrugs and polymer-macromolecule–carried drug-delivery systems. Prodrugs are pharmacologically inert forms of the active drug that must be converted to their active form (i.e., parent drug) by either a chemical or an enzymatic reaction at the site of action. As our understanding of active sites becomes clearer, this approach should lead to the production of drugs that have a targeting moiety built into the structure. Currently, several examples exist that show promise for site-specific drug delivery.

Polymer-macromolecule–carried drug-delivery systems are of two types: particulate and soluble macromolecular. Particulate drug-delivery systems, owing to their rapid clearance from the central circulation by the RES system, offer the greatest promise for use in combating diseases (e.g., tumors) of the RES system. Several of these systems (e.g., glucocerebroside glucosidase–encapsulated liposomes for the treatment of type I Gaucher's disease) are currently undergoing clinical trials. Various strategies to avoid uptake of particles by the RES have also been developed. This may provide opportunities to deliver drugs to cellular targets within the vasculature and to sites other than the RES.

Soluble macromolecular (natural and synthetic) systems are frequently used as lysosomotropic agents. Because of their ability to extravasate, they have been extensively explored for treating cancer and other remotely located diseases. The recent advent of the hybridoma technology and the progress made in identifying target-specific antibodies and ligands that enable ready target selectivity have provided additional impetus to design and develop site-specific delivery systems. Several of these systems have been proved very effective in animals, and it remains to be seen how these results will be translated in clinical trials; (e.g., SAMCNS in Japan and polyHMPA copolymer–anthracycline conjugates in the United Kingdom have been completed or are in progress).

As our understanding of the drug action and pathogenesis of various diseases becomes clearer, more rational approaches to the design of therapeutic systems with functions that selectively target the disease, or deliver the drug to its intended site of action, with no or with reduced side effects, will emerge. The advent of the control of gene expression has already provided several new classes of biopharmaceuticals, including peptidergic mediators and sequence-specific oligonucleotides, and it is important that they be delivered to their sites of action exclusively.

REFERENCES

1. P. Ehrlich, John Wiley & Sons, London, 1906. Chap. 36.
2. E. Tomlinson, J. Pharm. Pharmacol., 44 (Suppl. 1), 147 (1992).
3. E. Tomlinson, Int. J. Pharm. Technol. Prod. Manuf., 4, 49 (1983).
4. K. J. Widder, A. E. Senyei, and D. F. Ranney, Adv. Pharmacol. Chemother., 16, 213 (1979).
5. E. Tomlinson, (Patho)physiology and the temporal and spatial aspects of drug delivery, in *Site-Specific Drug Delivery. Cell Biology, Medical, and Pharmaceutical Aspects* (E. Tomlinson and S. S. Davis, eds.), John Wiley & Sons. Chichester, 1986, p. 1.
6. C. J. Vanoss, C. F. Gillman, P. M. Bronson, and J. R. Border, Immunol. Commun., 3, 329 (1974).
7. S. S. Davis, S. J. Douglas, L. Illum, P. D. E. Jones, E. Mak, and R. H. Muller, Targeting of colloidal carriers and the role of surface properties, in *Targeting of Drugs with Synthetic Systems* (G. Gregoriadis, J. Senior, and G. Poste, eds.). Plenum Press, New York, 1986, p. 123.
8. L. Illum, S. S. Davis, and P. D. E. Jones, Polym. Preprints, 27, 25 (1986).
9. L. Illum and S. S. Davis, Life Sci., 40, 1553 (1987).
10. K. Saito, J. Ando, M. Yoshida, M. Haga, and Y. Kato. Chem. Pharm. Bull., 36, 4187 (1988).
11. S. M. Moghimi, C. J. Porter, I. S. Muir, L. Illum, and S. S. Davis, Biochem. Biophys. Res. Commun., 177, 861 (1991).
12. M. J. Hsu and R. L. Juliano, Biochim. Biophys. Acta, 720, 411 (1982).
13. C. R. Hopkins, Site-specific drug delivery—cellular opportunities and challenges, in *Site-Specific Drug Delivery, Cell Biology, Medical and Pharmaceutical Aspects* (E. Tomlinson and S. S. Davis, eds.), John Wiley & Sons, Chichester, 1986, p. 27.

14. R. Duncan, H. C. Cable, F. Rypacek, J. Drobnik, and J. B. Lloyd, Biochem. Soc. Trans., 12, 1064 (1984).
15. R. Duncan, H. C. Cable, P. Rejmanove, and J. Kopecek, Biochim. Biophys. Acta, 799, 1 (1984).
16. T. Kooistra, A. Duursma, J. M. W. Bouma, and M. Gruber, Biochim. Biophys. Acta, 631, 439 (1980).
17. A. S. Harris, Biopharmaceutical aspects of the intranasal administration of peptides, in *Delivery Systems for Peptides* (S. S. Davis, L. Illum, and E. Tomlinson, eds.), Plenum Press, New York, 1986, p. 191.
18. L. Illum, N. F. Farraj, H. Critichley, and S. S. Davis, Int. J. Pharm., 46, 261 (1988).
19. W. A. J. J. Hermans, M. J. M. Deurloo, S. G. Romeyn, J. C. Verhoef, and F. W. H. M. Merkus, Pharm. Res., 7, 500 (1990).
20. A. N. Fisher, N. F. Farraj, D. T. O'Hagan, I. Jabbal-Gill, B. R. Johansen, S. S. Davis, and L. Illum, Int. J. Pharm., 74, 147 (1991).
21. A. Pusztai, Adv. Drug Deliv. Rev., 3, 215 (1989).
22. K. Matsuno, T. Schaffner, H. A. Gerbel, C. Ruchti, M. W. Hess, and H. Cottier, J. Reticuloendothel. Soc., 33, 263 (1983).
23. C. Damge, M. Aprahamian, G. Balboin, A. Hoetzel, V. Andrieu, and J. P. Devissaguet, Int. J. Pharm., 36, 121 (1987).
24. B. Tomlinson, Adv. Drug Deliv. Rev., 1, 87 (1987).
25. W. A. Ritschel, Methods Find. Exp. Clin. Pharmacol., 13, 205 (1991).
26. J. B. Dressman. P. Bas, W. A. Ritschel, D. R. Friend, A. Rubinstein, and B. Zhiv, J. Pharm. Sci., 82, 857 (1993).
27. W. A. Ritschel, Method. Find. Exp. Clin. Pharmacol., 13, 313 (1991).
28. V. H. L. Lee and A. Yamamoto, Adv. Drug Deliv. Rev., 4, 171 (1990).
29. S. Muranishi, Crit. Rev. Ther. Drug Carrier Syst., 7, 1 (1990).
30. S. S. Davis, J. Pharm. Pharmacol., 44 (Suppl. 1), 186 (1992).
31. H. P. Merkle, R. Anders, J. Sandow, and W. Schurr, Drug delivery of peptides: The buccal route, in *Delivery Systems for Peptide Drugs* (S. S. Davis, L. Illum, and E. Tomlinson, cds.), Plenum Press, New York, 1986, p. 159.
32. W. A. Ritschel, G. B. Ritschel, B. E. C. Ritschel, and P. W. Lucker, Methods Find. Exp. Clin. Pharmacol., 10, 645 (1988).
33. J. L. Richardson, P. S. Minhans, N. W. Thomas, and L. Illum, Int. J. Pharm., 16, 29 (1989).
34. S. S. Muranishi, K. Takada, H. Yoshikawa, and M. Murakami, Enhanced absorption and lymphatic transport of macromolecules via the rectal route, in *Delivery Systems for Peptide Drugs* (S. S. Davis, L. Illum, and E. Tomlinson, eds.), Plenum Press, New York, 1986, p. 177.
35. S. S. Davis and L. Illum, Colloidal delivery systems—opportunity and challenges, in *Site-Specific Drug Delivery: Cell Biology, Medical and Pharmaceutical Aspects* (E. Tomlinson and S. S. Davis, eds.), John Wiley & Sons, Chichester, 1986, p. 93.
36. W. J. Joyner and D. F. Kern, Adv. Drug Deliv. Rev., 4, 319 (1990).
37. K. Patrak and P. Goddard, Adv. Drug Deliv. Rev., 3, 191 (1989).
38. L. W. Seymour, Crit. Rev. Ther. Drug Carrier Syst., 19, 135 (1992).
39. D. F. Kern and J. A. Swanson, FASEB J., 3, A1390 (1989).
40. G. J. Arturson and K. Granath, Clin. Chim. Acta, 37, 309 (1972).
41. A. E. Taylor and D. N. Granger, Exchange of macromolecules across the microcirculation, in *Handbook of Physiology*, 6, *Microcirculation*, Part 1 (E. M. Renkin and C. C. Michel, eds.), Waverly Press, Baltimore, 1984, p. 467.
42. L. Ghitescu, A. Fixman, M. Simionescu, and N. Simionescu, J. Cell. Biol., 102, 1304 (1986).
43. J. Drobnik and F. Rypacek, Adv. Polym. Sci., 57, 2 (1984).
44. J. M. Yoffey and F. C. Courtice, *Lymphatics, Lymph and the Lymphomyeloid Complex*, Academic Press, London, 1970.
45. J. G. Hall, The lymphatic system in drug targeting: An overview, in *Targeting of Drugs. Anatomical and Physiological Considerations* (G. Gregoriadis and G. Poste, eds.), Plenum Press, New York, 1985, p. 15.
46. A. Boddy and L. Aarons, Adv. Drug Deliv. Rev., 3, 155 (1989).
47. A. Boddy, L. Aarons, and K. Petrak, Pharm. Res., 6, 367 (1989).
48. G. Levy, Pharm. Res., 4, 3 (1987).
49. P. K. Gupta and C. T. Hung, Int. J. Pharm., 56, 217 (1989).
50. R. E. Notari, Prodrugs kinetics: Theory and practice, in *Optimization of Drug Delivery* (H. Bundgaard, A. B. Hansen, and H. Koford, eds.), Munksgaard, Copenhagan, 1982, p. 117.
51. V. J. Stella and K. J. Himmelstein, J. Med. Chem., 23, 1275 (1980).
52. V. J. Stella and K. J. Himmelstein, Critique of prodrugs and site-specific drug delivery, in *Optimization of Drug Delivery, Alfred Benzon Symposium 17* (H. Bundsgaard, A. B. Hansen, and H. Kofod, eds.), Munksgaard, Copenhagen, 1982, p. 134.
53. C. R. Gardner and J. Alexander, Prodrug approaches to drug targeting: past accomplishments and future potential, in *Drug Targeting* (P. Buri and A. Gumma, eds.), Elsevier Science Publishers, Amsterdam, 1985, p. 145.
54. V. J. Stella, Prodrugs: An overview and definition, in *Prodrugs in Novel Drug Delivery Systems* (T. Higuchi and V. Stella, eds.), American Chemical Society, Washington, DC, 1975, p. 1.
55. E. B. Roche, ed., *Design of Biopharmaceutical Properties Through Prodrugs and Analogs*, American Pharmaceutical Association, Washington, DC, 1977.

56. G. C. Cotzias, M. H. VanWoert, and L. M. Schiffer, N. Engl. J. Med., 276, 374 (1967).
57. A. Hussain and J. E. Truelove, J. Pharm. Sci., 65, 1510 (1976).
58. S. Wilk, H. Mizoguchi, and M. Orlowski, J. Pharmacol. Exp. Ther., 206, 227 (1978).
59. D. R. Friend and G. W. Chang, J. Med. Chem., 28, 51 (1985).
60. V. J. Stella, T. J. Mikkelson, and J. D. Pipkin, Prodrugs: The control of drug delivery via bioreversible chemical modification, in *Drug Delivery Systems: Characteristics and Biomedical Applications* (R. L. Juliano, ed.), Oxford University Press, New York, 1980, p. 112.
61. R. Baurain, M. Masquelier, D. D.-D. Campeneere, and A. Trouet, J. Med. Chem., 23, 1171 (1980).
62. M. Masquelier, R. Baurain, and A. Trouet, J. Med. Chem., 23, 1166 (1980).
63. R K. Chakravarty, P. L. Carl, M. J. Weber, and J. A. Katzenellenbogen, J. Med. Chem., 26, 638 (1983).
64. N. Bodor and J. W. Simpkins, Science, 221, 65 (1983).
65. E. Shek, T. Higuchi, and N. Bodor, J. Med. Chem., 19, 113 (1976).
66. N. Bodor, Methods Enzymol., 112, 381 (1985).
67. N. Bodor and H. H. Farag, J. Med. Chem., 26, 528 (1983).
68. C. K. Chu, V. S. Bhadti, K. J. Doshi, J. T. Etse, J. M. Gallo, F. D. Boudinot, and R. F. Schinazi, J. Med. Chem., 33, 2188 (1990).
69. E. Palomino, Drugs Future, 15, 361 (1990).
70. M. E. Brewster, W. Anderson, and N. Bodor, J. Pharm. Sci., 80, 843 (1991).
71. N. Bodor and H. H. Farag, J. Pharm. Sci., 73, 385 (1984).
72. M. B. Yatvin, T. C. Cree, and I. M. Tegmo-Larsson, Theoretical and practical considerations in preparing liposomes for the purpose of releasing drug in response to changes in temperature and pH, in *Liposome Technology* (G. Gregoriaids, ed.), CRC Press, Boca Raton, FL, 1984, p. 157.
73. L. Illum and S. S. Davis, Passive and active targeting using colloidal carrier systems, in *Drug Targeting* (P. Buri and A. Gumma, eds.), Elsevier Science Publishers, Amsterdam, 1985, p. 65.
74. C. Chiles, L. W. Hedlund, R. J. Kubek, C. Harris, D. C. Sullivan, J. C. Tsai, and C. E. Putman, Invest. Radiol, 21, 618 (1986).
75. C. K. Kim, M. K. Lee, J. H. Han, and B. J. Lee, Int. J. Pharm., 108, 21 (1994).
76. B. M. Altura and T. M. Saba, *Pathophysiology of the Reticuloendothelial System*, Raven Press, New York, 1981.
77. I. Ahmad and T. M. Allen, Cancer Res., 52, 4817 (1992).
78. E. Hurwitz, A. Adler, D. Shouval, J. R. Takahashi, J. R. Wands, and M. Sela, Cancer Immunol. Immunother., 35, 86 (1992).
79. K. Affleck and M. J. Embleton, Br. J. Cancer, 65, 838 (1992).
80. L. W. Seymour, A. Al-Shamkhani, P. A. Flanagan, V. Subr, K. Ulbrich, J. Cassidy, and R. Duncan, Select. Cancer Ther., 7, 59 (1991).
81. G. Gregoriadis and E. D. Neerunjun, Biochem. Biophys. Res. Commun., 65, 537 (1975).
82. R. I. Juliano and D. Stamp, Nature, 261, 235 (1976).
83. G. Gregoriadis, N. Meehan, and M. M. Mah, Biochem. J., 200, 203 (1981).
84. G. Weissman, D. Bloomgarden, R. Kaplan, C. Cohen, S. Hoffstein, T. Collins, A. Gotlieb, and D. Nagle, Proc. Natl. Acad. Sci. USA, 72, 88 (1975).
85. M. R. Kaplan, B. Calef, T. Bercovivi, and C. Gitler, Biochim. Biophys. Acta, 728, 112 (1983).
86. K. J. Widder and A. E. Senyei, Magnetic microsphere: A vehicle for selective targeting of organs, in *Methods of Drug Delivery* (G. M. Ihler, ed.), Pergamon Press, New York, 1986, p. 39.
87. H. Sezaki, M. Hashida, and S. Muranishi, Gelatin microspheres as carriers for antineoplastic agents, in *Optimization of Drug Delivery* (H. Bundgaard, A. B. Hansen, and H. Kofod, eds.), Munksgaard, Copenhagen, 1982, p. 316.
88. M. B. Yatvin, J. N. Weinstein, W. H. Dennis, and R. Blumenthal, Science, 202, 1290 (1978).
89. M. B. Yatvin, W. Kreutz, B. A. Horowitz, and M. Shinitzky, Science, 210, 1253 (1980).
90. T. Kato, Encapsulated drugs in targeted cancer therapy, in *Controlled Drug Delivery* (S. D. Bruck. ed.), CRC Press, Boca Raton, FL, 1983, p. 189.
91. J. Kreuter and E. Liehl, J. Pharm. Sci., 70, 367 (1981).
92. P. Couvreur, Crit. Rev. Ther. Drug Carrier Syst., 5, 1 (1988).
93. R. Langer, Science, 263, 1600 (1994).
94. C. S. Maia, W. Mehnert, and M. Schafer-Korting, Int. J. Pharm., 196, 165 (2000).
95. M. T. Peracchia, E. Fattal, D. Desmaele, M. Besnard, J. P. Noel, J. M. Gomis, M. Appel, J. d'Angelo, and P. Couvreur, J. Controlled Release, 60, 121 (1999).
96. S. C. Yang, L. F. Lu, Y. Cai, J. B. Zhu, and C. Z. Ynag, J. Controlled Release, 59, 299 (1999).
97. M. Yokoyama and T. Okano, Nippon Rinsho (Jpn. J. Clin. Med.), 56, 3227 (1998).
98. E. Tomlinson and J. J. Burger, Monolithic albumin particles as drug carriers, in *Polymers in Controlled Drug Delivery* (L. Illum and S. S. Davis, eds.), Wright, Bristol, 1987, p. 25.
99. A. F. Yapel, U.S. Patent 4, 147, 747 (1979).
100. E. Edelman, J. Brown, J. Taylor, and R. Langer, J. Biomed. Mater. Res., 21, 339 (1987).
101. M. McCarthy, D. Soong, and E. Edelman, J. Controlled Release, 1, 143 (1984).
102. H. Hsu and R. Langer, J. Biomed. Mater. Res., 19, 445 (1985).

103. J. Kotsr, K. E. Noecker, and R. Langer, J. Biomed. Mater. Res., 19, 935 (1985).
104. P. K. Gupta and C. K. Hung, Int. J. Pharm., 59, 57 (1990).
105. M. N. Ravi Kumar, J. Pharm. Pharmaceu. Sci., 3, 234 (2000).
106. G. Gregoriadis, ed., *Liposome Technology*, Vol. 1–3, CRC Press, Boca Raton, FL, 1984.
107. G. Gregoriadis, ed., *Liposome Technology*, 2nd ed., Vol. 1–3, CRC Press, Boca Ralon. FL, 1993.
108. P. R. C. New, ed., *Liposome—A Practical Approach*, IRL Press, Oxford, 1990.
109. K. Yagi, ed., *Medical Applications of Liposomes*, Japan Scientific Press and Karger, Tokyo and Basel, 1986.
110. K. H. Schmidt. ed., *Liposomes as Drug Carriers*, Georg Thieme Verlag, Stuttgart, 1986.
111. G. Gregoriadis and A. C. Allison, eds., *Liposome in Biological Systems*, John Wiley & Sons, Chichester, 1980.
112. K. Maruyama, A. Mori, S. J. Kennel, M. V. B. Waalkes, G. L. Scherphof, and L. Huang, ACS Symp. Ser., 469, 275 (1990).
113. F. H. Roerdnik, T. Daemen, I. A. J. M. Bakker-Woundenberg, G. Storm, D. J. A. Crommelin, and G. L. Scherphof, Therapeutic utility of liposomes, in *Drug Delivery Systems and Fundamental and Techniques* (P. Johnson and J. G. L. Jones, eds.), Ellis Horwood, Chichester, 1987, p. 67.
114. F. Roerdink, J. Regts, T. Daemen, I. Bakker-Woundenberg, and G. Scherphof, Liposomes as drug carriers to liver macrophages, in *Targeting of Drugs with Synthetic Systems* (G. Gregoriadis. J. Senior, and G. Poste, eds.), Plenum Press, New York, 1985, p. 193.
115. G. Gregoriadis, J. Senior, B. Wolff, and C. Kirby, Fate of liposomes in vivo: Control leading to targeting, in *Receptor-Mediated Targeting of Drugs* (G. Gregoriadis, G. Poste, J. Senior, and A. Trouet, eds.), Plenum Press, New York, 1984, p. 243.
116. G. Lopez-Berestein, R. L. Juliano, K. Mehta, R. Mehta, T. McQueen, and R. L. Hopfer, Liposomes in antimicrobial therapy, in *Targeting of Drugs with Synthetic Systems* (NATO ASI- Series. Series A, Life Sciences; V. 113) (G. Gregoriadis, J. Senior, and G. Poste, eds.), Plenum Press, New York, 1985, p. 193.
117. S. M. Sugarman and R. Peres-Solar, Crit. Rev. Oncol. Hematol., 12, 231 (1992).
118. O. Alpar, Pharm. J., 246, 172 (1991).
119. G. Gregoriadis and A. T. Florence, Cancer Cells, 3, 144 (1991).
120. G. Gregoriadis, J. Antimicrob. Chemother., 28, 39 (1991).
121. J. Liliemark, Eur. J. Surg. Suppl., 561, 49 (1991).
122. F. Sozaka, Jr., Biotechnol. Appl. Biochem., 12, 496 (1990).
123. G. Lopez-Berstein, Antimicrob, Agents Chemother., 31, 675 (1987).
124. V. P. Torchilin, Crit. Rev. Ther. Drug Carrier Syst., 2, 65 (1985).
125. M. J. Hope, M. B. Bally, G. Webb, et al., Biochim. Biophys. Acta, 812, 210 (1985).
126. A. Gabizon, A. Dagan, D. Goren, Y. Barenholz, and Z. Funks, Cancer Res., 42, 4734 (1982).
127. L. D. Mayer, M. B. Bally, M. J. Hope, and P. R. Cullis, Biochim. Biophys. Acta, 816, 294 (1985).
128. V. Weissig, J. Lasch, and G. Gregoriadis, Pharmazie, 46, 56 (1991).
129. J. Senior and G. Gregoriadis, Biochim. Biophys. Acta, 1002, 58 (1989).
130. G. Poste, R. Kirsh, and T. Koestler, eds., *Liposome Technology. Targeted Drug Delivery and Biological Interactions*, Vol. 3, CRC Press, Boca Raton, FL, 1984.
131. P. E. Belchetz, I. P. Braidman, J. C. W. Crawly, and G. Gregoriadis, Lancet, 2, 116 (1977).
132. D. A. Tyrrel, B. E. Ryman, B. R. Keeton, and V. Dubowitz, Br. Med. J., 2, 88 (1976).
133. R. R. C. New, M. L. Chance, S. C. Thomas, and W. Peters, Nature, 272, 55 (1978).
134. C. R. Alving, E. A. Steck, J. W. L. Chapman, V. B. Waits, L. D. Hendricks, J. G. M. Swartz, and W. L. Hanson, Proc. Natl. Acad. Sci. USA, 75, 2959 (1978).
135. C. D. V. Black, G. J. Watson, and R. J. Ward, Trans. R. Soc. Trop. Med. Hyg., 71, 550 (1977).
136. I. A. J. M. Bakker-Woudenberg, A. F. Lokerse, F. H. Roerdnik, D. Regts, and M. F. Michel, J. Infect. Dis., 151, 917 (1985).
137. I. J. Fidler, The generation of tumoricidal activity in macrophages for the treatment of established mestastases, in *Cancer Invasion and Metastasis: Biologic and Therapeutic Aspects* (G. L. Nicolson and L. Milas, eds.) Raven Press, New York, 1984, p. 421.
138. S. Sone, S. Matsura, M. Ogawara, and E. Tsubura, J. Immunol., 132, 2105 (1984).
139. I. J. Fidler, S. Sone, W. E. Fogler, D. Smith. D. G. Graun, L. Tarcsay, R. J. Gister, and A. J. Schroit, J. Biol. Response Mod., 1, 43 (1982).
140. I. J. Fidler, A. Raz, W. E. Fogler, L. C. Hoyler, and G. Poste, Cancer Res. 41, 495 (1981).
141. L. Saiki, S. Sone, W. E. Fogler, E. S. Kleinerman, G. Lopez-Berestein, and I. J. Fidler, Cancer Res., 45, 6188 (1985).
142. L. Saiki and I. J. Fidler, J. Immunol., 135, 684 (1985).
143. S. Sone, P. Tandon, T. Utsugi, and M. Ogawara, Int. J. Cancer, 38, 495 (1986).
144. I. J. Fidler and A. J. Schroit, J. Immunol., 133, 515 (1984).
145. E. Mayhew and Y. Rustum, Biol. Cell, 47, 81 (1983).
146. R. R. C. New, M. L. Chance, and S. Heath, Antimicrob. Agents Chemother., 8, 371 (1981).
147. O. A. Rosenberg, V. Y. Berkreneva, L. V. Loshakova, S. P. Rezvaya, E. F. Davidenkova, and K. P. Hanson, Vopr. Onkol., 29, 56 (1983).

148. S. A. Burkhanov, V. A. Kosykh, V. S. Repin, T. S. Saatov, and V. P. Torchilin, Int. J. Pharm. 46, 31 (1988).
149. J. N. Weinstein, R. L. Magin, R. L. Cysyk, and D. S. Zaharko, Cancer Res., 40, 1388 (1980).
150. J. R. Tacker and R. U. Anderson, J. Urol., 127, 1211 (1982).
151. M. B. Yatvin, H. Muhensipen, W. Porschen, J. N. Weinstein, and L. F. Feinendegen, Cancer Res., 41, 1602 (1981).
152. C. Nicolau, A. L. Pape, P. Soriano, F. Fargette, and M. F. Juhel, Proc. Natl. Acad. Sci. USA, 80, 1068 (1983).
153. J. Szebeni, S. M. Wahl, G. V. Betageri, L. M. Wahl, S. Gartner, M. Popovic, R. J. Parker, C. D. V. Black, and J. N. Weinstein, AIDS Res. Hum. Retroviruses. 6, 791 (1990).
154. N. C. Philips, F. Skamene, and C. Tsoukas, J. AIDS. 4, 959 (1991).
155. M. Babincova, V. Altanerova, M. Lampert, C. Altaner, E. Machova, M. Sramka, and P. Babinec, Z. Naturforsch. C, 55, 278 (2000).
156. H. Pinto-Alphandary, A. Andremont, and P. Couvreur, Int. J. Antimicrob. Agents, 13, 155 (2000).
157. T. Velpandian, S. K. Gupta, Y. K. Gupta, N. R. Biswas, and H. C. Agarwal, J. Microencapsul., 16, 243 (1999).
158. J. A. Rogers and K. E. Anderson, Crit. Rev. Ther. Drug Carrier Syst., 15, 421 (1998).
159. A. J. Baillie, A. T. Florence, L. H. Muirhead, and A. Rogerson, J. Pharm. Pharmacol., 37, 863 (1985).
160. J. N. Israelachvili, S. Marcelja, and R. G. Horn, Q. Rev. Biophys. 13, 121 (1980).
161. C. A. Hunter, T. F. Dolan, G. H. Coombs, and A. J. Baillie. J. Pharm. Pharmacol., 40, 161 (1988).
162. H. Kiwada, H. Nimura, Y. Fujisaki, S. Yamada, and K. Kato, Chem. Pharm. Bull., 33, 753 (1985).
163. L. E. Echegoyen, J. C. Hernandez, A. E. Kaifer, G. W. Gokel, and L. Echegoyen, J. Chem. Soc. Chem. Commun., 863 (1988).
164. A. J. Baillie, Niosomes: A putative drug carrier system, in *Targeting of Drugs. Anatomical and Physiological Considerations* (G. Gregoriadis and G. Poste, eds.), NATO Series. Series A. Life Science, Vol. 155, Plenum Press, New York, 1988, p. 143.
165. M. N. Azmin, A. T. Florence, R. M. Handjani-Vila, J. F. B. Stuart, G. Vanlerberghe, and J. S. Whittaker, J. Pharm. Pharmacol., 3, 237 (1985).
166. M. N. Azmin, A. T. Florence, R. M. Handjani-Vila, J. F. B. Stuart, G. Vanlerberghe, and J. S. Whittaker, J. Microencapsul., 3, 95 (1986).
167. A. Namdeo and N. K. Jain, J. Microencapsul., 16, 731 (1999).
168. A Rogerson, Ph.D. thesis, University of Strathclyde, Glasgow, 1986; A. Rogerson. J. Cummings, and A. T. Florence, J. Microencapsul., 4, 321 (1987); A Rogerson, J. Cummings, N. Willmott, and A. T. Florence, J. Pharm. Pharmacol., 40, 337 (1988); D. J. Kerr, A. Rogerson, G. J. Morrison, A. T. Florence, S. B. Kaye, Br. Jr. Cancer, 58, 432 (1988).
169. A. J. Baillie, G. H. Coombs, T. F. Dolan, and J. Laurie, J. Pharm. Pharmacol., 38, 502 (1986).
170. M. K. Bijsterbosch and T. J. C. V. Berkel, Adv. Drug Deliv. Rev., 5, 231 (1990).
171. S. Eisenberg, J. Lipid Res., 25, 1017 (1984).
172. P. C. D. Smidt and T. J. C. V. Berkel, Crit. Rev. Ther. Drug Carrier Syst., 7, 99 (1990).
173. N. S. Damle, R. H. Seevers, S. W. Schwendner, and R. E. Counsell, J. Pharm. Sci., 72, 898 (1983).
174. M. Samadi-Baboli, G. Favre, E. Blancy, and G. Soula, Eur. J. Cancer Clin. Oncol., 25, 233 (1989).
175. S. Lestavel-Delattre, F. Martin-Nizard, V. Clavey, et al., Cancer Res., 52, 3629 (1992).
176. H. J. M. Kempen, C. Hoes, J. H. V. Boom, H. H. Spanjer, J. D. Lange, A. Langendoen, and T. J. C. V. Berkel, J. Med. Chem., 27, 1306 (1984).
177. J. Y. Scoazec and G. Feldman, Hepatology, 10, 627 (1989).
178. T. Takahashi. Crit. Rev. Ther. Drug Carrier Syst., 2, 245 (1985).
179. K. Ito, K. Kiriyama, T. Watanabe, M. Yamauchi, S. Akiyama, K. Kondou, and H. Takagi, ASAIO Trans., 36, M199 (1990).
180. M. F. Dean, H. Muir, P. F. Benson, L. R. Button, J. R. Batcheolor, and M. Bewica. Nature. 257, 609 (1975).
181. A. J. Matas, D. E. R. Sutherland, M. W. Steffes, R. L. Simmons, and J. S. Najarian, Science, 192, 892 (1976).
182. R. Baum, Chem. Eng. News, 72, 4 (1994).
183. R. Younoszai, R. L. Sorenson, and A. W. Lindal, Diabees, 19 (Suppl.), 406 (1971).
184. U. Spraundel, Res. Exp. Med., 190, 267 (1990).
185. G. M. Ihler and H. C. Tsang, Crit. Rev. Ther. Drug Carrier Syst., 1, 155 (1984).
186. M. Magnani, L. Rossi, M. D'ascenzo, I. Panzani, L. Bigi, and A. Zanella, Biotechnol. Appl. Biochem., 28, 1 (1998).
187. U. Benatti, E. Zocchi, M. Tonetti, et al., Pharmacol. Res., 21 (Suppl. 2), 27 (1989).
188. H. J. Leu, A. Wenner, and M. A. Spycher, VASA, 10, 17 (1981).
189. U. Zimmermann, Disch. Apoth. Zig., 122, 1170 (1982).
190. T. Kitao and K. Hattori, Cancer Res., 40, 1351 (1980).
191. M. M. Billah, J. B. Finean, R. Coleman, and R. H. Mitchell, Biochim. Biophys. Acta. 433, 54 (1976).
192. P. S. Lin, D. F. H. Wallach, R. B. Mikkelsen, and R. Schmidt-Ulrich, Biochim, Biophys. Acta, 401, 73 (1975).
193. A. Krantz, Y. Song, D. DeNagel, C. Hartmann, D. Bridon, J. Drug Target., 7, 113 (1999).
194. L. Gordon and A. J. Milner, Blood platelets as multifunctional cells, in *Platelets in Biology and Pathology*

(J. L. Gordon, cd.), Elsevier/North Holland Biomedical Press, Amsterdam, 1976, p. 3.
195. J. M. Weiss, N. Engl. J. Med., 293, 531 (1975).
196. Y. S. Ahn, J. J. Byrnes, and W. J. Harrington, N. Engl. J. Med., 298, 1101 (1978).
197. Y. S. Ahn, W. J. Harrington, J. J. Byrnes, L. Pall, and J. McCranic, JAMA, 249, 2189 (1983).
198. Y. S. Ahn, W. J. Harrington, J. J. Byrnes, A. S. Collin, M. L. Cayer, J. McCranie, and L. M. Pall, Blood, 58, 134 (1981).
199. N. S. Penney, Y. S. Ahn, and E. C. McKinney, Cancer, 49, 1944 (1982).
200. S. Y. Woo, R. S. Klappenbach, G. M. McCullars, D. M. Kerwin, G. Rowden, and L. F. Sinks. Cancer, 46, 2566 (1986).
201. A. W. Segal, M. L. Thakur, R. N. Arnot, and J. P. Lavender, Lancet, 2, 1056 (1976).
202. M. A. Gainey and I. R. McDougall, Clin. Nucl. Med., 9, 71 (1984).
203. S. Sixou and J. Teissie, Biochem. Biophys. Res. Commun., 186, 860 (1992).
204. G. M. Ihler, R. H. Glew, and F. W. Schnure, Proc. Natl. Acad. Sci. USA, 70, 2663 (1973).
205. U. Zimmermann, J. Vienken, and G. Pilwat. Bioclectrochem. Bioeng., 7, 332 (1980).
206. H. Sezaki and M. Hashida, Crit. Rev. Ther. Drug Carrier Syst., 1, 1 (1984).
207. J. Kopecek and R. Duncan, Poly(*N*-(2-hydroxypropyl)methacrylamide) macromolecules as drug carrier systems, in *Polymers in Controlled Drug Delivery* (L. Illum and S. S. Davis, eds.), Wright, Bristol, 1987, p. 152.
208. J. B. Lloyd, Soluble polymers as targetable drug carriers, in *Drug Delivery Systems. Fundamental and Techniques* (P. Johnson and J. G. Llyod, eds.), Ellis Horwood and VCH Verlagsgesellschaft, Chichester and Weinheim, 1987, p. 95.
209. K. Krishenbaum, R. N. Zuckermann, K. A. Dill, Curr. Opin. Struct. Biol., 9, 530 (1999).
210. D. C. Blakey, Acta Oncol., 31, 91 (1992).
211. K. E. Hellstrom, I. Hellstrom, and G. E. Goodman, Antibodies for drug delivery, in *Controlled Drug Delivery: Fundamental and Applications* (J. R. Robinson and V. H. Lee, eds.), Marcel Dekker, New York, 1987, p. 623.
212. K. Sikora, Monoclonal antibodies and drug targeting in cancer, in *Targeting of Drugs. Anatomical and Physiological Considerations* (G. Gregoriadis and G. Poste, eds.), Plenum Press, New York, 1987, p. 69.
213. V. R. Muzykantov, M. Christofidou-Solomidou, I. Balyasnikova, D. W. Harshaw, L. Schultz, A. B. Fisher, and S. M. Albelda, Proc. Natl. Acad. Sci. USA, 96, 2379 (1999).
214. Y. Arano, Y. Fujioka, H. Akizawa, M. Ono, T. Uehara, K. Wakisaka, M. Nakayama, H. Sakahara, J. Konishi, and H. Saji, Cancer Res., 59, 128 (1999).
215. A. Tai, A. H. Blair, and T. Ghose, Eur. J. Cancer, 15, 1357 (1979).
216. T. Ghose, J. Tai, A. Guclu, R. R. Ramam, and A. H. Blair, Cancer Immunol. Immunother., 13, 185 (1982).
217. G. F. Rowland, G. J. O'Neil, and D. A. L. Davies, Chemotherapy, 8, 11 (1977).
218. M. V. Pimm, R. A. Robins, M. J. Embleton, F. Jacobs, A. J. Markham, A. Charleston, and R. W. Baldwin, Br. J. Cancer, 61, 508 (1990).
219. M. K. Ghosh, D. O. Kildsig, and A. K. Mitra, Drug Des. Deliv., 4, 13 (1989).
220. L. Diang, J. Samuel, G. D. MacLean, A. A. Noujaim, E. Diener, and B. M. Longenecker, Cancer Immunol. Immunother., 32, 105 (1990).
221. F Hudecz, H. Ross, M. R. Price, and R. W. Baldwin, Bioconjug. Chem., 1, 197 (1990).
222. M. Page, D. Thibeault, C. Noel, and L. Dumas, Anticancer Res., 10, 353 (1990).
223. G. F. Rowland, R. G. Simmonds, J. R. F. Corvalan, et al., Protides Biol. Fluids, 30, 375 (1983).
224. G. P. Samokhin, M. D. Smirnov, V. R. Muzykantove, S. P. Domogatsky, and V. N. Smirnov, FEBS Lett., 154, 259 (1983).
225. D. L. Urdal and S. Hakomori, J. Biol. Chem., 255, 10509 (1980).
226. H. G. Eichler, S. Gasic, K. Bauer, A. Korn, and S. Bacher, Clin. Pharmacol. Ther., 40, 300 (1986).
227. M. A. Glukhova, S. P. Domogatsky, A. E. Kabakov, V. R. Muzykantov, O. I. Ornatsky, D. V. Sakharov, M. G. Frid, and V. N. Smirnov, FEBS Lett., 198, 155 (1986).
228. A. Trouet, D. D. Campeneere, R. Burain, M. Huybrechts, and A. Zeneberch, Desoxyribonucleic acid as carrier of antitumor drugs, in *Drug Carriers in Biology and Medicine* (G. Gregoriadis, ed.), Academic Press, London, 1979, p. 87.
229. A. Trouet, Carriers for bioactive materials, in *Polymeric Delivery Systems* (R. J. Kostelnik, ed.), Gordon & Breach, New York, 1978, p. 157.
230. C. Paul, J. Lliemark, U. Tidefelt, G. Gahrton, and C. Peterson, Ther. Drug Monitor., 11, 140 (1989).
231. A. Trouet, J. M. Jadin, and F. V. Hoof, Lysosomotropic chemotherapy in protozoal diseases, in *Biochemistry of parasites and Hosti–Parasites Relationships* (H. van den Bossche, ed.), North-Holland, Amsterdam, 1976, p. 519.
232. E. J. Franssen, R. G. van Amsterdam, J. Visser, F. Moolenaar, D. D. Zeeuw, and D. K. F. Meijer, Pharm. Res., 8, 1223 (1991).
233. T. Maack, V. Johnson, S. T. Kau, J. Figueiredo, and D. Siguelm, Kidney Int., 16, 251 (1979).
234. R. J. Kok, F. Grijpstra, R. B. Walthuis, F. Moolenar, D. de Zeeuw, D. K. Meijer, J. Pharmacol. Exp. Ther., 288, 281 (1999).
235. D. K. F. Meijer and P. V. D. Sluijs, Pharm. Res., 6, 105 (1989).

236. G. Molema, R. W. Jansen, R. Pauwels, F. Clerco, and D. K. F. Meijer, Biochem. Pharmacol., 40, 2603 (1990).
237. A. C. Roche, P. Midoux, V. Pimpancau, E. Negre, R. Mayer, and M. Monsigny, Res. Virol., 141, 243 (1990).
238. B. C. F. Chu and J. M. Whiteley, Mol, Pharmacol., 13, 80 (1977).
239. J. H. Han, Y. K. Oh, D. S. Kim, and C. K. Kim, Int. J. Pharm., 188, 39 (1999).
240. B. C. F. Chu and J. M. Whiteley, JNCI, 62, (1979).
241. J. M. Whiteley, Z. Nimec, and J. Galivan, Mol. Pharmacol., 19, 505 (1981),
242. L. Beijaars, G. Molema, B. Weert, H. Bonnema, P. Olinga, G. M. Goothuis, D. K. Meijer, and K. Poelstra, Hepatology, 29, 1486 (1999).
243. L. Fiume, C. Busi, and A. Mattioli, FEBS Lett., 153, 6 (1983).
244. P. J. Swart, L. Beljaars, M. E. Kuipers, C. Smit, P. Nieuwenhuis, and D. K. Meijer, Biochem. Pharmacol., 58, 1425 (1999).
245. J. M. Varga and N. Asato, Hormones as drug carriers, in *Targeted Drugs* (E. P. Goldberg, ed.), John Wiley & Sons, New York, 1983, p. 73.
246. A. D. Ross and D. M. Angaran, Drug Intell. Clin, Pharm., 18, 202 (1984).
247. L. Moleteni, Dextran as drug carriers, in *Drug Carriers in Biology and Medicine* (G. Gregoriadis. ed.), Academic Press, New York, 1979, p. 25.
248. E. Schacht, Polysaccharide macromolecules as drug carriers, in *Polymers, in Controlled Drug Delivery* (L. Illum and S. S. Davis, eds.), Wright, Bristol, 1987, p. 131.
249. I. Genta, P. Perugini, F. Pavanetto, T. Modena, B. Conti, and R. A. Muzzarelli, EXS., 87, 305 (1999).
250. S. Matsumoto, Y. Arase, Y, Takakura, M. Hashida, and H. Sezaki, Chem, Pharm. Bull., 33, 2941 (1985).
251. N. Schaschke, I. Assfatg_Machleidt, W. Machleidt, T. Lssteben, C. P. Sommerhoff, and L. Moroder, Bioorg. Med. Chem. Lett. 10, 677 (2000).
252. D. R. Friend and S. Pangburn, Med. Res. Rev., 7, 53 (1987).
253. W. C. Shen and H. J. P. Ryser, Mol. Pharmacol., 16, 614 (1979).
254. B. C. F. Chu and S. B. Howell, Biochem. Pharmacol., 30, 2545 (1981).
255. F. Zunino, G. Savi, F. Giuliani, R. Gambetta, R. Supinio, S. Tinelli, and G. Pezzoni, Eur, J. Cancer Clin. Oncol., 20, 421 (1984).
256. E. Hurwitz, M. Wilchek, and J. Pitha, J. Appl. Biochem., 2, 25 (1980).
257. P. Campbell, G. Glover, and J. M. Gunn, Arch. Biochem, Biophys., 203, 676 (1980).
258. J. Koecek, J. Controlled Release, 11, 279 (1990).
259. L. W. Seymour, K. O'Hare, R. Duncan, J. Strohalm, and K. Ulbrich, Br. J. Cancer, 63, 882 (1991).
260. J. Kopecek, B. Rihova, and N. L. Krinick, J. Controlled Release, 16, 137 (1991).
261. H. Maeda and Y. Matsumura, New tactics and basic mechanisms of targeting chemotherapy in solid tumors, in *Cancer Chemotherapy: Challenge for the Future* (K. Kimura. ed.), Excerpta Medical, Tokyo, 1989, p. 42.
262. Y. Matsumra, K. K. T. Yamamoto, and H. Maeda, Jpn. J. Cancer Res., 47, 852 (1988).
263. T. Konno and H. Maeda, Targeting chemotherapy of hepatocellular carcinoma: Arterial administration of SMANCS/Lipiodol, in *Neoplasm in the Liver* (K. Okada and K. G. Ishak, eds.), Springer-Verlag, New York, 1987, p. 343.
264. T. Konno, Targeting anticancer chemotherapy for primary and secondary liver cancer using arterially administered oily anticancer agents, in *Cancer Chemotherapy: Challenges for the Future* (K. Kimura, ed.), Excerpta Medica, Tokyo. 1987, p. 287.
265. H. Maeda, Adv. Drug Deliv. Rev., 6, 181 (1991).
266. H. Yamamoto, T. Miki, T. Oda, T. Hirano, Y. Sera, M. Akagi, and H. Maeda, Eur. J. Cancer. 26, 253 (1990).
267. M. Przybylski, E. Fell, H. Ringsdorf, and D. S. Zaharko, Makromol. Chem., 179, 1719 (1978).
268. D. S. Breslow, E. I. Edwards, and N. R. Newburg, Nature 246, 160 (1973).
269. D. M. Oh, H. K. Han, and G. L. Amidon, Pharm. Biotechnol., 12, 59 (1999).
270. V. Lenaerts and R. Gurny, eds., *Bioadhesive Drug Delivery Systems*, CRC Press, Boca Raton, FL, 1990.
271. K. Klokkers-Bethke and W. Fischer, J. Controlled Release, 15, 105 (1991).
272. G. Coppi, V. Iannuccelli, and R. Cameroni, Phar. Dev. Technol., 3, 347, (1998).
273. M. Saffran, G. S. Kumar, C. Savariar, J. C. Burnham, F. Williams, and D. Neckers, Science, 233, 1081 (1986).
274. E. P. Kakoulides, J. D. Smart, and J. Tsibouklis, J. Controlled Release, 54, 95 (1998).
275. E. P. Kakoulides, J. D. Smart, and J. Tsibouklis, J. Controlled Release, 52, 291 (1998)
276. R. Ito, Y. Machida, T. Sannan, and T. Nagai, Int. J. Pharm., 61, 109 (1990).
277. D. Wachsmann, J. P. Klein, M. Scholler, and R. M. Frank, Immunology, 54, 189 (1985).
278. D. T. O'Hagan, K. Palin, S. S. Davis, P. Arthursson, and I. Sjoholm, Vaccine, 7, 421 (1989).
279. D. T. O'Hagan, K. J. Palin, and S. S. Davis, Vaccine, 7, 213 (1989).
280. D. T. O'Hagan, D. Rahman, J. P. McGee, H. Jeffery, M. C. Davies, P. Williams, S. S. Davis, and S. J. Challacombe, Immunology, 73, 239 (1989).
281. S. J. Challacombe, D. Rahman, H. Jeffery, S. S. Davis, and D. T. O'Hagan, Immunology, 76, 164 (1992).

282. D. T. O'Hagen, D. Rahman, H. Jeffery, S. Sharif, and S. J. Challacombe, Int. J. Pharm., 108, 133 (1994).
283. J. F. Woodley, J. Drug Target., 7, 325 (2000).
284. B. D. Wigness, F. D. Dorman, T. D. Rhode, and H. Buchwald, ASAIO J., 38, M454 (1992).
285. H. Buchwald and T. D. Rhode, ASAIO J., 38, 772 (1992).
286. J. L. Salem, P. Micossi, F. L. Dumm, and D. M. Nathan, Diabetes Care, 15, 877 (1992).
287. J. L. Salem, Horm. Metab, Res., 24 (Suppl.), 144 (1990).
288. J. L. Salem and M. A. Charles, Diabetes Care, 13, 955 (1990).
289. P. J. Blackshear and T. D. Rhode, Horiz, Biochem. Biophys., 9, 293 (1989).
290. P. J. Blackshear, Implantable pumps for insulin delivery: Current clinical status, in *Drug Delivery Systems, Fundamentals and Techniques* (P. Johnson and J. G. Lloyd-Jones, eds.), Ellis Horwood, Chichester, 1987, p. 139.
291. J. M. Gallo, Y. Sanzgiri, E. W. Howerth, T. S. Winco, J. Wilson, J. Johnston, R. Tackett, and S. C. Budsberg, J. Pharm. Sci., 81, 11 (1992).
292. A. Poozetto, L. Fiume, B. Forzani, et al., Hepatology, 14, 16 (1991).
293. R. W. Jensen, J. K. Kruijt, T. J. V. Berkel, and D. K. Meijer, Hepatology, 18, 146 (1993).
294. L. Fiume, G. D. Stefano, C. Busi, and A. Mattioli, Biochem. Pharmacol., 47, 643 (1994).
295. P. Midoux, E. Negre, A. C. Roche, et al., Biochem. Biophys. Res. Commun., 167, 1044 (1990).
296. S. Kuchler, M. N. Graff, S. Gobaille, G. Vincendon, A. C. Roche, J. P. Delaunoy, M. Monsigny, and J. P. Zanetta, Neurochem. Int., 24, 43 (1994).
297. E. Negre, M. L. Chance, S. Y. Hanboula, M. Monsigny, A. C. Roche, R. M. Mayer, and M. Hommel, Antimicrob. Agents Chemother., 36, 2228 (1992).
298. Y. Kaneo, T. Tanaka, and S. Iguchi, Chem. Pharm. Bull., 39, 999 (1991).
299. T. J. V. Berkel, J. K. Kruijt, P. C. D. Smidt, and M. K.Bijsterbosch, Targeted Diagn. Ther., 5, 225 (1991).
300. V. Keegan-Rogers and G. Y. Wu, Cancer Chemother. Pharmacol., 26, 93 (1990).
301. E. J. Franssen, R. W. Jansen, M. Vaalburg, and D. K. Meijer, Biochem. Pharmacol., 45, 1215 (1993).

Chapter 17

Packaging of Pharmaceutical Dosage Forms

Thomas J. Ambrosio

Schering-Plough Research Institute, Kenilworth, New Jersey

The close relationship between a pharmaceutical preparation and its package is of major concern to the industrial pharmacist. Faulty packaging of pharmaceutical dosage forms can compromise the most stable formulation. Consequently, it is essential that the choice of immediate container materials for each formulation be made only after a thorough evaluation of the effect of these materials on the product's stability. This is accomplished by testing the container's effectiveness in protecting the product during extended storage under varying environmental conditions of temperature, humidity, and light.

Pharmaceutical packaging is the means of providing protection, presentation, identification and information, containment, and convenience to encourage compliance with a course of therapy. The period from product manufacture to ultimate use or administration lies within the product shelf life interval. Criteria for selecting a satisfactory packaging system for pharmaceutical products are established by addressing a checklist of basic considerations:

Which raw material (how fabricated, how processed) would be most appropriate as a package for a given dosage form or a particular product?

Considering the relative barrier and inertness properties of packaging materials, how will these factors affect the shelf life of the product packaged in it?

What methodology and experimental scheme could be used for predicting shelf life?

Would the packaging components contribute to any biological effects of the medication?

What controls and test procedures can be instituted to ensure reproducibility in the quality of the materials used in the packaging system?

What will the package integrity issues be? Can the mechanical, climatic, biological, and chemical hazards be addressed adequately by the packaging system?

I. GLASS—THE ABSOLUTE BARRIER

Glass has been the container of choice for pharmaceutical dosage forms because of its resistance to decomposition by atmospheric conditions or by solid or liquid contents of different chemical compositions [1]. Furthermore, by varying the chemical composition of glass, it is possible to adjust the chemical behavior and radiation protective properties of glass.

A. USP Classifications

The United States Pharmacopeia (USP) classifies glass containers as Types I, II, III, and NP according to the amount of alkali released from the glass when attacked by (or in intimate contact with) water under specified conditions [2]. Type I is a borosilicate glass, which releases the least amount of alkali; Type NP releases the most. Type II glass is a soda-lime glass that has been dealkalized by surface treatment of the finished container. The bulk composition of a Type II container is equivalent to Type III glass. The NP containers are fabricated from general-purpose soda-lime glass and can be used for packaging non-parenteral formulations.

Glass containers are either amber or "flint," which is the designation for a clear colorless container. The amber container provides for light resistance. Flint containers transmit light significantly from 300 nm upward in wavelength. Amber glass does not begin to transmit light to any appreciable extent until 470 nm. Since the photochemical activity of light radiation drops off with increasing wavelength, amber containers tend to offer better protection against light than flint glass. Therefore, amber glass can be used to package products subject to photodegradation.

Unfortunately, in some cases the newer, high-potency (and consequently, low-dosage) drugs can readily be affected by release of soluble alkali from glass containers [3]. A remedial measure for liquids and some semi-solids is to buffer the product whenever possible to offset pH changes due to release of alkali by glass. For pharmaceutical products, the USP designation can be used in selecting containers.

USP Type I can be used for all applications as it represents the most unreactive of the glasses available. Water for injection, unbuffered products, and those requiring terminal sterilization are most commonly packaged in Type I glass. While surface treatment is not usually required, it will further enhance the desirable characteristics of an already superior container. This enhancement may become especially important for small containers because of the high ratio of container surface area to the volume of the container contents. In most cases Type I glass is used to package products that are alkaline or will become alkaline prior to their expiration date. However, care must be exercised when selecting containers for solutions with a pH > 7 because even Type I glass may be attacked by alkaline solutions under certain conditions [4].

USP Type II can be used for products that remain below pH 7.0 for their shelf life. The suitability of Type II for small volume parenterals should be evaluated for unbuffered solutions on a case-by-case basis. Type II containers are frequently found to be suitable for a variety of large-volume parenterals due to the less stringent requirements imposed by their lower surface-to-volume ratios.

USP Type III has been found acceptable in packaging some dry powders that are subsequently dissolved to make a buffered solution and for liquid formulations that prove to be insensitive to alkali. Type III glasses are usually not used for those products that are sterilized in their final container. Type II glass containers can be dry heat sterilized and filled under aseptic conditions.

B. Other Factors

Other factors to be considered in the glass container selection process are:

- Thermal expansion properties, which may be important in some processing situations, such as freeze-drying. The physical design of the container also influences its resistance to thermal and mechanical shock.
- If a product is sensitive to particular ions such as barium or calcium, glass formulations are available where these are excluded.
- If the glass is to be sterilized by irradiation, a special formulation containing cerium oxide must be used to prevent discoloration of the container.

Some additional factors that influence glass container performance are:

- Container size and physical design: the concentration of materials leachable from glass decreases with increasing container size. The concentration of leached materials will increase with increasing surface-to-volume ratio for a given container size. In containers treated by the glass manufacturer, this extraction process can be significantly retarded [5].
- Methods of container fabrication:
  - Molded
  - Tubing reformed
- Container processing:
  - Storage conditions for containers before use
  - Washing procedure and pretreatment
  - Drying conditions
  - Sterilization prior to or after product fill
  - Closure design
  - Methods of sealing
- Product composition:
  - Type and concentration of ions present
  - pH
  - Physicochemical properties of drug and vehicles

II. ELASTOMERIC CLOSURES

An elastomeric closure is a packaging component that is, or may be, in direct contact with a drug product. Elastomer selection for parenteral packaging principally involves consideration of chemical, physical, and biological properties, with emphasis on the stability profile of the drug/container system. Typical elastomeric closure compositions are listed in Tables1–4. Although certain packaging applications frequently call to mind certain elastomer types, it is not feasible to prescribe specific

Table 1 Typical Elastomeric Formulation Ingredients

Elastomer	Base material
Curing agent	Form cross-links
Accelerator	Type and rate of cross-link
Activator	Efficiency of accelerators
Antioxidant	Antidegradant
Plasticizer	Processing aid
Filler	Physical properties
Pigment	Color

Table 2 Typical Thermoset Rubber Formulations

	PHR	%
Chlorobutyl	100	52.7
Calcined clay	75	39.6
Paraffinic oil	8	4.2
Titanium dioxide	2	1.1
Carbon black	0.25	0.13
Thiuram	0.35	0.18
Zinc oxide	3	1.6
Hindered phenol AO	1	0.53
Total	189.60	100.0

Table 3 Typical Thermoplastic Rubber Formulation

	PHR	%
Kraton G	100	71.4
Paraffinic oil	10	7.1
Calcined clay	30	21.5
Total	140	100.0

Table 4 Rubber-Curing Agents and Accelerators

Metal oxides
Resins
Peroxides
Amines
Dithiocarbamates
Thiurams
Sulfenamides
Thiazoles

elastomers for specific applications in all cases because of the multiplicity of product and end-use situations.

A. Mechanical Properties of Elastomers

For the most part, these are formulation-specific parameters and cannot be assessed on individual closures [6]. These include tensile strength, elongation at break, and modulus of elongation. These last two properties are important in compound selection in the area of coring and during needle penetration. The more an elastomer stretches before the needle punctures it, the smaller the core and resultant penetration hole.

Compression set and durometer hardness are also important mechanical properties. Compression set is defined as the amount by which an elastomer fails to return to its original thickness after being subjected to a standard compressive load or deflection for a specified time at a specified temperature. A low percent compression set typifies a more compression resistant elastomeric formulation. Compression set of a closure on a sealed vial is a factor in maintaining the sterility and potency of the drug itself.

Compression set of a plunger in a syringe or cartridge system is critical. The plunger fits snugly against the side of the barrel, maintaining a seal. If the compression set percentage is too high, there may be potential problems of leakage, loss of sterility, or potency loss. On the other hand, if the compression set percentage is too low, the break-loose force or the travel force may be too great. These can sometimes be adjusted with external lubricants prior to assembly. The detachment force of the plunger rod from the syringe plunger tip may also be too low.

In addition to normal compression set test conditions, usually 22 hours at 70 °C in a hot air oven, pharmaceutical elastomeric closures may be subjected to compression set conditions simulating steam sterilization cycles in an autoclave for 30 minutes at 121 °C. Also, sterilizing cycles employing ETO, radiation, or dry heat are used. Comparison data between formulations are used to develop compression set values that will identify potentially acceptable compounds under these conditions.

Durometer hardness is defined as the measure of resistance to indentation using either a macro- or microhardness tester. To the pharmaceutical drug manufacturer, hardness is important because of its relationship to ultimate mechanical properties—particularly modulus. In general, softer compounds of the same elastomer base have better coring and reseal properties, whereas harder compounds tend to process better on high-speed filling lines.

An additional consideration under mechanical properties is the characterization of formulation performance by measuring solvent resistance. This parameter is defined as the ability of an elastomeric closure to retain original mechanical and physical properties without undue dimensional change, decomposition or disintegration when immersed in solvents, or specific medical solutions, for specified times and temperatures. ASTM D 471–77 gives a procedure for determining the resistance of elastomeric vulcanizates to various solvents. Immersion tests are conducted under the specified conditions of time and temperature and the changes in mass, volume, dimensions, tensile strength, elongation, durometer hardness, or other pertinent physical characteristics are determined.

The ideal elastomeric closure is nonreactive physically and chemically, a complete barrier to vapor/gas permeation, easily penetrable via needle or spike, resealable, resistant to coring and fragmentation, and maintains package integrity at the seal surface.

B. Functional Properties of Elastomers

Coring is defined as the cutting of rubber from a closure during insertion of a hypodermic needle resulting in the production of elastomeric particles or fragments. Frictional testing of syringes determines the frictional characteristics of a contained closure called a plunger as it is started in motion (breakloose) and moved at a constant rate in the barrel of a syringe (extrusion pressure). Plunger movement should be profiled for each syringe system. It gives a measure of the performance of the amount, type, location, and uniformity of lubrication in the system as well as processing (sterilization) effects.

Vacuum retention determines the ability of an elastomeric closure to maintain vacuum in a container-closure system when vacuum retention is a requirement. In certain instances it impacts on the long-term stability of a parenteral system.

Needle penetration and resealability measures the force required to penetrate the target area of an elastomeric closure with a hypodermic needle and the ability of the closure to reseal when the needle is withdrawn.

Elastomers function as a barrier to either moisture or atmospheric gases (oxygen, nitrogen, and argon). This property is important in maintaining product integrity for lyophilized or liquid products subject to decomposition by water vapor or oxygen.

C. Rubber Control Techniques

1. Current Good Manufacturing Practices

Current good manufacturing practices (CGMPs) indicate that a parenteral manufacturer should confirm supplier certification on packaging components. The following characteristics are usually monitored for a specific elastomeric formulation:

Spectrophotometic identification of elastomer or pyrolyzate
Specific gravity
Percent ash where applicable
Ultraviolet spectrophotometry of extracts

2. Extractables from Elastomeric Closures

Procedures that facilitate the characterization of extractables from elastomeric closures are important to both manufacturers of closures and injectable drug products [7]. The closure manufacturer can find application in the assessment of closure lot-to-lot reproducibility, in development of extraction profiles for each closure, and as an additional means of establishing closure identification. The injectable drug manufacturer can apply these procedures during the preformulation and formulation phases of product development and as a means for setting specifications for incoming closures, particularly when known substances must be absent in order to assure product stability. In addition such methods are helpful in answering questions relating to functional group characterization or identification of major extractables that may arise during a product's shelf life.

By employing both instrumental and conventional analytical techniques on solvent extracts of an elastomeric closure formulation, extractables can be isolated, the inorganic ions determined quantitatively, and the organic components functionally characterized [8]. This information, together with additional work on the isolated fractions, can be used in the more difficult task of extractable identification, when desired or required.

Specification of acceptable limits on extractables is preferred when possible by regulatory authorities. At a minimum, a profiling of extractables using appropriate solvents is expected of pharmaceutical manufacturers.

3. Parenteral Package Integrity

It is recognized that physical and mechanical properties of a parenteral system affect seal integrity. However, physical and/or microbiological testing approaches may be used to challenge seal integrity or demonstrate that a seal has been achieved and is being maintained over the shelf life of the container system.

Among some of the test procedures that may be used for monitoring package integrity over time are dye immersion testing using either pressure or vacuum, seal force testing [9], to monitor initial residual seal force of a closure system as well as the value of the sealing force over time, and finally the monitoring of the performance of growth media–filled containers under different test conditions.

The microbial challenge can consist of:

1. Static aerosol challenge: Expose sealed containers to periodic challenge by generating aerosol containing the challenge organism
2. Static immersion challenge: Expose sealed containers to periodic challenge by immersion in a suspension of challenge organisms
3. Static ambient challenge: Expose sealed containers to ambient conditions and monitor periodically for evidence of microbial growth
4. Dynamic immersion challenge: Expose sealed containers to periodic challenge by immersion in a suspension of challenge organisms, with simultaneous additional stress of pressure/vacuum if warranted by the normal conditions of product storage

The duration of challenge stress may range from minutes to days (or longer), but usually shorter periods of time are used for severe challenges.

USP Chapters <87> and <88> describe Biological Reactivity Tests, In Vitro and In Vivo, for elastomerics, plastics, and other plastic materials with direct or indirect patient contact [2].

4. Advances in Closure Development

Recent advances in closure development include:

1. Ingredients
   - Elimination or reduction of ingredients such as:
     - MCBT—potential carcinogen
     - Sulfur curing agents
     - Carbon black polynucleararomatics
     - Sulfur/nitrogen-containing accelerators
     - Plasticizers
   - Reduction of metals
     - Al, Ca, Zn, Mg
     - Cd, Pb, Hg, hexavalent Cr
     - Reduction in total number of ingredients
2. Surface modifications

Coatings	Benefits
Teflon	More inert closure
Flurotech	Less lubrication required
Purcoat	Fewer particulates
Silicone	Improved machinability

   Warning: Package integrity may be compromised when using coated elastomers, especially for vacuum-sealed or gas-flushed vials [11].

3. Ready-to-use closures, precleaned and presterilized

   Precision injection molding where feasible, gamma radiation–resistant formulations, and improved production traceability and quality.

III. PLASTICS

The use of plastics for containers, closures, and medical devices evolved steadily in the second half of the twentieth century. Plastics are durable, easily molded into a variety of shapes, flexible, often unbreakable, and biocompatable in many applications.

As a group, plastics have been found to evoke a wide range of biological responses. Sources of these include polymers, additives, and fabrication agents. For the most part polymers are biologically inert, although they may contain unreacted monomers or polymers of low molecular weight or impurities from the synthetic process, such as catalysts and residual solvents. The additives, which represent a large group of low molecular weight substances, are more easily extractable and may constitute the major reason for undesirable effects.

The fabricating agents include adhesives and printing inks. The former are widely used in converting different webs into laminates, for sealing purposes, and for the attaching of labels; both are compounded with solvents and other low molecular weight substances that can migrate through plastic. Typical plastic additives are listed in Table 5.

The Code of Federal Regulations, Title 21, Drugs, Current Good Manufacturing Practice in Manufacture, Processing, Packaging or Holding requires that "containers, closures and other component parts of drug packages are suitable for their intended use in that they are not reactive, additive or absorptive to an extent that significantly affects the identity, strength, quality or purity of the drug and furnish adequate protection against its deterioration or contamination."

Factors responsible for plastic properties are:

- Chemical structure
- Molecular weight
- Crystallinity and orientation
- Cross-linking
- Addition of other agents

Some of the most important problems that can arise from the use of plastic containers or laminations for

Table 5 Plastic Additives

Type	Purpose	Examples
1. Lubricants	Improve processibility	Stearic acid Paraffin waxes PE waxes
2. Stabilizers	Retard degradation	Epoxy compounds Organotins Mixed metals
3. Plasticizers	Enhance flexibility, resiliency, melt flow	Phthalates
4. Antioxidants	Present oxidative degradation	Hindered phenolics (BHT) Aromatic amines Thioesters Phosphites
5. Antistatic agents	Minimize surface static charge	Quaternary ammonium compounds
6. Slip agents	Minimize coefficient of friction, especially polyolefins	
7. Dyes, pigments	Color additives	

packaging of pharmaceutical preparations are described in the following sections.

A. Sorption

Sorption is defined as the bonding of a solute to a plastic. It is a physicochemical phenomenon related to the properties of the plastic and the chemical structure of the drug or other soluble components of the preparation. Interactions of this type can be determined by measuring the loss of the solute to the plastic at equilibrium under constant temperature conditions [11].

The high level of potency of many new drugs results in the preparation of relatively dilute dosage forms, so that any appreciable losses due to sorption can be of therapeutic significance. Factors that have been implicated as determinants in the degree of sorption include pH, solvent system, concentration of solute, temperature, and chemical structure of the polymer. A comprehensive, stability testing program will easily pick up drug loss in containers and alert researchers to the need for substituting a more satisfactory material for the package.

B. Desorption

Desorption, or the leaching of plastic components into the contents of the container, has received a great deal of attention, particularly with respect to parenteral and ophthalmic preparations. The potential toxicity of extractives has been questioned and has led to the adoption of various tests in the USP (<87>, <88>, and <381>) and specifications by regulatory authorities [13].

With liquid and semi-solid dosage forms, the rate and the extent of desorption are influenced by the solvent system of the preparation, pH, and temperature conditions during processing and storage. If a severe problem exists, it will usually manifest itself via an outward sign, such as container collapse, product discoloration, or precipitation [14].

C. Permeation

Consideration of the stability of dosage forms in blister packages, plastic containers, or laminations immediately brings into focus the possibility of permeability of moisture, gases, and light. Excessive loss or gain of water, oxygen, or volatile organic compounds can cause deterioration of the product, both chemically and/or physically. In evaluating a container, the acquisition of permeability data on a particular product is a definite requirement before accepting it for use [15].

Although each composition should be considered individually, water and gas penetration reactions for solid dosage forms are such that penetrants will tend to move towards the package contents with potential implications for oxidative degradation, physical changes in the dosage form, or an improved medium for microbiological growth.

In liquid preparations containing organic solvents, drug concentration changes can occur through loss of solvent to the atmosphere. Similarly, flavors and aromas in formulations may diminish in strength as volatile components pass out of the preparation.

D. Photodegradation

Although the problem of photodegradation with pharmaceutical preparations is restricted to those drugs that are sensitive to radiation energy and only certain dosage forms are apt to be exposed to ultraviolet (UV) light, consideration must be given to the transparency of polymers to the spectrum in the 300–400 nm range. Functional groups in most polymers, such as carbonyls (C=O) and aromatic rings, absorb UV light and thereby initiate an unstable state of excitation. Resulting degradation products of the carbonyl, hydroxyl, and peroxide types tend to increase UV absorption and accelerate the reaction. In addition to the direct effect of UV absorption on drugs, chemical and physical changes in the polymer itself can influence the stability of the packaged medicament

[14]. If a product is light sensitive, appropriate measures to protect it must be taken. This can take the form of addition of opacifying agents to the plastic, use of aluminum foil laminations, or employing light-resistant secondary packaging.

E. Polymer Modification

Interactions affecting the properties of the plastic container, as a consequence of contact with the drug preparation, are also of importance. To a large extent, the protective or functional aspects of a plastic container are directly related to its mechanical properties. While this can be satisfactory initially, changes resulting from interactions can occur gradually and require evaluation as part of the stability testing program.

Polyethylene and polystyrene are examples of plastics subject to environmental stress cracking. Crack resistance tests have shown that surfactants, alcohols, organic acids, vegetable and mineral oils, and ethers provide an active environment for stress cracking of polyethylene. Table 6 lists typical sterile devices and plastic materials used to fabricate them, while Tables 7–9 list the potential effects of sterilization processes on polymeric materials. The effect of gamma irradiation on elastomeric closures has been studied by the Parenteral Drug Association [15].

Table 6 Parenteral Drug Administration Devices

Sterile device	Plastic material
Containers for blood products	Polyvinyl chloride
Disposable syringes	Polycarbonate Polyethylene Polypropylene
Irrigating solution containers	Polyethylene Polypropylene Polyvinyl chloride
i.v. Infusion fluid containers	Polyethylene Polypropylene Polyvinyl chloride
Administration sets	Nylon (spike) Polyvinyl chloride (tubing) Polymethylmethacrylate (needle adapter) Polypropylene (clamp)
Catheter	Teflon Polypropylene Thermoplastic elastomers

Table 7 Gas Sterilization—Effects on Polymeric Materials

Advantage: low temperature sterilization
Considerations:
- ETO reactivity with polymer/product
- ETO penetration/aeration varies with polymer
- ETO and degradation product toxicity
- Impact on seal integrity

Table 8 Steam Sterilization—Effects on Polymeric Materials

Curling/aging effect
Viscoelastic effects and impact on functionality
Solubility changes of polymer
Dimensional effects
Moisture content in polymer

Table 9 Ionizing Radiation—Effects on Polymeric Materials

Free radical and excited ion formation
Bond scission/cross-linking
Cosmetic effects
Drug/polymer reactions
Effects vary with geometry/additives

Recent advances in plastics development include:

Fewer extractables
Greater biocompatibility
Cleaner materials
Specialty laminates
Gamma irradiation resistance

IV. METAL

Materials used for various pharmaceutical drug-delivery systems include tin-plated steel, mild steel, stainless steel, tin-free steel, and aluminum and its various alloys.

A. General Properties

Metal is strong, opaque, and impermeable to moisture, gases, odors, light, bacteria, etc. It is resistant to high and low temperatures. Malleable and ductile, metal is usually used in thin sections.

B. Disadvantages

Metal is not inert and can be attacked by acids and alkalies. It will corrode unless coated or lacquered.

C. Cost

Tin is relatively expensive. Strength and handling can be improved by corrugations, knurling, etc.

D. Container Fabrication

Multipiece built-up containers rely on a variety of seams: lap, butt, locked, single and double seaming.

E. Seam Treatment

Seams can be soldered, welded, cemented, treated with solutions, compound lined, dry, etc. Seams can be one piece drawn, stamped, or pressed. They may be drawn and wall ironed (DWI) or drawn and redrawn (DRD). Seams may be treated by impact extrusion (rigid and flexible, e.g., collapsible aluminum tubes are annealed).

F. Aluminum Foil

Foil 25 μm (0.001 inch) and above is generally accepted as commercially pinhole-free. Thinner gauges contain various levels of pinholes. It should be noted that flex cracking of aluminum foil during the packaging operation or as a result of shock and vibration in transit is not to be considered pinholing. Pinholes produced during the fabrication of the aluminum foil sheet are usually sandwiched between plies of other materials to form a composite lamination. Therefore, in most cases, the pinholes are covered with multiple layers of heat seal and other coatings and contribute minutely to vapor or gas transmission.

Aluminum foil is manufactured by an initial hot rolling to give foil stock, which is then cold rolled, finishing by the rolling of two plies together, which are subsequently separated to give foil plies down to 6 μm. These thin gauges have a dull and bright side. Foil has to be annealed to overcome the work-hardening property to give a soft foil. Hard foil (for blister packs) of 18–25 μm also exists. Special foils can be obtained by alloys with magnesium or manganese.

G. Decoration and Protective Coatings

Most metals receive a base coat of enamel (or occasionally paint), which is baked on. Printing then takes place on the enamel coating by offset lithography, dry offset letterpress, and occasionally other processes.

Protective coatings and lacquers may be applied as a roller or spray coating, usually based on vinyl, epoxy, polyester, phenol-alkyd resin, or wax coatings.

H. Traditional Choice for Topical Preparations

Metal tubes constructed of a single material can be tested readily for stability with a product. Tubes with a coating, however, present additional problems, since it must be established that the coating material is inert for the preparation and that it completely covers the underlying material. In addition, the coating must be evaluated for resistance to cracking and solvents. Aluminum tubes, though quite popular, have demonstrated reactivity with fatty alcohol emulsions, mercurial compounds, and preparations outside a pH range of 6.5–8.0. Nonreactive, epoxy linings have been found to make aluminum tubes more resistant to attack.

I. Other Metal Applications

Other applications for metals include:

Cans, pails, boxes, including aerosols
Closures
Aluminum foil, laminates, labels
Barrels, kegs, and drums
Crates and boxes
Metal strapping and banding

V. PAPER AND BOARD

A. Composition

Paper and board are composed of cellulose obtained by the mechanical or semi-chemical treatment of vegetable fibers (pulp) derived from various sources like wood, hemp, cotton, etc. In some cases waste and regenerated paper is used.

The chemical processes provide for a purer form of pulp, with the removal of lignin, certain other undesirable chemicals, better fiber control, and fewer fiber clumps or bundles. Two chemical processes are in general use—the sulfate and sulfite systems. The final quality of the cellulose fiber is controlled by the beater and refiner stages. Various fillers, coloring agents, and sizing can be added at the beater stage. Whether paper or board is ultimately produced depends on the final machine used. Two basic types exist: Fourdrinier machines (single or twin wires) and cylinder machines. Both paper and board show a grain direction related to the orientation of the fibers in the machine (MD) and cross (CD) directions. (*Note*: Wood usually consists of

50% cellulose fibers, 30% lignin, 16% carbohydrates, and 4% others, such as proteins, resins, and fats.)

B. Properties of Paper and Board

Paper and board products are nontoxic, low cost, and from a natural renewable source. These cellulose products have good rigidity and strength, but properties change according to moisture content (fibers expand or contract). They are readily printable by virtually all processes. The finished products are generally opaque but can be translucent (glassine, vegetable parchment). They is readily torn (easier in machine direction). Paper has some compression properties. It has no barrier properties and can have high or controlled porosity unless modified, coated, laminated, etc. Paper cannot be heat-sealed unless coated. It has poor transparency and gloss compared with plastic films, but these properties can be improved by special treatments. Paper has grain direction resulting from the way individual fibers are laid down. Its dimensional stability is poor as it expands and contracts as moisture passes in or out.

C. Conversion Processes for Paper/Board-Based Materials

Paper can be coated, cut, creased, glued, and laminated to paper, plastics, or foil. It can only be molded as pulp, i.e., pulpboard containers produced by suction or pressure operations. It cannot be molded in the plastic sense [16].

Corrugated materials involving several plies of paper consist of facings and steamed and formed layer(s) of corrugated paper. They may exist as single-faced or double-faced (a, b, c, e flute types) double-wall or triple-wall materials. The latter contain two and three corrugated layers.

Solid board materials may be converted into collapsible or rigid cartons or rigid fiberboard (outers). International codes exist for solid and corrugated fiberboards in terms of design (style). These cases are specified by style, internal dimensions, board grade, and quality.

D. Other Packages Using Paper-Based Materials

These products include:

- Wrapping materials
- Fiber drums
- Certain composites—spiral and convolute wood containers
- Multiwall paper sacks, bags, and bales
- Lined carton systems, bag in box, etc., plus a range of packaging components
- Labels
- Sealing tapes (e.g., gummed tape)
- Cards, display cards, divisions and liners, packaging leaflets and inserts
- Laminates

E. Regenerated Cellulose

Regenerated cellulose film (RCF) is basically a form of cellulose. Wood chips are immersed in a caustic solution and, after a maturation period, dissolved in carbon disulfide. This solution is subsequently extruded through a die into an acid solution, where regeneration occurs. The resulting film is then washed and plasticized with various glycols and humectants.

RCF itself is not a good barrier, nor can it be heat-sealed. Barrier and heat-sealing are conferred by coatings of nitrocellulose or polyvinylidene chloride on one or both sides. RCF has poor dimensional stability due to moisture loss or gain. Its principal use is in laminates and over wrapping.

The original trade name Cellophane is frequently misused generically, as other brand names for regenerated cellulose film also exist (Rayophane, Diophane, etc.).

VI. SPECIAL PACKAGING

A. Tamper-Resistant Packaging

One of the central features of tamper-resistant regulations [17] is the basis requirement for a tamper-resistant package. This section reads in part:

> A tamper-resistant package is one having an indicator or barrier to entry which, if breached or missing, can reasonably be expected to provide visible evidence to consumers that tampering has occurred. To prevent the substitution of the tamper-resistant feature after tampering, the indicator or barrier to entry is required to be distinctive by design or by the use of an identifying characteristic. A tamper-resistant package may involve an immediate (container and closure) system or a secondary (container or carton) system or any combination of systems intended to provide a visual indication of package integrity. The tamper-resistant feature must remain intact when handled in a reasonable manner during manufacture, distribution, and retail display.

Another key feature of the regulations requires labeling. This provision reads in part:

> Each retail package is required to contain a statement that is prominently placed so that consumers are alerted to the specific tamper-resistant feature of the package. The labeling statement is required to be so placed that it will be unaffected if the tamper-resistant feature of the package is breached or missing.

This labeling requirement recognizes that the last line of defense in tampering is the consumer. The consumer must have his or her attention directed to the specific feature intended to indicate tampering. If the consumer is not aware of the feature, irrespective of its physical characteristics, the consumer remains unprotected. The three elements of tamper resistance are the label statement, the indicator/barrier, and the distinctive by design feature for the indicator/barrier.

In the year 2000 approximately 12% of our population was over 65 years old. By 2020 almost 16% of the population will be over 65. The question of "elderly access" has been raised [18]. Both the regulatory and the industrial communities must address the needs of senior citizens, as well as those of the handicapped.

B. Child-Resistant Packaging

In 1970 the Poison Prevention Packaging Act was passed. It provides for "packaging designed and constructed to be difficult for young children to open within a reasonable time and that is not difficult for adults to use properly." Establishing child-resistance effectiveness in a flexible unitized package is considerably more complex and, in certain circumstances, more difficult than doing so with a child-resistant cap on a bottle [21].

The Poison Prevention Packaging Act of 1970 outlines two distinctly different protocols for establishing child-resistant effectiveness in these two types of packaging. In the case of a bottle package, the protocol is relatively uncomplicated and straightforward in requiring that a specific percentage of test children not be able to open the package even after being instructed about how to do so. Table 10 lists the criteria for the tests. Table 11 addresses the child test protocol for oral solids. Table 12 addresses the adult test protocol. Table 13 gives the adult test for torque-dependent closures. Table 14 gives a list of categories of products requiring child-resistant packaging.

The unitized package protocol established similar numerical limits, but then added the definition of what constitutes a toxic amount of product for a 25 lb child. For aspirin, eight tablets were determined to be the realistic package "failure criteria." The failure

Table 10 Child-Resistant Packaging Criteria for Consumer Safety Commission Protocol (CPSC)

Criteria	Application
CPSC Child Test	Oral solids
CPSC Adult Test	Oral liquids

Table 11 Child Test Protocol

Panel	200 children (50% male, 50% female) Ages 42–51 months Tested in pairs
Test	5 minutes no instructions 5 minutes with demonstration
Criteria	85% pass first 5 minutes 80% pass second 5 minutes
Access dose	Dose to seriously injure a 25 lb child

Table 12 Senior Adult Test Protocol

Number of adults	100 (70% female, 30% male)
Ages	50 – 70 years
Time (2)	5 minutes and 1 minute
Criteria for pass	90% must open and close properly

Table 13 Single Adult Use Effectiveness[a]

100 senior adults (50 – 70 years old)
All apparently closed units from the 1-minute opening and closing test are then tested with children
All packages that are opened in excess of 20% count against the SAUE (senior adult use effectiveness)
Performance standard remains at 90% or greater

[a]Used for torque-dependent threaded closures.

Table 14 Products Requiring Child-Resistant Packaging

OTC (by concentration)
Aspirin
Iron
Acetaominophen
Rx
Prescription trade products intended for direct pharmacist dispensing
Exempt
Physician free samples
Preapproved CPSC exemptions

criteria vary considerably for other products. For some highly potent products, a package that might allow a child access to a single tablet might be considered injurious.

Regulations are in effect internationally. This area of packaging is being targeted for harmonization so that a uniform standard can be adhered to.

C. Compliance Packaging

As a direct response to the profound negative impact that a high rate of noncompliance has on therapeutic efficacy and total health care costs, some pharmaceutical manufacturers have taken steps to develop compliance packaging for some products prescribed for ambulatory patients. Compliance packaging [20] holds promise as a significant patient-education tool when health professionals combine it with personalized patient counseling and well-written medication instructions. Well-controlled cost-effectiveness studies are needed to determine the impact of compliance packaging on reducing total health care costs.

Compliance packaging can be defined as a prepackaged unit that provides one treatment cycle of the medication to both the pharmacist and the patient in a ready-to-use package. This innovative type of packaging is usually based on blister packaging using unit-of-use dosing. The separate dosage units and separate days are usually indicated on the dosage cards to help remind the patient when and how much of the medication to take. Compliance packaging has two primary purposes: to serve as a patient-education tool for health professionals and to make it easier for patients to remember to take their medications correctly at home [21]. The ideal compliance package will be developed according to patient education guidelines and will contain targeted patient instructions to help improve patient compliance with the specific medication.

Compliance packaging for ambulatory patients is distinctly different from prepackaging. Both systems use prepackaged medications, and each unit contains a predetermined number of doses in either strip packs or blister packs. The units are directly dispensed to the patient. Obviously, such a system for ambulatory patients requires agreement among health professionals on the prescribed dosage and length of the therapy. Compliance packaging is basically one step beyond prepackaging and incorporates dosage and treatment instructions to help the patient manage the prescribed medication regimen correctly.

Packaging that is developed according to patient education principals can serve as a strong reminder or motivational aid to the patient. The "complete package," a new concept recently proposed, is the most advanced type of compliance packaging. The proponents of this concept recommend that pharmaceutical companies expand their definition of a "product" beyond that of the medication. The complete package consists of the medication plus the complete set of compliance packaging and the educational materials necessary to help the patient obtain the desired therapeutic outcome.

There are many successful examples of compliance packaging in the marketplace. These include oral contraceptives, unit-of-use packaging for steroids, "convenience paks," and blister packaging systems that incorporate reminder and information leaflets (the MACPAC).

VII. ANALYSIS AND CONTROL OF PACKAGING MATERIALS

Present-day instrumental analytical methods lend themselves quite well to the identification, control, and evaluation of packaging materials. There are also precise techniques for measuring the physical and functional characteristics of packaging components.

Most nondestructive test methods involve more than visual inspection of surfaces. Nearly every basic principle of physics has been used to obtain the necessary information concerning the properties of finished packaged products. The great majority of methods rely upon mechanical measurements or upon a flow or transfer of energy. There are a variety of instrumental test methods, which utilize some form of energy transfer to identify, classify, and control packaging materials and/or components of functioning packaging systems. Although not all the techniques used in testing packaging material are nondestructive, one can sense where emerging technologies are proceeding in that direction for better quality assurance.

The principal instrumental techniques employed for applied packaging controls are:

Spectrophotometry
Chromatographic methods
Thermal analysis techniques
Gas transmission analysis
Physical test methods
Miscellaneous techniques

A. Spectrophotometry

Spectroscopy applied to packaging materials is most often used as a technique for identification.

In the early 1960s multiple internal reflectance spectroscopy (MIR) was developed. It relies on the principle that when a beam of radiation is internally reflected from the surface of a crystal, part of the radiation passes outside of the surface of the crystal during the reflection process. When a sample touches the reflection surface, it will absorb at its characteristic wavelength. Thus, the reflected radiation is attenuated at the absorbing frequencies of the sample and an infrared spectrum is obtained. Penetration of the sample by the beam is of the order of a few μm and can be varied by altering the angle of incident radiation. Since absorption takes place only at the interface of the sample and the crystal, the process is independent of sample thickness. MIR is useful not only in coating identification but also in evaluating the effects of long-term storage on the coatings. The effects of temperature, humidity, and aging can be conveniently monitored without altering the sample. Surface phenomena such as color changes, plasticizer blooming, or excessive oxidation can also be evaluated [14].

MIR techniques have simplified obtaining infrared spectra of many materials important in packaging. These include rubber, plastics, laminations, and components of these materials that find use in pumps, sample packages, and devices. The combination of MIR and computerized pattern recognition techniques can be used for differentiating and classification of flexible packaging polymers such as polyvinyl chloride (PVC), polyvinylidene chloride (PVdC), acrylonitrile (Barex), and CTFE (Aclar) [22].

B. Chromatographic Methods

Chromatographic methods of all types have demonstrated utility in package control. Studies on sensorially and toxicologically important residues have shown that contact of polymers with such substances in the normal manufacturing process results in measurable sorption or retention, even under the extremes of commercial conditions used for their removal. Methodology developed for the determination of such residues is documented and in wide use [23].

C. Thermal Analysis Techniques

The characterization of polymer systems important to packaging is, of course, essential to their development. Some of the most powerful techniques for studying polymers conveniently and rapidly come under the heading of thermal methods of analysis. Manufacturers and end users can see to it that their packaging materials meet specified levels of oxidative resistivity and can check whether each lot meets established specifications. The scope of applicability offered by thermal method of analysis is still uncertain with respect to packaging as a practical process control mechanism.

In the broadest sense, thermal analysis (TA) measures physical changes in a material as a function of temperature. TA instruments measure variables in a sample such as heat flow, weight, dimensions, etc. A typical "fingerprint" of a compound might be the endothermic peak on a thermogram indicating a sample's crystalline melt.

D. Gas Transmission Analysis

The development of diffusometers for research and quality control for the packaging materials industry represents a substantial analytical breakthrough. Instrumentation is available for measuring oxygen, water vapor, carbon dioxide, and ethylene oxide permeation through sheet materials and complete packages. This provides the advantage of testing folds, creases, seals, printing, closures, and other imposed package features of ambient temperature with no pressure differentials.

E. Leak Detection

Instrumentation exists that reveals pinhole leaks or cracks by detecting a tracer gas which escapes when the package is placed in a partial vacuum [11]. In addition to their normal contents, therefore, packages to be tested must contain an easily identifiable tracer gas. It is desirable that this gas be inexpensive, nontoxic, inert, and easy to detect. Carbon dioxide (CO_2) is one gas that meets these general requirements.

F. Physical Test Methods

Physical test methods also have a place in defining and controlling package performance. The functional properties of packaging materials are dependent upon friction or slip characteristics, tensile, tear or impact strength, and the heat seal peel energy. The generation of seal strength curves provides for control of incoming laminated materials and guidelines for production processing conditions.

Versatile instruments are designed to accurately apply compression or tensile forces as a function of time and distance and record the results graphically. These are adaptable to a wide variety of applications in research, development, and packaging control.

In the manufacture of disposable syringes such an instrument will permit measurement of the forces required to start the plunger in motion (breakthrough force), force required to expel the contents, and changes in these forces as a result of interaction of the drug with the package. The instrument will permit detection of problems resulting from variations in the dimensions or properties of the plastic or rubber, loss of lubricity between the plunger and the barrel, physical deterioration of any of the package components as a result of interaction with the drug, or environmental insult. Such changes can be detected very early by use of physical profiling and be useful in predicting the ultimate performances of the package [24].

G. X-Ray Fluorescence Analysis

X-ray fluorescence analysis is a nondestructive method to analyze rubber materials qualitatively and quantitatively. It is used for the identification as well as for the determination of the concentration of all elements from fluorine through the remainder of the periodic table in their various combinations. X-rays of high intensity irradiate the solid, powder, or liquid specimen. Hence, the elements in the specimen emit X-ray fluorescence radiation of wavelengths characteristic to each element. By reflection from an analyzing crystal, this radiation is dispersed into characteristic spectral lines. The position and intensity of these lines are measured.

H. Other Methods

The Flexible Packaging Association (1090 Vermont Avenue, N.W., Suite 500, Washington, DC) provides a number of procedures for testing flexible packaging materials as well as completed packages fabricated for the medical industry.

The American Society for Testing and Materials (ASTM) has many test procedures for the characterization of packaging materials. These methods are available individually or in specific books of ASTM standards. A list of typical tests may be found in Table 15.

Table 15 Typical Test Procedures for Packaging Materials

General	
Melt Index Test (MFI—melt flow index)	ASTM D 1238
Capillary rheometer test	D 3835
Density	D 792
Mold shrinkage	D 955
Water absorption	D 570
Optical	
Transmittance	D 1003
Haze	D 1003
Gloss	D 523
Mechanical	
Tensile properties	(various[a] D 638)
Compressive properties	D 695
Flexural properties	(various[a] D 790)
Notched Izod impact rest	D 256
Tensile impact test	D 1822
Rockwell hardness test	D 785
Torsion stiffness test (temperature related)	D 1043
High-speed puncture test	D 3763
Gardner dart Impact	D 3029
Burst strength	D 774
Taber abrasion resistance	D 1044
Shear strength	D 732
Tear strength	D 624
Folding endurance	D 643
Drop height to break	D 2436

[a]It should be noted that tensile and flexural properties can be measured at various values, i.e., tensile strength, at yield and break, elongation at break, flexural modulus, flexural strength, etc.

VIII. BLISTER AND STRIP PACKAGING

A. The Blister Package

Blister packages for pharmaceuticals consist of two basic packaging components: lidding material and forming films. The lidding material consists of a supporting material, e.g., aluminum that has a heat seal lacquer on one side to act as a sealing agent, and on the other side an assortment of other layers depending on the end requirements of the blister package (tamper-evident, child resistance, or simple unit dose delivery). The side coated with the sealing agent faces the product and the forming films. The forming film can be a monolayer sheet of PVC or a composite of other materials or coatings to increase the water vapor barrier effect.

The forming film or composite is the packaging component that receives the dosage form in deep-drawn pockets. Plastic forming films such as PVC, polypropylene (PP), and polyester (PET) can be thermoformed, but other formable structures containing aluminum are cold formed. Forming films are usually colorless and transparent. However, when light resistance is required, light-protective or opaque forming films can be employed.

Rigid PVC is currently the most widely used forming film because of its ideal thermoforming characteristics. A typical thickness before thermoforming is 250 μm (10 mil). PVC does not provide a good barrier for moisture-sensitive products. When better barrier properties are required in a thermoformable blister, PVC is laminated or coated with other materials. Because of environmental issues, other materials such as PP compete for blister usage with PVC. In the medical device industry it has been completely replaced by materials such as PET.

PVdC-coated PVC increases the sheet's water-vapor permeability resistance by a factor of 5–10. The coating is applied at different loadings per square meter of PVC sheet. The coating is applied on one side and usually faces the product and lidding material. Stability studies will establish whether interactions with the product are taking place. This is usually indicated by discoloration of the blister or the product.

Laminated sheets made from PVC bonded to chlorotrifluoroethylene (CTFE) have the lowest water-vapor permeability of all the materials used in blister packaging. Compared to 250 μm PVC sheet, a lamination of 200 μm PVC–19 μm CTFE (8 mL PVC–0.8 mL CTFE) has a 15-fold lower water-vapor permeability. There are many grades of CTFE available with more or less barrier and ease of formability. Figure 1 shows the difference between flat sheet and formed blister moisture permeabilities.

There has been a considerable effort to replace PVC with PP as a support material for blister packaging. Its moisture-barrier properties are comparable to PVdC-coated PVC in some cases. However, the processing properties of PP pose a problem. The narrow temperature range required for thermoforming PP and the temperature of the subsequent cooling process must be precisely controlled. PP packages are not as rigid as those made from PVC and PVC composites. Therefore, machinability of blister packaging made from PVC and PVC composites is not as problematic.

PET competes effectively with PVC in medical packaging because of its strength and superior resistance to sterilizing effects. However, it is a poor moisture-vapor barrier and its enhancement by PVdC is not viable because of environmental concerns about plastics that contain chlorine.

Nylon, aluminum, PVC (OPA-aluminum-PVC) composites offer functional alternatives to traditional thermoformed materials. With a laminate structure of 25 μm OPA, 45 μm aluminum, with 60 μm PVC (1 mL OPA–1.8 mL aluminum–2.4 mL PVC), it is possible to almost completely eliminate water-vapor permeability [25].

Replacing PVC with PP allows compliance with environmental standards in some pharmaceutical markets. These materials are cold formed instead of being thermoformed. Such packages require more packaging materials than thermoplastic plastic films for the packaging of the same number and same size of tablets or capsules.

Lidding substrates are required to be sealed to the preformed blister materials. An essential component of lidding material is a coating suitable for heat sealing. The heat sealing lacquers used must comply with FDA standards set forth in the Code of Federal Regulations (CFR) for indirect food additives.

Adhesives and coatings in food-packaging applications are regulated because they are considered to be indirect food additives. This designation acknowledges the possibility of migration between package components and food items. The Code of Federal Regulations addresses indirect food additives in the following parts of Title 21:

- Part 174—Indirect food additives: General provisions
- Part 175—Indirect food additives: Adhesives and components of coatings
- Part 176—Indirect food additives: Paper and paperboard components
- Part 177—Indirect food additives: Polymers
- Part 178—Indirect food additives: Adjuvants, production aids, and sanitizers

These coatings must precisely match chemically the respective forming films (PVC, PP, or PET). A permanent sealing effect between lidding and forming film must exist under all climates. The sealing strength of the blister must fall within predetermined tolerances for the package to be functional.

Package access can be varied through selection of various lidding structures. The use of simple hard or soft tempered foils permits the classical push through feature of blister packages. When paper is laminated onto the aluminum, the product is accessed by peeling off the lidding material. For child resistance, PET is added to the paper-foil lamination. Child resistance is achieved by peeling off the lidding prior to pushing out the dosage form.

Laminates used in strip packaging are combinations of various plies created to obtain the properties not provided by one material alone. They use a minimum amount of materials and are cost-effective. However, they conflict with certain environmental issues, because recycling or reuse is virtually impossible. Examples of widely used laminations are polyester/foil/

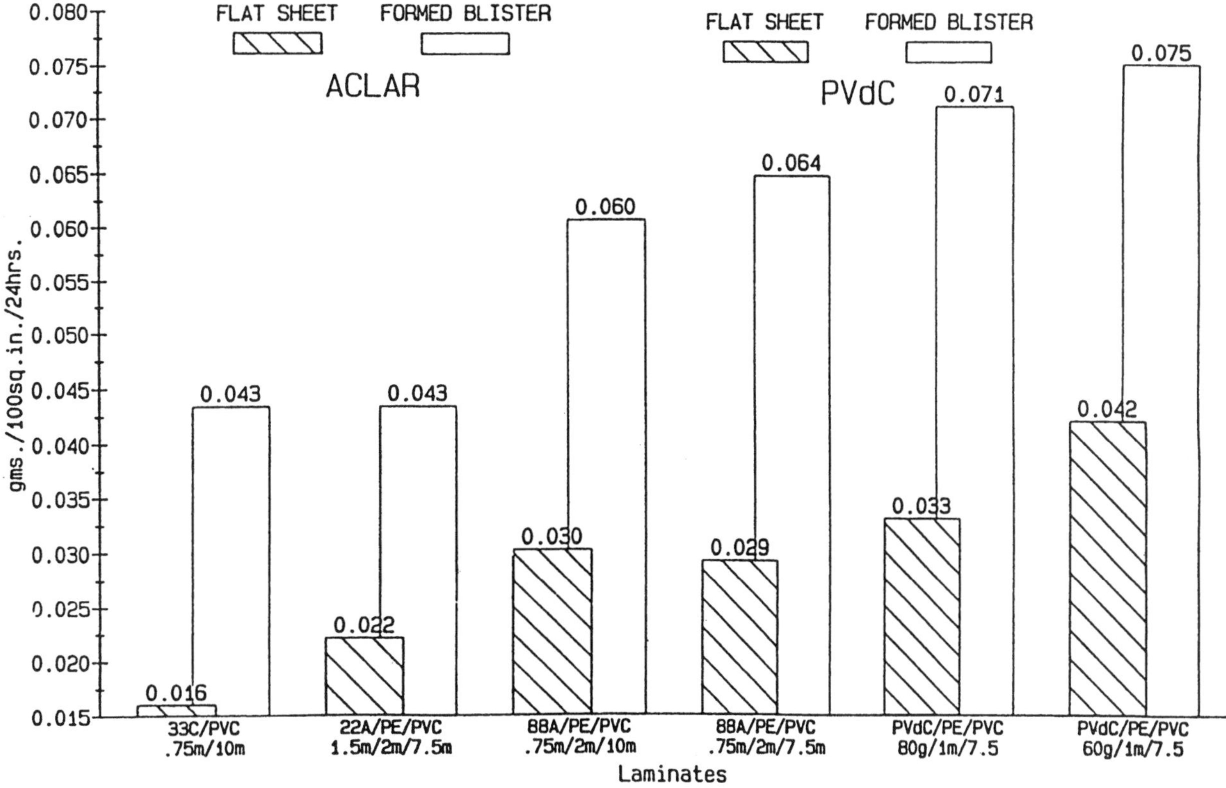

Fig. 1 Flat sheet and formed blister moisture permeabilities.

polyethylene or paper/foil/surlyn. In these constructions polyester provides child resistance, paper provides surface printability, foil provides a barrier to moisture, oxygen, and light, and polyethylene or surlyn gives heat sealability to the structure.

B. Strip Packaging

Strip packages represent an alternative form of packaging for unit-dose medication. Strips can be produced from single- or multiple-ply laminated materials provided the two inner plies can be sealed by heat or pressure (e.g., cold self-adhesive seals). Materials can range from relatively permeable plies to those that incorporate a foil ply of sufficient thickness and effectiveness of seal so that an individual hermetic seal is produced for each dosage. Strip packages are produced at lower speeds and occupy greater volume than blisters.

Strip designs are very basic as the emerging units are either square or rectangular strips. The pocket area is critical to the diameter, shape, and thickness of the product. The pocket area is extended when the product is inserted. If the pocket is too tight, tearing, perforation of the pocket periphery, or wrinkling of the seal area may occur. If the seal area is likely to wrinkle or crease, then wider seals may be necessary. It should be noted that laminates are versatile and include both thermoplastic and other materials such as paper and foil. They allow for printing and coating to enhance the function of the package. Laminates can be assembled using a variety of adhesives, which provide good resistance to delamination during a product's shelf life. The average lamination for solids or semisolids possesses adequate rigidity, too, for processing in secondary packaging operations.

The cylindrical-type sealing process for strip packaging does not usually have a cooling cycle or quench surface, hence any pull on the seal ply will tend to weaken the seal while the sealant is still pliable. Therefore, it is desirable that the sealant have good hot tack or a high melt viscosity at processing temperatures. Hot tack is generally accepted to mean the adhesion quality of the sealant from the moment it leaves the seal head and the time it returns to its set or permanent condition.

Thus, any laminate may consist of plies selected from paper, polyester, numerous other plastic films, foils, coatings, adhesive layers, metalization, etc. The choice of laminate structure is usually governed by technical requirements, cost of base materials, cost of lamination processes, cost of printing cylinder and process, and the amount of laminate required (quantity), the yield from which the cost per area of laminate is derived.

IX. PACKAGE-RELATED CONTENTS IN THE OFFICIAL COMPENDIA

A. General Notices and Requirements Regarding Preservation, Packaging, Storage and Labeling

Definitions are available for the following [2]:

1. **Container**
   - Tamper-resistant packaging
   - Light-resistant container
   - Well-closed container
   - Tight container
   - Hermetic container
   - Single-unit container
   - Single-dose container
   - Unit-dose container
   - Unit-of-use container
   - Multiple-use container
2. **Labeling**
   - Amount of ingredient per dosage unit
   - Use of leading and terminal zeros
   - Labeling of salts of drugs
   - Labeling vitamin-containing products
   - Labeling parenteral and topical preparations
   - Labeling electrolytes
   - Labeling alcohol
   - Special capsules and tablets
   - Expiration date
3. **Storage Temperature**
   - Freezer
   - Cold
   - Cool
   - Room temperature
   - Controlled room temperature
   - Warm
   - Excessive heat
   - Protection from freezing
4. **Storage under Nonspecific Conditions**

B. General USP Chapters on Physical Tests and Determinations

General chapters on physical tests and determinations are included in Table 16.

C. Pharmacopeial Forum Articles [26]

Pharmacopeial Forum's list of in-process revision draft articles for consideration [31] include the following chapters relevant to pharmaceutical packaging:

Chapter 1118 Monitoring Devices—Time, Temperature and Humidity
Chapter 1141 Packaging, Storage, and Distribution of Pharmaceutical Articles
Chapter 1146 Packaging Practice—Repackaging a Single, Solid, Oral Drug Product into a Unit Dose Container

D. Interchangeability of Packaging Materials

Chapter 661 of the USP provides criteria for the interchangeability of low- and high-density polyethylene for dry, oral dosage forms. In addition, there are standards for polyethylene terephthalate bottles and polyethylene terephthalate G bottles. USP criteria for interchangeability are listed in Table 17. These criteria allow usage of alternate materials in the same plastic class to be used prior to obtaining prior stability data.

The USP is continuing to seek other materials for which acceptable criteria for interchangeability can be established. These include polypropylene for dry, oral solids and ophthalmic liquid products. Additional criteria may be established for substituting replacement resins for closures.

Table 16 General Chapters on Physical Tests and Determinations

Chapter	Topic
1	Injections
601	Aerosols
661	Containers
671	Containers Permeation
691	Cotton
698	Deliverable Volume
751	Metal Particles in Ophthalmic Ointments
1078	Principles of Good Manufacturing Practices for Bulk Pharmaceutical Excipients

Table 17 Criteria for Interchangeability

	Physicochemical tests—plastics	Polyethelene containers	PET and PETG bottles
Applicability	All plastics	Dry oral dosage forms	Liquid oral
Extractant	H_2O (6.67 Mohm) at 70° Hexane at 50°	H_2O and ETOH at 70° Hexane at 50°	H_2O, 50% ETOH (PET), 25% ETOH (PETG) *n*-heptane 49° for 10 days
Sample size	120 cm^2 for 20 mL extractant	60 cm^2 20 mL	Entire bottle 90% full
Blank	H_2O	Not specified	H_2O
Nonvolatile residue	< 15 mg	< 12 mg H_2O < 75 mg for ETOH < 100 mg for hexane-PE < 350 mg for hsexane-HDPE	No test
Residue on ignition	< 5 mg	No test	No test
Heavy metals	< 1 ppm in 10 min	Same as plastics	Same as plastics
Buffering capacity	NMT 10 mL >blank	No test	No test
Multiple internal reflectance	No test	Same as USP std.LDPE or HDPE	Same as USP std. of PET or PETG
Thermal analysis	No test	Same as USP stds. endotherm and exotherm units – 6° (HDPE), and 8° (LDPE)	Same as USP stds. endo and exo limits—9((PET), none for PETG, glass transition within 4° (PET), 6° (PETG)
Light transmission	No test	Meets requirements under "*Light Transmission.*"	Same as PE
Water vapor permeation	No test	HDPE—NMT 1 of 10 > 10 mg None > 25 mg LDPE—NMT 1 of 10 > 20 mg None > 30 mg.	Tight if: NMT 1 of 10 > 100 mg/d/L: none > 200 mg
Total terephthaloyl moieties	N/A	N/A	<1 ppm ETOH + heptane
Ethylene glycol	N/A	N/A	< 1 ppm

Note: All temperatures are °C.

Table 18 Examples of Packaging Concerns for Common Classes of Drug Products

Degree of concern associated with the route of administration	Likelihood of packaging of component—dosage form interaction		
	High	Medium	Low
Highest	Inhalation aerosols Injectables	Sterile powders Injection	
High	Ophthalmic solutions Transdermal patches Nasal aerosols		
Low	Topical solutions Oral solutions	Topical powders Oral powders	Oral tablets Capsules

The regulatory authorities in the United States have issued interim guidelines for the interchangeability of blister packaging materials. The initial suggested criterion for consideration is:

> "a change in container closure system of unit dose packaging (blisters) for non-sterile solid dosage forms is permitted as long as the new package provides the same or better protective properties and any new primary packaging component materials have been used in and been in contact with CDER approved products of the same type." Examples of packaging concerns for common classes of drug products are listed in Table 18.

X. IN SUMMARY

Packaging of pharmaceutical dosage forms and medical devices have many requirements in common with other commercial products. Package design must address the finished products' needs, including:

Physical and chemical properties of the product
Deteriorating factors in the environment
Process requirements
Package machine operation
Storage and distribution requirements
Distribution flow and timing
Methods of distribution

Successful packaging can be achieved when all factors in the system are addressed adequately.

REFERENCES

1. F. R. Bacon. Glass Indust., 49, 438 (1968).
2. *The United States Pharmacopeia*, 24th Revision. United States Pharmacopeial Convention, Inc., Rockville, MD, 2000.
3. S. J. Borchert, M. M. Ryan, R. L. Davison and W. Speed. J. Parenter. Sci. Technol., 43, 67, 1989.
4. Glass containers for small volume parenteral products: Factors for selection and test methods for identification. Parenteral Drug Association Inc., Technical Methods Bulletin No. 3, 1982.
5. S. J. Borchert and R. J. Maxwell. ESCA depth profiling studies of borosilicate glass containers. J. Sci. Technol., 44, 154, 1990.
6. Elastomeric closures: Evaluation of significant performance and identity characteristics. Parenteral Drug Association Inc. Technical Methods Bulletin No. 2.
7. Extractables from elastomeric closures: Analytical procedures for functional group characterization/identification. Parenteral Drug Association Inc. Technical Methods Bulletin No. 1.
8. C. J. Milano and L. Bailey. Evaluation of current compendial physiochemical test procedures for pharmaceutical elastomeric closures and development of an improved HPLC procedure. J. Parenter. Sci. Technol., 53, 202 (1999).
9. D. K. Morton and N. G. Lordi, J. Parenter. Sci. Technol., 42, 57 (1988).
10. L. IIlum and H. Bundgaard. Sorption of drugs by plastic infusion bags. Int. J. Pharm., 10, 339 (1982).
11. D. K. Morton, N. G. Lordi and T. J. Ambrosio. Quantitative and mechanistic measurements of container/closure integrity: leakage quantitation. J. Parenter. Sci. Technol., 43, 88 (1989).
12. R. W. Jahnke, J. Kreutner and G. Ross. Content/container interactions: phenomenon of haze formation on reconstitution of solids for parenteral use. Int. J. Pharm., 77, 47 (1991).
13. H. Vromans and J. A. Van Laarhoven. Study on water permeation through rubber closures of injection vials. Int. J. Pharm., 79, 301 (1992).
14. I. Jagnandan, H. Daun, T. J. Ambrosio and S. G. Gilbert. Isolation and identification of 3,3,5,5-tetrabis(tert-butyl) stilbenequinone from polyethylene closures containing titanium dioxide and butylated hydroxy toluene. J. Pharm. Sci., 68, 916 (1979).

15. Effects of gamma irradiation on elastomeric closures. Technical Report No. 16. Parenter. Sci. Technol., 50, 1 (1992).
16. G. Erickson. Paperboard cartons: more than just boxes. Pharm. Med. Packaging News, 6, 32 (1998).
17. FDA, Title 21 of Code of Federal Regulations (CFR).211.132, 1990.
18. E. Swain. Senior friendly blisters. Pharm. Med. Packaging. News, 8, 16 (2000).
19. H. Forcino. Child resistant closures: Do you pass the test? Pharm. Med. Packaging News, 4, 41 (1996).
20. D. L. Smith. Compliance packaging: A patient education tool. Am. Pharm. NS, 29, 42 (1989).
21. D. Allen. Compliance packages recognized for excellence. Pharm. Med. Packaging News, 8, 10 (2000).
22. H. Liu. Classifications of PVC for pharmaceutical blister packaging using pattern recognition techniques. Ph.D. dissertation, Rutgers University, New Brunswick, NJ, 1998.
23. T. Mundry, T. Schurreit and P. Surmann. The fate of silicone oil during heat-curing glass siliconization—changes in molecular parameters analyzed by size exclusion and high temperature gas chromatography. J. Parenter. Sci. Technol., 54, 383 (2000).
24. Elastomeric closures: Evaluation of significant performance and identity characteristics. Parenteral Drug Association Inc., Technical Methods Bulletin No. 2.
25. D. Allen. High barrier materials for blister packaging. Pharm. Med. Packaging News, 8, 37 (2000).
26. Pharmacopeial Forum 26:481, 803 (2000).

Chapter 18

Optimization Techniques in Pharmaceutical Formulation and Processing

Joseph B. Schwartz

Philadelphia College of Pharmacy, Philadelphia, Pennsylvania

Robert E. O'Connor

Pharmaceutical Sourcing Group Americas, a division of Ortho-McNeil Pharmaceutical, Bridgewater, New Jersey

Roger L. Schnaare

Philadelphia College of Pharmacy, Philadelphia, Pennsylvania

I. INTRODUCTION

A significant portion of this book is devoted to the concepts involved in formulating drug products in their various forms. Physical, chemical, and biological properties all must be given due consideration in the selection of components and processing steps for that dosage form. The final product must be one that meets not only the requirements placed on it from a bioavailability standpoint, but also the practical mass production criteria of process and product reproducibility. In the current regulatory climate, formulation and process justification is a requirement for preapproval inspections for all new drug applications. In fact, development reports for both formulation and process are reviewed during these inspections. It is in the best interest of the pharmaceutical scientist to understand the theoretical formulation and target processing parameters, as well as the ranges for each excipient and processing parameter. Optimization techniques provide both a depth of understanding and an ability to explore and defend ranges for formulation and processing factors. With a rational approach to the selection of the several excipients and manufacturing steps for a given product, one qualitatively selects a formulation. It is at this point that optimization can become a useful tool to quantitate a formulation that has been qualitatively determined. Optimization is not a screening technique.

The word "optimize" is defined as follows: to make as perfect, effective, or functional as possible [1]. The last phrase, "as possible," leads one immediately into the area of decisions making, since one might ask: (a) perfect by whose definition; (b) for what characteristics; and (c) under what conditions? The term "optimization" is often used in pharmacy relative to formulation and to processing, and one will find it in the literature referring to any study of the formula. In developmental projects, one generally experiments by a series of logical steps, carefully controlling the variables and changing one at a time until a satisfactory system is produced. If the experimenter had sufficient help or sufficient time, he or she would eventually perfect the formulation, but under the circumstances the "best" one is often simply the last one prepared. It is satisfactory, but how close is it to the optimum, and how does the experimenter know?

No matter how rationally designed, the trial-and-error method can be improved upon. It is the purpose of this chapter to discuss the general principles behind the techniques of optimization and to review the specific techniques that have been applied to pharmaceutical systems.

II. OPTIMIZATION PARAMETERS

A. Problem Types

There are two general types of optimization problem: constrained and unconstrained. Constraints are restrictions placed on the system by physical limitations or perhaps by simple practicality (e.g., economic considerations). In unconstrained optimization problems there are no restrictions. For a given pharmaceutical system one might wish to make the hardest tablet possible. The constrained problem, on the other hand, would be stated: make the hardest tablet possible, but it must disintegrate in less than 15 minutes.

Within the realm of physical reality, and most important in pharmaceutical systems, the unconstrained optimization problem is almost nonexistent. There are always restrictions that the formulator wishes to place or must place on a system, and in pharmaceuticals, many of these restrictions are in competition. For example, it is unreasonable to assume, as just described, that the hardest tablet possible would also have the lowest compression and ejection forces and the fastest disintegration time and dissolution profile. It is sometimes necessary to trade off properties, that is, to sacrifice one characteristic for another. Thus, the primary objective may not be to optimize absolutely (i.e., a maxima or minima), but to realize an overall pre selected or desired result for each characteristic or parameter. Drug products are often developed by teaching an effective compromise between competing characteristics to achieve the best formulation and process within a given set of restrictions.

An additional complication in pharmacy is that formulations are not usually simple systems. They often contain many ingredients and variables, which may interact with one another to produce unexpected, if not unexplainable, results.

B. Variables

The development of a pharmaceutical formulation and the associated process usually involves several variables. Mathematically, they can be divided into two groups. The independent variables are the formulation and process variables directly under the control of the formulator. These might include the level of a given ingredient or the mixing time for a given process step. The dependent variables are the responses or the characteristics of the in-progress material or the resulting drug delivery system. These are a direct result of any change in the formulation or process.

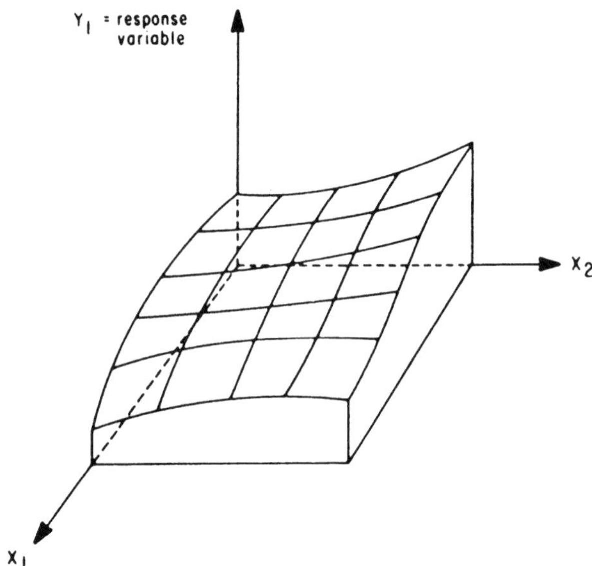

Fig. 1 Response surface representing the relationship between the independent variables X_1 and X_2 and the dependent variable Y_1.

The more variables one has in a given system, the more complicated becomes the job of optimization. But regardless of the number of variables, there will be a relationship between a given response and the independent variables. Once this relationship is known for a given response, it defines a response surface, such as that represented in Fig. 1. It is this surface that must be evaluated to find the values of the independent variables, X_1 and X_2, which give the most desirable level of the response, Y. Any number of independent variables can be considered; representing more than two becomes graphically impossible, but mathematically only more complicated.

III. CLASSIC OPTIMIZATION

Classic optimization techniques result from application of calculus to the basic problem of finding the maximum or minimum of a function. The techniques themselves have limited application, but they might be useful for problems that are not too complex and do not involve more than a few variables. The concept, however is important.

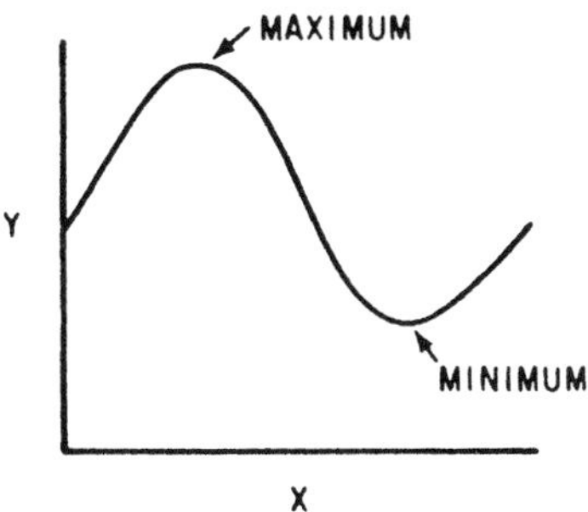

Fig. 2 Graphic location of optimum (maximum or minimum).

The curve in Fig. 2 might represent the relationship between a response Y and a single independent variable X in a hypothetical system, and since we can see the whole curve, we can pick out the highest point or lowest, the maximum or minimum. Use of calculus, however, makes the task of plotting the data or equation unnecessary. If the relationship, that is, the equation for Y as a function of X, is available [Eq. (1)]:

$$Y = f(X) \tag{1}$$

we can take the first derivative, set it equal to zero, and solve for X to obtain the maximum or minimum. For many functions of X, there will be more than one solution when the first derivative is set equal to zero. The various solutions may all be maxima or minima, or a mixture of both.

There are also techniques to determine whether we are dealing with a maximum or a minimum, that is, by use of the second derivative. And there are techniques to determine whether we simply have a maximum (one of several local peaks) or the maximum. Such approaches are covered in elementary calculus texts and are well presented relative to optimization in a review by Cooper and Steinberg [2].

When the relationship for the response Y is given as a function of two independent variables, X_1 and X_2,

$$Y = f(X_1, X_2) \tag{2}$$

the problem is slightly more involved. Graphically, there are contour plots (Fig. 3) on which the axes represent the two independent variables, X_1 and X_2, and the contours (analogous to elevations, as on a contour map) represent a specific level of Y. Again, we can select an optimum graphically. Mathematically appropriate manipulations with partial derivatives of the function can locate the necessary pair of X values for the optimum.

The situation with multiple variables (any more than two) becomes graphically impossible. It is still possible by mathematics, but very involved, making use of partial derivatives, matrices, determinants, and so on. The reader is referred to optimization texts for further details. Because of the complications involved and because the classic calculus methods apply basically to unconstrained problems, more practical methods are generally used.

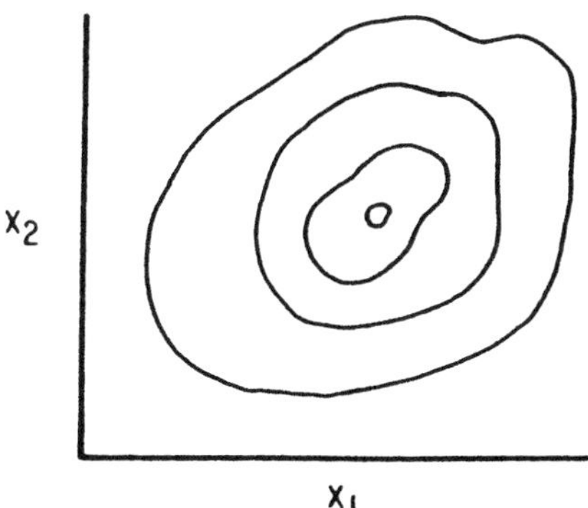

Fig. 3 Contour plot. Contours represent values of the dependent variable Y.

IV. STATISTICAL DESIGN

The techniques most widely used for optimization may be divided into two general categories: one in which experimentation continues as the optimization study proceeds, and another in which the experimentation is completed before the optimization takes place. The first type is represented by evolutionary operations and the simplex method, and the second by the more classic mathematical and search methods. (Each of these is discussed in Sec. V.)

For the techniques of the second type, it is necessary that the relation between any dependent variable and the one or more independent variables be known. To obtain the necessary relationships, there are two possible approaches: the theoretical and the empirical.

If the formulator knows a priori the theoretical equation for the formulation properties of interest, no experimentation is necessary. However, much of the work in pharmaceutics has been in the pursuit of such relationships, and to our knowledge most have not been determined. Therefore, it remains the task of the formulator to generate the relationships between the variables for the particular formulation and process.

In a text on experimental design, Davis states [3]:

> Theoretically, the behavior of chemical reactions, or for that matter the behavior of any system, is governed

> by ascertainable laws, and it should be possible to determine optimum conditions by applying such laws. In practice, however, the underlying mechanisms of the system are frequently so complicated that an empirical approach is necessary.

To apply the empirical or experimental approach for a system with a single independent variable, the formulator experiments at several levels, measures the property of interest, and obtains a relationship, usually by simple regression analysis or by the least-squares method. In general, however, there is more than one important variable, so the experimenter must enter into the realm of "statistical design of experiments and multiple linear regression analysis." Statistical design and multiple linear regression analysis are separate and rather large fields, and, again, the reader is referred to appropriate texts [3–5,40]. The concept of interest to the pharmacist planning to utilize optimization techniques is that there are methods available for selecting one's experimental points so that (a) the entire area of interest is covered or considered, and (b) analysis of the results will allow separation of variables (i.e., statistical analysis can be performed, which allows the experimenter to know which variable caused a specific result).

One of the most widely used experimental plans is that of the factorial design, or some variation of it (two of the techniques in the following section utilize it). By multiple regression techniques, the relationships between variables, then, are generated from experimental data, and the resulting equations are the basis of the optimization. These equations define the response surface for the system under investigation.

V. APPLIED OPTIMIZATION METHODS

There are many methods that can be, and have been, used for optimization, classic and otherwise. These techniques are well documented in the literature of several fields. Deming and King [6] presented a general flowchart (Fig. 4) that can be used to describe general optimization techniques. The effect on a real system of changing some input (some factor or variable) is observed directly at the output (one measures some property), and that set of real data is used to develop mathematical models. The responses from the predictive models are then used for optimization. The first two methods discussed here, however, omit the mathematical-modeling step; optimization is based on output from the real system.

A. Evolutionary Operations

One of the most widely used methods of experimental optimization in fields other than pharmaceutical technology is the evolutionary operation (EVOP). This technique is especially well suited to a production situation. The basic philosophy is that the production

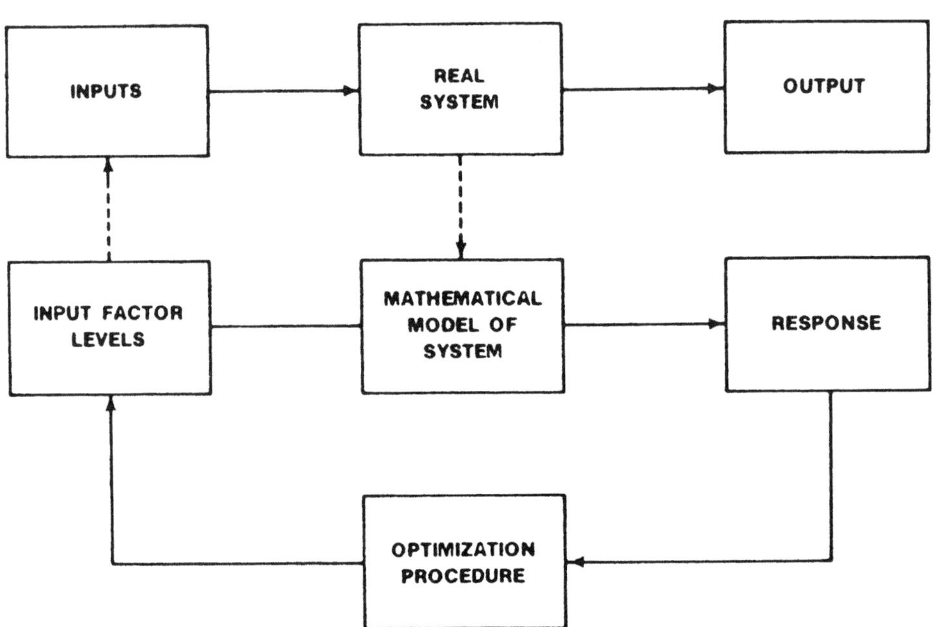

Fig. 4 Flowchart for optimization.

procedure (formulation and process) is allowed to evolve to the optimum by careful planning and constant repetition. The process is run in a way such that it both produces a product that meets all specifications and (at the same time) generates information on product improvement.

By this method the experimenter makes a very small change in the formulation or process but makes it so many times (i.e., repeats the experiment so many times) that he or she can determine statistically whether the product has improved. If it has, the experimenter makes another change in the same direction many times and notes the results. This continues until further changes do not improve the product or perhaps become detrimental. The experimenter then has the optimum—the peak.

In an industrial process, this large number of experiments is usually not a problem, since the process will be run over and over again. The application of this technique to tablets has been advocated by Rubinstein [7]. It has also been applied to an inspection system for parenteral products [8].

In most pharmaceutical situations, however, there is often insufficient latitude in the formula or process to allow the necessary experimentation. The pharmaceutical industry is subject to regulatory constraints that make EVOP impossible to employ in validated production processes and, therefore, impractical and expensive to use. Moreover, EVOP is not a substitute for good laboratory-scale investigation and, because of the necessarily small changes utilized, is not particularly suitable to the laboratory. In pharmaceutical development, more efficient methods are desired.

B. The Simplex Method

The simplex approach to the optimum is also an experimental method and has been applied more widely to pharmaceutical systems. Originally proposed by Spendley et al. [9], the technique has even wider appeal in areas other than formulation and processing. A particularly good example to illustrate the principle is the application to the development of an analytical method (a continuous flow analyzer) by Deming and King [6].

A simplex is a geometric figure that has one more point than the number of factors. So, for two factors or independent variables, the simplex is represented by a triangle. Once the shape of a simplex has been determined, the method can employ a simplex of fixed size or of variable sizes that are determined by comparing the magnitudes of the responses after each successive calculation. Figure 5 represents the set of simplex movements to the optimum conditions using a variable size technique.

The two independent variables (the axes) show the pump speeds for the two reagents required in the analysis reaction. The initial simplex is represented by the lowest triangle; the vertices represent the spectrophotometrie response. The strategy is to move toward a better response by moving away from the worst response. Since the worst response is 0.25, conditions are selected at the vortex, 0.6, and, indeed, improvement is obtained. One can follow the experimental path to the optimum, 0.721.

For pharmaceutical formulations, the simplex method was used by Shek et al. [10] to search for an optimum capsule formula. This report also describes the necessary techniques of reflection, expansion, and contraction for the appropriate geometric figures. The same laboratories applied this method to study a solubility problem involving butoconazole nitrate in a multicomponent system [11].

Bindschaedler and Gurny [12] published an adaptation of the simplex technique to a TI-59 calculator and applied it successfully to a direct compression tablet of acetaminophen (paracetamol). Janeczek [13] applied the approach to a liquid system (a pharmaceutical solution) and was able to optimize physical stability. In a later article, again related to analytical techniques, Deming points out that when complete knowledge of the response is not initially available, the simplex method is probably the most appropriate type [14]. Although not presented here, there are sets of rules for the selection of the sequential vertices in the procedure, and the reader planning to carry out this type of procedure should consult appropriate references.

C. The Lagrangian Method

This optimization method, which represents the mathematical techniques, is an extension of the classic method and was the first, to our knowledge, to be applied to a pharmaceutical formulation and processing problem. Fonner et al. [15] chose to apply this method to a tablet formulation and to consider two independent variables. The active ingredient, phenylpropanolamine HCl, was kept at a constant level, and the levels of disintegrant (corn starch) and lubricant (stearic acid) were selected as the independent variables, X_1 and X_2. The dependent variables include tablet hardness, friability, volume, in vitro release rate, and urinary excretion rate in human subjects.

This technique requires that the experimentation be completed before optimization so that mathematical

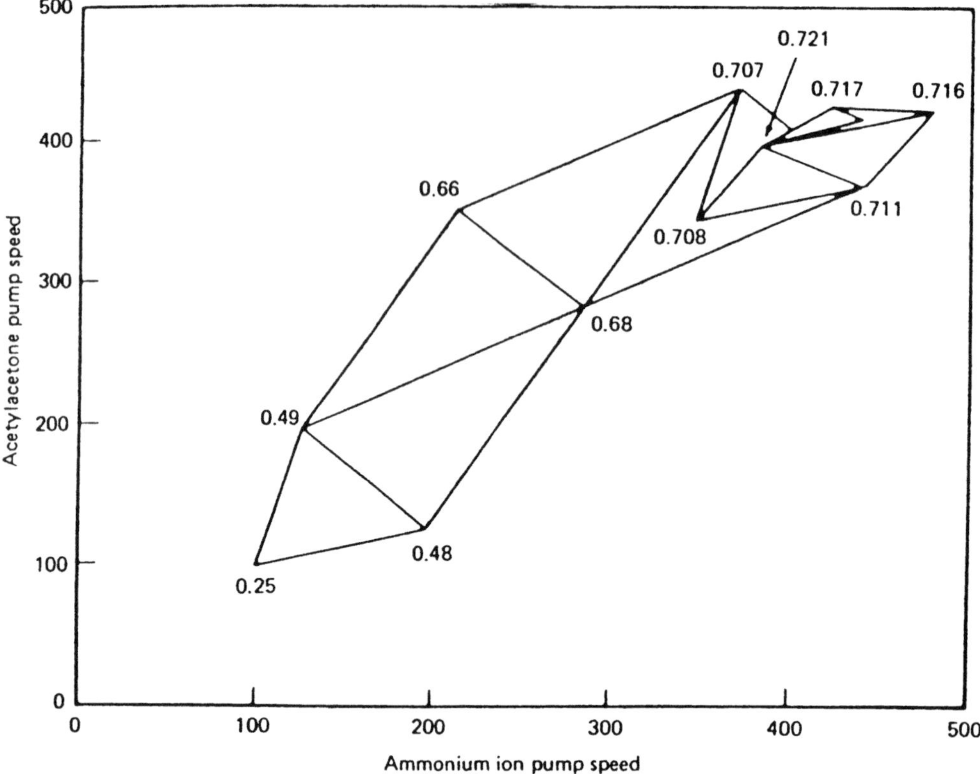

Fig. 5 The simplex approach to optimization. Response is spectrophotometric reading at a given wavelength. (From Ref. 6.)

models can be generated. The experimental design here was a full 3^2 factorial, and, as shown in Table 1, nine formulations were prepared. Polynomial models relating the response variables to the independent variables were generated by a backward stepwise regression analysis program. The analyses were performed on a polynomial of the form

$$y = B_0 + B_1X_1 + B_2X_2 + B_3X_1^2 + B_4X_2^2 + B_5X_1X_2 + B_6X_1X_2^2 + B_7X_1^2X_2 + B_8X_1^2X_2^2 \quad (3)$$

and the terms were retained or eliminated according to standard stepwise regression techniques. In Eq. (3), y represents any given response and B_i represents the regression coefficient for the various terms containing

Table 1 Tablet Formulations

	Ingredient per tablet (mg)			
Formulation no.	Phenylpropanolamine HCl	Dicalcium phosphate · $2H_2O$	Starch	Stearic acid
1	50	326	4 (1%)	20 (5%)
2	50	246	84 (21%)	20
3	50	166	164 (41%)	20
4	50	246	4	100 (25%)
5	50	166	84	100
6	50	86	164	100
7	50	166	4	180 (45%)
8	50	86	84	180
9	50	6	164	180

Source: Ref. 15.

levels of the independent variables. One equation is generated for each response or dependent variable.

A graphic technique may be obtained from the polynomial equations, as represented in Fig. 6. Figure 6a shows the contours for tablet hardness as the levels of the independent variables are changed. Figure 6b shows similar contours for the dissolution response, $t_{50\%}$. If the requirements on the final tablet are that hardness be 8–10 kg and $t_{50\%}$ be 20–33 min, the feasible solution space is indicated in Fig. 6c. This has been obtained by superimposing Fig. 6a and b, and several different combinations of X_1 and X_2 will suffice.

Slightly different constraints are used to illustrate the mathematical technique. In this example, the constrained optimization problem is to locate levels of stearic acid (X_1) and starch (X_2) that minimize the time of in vitro release (y_2) such that the average tablet volume (y_4) did not exceed 9.422 cm^2 and the average friability (y_3) did not exceed 2.72%.

To apply the Lagrangian method, this problem must be expressed mathematically as follows:

$$\text{Minimize } y_2 = F_2(X_1, X_2) \quad (4)$$

such that

$$y_3 = f_3(X_1, X_2) \leq 2.72 \quad (5)$$

$$y_4 = F_4(X_1, X_2) \leq 0.422 \quad (6)$$

and

$$5 \leq X_1 \leq 45 \quad (7)$$

$$1 \leq X_2 \leq 41 \quad (8)$$

Equations (7) and (8) serve to keep the solution within the experimental range.

The foregoing inequality constraints must be converted to equality constraints before the operation begins, and this is done by introducing a slack variable q, for each. The several equations are then combined into a Lagrange function F, and this necessitates the introduction of a Lagrange multiplier, λ, for each constraint.

Then, following the appropriate steps (i.e., partial differentiation of the Lagrange function) and solving the resulting set of six simultaneous equations, values are obtained for the appropriate levels of X_1 and X_2, to yield an optimum in vitro time of 17.9 mm ($t_{50\%}$). The solution to a constrained optimization program may depend heavily on the constraints applied to the secondary objectives.

oA technique called *sensitivity analysis* can provide information so that the formulator can further trade off one property for another. For sensitivity analysis the formulator solves the constrained optimization problem for systematic changes in the secondary objectives. For example, the foregoing problem restricted tablet friability, y_3, to a maximum of 2.72%. Figure 7 illustrates the in vitro release profile as this constraint is tightened or relaxed and demonstrates that substantial improvement in the $t_{50\%}$ can be obtained up to about 1–2%. Subsequently, the plots of the independent variables, X_1 and X_2, can be obtained as shown in Fig. 8. Thus the formulator is provided with the solution (the formulation) as he changes the friability restriction.

The several steps in the Lagrangian method can be summarized as follows:

1. Determine objective function.
2. Determine constraints.
3. Change inequality constraints to equality constraints.
4. Form the Lagrange function, F:
   a. One Lagrange multiplier λ for each constraint
   b. One slack variable q for each inequality constraint
5. Partially differentiate the Lagrange function for each variable and Set derivatives equal to zero.
6. Solve the set of simultaneous equations.
7. Substitute the resulting values into the objective functions.

Although many steps in the procedure may be carried out by computer, the application requires significant mathematical input from the person involved.

Buck et al. [16] expanded on the previous work and proposed that the statistical design technique can be incorporated into an overall management philosophy for proposed product design. The authors discussed four phases in this philosophy, which are defined as (a) a preliminary planning phase, (b) an experimental phase, (c) an analytical phase, and (d) a verification phase. They include case studies of a tablet design and a suspension design to illustrate the efficient and effective procedures that might be applied. Representation of such analysis and the available solution space is shown for the suspension in Figs. 9 and 10.

D. Search Methods

In contrast with the mathematical optimization methods, search methods do not require continuity or differentiability of the function—only that it be

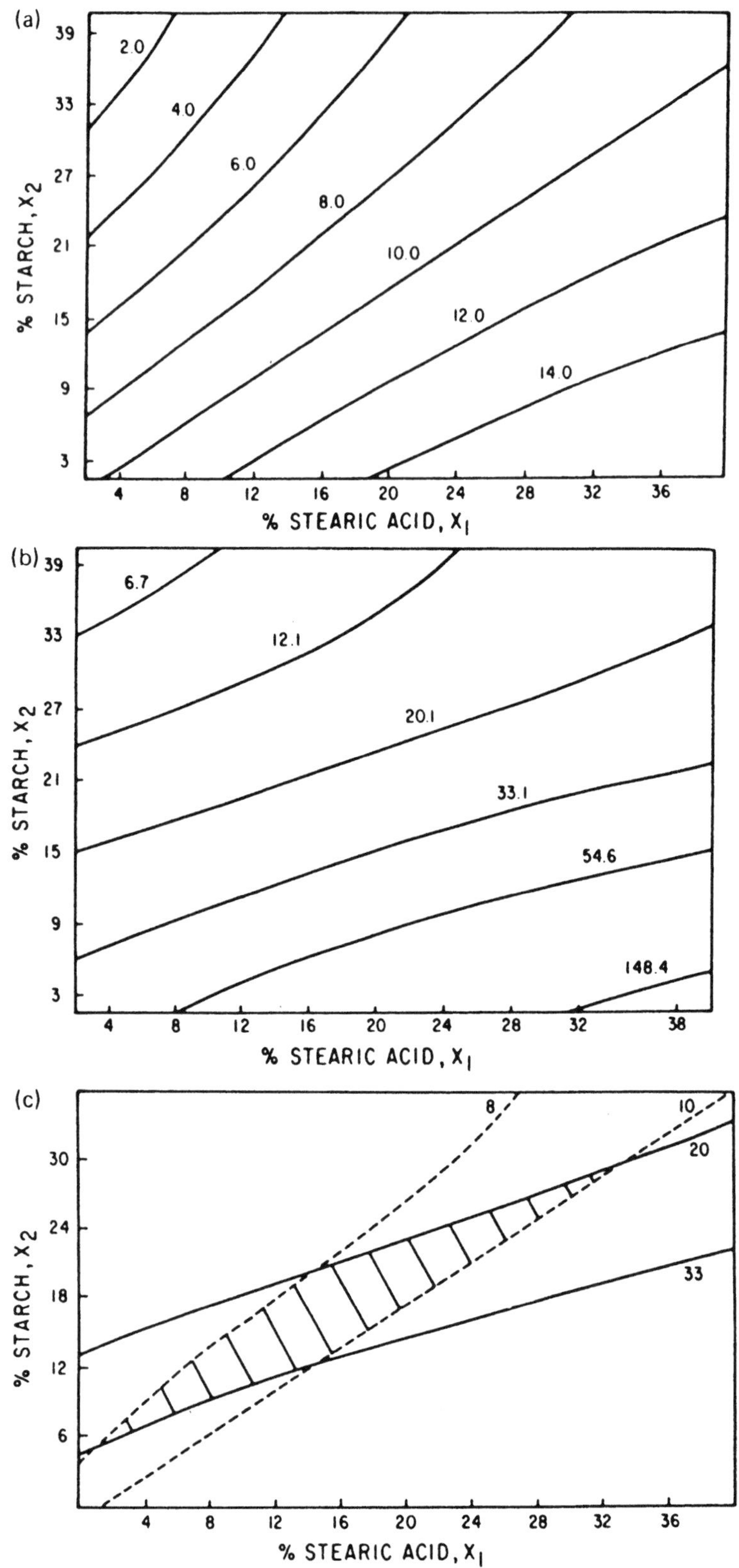

Fig. 6 Contour plots for the Lagrangian method: (a) tablet hardness; (b) dissolution ($t_{50\%}$); (c) feasible solution space indicated by crosshatched area. (From Ref. 15.)

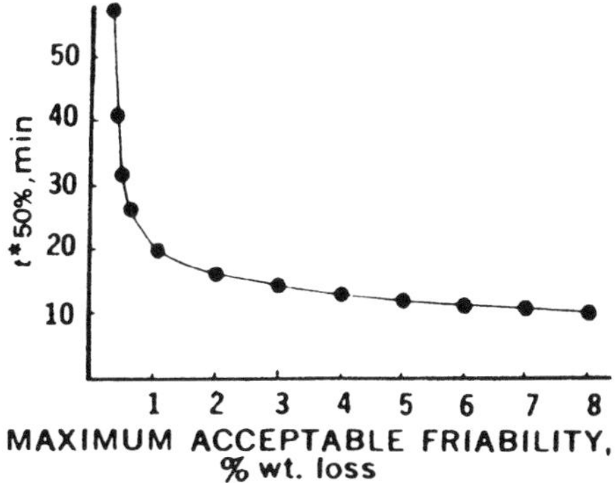

Fig. 7 Optimum in vitro $t_{50\%}$ release rate as a function of restrictions on tablet friability. (From Ref. 15.)

computable. In these methods the response surfaces, as defined by the appropriate equations, are searched by various methods to find the combination of independent variables yielding the optimum.

Although the Lagrangian method was able to handle several responses or dependent variables, it was generally limited to two independent variables. A search method of optimization was also applied to a pharmaceutical system and was reported by Schwartz et al. [17]. It takes five independent variables into

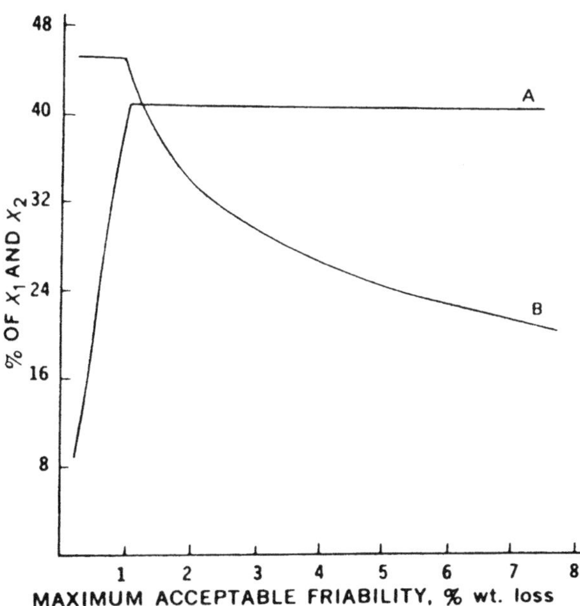

Fig. 8 Optimizing values of stearic acid and starch as a function of restrictions on tablet friability: (A) percent starch; (B) percent stearic acid. (From Ref. 15.)

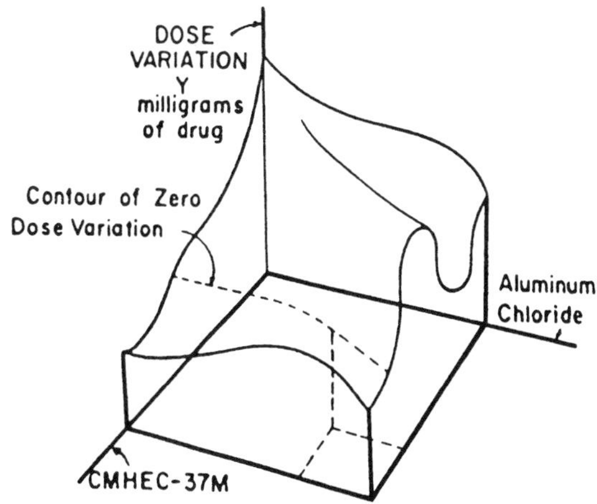

Fig. 9 Response surface concept and results of the second case study. (From Ref. 16.)

account and is computer-assisted. It was proposed that the procedure described could be set up such that persons unfamiliar with the mathematics of optimization and with no previous computer experience could carry out an optimization study.

The system selected here was also a tablet formulation. The five independent variables or formulation factors selected for this study are shown in Table 2. The dependent variables are listed in Table 3. Since each dependent variable is considered separately, any number could have been included.

The experimental design used was a modified factorial and is shown in Table 4. The fact that there are five independent variables dictates that a total of 27 experiments or formulations be prepared. This design is known as a five-factor, orthogonal, central, composite, second-order design [3]. The first 16 formulations represent a half-factorial design for five factors at two levels, resulting in $\frac{1}{2} \times 2^5 = 16$ trials. The two levels are represented by $+1$ and -1, analogous to the high and low values in any two-level factorial design. For the remaining trials, three additional levels were selected: zero represents a base level midway between the aforementioned levels, and the levels noted as 1.547 represent extreme (or axial) values.

The translation of the statistical design into physical units is shown in Table 5. Again the formulations were prepared and the responses measured. The data were subjected to statistical analysis, followed by multiple regression analysis. This is an important step. One is not looking for the best of the 27 formulations, but the

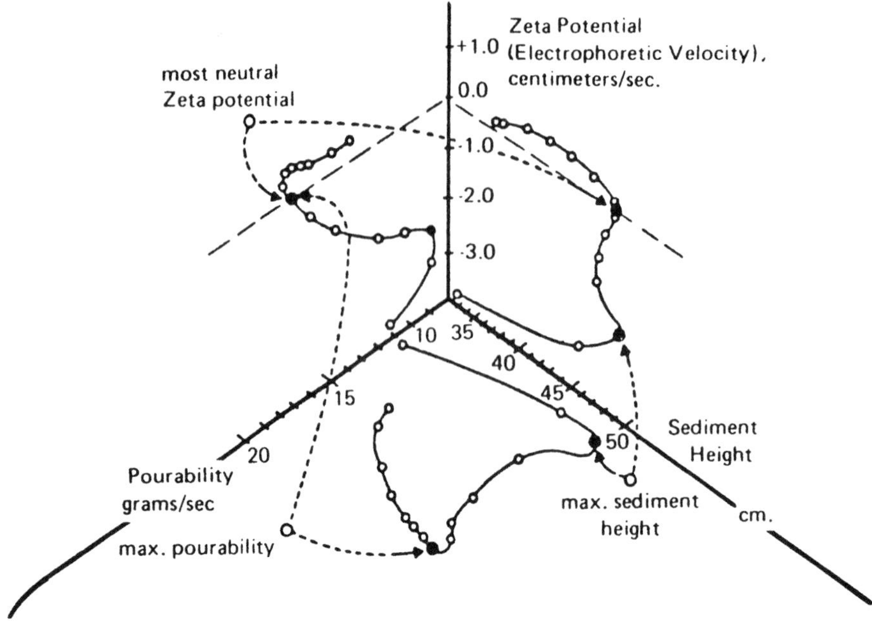

Fig. 10 Secondary properties of various suspensions yielding zero dose variation. (From Ref. 16.)

"global best." The type of predictor equation used with this type of design is a second-order polynomial of the following form:

$$Y = a_0 + a_1X_1 + \cdots + a_5X_5 + a_{11}X_1^2 + \cdots + a_{55}X_5^2 + a_{12}X_1X_2 + a_{13}X_1X_3 + \cdots + a_{45}X_4X_5 \quad (9)$$

Table 2 Formulation Variables (Independent)

X_1	Diluent ratio
X_2	Compressional force
X_3	Disintegrant level
X_4	Binder level
X_5	Lubricant level

Table 3 Response Variables (Dependent)

Y_1	Disintegration time
Y_2	Hardness
Y_3	Dissolution
Y_4	Friability
Y_5	Weight uniformity
Y_6	Thickness
Y_7	Porosity
Y_8	Mean pore diameter

where Y is the level of a given response, a_{ij} the regression coefficients for second-order polynomial, and X_i the level of the independent variable. The full equation has 21 terms, and one such equation is generated for each response variable. The usefulness of the equation is evaluated by the R^2 value, or the index of determination, which is an indication of the fit. In most cases the fit was satisfactory, and the equations were used. One possible disadvantage of the procedure as it is set up is that not all pharmaceutical responses will fit a second-order regression model. In fact, further analysis was attempted, and the results indicated that one of the responses was adequately described by a modified third-order model (inter-action terms were eliminated.) However, a significant advantage of the digital system utilized is that it can be modified to accept other mathematical models—another order polynomial, any other empirical relationship, or a mathematical model based on first principles.

For the optimization itself, two major steps were used: the feasibility search and the grid search. The feasibility program is used to locate a set of response constraints that are just at the limit of possibility. One selects the several values for the responses of interest (i.e., the responses one wishes to constrain), and a search of the response surface is made to determine whether a solution is feasible. For example, the constraints in Table 6 were fed into the computer and were relaxed one

Table 4 Experimental Design

Trial	Factor level in experimental units				
	X_1	X_2	X_3	X_4	X_5
1	−1	−1	−1	−1	1
2	1	−1	−1	−1	−1
3	−1	1	−1	−1	−1
4	1	1	−1	−1	1
5	−1	−1	1	−1	−1
6	1	−1	1	−1	1
7	−1	1	1	−1	1
8	1	1	1	−1	−1
9	−1	−1	−1	1	−1
10	1	−1	−1	1	1
11	−1	1	−1	1	1
12	1	1	−1	1	−1
13	−1	−1	1	1	1
14	1	−1	1	1	−1
15	−1	1	1	1	−1
16	1	1	1	1	1
17	−1.547	0	0	0	0
18	1.547	0	0	0	0
19	0	−1.547	0	0	0
20	0	1.547	0	0	0
21	0	0	−1.547	0	0
22	0	0	1.547	0	0
23	0	0	0	−1.547	0
24	0	0	0	1.547	0
25	0	0	0	0	−1.547
26	0	0	0	0	1.547
27	0	0	0	0	0

Source: Adapted from Ref. 17.

at a time until a solution was found. The first feasible solution was found at disintegration time = 5 min, hardness = 10 kg, and dissolution = 100% at 50 min: This program is designed so that it stops after the first possibility; it is not a full search. The formulation obtained may be one of many possibilities satisfying the constraints.

The next step, the grid search, is essentially a brute-force method in which the experimental range is divided into a grid of specific size and methodically searched. The method is called an exhaustive grid search. From an input of the desired criteria, the program prints out all points (formulations) that satisfy the constraints.

The purpose of the preliminary step of the feasibility program is simply to limit the number of solutions in the grid search. In addition to providing a printout of each formulation, the grid search program also gives the corresponding values for the responses. At this point, the experimenter can trade off one response for another, and the fewer possibilities there are, the easier the job. Thus, the best or most acceptable formulation is selected from the grid search printout to complete the optimization.

The two steps just discussed require that one or more responses be constrained, and a question may arise as to which ones to select. The formulator may have certain basic constraints, such as a minimum hardness value, but it is nevertheless important to know which property or properties can be used to distinguish between the available choices. Generally, this is done by an educated guess, based on experience with the system and with pharmaceutical systems in general.

Table 5 Experimental Conditions

Factor	−1.547 eu	−1 eu	Base 0	+1 eu	+1.547 eu
X_1 = Calcium phosphate/ lactose ratio (1 eu = 10 mg)	24.5/55.5	30/50	40/40	50/30	55.5/24.5
X_2 = compression pressure (1 eu = 0.5 ton)	0.25	0.5	1	1.5	1.75
X_3 = Corn starch disintegrant (1 eu = 1 mg)	2.5	3	4	5	5.5
X_4 = Granulaitng gelatin (1 eu = 0.5 mg)	0.2	0.5	1	1.5	1.8
X_5 = Magnesium stearate (1 eu = 0.5 mg)	0.2	0.5	1	1.5	1.8

Source: Ref. 17.

Table 6 Specifications for Feasibility Search

Variable	Constraint	Experimental range[a]
Disintegration time (min)	1(1)[b]	1.33–30.87
	3(2)	
	5(3)	
Hardness (kg)	12(1)[b]	3.82–11.60
	10(2)	
	8(3)	
Dissolution (% at 50 min)	100(1)[b]	13.30–89.10
	90(2)	
	80(3)	

[a]It is possible to request values for a response that are more desirable than any data obtained in the set of 27 experiments.
[b](1) = first choice.

However, there is a mathematical method for selecting those variables that best distinguish between formulations—those variables that change most drastically from one formulation to another and that should be the criteria on which one selects constraints. A multivariate statistical technique called *principal component analysis* (PCA) can effectively be used to answer these questions. PCA utilizes a variance-covariance matrix for the responses involved to determine their interrelationships. It has been applied successfully to this same tablet system by Bohidar et al. [18].

In addition to the programs to select the optimum discussed previously, graphic approaches are also available and graphic output is provided by a plotter from computer tapes. The output includes plots of a given response as a function of a single variable (Fig. 11) or as a function of all five variables (Fig. 12). The abscissa for both types is produced in experimental units, rather than physical units, so that it extends from −1.547 to +1.547 (see Table 5). Use of the experimental units allows the superpositioning of the single plots (see Fig. 11) to obtain the composite plots (see Fig.12).

An infinite number of these plots is possible, since for each curve represented, four of the five variables must remain constant at some level. This is analogous to a partial derivative situation, and the slope of any one graph does indeed represent a partial derivative of the response for one of the independent variables. It will change, depending on the level of the other four variables.

Contour plots (Fig. 13) are also generated in the same mariner. The specific response is noted on the graph, and, again, the three fixed variables must be held at some desired level. For the contour plots shown, both axes are in experimental units (eu). This technique is automated so that a formulator with no previous computer experience and no familiarity with the mathematics of optimization can follow the steps necessary to complete such a study. Those steps may be summarized as follows:

1. Select a system.
2. Select variables:
   a. Independent
   b. Dependent
3. Perform experiments and test product.
4. Submit data for statistical and regression analysis.
5. Set specifications for feasibility program.
6. Select constraints for grid search.
7. Evaluate grid search printout.
8. Request and evaluate:.
   a. "Partial derivative" plots, single or composite
   b. Contour plots

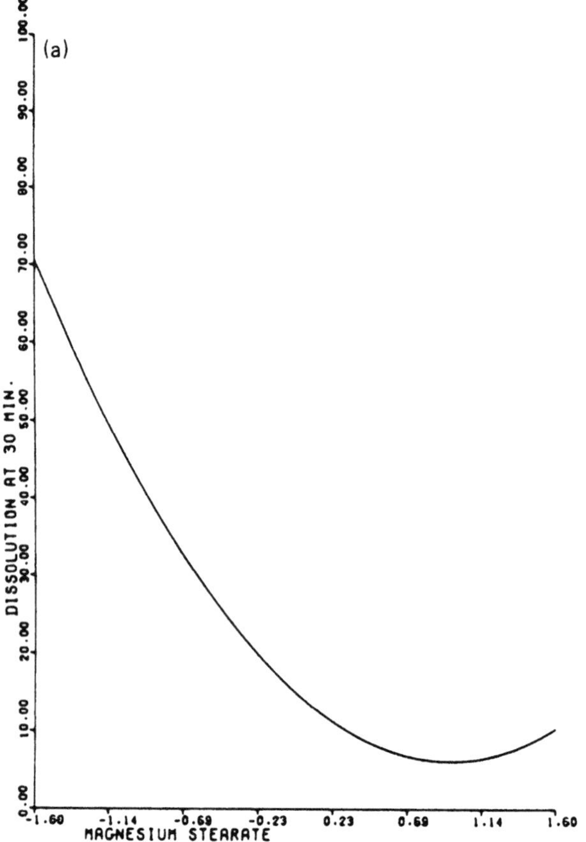

Fig. 11 Computer-generated plots for a single variable.

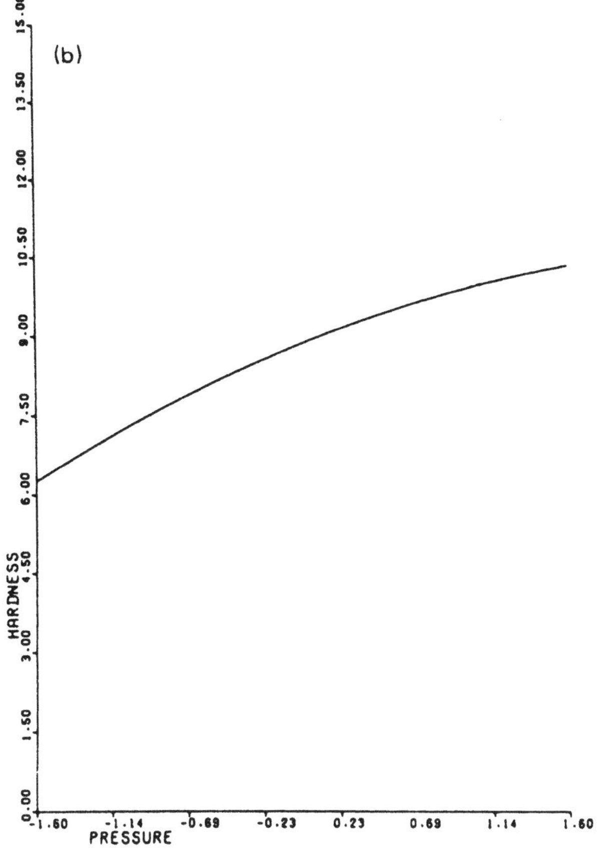

Fig. 11 (continued).

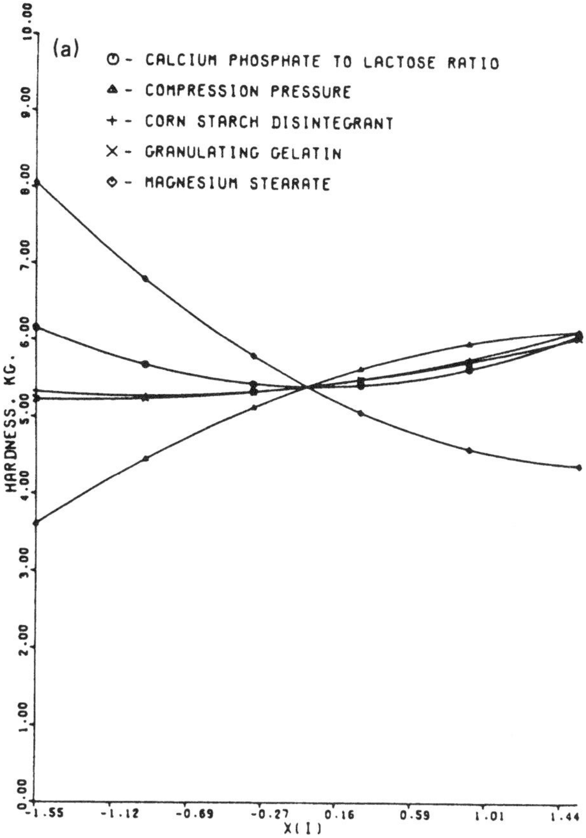

Fig. 12 Computer-generated composite plots.

The last step, which concerns the graphic techniques, may be requested at any time after the regression analysis has been performed and will probably be appropriate at several different stages of a project.

The key to successful application of the experimental optimization techniques is based on adequate experimental design. A system based on this experimental design (see Table 4), but utilizing a special analog computer for analysis, was presented by Claxton [19] as the Firestone Computer/Optimizer.

This approach demonstrates that use of only a part of this procedure will represent a step forward over the trial-and-error method of formula and process modification. It is not always necessary to carry these studies to completion. For example, once the designed experimentation has been completed, one might be able to accomplish the task simply by analyzing the graphs; therefore, further mathematical treatment or search programs will not be necessary. Some of the examples in the following section illustrate this fact.

E. Canonical Analysis

Canonical analysis, or canonical reduction, is a technique used to reduce a second-order regression equation, such as Eq. (9), to an equation consisting of a constant and squared terms, as follows:

$$Y = Y_0 + \lambda_1 W_1^2 + \lambda_2 W_2^2 + \lambda_3 W_3^2 + \cdots \tag{10}$$

The technique allows immediate interpretation of the regression equation by including the linear and interaction (cross-product) terms in the constant term (Y_0 or stationary point), thus simplifying the subsequent evaluation of the canonical form of the regression equation. The first report of canonical analysis in the statistical literature was by Box and Wilson [37] for determining optimal conditions in chemical reactions. Canonical analysis, or canonical reduction, was described as an efficient method to explore an empirical response surface to suggest areas for further experimentation. In canonical analysis or canonical reduction, second-order regression equations

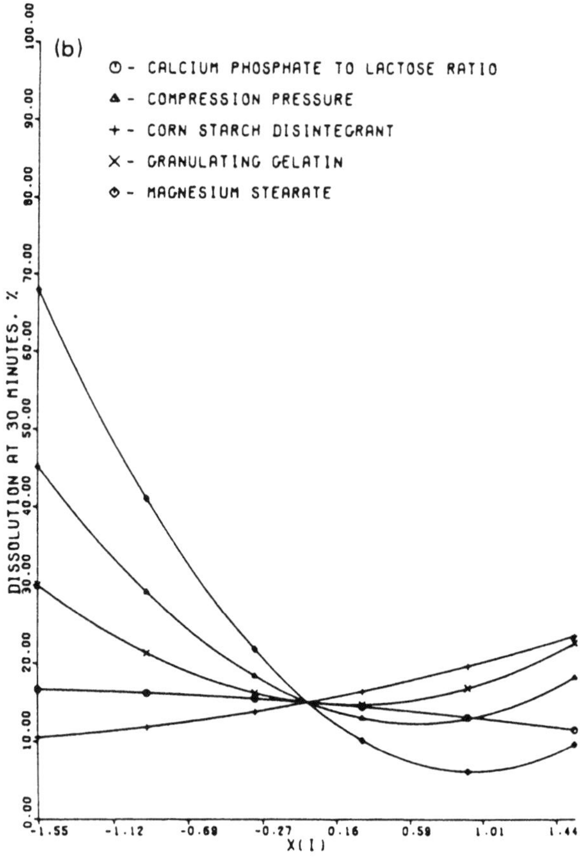

Fig. 12 (continued).

are reduced to a simpler form by a rigid rotation and translation of the response surface axes in multidimensional space, as shown in Fig. 14 for a two-dimension system. This mathematical technique, which makes use of eigenvalues and eigenvectors, is based in matrix algebra and is described in textbooks on response surface methodology [38,39].

A reported application of canonical analysis involved a novel combination of the canonical form of the regression equation with a computer-aided grid search technique to optimize controlled drug release from a pellet system prepared by extrusion and spheronization [28,29]. Formulation factors were used as independent variables, and in vitro dissolution was the main response, or dependent variable. Both a minimum and a maximum drug release rate was predicted and verified by preparation and testing of the predicted formulations. Excellent agreement between the predicted values and the actual values was evident for the four-component pellet system in this study.

VI. OTHER APPLICATIONS

In the last few years, optimization techniques have become more widely used in the pharmaceutical industry. Some of these have appeared in the literature, but a far greater number remain as "in-house" information, using the same techniques indicated in this chapter, but with modifications and computer programs specific to the particular company. An excellent review of the application of optimization techniques in the pharmaceutical sciences was published in 1981 [20]. This covers not only formulation and processing, but also analysis, clinical chemistry, and medicinal chemistry.

Designed experimentation, involving mostly some type or modification of factorial design, has been used to study many different types of formulation problems. These include a pharmaceutical suspension [21], a controlled-release tablet formulation [22], and a tablet-coating operation [23]. In the latter case, Dincer and Ozdurmus studied an enteric film coating and utilized the steepest descent graphic method to select the optimum.

Adaptation of the modified factorial techniques to desktop computers has also been accomplished [24, 25]. Down et al. [25] presented this concept and applied the programs to a tablet problem. The statistics involved were presented in some detail. A similar design was also used to study a high-performance liquid chromatography (HPLC) analysis [26]. In an unusual application, optimization techniques were even used to study the formulation of a culture medium in the field of virology [27].

Other applications of the previously described optimization techniques are beginning to appear regularly in the pharmaceutical literature. A literature search in *Chemical Abstracts* on process optimization in pharmaceuticals yielded 17 articles in the 1990–1993 time-frame. An additional 18 articles were found between 1985 and 1990 for the same narrow subject. This simple literature search indicates a resurgence in the use of optimization techniques in the pharmaceutical industry. In addition, these same techniques have been applied not only to the physical properties of a tablet formulation, but also to the biological properties and the in-vivo performance of the product [30,31]. In addition to the usual tablet properties the authors studied the following pharmacokinetic parameters: (a) time of the peak plasma concentration, (b) lag time, (c) absorption rate constant, and (d) elimination rate constant. The graphs in Fig. 15 show that for the drug hydrochlorothiazide, the time of the plasma peak and the absorption rate constant could, indeed, be

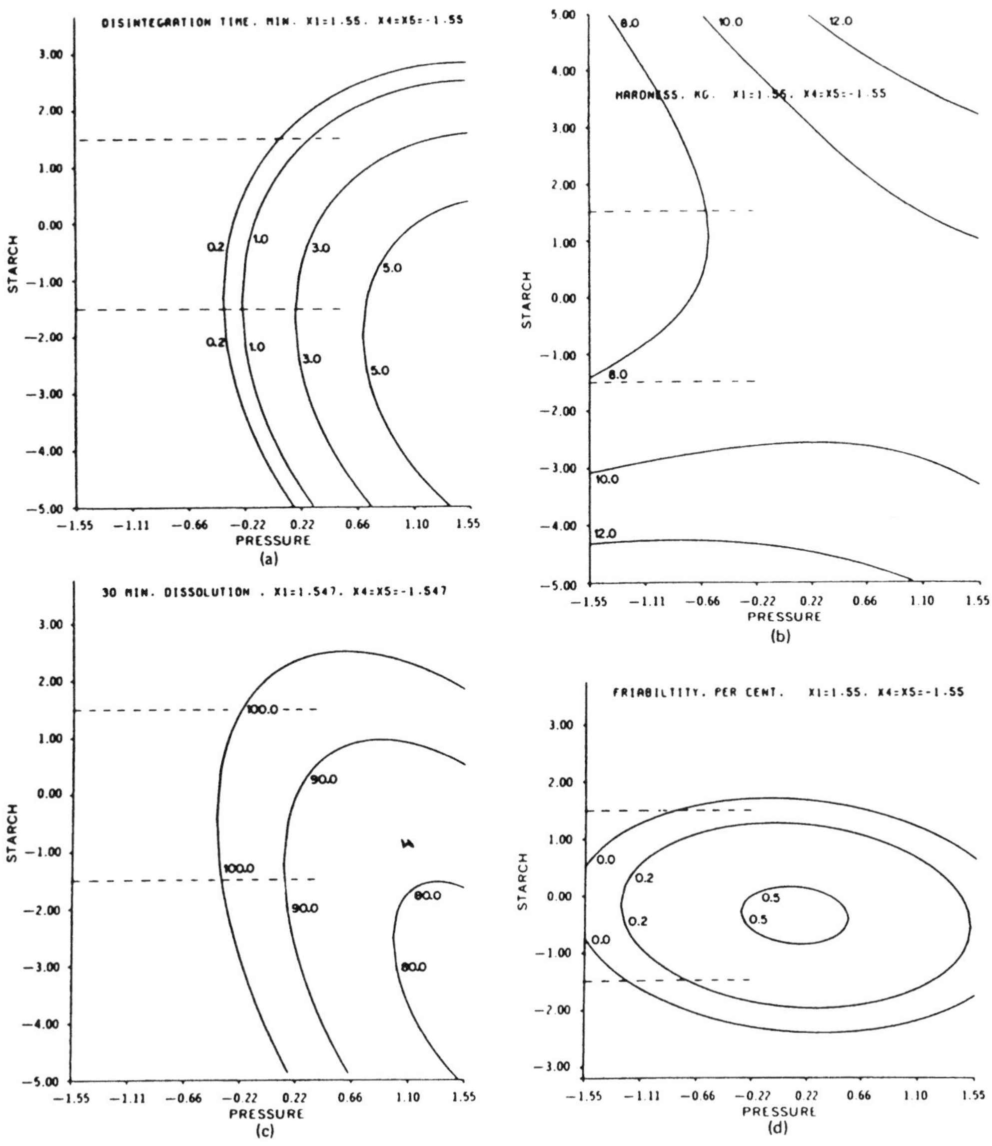

Fig. 13 Contour plots for (a) disintegration time; (b) tablet hardness; (c) dissolution response (%); (d) tablet friability as a function of disintegrant level and compressional force. Dashed lines on ordinate denote limits of experimental range (−1.547 to +1.547 eu; see text for details).

controlled by the formulation and processing variables involved.

VII. COMPUTERS AND SYSTEMS

It is obvious that the use of computers will facilitate the data analysis steps in the procedures discussed and will be needed for any mathematical analysis or search methods. In fact, a textbook has appeared describing the practical application of computer-aided optimization and provides direction for the implementation of these techniques to formulation [41]. Most of the examples presented have made use of computers in some way, and a few were completely performed by computer.

Several companies have adapted these experimental analysis techniques to computer software, but have kept the programs in-house. Representatives of a few

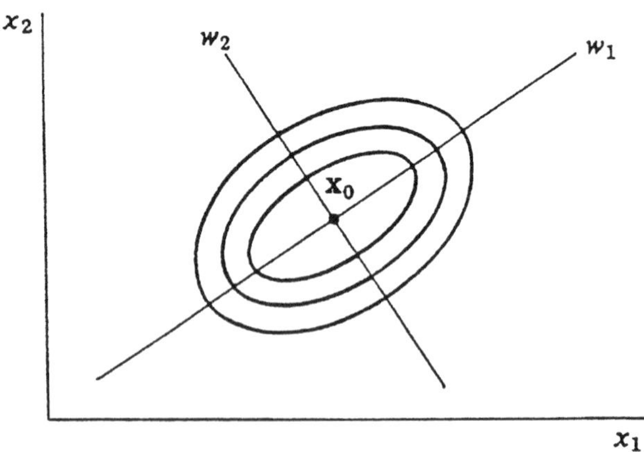

Fig. 14 Two-dimensional representation of the rigid rotation and translation involved in canonical analysis.

have, in fact, presented data at various conferences [24,32–34]. However, there are several commercially available programs that may be bought or licensed and several courses in experimentation address this subject.

The interested reader might be alerted to courses offered by the American Chemical Society, Dupont Corporation, or the Foremost Corporation. Some of these programs offer the use of statistical or response surface software. Specific computer packages are also available through Statistical Analysis Systems (SAS), IBM, and RS/Discover (RS1), which are designed for mainframe computers. The number of software packages available for standard desk-top office computers is large and is expected to increase. Several software packages—eCHIP, XStat, JMP, and Design Expert—are commonly used in the pharmaceutical industry, but these titles do not provide a complete list of available programs.

VIII. CONCLUDING REMARKS

As the list of applications illustrates, the techniques of optimization are not limited to tablets or even to solids. Any dosage form and any process should be amenable to this type of experimentation and analysis. From the most simple formulation to the most complicated one, there are ingredient levels and processing steps that can be varied, and any information on the result of such variation should be useful to the formulator.

Properly designed experimentation and subsequent analysis can not only lead to the optimum or most desirable product and process, but, if carried far enough, can shed light on the mechanism by which the independent variables affect the product properties. There are appropriate statistical techniques involving the use of selective regression analysis by which such analyses can be carried out [35]. Because this technique answers the question, "What independent variables most affect each response studied?" the application to selection of critical formulation and processing variables is obvious. This could provide supporting statistical evidence for the identification of critical variables in today's regulatory environment.

By appropriate analysis and generation of model (regression) equations (which are continuous), the formulator is able to select not the best of the formulations experimentally prepared, but the best within an experimental range; the optimum may be a combination of ingredients that the formulator has never prepared (and might never think to prepare). In the 30 years since the techniques of optimization were introduced to the pharmaceutical literature, the number of published studies on delivery systems has grown exponentially. There are numerous examples of the use of design of experiments, related statistical analysis, response surface methodology, and other methods for optimization in the recent literature. In many cases the techniques are used to study the variables in a system, rather than make any major changes.

Franz et al. [42] reviewed these techniques completely, along with statistical screening techniques and other experimental methods, with an excellent list of publications. A few selected publications from the recent literature demonstrate the wide variety of formulation and processing problems to which these techniques can be applied and the varying methods selected for optimization.

Porter et al. [43] applied the method to study the process variables in the tablet-coating operation. Remon et al. [44] studied high shear granulation and microwave drying to minimize dust production along with other responses using design of experiments, specifically a central composite design. Pujari and Chandra [45] reported on riboflavin production, optimizing the culture growth media via Plackett-Burmann screening methodology followed by factorial design.

Wu et al. [46] used the approach of an artificial neural network and applied it to drug release from osmotic pump tablets based on several coating parameters. Gabrielsson et al. [47] applied several different multivariate methods for both screening and optimization applied to the general topic of tablet formulation: they included principal component analysis and

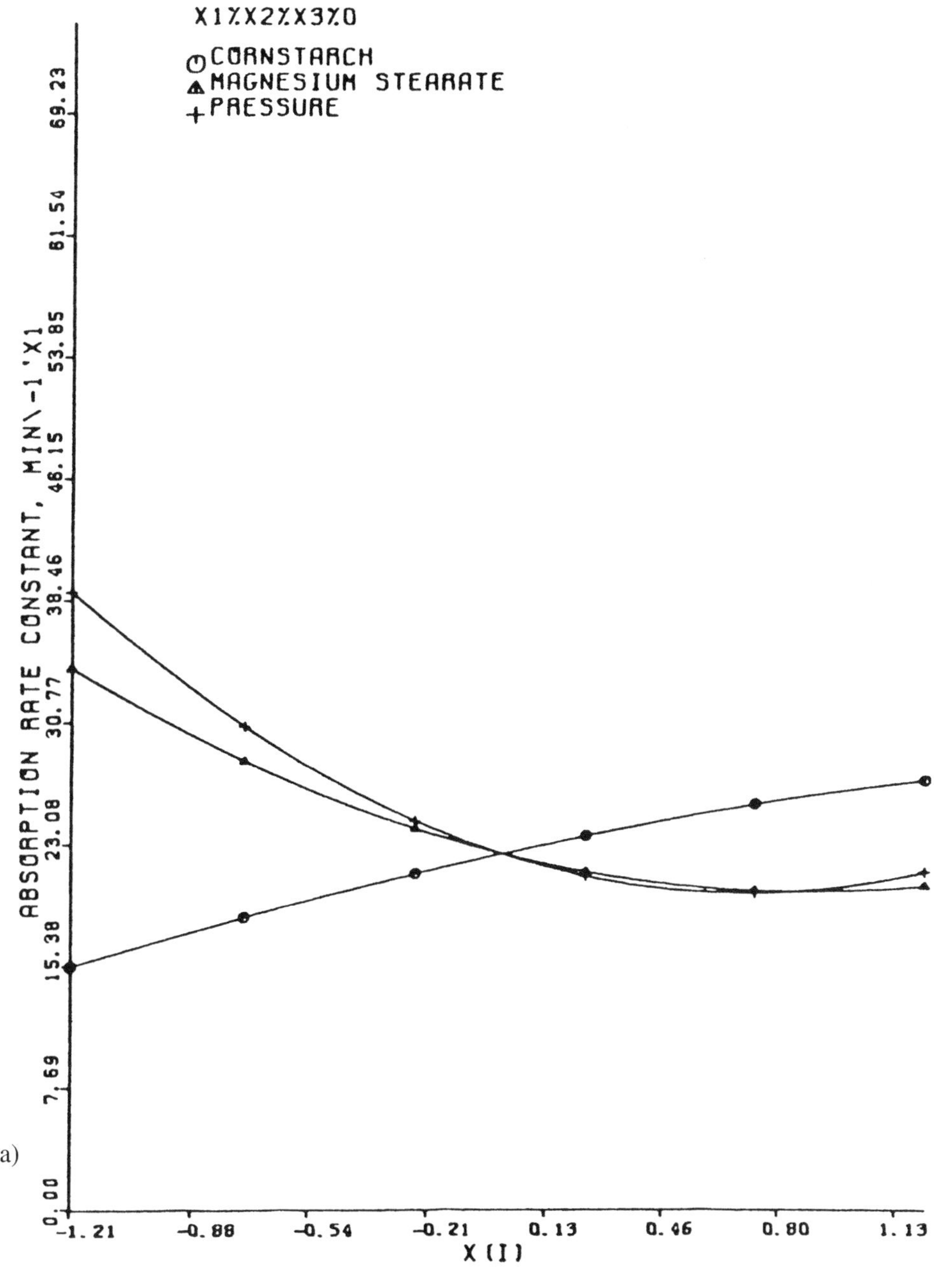

Fig. 15 Computer plots for (a) absorption rate constant and (b) time of plasma peak. (From Ref. 31.)

factorial design. Marti-Mestres et al. [48] studied submicron emulsions with sunscreens using simplex centroid design. Shiromani and Clair [49] performed a statistical comparison of high shear versus low shear granulation using a common formulation and a central composite design.

These techniques of optimization can be useful, even if selecting the optimum is not the primary objective. The formulator may have no intention of drastically changing a given formulation. Many times a very small change in processing or ingredient level can dramatically improve a particular property. The use of such information in "troubleshooting" situations has been demonstrated [36].

The independent variables have been, or should have been, selected by the formulator, and there is no substitute for experience. Experience with the system or with pharmaceutical systems in general can guide

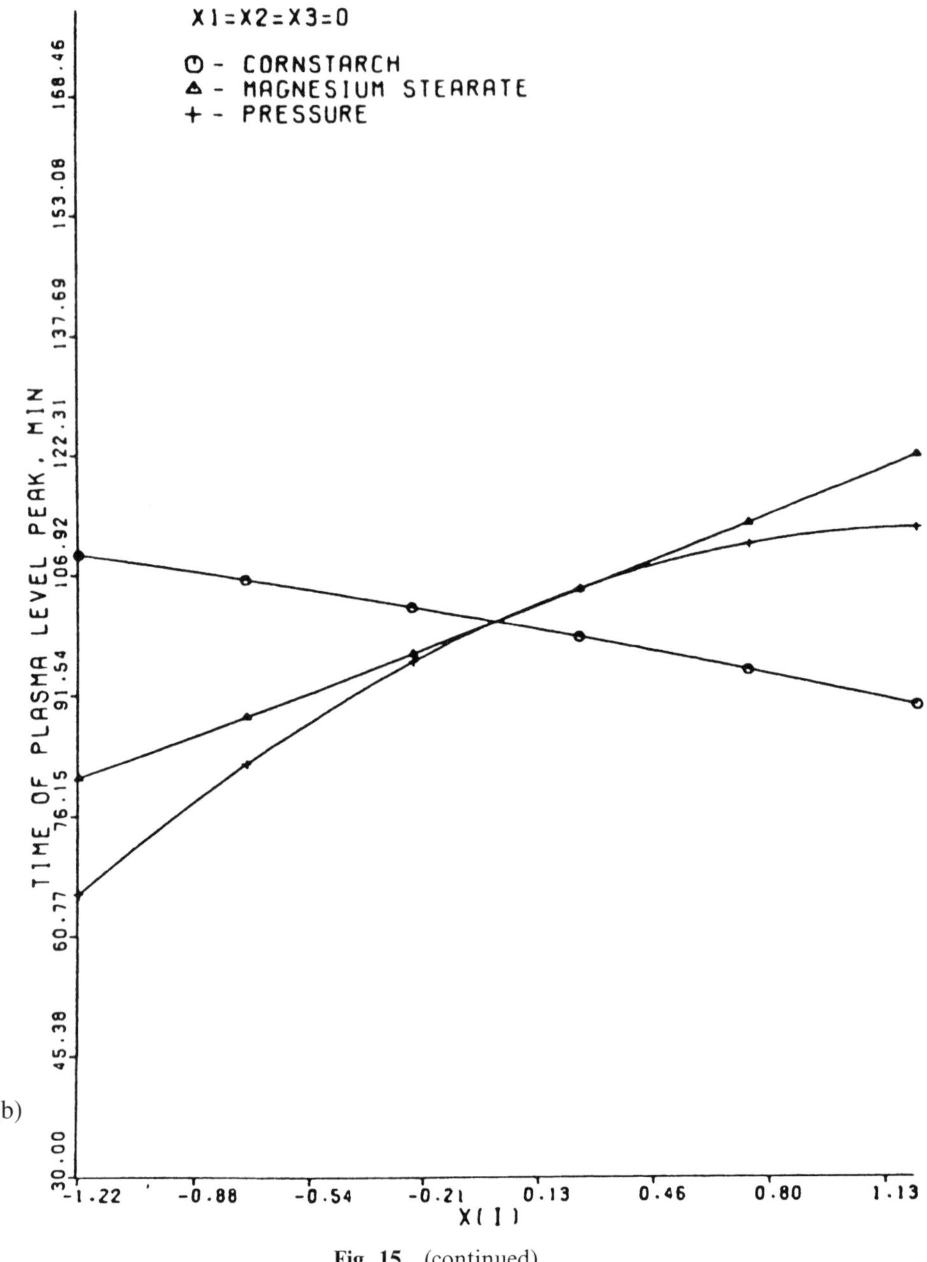

Fig. 15 (continued).

the formulator to select those variables most likely to have an effect on those levels which are most practical. The results of an optimization study, especially the graphic output, can give direction for product improvement—no matter why the improvement is necessary or desirable.

Once experimental data have been collected and relationships generated by regression analysis (or even derived from first principles), the formulator has many options available for subsequent analysis, These need not be restricted to mathematical techniques or to elaborate computerized systems.

A side benefit of this designed type of experimentation is its potential usefulness in product and process validation. The subject of validation is of great interest to those in the operations area, but if approached rationally, validation must begin in the product development phase. The designs usually selected lend themselves to the concept of processing limits and "challenge." The resulting data can be applied to scale-up, can aid in the transfer of information to the operations area, and should be the basis of the protocol design for validation.

The emphasis, once again, is that appropriate statistical design is an important consideration. For a formulator planning such a study, it should be noted that the independent variables can be anything that he or she can quantitate and control; and the dependent variables can be anything that he or she can quantitate. From the data resulting from the required number of experiments, one is able to generate a mathematical model to which the appropriate optimization technique is applied (e.g., graphic, mathematical, or the search method).

The final conclusion is the ultimate benefit: The more the formulator knows about a system, and the better that he or she can define it, the more closely it can be controlled.

REFERENCES

1. *Webster's New Collegiate Dictionary*, G. & C. Merriam, Springfield, MA, 1974.
2. L. Cooper and D. Steinberg, *Introduction to Methods of Optimization*, W. B. Saunders, Philadelphia, 1970.
3. O. L. Davis (ed.), *The Design and Analysis of Industrial Experiments*, Macmillan (Hafner Press), New York, 1967. [2nd ed., Longman, Harlow, Essex, England, 1978.]
4. W. G. Cochran and G. M. Cox, *Experimental Designs*, John Wiley & Sons, New York, 1957, Chap. 8A.
5. G. E. P. Box, W. G. Hunter, and I. S. Hunter, *Statistics for Experimenters: An Introduction of Data Analysis and Model Building*, John Wiley & Sons, New York, 1978.
6. S. N. Deming and P. G. King, Res./Dev., p. 22, May (1974).
7. M. H. Rubinstein, Manuf. Chem. Aerosol News, p. 30, Aug. (1974).
8. T. N. DiGaetano, Bull. Parenter. Drug Assoc., 29, 183 (1975).
9. W. Spendley, G. R. Hext, and F. R. Himsworth, Technometrics, 4, 441 (1962).
10. E. Shek, M. Ghani, and R. Jones, J. Pharm. Sci., 69, 1135 (1980).
11. S. T. Anik and L. Sukumar, J. Pharm. Sci., 70, 897 (1981).
12. C. Bindschaedler and R. Gurny, Pharm. Acta Helv., 57(9), 251 (1982).
13. D. Janeczek, M. S. thesis, Philadelphia College of Pharmacy and Science (1979).
14. S. L. Morgan and S. N. Deming, Anal. Chem., 46, 1170 (1974).
15. D. E. Fonner, Jr., J. R. Buck, and G. S. Banker, J. Pharm. Sci., 59, 1587 (1970).
16. J. R. Buck, G. E. Peck, and G. S. Banker, Drug Dev. Commun., 1, 89 (1974–75).
17. J. B. Schwartz, J. R. Flamholz, and R. H. Press, J. Pharm. Sci., 62, 1165 (1973).
18. N. R. Bohidar, F. A. Restaino, and J. B. Schwartz, J. Pharm. Sci, 64, 966 (1975).
19. W. E. Claxton, paper presented to the Industrial Pharmaceutical Technology Section, American Pharmaceutical Association, Academy of Pharmaceutical Sciences, San Francisco meeting, Mar. 1971.
20. D. A. Doornbos, Pharm. Weekbl. Sd. Ed., 3, 33 (1981).
21. J. L. O'Neill and R. E. Dempski, through J. Soc. Cosmet. Chem., 32, 287 (Sept./Oct. 1981).
22. M. Harris, J. B. Schwartz, and J. McGınity, Drug Dev. Intl. Pharm., (in press).
23. S. Dincer and S. Ozdurmus, S. Pharm. Sci., 66, 1070 (1977).
24. D. R. Savello. K. J. Koenig, K. R. Nelson, J. B. Schwartz, and C. G. Thiel, paper presented to the American Pharmaceutical Association, Academy of Pharmaceutical Sciences. Atlanta meeting. Nov. 1975.
25. G. R. B. Down. R. A. Miller, S. K. Chopra, and J. F. Millar, Drug Dev. Iid. Pharm. 6, 311 (1980).
26. M. L. Cotton and G. R. B. Down, J. Chromatogr., 259, 17 (1983).
27. E. M. Scattergood, J. B. Schwartz, M. O. Villarejos, W. J. McAleer, and M. R. Hilleman. Drug Dev. Ind. Pharm., 9, 745 (1983).
28. R. E. O'Connor, N. R. Bohidar, and J. B. Schwartz, Optimization by Canonical Analysis Applied to controlled Release Pellets, Abstracts of the 1st National AAPA Meeting. Washington, DC. Nov. 2–6, 1986.
29. R. E. O'Connor, The Drug Release Mechanism and Optimization of a Microcrystalline Cellulose Pellet System, Ph.D. dissertation, Philadelphia College of Pharmacy & Science, 1987.
30. A. N. Karabelas, R. W. Mendes, and J. B. Schwartz, paper presented to the Industrial Pharmaceutical Technology Section, American Pharmaceutical Association, Academy of Pharmaceutical Sciences, San Antonio meeting, Nov. 1980.
31. J. B. Schwartz, J. Soc. Cosmet. Chem., 32, 287, Sept/Oct. (1981).
32. A. R. Lewis and R. Poska, paper presented to the Midwest Regional IPT meeting, American Pharmaceutical Association, Academy of Pharmaceutical Sciences, May 1981.
33. D. R. Savello, Workshop presentation, American Pharmaceutical Association, Academy of Pharmaceutical Sciences, Las Vegas meeting, April 1982.
34. S. E. Brown, paper presented at RxPo Conference, New York, June 1984.
35. N. R. Bohidar, F. A. Restaino, and J. B. Schwartz, Drug Dev. Ind. Pharm., 5, 1975 (1979).
36. J. B. Schwartz, J. R. Flamholz, and R. H. Press, J. Pharm. Sci., 62, 1518 (1973).

37. G. E. P. Box and K. B. Wilson, S. R. Statist. Soc. Ser. B, (Methodological), 13, 1 (1954).
38. G. E. P. Box and N. R. Draper, *Empirical Model Building and Response Surfaces*, John Wiley & Sons, New York, 1987.
39. R. H. Myers, *Response Surface Methodology*, Allyn & Bacon, Boston, 1971.
40. D. G. Kleinbaum, L. L. Kupper, and K. E. Muller, *Applied Regression Analysis and Other Multi-variate Methods*, PWS-Kent, Boston, 1988.
41. A. H. Bohl (ed.), *Computer-Aided Formulation*, VCH, New York, 1990.
42. R. M. Franz, D. M. Cooper, J. E. Brown, and A. R. Lewis, in: *Pharmaceutical Dosage Forms: Disperse Systems*, Vol. 1, 2nd ed., Marcel Dekker, New York, 1996.
43. S. C. Porter, R. P. Verseput, and C. R. Cunningham, Pharm. Tech., 21(10), 60 (1997).
44. F. Kiekens, M. Cordoba-Diaz, and J. P. Remon, DDIP, 25(12), 1289 (1999).
45. V. Pujari and T. S. Chandra, Proc. Biochem., 36, 31 (2000).
46. T. Wu, W. Pan, J. Chen and R. Zhang, DDIP, 26(2), 211 (2000).
47. J. Gabrielsson, A. Nystrom, and T. Lundstedt, DDIP, 26(3): 275 (2000).
48. G. Marti-Mestres, F. Niellood, R. Fortune, C. Fernandez, and H. Maillols, Drug Dev. Ind. Pharm., 26(3), 349 (2000).
49. P. K. Shiromani and J. Clair, Drug Dev. Ind. Pharm., 26(3), 357 (2000).

Chapter 19

Food and Drug Laws that Affect Drug Product Design, Manufacture, and Distribution

Garnet E. Peck

School of Pharmacy, Purdue University, West Lafayette, Indiana

Rolland Poust

Pharmaceutical Services Division, College of Pharmacy, University of Iowa, Iowa City, Iowa

I. IMPACT OF THE FOOD AND DRUG LAWS

A. Historical Perspective: Effect of the 1906 Act on Drug Product Distribution

The establishment of a set of laws to control the purity of the food and drink offered to the public can be traced back in history to 1202, when King John of England issued the first English food law, which included the prohibition of the adulteration of bread with such ingredients as ground peas or beans [1]. The earliest history of food law in the United States occurred as follows:

1784	Massachusetts enacted the first general food law in the United States
1848	The Import Drugs Act—the first federal statute to ensure the quality of drugs—was passed when quinine used by American troops in Mexico to treat malaria was found to be adulterated
1850	California passed a pure food and drink law 1 year after the Gold Rush
1879–1905	During these 25 years, more than 100 food and drug bills were introduced into Congress
1879	Chief Chemist Peter Collier, Division of Chemistry, U.S. Department of Agriculture, began investigating food and drug adulteration; the following year he recommended enactment of a national food and drug law

Harvey Wiley, who became the chief chemist of the U.S. Bureau of Chemistry in 1883, is generally considered to be the father of the original U.S. pure food and drug laws. His life's work was concerned with food and drug adulteration. He not only championed the first Federal Food, Drug and Cosmetic Act, but he can also be considered the federal government's first strong consumer advocate [2]. In the eighteenth and nineteenth centuries in the United States, drugs of very dubious quality, as well as many quack or patent remedies that ranged from valueless, to harmful, to addicting, were distributed and sold totally without control.

In 1902 Congress passed the Biologics Control Act, which licensed and regulated the interstate sale of serums and vaccines used to prevent and treat diseases in humans. The effect of this would seem obvious because, after much discussion before the Committee on Interstate and Foreign Commerce, the final result was passage of the Federal Food, Drug, and Cosmetic Act of 1906 [2]. This bill was signed into law by President Theodore Roosevelt on June 30, 1906 [3]. The Meat

Inspection Act was also passed that same day. This was the result of shocking disclosures of unsanitary conditions in meatpacking plants. It is obvious that numerous problems did exist in the food and drug supply of the United States before the twentieth century. They were not simply centered around dangerous preservatives and dyes in, and adulteration of, foods and alcoholic beverages, as well as totally unfounded claims and worthless or dangerous patent medicines, but included problems in the total distribution and control of the safety, purity, and quality of all foods and drugs supplied to the public.

The next important drug-related law was the Caustic Poison Act of 1927, which required warning labels and antidotes on 10 dangerous or corrosive substances sold for household use [1]. As we reflect on the history of the food and drug laws, we find that changes came about because of accidents or improper use of substances in drug products or active agents being used without adequate testing. Selected and probably rare episodes of negligence on the part of a few pharmaceutical manufacturers led to new drug laws or amended laws. Both the 1938 law and the 1962 amendments were triggered in this manner. In 1937, a new wonder drug, sulfanilamide, was formulated into an elixir that contained ethylene glycol, rather than propylene glycol, with the result that at least 107 people died [4]. The resulting public outcry led, at least in part, to the major revision of the Federal Food, Drug, and Cosmetic Act the following year. This 1938 act contained the following new provisions [5]:

- Extended coverage to cosmetics and devices
- Required predistribution clearance for safety of new drugs
- Eliminated Sherley Amendment requirement to prove intent to defraud in drug-misbranding cases
- Provided for tolerances for unavoidable poisonous substances
- Authorized standards of identity, quality, and fill of container for foods
- Authorized factory inspections
- Added the remedy of court injunction to previous remedies of seizure and persecution

This revision not only concerned itself with new drug substances, but was extended to cosmetics and devices.

Trade associations and the compendia also played an important role in drug product control and quality during the nineteenth and twentieth centuries. The *United States Pharmacopeia* (USP) and *National Formulary* (NF) established standards of potency and purity for the most commonly used drugs and drug products. The first USP was issued in 1833 and the first NF was published in 1887 [6]. In the early 1900s two trade associations existed that were to benefit the industry and attempt to bring them together on common causes. These two trade associations were the American Drug Manufacturers Association and the American Pharmaceutical Manufacturers Association. In 1924 a committee was formed between these two organizations, which was known as the Contact Committee. This committee's purpose was to examine the need of the pharmaceutical industry for standards, tolerances, and test methodology for tablet and parenteral products [7]. This Contact Committee later formed the quality control section of the Pharmaceutical Manufacturers Association, which was the union of both original associations concerned with pharmaceutical manufacturing. This represented the industry's own attempts to better control the manufacture of drug products by establishing better standards and test methods. Standards were issued in a loose-leaf publication entitled *Pharmaceutical Standards Including Tolerances and Methods of Analyses*, first issued in 1924 and revised over the following 2 years to be more closely linked to the official compendia (USP and NF). The Contact Committee served as the sounding board for drug product quality for a number of years.

In 1940, the U.S. Food and Drug Administration (FDA) was transferred from the U.S. Department of Agriculture to the Federal Security Agency, after which the First Commissioner of Food and Drugs was named [1]. In 1945 the Food, Drug, and Cosmetic Act was amended to require the certification of the safety and efficacy of penicillin. The act has since been amended many times over the years to include all antibiotics and antibiotic products. The next major revision came in 1951 in the form of the Durham-Humphrey Amendment, which required the labeling of prescription items as follows: "Legend drugs may not be dispensed without a prescription from a physician, dentist, or other designated practitioner." In 1955, it was recommended that FDA expand its facilities to improve its educational and informational programs. Citizen input provided some of the impetus to have this done. In 1960 the color additive amendments were enacted, which allowed FDA to establish by regulations the conditions of safe use of color additives in foods, drugs, and cosmetics and to require manufacturers to perform the necessary studies to establish safety. As happened previously following a serious drug toxicity episode, new legislation passed in 1962, known as the Kefauver–Harris Drug Amendments, required a much greater degree of safety assurance and strengthened the new drug clearance procedures. This legislation was a result of the use of thalidomide in Western Europe, Canada, and, to a limited extent, the United States, on a clinical trial. This particular drug substance produced malformed babies when taken by pregnant women. However, it should be noted that the Pharmaceutical Manufacturers Association was also very active during this time in trying to improve the law. For example, in May 1961 they issued a document entitled *Principles of Control of Quality in the Drug Industry*. This combined the thoughts of many of the manufacturers and their concern over improving drug product quality [7]. From this point on, drugs and drug products for distribution in the United States were required to show clear evidence of safety, effectiveness, and high quality and to be manufactured by prescribed procedures—as regulated by law, but also as intended by the major drug manufacturers.

B. Functions and Organization of the Federal Food and Drug Administration

FDA was created to administer the Federal Food, Drug, and Cosmetic Acts and their various amendments. Currently, this agency functions within the U.S. Department of Health and Human Services. Figure 1 outlines the major divisions of FDA. As shown in the figure, the Commissioner has reporting to him or her a number of associate commissioners, who are responsible for various centers, which, in turn, have responsibility for the various types of products that currently come under FDA regulations. FDA also has several offices that are concerned with various functions of the agency. The Office of Regulatory Affairs, for example, is concerned with inspection of manufacturing facilities and assurance that they are adhering to that section of the regulations entitled Current Good Manufacturing Practices (GMPs). These manufacturing practices are summarized later in this chapter. Figures 2 and 3 give detailed outlines of the Centers for Drug Evaluation and Research, and Biologics Evaluation and Research, respectively, which are the FDA divisions having the greatest relevance to most pharmacists in their professional practice. These centers are the FDA divisions responsible for the approval of all new human prescription drugs marketed in the United States; the reevaluation of older drugs; and evaluation, approval, and control of over-the-counter (OTC) drugs (i.e., drugs sold without prescription); it is basically concerned with the regulation of the manufacture, distribution, and sale of all drugs involved in interstate commerce. The Center for Medical Devices and Radiological Health (see Fig. 1) has become more prominent in the regulatory area. As new regulations are promulgated to govern medical devices and diagnostic aids, this center will have an increasing impact on pharmacy practice, especially in the hospital field.

Figure 4 shows the functional units of the Center of Veterinary Medicine. Many pharmacy practitioners are also involved in the drugs controlled by this unit of FDA and may have occasion to communicate with it.

Figures 1–4 came from the FDA website (www.fda.gov). The names of the various directors listed in the table change with time, but the current directors can be identified at any time by visiting the website. The FDA website is very extensive and provides quick access to pharmacists and researchers on contemporary topics through *FDA News*, the FDA's news publication, or through such headings as current recalls, product alerts, and numerous other topics. Their massive A-to-Z index provides a comprehensive review of the many subjects covered. A complete chapter-by-chapter listing of all current regulations enforced by the U.S. FDA is provided together with pending regulations. All readers of this chapter are encouraged to make a quick visit to the website to develop a sense of the wide range of interesting and informative topics there, together with an appreciation of the site for drug information.

II. LAWS GOVERNING EVALUATION OF NEW DRUG PRODUCTS

A. Claimed Investigational Exemption for a New Drug

When the Federal Food, Drug, and Cosmetic Act of 1938 was passed, a new era of drug product development began. It was the beginning of a requirement for the preclearance of a drug product before it's marketing. The act required the assurance of safety and stated minimum requirements for manufacturing and quality control. It provided only 60 days for review by FDA before the distribution of any new drug product [8]. The 1962 Kefauver–Harris Amendments to the act required greatly increased information concerning the safety, effectiveness, manufacture, and controls of drug products [1]. For the first time it was also necessary for a drug firm or other organization interested in a new drug substance to inform FDA of the intent to test the drug in humans. The document to initiate a human study involving a new drug (which includes not only

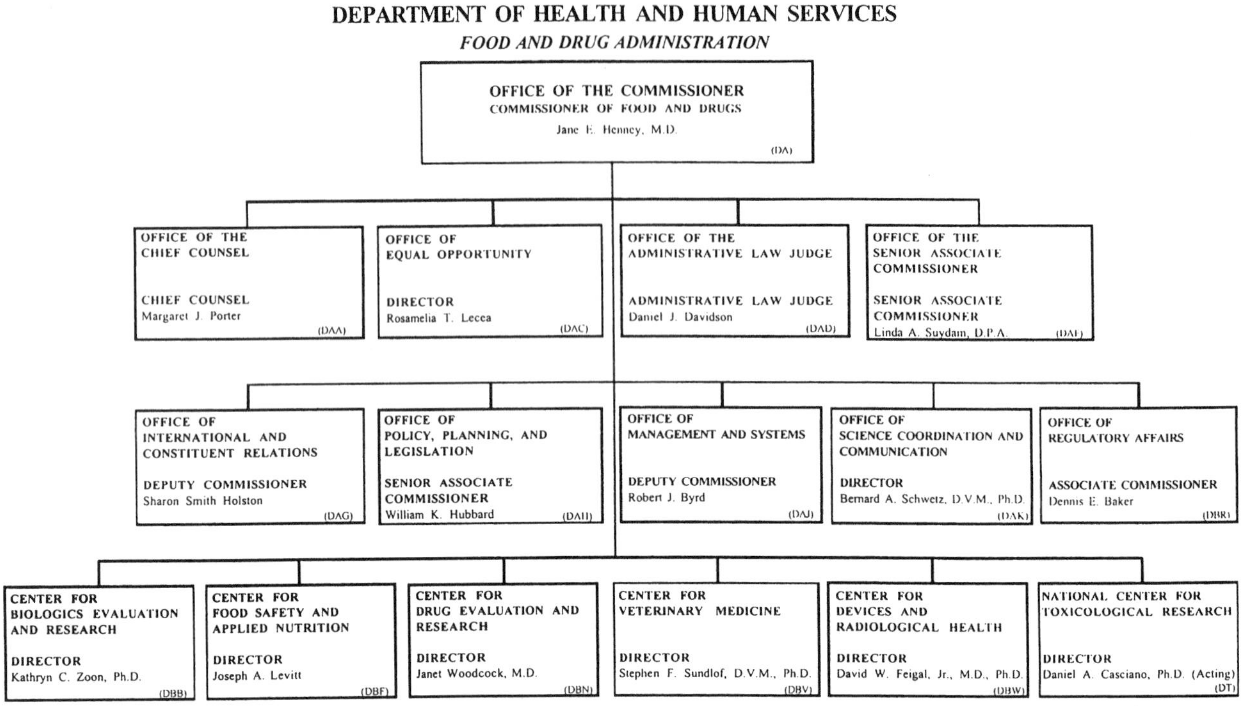

DEPARTMENT OF HEALTH AND HUMAN SERVICES
FOOD AND DRUG ADMINISTRATION

OFFICE OF THE COMMISSIONER
COMMISSIONER OF FOOD AND DRUGS
Jane E. Henney, M.D.
(DA)

OFFICE OF THE CHIEF COUNSEL
CHIEF COUNSEL
Margaret J. Porter
(DAA)

OFFICE OF EQUAL OPPORTUNITY
DIRECTOR
Rosamelia T. Lecea
(DAC)

OFFICE OF THE ADMINISTRATIVE LAW JUDGE
ADMINISTRATIVE LAW JUDGE
Daniel J. Davidson
(DAD)

OFFICE OF THE SENIOR ASSOCIATE COMMISSIONER
SENIOR ASSOCIATE COMMISSIONER
Linda A. Suydam, D.P.A.
(DAI)

OFFICE OF INTERNATIONAL AND CONSTITUENT RELATIONS
DEPUTY COMMISSIONER
Sharon Smith Holston
(DAG)

OFFICE OF POLICY, PLANNING, AND LEGISLATION
SENIOR ASSOCIATE COMMISSIONER
William K. Hubbard
(DAH)

OFFICE OF MANAGEMENT AND SYSTEMS
DEPUTY COMMISSIONER
Robert J. Byrd
(DAJ)

OFFICE OF SCIENCE COORDINATION AND COMMUNICATION
DIRECTOR
Bernard A. Schwetz, D.V.M., Ph.D.
(DAK)

OFFICE OF REGULATORY AFFAIRS
ASSOCIATE COMMISSIONER
Dennis E. Baker
(DBR)

CENTER FOR BIOLOGICS EVALUATION AND RESEARCH
DIRECTOR
Kathryn C. Zoon, Ph.D.
(DBB)

CENTER FOR FOOD SAFETY AND APPLIED NUTRITION
DIRECTOR
Joseph A. Levitt
(DBF)

CENTER FOR DRUG EVALUATION AND RESEARCH
DIRECTOR
Janet Woodcock, M.D.
(DBN)

CENTER FOR VETERINARY MEDICINE
DIRECTOR
Stephen F. Sundlof, D.V.M., Ph.D.
(DBV)

CENTER FOR DEVICES AND RADIOLOGICAL HEALTH
DIRECTOR
David W. Feigal, Jr., M.D., Ph.D.
(DBW)

NATIONAL CENTER FOR TOXICOLOGICAL RESEARCH
DIRECTOR
Daniel A. Casciano, Ph.D. (Acting)
(DT)

Fig. 1 Organizational chart for the U.S. Food and Drug Administration.

new drug substances, but also new dosage forms for existing drugs) is known officially as a Notice of Claimed Investigational exemption for a New Drug (Form FD 1571), also often called the IND. These regulations appear in Section 505 of the act [9]. A "new drug" is one not presently recognized by experts in the field of clinical pharmacology as having been established to be safe and effective based on currently available clinical evidence. All the definitions for a new drug appear in the *Code of Federal Regulations* for a new drug entity [10].

The "newness" of a drug may consist of:

1. The newness for drug use of any substance that composes such drug, in whole or in part, whether it be an active substance or an excipient, carrier, coating, or other component
2. The newness for a drug use of a combination of two or more substances, none of which is a new drug
3. The newness for drug use of the proportion of a substance in a combination, even though such combination containing such substance in other proportion is not a new drug
4. The newness of use of a drug in diagnosing, curing, mitigating, treating, or prevention a disease, or to affect a structure or function of the body, even though such drug is not a new drug when used in another disease or to affect another structure or function of the body
5. The newness of a dosage, or method of duration of administration or application, or other condition of use prescribed, recommended, or suggested in the labeling of such drug, even though such drug when used in other dosage, or other method or duration of administration or application, or different condition, is not a new drug

To determine whether human testing for a new drug or new drug product is reasonable, it is first necessary to conduct preclinical studies and to submit the IND. The necessary information needed to prepare the IND is outlined in Table 1. The IND is to contain information on appropriate prior animal studies for safety evaluation, any available clinical data, adequate drug identification and manufacturing instructions, and a detailed outline of the proposed clinical study, routs of administration, approximate number of patients to be used, and an estimate of the length of treatment and an environmental impact statement.

After the IND has been filed with FDA and the date of receipt noted, a 30-day waiting period is needed

DEPARTMENT OF HEALTH AND HUMAN SERVICES
FOOD AND DRUG ADMINISTRATION
CENTER FOR DRUG EVALUATION AND RESEARCH

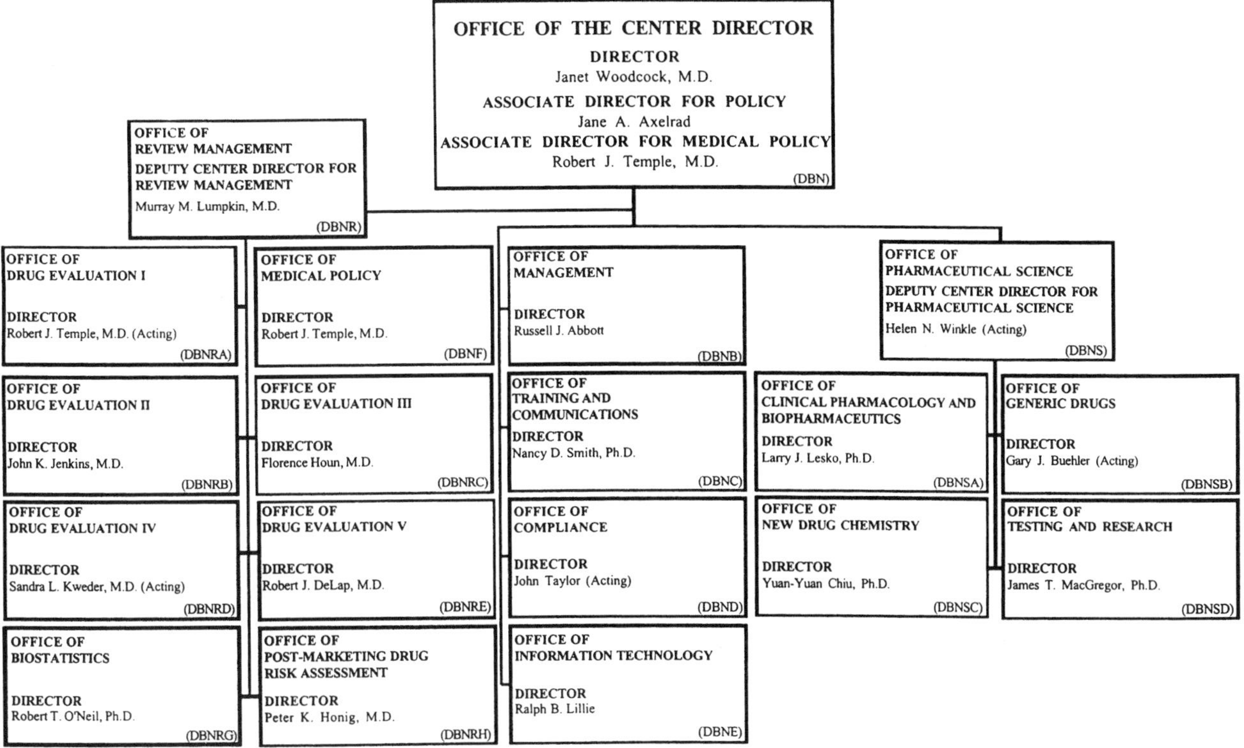

Fig. 2 Organizational chart for the Center for Drug Evaluation and Research.

before the initiation of the studies by the sponsor. Following this period, and if no objections have been raised by FDA, the drug may be shipped to the clinical investigators, as long as the label bears the statement "Caution: New Drug—Limited by Federal (or United States) Law to Investigational Use." The sponsor must maintain records of distribution of the new drug for 2 years after approval of the drug for use; if not approved, the records must be retained for 2 years after the last shipment and delivery to investigators. Pharmacists in institutional settings are often assigned responsibility for this record keeping. An additional important point of the 1962 amendment was the requirement that FDA be informed if and when a study was stopped and for what reasons. Before this time, no record was made of any clinical study until the time came to apply for a new drug release.

The clinical evaluation of a new drug is divided into three phases. The first phase of human testing considers what chemical actions a drug has, how it is absorbed by the body, and a safe dosage range [10]. Normally, fewer than 10 individuals are used as subjects, and these individuals are usually normal rather than ill or diseased persons. This Phase I is used to describe the human pharmacology of the drug and the preferred route of administration. Phase II studies involve the dosing of a limited number of patients for treatment or prevention of the disease of interest. This step preliminarily evaluates the effectiveness of the drug. The amount of animal toxicity testing will increase if the drug appears to be a favorable candidate for extended study. Phase III studies are the next step, during which the drug is assessed for its safety, effectiveness, and the most desirable dosage for the disease to be treated, and the results are collected and verified in a large number of patients (from several hundred to thousands).

The sponsor is required to obtain statements from the clinical investigators describing his or her qualifications to take part in the proposed studies. Reference

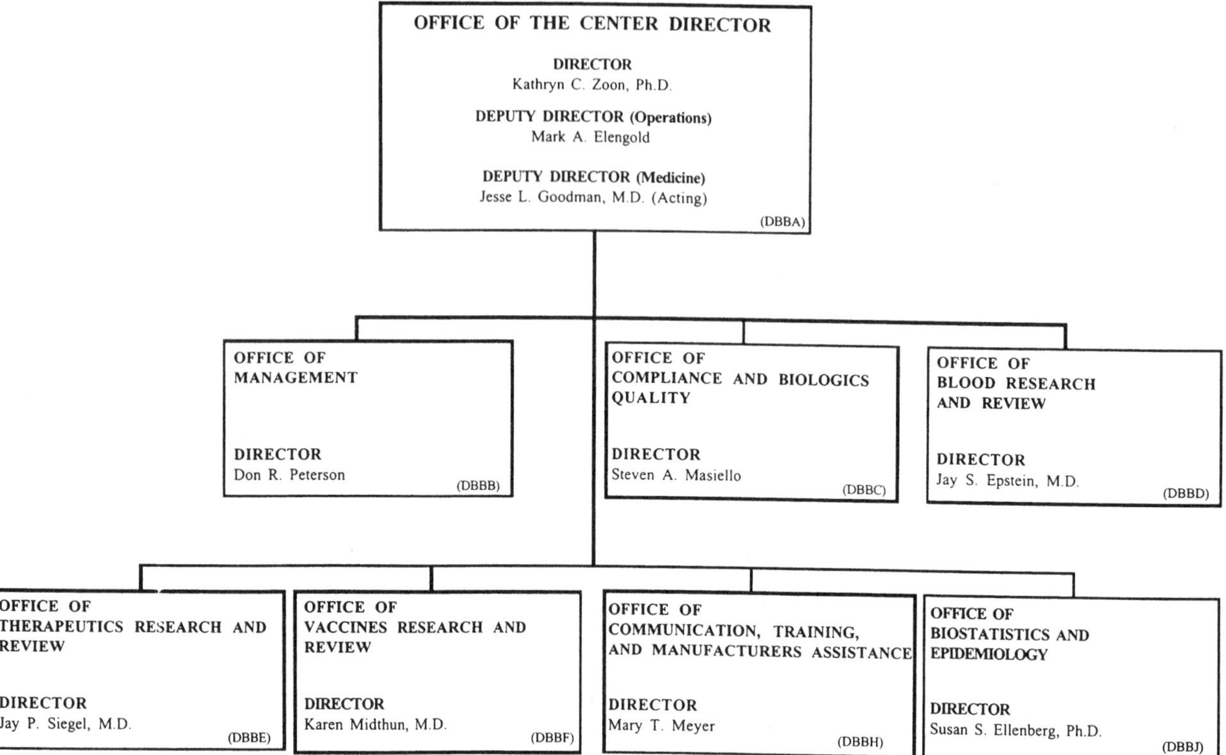

Fig. 3 Organizational chart for the Center for Biologics Evaluation and Research.

to the "*review committee*" in this document is to the institutional human review committee of the hospital or other facility where the study will be undertaken. Note that both documents require that the investigator certify that all subjects (patients), whether used as controls or test subjects, be notified that they are receiving drugs being used for investigational purposes, and that their consents be obtained.

B. New Drug Application

Once a new drug substance, or anything that is by definition a new drug, has been through Phase III (i.e., the clinical trial) and the appropriate data accumulated, a document is prepared entitled "*New Drug Application*" (*NDA Form 356H*). The data must normally be obtained under a specific IND that has permitted the gathering of information about acute and chronic toxicity, extended clinical pharmacology, full-scale clinical evaluation, complete product design and manufacturing methods, complete package design, and complete labeling requirements.

Because of today's myriad regulations, the NDA submission has become a compilation of information that could be compared in size with any one of the well-known encyclopedias. Before 1962, only a few volumes were necessary for an NDA submission [11]. Today it is not uncommon for this justification to consist of as many as 200 volumes of information (see Table 2). It is important for the pharmacy and medical practitioner to have some sensitivity to the many requirements and high cost placed on manufacturers who develop and market new drugs (especially new drug substances) today.

Some of the elements of the NDA are of particular significance to the pharmacist. For example, in the statement on labeling it is necessary for manufacturers to abstract from their clinical summaries that which is both recommended for the description of the use of the drugs and that which is necessary for the warning or

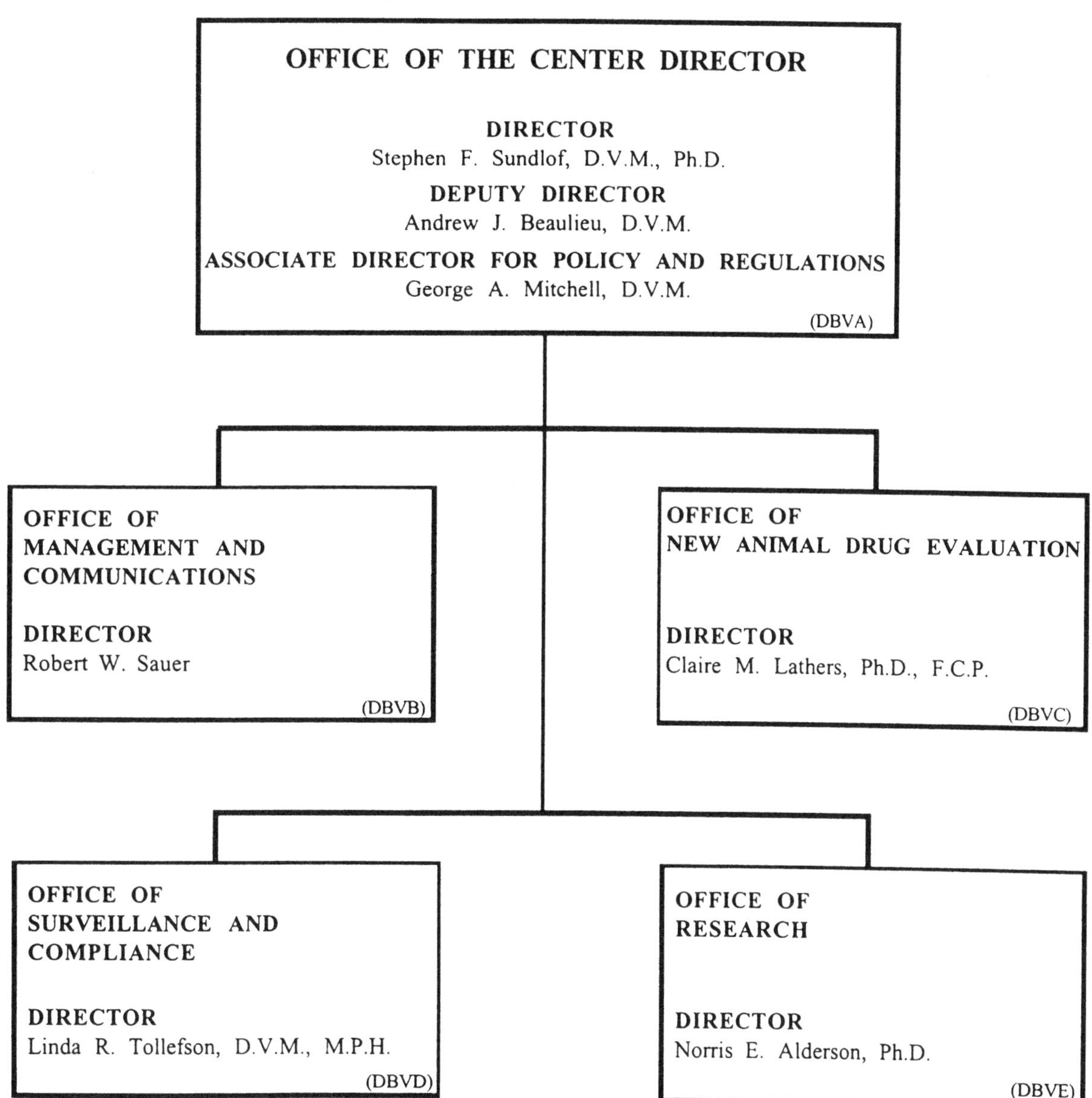

Fig. 4 Organizational chart for the Center for Veterinary Medicine.

cautions needed for the administration of the new products. The labeling, which includes the package insert, must assist all professionals in the proper administration and use of new drugs. The labeling is also approved by FDA to ensure that only those uses verified in the clinical studies are recommended [12]. Drug companies may not legally advocate use of their product for any other purpose.

Other points that are of great significance to the manufacturer and, in turn, to the physician and

Table 1 Components of a Notice of Claimed Investigational Exemption for a New Drug (IND)

1. Best available descriptive name of the drug product and how it is to be administered
2. Complete list of components of the drug product
3. Quantitative composition of the drug product
4. Description of the source and preparation of any new drug substance used as a component
5. Description of the methods, facilities, and controls used to prepare and distribute the drug product
6. Information available from preclinical investigations and any clinical studies that may have been conducted
7. Copies of any labels or labeling to be used in the study
8. Scientific training and experience to qualify the investigators
9. Complete information of each investigator, including training and experience
10. Outline of any phase or phases of the planned clinical investigation
11. Assurance that the Food and Drug Administration will be notified if the studies are discontinued
12. Assurance that investigators will be notified if a new drug application is approved or the studies discontinued
13. Explanation of why a drug product must be sold during a study
14. Agreement not to start a study for 30 days after notice of receipt of IND by Food and Drug Administration

pharmacist, include the exact production methods used, the facilities and controls used, and the overall processing and packaging of any new drug substance. The NDA requires full descriptions of all of these elements to ensure safe and effective marketed drug products. These descriptions are so detailed in the original NDA that even drying temperatures for tablets prepared by wet granulation must be closely adhered to in all subsequent manufactured lots. The NDA will contain descriptions of the exact equipment and processes and the specifications of all drugs and excipients that are used for manufacture of the product. At a later date, if these are modified, the manufacturer may be required to submit a supplement to the NDA, which verifies that no quality features of the product (such as bioavailability) have been altered.

Many products have specific packaging requirements owing to inherent problems in their physical, chemical, and possibly biological stability. For this reason detailed information must be given for the packaging of any new drug covered by an NDA. The pharmacist or physician should be aware of the extensive research that goes into package selection to satisfy FDA. Any repackaging of a drug product should, as a rule, attempt to place the product in a package that is at least as protective as the one from which it was removed.

Table 2 Components of a New Drug Application (Drugs for Human Use)

1. Table of contents
2. Summary
3. Evaluation of safety and effectiveness
4. Copies of the label and all other labeling to be used for the drug
5. A statement as to whether the drug is (or is not) limited in its labeling and by this application to use under the professional supervision of a practitioner licensed by law to administer it
6. A full list of the articles used as components of the drug
7. A full statement of the composition of the drug
8. A full description of the methods used in, and the facilities and controls used for, the manufacture, processing, and packing of the drug
9. Samples of the drug and articles used as components
10. Full reports of preclinical investigations that have been made to show whether or not the drug is safe for use and effective in use
11. List of investigators
12. Full reports of clinical investigations that have been made to show whether or not the drug is safe for use and effective in use
13. If this is a supplemental application, full information on each proposed change concerning any statement made in the approved application

Another important section of the NDA is a full report of all preclinical investigations of the new drug substance or new drug. These investigations ensure safety and efficacy of the new drug. No animal study, large or small, can be unreported. There have been instances in the past in which some animal data were not reported, and problems resulted later when the drug was administered to humans. Ideally, the more animal data from chronic studies that are gathered, the better indication one will have of the drug's prospective safety in humans. This information can be as important as the clinical work in patients to demonstrate safety.

Of ultimate importance are the full reports of the clinical studies in humans and their results. These data will be treated statistically for their validity. The number of studies for a specific compound or combination of compounds will vary with the type of drug being tested, as will the number of tests needed to appraise relative or absolute safety and to clearly demonstrate efficacy. The basic requirement is the proof of safety and efficacy of the product being submitted under the NDA system. A drug that does not contribute to therapy, such as a new antihistamine that does not demonstrate greater safety or efficacy, or both, compared with drugs already on the market, will have a difficult or impossible time achieving approval.

After the new drug application has been compiled, it is forwarded to FDA, where it receives a specific identification number and is submitted to a scheduled review. In recent years, extensions of the schedule limits have been the rule, rather than the exception, for FDA to complete its review. These extensions are generally for a specific number of days or months. Once reviewed by FDA, a response is returned to the sponsor that generally contains numerous questions concerning the application. The sponsor will then attempt to satisfy the questions raised and resubmit the application for review by FDA. This process may be repeated for as long as a few months to several years, until the agency is convinced that the drug is, in fact, safe and effective. Once so proved, permission is granted to the sponsor to manufacture and distribute the product to the public. Currently, the period from the time of synthesis of a compound, or its isolation, to its release for marketing is generally 10 years or longer, at a total development cost approaching a half billion dollars.

C. Drug Efficacy Study

In 1966, the FDA Commissioner approached the Division of Medical Sciences of the National Academy of Sciences–National Research Council (NAS–NRC) for assistance in reviewing drugs that had been marketed under NDAs approved during the period 1938–1962 [13]. There were approximately 7000 drug formulations in this category, and of these about 4000, containing 300 distinctly different medicinal agents, were still being marketed. Since these drugs had been approved under the old law, which did not include the new requirement of the 1962 amendments that the drug clearly demonstrate effectiveness, James Goddard, sought the help of the NAS–NRC to establish review committees to undertake this formidable review task. To proceed in this undertaking, a Policy Advisory Committee was first formed, whose members needed to become acquainted with major medical, legal, and industrial problems in the field of drugs. Early in the development of the study, it was recognized that a system of evaluating panels would have to be established. Twenty-seven panels were originally formed. Later, additional panels were added as the need arose. Some of the panels formed concerned themselves with drugs used in allergy, anesthesiology, antineoplastic and cardiovascular therapy, dermatology, and other specific fields of medicine or drug therapy. Guidelines were established by the Policy Advisory Committee for the review activities of the panels, and appropriate individuals representing various scientific and professional disciplines were appointed to the panels. By October 1966 the review program was formerly organized and in operation. The type of products reviewed included single-drug entities, as well as products containing two or more active ingredients. Extensive duplication of products was most evident in the antibiotic, antihistamine, and antihypertensive areas.

One of the major problems in initiating the study was to attempt to establish a categorical rating of effectiveness. FDA developed four effectiveness categories: (a) effective, (b) probably effective, (c) possibly effective, and (d) ineffective. In a little more than 2 years, a large amount of data was collected on more than 80% of the drugs currently on the market. The results of the NAS–NRS study and the effectiveness categorization of various products were periodically published by FDA in the *Federal Register* (the official publication of the federal government for all notices, proposed rules, and regulations). In many cases, time was given for a response by the companies affected by the results of this study. Some of the results were (a) the immediate removal of products currently marketed, (b) the recognition that certain clinical studies were required to verify or establish effectiveness under the new law and according to past product claims, and (c) the recognition that directions or labeling of certain products were poorly organized, repetitive, outdated, evasive, and oriented to the promotion of products.

As one broad positive impact of this study, it was recognized that package inserts needed to be brought up to modern standards of accurate and objective drug information. Several products were voluntarily removed from the marketplace by manufacturers who were unable or unwilling to establish the necessary proofs of efficacy. Some of the types of products that ceased to exist following this review were antibiotic-containing troches and lozenges for the treatment of minor sore throat; antibiotic, antihistamine, and analgetic/antipyretic combinations for treatment of colds and influenza; and many other drug combination products. This review was undoubtedly beneficial to the public, in that more stringent principles of rational therapeutics were applied.

D. Abbreviated New Drug Application

A detailed description of the concept of an Abbreviated New Drug Application (ANDA) was published in the *Federal Register* of June 20, 1975 [14]. The ANDA represents a form of new drug application in which certain information is not needed because previously acquired data has been filed with FDA. In the ANDA procedure, FDA's intent is to minimize duplication of effort in preparing applications for drugs about which some of the needed information is already available, while assuring that the new product will be equivalent to established marketed products. Normally, the information allowed to be omitted relates to preclinical and clinical studies pertaining to the safety and effectiveness of the active ingredient(s) that have been on the market for many years. Since many of the items are established generic drugs, it is unnecessary to reverify their efficacy. It may simply be necessary to have assurance that the manufacturing procedures, specifications, and labeling are adequate. In other cases it will be necessary to demonstrate the bioequivalence of the new product relative to currently available standard products or to the original NDA-approved product.

In addition to a description of the manufacturing method, packaging, and stability data, the ANDA requires only the following: a description of the components and composition of the dosage form to be marketed; brief statements that identify the place where the drug is to be manufactured; the name of the supplier of the active ingredients; assurance that the drug will comply with appropriate specifications; facilities used in the manufacture and packing; certification that the drug will be manufactured in compliance with current GMP, as defined by regulation; labeling; and—when so specified—data adequate to assure the drug's biological availability [15].

In selecting drugs suitable for the ANDA, one considers the characteristics of the drug, method of use, method of manufacture and packaging, stability, extent of use, safety and potency, and past history. Difficulties or known problems in any of these areas usually prevent the drug from being included in the abbreviated new drug procedure category. For example, the limited information included in an abbreviated application would not be sufficient to permit FDA to conclude that a high-potency drug that requires extremely careful handling during manufacture is suitable for marketing. The same is true of a drug for which the container plays a critical part in its administration, for instance, a metered aerosol. The purpose of the ANDA procedure is thus to eliminate unnecessary and costly animal and human experimentation, to assist manufacturers in attempting to market duplication drug products, and to make all drug substances not covered by patents readily available to the consumer in a competitive market.

In 1984, an amendment to the Food, Drug, and Cosmetic Act was passed entitled the Drug Price Competition and Patent Term Restoration Act of 1984 [19]. This revised the ANDA procedure and permitted the approval of post-1982 drugs once the patent of the innovator had expired. This has also become known as the Waxman–Hatch Amendment. As a result of this amendment many generic products have been placed on the market, with a minimum amount of clinical effort but with the establishment of the physical and chemical equivalency to marketed products [20]. The amount of bioequivalency study necessary under an ANDA will vary with the particular drug product. This act was also tied into the Patent Restoration Act, which allows an extended time to be given to innovator firms for new drug substances. Although this amendment may allow numerous companies to get into the generic manufacturing of drugs, the act is specific about the requirements, and only those who can document adequately their ANDA will be permitted to distribute the drugs in the marketplace. This is also an important application of the current good manufacturing practices and their importance to drug products and drug product distribution.

III. LAWS GOVERNING PREPARATION AND DISTRIBUTION OF EXISTING PRODUCTS

A. Current Good Manufacturing Practices

On June 20, 1963, FDA published new regulations governing "current good manufacturing practices" (GMP) in the "manufacturing, processing, packaging, and holding of finished pharmaceuticals" [16]. These regulations represented an official step in the interpretation of GMP and quality-control functions of a pharmaceutical operations. They also recognized the potential for innovation and made allowances for such developments as automatic, mechanical, or electronic equipment to be used in the production of drugs, provided adequate controls are available to verify the production operation.

The section on current GMP of the *Code of Federal Regulations* (revised as of April 1, 1985) is divided into two parts [17]. The first is Part 210: "Current Good Manufacturing Practices in Manufacturing Processing, Packaging, or Holding of Drugs: General" This section defines or refers to other sections of the law for definitions. It includes definitions of what a "component" is, what a "batch" is, what the term "lot" means, what the use of lot number or control number is, what an "active ingredient" means as to its application in a dosage form for either humans or animals, what the term "inactive ingredient" means, what the term "materials approval unit" means, and what the term "strength" means. It is very important that in this last item some basic concepts of concentration of the drug substance have been clearly defined. The examples used include weight/weight, weight/volume, or unit-dose/volume basis; it is accepted that the therapeutic activity of the drug substance is indicated based on laboratory and controlled clinical data. The second section, Part 211, is entitled "Current Good Manufacturing Practices for Finished Pharmaceuticals." This section is subdivided as follows [18]:

Subpart A: General Provisions
Subpart B: Organization and Personnel
Subpart C: Buildings and Facilities
Subpart D: Equipment
Subpart E: Control of Components and Drug Product Containers and Closures
Subpart F: Production and Process Controls
Subpart G: Packaging and Labeling Control
Subpart H: Holding and Distribution
Subpart I: Laboratory Controls
Subpart J: Records and Reports
Subpart K: Returned and Salvaged Drug Products

To help understand the current good manufacturing practices (CGMP), the following general comments will be made concerning several of the subparts of the regulations. It is hoped that by giving these explanations, the reader will be able to better understand where the regulations fit into the control of the manufacture of those products being dispensed and distributed to the consumer. For more details of these regulations, the reader is to refer to Section 21, Food and Drug *Code of Federal Regulations*, Part 211.

Section 211.1: Scope of the Regulations

For all pharmaceutical products, it must first be assured that the drugs will be prepared under conditions that will assure them to be safe and to have the identity and strength as stated by the manufacturer. The regulations require a complete description of all that is involved with the manufacture of the dosage form.

Section 211.25: Personnel

In this section, the personnel responsible for directing the manufacture and control of the drugs and drug products are described. They must be of a sufficient number and have an educational background, which may be of a formal nature or of a training nature, or a combination of the two, so that they can make appropriate decisions on the safety and identity of the products being produced by the manufacturer or agency. It is imperative that they understand all manufacturing and control procedures to be performed that will ensure the preparation of quality products and that they clearly understand their respective functions.

It is further stated that any individuals who have an apparent illness or open lesions that could in any way affect the safety and quality of drugs shall be excluded from direct contact with the pharmaceutical products being prepared. It may be necessary to assign these individuals temporarily to other duties until they are in satisfactory health. It is imperative that the employees be instructed to report any of the foregoing conditions to their supervisors. The supervisory personnel have additional responsibility to ensure that this requirement is met.

Section 211.42 to .58: Buildings

It is evident that buildings used for the manufacture, processing, packaging, labeling, or holding of drug products should be clean and kept in an orderly manner. The law, however, is much more specific and states that space provisions must be made and gives certain general instructions on space utilization, as for the following:

1. The appropriate place of equipment and materials to minimize the risk of mix-ups between different drugs and all that is required to prepare a product (should also provide for the minimizing of cross-contamination)
2. The receipt, storage, and holding of all substances for a pharmaceutical product before release for use
3. The holding and storage of rejected materials
4. The storage of all items needed in pharmaceutical production
5. The obvious space for manufacturing and processing operations
6. The packaging and labeling operations to be done in close proximity to other packaging and labeling operations
7. The storage of finished products to be very well provided for
8. The control and production laboratory operations to be considered as important as any other space commitment

The law also specifies the type of lighting, ventilation, and screening required to control the environment of the facility, together with other steps to assure that certain areas shall be protected from microbial contamination or dust or be maintained at special humidity and temperature conditions. These requirements are in order to:

1. Minimize contamination of products. This contamination may come from other products being made either in the same building or nearby
2. Endeavor to minimize microbial contamination from one area to another, regardless of the dosage form being prepared. We now see greater emphasis of this on nonsterile products as well as products that are intended to be sterile
3. Provide storage conditions that will maintain raw materials and finished products in a stable form

Other general provisions are as follows:

1. Locker facilities must be provided for the employees such that they can prepare themselves adequately for the duties to be performed in their specific work areas
2. Suitable water must be available, continuously under pressure from a system free of defects, so that any water used has not been contaminated in any way. There shall also be a good system of drains within the entire operation.
3. When needed, suitable housing shall be provided for the care of any laboratory animals needed
4. There must be a safe and sanitary procedure for the disposal of sewage, trash, and other materials that could cause contamination of the building or the immediate surroundings. It should be noted that in 1967 the Pharmaceutical Manufacturers Association established sound sanitary rules and regulations for all the member firms

Section 211.63 to .72: Equipment

"Equipment used for the manufacture, processing, packaging, labeling, holding, testing, or control of drugs shall be maintained in a clean and orderly manner and shall be of suitable type, size, construction, and location to facilitate cleaning, maintenance, and operation for its intended purpose." The equipment should:

1. Be so constructed that all surfaces that come into contact with a drug product shall not be reactive, additive, or absorptive
2. Be so constructed that any substances required for operation of the equipment, such as lubricants or coolants, do not contact drug products
3. Be so constructed and installed to facilitate adjustment, disassembly cleaning, and maintenance to assure the reliability of control procedures, uniformity of production, and exclusion from the drugs of contaminants from previous and current operations
4. Be of suitable type, size, and accuracy for any testing, measuring, mixing, weighing, or other processing or storage operations

Section 211.100 to .115: Production and Process Control

"Production and control procedures shall include all reasonable precautions, indicating the following, to assure that the drugs produced have the safety, identity, strength, quality, and purity they purport to possess."

1. Each significant step in the process, such as the selection, weighing, and measuring of components, the addition of ingredients during the process, weighing and measuring during various stages of the processing, and the determination of the finished yield shall be performed by a competent and responsible person and checked by a second competent and responsible person. The written record of the significant steps in the process shall be identified by the person performing these tests and by the person charged with checking these steps
2. It is necessary that all containers, production lines, and equipment be properly identified to ensure batch integrity and the stage or location during processing
3. To minimize and essentially eliminate contamination, and to liminate mix-ups, equipment, utensils, and containers are to be thoroughly cleaned and adequately stored
4. If products are to be of a sterile nature or their requirements are such that these should be free of objectionable microorganisms, precautions must be taken to aid in this final goal
5. All precautions that might contribute to cross-contamination of drugs during manufacture or storage must be taken
6. In-process controls, such as the checking of weights and disintegration or dissolution of tablets, satisfactory mixing, appropriate suspension preparation, or clarity of solutions must be conducted to ensure appropriate product content uniformity and performance
7. A sufficient number of samples of various dosage forms should be tested to see if they meet product specifications
8. This section requires the review and approval of all production and control records before the release or distribution of any batch. If any unexplainable discrepancy cannot be resolved, a thorough investigation is required, terminating in a written report of the investigation
9. This section concerns itself with returned goods. It should be obvious to all handling drug products that it is absolutely necessary to be able to identify and evaluate products that may be either returned to stock or reprocessed. If neither of these is capable of being done, the material should be destroyed. There is no room for uncertainty
10. This section concerns itself with asbestos-containing or other fiber-releasing filters. Current technology, as well as current feelings on these items, accepts the fact that such release of fibers should not happen, especially for parenteral injections for humans; hence, the need for different types of filter media. However, it would be well to concern ourselves with any filter media that release fibers, and a recommendation is that "a fiber is defined as any particle with length at least three times greater than its width." As new filter media become available, we anticipate that this difficulty will be eliminated

This section specifically concerns itself with filters that must be used that do release fibers. It is noted that an additional filter with a maximum pore size of either 0.2 or 0.45 μm must also be used to finish the filtration. This is an absolute requirement with asbestos filters used because of the total concept of safety and effectiveness of the drug. This section simply sets the time limit for instituting good filtration procedures for parenteral products.

Section 221.80 to .94: Control of Components and Drug Product Containers and Closures

The section on components deals with all materials that may be used in the manufacture, processing, and packaging of drug products, plus materials used for maintenance of the building and equipment. They must be stored and handled in a "safe, sanitary, and orderly manner." These precautions are needed to prevent mix-ups and cross-contamination of drugs and drug products. All items should be held until they have been sampled and tested according to the company's specifications and not released until the tests have been completed. In this section it is required that:

1. A check should be made of the container of a component to see whether it has been damaged or contaminated. This is done by visual inspection
2. Samples should be taken that are representative of each lot. Samples of components that may be susceptible to insect infestation or similar contamination should be carefully examined
3. Further sampling should be carried out to ensure potency, lack of microbiological contamination, identity, and the like. It should be noted that because of the above, approved components must therefore be stored to prevent contamination, and that the oldest stock should be used first, and that rejected

components should be so identified for appropriate disposal

4. Records should be maintained to ensure the identity, the supplier, the lot number, the date of receipt, and the decision whether to accept or reject, and an inventory scheme for each component

A specific statement then is given that requires that a reserve sample be retained for all required tests and that it should be available for at least 2 years after distribution of the last drug lot that utilized the components or 1 year after a stated expiration date of the finished product.

Section 211.122 to .137: Product Containers and Their Components

This section requires written procedures for identifying and storing of all items involved with packaging. It also describes how labels are to be prepared and stored. Strict regulation is enforced concerning labeling and how this material is issued within a pharmaceutical operation or a repackaging operation. This should be noted, since there are times when a large pharmacy may be involved with relabeling. Reference should be made to these regulations for guidance in the design of an operation such as repackaging. This section also discusses the expiration dates required for drug products so that they meet the standards of identity, strength, quality, and purity at the time of use.

Section 211.160 to .176: Laboratory Controls

The backbone of the laboratory control system rests on the philosophy used to establish sound and appropriate specifications, standards, and test procedures to ensure drug product quality. Some of the components of this section of the law are as follows:

1. The laboratory should maintain the master records for all lots of incoming raw material as well as finished product. Samples should be retained by the laboratory for immediate identification or future reference, which constitutes a reserve sampling system
2. The master records should also indicate the sampling and test procedures involved with in-process control and sampling procedures for finished drug products
3. Provisions should be made for checking the identity and strength of drug products for all active ingredients and, where applicable, sterility, pyrogenicity, and minimal contamination of ophthalmic ointments by "foreign particles and harsh or abrasive substances." It is also important that for sustained-release products a satisfactory laboratory method be available to ensure that release specifications are met
4. This section also concerns itself with the ability to review laboratory test procedures and laboratory instruments used. It is stressed that reserve samples of marketed products must be retained in their original containers for at least 2 years after the final distribution of a lot or at least 1 year after the drug's expiration date. In this same light, laboratory data for each batch or lot of drug should be retained for these time periods
5. This section requires that animals used for quality control purposes must be maintained in the proper manner and records kept for their identity and for their use
6. An important element was subsequently added to this section which concerned the contamination of products by penicillin, especially when a firm manufacturers both penicillin-containing and non–penicillin-containing products. It is established in the regulation that there may not be more than 0.05 unit of penicillin G per single dose of any drug when it is to be injected, or no more than 0.5 unit of penicillin G for drugs taken orally. This has led many companies to establish separate facilities for the preparation of penicillin-containing products

Because of the success of the CGMP laws, a new line of thought was developed that involved the subject of good laboratory practices. On December 22, 1978, the regulations entitled "Non-clinical Laboratory Studies" were issued in the *Federal Register* [21]. These regulations, which became known as Good Laboratory Practice, are involved in the evaluation of nonclinical laboratory studies.

The purpose of the regulations was to ensure proper operation of laboratories that generated data to support either INDs or NDAs. In particular, they addressed animal studies, including animal care and animal accountability. They also involved the equipment used to do the various procedures for analysis and the maintenance and calibration of the equipment. In general, these regulations now cover the operation of the laboratories and how the data are collected and stored. This ensures that good laboratotory procedures are followed during all the various studies.

B. Over-the-Counter Human Drugs

In the *Code of Federal Regulations*, Title 21, Part 330 outlines the general information for the regulations covering OTC human drug products that are generally recognized as safe and effective and not misbranded. Any product that fails to conform to the conditions outlined for the products would be in regulatory violation. In this section, monographs have been prepared for various classes of drugs and the conditions that should be met for their distribution. It is noted that the products must be manufactured in compliance with CGMP.

This section and those that immediately follow outline what has been approved for use and the necessary warnings for these OTC drugs. The categories that have been designated in the OTC area are antacids, laxatives, antidiarrhea products, emetics, antiemetics, antiperspirants, sunburn prevention and treatment products, vitamin-mineral products, antimicrobial products, dandruff products, oral hygiene products, hemorrhoidal products, hematin-ics, bronchodilator and antiasthmatic products, analgesics, sedatives and sleep aids, stimulants, antitussives, allergy treatment products, cold remedies, antirheumatic products, ophthalmic products, contraceptive products, miscellaneous dermatological products, dentifrices and dental products, and miscellaneous. The last category covers all OTC products that do not fall into any specific therapeutic category.

Materials that are under the OTC classification must be reviewed by the appropriate FDA division to evaluate elements concerning labeling, quantities of active ingredient, animal safety data, human safety data, and other elements that would support the marketing of the appropriate products.

Following this section of the regulations, other parts are given for specific categories, such as Part 331—"Antacid Products of Over-the- Counter Human Use." In the monograph, such items are addressed as active ingredients, tests and procedures, and labeling. Very specific information is given on how materials are categorized and what tests are used for their evaluation. A manufacturer of these particular types of products would have to comply with all points as stated in the regulations. This is to ensure that appropriate products are in the marketplace and that they have been satisfactorily labeled. Depending on the monograph, appropriate warning labels are necessary to ensure safety for the consuming public. This might include,"avoid alcoholic beverages while taking this product," "do not take this product if you are taking sedatives or tranquilizers without first consulting your doctor," and so forth. Other appropriate precautions would be noted and would be required on the labeling. It is very important when working with patients that, if it is necessary to draw attention to caution labels, this be done at the time of presenting prescription information to the consumer.

C. The FDA Recall System

One of the important functions of FDA is its responsibility to the American consumer to ensure that defective or hazardous products will be immediately removed from distribution and the marketplace. The principal legal procedure that is followed is to remove from commerce, through seizure, any product that is deemed unsafe. When the recall system was first initiated, it did not have a well-defined mechanism for either seizure or voluntary removal of products found defective from the marketplace. This lack of ability to recall products was evident in the late 1930s when the famous "elixir of sulfanilamide," which killed more than 100 people (see Sec. I), had to be found and returned to the manufacturer [6]. This situation initiated considerations of a better recall system. Also, there was no clear legal statement on a recall system; it was simply an accepted concept in the food and drug industry. The recall procedure increased in usage during the 1960s, and in 1967 FDA started to publish a weekly recall list. In 1971 FDA refined the procedure and stated that two types of recalls should be defined [22]:

1. Products that were an immediate threat to public safety
2. Products that may have or could be of potential hazard

On further investigation by an internal FDA task force, the following recall definitions were established in 1973, which seemed to better define the types of product defects that currently are being found. The recalls are now divided into the following three classes.

Class I recalls are those that have been judged to present a serious threat to the health of the consumer. Examples of this type of recall include brewers' yeast tablets (product contaminated with *Salmonella*), defective pacemakers (electronically unsafe), and numerous cases of mislabeling of drug substances, such as the belladonna alkaloids [20].

Class II recalls are those in which the use of or exposure to a product found in violation of the law may cause a temporary health problem that is reversible, or in which the situation would not cause serious adverse health consequences. Examples of this type of recall would include uncertainty of the sterility of an injectable product, *Salmonella* contamination of various types of oral dosage forms, inadequate directions for use, and improper buffering of solution for injection [20].

Class III recalls are those that involve violations of the law, but for which a health hazard is remote. Examples in this case include insect parts or droppings in flour, the marketing of a product without an approved NDA, unacceptable disintegration or dissolution of tablets, or swollen cans of certain food products [23].

To obtain weekly information on drug recalls, the practitioner should follow various professional association journals or newsletters for this information (i.e., Ref. 23). It should be noted that it is possible to receive information on both drug recalls and new drug approvals by following the USP DI monthly supplements [24]. This is an excellent reference also for drug information for health professionals and patients. It is important to be aware of drug recalls as well as to know the new drug products entering the marketplace. As reported previously, FDA also maintains a website that reports drug recalls as well as much other useful information [267].

Every practicing pharmacist has a responsibility to follow the recall lists to ensure that all listed products are immediately removed from the distribution system. This should be a concern of all practitioners to be taken on as a direct obligation within his or her professional capabilities.

D. Tamper-Resistant Packaging

On November 5, 1982, regulations were issued in the *Federal Register* concerning the use of tamper-resistant packaging for OTC drugs, which included certain human drugs, cosmetic products, contact lens solutions, and solid dosage forms. This was due to the unfortunate poisoning that took place in Chicago beginning on September 30, 1982, and that was followed by a number of other cases in the ensuing weeks involving tampering with Tylenol after distribution to retail settings [25].

A *tamper-resistant package* is defined as "one having an indicator or barrier to entry, which if breached or missing, can reasonably be expected to provide visible evidence to consumers that tampering has occurred." Because of the tragedy of 1982, this evidence on over-the-counter products was very important to tablets, capsules, certain liquids, and other substances that would be detrimental to the public if tampered with. Unfortunately, it did not stop, and during 1985 further tampering cases occurred. Further efforts were made to improve packaging to help prevent this unfortunate happening.

Packages considered to be tamper-resistant are defined as follows: film wrappers; blister or strip packs; bubble packs; shrink seals and bands; foil, paper, or plastic pouches; bottle seals; tape seals; breakable caps; sealed tube; sealed carton; and aerosol containers. These and other designs are currently being used in an attempt to product tamper-resistant packaging for the consumer. Products must contain a label indicating to the consumer the existence of a specific tamper-resistant mechanism. Tamper resistance for OTC products is an aim of the industry to protect the public. It must be understood that absolute tamper-proofing is impossible. Only through proper education of the consumer can we ensure adequate package protection. The pharmacist in contact with the public has an opportunity to educate them further in the proper use of OTC products.

IV. FURTHER CONSIDERATIONS

This chapter has summarized current federal regulations that affect the manufacture and distribution of pharmaceutical products. Other U.S. agencies are involved with the manufacture of pharmaceutical products, including the Occupational Safety and Health Administration (OSHA) and the Environmental Protection Agency (EPA). For the clinical practitioner, there are also laws involving the cost of drug distribution and selection, which include Maximum Allowable Costs (MAC) and other federally sponsored funding programs. Thus, we see that both the pharmaceutical manufacturer and the clinical pharmacist must be continuously observant of changes in federal and state regulations.

REFERENCES

1. *Milestones in U.S. Food and Drug Law History*, Publ. (FDA) 73–1018, U.S. Dept. of Health, Education, and Welfare, Food and Drug Administration, Washington, DC, 1972.
2. H. W. Wiley and H. W. Wiley, *The History of a Crime Against the Food Law*, Washington, DC, 1929, p. 1.

3. H. W. Wiley and H. W. Wiley, *The History of a Crime Against the Food Law*, Washington, DC, 1929, p. 56.
4. H. A. Toulmin, *A Treatise on the Law of Foods, Drugs, and Cosmetics*, 2nd ed., W. H. Anderson, Cincinnati, Ohio, 1963, p. 13.
5. H. A. Toulmin, *A Treatise on the Law of Foods, Drugs, and Cosmetics*, 2nd ed., W. H. Anderson, Cincinnati, Ohio, 1963, p. 19.
6. A. Hecht, FDA Consumer, p. 25 (Oct. 1977).
7. *Fifty Years of Quality Assurance in the Pharmaceutical Industry*, Pharmaceutical Manufacturers Association, Washington, DC, 1974.
8. C. Kumkumian, Manufacturing and Controls: Guidelines for IND's and NDA's, paper presented at the 15th Annual International Industrial Pharmacy Conference, University of Texas, Austin, 1976.
9. Federal Food, Drug, and Cosmetic Act as amended, Aug. 1991.
10. *Code of Federal Regulations*, Title 21, *Food and Drugs*, Part 310.3, Apr. 1, 1998.
11. M. Pernarowski and M. Darrach (eds.), *The Development and Control of New Drug Products*, Evergreen Press, Vancouver, BC, Canada, 1972, pp. 118–120.
12. *Code of Federal Regulations*, Title 21, *Food and Drugs*, Part 312, pp. 62–97, Apr. 1, 1998.
13. *Drug Efficacy Study: A Report to the Commissioner of Food and Drugs*, National Academy of Sciences, National Research Council, Washington, DC, 1969.
14. Fed. Reg. 40, 26142 (1975).
15. L. Geismer, FDA Pap., Dec. 1970 to Jan. 1971 (1971).
16. Kefauver-Harris Amendments, *Public Law (PL) 87-781*, 87th Congress, Oct. 10, 1962.
17. *Code of Federal Regulations*, Title 21, *Food and Drugs*, Part 210, Apr. 1, 1998.
18. *Code of Federal Regulations*, Title 21, *Food and Drugs*, Part 211, Apr. 1, 1998.
19. Drug price competition and patent term restoration act of 1984, *Public 98-417*, 98 Stat. 1585-1605, Sept. 24, 1984.
20. W. M. Troetel, How new drugs win FDA approval, U.S. Pharm. (Nov. 1986).
21. Fed. Reg., 43, 59985 (1978).
22. Statement of FDA recall policy, by A. M. Schmidt (Commissioner, Food and Drug Administration), Sept. 21, 1973.
23. Pharm. Wk., American Pharmaceutical Association, Washington, DC, 1996.
24. *USP DI and Supplements*, United States Pharmacopeial Convention, Washington, D.C., 1998.
25. Fed. Reg., 47, 50441 (1982).
26. www.fda.gov.

Chapter 20

European Aspects of the Regulation of Drug Products with Particular Reference to Development Pharmaceutics

Brian R. Matthews

Alcon Laboratories (UK) Ltd, Hemel Hempstead, United Kingdom

I. INTRODUCTION

In this chapter, the regulatory requirements relating to data on development pharmaceutics and process validation will be discussed. The discussion will be limited to Marketing Authorization Applications (MAAs) for the European Economic Area and many central and eastern European countries.

The reader may wonder why process validation is included. This is simply a matter of consideration of the content of guidelines issued in the past that relate to development pharmaceutics. The first such pan-European guideline, adopted by the Committee for Proprietary Medicinal Products (CPMP) in 1988, included advice on both development pharmaceutics and process development. Later versions of the guidelines on development pharmaceutics and on process development have addressed these topics separately, but the historical and practical perspectives suggests that both need to be discussed here.

European regulatory requirements are based on legal requirements, which are, in the pharmaceutical sector, now effected at the European level by means of Regulations (which are directly binding on the concerned parties) and Directives (which are binding on the member states to which they are addressed in terms of the effect to be achieved, but which allow a degree of freedom as to the precise method of national implementation) and in guidance (often included in "Notes for Guidance" and occasionally in "Points to Consider" and "Concept Papers").

The requirements in Directives (and Regulations) are therefore binding. They are legal requirements, although technically compliance is the responsibility of the member states. Of course it is also expected that others will meet the requirements, too. However, as will be seen below, the legislative texts tend to be worded in general terms. Their interpretation is to a large extent dependent upon the content and interpretation of the various guidelines.

There is a large number of available guidelines. These cover a very wide range of topics, and the company submitting an application for a pharmaceutical product should be aware of the contents of these documents and how they interact with other guidelines as well as the interpretation of the legislative requirements. It is necessary to be aware of the impact of guidelines in all areas within the pharmaceutical sector and, in some cases, within the medical device sector. Some of these effects are not obvious from the titles of the documents.

However, it is nonetheless true to say that the contents of guidelines is advisory and that it is possible in justified cases to deviate from them. But in order to justify deviations it is first necessary to know the current thoughts of the regulatory authorities on a particular topic. How can this be done?

In the case of European legislation there is a published information source that contains many of the relevant documents. This is the hard copy or electronic version of the multiple volumes of *The Rules Governing Medicinal Products in the European Union*. The most convenient way to obtain these documents—which will eventually consist of nine volumes, some of which will have several parts—is via the internet. The available volumes can be found by way of the following web address: http://dg3.eudra.org/eudralex/index.htm. The volumes relevant for human medicinal products are:

Volume 1—Pharmaceutical legislation
Volume 2—*Notice to Applicants* (consisting of Parts 2A, 2B, and 2C)
Volume 3—Guidelines (consisting of Parts 3A, 3B, and 3C)
Volume 4—Good Manufacturing Practices
Volume 9—Pharmacovigilance (not posted at the web site and not available in hard copy at the date of writing—September 2000)

Unfortunately, this is not a complete set of the current documents. Certain additional legal requirements have been posted separately at the Enterprise Directorate General web site (still named after the former Directorate General III) http://dg3.eudra.org, and it would be worth visiting the archives at that site to trace such documents, e.g., relating to the additional requirements relating to transmissible spongiform encephalopathies, which were introduced in 1999, and to the latest interpretation of issues concerned with essential similarity (which is important for generic and other products that do not qualify as "new molecular entities").

There is also a large number of additional guidelines and other documents at the web site of the CPMP, the Committee for Veterinary Medicinal Product (CVMP), and the European Medicines Evaluation Agency (EMEA). (These can be found at http://www.eudra.org.) The guidelines and related documents are available from a number of web pages, e.g., relating to the International Conference on Harmonization (ICH) and from the various Working Parties of the CPMP—Quality (QWP), Safety (SWP), Efficacy (EWP), and Biological/Biotechnological (BWP).

The reason for including the CVMP in this list is that a number of the documents at their web sites are more recent versions of the equivalent human guidance at the CPMP site. Thus, it is possible to get a feel for the newest developments in particular fields (although those aspects relating exclusively to veterinary products can be disregarded if the reader is interested only in products for human use).

Finally, some further documents have been developed by the separate inspectors' groups (which report via the European Union's Pharmaceutical Committee), and these can be found in the "What's New" or the "Archive" section of the Enterprise DG web site.

Guidelines and directive requirements are worded generally, without sufficient detail to allow an interpretation of what is actually wanted by the regulatory agencies in a particular case. How can the interested manufacturer determine what the current practical requirements of the regulatory agencies are?

One way is to take account of his own practical experience with recent applications to the relevant regulatory agencies: What new regulatory questions have been asked recently? Has the nature of questions on known topics changed recently? How will this potentially affect the current development projects? However, the extent of experience of this sort might be limited, and there is another source of useful regulatory intelligence—the published European Public Assessment Reports (EPARs) at the EMEA web site (cited above) for applications that have been processed through the Centralized procedure and possibly at the various European agency web sites in connection with applications that have been processed through the Mutual Recognition procedure (although the number of published assessment reports from this source was very limited at the time of writing). (National assessment reports are not available to the public at the time of writing.)

In this chapter, the discussion will be limited to medicinal products, meant for humans, that contain chemically synthesized active ingredients. Different or additional requirements might apply in the case of radiopharmaceuticals, blood products, biological products, biotechnology products, herbal products, and homoeopathic products. For these more specialized topics, the contents of this chapter may provide some relevant information, but interested readers should seek additional information from the relevant guidelines.

The text will be based on an interpretation of the legislative requirements and will include consideration of many of the available guidance documents. In addition, consideration has also been taken of published EPARs and the author's own experience of the European regulatory system (which extends over some 25 years). In case of doubt or disagreement, readers are referred to the original texts of the legislation, notes for guidance, and EPARs.

II. LEGAL BASIS OF MARKETING AUTHORIZATIONS IN THE EUROPEAN ECONOMIC AREA (EEA)

A. Application Procedures by Which a Marketing Authorization May Be Obtained

There are three procedures by which pharmaceutical products may gain a marketing authorization in the EEA. These are the National, Mutual Recognition, and Centralized procedures.

The first of these can be used when a product is to be marketed in a single country. It can be used for any type of application except for certain types of biotechnology-based items. Having been approved in one country, in most cases an application to a second country will trigger the Mutual Recognition procedure in other concerned countries. There are certain exceptions to this, e.g., where a product has different "summaries of product characteristics" (SmPCs) in different countries, and these have not been subjected to a harmonization procedure. Line extensions to such products could also remain subject to national procedures.

The Mutual Recognition procedure can also be used for most types of application and is based on a product being approved in one country and a request for this to be mutually recognized by the regulatory agencies in other EEA countries in which the manufacturer/market authorization holder wishes to sell the product. The practice of the member states is that such applications are rarely accepted without some additional questions being asked. When such additional questions are asked, there is a very short time period for the applicant to answer them. Any problems that arise are considered not only by the originating member state (i.e., the agency in the country whose original approval has formed the basis for the Mutual Recognition application) and the concerned member states (i.e., the agencies that have been asked to accept it as valid in their country) but also the Mutual Recognition Facilitation Group (which meets regularly at the offices of the EMEA in London on the Monday before CPMP meetings). Successful applications are valid in the concerned member states. The approval can be extended to other member states by undertaking another Mutual Recognition application.

The final option is the Centralized Procedure. This is available for a defined list of product types (included in an Annex to the relevant Regulation) and for Orphan Drugs as defined by the Orphan Drug Committee. This procedure involves the appointment of members of the CPMP as rapporteur and co-rapporteur. These persons are then responsible for the preparation of an assessment report. In practice, the authors of the assessment report are initially members of staff of the regulatory agencies, usually those from which the rapporteur and co-rapporteur come. Two initial assessment reports and two draft lists of questions are prepared and later consolidated into a single assessment report and a single list of question after discussion and input from the members of the CPMP. Additional information can be provided by the applicant, and there is a defined appeal mechanism. In the case of products for which the CPMP reaches a positive "Opinion," the European Commission (specifically the pharmaceutical sector of the Enterprise Directorate General) converts the Opinion to a Decision (which is legally binding) after seeking the input of the member states. Centralized procedure approvals are valid in all member states of the European Economic Area.

B. Legal Basis for Applications

The basis for applications will follow the principles laid down in basic European level legislation for the pharmaceutical sector. This is more or less common regardless of the actual mechanism used to gain an approval. The basic requirements for pharmaceutical marketing authorization applications are laid down in Directive 65/65/EEC (as amended). There are no *specific* requirements for pharmaceutical development or process validation included in the text of that document.

C. Legislative Requirements for Data on Development Pharmaceutics

With respect to development pharmaceutics data, the requirements stated in Directive 75/318/EEC (as amended) are included in the Annex to that document at Part 2 A 4 (page 20 of the *Rules Governing Medicinal Products in the European Union*, Volume 1, *Pharmaceutical Legislation: Medicinal Products for Human Use*). With respect to the general requirement for pharmaceutical products this states: "4.1 An explanation should be provided with regard to the choice of composition, constituents and container and the intended function of the excipients in the finished product. This explanation shall be supported by scientific data on development pharmaceutics. The overage, with justification thereof, should be stated." This, then, is the legal requirement. Needless to say, there is a considerable amount of additional information in other places to expand on this rather bland statement.

There is one additional general requirement included in Directive 75/318/EEC as amended, which affects all parts of the pharmaceutical section of the dossier. This is a blanket requirement that all analytical methods are to have been adequately validated and the validation data included in the submission. This applies to all analytical methods including those used in connection with preclinical and clinical parts of the dossier. Additional guidance on how to meet these requirements is included in the two notes for guidance developed on the topic of analytical validation through the ICH process, available at the EMEA web site or at the Commission's web site, mentioned earlier.

III. THE REQUIREMENTS: FORMAT AND CONTENT OF APPLICATIONS

A. Notice to Applicants

Three volumes of information on the format and content of applications for marketing authorization and relevant regulatory guidelines have been prepared by the Commission (Enterprise Directorate General) and published as the *Notice to Applicants*. These volumes do not have legal force, but applications that fail to follow their prescriptions can be returned to applicants as invalid.

Included in these three volumes are the suggested format for applications, the sequence of their presentation, and other guidance relating to applications. This is laid down in some detail for the four parts of the application: Part I (including the application form, labeling and product information, and Expert Reports); Part II (data on the pharmaceutical and manufacturing aspects of the application); Part III (the nonclinical data); and Part IV (the clinical data). There are also suggested formats for the various parts of the Expert Report and some suggested layouts for the tabulated parts of that document.

The Expert Report is a particular requirement of the European pharmaceutical regulatory system. It is intended that the Expert Report submitted by the applicant should include an accurate summary of the supporting evidence for the application and that it should also include a critical discussion of that information. Expert reports were originally required when a requirement for an Assessment Report was imposed on the member states: the intention was that the Expert Report should form the basis for that Assessment Report.

The requirements laid down for Part II, which relate to development pharmaceutics, include:

1. An explanation for the choice of the formulation, for its composition, the ingredients used, and the container employed, supported by the necessary data on development pharmaceutics.
2. A statement of any overages present in the product and a justification for them.
3. Detailed development pharmaceutics data where relevant studies have been undertaken—e.g., in vitro dissolution studies.

The pharmaceutical part of the Expert Report is expected to include a discussion of the following points (which suggests that the list above is intended to cover the same material):

1. The choice of the dosage form and the formulation and its suitability for the intended indications for use.
2. Those aspects critical to the in vivo bioavailability of the product and routine control tests proposed to ensure that the product has consistent bioavailability from batch to batch. Where a product has low in vivo absorption, the evidence should be discussed and a conclusion reached as to whether this is due to intrinsic properties of the active ingredient(s) or whether it is related to the properties of the dosage form concerned. In the case of products intended to have a nonsystemic effect, the potential for systemic absorption may need to be considered. This may involve specific studies to determine the levels of the active ingredient(s) in the blood, plasma, urine, or feces and a discussion of the clinical significance of those results.
3. The choice of the excipients and their concentration, including their function (e.g., antimicrobial preservatives, antioxidants...). In the case of antimicrobial preservatives, data are expected on the preservative efficacy in products on storage, including after reconstitution or dilution and during the period of use.
4. Relevant issues relating to the use of chiral active ingredient(s).

An examination of the draft formats for the data summaries in the pharmaceutical Expert Report gives some additional insight into the nature of the required discussion.

The section on the choice of the composition of the product is expected to discuss the optimization of the amounts of the various substances included in the product. Appropriate data are also required for the compatibility of the pharmaceutical product with other products with which it is intended to be used, such as diluents or reconstitution media for injection products, as well as information on the compatibility of the product with its container-closure system.

The information on the immediate packaging material should include the type of materials used, the construction of the packaging system and its specification (supported by batch analytical results), as well as a summary of the development studies relating to the packaging. With respect to process validation, it is required that the applicant discuss the experimental work undertaken to ensure that the proposed manufacturing procedures will consistently provide product of the desired quality. Particular emphasis is placed on process validation where a nonstandard method of manufacture is used and for those steps of the manufacturing process which are critical for the product. Experimental data will normally be required relating to the manufacturing process, including a demonstration that when materials of the stated quality are used with the types of manufacturing equipment specified this will consistently result in the production of product of the desired quality.

All of these topics are discussed in more detail below.

B. The Common Technical Document

Readers may also be aware that under the auspices of the ICH a document is being developed on the organization of the Common Technical Document. It is intended that this will result in a common format (and, to at least some extent, content) of marketing authorization applications in the jurisdictions of those party to the ICH process (Japan, the EEA, and the United States). At the time of writing, a draft document had been circulated for comment. When adopted and implemented, this will result in a considerable amendment to the format and sequencing of information in a marketing authorization application.

Biopharmaceutical issues to be addressed will include a discussion of the pharmaceutical development process as it relates to in vivo and in vitro performance and the general approach taken concerning bioavailability, bioequivalence, and in vitro dissolution profiles. There should be a comparative analysis of relevant studies—objectives, study design, conduct, outcome, and data analyses. The effects of formulation changes (including different strengths of product and the proportionality of biopharmaceutical characteristics) will need to be considered in relation to possible changes in bioavailability and bioequivalence, particularly for products with more complex manufacturing processes. Changes between clinical study formulations and marketing formulations will need to be considered. The effects of food (type and timing) will need to be discussed. Affects should be considered in terms of C_{max}, T_{max}, $T_{\frac{1}{2}}$, AUC, and CL, as appropriate, with reports of the mean ratios of the test and reference formulations for C_{max} and AUC (with 90% confidence intervals).

Other development studies that will need to be considered include the choice of the dosage form and formulation in terms of the route of administration and the usage (and usage instructions) being suitable. The choice of the container-closure system and any dosing device also needs to be considered in this context. Data may be derived from the literature or from specific studies.

The choice of the excipients, their intended function, and their concentration will need to be considered in relation to those characteristics that may affect product performance.

The product manufacturing process will need to be discussed in terms of the process attributes that may influence batch reproducibility, product performance, and product quality. The selection of the process, its optimization, and its validation will need to be considered, especially for identified critical aspects. Particular attention will need to be paid to the choice of sterilization and aseptic processing methods and their validation, which will have to be explained and justified. Novel processes or technologies will need extensive discussion. Packaging operations that might affect product quality will also be important. Validation and evaluation studies will need to be reported, with particular attention being applied to critical stages. Where the validation process is still ongoing, a "process validation protocol" will need to form part of the supporting data. There should be a discussion of significant changes that have occurred in the manufacturing processes during the development of the product, including any changes in the manufacturing sites. All phases of development from laboratory scale through pilot scale to production scale will need to be considered.

Any overages will need to be declared, discussed, and justified. Reprocessing proposals will need to be justified.

Physicochemical characteristics of the formulation will need to be considered, including pH, ionic strength, dissolution performance, redispersion, reconstitution, particle size distribution, aggregation, effects of polymorphism of the active ingredient, and rheological characteristics as appropriate.

Microbiological aspects will need to be discussed, but the amount of information will depend on the type of product. For nonsterile products there will need to be a description of the microbiological attributes of the product and, if appropriate, a rationale for not performing microbial limit tests. For preserved products the selection of the antimicrobial preservatives will need to be discussed and the effectiveness of the selected system demonstrated. For sterile products there will need to be appropriate process validation data and information on the integrity of the container-closure system.

Under the active ingredient (drug substance) proposals information on compatibility of the active ingredients and excipients (and of active ingredients with other active ingredients in the case of combination products) will need to be included in the information on the active ingredient. This will also include discussion of the key physicochemical characteristics that might affect product performance, e.g., water content, solubility characteristics, particle size distribution, and polymorphic and solid-state characteristics. The manufacturing/synthetic processes will need to be described together with any modifications during the development process (including route of synthesis and manufacturing site). The development from initial synthesis through all stages of scale-up will need to be considered.

Primary container-closure system–related data will need to cover storage, transportation, and use. The choice of materials of construction, their description, and the ability of the container-closure system to protect from moisture and/or light will need to be considered. The compatibility of the container-closure and its contents will need to consider sorption, leaching, and safety. The performance of the container-closure system will also need to be considered in terms of dose delivery from any associated device that is to be supplied as part of the product. Container-closure components will require adequate specifications covering description, identification, critical dimensional tolerances, and test methodology (including pharmacopeial and noncompendial methods). More data are likely to be required for liquid or semi-liquid products than for solid dosage forms. In the latter, product stability data and container-closure system specifications may suffice.

Less information will be required for nonfunctional secondary packaging. More information will be required where the secondary packaging has a function to perform.

IV. EUROPEAN GUIDELINES

A. Development Pharmaceutics

There are four relevant guidelines relating to development pharmaceutics. These are usually identified by the document number in Volume 3a of the *Rules Governing Medicinal Products* or the adopted document number at the CPMP or the CVMP. The identifiers for these four guidelines are: 3AQ1a (adopted by the CPMP in April 1988—this also included process development in the same guideline), CPMP/QWP/155/96 (adopted by the CPMP in January 1998), CPMP/QWP/054/98 corr (adopted by the CPMP in February 1999), and EMEA/CVMP/315/98 final (adopted by the CVMP in August 1999). In the following discussion the contents of the development pharmaceutics guidelines will be considered first, and then any more specific guidelines will be considered under the appropriate subheading.

In the earliest development pharmaceutics guideline it was indicated that development pharmaceutics studies *may be needed* to support a marketing authorization application. Subsequent documents have made it clear that such data *will be expected* to form part of the application.

The expectation is that the development pharmaceutics section of the application will establish why the type of dosage form and the formulation proposed would be satisfactory for the purposes specified in the application. It would identify formulation and manufacturing aspects (especially sterilization processes) critical for batch reproducibility and establish the routing monitoring requirements necessary to ensure this. There is specific comment on the inappropriateness without justification of developing unpreserved products for multiple use where the product does not possess adequate inherent preservative efficacy. The European Pharmacopoeia also has some general advice on the formulation of sterile products which are produced using aseptic processes (e.g., permitting the inclusion of a preservative in certain cases).

Development pharmaceutics information is intended to cover a number of aspects related to the active ingredient(s), excipients, container-closure system, and the finished (drug) product. These aspects will be considered individually below.

Development studies are not normally considered to fall within the system of good manufacturing practice

(GMP) controls and inspection, although where appropriate these requirements should be complied with. Manufacture of the finished dosage form should always be GMP compliant. There are also proposals for GMP compliance for active ingredient manufacture, which have been submitted for comment by the Enterprise Directorate General and under the auspices of the Pharmaceutical Inspection Convention–Pharmaceutical Inspection Co-operation Scheme (PIC-PIC/S) and the ICH process.

Active Ingredient Aspects

The compatibility of the active ingredient with other active ingredients and excipients should be demonstrated. Preformulation study reports often provide useful relevant information. Preliminary stability study reports may be used as supporting data.

The physical characteristics should be considered (in combination as appropriate) in relation to the proposed dosage form and route of administration. Factors to be considered extend to solubility characteristics, crystal form and properties, moisture or solvent content, particle size and size distribution (which may affect bioavailability, content uniformity, suspension properties, stability, and preclinical or clinical acceptability), polymorphism, etc.

Where a physical characteristic is variable from batch to batch of the raw material, it might be necessary to control identified parameters that are critical to product quality. The control specification and method may be included in the active ingredient specification or by other means.

The active ingredient specification may need to include specific relevant tests that relate to the use of the material in particular products. These may be in addition to any relevant pharmacopeial monograph specifications.

Excipients and Other Additives/Nonactive Ingredients

The incorporation of certain excipients in products is deemed to be undesirable. Examples are the inclusion of mercurial preservatives, the inclusion of benzyl alcohol in parenteral products for use in children, the use of benzoic acid esters in injections, and the inclusion of sulfites and metabisulfites in products in general. If it is intended to use any of these materials, then a full justification will be required.

The function of each excipient is to be explained and the inclusion of the material justified. Compatibility data should establish the suitability of the combination of excipients. A specific example is included in the guidelines on the justification for the inclusion of combinations of antimicrobial preservatives in multiple preservative systems. Supporting stability studies may suffice. Other types of excipient that may require specific discussion include antioxidants (and their effectiveness over the unopened shelf life and the in-use period with sufficient activity shown to be present at the end of these periods), surfactants, solvents, chelators, permeability enhancers, tablet lubricants, release moderators, etc.

Where an unusual excipient is chosen, or where an established excipient is chosen for a dosage form that results in its administration by a novel route of administration, then additional data will need to form part of the application. In effect, a novel excipient will need to be supported by data similar to those required for a new drug, with full supporting data including composition, function, and safety. Novel excipients include the components of the matrix in prolonged release products, new propellants, and new permeability enhancers. The exception to this need for extensive supporting data would be for a material already approved for food use and administered by the oral route or a material already approved for cosmetic use with a topical route of administration. In all cases the quality of the excipients has to be described adequately and shown to be satisfactory (which will depend on its role).

Particular attention needs to be given to antimicrobial preservatives (see also below), which should be shown to be effective in appropriate tests to demonstrate antibacterial and antifungal activity using the European Pharmacopoeia (Ph Eur) test method. It is normally expected that products will meet the 'A' criteria unless other performance characteristics—e.g., meeting or exceeding the 'B' criteria—can be justified. Additional data will normally be expected to demonstrate that the product is adequately preserved for its proposed shelf life (unopened) and in simulated in-use conditions (including any dilution or reconstitution and also taking into account the method and frequency of sample removal from the pack), although for the latter purpose the Ph Eur test procedure may need to be amended to include additional challenges and additional sampling points. From the latter data (and associated chemical stability data), an in-use shelf life should be proposed. This should be chosen carefully, in line with recommendations of the Ph Eur for specific product types, and should be as short as possible, taking into account patient convenience and safety.

Where a large pack size is provided, it might be necessary to undertake more extensive in-use testing and/or to restrict the in-use shelf life once the container has been opened. In addition to preservative efficacy testing the chemical stability of antimicrobial preservatives should also be investigated over the unopened and in-use shelf lives of the product.

In addition to the information relating to excipients in the development pharmaceutics guidelines there are two guidelines that specifically address excipients in pharmaceutical products—3AQ9a (adopted February 1994) and EMEA/CVMP/004/98 Final (adopted February 1999). These expand on the information in the development pharmaceutics guidelines.

Excipients should be listed in the composition using their Ph Eur name (or one from another national pharmacopeia from an EEA member state), the International Nonproprietary Name, or an exact scientific designation, other than for materials such as preservatives or coloring agents which can be identified by an E-number. Third country pharmacopeial names may be acceptable. Coloring matter is subject to the provisions of specific legislation in the EEA.

In the case of an excipient that contains a mixture of constituents, qualitative and quantitative details of the composition should be provided (other than for flavoring or aromatic products, which must state the information only qualitatively provided there is a suitable method for ensuring consistency of composition and of the presence of the main ingredients and any carriers, with relevant references to purity criteria such as those established by the World Health Organization Food and Agriculture Organization).

Where chemically transformed components that could be confused with nontransformed materials are used, the nomenclature should differentiate the two materials adequately— e.g., modified starch. Where mixtures of chemically related compounds are used, the nature and content of each component should be listed, identifying technological characteristics relevant to the dosage form and stating any additives present. Ready-mixed excipients such as direct compression mixtures and film coating compounds should give a qualitative and quantitative composition and the relevant specifications (using monograph specifications as far as possible).

For materials of natural origin, information should be given relating to chemical treatments and other processes used to obtain and purify the material as well as information on any special characteristics. Particular consideration should be given to decomposition products, specific impurities, chemicals used in the processing and any residuals, and any necessary sterilization or decontamination processes. For materials of animal or human origin special consideration will need to be given to transmissible spongiform encephalopathies and other issues arising from risks of transmission of adventitious agents. For such materials information is likely to be required on the preparation and control of the material, and the name of the manufacturer and site of manufacture may be required.

Where there is a Ph Eur or national pharmacopeial specification for the excipient, this should be applied. Third country pharmacopeial specifications may also be acceptable. Routine tests and specifications should be stated. Function-related specifications should be included.

For pharmacopeial materials scientific data are not normally required in the application provided that the method of production is such that uncontrolled impurities will not be present in the material. Otherwise the impurities concerned should be declared and appropriate specifications and test methods put forward.

For nonpharmacopeial materials a full specification should be included in the application. This should include appropriate tests and requirements for physical characteristics, identification, relevant purity tests, and performance-related tests. Characteristics likely to influence bioavailability of the finished product should be controlled. Routine tests and specifications should be described. Methods should be validated. The material should be fully characterized, with full data on the chemistry concerned and including consideration of the safety of the excipient. Any relevant European Directive requirements or other international specifications should be met, but additional requirements might apply depending on the intended use of the product—e.g., for materials to be used in sterile products.

Microbial contamination issues are particularly significant for excipients to be used in sterile products.

With the exception of antimicrobial preservatives and antioxidants (see below) and coloring matter (for which an identity test should be available), it is not normally necessary to test for the presence of excipients in finished products.

Antioxidants and antimicrobial preservatives are the subject of a further specific guideline (CPMP/CVMP/QWP/115/95, adopted July 1997). These materials are designed to be aggressive, and there are certain risks associated with their use. They are used, respectively, to (a) reduce the rate or extent of oxidation of active ingredients or other ingredients or to (b) reduce, inhibit, or prevent proliferation of microbial contaminants in finished products during storage and use, especially for products intended to be used on more than one occasion. In both cases it is necessary for the application to include a reason for the incorporation of the antioxidant and/or antimicrobial preservative in the formulation and to show that the intended activity is achieved. Their inclusion is not an alternative to the optimization of the formulation or the manufacturing process, nor is it an alternative to the application of GMPs.

Where antioxidants or antimicrobial preservatives are used, the finished product release specification will need to include identification tests and assays for these two types of excipient. The shelf life specification should also include a specification for assay for antimicrobial preservatives. Stability data will be required for both antioxidants and antimicrobial preservatives in the finished product, and in addition the preservative efficacy of the formulated product should be examined over its shelf life and by means of appropriate in-use stability tests. Preservative efficacy data should also be presented at the lower limit of the preservative assay.

Antioxidants should be used only when it can be shown that their incorporation cannot be avoided by appropriate manufacturing methods or packaging. Their intended performance in the product should be clearly stated—e.g., whether for the benefit of the active ingredient or an excipient. Their efficacy can depend on their nature, their concentration (subject to safety considerations), when they are incorporated in the manufacture of the finished product, the container, and the formulation (particularly their compatibility with other constituents). All of these issues should be addressed. Their activity should also be determined in the finished product under conditions simulating the use of the product. The extent of degradation should be determined with and without the antioxidant.

Aqueous products that are at greatest risk from microbial spoilage include solutions, suspensions, and emulsions for repeated oral, parenteral, or external use and include critical products such as multidose injections and eye drops. Unpreserved products without adequate antimicrobial efficacy should not be presented in containers intended for use on more than one occasion unless justified. When antimicrobial preservatives are used, their efficacy has to be demonstrated using the Ph Eur test for antimicrobial preservative efficacy. Factors to be taken into account in designing a preserved product include the nature of the preservative, its concentration in the product, the physical and chemical characteristics of the product (particularly its pH), the pack design, and the storage conditions.

Composition of the Finished Product

This section of an application includes the full details of the composition of the product including any materials that do not appear in the final dosage form—e.g., solvents. Consideration also has to be given to the therapeutic activity of the product, the posology (dosing), and the route of administration.

Any overages included in the manufacturing formula have to be stated. Overages may be included to cover potential manufacturing losses (in which case there should be no excess of the material in the finished product and the release specification should not reflect the inclusion of an overage). They may also be present to allow for product stability issues. The inclusion of overages is now positively discouraged because of the risk of overdosing if a product containing an overage is consumed shortly after its release to the market. In any case, where the inclusion of an overage is justified it should not exceed 10% of the nominal content of active ingredient. The inclusion of overages should not be proposed for inherently unstable formulations (when a shorter shelf life or even reformulation might be more appropriate), or where the analytical procedures are imprecise or inaccurate, or where they are required because the manufacturing processes are sub-optimal.

The development pharmaceutics section should also include consideration of possible overdosing of the active ingredient that might arise from normal use of the dosage form—e.g., deposition of drug substance from a metered dose inhalation product in the mouth.

Liquid and Semi-solid Dosage Forms

The development pharmaceutics discussion for liquid and semi-liquid dosage forms may need to pay particular attention to the following points or issues as well as the general points listed above.

The effect of pH within the range specified in the product specification should be considered with respect to possible effects on antimicrobial efficacy and on long-term stability. The bioavailability might also be affected. The physiological implications of pH may need to be discussed. Where appropriate, the inclusion of buffer systems may need to be considered to maintain a narrow pH range. Other general aspects to be considered include the ease of dissolution or redispersion, particle size and particle size distribution, aggregation, and rheological properties.

For parenteral products specific consideration needs to be included for tonicity adjustment, emulsion globule size, ease of resuspension and sedimentation rate, particle size and particle size distribution, viscosity and syringeability, and crystal form changes. Full consideration should be included of the proposed instructions for dilution or reconstitution of products and of compatibility with the proposed solvents or diluents. This should include a demonstration that the proposed storage temperature and extremes of concentration are suitable.

The preservation efficacy aspects of parenteral products are particularly important for those products that are permitted to contain preservatives. This is not allowed for large-volume injections or for any product gaining access to the cerebrospinal fluid or for intra- or retro-ocular injection (according to the Ph Eur). Unpreserved products should be labeled to state this unequivocally.

Solid Dosage Forms

Issues relating to chemical incompatibility and instability may be less significant for solid dosage forms compared with liquid and semi-solid preparations.

For modified- and immediate-release solid dosage forms, data are usually expected from appropriate dissolution and disintegration studies. These should be used to justify whether or not stability tests and routine batch testing should include dissolution and/or disintegration tests. This, in turn, will depend on the dosage form, the route of administration, whether the active ingredient is intended for immediate or modified release, etc. Normally it is expected that individually validated limits will be applied to each batch of product for oral solid dosage forms and suppositories, for example. These tests may be applied on the finished product or at some intermediate stage of manufacture—this to be considered on a case-by case-basis. The omission of disintegration testing may be proposed if a dissolution test of appropriate discriminating power is included in the batch release specification.

The test apparatus chosen for disintegration testing and dissolution testing should be one of those described in the Ph Eur unless another pharmacopoeial or a noncompendia method can be justified. The test conditions and the proposed release rates should be justified in terms of batch reproducibility.

Appropriate account needs to be taken of in vivo bioavailability data, and, where feasible, an in vivo–in vitro correlation should be established, particularly where the active ingredient has a narrow therapeutic window. It is, however, recognized in the guidelines that the establishment of an in vitro–in vivo correlation is difficult due to a number of factors. It should nonetheless be usual practice to investigate the dissolution characteristics of products during the development process and then to decide on the relevance of the test to the in vivo performance of the product. For immediate-release products development and stability data may provide a justification for not including routine finished product, tests or confirm their need. In the case of modified release products, tests will normally be required and the test conditions and release rates proposed will need to be justified (batch reproducibility) taking into account in vivo study results. This is discussed further below.

Additional studies may be required where there are significant changes introduced during the product development process into the dosage form (e.g., from capsules to tablets), the composition of the product, its manufacturing method or site of manufacture, the manufacturing equipment used, or where there have been significant changes to the control tests on the active ingredient or finished product.

The homogeneity of the product should be addressed. The adequacy of mixing processes should be shown (and confirmed with appropriate process validation data) and potential segregation discussed (as affected by surface properties, crystallinity, particle size, etc.). The Ph Eur uniformity of content requirements should apply to the dosage forms and uniformity of distribution needs to be shown between batches and within batches. The need for appropriate routine tests as part of the release specification should be discussed.

Half-unit doses are discouraged for tablets. Where it is possible to justify a half-unit dosage, then additional information will be required for dose uniformity within the halves and on the breakability of the dosage form in patient use conditions.

Where the instructions for use of the product involve admixture or dilution with drinks or other materials, appropriate compatibility data will be required. Factors to consider include ease and rate of dissolution, homogeneity, chemical and physical stability over the period of use, particle size, etc.

Transdermal Patches

The development pharmaceutics section of the application should address the clinical need for a transdermal delivery system and the appropriateness of the active ingredient for this type of product based on its physicochemical characteristics, potency, and compatibility with the other components of the product. In particular, the compatibility with the adhesive and the matrix reservoir (as relevant) should be addressed. In vitro studies on the release characteristics for the active ingredient from the finished product should be reported based on suitable diffusion cell studies with a relevant and justified barrier membrane. These should define the acceptable release characteristics and thus define transmission rate characteristics.

Additional guidance on the development pharmaceutics aspects of this type of product is included in document CPMP/QWP/604/96, adopted July 1999. This emphasizes the need for information on the rationale for the design of the product—e.g., therapeutic benefit, pharmacokinetics, and physical properties of the active ingredient.

The information included in the application should include a description of the product (including materials used and their function, dimensions and tolerances, compatibility data for the constituents, manufacturing method including solvents used and their residual levels, process development, drug load and total amount of active ingredient released, and the proportionality of different strengths). Local tolerance, waterproofness, and occlusiveness may need to be considered. The potential for precipitation or crystallization of the active ingredient during use of the product should be discussed and any potential impact on drug absorption indicated.

The product specification should include a measure of uniformity of content and a dissolution test following the release of the active ingredient until steady state is achieved (or justifying shorter periods of testing). Where possible, the dissolution specification (often expressed as quantity of active ingredient released per unit area of surface per unit time) should be related to the results obtained from batches found to be acceptable in clinical studies. In these tests six units should be tested for dissolution characteristics and the mean value stated with a measure of variability.

Pressurized Metered Dose Preparations for Inhalation

In the case of suspension products of this type, the function should be considered based on the particle size of the active ingredient. The combination of active ingredient, propellant, co-solvent, and surfactant should be investigated. Potential for extraction and other interactions with the container system parts (including the valve mechanism) should be reported. Studies should be reported on the delivery and the deposition of active ingredient using a Ph Eur test method. This should be reflected in the specification and, if possible, an in vivo–in vitro correlation established. Uniformity of content between doses should also be established.

Dry Powders for Inhalation

Factors affecting the mix of active ingredients and excipients should be discussed. These should include particle size and shape, rugosity, charge, flow properties, and water content. Since the dose delivery for these products is dependent on air flow characteristics, an attempt should be made to establish an in vivo–in vitro correlation.

Additional guidance is included in document CPMP/QWP/158/96, adopted June 1998. This includes information requirements on the formulation, development pharmaceutics, and process validation. Different types of product are identified—those based on single dose predispensed systems and those that use some kind of reservoir. The issues arising from different efficacies in the delivery of the active ingredient by different types of product are raised—the delivery of appropriate amounts of fine-powder active ingredient to achieve the same therapeutic effect may be achieved using different labeled doses. Therapeutic equivalence of different products needs to be established by in vivo studies. Where products are not intended to be interchangeable this should be indicated in the SmPC. In vitro data on deposition of active ingredient (e.g., in a multistage impactor) are not normally sufficient to demonstrate the clinical equivalence of different products.

The formulation of this type of product usually employs a small number of ingredients and sometimes only the active ingredient. Particle size and particle size distribution, rugosity, and particle charge should be considered for all ingredients, and the specific grade of excipients should be stated. The excipients should be sourced from a single supplier (with data to demonstrate the suitability of different batches of material), but if multiple sources are used, additional data will be required to establish the suitability of different batches from each supplier.

In the case of reservoir systems that rely on the cohesivity of the blend due to interparticle interactions, studies are required on vibrational stability in simulated storage, transport, and use tests, including determination of the effects of elevated temperature and humidity.

A multipoint specification for size of all ingredients (and granules if relevant) should be established. The test method can be an impaction test or another validated method (e.g., laser diffraction). The limits proposed should be based on studies at the extremes of the range under consideration using in vivo studies and multistage impactors (e.g., that described in the Ph Eur). In addition, the flow properties of the ingredients and mixes and other relevant physical characteristics should be discussed. Disaggregation of the formulated product on inhalation should be addressed.

The delivery system needs to be discussed. This will include consideration of surface charges of the particles and of the device, the development of charges during filling of the product and during in-use streaming, and any relevant changes in effective particle size. Where the prototype device differs from the production device, additional data may be required. Dose uniformity and fine particle assessments at the relevant air flow rates should be reported.

The effect of the device on air flow resistance and the ability of patients to achieve the necessary air flow rate for proper use of the product should be considered. The in vitro test method should also take this into account since the results obtained may be dependent on air flow characteristics.

Data should be provided on uniformity of delivered dose using the Ph Eur method. Products should be able to attain a range of nominal ±20% or better. The specification should be based on data from satisfactory clinical batches of product, taking into account the tolerances of the device and the batch variability for lots used in clinical studies.

The multistage impactor should be used for development studies into particle size assessment. Routine tests may be based on a two-stage impactor provided that this has been validated against performance in a multistage impactor.

Process validation should address issues concerned with the mixing process, the filling process, and derived physical tests.

Modified-Release Products

There are two specific guidelines on prolonged-release oral dosage forms (3AQ10a, adopted November 1992) and on modified-release products—oral dosage forms and transdermal dosage forms (CPMP/QWP/604/96, adopted July 1999). The advice in the two documents differs in a number of ways.

The development pharmaceutics section of the application should include information on the basis for the development of a modified-release product—e.g., the rationale, objectives, relevant pharmacokinetics of the active ingredient, therapeutic justification, physicochemical characteristics of the active ingredient (solubility with pH, partition coefficient, particle size, polymorphism), how modified release is achieved and detailed information on release-controlling excipients, whether the product is a single unit or a multi-unit system, relevant release kinetics and mechanism. The use of half-unit doses is not considered to be good practice and if proposed will need to be justified.

The information requirements for products such as prolonged-release oral dosage forms will depend on whether or not it has been possible, during the development of the product, to establish an in vivo–in vitro correlation between clinical data and dissolution studies. In vivo–in vitro correlations should be attempted using product at different stages of development, but bioavailability and pharmacokinetics data from pivotal clinical studies using at least pilot-scale production materials and possibly routine production material are particularly important. Where it is not possible to establish an in vivo–in vitro correlation, additional data will be required to compare the bioavailability of product developed at laboratory scale, pilot scale, and production scale. In the absence of an in vivo–in vitro correlation, the dissolution test will be a quality control tool rather than a surrogate marker for in vivo performance of the product.

Three types of in vivo–in vitro correlation are described in the guidelines (to which interested readers are referred).

Dissolution test data will be required in all cases (and for all strengths of product) for development and routine control and should be based on the most suitable discriminatory conditions. The method should discriminate between acceptable and unacceptable batches based on in vivo performance. Wherever possible Ph Eur test methods should be used (or alternatives justified). Test media and other conditions (e.g., flow through rate or rate of rotation) should be stated and justified. Aqueous media should be used where possible and sink conditions should be maintained. A small amount of surfactant may be added where necessary to control surface tension or for active ingredients of very low solubility. Buffer solutions should be used to span the physiologically relevant range—the current advice is over pH 1–6.8 or perhaps up to pH 8 if necessary. Ionic strength of media should be reported. The test procedure should employ six dosage forms (individually) with the mean data and a measure of variability reported.

The dissolution specification for prolonged-release dosage forms should cover a minimum of three points: one to ensure that dose-dumping does not occur (early, typically 20–30% release), one to confirm compliance with the dissolution curve profile (around 50% release), and one to ensure that the majority of the dose has been released (often more than 80% released). The robustness of the test procedure should be considered (e.g., to temperature, pH, and rotational speed).

Rather different requirements apply to delayed-release products (such as gastroresistant capsules, tablets, and granules). The development pharmaceutics section of the application for such products should discuss the rationale for delayed release, e.g., gastric mucosa protection, protection of the active ingredient from the gastric contents, or intended release at a specific segment of the gastrointestinal tract. The excipients used to achieve gastroresistance should be stated.

Single-unit gastroresistant dosage forms are discouraged on the basis of unpredictable gastric residence time and the higher risks of dose-dumping. Disintegrating multiple-unit dosage forms are preferred. The exceptions to this need to be justified (e.g., products intended to target colonic release). In any case, studies should be reported on uncontrolled release of the active ingredient by diffusion mechanisms in the gastric medium.

The Ph Eur test procedure for gastroresistance should be applied. Two media should be used, e.g., at pH 2 for one hour to detect possible damage to the gastroresistant coating and to detect active ingredient diffusion (with a limits of 10% release of active ingredient) and at pH 6.8 to simulate transfer to the intestinal segment (with complete release). Biostudy results should be reported to confirm acceptable in vivo performance.

Medicinal Gases

There is a draft guideline that includes information relating to the quality aspects of medicinal gases (CPMP/QWP/1719/00 draft, released for comment in July 2000). This includes several points of relevance to the description of the product and to development pharmaceutics.

In the description of the product considerable attention should be paid to the container and valves and associated issues. Materials of construction, dimensional controls, container suppliers, valves and their suppliers, and the design limitations of the container should be discussed.

The development pharmaceutics section should include a discussion of the properties of the gas or mixture of gases in relation to their intended presentation and use. For single gases that have been in use for a long period, bibliographical data (effectively a history of the development of the gas pressure equipment) will often suffice. In other cases compatibility of the gas with its container and other equipment necessary for its use will need to be addressed. Gas compatibility with new materials and valves will be of particular importance. Consideration should also be given to the practicality and safety of use and storage of large cylinders.

With mixtures of gases it should be indicated if any of the constituents should be considered as excipients. The physical and chemical compatibility of the different gaseous components should be demonstrated and properties of liquefied materials considered. Where superimposed liquid layers are present issues relating to the level of the outlet of the dispensing system should be described and mastered, as should the homogeneity of the gas mixture under different conditions of storage, transport, and use. Where necessary (e.g., for a mixture of a liquefied gas and a permanent gas), a frost exposure indicator may be required together with a cylinder thermal protection system and a rehomogenization procedure.

Containers and Packaging Materials

The choice of the primary packaging should be justified. This should include consideration of the safety of the packaging for the patient and user. Account should be taken of the optimal sterilization method for the finished product.

The integrity of the container and its closure should be discussed. Factors such as child resistance or *tamper evidence*, etc., should be discussed. The PhEur includes a requirement for certain types of product to be supplied in *tamper proof* container-closure systems—which is not possible if the product is to be used by a patient!

The possibility of container-closure interactions should be considered, taking into account any admixture and dilution of products. Sorption of active ingredients and excipients should be considered as should leaching of container-closure components over the shelf life. Studies should extend to simulation of use. Pack components, administration devices (e.g., giving sets), and label adhesives should be considered.

Fragmentation and self-sealability of closures should be considered taking into account the maximum probable individual occasions on which the contents of the container may be withdrawn over the lifetime of the product. There is some confusion at the time of writing concerning suitable test methods for this. It was intended that these would be developed by the European Standardization Committee (CEN), but at the time of writing it appeared that they would be reintroduced into the Ph Eur based on earlier requirements.

Where there is a dosing device provided with the product, the dose reproducibility and accuracy should be demonstrated. Examples include dropper devices, dose-measuring devices, and pen injectors. The instructions for use should also be discussed for such devices and may be particularly important for devices such as two-chamber cartridges and the like containing suspension products. It might be necessary to discuss how dosing devices meet the relevant Essential Requirements of the Medical Device Directives with reference to appropriate and relevant harmonized and other European (EN) and International Standards Organization (ISO) standards.

In addition to the various advice included in the development pharmaceutics guidelines there is also a specific guideline on plastic primary packaging materials (3AQ10a, adopted February 1994), which describes general requirements for all plastic containers but pays particular attention to those for parenteral and ophthalmic use.

For nonparenteral/ophthalmic use the plastics should meet the requirements of relevant EU food use legislation, and if the material has not been so approved then toxicology data will be required. If the container is to be used for ophthalmic or parenteral products then compliance with the relevant requirements of the Ph Eur or other relevant member state pharmacopeial requirements will be required or "appropriate" additional data provided.

Where polymers, etc., are approved for food use, the available toxicology data should be provided. Additional information is required on the source of the polymer, its conversion, and the manufacturers involved for parenteral and ophthalmic uses.

The information on the container and the development pharmaceutics is to cover the qualitative composition (polymeric and other), closure type and method of operation, tightness of the closure, dosing device information, tamper evidence and child resistance, stability of the product in the container, the method of administration of the medicinal product, any sterilization procedures, the ability of the container to protect the contents from external factors, container-closure-contents interactions, etc. Migration studies are required, depending on the type of product. The use of simulated extractants is not encouraged and can be used as predictive evidence only. Leaching studies should try to determine the likelihood of removal of antioxidants, monomers and oligomers, plasticisers, mineral compounds (e.g., of calcium, barium, or tin), catalysts, processing aids, or other additives from polymer components of the container-closure system.

In-Use Stability Testing

There are three documents that give guidance on the design and conduct of in-use stability tests: the EMEA/CVMP/127/95 final (adopted March 1996), CPMP/QWP/2570/98 (a concept paper adopted in November 1998) and CPMP/QWP/2934/99 draft (released for comment in December 1999). The studies undertaken may be discussed in the development pharmaceutics or the stability section of the dossier.

The purpose of in-use stability studies is to establish the period for which a product intended to be used on more than one occasion may be used after reconstitution or dilution or the withdrawal of the first dose from the container without adversely affecting the integrity of the product and with the product retaining acceptable quality characteristics. This type of test can be applied to any multiple use product (e.g., sterile products in multiple-use containers, powders or granules including those used to produce oral solutions or suspensions) but is likely to be of particular importance in the case of products that are manufactured with an inert headspace gas, for products containing antioxidants to protect an active ingredient that is liable to oxidative decomposition, and for products that contain a volatile antimicrobial preservative.

Specific in-use studies may be indicated if instability is identified in the conventional stability studies and for nonsterile products with an in-use shelf life of more than one month.

The application should state the rationale for the design of the in-use stability tests performed. The procedures used should be fully validated. One key factor is that the test should simulate the use of the product as far as practicable. This should include any reconstitution or dilution prior to use. Aliquots should be removed in an appropriate manner following, as far as possible, the usage pattern that will be encountered in practice. Physical (color, clarity, closure integrity, particulate matter, and particulates/particle size), chemical (assays for active ingredient, antioxidants and antimicrobial preservatives, degradation product levels, pH), and microbiological (total viable count and antimicrobial preservative efficacy using single-challenge and multiple-challenge procedures) properties should be determined.

Product manufactured at pilot scale should be used for in-use stability tests if possible, and it should be in the container-closure system intended for marketing (using the container size likely to offer the greatest challenge) together with any administration device that will normally be used with it. A minimum of two batches of product should be tested, one of which should be towards the end of its shelf life should there be any suggestion of significant change in the chemical characteristics. Product should normally be stored at 25°C/60% relative humidity for the duration of the test unless the storage conditions recommended for patient use suggest alternative storage conditions, which should then be justified. The results should be summarized, tabulated, and evaluated with a conclusion. Any anomalous results should be discussed. A maximum recommended in-use shelf life should be based on these results.

B. Process Validation

Relevant information is included in documents with the following references: 3AQ1a (adopted April 1988), CPMP/QWP/155/96 (January 1998), CPMP/QWP/054/98 corr (February 1999), EMEA/CVMP/315/98 (August 1999), and EMEA/CVMP/065/99 Final (February 2000).

General Issues

The purpose of this section of an application is to establish that the proposed manufacturing process is suitable and that it will yield consistently product of the desired quality. The concept is closely related to GMP and the detail of conventional manufacturing process validation may not be required. However, data will normally be required for nonstandard manufacturing processes (particularly nonstandard sterilization processes) and for those aspects of manufacture that are critical in terms of product quality, e.g., in the manufacture of modified-release products the quality, safety, or efficacy of which will be affected by the method of manufacture.

The choice of the method of manufacture should be explained. Its justification should be included in the development pharmaceutics section of the application. The method should be shown to be suitable for the preparation of a dosage form with the desired quality using starting materials of the appropriate quality. Process development studies should be included that address process optimization and process validation and that identify particular microbial quality requirements.

In addition to the older guidelines, there is a draft document on process validation, CPMP/QWP/848/96 draft, released for comment in September 1999.

Process validation is intended to show and document that the process described, when operating within the designated parameters, will produce product of the appropriate quality and demonstrate that the manufacturing process is under full control. Process validation should extend from laboratory-scale and preformulation studies (say $\frac{1}{100}$ to $\frac{1}{1000}$ of production scale) to formulation to pilot-scale manufacture (say $\frac{1}{10}$ production scale) to full industrial-scale manufacture, with a clear, logical, and continuous path between these stages. The magnitude of scale-up at each stage should not normally exceed a factor of 10.

Therefore, there is a clear link between the development pharmaceutics section and those on manufacture of the finished product and finished product specifications and control tests. From the development studies there will be understanding of the drug substance and the composition of the product and manufacturing process, with critical steps of the manufacturing process being identified. These critical variables should then be examined to determine the degree to which they need to be controlled to ensure batch-to-batch consistency of the finished product. This can be determined by stressing the manufacturing system to demonstrate its robustness and the limits of tolerance. This information is then fed into the method of manufacture and the process validation procedure and will be reflected in some aspects of the finished product specification.

Industrial-scale manufacturing data may not be available at the time of submission of the application. In such cases a validation protocol (details of which are included in the draft guideline) should be included in the submission.

Particular attention should be paid to "nonstandard" production technologies including nonstandard methods of sterilization, sterile filtration and aseptic processing, lyophilization, microencapsulation, and certain critical mixing and coating operations. With such processes pilot-scale manufacture may not be predictive of industrial scale manufacture, and data on three full-scale production batches may be required in the application.

For all products there is a need to submit some data on process validation, but the amount and its nature and complexity will depend on the particular product and the proposed manufacturing procedures.

Another relevant guideline is that on manufacture of the finished product, CPMP/QWP/486/95 reissue (adopted April 1996). This includes a number of more detailed points relating to the manufacturing process, some of which should be taken into account in the development pharmaceutics and process validation sections of an application.

The guideline confirms that GMP applies but that only those aspects specific to the product need be included in the MAA.

The complete manufacturing chain is to be described in the MAA. Variable or alternate batch sizes need to be justified. All ingredients need to be declared in the manufacturing formula, including those that are removed during the production process (e.g., solvents) and those that are not always used (e.g., sodium hydroxide and hydrochloric acid for pH adjustment). Experience also suggests that ranges for the amounts of all ingredients need to be stated: these can start at 0 in appropriate cases.

Upper and lower acceptance limits are expected for all ingredients—these would normally be nominal $\pm5\%$ for active ingredients and nominal $\pm10\%$ for excipients, with wider ranges being individually justified. Where factorization is used, the details should be included, together with information on total mass adjustment if necessary. Overages need to be stated and justified in the development pharmaceutics section.

There is general advice that the manufacturing process should be described but not so comprehensively as to necessitate frequent variation application for relatively minor changes. The details submitted in the application are binding and will need formal approval before they can be changed. Manufacturers are expected to have an appropriate change control system to ensure that this is undertaken appropriately.

Manufacturing validation data, which should aim to identify the critical process steps, especially for nonstandard manufacturing processes such as for new dosage forms, should be discussed in the development pharmaceutics section of the application. Validation data may be accepted based on closely related products. In-process control tests and acceptance limits should be included for any aspect where conformity with the finished product tests cannot otherwise be guaranteed (e.g., mixing, granulation, emulsification and nonpharmacopeial sterilization processes).

Details of the specific types of apparatus need not normally be given except for nonstandard processes. A flow chart of the manufacturing operation and the in-process controls (and acceptance limits) is required. Proposals for alternative processes will need to be supported by appropriate data to show that the finished products resulting from these are consistent with the finished product specification. Certain manufacturing operations such as mixing may require additional information on quality parameters monitored during production and prior to batch release. Appropriate quality parameters should be included in the finished product specification regardless of the outcome of validation studies (e.g., content uniformity for solid and semi-solid products).

The sterilization processes described in the Ph Eur are preferred, especially terminal sterilization in the final container: alternative processes have to be justified. All sterilization processes will need to be described and appropriate in-process controls and limits included. Where Ph Eur prescriptions are followed, there should be a statement to this effect in the application. Most of this information should be discussed in the development pharmaceutics section. Reference is made to the specific guidelines on ethylene oxide sterilization and irradiation sterilization, which are discussed further below. The possibility of parametric release for terminal processes such as saturated steam and irradiation is mentioned (see below). For all sterile products there should be a sterility requirement included in the finished product specification regardless of the outcome of validation studies.

For terminal heat processes at 121°C/15 minutes (steam) or 160°C/120 minutes (dry heat), the information required includes time, temperature, and acceptance limits for in-process controls. Validation data are not normally required, but may be requested. For other process conditions, additional information will be required, such as in-process controls and acceptance limits, presterilization bioburden data, and sterility assurance level validation data.

In the case of ethylene oxide sterilization, rather more detail is included on the information expected in an MAA: description of the sterilizer and associated facilities, the gas concentration used, bioburden monitoring and limits prior to exposure to gas, gas exposure time, temperature and humidity prior to exposure and during the exposure cycle, and the conditions under which ethylene oxide desorption is undertaken.

Where sterilization by filtration is used, more information will be required. The maximum acceptable bioburden limit prior to sterilization filtration is to be provided and should be not more than 10 cfu per 100 mL (if necessary with a prefiltration to achieve this), with due account taken of the volume to be filtered and the validated capacity of the filter. (Ingredients should be controlled, e.g., to not more than 100 cfu per g or per mL; the water used for the manufacture of sterile products should be controlled to 1 cfu per 100 mL.) The type of filter and its nominal pore size should be stated—pore sizes of up to 0.22 μm will be accepted without further justification. The guideline suggests that media fill data are normally considered to be in the realms of GMP, although data may be requested. Experience suggests that it is worth providing such data in the application.

Where toxic gases or solvents have been used in the manufacturing process, validation data on their removal and relevant release and shelf life specifications and acceptance limits should be included in the dossier (taking into account the ICH guidelines on residual solvents and the CPMP guideline on ethylene oxide usage). These can be discussed in the development pharmaceutics section or elsewhere.

Cleaning of primary packaging material is normally considered to be a GMP issue, although data may be requested. Sterilization processes applied to packaging materials need to be described in the application in the normal manner.

Reprocessing and production area cleanliness are normally GMP issues, although information may be requested.

Sterilization Processes

For sterile products, particular attention should be paid to the choice of an appropriate method of sterilization. Wherever possible a terminal sterilization process should be applied to the product in its final container-closure system, as suggested in the Ph Eur. The preferred options include steam sterilization, dry heat sterilization, and irradiation using the Ph Eur listed conditions (saturated steam at 121°C for 15 minutes; dry heat at 160°C for 120 minutes; irradiation with an absorbed dose of not less than 25 kGy). Where these cannot be used, the application must include justification for the alternative procedure adopted on the understanding that the highest achievable sterility assurance level should be achieved in conjunction with the lowest practicable level of presterilization bioburden. There is guidance in the form of "decision trees" as to the preferred options for sterilization method to be applied:

1. Aqueous products: moist heat at 121°C/15 minutes; then moist heat to achieve a F_0 value of not less than 8 minutes to achieve a sterility assurance level of 10^{-6}; then aseptic filtration and aseptic processing; then the use of presterilized components and aseptic compounding and assembly
2. Nonaqueous liquids, semi-solids, and dry powders: dry heat at 160°C/120 minutes; then dry heat under alternative conditions of time and temperature to achieve a sterility assurance level of 10^{-6}; then an alternative to dry heat, e.g., ionizing radiation with a minimum absorbed dose of not less than 25 kGy; then a validated alternative irradiation dose (according to ISO 11137); then aseptic filtration and aseptic processing; and then the use of presterilized components and aseptic compounding or filling

Justifications for the use of nonstandard (i.e., nonpreferred or nonpharmacopeial) methods of sterilization may include the heat instability of the active ingredient or an essential excipient. The choice of a method based on filtration through a microbial retentive filter and/or aseptic assembly should be justified, and the appropriate in process controls (including bioburden controls on active ingredients, excipients, bulk solutions, process time constraints etc) discussed in detail in the application. Commercial considerations should not form part of the argument for the application of a nonstandard sterilization process. The highest possible sterility assurance level should be achieved.

The packaging material should normally be selected so as to allow the optimal sterilization process to be applied to the product as a whole. However, factors other than the method of sterilization have to be taken into account in selecting a container material, such as the route of administration and patient convenience and compliance. Where the choice of container-closure precludes the use of terminal processing in the final container, the application should include appropriate documentation to explain and scientifically justify such a choice. The guidelines indicate that in such cases it is still the manufacturer's duty to continue the search for alternative containers that would allow terminal processes while providing the necessary product characteristics.

In addition to the general guidelines on sterilization issues, there are two specific guidelines: on the use of ethylene oxide sterilization (3AQ3a, adopted in 1994) and on irradiation sterilization (3AQ4a, adopted in 1992).

Ethylene oxide is used in the manufacture of raw materials and can be used to sterilize the surface of finished products and containers. Unfortunately, ethylene oxide is a genotoxic carcinogen and its use is not accepted without justification. In any event, tight controls are required on residues of ethylene oxide and its halohydrin-related substances. For raw materials the amount of these residues is limited to 1 and 50 μg/g, respectively; for finished products 1 and 50 μg/g, respectively (with any affected ingredients subject to the control limits for raw materials); and for containers, based on simulated use, 1 and 50 μg/mL container volume, respectively.

Irradiation may be used for microbial decontamination, sterilization, or other treatments. It can be used on starting materials, packaging materials, intermediate products, bulk products, or finished products. Details are required of the plant in which the process will be undertaken and also of the precise details of the facility, the process, and its validation. Data are required on presterilization bioburden over several batches with information on the types of organism and their radiation resistance. Inactivation curves should be generated. The possibility of radioisotope formation should be considered for electron beam irradiation at 10 MeV or more. The effect of loading patterns should be investigated and appropriate dose mapping data provided. Appropriate standard operating procedures relating to load patterns, products to be irradiated, and dosimeter type and position should form part of the submission. Additional information on the operational parameters of electron beam facilities will be required.

Parametric Release

There are two relevant proposals at the time of writing: CPMP/QWP/3015/99 draft (released for comment March 2000) and ENTR/6270/00 proposal (released for comment April 2000) from the Inspectors Group and the Pharmaceutical Inspection Convention–Pharmaceutical Inspection Cooperation Scheme (PIC-PIC/S).

The Ph Eur mentions the possibility of parametric release for certain terminal sterilization processes (saturated steam, dry heat and irradiation) where sterilization parameters can be accurately monitored and recorded and controlled. Much of the information in the two draft documents relates to parametric release of sterile products, but the possibility of parametric release of other quality parameters is also raised (e.g., for eliminating or reducing raw materials testing based on manufacturing and supply chain controls, tableting processes, and for in-process controls and analytical chemistry testing).

Parametric release is a system that gives assurance that the product is of the intended quality based on the information collected during the manufacturing process and on compliance with specific GMP requirements. Its use is based on successful validation of the manufacturing process and review of the documentation relating to the process monitoring. This concept has a wide scope and can reduce, or eliminate, routine testing of raw materials, routine in-process testing, and routine finished product testing. However, its application requires a high level of compliance with GMPs for the whole scope of operations undertaken by the manufacturer concerned together with a commitment to maintain a rigorous quality system. For application of parametric release to a particular process, adequate information will need to be available on the development and optimization of the process, its robustness, the validation data (identifying critical parameters), the reliability of the process controls, detailed acceptance criteria, and clearly defined procedures, as well as experience of its use (historical batch data). In addition, historical compliance with GMPs will be required.

Acceptance of parametric release will be on a product-by-product basis and will involve specific inspections attended by both inspectors and assessors from the regulatory agency concerned.

Currently the main application of interest for parametric release is to replace the sterility test as a control method in appropriate cases (given the limited value of that test to predict sterility assurance due to statistical considerations, although it is also pointed out that a sterility test provides a final opportunity to identify a major failure, although other means should provide a more reliable way of detecting such failures). The concept is applicable to well-founded methods of sterilization where the product stability is known and development data have identified the critical process parameters. The measured parameters should be such as to ensure that correct processing of the batch provides sufficient assurance that the sterility assurance level intended has been achieved.

In the case of heat sterilization processes, the supporting data required include heat distribution and heat penetration studies (usually at least three runs at the minimum process parameters), with calculation of heat equivalents (F_0) and biological validation such as information on the type and heat resistance of bioburden organisms. Chemical indicators may be used in addition. Appropriate in-process controls may be expected, e.g., presterilization bioburden (including type, number, and heat sensitivity of the organisms present), cycle parameter monitoring, and verification that the load has been processed. Information will also be required on any bioindicators used (D-value, z-value, type, and stability).

In the case of irradiation sterilization, the minimum absorbed dose is generally accepted at 25 kGy. Lower doses will require a low level of bioburden (checked routinely) and adequate validation data. Compliance with the requirements of the GMP guideline on irradiation sterilization is also expected.

Even where it is possible to omit routine or even any sterility testing of finished product, the sterility requirement should be retained in the finished product specification.

The draft guidelines give considerable information on how an applicant can submit relevant data to request parametric release. However, since this is unlikely to be accepted until considerable manufacturing experience of the product concerned has been gained, it is probable that this will be submitted as a later variation application rather than in an initial marketing authorization application.

V. EXPERIENCE WITH REGULATORY APPLICATIONS

A. Introduction

This part of the chapter is based on consideration of the published EPARs at the EMEA's web site. At the time of writing there were more than 60 EPARs available. The contents of the pharmaceutical assessment section of each of these were examined, and detailed notes were made from more than 50 of those documents. The amount of information in the different EPARs varies considerably. Some have specific sections with the heading "development pharmaceutics," while others include relevant information in the text without a heading. In some cases there are simple statements to the effect that satisfactory pharmaceutical development data were submitted. Therefore, an attempt has been made to glean information of a general nature, and this will be presented as a discussion of relevant topics by dosage form.

B. Tablets, Hard Gelatin Capsules, Soft Gelatin Capsules, and Granules

All of the products considered in detail were immediate-release dosage forms.

The physicochemical characteristics of the active ingredient in relation to the dosage form and the suitability for its intended purpose was discussed in several EPARs, particularly relating to the solubility characteristics and absorption from the gut. The compression characteristics were also mentioned in some EPARs. The possible effects of different polymorphs or evidence that only a single polymorph is used are addressed as appropriate. Different amorphous or crystalline forms are also discussed. Where affecting the dosage form, selection properties such as unpleasant taste or smell are mentioned.

Several of the active ingredients were chiral, and the nature of the material used in the marketed product—racemate or single isomer—was considered and chiral stability issues discussed.

Where there are existing pharmacopeial specifications for active ingredients in the Ph Eur or the pharmacopeia of a member state, these will be expected to apply. Other pharmacopeial specifications or in-house specifications may be used in other cases. The same is true for excipients where harmonized specifications are mentioned. Particular quality requirements related to a particular application are discussed, e.g., particle size control requirements.

Compatibility of the excipients and active ingredient is addressed (but often with little detail). Formulation optimization and excipient ranges may be included in the discussion. The inclusion of antioxidants in the formulation is discussed as appropriate.

Product bioavailability is mentioned, especially where it is low. Where there are differences between the formulations tested for bioavailability during the development process and the formulation to be marketed, there is considerable discussion of the data provided on the bioequivalence of the different products and/or formulations. This is particularly so where, for example, early clinical studies were undertaken with capsules but the marketed dosage form is to be a tablet. Bioequivalence data and pharmacokinetic data (e.g., in crossover studies) and comparative dissolution studies are usually reported. This is particularly significant where the different strengths of the final products are not achieved by using different quantities of the same granulate formulation. Process optimization may also be addressed in such cases.

Comparative bioavailability data are discussed where a number of different dosage forms/routes of administration have been used during the development process, e.g., tablets, capsules, oral solutions, granules, and injections.

Where affected excipients are used—particularly when of bovine origin—including lactose, gelatin, stearic acid/stearates, etc., a statement of compliance with the current requirements relating to transmissible spongiform encephalopathies is included in the EPARs.

The development of new dosage forms such as rapidly dispersible tablets are discussed in some detail.

The manufacturing process is sometimes discussed in terms of the characteristics of the active ingredient, e.g., the need for nonaqueous granulation processes, the need for controlled humidity in the manufacturing environment. The number of different manufacturing sites requested is mentioned in the assessment reports. Special manufacturing processes such as extrusion/spheronization are mentioned in the EPARs.

A few products have declared overages of active ingredient, which have been justified. In the case of some other product types, the initial inclusion of overages and their subsequent removal is mentioned.

Where scored tablets are provided, there is often discussion of the suitability of the product for half-tablet dosing. This includes data on content uniformity and on the suitability of the finished product for subdivision—e.g., hardness specifications, data on ability to subdivide.

For granules and the like with a dose-delivery system, there is discussion of the accuracy of dosing and the suitability of the delivery system, taking into account the recommended dosing instructions for the product.

The packaging systems used were discussed in some detail in several EPARs. The number of products requiring a desiccant of some type is quite a high proportion of the total. In many cases both blister packs (of various compositions) and bottles (glass or plastics) were used for the same product. Effectiveness in protecting light-sensitive active ingredients and products is mentioned in the EPARs. Child resistance and tamper evidence is also mentioned.

C. Parenteral Products (Injections, Powders for Injection, Concentrates for Injection, Sterile Implants)

Issues similar to those discussed above for other dosage form types arise from the active ingredients and excipients proposed for use.

Where a compromise is reached between product pH and optimal stability pH, this will be discussed in the EPAR. Particular discussion will be included where the formulation is unusual in terms of co-solvents and/or stabilizers.

Particular attention is paid to the presentation of the product, especially for lyophilized products, which need to be reconstituted prior to use. The use of an ampule presentation of a freeze-dried product was not well received. Where products are reconstituted or diluted before use, this process is discussed and stability of the resulting solution or suspension in the administration medium considered. Information is included where diluents are provided with dried formulations of active ingredient, including their presentation (e.g., prefilled syringe, vial, or ampule). The media used for the generation of stability data is mentioned, especially for large-volume infusions, e.g., where 0.9% sodium chloride infusion, 5% glucose infusion, and possibly others such as lactated Ringers infusion are used. The period for which chemical stability for the use of such products has been shown will be mentioned and the final labeling text included in the EPAR. (Note that in the European context the "labelling" is usually taken to be the text that appears on the product label. Other documentation such as information leaflets and practitioner information has separate headings. Advertising materials are not part of MAAs, but in many cases the pharmaceutical authorities monitor it separately.)

The availability of unpreserved and preserved dosage forms is considered. Mention is made of formulation changes necessitated by multidose products. The need for adequate antimicrobial preservative efficacy can be discussed if this was an issue during product development.

Container composition and tamper evidence is discussed in the EPARs. There is also discussion of containers in cases where special systems such as two-compartment cartridges are used. Any particular points relating to multiple withdrawals of doses from the container will also be included. Special issues relating to pen injectors will be included.

Where terminal processing is not possible, the justification for alternative sterilization methods will be included in the EPAR, or at least a statement to the effect that sterile filtration/aseptic processing will be used. Presterilization bioburden issues that arose during the assessment will be included in the EPAR.

In the case of a novel product such as an intraocular implant, considerable discussion is included in the EPAR concerning the development, manufacture, and control of the product. In the particular case of one product, there is also discussion of the product's compliance with relevant medical device essential requirements.

D. Other Dosage Forms

There are two EPARs for eyedrops. Specific issues considered for these include container composition and tamper evidence, the optimization of the formulation and manufacture, preservative and preservation issues, and justification for the use of nonterminal sterilization processes. Many of the points concerning active ingredients and excipients are similar to those discussed above. Changes in formulation during the development process (e.g., for carbomers or surfactants) are mentioned. Particle size controls for suspension products are discussed.

A number of oral solution or suspension products are included in the EPARs. Apart from the usual points of consideration for active ingredients and excipients, particular mention is made of possible precipitation of active ingredient when a solution is in use, the inclusion of excipients having a major impact on bioavailability, the need for flavoring to mask the taste of the active ingredient, relative potency compared with other routes of administration, preservation issues, dosing devices and the precision and accuracy of the dose delivered, and bioequivalence where formulations have been modified during the development process.

VI. DOCUMENTS USED TO PREPARE THIS CHAPTER

A. Legislation

Rules Governing Medicinal Products in the European Union, Volume 1, *Pharmaceutical legislation—Medicinal products for human use*
Commission of the European Communities, Luxembourg, 1998
Also available at the Enterprise Directorate General's internet site at http://dg3.eudra.org.

Directive 65/65/EEC (pages 3–12)
Directive 75/318/EEC (pages 13–40)

B. Commission Guidance on the Format and Content of Applications for Marketing Authorization

Rules Governing Medicinal Products in the European Union, Volume 2, *Notice to applications—Medicinal products for human use*
Volume 2A *Notice to applicants—Medicinal products for human use—Procedures for marketing authorisation*
Volume 2B *Notice to applicants—Medicinal products for human use—Presentation and content of the dossier*
Volume 2C *Notice to applicants—Medicinal products for human use—Regulatory guidelines* Commission of the European Communities, Luxembourg, 1998/1998/1999 (and amendments)
Also available at the Enterprise Directorate General's internet site (cited above).

C. Guidelines

Guidelines Included in Rules Governing Medicinal Products

Rules Governing Medicinal Products in the European Union, Volume 3A, *Guidelines—Medicinal products for human use—Quality and biotechnology*

3AQ1a *Development pharmaceutics and process validation* (pages 3–10)
3AQ2a *Manufacture of the finished dosage form* (pages 11–18)
3AQ3a *Limitations to the use of ethylene oxide in the manufacture of medicinal products* (pages 19–22)
3AQ4a *The use of ionising radiation in the manufacture of medicinal products* (pages 23–30)
3AQ9a *Excipients in the dossier for application for marketing authorisation of a medicinal product* (pages 67–74)
3AQ10a *Plastic primary packaging materials* (pages 75–82)
3AQ13a *Validation of analytical procedures—methodology* (pages 107–118)
3AQ14a *Validation of analytical procedures—definitions and terminology* (pages 119–126)
3AQ19a *Quality of prolonged release oral solid dosage forms* (pages 167–74)

Volume 3, *Guidelines—Medicinal products for human use—Efficacy*

3CC29a *Investigation of chiral active substances* (pages 381–392)

Volume 4, *Good manufacturing practices*

Annex 12 *Use of ionising radiation in the manufacture of medicinal products* (pages 113–118)

*Guidelines Published by the CPMP and CVMP and the Commission**

These documents are available from relevant trade associations, some professional associations, such as BIRA and DIA, by subscription to schemes such as Euro Direct, operated by the UK Medicines Control Agency, and via the internet at http://www.eudra.org (or http://dg3.eudra.org for the item marked*).

CPMP/QWP/155/96 *Note for guidance on development pharmaceutics* (January 1998)

EMEA/CVMP/315/98 final *Development pharmaceutics for veterinary medicinal products* (August 1999)

CPMP/QWP/054/98 corr *Annex to note for guidance on development pharmaceutics—Decision trees for methods of sterilisation* (February 1999, amended after February 2000)

EMEA/CVMP/065/99 final *Decision trees for the selection of sterilisation methods* (February 2000)

EMEA/CVMP/004/98 final *Note for Guidance—Excipients in the dossier for application for marketing authorisation for veterinary medicinal products* (February 1999)

CPMP/CVMP/QWP/115/95 *Note for guidance on inclusion of antioxidants and antimicrobial preservatives in medicinal products* (July 1997)

EMEA/CVMP/127/95 final *Note for guidance—In-use stability testing of veterinary medicinal products (March 1996)*

CPMP/QWP/2570/98 *Concept paper on the development of a CPMP note for guidance on in-use stability testing of non-sterile human medicinal products* (November 1998)

CPMP/QWP/2934/99 draft *Note for guidance on in-use stability testing of human medicinal products* (released for comment December 1999)

CPMP/QWP/598/99 draft *Note for guidance on process validation* (released for comment September 1999, also issued under CVMP reference EMEA/CVMP/598/99 draft)

CPMP/QWP/486/95 *Note for guidance on manufacture of the finished dosage form* (reissued April 1996)

CPMP/QWP/2431/98 *Concept paper on the development of a CPMP note for guidance on parametric release* (November 1998)

CPMP/QWP/3015/98 draft *Note for guidance on parametric release* (released for comment April 2000)

ENTR/6270/00 * *Proposal for an Annex 17 to the EU Guide to Good Manufacturing Practice: Parametric release* (released for comment April 2000)

CPMP/ICH/2887/99 *Note for guidance on Organisation of Common technical document Draft consensus guideline* (released for comment July 2000)

Chapter 21

Pediatric and Geriatric Aspects of Pharmaceutics

Michele Danish

St. Joseph Health Services, Providence, Rhode Island

Mary Kathryn Kottke

Cubist Pharmaceuticals, Inc., Lexington, Massachussets

I. INTRODUCTION

A. Classification of Age Groups

Definition of Pediatric Age Groups

The rapid physical maturation that occurs between birth and adulthood is well known. Logically, it would be anticipated that these changes would result in altered responses to xenobiotics. Within the first 5 years of life 95% of children have been prescribed medications. Yet in 1977 only one third of the new molecular entities that have potential usefulness in pediatric patients had pediatric labeling at the time of approval.

In its continuing effort to improve the safety and efficacy of drugs in the pediatric population, the U.S. Food and Drug Administration (FDA) has defined five subgroups of this population based on age. Each subgroup is not homogeneous but does contain similar characteristics that are considered milestones in growth in development. The FDA classifications are listed in Table 1.

Age classifications do not provide an ill-inclusive method for establishing pediatric doses. Based on current knowledge, the most accurate pediatric doses are determined utilizing both weight and age. Dosing based on surface area has been shown to have no practical advantages for the general pediatric population [1].

The classification listed in Table 1 will be utilized throughout this chapter. Caution must be exercised when referring to observations in the neonatal period, however, since premature and/or very low birth weight neonates often have drug responses and disposition significantly different from those of full-term neonates. These differences will be clearly identified in the text.

Definitions of Elderly

Old age has been defined as the "advanced years of life when strength and vigor decline" [2]. Although this definition appears to be quite ambiguous, one realizes that it is necessarily so because the aging process itself is subject to a large amount of interindividual variation [3,4]. This means that when comparing studies of a "young adult" population with studies of an "elderly"

Table 1 FDA Classification by Age of the Pediatric Population

Age group	Description
Intrauterine	Conception to birth
Neonate	Birth to 1 month
Infant	1 month to 2 year
Child	2 year to oneset of puberty
Adolescent	Onset of puberty to adult

Table 2 Eligibility, by Age, for Federally Funded Programs

Age criteria	Program
60	Older Americans Act Title VII
62	Housing and urban development
65	Medicare Program Title XVII
70	Mandatory retirement age

population, one will find the variance to be much greater in the elderly group. For instance, many readers probably know of a 65-year-old who "doesn't look a day past 50." whereas others may have made the acquaintance of a 50-year-old who is exceedingly frail.

Chronological Age. Because of this wide variation within the elderly population, it is difficult to devise a "catch-all" age one must attain to be considered elderly. Within the government, there also appears to be a problem of consistently defining this age group. Table 2, which lists a variety of federally funded programs and their corresponding age criteria, illustrates this point quite well. Table 3 lists what seems to be one of the better classification systems that has been devised [5]. As well as being the system currently used by the U.S. Bureau of the Census, it is often implemented in studies that specifically deal with elderly populations [6,7].

Biological and Functional Age. To compensate for this wide variation noted among older populations, researchers have attempted to assess age in terms of biological or functional age. This basically involves combining a variety of factors, such as physiological, psychological, and intellectual parameters, to develop a *functional age* that would serve as the older counterpart of *developmental age*, which is used when assessing neonatal development [3,4,8]. The derivation of biological and functional age is quite complex, and although many interesting approaches to this problem have been studied, no one derivation has been universally accepted [3,8].

Table 3 Commonly, Utilized Age Classification System

Age(yr)	Category
65–74	Young–old
75–84	Middle–old
85	Old–old

Soruce: Ref. 5.

II. THE PEDIATRIC POPULATION

A. The Effects of Maturational Changes on Drug Disposition

Traditionally, drug dosing in infants and children has been based on age or weight ratio reduction of the adult dose. Data compiled in the past 30 years on maturational changes in organ function have allowed us to gain a much greater appreciation of the differences in drug disposition in pediatrics when compared with adults. Numerous review articles have addressed in detail clinical pharmacokinetics in infants, and children [9–14]. In this chapter we will highlight the changes that are pertinent in the development of pediatric dosage forms.

Absorption

Age affects the capacity of all the physiological functions of the gastrointestinal tract. Gastric acid output follows a biphasic pattern in neonates, with the lowest gastric acid output observed between 10 and 30 days. Gastric acid output approaches adult values by 3 months of age. Acid output on a kilogram basis, is similar to adult levels by 24 months of age [15]. Enteral feedings influence gastric acid secretion [16]. This suggests that hospitalized neonates receiving only parenteral nutrition will be relatively achlorhydric. This hypothesis is supported by reports of increased absorption of acid-labile drugs in the newborn period [10].

Gastric-emptying time and intestinal transit time are erratic in neonates. Gastric-emptying time is influenced by gestational and postnatal age and the type and frequency of feeding [17]. Although there is some controversy over the postnatal age at which adult patterns of gastric emptying are attained, it is generally accepted that adult values are reached by 6–8 months of age. There have been reports of erratic absorption of sustained-release products in children up to 6 years of age [18]. The possible role of gastric emptying on this clinical finding is unknown.

The first-pass effect has not been extensively evaluated in infants and children. The maturational rate of metabolic pathways would be directly related to the oral bioavailability of a drug subject to first-pass effect. Drugs that undergo glucuronidation during enterohepatic recirculation may have altered systemic availability in children up to approximately 3 years of age because of delayed maturation of conjugation.

Pancreatic enzyme activity is very low in premature neonates. Lipase activity increases 20-fold in the first 9 months of life. Since concentration of bile salts is also low, it is anticipated that lipid-soluble drugs would be poorly absorbed in early infancy.

Colonization and metabolic activity of gastrointestinal bacterial flora do not approach adult values until 2–4 years of age [19]. This has resulted in increased bioavailability of digoxin in infants and young children.

Drugs absorbed by active transport mechanisms appear to have a delayed rate, but not extent of absorption, in the neonatal period [20]. The absorption of vitamin K depends, to some extent, on the development of intestinal flora.

Drug absorption is highly variable in neonates and infants [21,22]. Older children appear to have absorption patterns similar to adults unless chronic illness or surgical procedures alter absorption. Differences in bile excretion, bowel length, and surface area probably contribute to the reduced bioavailability of cyclosporine seen in pediatric liver transplant patients [22a]. Impaired absorption has also been observed in severely malnourished children [22b]. A rapid GI transit time may contribute to the malabsorption of carbamazepine tablets, which has been reported in a child [23]. Selection of a more readily available bioavailable dosage form, such as chewable tablets or liquids, should be promoted for pediatric patients.

Distribution

Significant changes occur in percent total body water, albumin, alpha-1 acid glycoprotein concentration, and fat composition from the neonatal period through adulthood [24]. The most rapid changes occur during the first month of life [25,26], with values approaching adult levels by one year [24]. Adult levels of total body water and extracellular water are reached in adolescence [12]. Malnourished children, who represent 40% of the pediatric population living in developing countries, have significantly reduced concentrations of albumin and alpha-1 acid glycoprotein [22b].

Metabolism

Drug metabolic activity cannot be reliably predicted from gestational or postnatal age. The most noticeable changes occur in the first year of life and again at puberty. Parental exposure to inducing agents, nutritional status, and hormonal changes all play a role in metabolic activity. An added consideration is the fact that neonates requiring medications are often subject to other medical and surgical interventions that may influence drug disposition by liver [27]. The underlying genetic pattern of enzymatic activity must also be considered in the assessment of dose-related effects [27a].

In general, phase I reactions, such as oxidation and *n*-demethylation are delayed in the neonate but are fully operational at or above adult levels by 4–6 months of age in the full-term neonate [27a–30]. Conjugation pathways, such as glucuronidation, do not approach adult values until 3 or 4 years of age. Sulfation activity does appear to reach adult levels in early infancy. For drugs that are subject to metabolism by both pathways, such as acetaminophen, the efficient activity of the sulfation pathway allows infants and children to compensate for low glucuronidation ability [31]. The elimination of other compounds in which sulfation (e.g., chloramphenicol) is not an alternative pathway are subject to prolonged elimination half-lives [32].

Infants and children older than 1 year of age are considered to be very efficient metabolizers of drugs and may actually require larger doses than those predicted by weight adjustment of adult doses or shorter dosing intervals [33]. On the basis of metabolic activity, sustained-release formulations would appear to be ideal for children 1–10 years old, if bioavailability issues prove not to be problematic. The ability to clear drugs in critically ill children may be severely compromised; therefore, dosing in this subgroup of patients requires careful titration [34].

Metabolic activity declines with the onset of adolescence. After puberty, adolescents metabolize drugs at a rate similar to adults [27a,35].

Renal Excretion

The renal excretion of drugs depends on glomerular filtration, tubular secretion, and tubular absorption. A twofold increase in glomerular filtration occurs in the first 14 days of life [36]. The glomerular filtration rate continues to increase rapidly in the neonatal period and reaches a rate of about 86 mL/min per 1.73 m^2 by 3 months of age. Children 3–13 years of age have an average clearance of 134 mL/min per 1.73 m^2 [37]. Tubular secretion approaches adult values between 2 and 6 months [11]. There is more variability observed in maturation of tubular reabsorption capacity. This is likely linked to fluctuations in urinary pH in the neonatal period [38].

Summary

It is evident from the foregoing discussion that the greatest effects of maturation on drug disposition are observed in the first 6 months of life. However, individual variation in maturation in the first 3 years necessitates individual monitoring in both the ill neonate and the young child. Pediatric-dosing formulations that readily provide for small increments or de creases in single doses would greatly facilitate dosing in this age group.

B. Pharmacodynamic Differences Observed In Pediatric Patients

It has been generally assumed that therapeutic serum drug concentration ranges based on data obtained in adults were applicable to children. However, in many instances, when drug response is studied in children, differences in drug distribution and metabolism and in receptor sensitivity rendered this assumption invalid [39].

Receptor Sensitivity and Response

Age-related variations in central nervous system (CNS) neurotransmitter production and receptor sensitivity are the most likely explanations for the pharmacodynamic differences observed between children and adults following administration of psychotropic medications [39a]. Children have lower phenobarbital ratios than adults, and the ratio increases with gestational age [40,41]. Conversely, a lower therapeutic range for children has been identified for cyclosporine, phenytoin, and digoxin [42].

Age does not significantly affect plasma concentrations or disposition of ibuprofen; however, investigators have determined that the onset of antipyresis and maximum antipyretic effect is greater in children less than one year old as compared to children older than 6 years [43]. The authors hypothesized that this accelerated response was related to the greater relative body surface area of the young child. It should be noted that cystic fibrosis patients do have a higher clearance of ibuprofen [43a].

Adverse Reactions

Adverse reactions to drugs differ in both type and incidence in the pediatric population. Because of immature metabolic pathways, infants and children may have different metabolic patterns than adults. This at least partially explains why neonates require lower theophylline serum concentrations for the treatment of neonatal apnea and why the incidence of hepatotoxicity following acetaminophen overdose is much lower in young children than in adults [44,45]. Antibiotic adverse effects unique to the pediatric population may be due to immature metabolic pathways [46] or their effect on bone development [47]

Differences in receptor sensitivity have been offered to explain the spectrum of unexpected drug responses observed in children. Neonates and young children are at increased risk to experience paradoxical CNS stimulation following antihistamine administration. Symptoms observed in pediatric cases of acute overdose include hallucinations, excitation, and seizures. A physiological explanation for this reaction has not been identified. Antihistamines should not be included in over-the-counter (OTC) cough and cold products recommended for infants and young children.

Resistance to drug toxic effects has also been observed in children. The incidence of aminoglycoside toxicity has been reported to be much lower in infants and children than in adults [39,48]. Diminished tissue sensitivity has been suggested as an explanation.

The high reported incidence of gastrointestinal abnormalities in children receiving nonsteroidal agents was also unexpected [49]. It was anticipated that they would be more resistant to gastrointestinal injury than adults.

The incidence of reported adverse drug reaction (ADR) hospital admissions in pediatrics ranges from 1.8 to 3.2%. This is lower than the incidence observed in the general population and may be the result of differences in organ function or of a reduced level of drug exposure in children [50]. In a survey of outpatients, the incidence of adverse events in children was similar to adults [51]. A significant number of the adverse event reports were related to excessive responses to OTC drug products; this implies that inappropriate dosing may contribute to the high frequency of adverse effects. More precise dosing instructions on the labelling of OTC products intended for use in the pediatric population may alleviate this problem.

C. Drug-Delivery System and Compliance Issues

Inactive Ingredients

Over 760 excipients have been approved by FDA for use as "inactive ingredients" in drug products. The FDA Division of Drug Information Resources compiles a list of all inactive ingredients in approved prescription drug products in the *Inactive Ingredient Guide*. FDA requires the listing of excipients in pharmaceuticals other than oral. The labeling of inactive ingredients in oral drug products is voluntary. The reported incidence of adverse drug reactions to excipients is much lower than the incidence reported with active drug. This may be due to several factors, including the generally safe nature of the excipients, the low concentration found in single doses, or lack of identification of an excipient as a causative agent.

Selecting excipients for incorporation into a drug product for human consumption is complex. In selecting excipients for drug products intended for use in the pediatric population, additional cautions must be taken. Several subgroups of the pediatric population who are likely to be hospitalized and receive both oral and parenteral drug products have been identified as being particularly susceptible to excipient reactions. Serious events have been reported in low birth weight neonates and infants, asthmatics, and diabetics. Reactions have ranged from dermatitis to seizures and death [52,53]. Table 4 lists the excipients that have been reported to cause adverse events in the pediatric population.

Many of these reactions are related to the quantity of excipient found in a dosage form. Benzyl alcohol benzalkonium chloride, propylene glycol, lactose, and polysorbates are all associated with dose-related toxic reactions [52–54]. Large-volume parenterals containing 1.5% benzyl alcohol as a preservative have caused metabolic acidosis, cardiovascular collapse, and death in low birth weight premature neonates and infants. The cumulative dose of benzyl alcohol ranged from 99 to 234 mg/kg per day in these patients [55,56]. Dose-related adverse effects to excipients are of particular concern in the preterm, low birth weight infant because of the known immaturity of hepatic and renal function in this population.

Dose-related reversible CNS effects have also been reported in children receiving long-term therapy in which propylene glycol was a cosolvent [57].

Dyes. Dose does not appear to be a factor in patient reaction to dyes. The mandatory labeling of the azo dye tartrazine (FD&C yellow No. 5) in OTC and prescription medications [58] has focused the attention of pharmaceutical manufacturers and the consumer on the potential danger of dyes in susceptible individuals.

Hypersensitivity reactions have been reported with several azo dyes, particularly FD&C Yellow No. 5 and No. 6. Tartrazine-induced bronchoconstriction is commonly considered a cross-reaction to aspirin in sensitive asthmatics, although urticaria has been reported in other patient populations [59]. In a double-blind challenge involving aspirin-sensitive asthmatics, hypersensitivity to dyes was only 2%[60]; however, numerous case reports involving azo dyes suggest caution when using a drug containing an azo dye in asthmatics [61]. Non-azo dyes are considered to be weak sensitizers.

The association of dye content with hyperactivity in children remains controversial and unproved.

Sweeteners. Sweeteners are commonly included in pediatric formulations to increase palatability.

Sucrose is still the most popular sweetener. Chewable tablets may contain 20–60% sucrose, and liquid

Table 4 Excipients Reported to Cause Adverse Reactions in Children

Name	Route of administration	Reaction	Ref.
Azo dyes (tartrazine)	Oral	Urticaria. bronchoconstriction, angioedema	100 101
Benzalkonium Cl	Oral, inhalation, topical	Bronchoconstriction	102 103
Benzyl alcohol	IV	Metabolic acidosis, neurotoxicity	55 56
Lactose	Oral	Lactose intolerance, prolonged diarrhea	104 105
Parabens	Oral. IV	Hypersensitivity	106
Polysorbate 80 and 20/tocopherol	IV	Liver and kidney failure in low birth weight infants	107
Propyl gallate	Oral	Methemoglobinemia	108
Propylene glycol	Oral. IV. topical	Seizures. hyperosmolality, contact dermatitis	57 109
Thiomersal	Topical. otic, IM	Hypersensitivity, mercury toxicity	110 111 112

preparations may contain up to 85% sucrose. In a survey of sweetener content of 107 pediatric antibiotic liquid preparations. Only four were sucrose-free [62]

The sucrose content of oral liquids may cause significant problems when these products are prescribed for long-term therapy (e.g., asthma, seizure control, recurrent infections). Oral liquid preparations can represent a substantial carbohydrate load to children with labile diabetes, particularly if a child is ingesting more than one liquid medication with a high sugar content.

A wider problem exists with the possible role of liquid medications in dental caries formation [63]. The extent of acid production in the oral cavity is closely related to caries formation. In a study of liquid medication, investigators have observed that medications with sucrose concentrations higher than 15% were able to significantly lower pH; there was an inverse relation between sucrose content and a decrease in oral cavity pH [64]. In a comparison of sorbitol and sucrose-sweetened liquid iron preparations, only sucrose-containing products produced a significant decrease in oral cavity pH [65].

Viscous formulations with a high-sucrose content are especially prone to contribute to caries formation because of their prolonged contact time in the oral cavity.

Sorbitol is a polyhydric alcohol, with a high caloric content. In a survey of 129 oral liquid dosage forms stocked at a large university teaching hospital, 42% contained sorbitol [66]. The sorbitol concentration in the identified products varied from 3.5 to 72% w/v (0.175–3.6 g/mL).

Sorbitol is an appropriate substitute for children whose sucrose intake must be restricted. Although it is prepared by hydrogenation of glucose or corn syrup, sorbitol does not require insulin for metabolism [67]. It is considered to have very low cariogenic potential because it is not fermented by salivary bacteria. Sorbitol is a hyperosmotic laxative, and diarrhea has been reported in children receiving only 9 g/dav [68]. In patients with sorbitol intolerance, abdominal cramping and diarrhea may occur with even lower daily ingestion. When the active ingredient produces similar adverse gastrointestinal (GI) effects, it is difficult to identify the causative agent. Acetaminophen elixir, theophylline elixir, valproic acid syrup, and cimetidine and hydralazine solutions contain sorbitol; all have been reported to cause osmotic diarrhea in children.

Special consideration for sorbitol content is necessary for diabetic patients. Diabetics tend to have altered GI motility and ingest sorbitol from many food sources in addition to medications.

Both solid and liquid dosage forms may contain saccharin. Saccharin is a nonnutritive sweetening agent, which is 300 times as sweet as sucrose. In a survey of sweetener content of pediatric medications, seven out of nine chewable tablets contained saccharin (0.45–8.0 mg/tablet) and sucrose or mannitol. Seventy-four of the 150 liquid preparations investigated contained saccharin (1.25–33 mg/5 mL) [62]. Saccharin is a sulfanamide derivative that should be avoided in children with sulfa allergies [54].

It is recommended that daily saccharin intake be maintained below 1 g because of a risk of bladder cancer. A lifetime daily diet containing 5–7.5% saccharin has induced bladder tumors in rats [69]. However, it is probable that saccharin is only a very weak carcinogen in humans. The amount contained in pharmaceutical preparations is well below the recommended maximum human daily intake.

Because of the high incidence of lactose intolerance in the general population, lactose is not recommended as a sweetener for pediatric populations [70]. Aspartame, a phenylalanine derivative, is incorporated in many chewable tablets and sugar-free dosage forms. Aspartame-containing products should be avoided in children with autosomal recessive phenylketonuria [54].

Vehicle Selection

Ethanol has long been employed as a solvent in pharmaceuticals. Since it also acts as a preservative and flavoring agent, it is second only to water in its use in liquid preparations. It has also been suggested that it may enhance the oral absorption of some active ingredients [71].

Hepatic metabolism of ethanol involves a nonlinear saturable pathway. Young children have a limited ability to metabolize and thereby detoxify ethanol. Ethanol intoxication has been recorded in children with blood levels as low as 25 mg/dL. Alcohol has a volume of distribution of approximately 0.65 L/kg. Ingestion of 20 mL of a 10% alcohol solution will produce a blood level of 25 mg/dL in a 30 pound child. The American Academy of Pediatrics (AAP) Committee on Drugs recommends that pharmaceutical formulations intended for use in children should not produce ethanol blood levels of >25 mg/dL after a single dose.

In general, manufacturers have voluntarily complied with the recommendations. In 1992 the

Nonprescription Drug Manufacturers Association established voluntary limits for alcohol content of nonprescription products [72]:

1. A maximum of 10% alcohol in products for adults and teens, 12 years old and over
2. A maximum of 5% alcohol in products intended for children 6–12 years of age
3. Less than 0.5% alcohol content for products intended for children less than 6 years of age

Extemporaneous production of pediatric dosage forms is commonly undertaken in hospitals. Without the sophisticated formulation capabilities of pharmaceutical manufacturers, alcohol-based vehicles have been recommended for extemporaneous preparation of liquid dosage forms [73]. There is a critical need to conduct research studies to assist the pharmacist in replacing current formulations with stable, alcohol-free preparations [74].

Administration Considerations in Dosage Form Development

Oral Administration. Oral administration is the preferred route of administration. There is a general consensus among pediatricians and parents that children younger that 5 years of age have great difficulty with, or are unable to swallow, a solid oral dosage form. Manufacturers, therefore, have developed liquid formulations for many of the commonly used pediatric products. The liquid dosage form, however, is not free of problems. Liquid products are often unstable and have short expiration dates; accurate measurement and administration of the prescribed dose is also a problem, especially in infants.

Chewable tablets and sprinkle capsule formulations have been very well received by both patients and their parents for use in children with full dentition (older than 3 years, [75–77]. This is potentially a very fruitful area for future research and development. Pharmaceutical preparations developed for administration to young children need to have consistent bioavailability when administered with food [78].

Rectal Administration. The administration of drugs by a solid rectal dosage form (i.e., suppositories) results in a wide variability in the rate and extent of absorption in children [79]. This fact, coupled with the inflexibility of a fixed dose, makes this a route that should not be promoted for pediatric patients. At least one death involving a 7-month-old infant can be directly attributed to the use of solid rectal dosage form of a therapeutic dose of morphine [80].

Rectal administration of a drug is considered unacceptable by adolescents and various ethnic groups.

Transdermal Administration. The development of the stratum corneum is complete at birth and is considered to have permeability similar to that of adults, except in preterm infants [81]. Preterm neonates and infants have an underdeveloped epidermal barrier and are subject to excessive absorption of potentially toxic ingredients from topically applied products.

No transdermal products have been marketed for use in the pediatric population. The development of transdermal products in pediatric doses could be very beneficial for children who are unable to tolerate oral medications.

Parenteral Administration. Absorption of medication following an intramuscular (IM) injection is often erratic in neonates owing to their small muscle mass and an inadequate perfusion of the intramuscular site [13,82]. In a study of infants and children 28 days to 6 years of age, the IM administration of chloramphenicol succinate produced serum levels that were not significantly different from intravenous administration [83]. However, the bioavailability of most drugs administered intramuscularly has not been evaluated in the pediatric population. In addition to bioavailability issues, there are other concerns specific to pediatrics with the IM administration of drugs. The volume of solution injected is directly related to the degree of pain and discomfort associated with an IM injection. Manufacturers' recommendations for reconstitution of IM products often result in a final volume that is excessive for a single injection site in a child's smaller muscle mass, thereby requiring multiple injections and a significant degree of discomfort for the patient. If a smaller volume is used for reconstitution, the problems of drug solubility and high osmotic load at the site of injection must be addressed [84,85]. The inclusion of a local anesthetic, such as lidocaine, as part of the reconstituted product is often necessary [84,85,85a].

In a report from the Boston Collaborative Drug Surveillance Program, pediatric nurses have reported a much higher frequency of complications from IM injections than that observed in the adult population. Twenty-three percent of pediatric nurses surveyed had observed complications (local pain, abscess, hematoma) versus a rate of 0.4% reported in adult patients [86]. Serious complications, such as paralysis from infiltration of the sciatic nerve, quadriceps myofibrosis, and accidental intra-arterial injection, are usually the result of the difficulty in placement of an intramuscular injection in children.

The major problem with the intravenous route in children is dosing errors. Because of the unavailability of stock solutions prepared for pediatric doses, errors in dilution of an adult stock solution have resulted in 10- to 20-fold errors in administered doses [87,88]. A secondary problem is the maintenance of patent intravenous lines in infants and nonsedated children.

Pulmonary Drug Delivery. Endotracheal drug delivery is a very effective method of administering emergency medications (i.e., epinephrine, atropine, lidocaine, naloxone) to children when an intravenous line is not available. To optimize drug delivery to the distal portions of the airway, the drug must be administered rapidly, using an adequate volume of diluent: 5–10 mL in young children; 10–20 mL for adolescents [89].

Pressurized inhalation products have also been very successfully employed in the pediatric population to provide a drug directly to the desired site of action, the lung. These products are designed to deliver a unit dose at high velocity with small particle size, the ideal conditions for drug delivery to distal airways [90]. Many new inhaler devices are currently in development. Chlorofluorocarbon-free formulations, using hydrofluoroalkane as the propellant, are under investigation. These new devices offer the potential for increased fine particle mass and improved intrapulmonary deposition [90a].

The use of the aerosol route for delivery of antibiotics for pulmonary infections remains controversial. The majority of pediatric studies have been conducted in children with cystic fibrosis. In these patients distribution of the antibiotic to the desired tissue site is impeded because of the viscosity of the sputum in patients with acute exacerbations of their pulmonary infections [91,92]. Long-term studies have demonstrated preventive benefits of aerosolized antibiotics in children with cystic fibrosis who are colonizing *Pseudomonas aeruginosa* in their lungs but are not acutely ill [93,94]. Cyclic administration of tobramycin administered by nebulizer has received FDA approval [95].

Systemic treatment via the respiratory tract needs further study to determine its usefulness.

Compliance Issues: Taste Preference and Palatability

Written and verbal education of parents, midtherapy reminders, and special packaging have all been employed to improve compliance to prescribed dosing regimens for pediatric patients [95]. Two factors make taste preference and palatability critical considerations in pediatric compliance.

The dosage forms most commonly employed for pediatric formulations are liquids and chewable tablets. A perceived unpleasant taste is much more evident with these dosage forms than when a drug is administered as a conventional solid oral dosage form. Second, it is widely believed that children younger than the age of 6 years have more acute taste perception than older children and adults. Taste buds and olfactory receptors are fully developed in early infancy. Loss of taste perception accompanies the aging process.

Smell, taste, texture, and aftertaste, therefore, are important factors in the development of pediatric dosage forms. In a study of six brands of OTC chewable vitamins, flavor type and intensity, soft texture, and short aftertaste were critical factors in product preference. The flavor and texture attributes of the best-selling product were significantly different from the other brands [97].

There are at least 26 different flavorings used in pediatric antimicrobial preparations [70]. Cherry is the most commonly used flavoring, although a blind taste comparison found that other flavorings, such as orange, strawberry, and bubble gum, are well accepted in pediatric antimicrobial suspensions [98].

In many circumstances it may be difficult to mask the unpleasant taste of the active ingredient. Regardless of flavoring used, parents consistently report that children prefer cephalosponin products to penicillin suspensions [98].

D. Future Directions

Effective and safe drug therapy for newborns, infants, and children depends on knowledge of pediatric pharmacokinetics and pharmacodynamics and knowledge of the drug formulation and delivery issues specific to this population.

In 1999, FDA regulations became effective requiring new drugs and biologics that are therapeutically important for children to have label information on safe pediatric use [99]. This rule also allows FDA to require pediatric testing of already-marketed drugs when the drug is frequently prescribed for children. This regulation will spur pediatric research and increase the availability of information for pediatric prescribers.

There has been tremendous progress in the identification of pharmacokinetic and pharmacodynamic parameters in chronically ill infants and children.

Pharmacokinetic and pharmacodynamic issues in the acutely ill child have been sporadically addressed and deserve further evaluation.

The critical void in pediatric drug therapy now lies in effective drug-delivery systems. Some inroads have been made in the manufacturing of pediatric dosing systems, particularly OTC preparations. There needs to be a redirection of the focus in nonparenteral drug formulations towards pediatric dosage forms with proven stability and bioavailability that can be easily and accurately administered to infants and children.

III. THE ELDERLY POPULATION

A. Diminution of Physical Function and its Effects on Drug Disposition

Within the medical community it has been acknowledged that elderly patients often respond to drug therapy differently from their younger counterparts. Aside from alteration of various pharmacokinetic and pharmacodynamic processes, elderly patients tend to suffer from a number of chronic conditions and, thus, have more complex dosage regimens. Additionally, a variety of physical limitations prevalent among the elderly may hinder their ability to self-administer medication.

Most of those involved in health care administration agree that elderly patients are the primary consumers of drug products. The actual extent to which this occurs is shown quite clearly in Fig. 1, which lists by age group the distribution in the United States of the "drug mentions" those medications that have been "prescribed, recommended or given in any medical setting by a private physician") [113]. As is shown in this figure, in 1996 those older than age 65, henceforth "the elderly," account for more than 26% of the drug mentions in the United States. Thus, although the elderly constitute only 12% of our population, they are the biggest consumers of drug-related products [113,114].

The effects of aging on drug disposition is one aspect of drug-taking behavior among the elderly that has been researched by individuals within both the medical and pharmaceutical fields. Before discussing the actual changes that occur with aging, two points must be stressed. First, because of wide variation among older individuals, it is very difficult to quantify the extent of changes that occur within this population. Second, most of these changes are related to the fact that, with increasing age, there is an overall decrease in the capacity of homeostatic mechanisms to respond to physiological changes.

Pharmacokinetics

During the past decade, numerous articles reviewing the effects of aging on pharmacokinetic processes (i.e., absorption, distribution, metabolism, and elimination) have been published [115–124h]. An outline of the observations made in these reports is supplied in Table 5. The absorption process is the only process that will be covered in depth in this chapter, as this is the process that can most easily be manipulated through formulation techniques.

First of all, there is a decrease in gastric secretion that causes the elevated pH that has been noted in elderly patients [116–127]. This condition is commonly referred to as hypochlorhydria or, in severe cases,

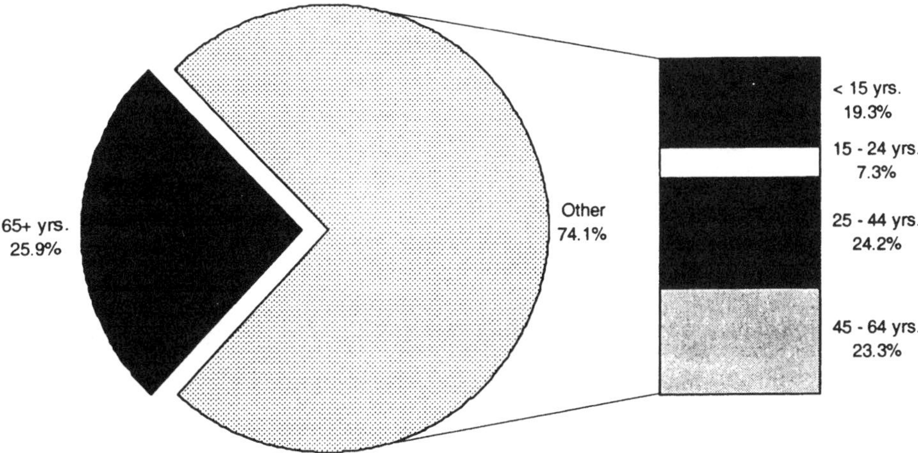

Fig. 1 Percent distribution of drug mentions, by age: United States, 1995–1996. (From Ref. 113)

Table 5 Changes in Pharmacokinetic Processes Observed with Aging

Process	Changes	Effects
Absorption	↓ Intestinal blood flow ↑ Gastric pH ↓ Active absorption ↓ GER?	↓ Rate of absorption
Distribution	↓ Cardiac output ↑ Fat/lean body mass ↓ Serum albumin concentration	↓ V_d water-soluble drugs ↑ V_d lipid-soluble drugs ↑ V_d protein-bounde drugs
Metabolism	↓ Hepatic blood flow ↓ Liver size ↓ Phase I metabolism ↑ Incidence liver dysfunction	↑ $t_{1/2}$ hepatically extracted drugs
Elimination	↓ Renal blood flow ↓ GFR ↓ ARTS ↓ No. functioning nephrons	↑ $t_{1/2}$ renally excreted drugs

Abbreviations: GER. gastric-emptying rate: V_b volume of distribution: $f_{t,2r}$ half-life: GFR, glomerular filtration rate: ARTS: active renal tubular secretion.

achlorhydria and may be the result of atrophic gastritis [123,126–128]. It may have a substantial effect on a formulation if an enteric-coated product or a weakly acidic or weakly basic drug is being considered. In the former case, the increased pH may cause the contents of the formulation to be prematurely released in the stomach, rather than in the small intestine and may lead to excessive gastrointestinal irritation. The elevated pH that exists within the stomach may also result in incomplete absorption of weakly acidic compounds from the stomach and decreased rate of absorption of poorly soluble weak bases. The reduced gastric blood flow that has been noted in elderly patients may hinder the rate of absorption [116,117,123,126,127]. In most instances, this decrease in the rate of absorption does not necessarily cause a decrease in the extent of absorption. In fact, only those compounds that are actively absorbed (e.g., riboflavin) have a decreased rate of absorption [126,128]. Drugs that are degraded in the acidic environment of the stomach (e.g., penicillin), however, may actually have an increased extent of absorption in elderly patients because less acid is available to degrade the drug before absorption.

There appears to be an ongoing dispute over whether or not gastric-emptying rate (GER) and GI motility are affected by the aging process [116,117, 124,126,129–134a]. Most studies tend to suggest that there is, indeed, a decrease in GER as the body ages. As GER is the primary physiological determinant of the rate of absorption of solid oral dosage forms, one can see that a decrease in GER may result in a subsequent decreased rate of absorption, particularly when coupled with the compromised blood flow to the GI track also noted in elderly patients. Additionally, unpredictable GER has a significant influence on extended-release formulations, as it becomes difficult to predict whether or not acceptable blood levels will be obtained [123]. To circumvent the possible problems that may arise from a decrease in GER, a liquid or readily disintegrating formulation may be used.

Pharmacodynamics

Although there are several reviews assessing the changes in pharmacodynamics prevalent among the elderly population, this area has not been as widely studied as have changes occurring in pharmacokinetic processes [115–117,119a,124d]. In Table 6 some of the major changes that have been evaluated in elderly patients are listed.

The decrease in the ability of the aging body to respond to baroreflexive stimuli can result in very serious consequences for elderly patients [115–117]. Because of this decrease in sensitivity and the decreased cardiac output witnessed in elderly patients, they are predisposed to the effects of orthostatic hypotension that can occur when one is taking antihypertensive medication (e.g., prazosin). Indeed, the fact that elderly persons are prone to accidental falls may be due to this change in sensitivity [115–117].

Decreases in β_1-receptor response were investigated when it was found that elderly patients taking

Table 6 Pharmacodynamic Changes Observed with Aging

Decrease baroreflex sensitivity
Decrease β_t-receptor response
Decrease α_2-receptor response
Increase sensitivity to barbiturates
Decrease glucose tolerance

β-adrenergic blockers (e.g., propranolol) were experiencing the ADRs associated with these medications, but they were not obtaining the proper therapeutic response (i.e., decrease in heart rate) [115–117]. Whether the exact mechanism for this decreased response is due to a decrease in affinity or a decrease in the number of receptors has yet to be conclusively determined [115].

The changes in α_2-receptor response observed in some elderly patients have not yet been found to have any clinical significance. Theoretically, this decrease should result in an increase in the amount of norepinephrine being released from nerve terminals, but this has not yet been demonstrated [115,116].

The incidence of diabetes and decreased glucose tolerance among the elderly is well documented [116,135–137]. Because of this, formulators should make every attempt to avoid using any sugar-containing excipients in their production processes.

Absorption Within the Oral Cavity

When dealing with oral dosage forms, it is important to study the various changes occurring within the oral cavity, particularly if a buccal or sublingual formulation is being considered. Table 7 lists the changes within the oral cavity that have thus far been elucidated [124,127,138–144]. It is very important to note that there is a decrease in the capillary blood supply to the oral mucosa. This may make it difficult to predict accurately the absorption rates that will occur when using sublingual and buccal formulations in the elderly age group. Additional changes occurring in and about the oral cavity will be discussed at length later in this chapter.

Table 7 Changes in and About the Oral Cavity Observed with Aging

Mucosa	Drier
	Increase Susceptibility to injury
	Decrease capillary blood supply
Muscle	Decrease bulk and tone
	Decrease masticatory efficiency
Salivary glands	Decrease resting secretory rate
	Increase viscosity of saliva
	Decrease enzyme activity of saliva
Miscellaneous	Decrease number of taste buds
	Increase dysfunction and cancer

Percutaneous Absorption

With the increasing acceptance of transdermal formulations by the pharmaceutical industry and the trend toward an aging population that is occurring in our nation, it is vital that the effects of aging on percutaneous absorption be evaluated. Certainly, elderly patients are the primary users of such drug-delivery systems (e.g., Transderm Nitro; Nitro Dur II), so the need for assessment of percutaneous absorption in the elderly should be emphasized. In light of this, it is surprising to find that there have been relatively few studies published that specifically address percutaneous absorption in the elderly [145,146]. Table 8 provides an outline of changes in characteristics of the skin that occur with aging [145–148].

Researchers assessing the various factors surrounding percutaneous absorption (e.g., permeation and clearance) have theorized that, although there is an increase in the rate of permeation through aging skin, substances that permeate through the skin have a slower rate of removal into the general circulation and, thus, distribution may be incomplete [145,146]. Unfortunately, there appear to be few published reports addressing this phenomenon. Studies that do specifically evaluate percutaneous absorption in the elderly have used only one compound, testosterone, in their analyses [145,146]. Therefore, before formulating drugs for transdermal delivery in the elderly, changes in percutaneous absorption that occur on aging should be assessed further.

Physical Limitations

Table 9 lists the top 10 chronic conditions prevailing in the elderly population [136]. Many of these conditions severely limit the range of activities that one can

Table 8 Changes in Skin Characteristics Observed with Aging

Dry skin
Loss of elasticity
Impaired wound healing
Deletion and derangement of small blood vessels
Increase permeation to water and some chemicals
Decrease clearance into blood stream
Decrease absorption?

Table 9 Top 10 Chronic Conditions in the United States, 1990–1992

Rank	All persons	65–74 yr	≥75 yr
1	Orthopedic impairment	Arthritis	Arthritis
2	Chronic Sinusitis	Hypertension	Hearing impairment
3	Arthritis	Hearing impairment	Hypertension
4	Hypertension	Heart disease	Heart disease
5	Allergies	Orthopedic impairment	Orthopedic impairment
6	Hearing impairment	Chronic sinusitis	Cataracts
7	Heart disease	Cataracts	Chronic sinusitis
8	Chronic bronchitis	Diabetes	Visual impairment
9	Asthma	Tinnitus	Diabetes
10	Headache	Allergies	Tinnitus

Source: Ref. 136.

perform (Fig. 2) [135,136]. Indeed, researchers have studied, in depth, the extent to which age limits one's activities of daily living (ADL) [114,135,137,149,150]. Moreover, some of these conditions, such as arthritis and impaired vision, impair the patient's ability to accurately self-administer medication.

Dexterity. Dexterity may be impaired in the elderly for a variety of reasons, such as the following: (a) over 43% of the elderly suffer from some form of arthritis [136]; (b) many elderly experience tremors associated with Parkinsonism or other neurological disorders; and (c) frailty and weakness are prevalent in many elderly patients. In fact, the National Institute on Aging has been conducting a comprehensive study to assess all of the characteristics common among the elderly. This study reveals that at least 13% of the elderly have some difficulty in handling small objects (e.g., tablets) [149]. Another government study reports that more than 4% of the elderly experience difficulty preparing their own meals and, therefore, are likely to encounter problems when self-administering medication [137].

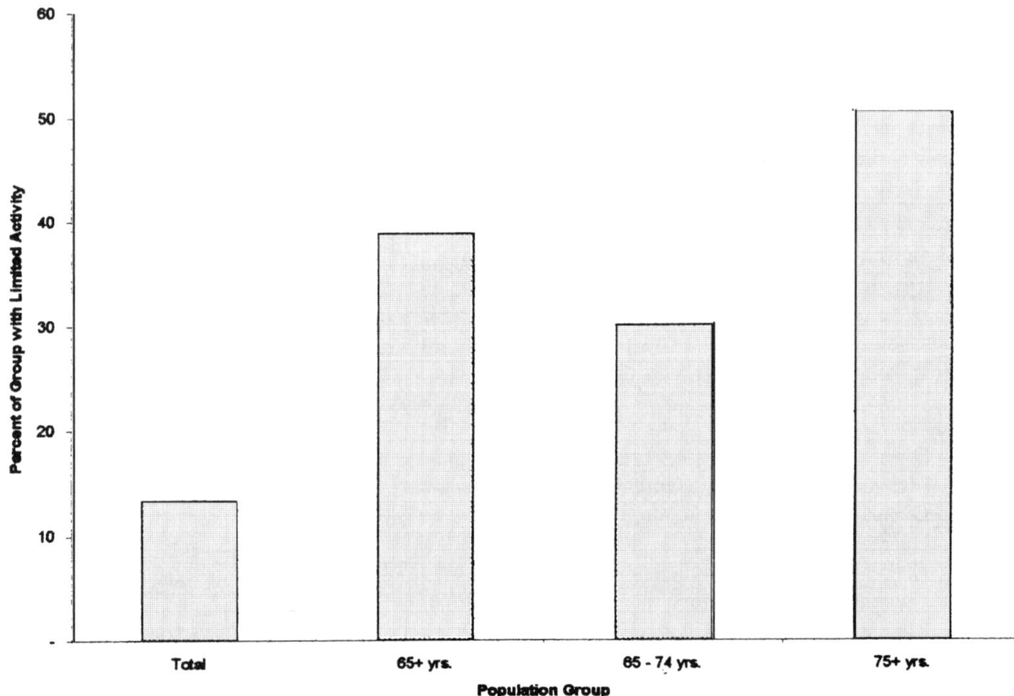

Fig. 2 Limitation of activity caused by chronic conditions: United States, 1997. (From Ref. 114.)

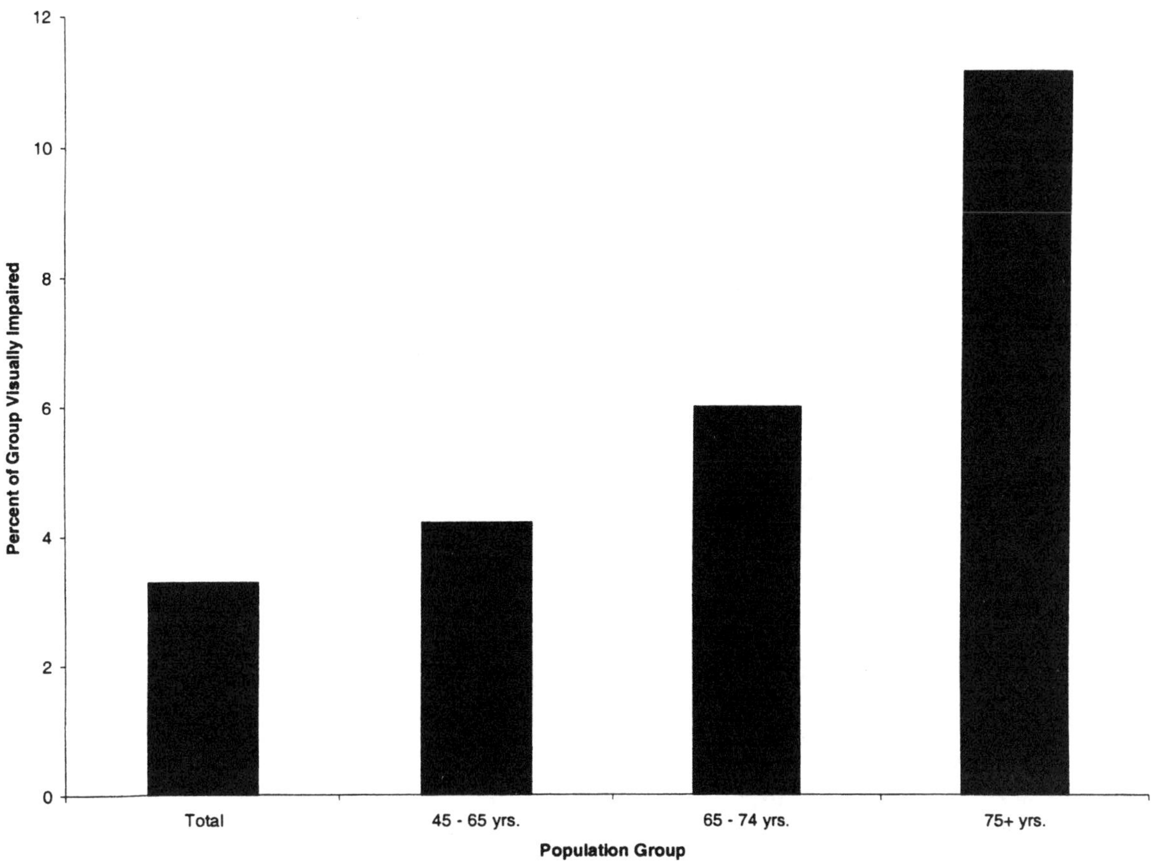

Fig. 3 Incidence of visual impairment, by age: United States, 1992. (From Ref. 136.)

Vision. Many people experience visual decline as they age (Fig. 3) [135]. Impaired vision may also hinder one's ability to self-administer medication. Listed in Table 10 are some of the effects that are associated with impaired vision in the elderly. Some of the processes of self-administration that are affected by impaired vision are as follows: (a) the ability to accurately measure liquids; (b) the ability to correctly read instructions; and (c) the ability to differentiate between various types of medications (both the labeling of these drugs and their physical characteristics) [137,151–153].

Table 10 Some Visual Declines Observed with Aging

General acuity
Peripheral vision
Ability to see in low light levels
Ability to see highly reflective surfaces in bright light
Ability to discriminate between colors
Ability to adapt to darkness

Swallowing and Chewing. In addition to those changes occurring in the oral cavity (see Table 6), there are other factors that may inhibit an elderly patient's ability to both swallow and chew. For instance, xerostomia, or dry mouth, is a condition that is prevalent among older people. Xerostomia may be caused by any one of the following conditions: (a) elderly patients often do not consume adequate amounts of liquid and are thus dehydrated; (b) many elderly patients "mouth breathe" because of asthma or other respiratory diseases; and (c) elderly patients often take medications having anticholinergic side effects (e.g., antidepressants and neuroleptics) [142,143,154–156]. Patients experiencing xerostomia often have difficulty swallowing tablets or capsules because they tend to adhere to the esophageal mucosa when it is dry [124,127,157–161]. In addition, esophageal lesions are common among the elderly and may affect a patients ability to swallow; this is compounded by the inhibition of peristalsis by the weakened esophageal musculature [127,129]. The ability of elderly patients to chew is also compromised

[127,138,139,144], perhaps as a result of the decreased bulk and tone of the oral musculature as one ages [144]. Additionally, it has been estimated that 50% of all elderly persons in the United States are fully edentulous (i.e., toothless) [127,139]. The absence of teeth not only hinders one's ability to chew, it also changes the bacterial flora within the oral cavity from predominantly anaerobic to aerobic [127].

B. Dosing Considerations Determined by Alterations in Physiology with Aging

The pharmacokinetics of each compound should be determined when one is deciding which drug candidates to use in designing formulations for the elderly (See Table 3). For instance, some medications have an increased half-life in older adults, either because these drugs undergo extensive hepatic metabolism (e.g., diazepam, verapamil, and pentazocine), or because they are excreted primarily by the kidneys (e.g., lithium aminoglycosides, and digoxin) [114–120,124e]. In addition, drugs that are highly protein-bound (e.g., warfarin) may be the cause of serious adverse reactions among elderly patients because of the decreased concentration of serum albumin in these patients and the subsequent rise in circulating "free" drug [114–120, 124f]. So, if the pharmacokinetic behavior of the drug is known to change in elderly patients, it may be wise to avoid such drugs or to adjust the dosage accordingly. A guide has been recently published that lists a number of suggestions for dosing regimens in the geriatric patient [162].

C. Drug-Delivery Systems and Compliance Issues

The changes experienced in aging may affect a patient's ability to use some of the drug-delivery systems existing today. It should be kept in mind, however, that within the context of this chapter, a drug-delivery system is not merely a novel dosage form: it is the dosage form with its container, labeling, *and* any other information supplied with the medication to the user.

Dosage Form Preferences

Solid oral dosage forms, particularly tablets, are the preferred type of formulation in the United States. Not only are these products widely accepted by consumers, but they are also relatively cheaper to develop and manufacture than oral liquids or suspensions, parenterals, or suppositories. Figure 4 shows, quite clearly, that even the elderly primarily make use of solid oral dosage forms [162].

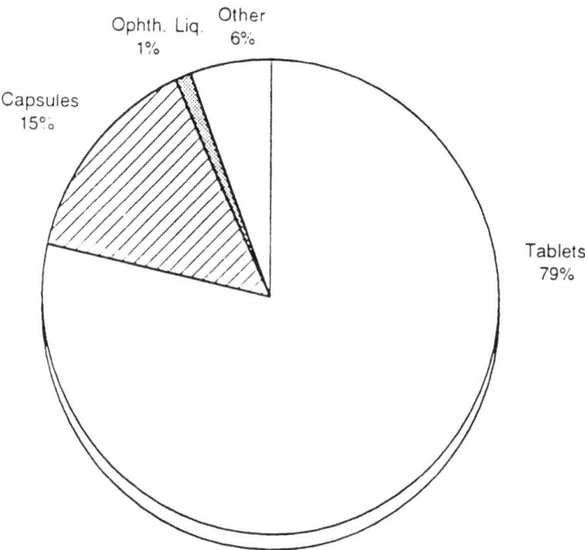

Fig. 4 Dosage forms commonly used by elderly patients. (From Ref. 162.)

Oral Dosage Forms.

Chewable Tablets. It has already been noted that most elderly patients experience a decrease in their ability to chew efficiently [125,137,138,143]. Therefore, by virtue of their design, chewable tablets are not often recommended for use by elderly patients (particularly those who are edentulous) 155–163,164]. Most chewable formulations also rely on an adequate amount of chewing action to obtain full release of their ingredients (e.g., chewing promotes the foaming action provided by some chewable antacid products). So, aside from being difficult form the elderly patient to use, full benefit of a chewable dosage form may not be achieved by these patients. Additionally, the use of chewable tablets by denture wearers may cause local irritation in the oral cavity [155].

Sublingual and Buccal Tablets. Although sublingual and buccal tablets (e.g., nitroglycerin or isosorbide) are used by many elderly patients, few, if any, researchers have determined the effects that aging may have on the bioavailability of these dosage forms [136–142]. Patient acceptance of these types of formulations must also be considered. Elderly patients who suffer from dry mouth conditions may find sublingual or buccal tablets irritating and may refuse to use such medications. Another problem may involve demented or contrary patients who may feel foreign objects inside their mouths and pull the tablets out before the active ingredients have been released from the formulation.

Capsules. A number of scientists have investigated the effect of formulation on esophageal transit and have found that capsules tend to adhere to the esophageal mucosa more often than any other type of oral dosage form [157–160]. Moreover, due to the conditions of xerostomia and hindered swallowing that are prevalent among the elderly, mucosal adherence of capsules in these patients may be more pronounced [125,127,141, 153–155]. In light of these observations, the use of capsules by older patients may not be advisable. This is an extremely important consideration if the drug to be delivered is one that is known to cause esophageal ulceration (e.g., tetracycline or aspirin) [159].

Liquids and Suspensions. Most liquid formulations are not packaged in unit-dosage form. Therefore, before administration, the proper amount of medication to be taken for each dose must be measured. This additional requirement may compound any difficulties a patient may have in following a prescribed schedule. Patients suffering from visual impairment, arthritis, or tremors associated with neurological disorders are particularly likely to become frustrated with this type of formulation. Visual impairments make it difficult, if not impossible, for many elderly patients to measure the prescribed amounts of medication accurately. Impaired dexterity, owing to tremors or arthritis, may have effects on a patient's ability to hold both a spoon and a bottle at the same time while pouring out the desired amount of liquid.

Additional difficulties are encountered by elderly patients if a medication is in the form of a suspension. Problems may occur because a patient cannot see, or disregards, the words "Shake Well" on the label or is not able to exert the amount of agitation necessary to provide a uniform suspension. Certainly, unevenly distributed amounts of active ingredients throughout a suspension may result in serious consequences for a patient in terms of either under- or overdosing.

Transdermal Delivery Systems. Although transdermal drug delivery may offer a means of increasing compliance among elderly patients, it has yet to be determined whether or not changes exist between the bioavailability of such products when administered to elderly patients versus young adults. Indeed, there may be a decrease in the absorption of compounds that are transdermally delivered to elderly patients [143–146]. Still, some may prefer the transdermal design and may opt to perform all the preliminary investigations necessary to quantify percutaneous bioavailability in older patients. If this route is chosen, one should keep in mind that transdermal products formulated around these changes may be applicable to only the older patients for whom the product have been designed. Such products may have differing release characteristics in the rest of the population. Therefore, it is possible that these products, which will probably require lengthy preliminary studies, will be able to be used effectively by only a limited portion of the population.

Parenteral Dosage Forms and Invasive Devices. Parenteral and invasive devices provide the distinct advantage of the delivery of medication directly into the bloodstream or at the site of action. Additionally, these methods result in assures patient compliance because, in most cases, an individual other than the patient is responsible for the administration of medication by these means. Unfortunately, this attribute is counteracted by numerous problems that are illustrated in Table 11.

In this table, it can be recognized that there are problems inherent in these types of formulations from both the patient's and the manufacturer's point of view. This is why most pharmaceutical companies make attempts to avoid these types of dosage forms, if at all possible. However, with the advent of biotechnological products, which often do not lend them, selves to "conventional" dosage formulations, parenteral and invasive measures may be the only answer.

Alternative Delivery Systems

Although elderly patients seem to experience difficulties with the above-mentioned drug-delivery systems, other systems are currently available that may be more suited to the needs of these patients. Although most of these systems are not specifically designed for the geriatric community, they may offer aid to this group of patients. This may be accomplished through the use of dosage formulations or packaging designs that are easier to handle or by supplying patients with devices

Table 11 Possible Problems Associated with Parenteral Delivery

Cost to patient and manufacturer
Patient discomfort
Risk of infection
Administration by trained personnel required
Limitations on particle size
Sterilization necessary
Prone to chemical, mechanical, and microbial instability
Complex manufacturing processes
Cumbersome and fragile packaging

or information that will enable them to better follow their prescribed dosing regimen.

Compliance Aids. Many pharmacists and physicians have recognized that most elderly patients have complicated dosing schedules and need some sort of reminder that will help them keep track of their prescribed regimens [115,154,155,160,164–173]. This can be achieved through several methods. First, various types of packages, such as Dosett Trays, Calendar-Paks, and Patient Med Paks, can be prepared by pharmacists [167,169,174–176]. These packages are usually devised so that all of the medications that have been prescribed to be taken at a specified time are packed together. For instance, all the medications that are to be taken before breakfast are placed in the same container, and all those to be taken 1 hour after breakfast are placed in another container. Labeling for each container should specify the time at which its contents are to be taken, as well as a list of each individual medication it holds. In an effort to promote this type of packaging, the *United States Pharmacopeia* (USP) has set guidelines for pharmacists to follow when preparing Patient Med Paks [176]. In this manner, the USP has provided the pharmacist with a means to help out those patients with complex-dosing schedules and still comply with official-labeling criteria (i.e., it is not standard practice to supply more than one drug in a single container). Another way in which pharmacists and physicians can help patients regulate their dosing schedules is by supplying them with drug-reminder cards [115,167,171,172]. The concept for the cards is essentially the same as that for the labels on the packaging just described (i.e., time of day and all medications to be taken at that time). Various modifications of this design can be made, such as including the physical characteristics of each medication or providing stickers to be placed on the card and on its corresponding container (i.e., one sticker is placed on the prescription bottle and the other sticker is placed next to the medication's name on the reminder card) [171,172].

Unfortunately, both the drug-reminder cards and packaging methods described here must be made for each patient on an individual basis, and some people are not willing to take the extra time needed to prepare these systems.

Oral Dosage Forms. The advantages of oral dosage formulations have already been discussed. It appears that this route of delivery is preferred by physician, patients, and manufacturers alike. The relatively low cost of oral dosage forms makes them a particularly attractive means of drug delivery for those patients, such as the elderly, who may be economically depressed [177]. These dosage forms are also comparatively easier to formulate, package, and ship than other types of dosage forms [179]. Moreover, changes in pharmacokinetic parameters among the elderly have been assessed only in those formulations that are oral or parenteral in nature [115–125]. Therefore, it is appropriate to focus on oral dosage formulations for drug delivery in the elderly.

Granules. Granules are one type of oral formulation of which use among the elderly is warrented [163,164]. This type of dosage form not only circumvents the difficulty in swallowing that may be encountered by older patients, but it also provides the patient with a certain amount of rehydration. As the elderly are often dehydrated, this is a feature that should not be overlooked. More importantly, medications that have been dispersed in a liquid are not likely to be affected by changes in gastric-emptying rate that may occur in older patients.

Problems may still arise because granules may be supplied in either unit-dose packages or in bulk containers. If unit-dose packages are used, patients with impaired manual dexterity may have difficulty opening the packets. With bulk containers, most of the handling problems associated with administering liquid formulations that have been discussed can occur. However, bulk containers do offer the advantage of dosage flexibility that cannot be realized with other solid dosage formulations.

Coated Tablets. Investigators studying the effects of dosage formulation on esophageal transit have concluded that coated tablets are less likely to adhere to the esophageal mucosa than other solid dosage forms (e.g., uncoated tablets or capsules) [155,157–160]. In addition, this effect may be complemented by the use of oval-shaped tablets, commonly referred to as "caplets" [159–161]. This type of tablet offers advantages over uncoated tablets and capsules, especially in those patients who have difficulty swallowing. Still, it is imperative that physicians and pharmacists instruct patients to take their medications with a full glass of water because esophageal adherence is still possible in those patients who are dehydrated.

Effervescent Tablets. Effervescent tablets are another means of supplying medications to the elderly. This type of formulation provides the patient with an easy-to-swallow product that is aesthetically pleasing (i.e., forms a clear solution, rather than a cloudy suspension). However, pharmaceutical chemists are well aware of the problems that exist when preparing effervescent formulations. These problems may be partly solved by certain advances in pharmaceutical technology that allow direct compression of all excipients necessary to form such tablets [180–182]. Although this makes the manufacture of such products easier, stability problems still exist because these formulations must be adequately protected against moisture. As with granules, the type of packaging required for effervescent tablets can be a problem for those patients with impaired manual dexterity. Moreover, and perhaps more importantly, the high sodium content necessary to manufacture effervescent products may have serious implications when used by patients with hypertension or congestive heart failure.

Dispersion or Soluble Tablets. The trend toward formulation of dispersible tablets is evident in Europe [183,183c] and is becoming more commonplace in the United States with OTC preparations available in the form of the following technologies: Zydis® (Scherer DDS); LYoc®(Farmalyyoc); WOW® Tab (Yamanouchi); FlashDose® (Fuisz Technologies); OraSolv®(CIMA); and DuraSolv® (CIMA). These tablets are either placed in the mouth where they quickly dissolve or placed in a glass of water prior to ingestion. As with granules and effervescent tablets, dispersible tablets offer the patient a dosage form that is both portable and easy to swallow.

A challenge faced by formulators designing dispersible tablets is the ability to develop a formulation that rapidly disintegrates and is able to withstand shipping processes. In addition, this type of tablet should form a uniform and somewhat stable suspension when dispersed in water. An interesting answer to this challenge is the design of a "porous table" [184–184b], in which a volatizable solid (e.g., urethane or ammonium bicarbonate) is added to a standard, directly compressible formulation. After the tablets have been compressed, the volatilizable solid is removed by a freeze-drying or heating process. Water easily penetrates through the pores and promotes rapid disintegration of the tablets produced in this manner. Thus, these tablets are able both to maintain their mechanical strength and to provide rapid disintegration or dispersion of product. Lyoc® and Zydis® tablets both use freeze-drying technologies.

Gel Peparations. Some Japanese investigators are promoting the use of jelly-like preparations to help elderly patients overcome their difficulty in swallowing conventional tablets and capsules [184c–184e]. These dosage forms rely on gelation of materials such as sodium casseinate, glycerogelatin, dried gelatin gel powder, and silk fibroin.

Tiltabs.® Tiltab tablets represent one of the few dosage formulations that has been developed expressly to meet the needs of patients with impaired dexterity [185]. Marketed by Smith, Kline & French Laboratories, Ltd. in several European countries, the novelty of the Tiltab design is its irregular shape that prevents it from lying flat. Apparently, tablets manufactured in this fashion are easier to handle by those with impaired dexterity. Moreover, these tablets are readily identifiable by patients so that differentiation from other medication is facilitated. Other innovations like this are needed for drug-delivery systems with the particular needs of the geriatric patient in mind.

Concentrated Oral Solutions. Presentation of a drug may be made in the form of a concentrated solution that allows the entire dose to be held within a volume of less than 5 mL (e.g., Intensol® Concentrated Oral Solutions, Roxanne). This opens up another means of providing medication to the aged, infants, or any other patients experiencing difficulties swallowing. Such preparations can be mixed with food or drink. Taste and poor solubility are problems that may set limits on the number of successful formulations that can be prepared in this way. Also, small errors in the measurement of such preparations represent large errors in dosing.

Taste Preferences in Oral Dosage Forms

Changes in elderly patients' abilities to taste various substances do not necessarily affect the ease or difficulty of administration of medications, but these changes do have an effect on the patients' acceptance of a product. For instance, although it may be easier for patients to swallow liquid medications, they may find the taste or smell of the product so objectionable that they will refuse to take any medication prepared in this manner. Indeed, even some solid dosage forms carry with them objectionable tastes or odors that result in limitation of patient acceptance. Although there have been few studies assessing elderly patients' taste preferences, these reports have indicated that differences in taste preference and perception do exist between elderly and young adult populations [127,134,138,186,187]. It has been determined that, although the number of taste buds declines with age, thresholds for certain tastes are affected, whereas others are not. Unfortunately, reports of taste threshold changes among the elderly are contradictory, and it is difficult to ascertain what changes really do occur [127,134,138,186.187]. Current reports claim that these changes in taste thresholds are not due to the aging process, per se, but to medications that the patient may be taking [138,187]. For example, it appears that an increased concentration of sour compounds must exist in order to be detected by patients taking medications [187].

Package and Label Design

One of the most important aspects of drug-delivery design for the elderly is the presentation of the package and its label. If the patient is unable to open a package or cannot read a label properly, even the best dosage formulation design will be unsuccessful [176]. For prescription medications the package design is difficult to control, because the container supplied by the manufacturer is not necessarily the container in which the medicine will be dispensed by the pharmacist. But pharmacist selection of special packaging is a prospect open to most drugs whenever elderly-friendly packaging is in hand. The OTC products, in partial contrast, provide a manufacturer with the opportunity to make substantial changes in the design of packages and their labels. When developing a design, it is important to always keep in mind that impaired dexterity and visual decline are prevalent among the elderly. Listed in Table 12 are some suggestions that may be useful when designing a product's label [152,153,165,166,188,189].

In terms of the package itself, it is difficult to devise a package that is both childproof and tamperproof and still able to be opened easily by someone with impaired dexterity, it has been suggested that packaging a medication in unit-dose Calendar-Paks may increase patient compliance [8]. The problem is that other studies have shown that most elderly patients encounter difficulties when attempting to open this type of packaging (blister packaging) [167,175]. Additionally, this type of packaging (i.e., C-Paks and the like) for OTC products may be unacceptable to the Federal Trade Commission and FDA, as it promotes the daily use of the product. So, it is apparent that different types of packaging are needed, depending on whether a drug is for OTC or prescription-only use.

Table 12 Suggestions for Labels Designed to be Used by Elederly Patients

Avoid pastels
Use matte surfaces to minimize glare
Light colors on dark background are more visible than dark colors on light background
Use distinct spacing between letters
Increase height and thickness of letters
Use additional labels that explain purpose of medication[a]

[a] This type of label is required on drugs dispensed in Denmark.

IV. PHARMACEUTICAL FACTORS IN ORAL DOSAGE FORMULATIONS FOR SELECT POPULATIONS

Before the start of any formal laboratory work, the characteristics of the drug and excipients to be used must be considered. When performing this evaluation, it is necessary to keep in mind all of the pharmacokinetic and physical changes experienced by the elderly and pediatric population.

A. Particle Size

The relevance of particle size to solid dosage formulations has been determined by a number of individuals [54,190–196]. As is illustrated in Table 13, particle size affects the solid dosage formulation in numerous ways. For instance, particle size can have a profound effect on the dissolution of a formulation within the GI tract. This is most notably characterized by the Noyes-Whitney equation:

$$\frac{dm}{dt} = \frac{DS}{h(C_s - C)}$$

where

M = mass of drug dissolved
t = time
D = diffusion coefficient of drug
S = effective surface area of drug particles
h = stationary layer thickness
C_s = concentration of solution at saturation
C = concentration of solute at time t

As decreases in particle size produce increases in surface area, S, it becomes evident that particle size reduction provides an increase in the rate of dissolution

Table 13 Processes in Solid Dosage Formulation Affected by Particle Size

Disintegration
Dissolution
Flowability
Compressibility
(Gastrointestinal bleeding)

(dM/dt). When one remembers that elderly patients are likely to have decreased GER, one can see that increased dissolution rates are particularly desirable in these patients because once the formulation is in solution, GER is no longer able to limit significantly the rate of absorption [123,131,164].

Particle size impacts on aspirin-induced GI blood loss [195,196]; gastrointestinal micro-bleeding decreases as the particle size of the formulation declines [195,196]. In theory, this occurs because the time during which the aspirin particles are in contact with the GI mucosa is shortened as a result of the decreased particle size of the formulation and, subsequently, the increased rate of dissolution [190,195,196]. Clearly then, given the effects on dissolution and GI erosion, formulations with smaller particle size are desired. However, if the particle size is too small, problems may arise in the handling of the powder during manufacture, and its flow properties may be impeded, leading to poor dosage uniformity [195,196].

B. pK_a and Stability

As the acid content within the GI tract is known to change as the body ages, it is also important to evaluate the dissociation constant(s) (K_a) of the drug(s) to be used. From the Henderson-Hasselbach equation of weak acids:

$$\mathrm{pH} = \mathrm{p}K_a + \log\left(\frac{[\mathrm{salt}]}{[\mathrm{acid}]}\right)$$

it is apparent that changes in pH cause the proportions of drug that are ionized (salt) and nonionized (acid) to change. Since most compounds dissolve more readily when they are in the ionized form, it can be theorized that conversion of drugs with poor solubility to their salt form facilitates their rate of dissolution. Indeed, Hoener and Benet have modified the Noyes-Whitney equation so that it includes the effects of pH and pK_a, on the rate of dissolution [197]. For weak bases, this equation is defined as

$$\frac{dM}{dt} = \left(\frac{DS}{h}\right)\left[C_s\left(1 - \frac{[\mathrm{H}^+]}{K_a}\right) - C_g\right]$$

where

C_s = concentration of solution at saturation
C_g = concentration of drug in the GI tract
$[\mathrm{H}^+]$ = H^+ concentration in the GI tract
K_a = dissociation constant of drug

This further serves to illustrate the tact that, as pH increases, poorly soluble, weak bases are more likely to exist in the nonionized form and, thus, have a decreased rate of dissolution. Since gastric pH is elevated in most elderly patients, products containing weak bases that are meant to be used in this population should be formulated with these changes in mind.

Although not exclusively relevant to the design of drug-delivery systems for an elderly or pediatric population, the stability of drug(s) and excipient(s) used within a formulation may have a dramatic effect on the final product. If there are instabilities inherent in the materials used in the formulations, these problems are most often translated to the final product. Instability may be physical, chemical, or microbial. When one is dealing with solid dosage forms, physical and chemical instabilities often occur. Instability may be due to decomposition of an active ingredient through hydrolysis or oxidation, or it may be a result of incompatibilities that exist between a drug and the excipients being used. The use of materials that are polymorphic (i.e., have more than one type of molecular orientation in the solid state) may also be the cause of instability within a formulation (e.g., dissolution and absorption rates differ among the various polymorphs of a material). Additionally, if drug-recipient interactions are not carefully evaluated, tablet hardening and an accompanying decreased rate of dissolution may result as the tablets age (e.g., dibasic calcium phosphate and ascorbic acid).

C. Disintegration

To provide the rapid rate of disintegration that is required to achieve efficient dispersion from tablets, the addition of a disintegrating agent is necessary. Such agents enable a formulator to produce a tablet that will quickly disintegrate when placed in a liquid. In addition, the use of suspending agents or surfactants may be desired so that more stable suspensions can be formed. In choosing these agents, it should be remembered that most elderly patients are unable to handle large loads of sodium. Therefore, compounds such as sodium starch glycolate may be inappropriate for use by these patients.

D. Compressibility and Flow

To produce tablets that are uniform in weight and content and exhibit a certain degree of mechanical strength, one needs a mixture of powders with (a) good flow properties; (b) a minimum tendency for segregation, and (c) the ability to be compressed. To achieve these ends, granulation with other excipients is often necessary.

Segregation can be minimized by ensuring that all particles within a mixture have approximately the same size and density [191–194]. The flow of particles, however, is a bit more complex. On the other hand, mixtures of small granule size (800 μm) have the propensity to produce tablets with minimal dosage variation. But if the particle size becomes too small (<14 μm), flow through an orifice (e.g., a tablet press hopper) becomes impaired because the cohesive forces between the particles are of the same magnitude as the gravitational forces being imparted on the powder bed. The restricted flow may be improved by the addition of glidants, such as magnesium stearate or talc, but most of these agents are hydrophobic and may impair the tablet's ability to disperse. Superfine, high molecular weight polyethylene glycols (PEGs), which are water-soluble, have been proposed for use as lubricant-glidant in tablet formulation [180]. PEGs may then provide the formulator with an agent that is both lubricating and hydrophilic and, as such, may be a viable choice for use in the formulation of dispersible tablets.

Another factor that impacts on tablet formation is the ability, or inability, of powders to be compressed. The ability of materials to be compressed may be due to the following: (a) compression force, (b) particle size, and (c) deformation processes. Obviously, by increasing the force of compression, one can, in theory, increase the mechanical strength of the compact. There is some evidence suggesting that the strength of the tablet may be increased by using granulations of smaller particle size [191–194]. Here again, this increased strength must be balanced with the ability of the powder bed to flow evenly through a hopper. Also, for suitable compacts to be formed, a material must exhibit a certain amount of plastic (i.e., permanent) deformation [198]. Powders that undergo more elastic than plastic deformation will lose their structure after ejection from the tablet die. Therefore, if one is using a material that does not undergo a significant amount of plastic deformation, additional processing steps are necessary so that a stable structure can be produced.

It becomes evident that a variety of factors need to be considered when designing tablet formulations. In addition, certain compromises between these parameters must be made, because it is nearly impossible to meet all specifications with the same process variables.

E. Salt and Sucrose Content

The increased incidence of glucose intolerance, congestive heart failure, and hypertension among elderly patients make them particularly sensitive to levels of sucrose and sodium. Those involved in the manufacture of antacids are well apprised of this as they are required to carry a precautionary statement on the level of those products that contain more than 5 mEq of sodium per dose [155,156,164].

Additionally, when reviewing the various liquid preparations available in the OTC market today, one can see that many of these products are now sugar- or sodium-free or both. Indeed, decreased sodium and sugar levels are beneficial to the entire population. This would seem to suggest that every effort should be made to keep sodium and sucrose contents to an absolute minimum in products intended for use in older patients.

F. Conclusions

It is evident that numerous conditions exist that separate the elderly from young adults. Moreover, some of these conditions have a substantial impact on the use of drug-delivery systems by elderly patients. With the ever-increasing proportion of elderly patients in our population, it is surprising that relatively few special products are marketed to accommodate the needs of these patients in terms of drug-delivery design.

REFERENCES

1. G. Maxwell. Pediatric drug dosing. Drugs. 37, 113 (1989).
2. D. B. Guralnik (ed.). *Webster's New World Dictionary of the American Language*, 2nd ed., Simon & Schuster, New York, 1986.
3. R. C. Adelman. Definition of biological aging, in *Second Conference on the Epidemiology of Aging*, (S. G. Haynes and M. Feinleib, eds.), U.S. Government Printing Office. Washington. DC, 1980.
4. P. T. Costa and R. R. McCrae, Functional age: A conceptual and empirical critique, in *Second Conference on the Epidemiology of Aging* (S. G. Haynes and M. Feinleib, eds.), U.S. Government Printing Office, Washington, DC, (1980), pp. 23–32.
5. G. L. Maddox, ed., *The Encylopedia of Aging*, Springer, Publishing, New York, 1987.
6. R. N. Butler. Current definitions of aging, in *Second Conference on the Epidemiology of Aging* (S. G. Haynes and M. Feinleib. eds.), U.S. Government Printing Office, Washington, DC, 1980, pp. 7–13.
7. R. Temple, The clinical investigation of drugs for use by the elderly, J. Geriatr. Drug Ther., 2, 33 (1988).
8. E. D. Sumner, General considerations, in *Handbook of Geriatric Drug Therapy for Health Care Professionals*, Lea & Febiger, Philadelphia, (l983), pp. 1–9.

9. S. Yaffe and M. Danish, Problems of drug administration in the pediatric patient, Drug Metab. Rev., 8, 303 (1978).
10. B. Assael, Pharmacokinetics and drug distribution during postnatal development, Pharmacol. Ther. 18, 159–197 (1982).
11. C. Stewart and E. Hampton, Effect of maturation on drug disposition in pediatric patients, Clin. Pharm. 6, 548–64 (1987).
12. B. Anderson, A. McKee, and N. Holford, Size, myths and clinical pharmacokinetics of analgesia in paediatric patients, Clin. Pharmacokinetics, 33(5), 313 (1997).
13. R. Loebstein and G. Koren, Clinical pharmacology and therapeutic monitoring in neonates and children, Pediat. Rev., 19(12), 423 (1998)
14. M. Danish and S. Rosenbaum, Dosing considerations for non-prescription drugs in infants and children, Clin. Res. Regul. Affairs, 9, 89 (1992).
15. J. Deren, Development of structure and function of the fetal and newborn stomach, Am. J. Clin. Nutr., 24, 144 (1971).
16. P. Hyman. E. Feldman, and M. Ament, Effect of external feeding on the maintenance of gastric acid secretory function, Gastroenterology, 84, 341 (1983).
17. M. Gupta and Y. Brans, Gastric retention in neonates, Pediatrics, 62, 26 (1978).
18. L. Hendeles, R. Iafrate, and M. Weinberger, A clinical and pharmacokinetic basis for the selection and use of slow release theophylline products, Clin. Pharmacokinet., 9, 95 (1984).
19. L. Linday, J. Dobkin, and T. Wang, Digoxin inactivation by the gut flora in infancy and childhood, Pediatrics, 544 (1987).
20. W. Jusko, G. Levy, and S. Yafft, Effect of age on intestinal absorption of riboflavin in humans, J. Pharm. Sci., 59, 487 (1970).
21. G. Heimann, External absorption and bioavailability in children related to age, Eur. J. Clin. Pharmacol., 18, 43 (1980).
22. L. Pedersen-Bjergaard and K. Petersen, Oral absorption of piyampicillin and ampicillin in young children, Clin. Pharmacokinet., 2, 451 (1977).
22a. G. Cooney, K. Habucky, and K. Hoppu, Cyclosporine pharmacokinetics in paediatric transplant recipients, Clin. Pharmacokinetics, 32(6), 481 (1997).
22b. D. Murry, L. Rwa, and D. Poplack, Impact of nutrition on pharmacokinetics of anti-neoplastic agents, Int J Cancer Suppl., 11, 48 (1998).
23. J. Gilman, M. Duchown, T. Resnick and E. Hershorin, Carbamazepine malabsorption: A case report, Pediatrics, 82, 518 (1988).
24. B. Friss-Hansen, Body water compartments in children during growth and related changes in body composition, Pediatrics, 28, 169 (1961).
25. R. Heimler, B. Doumas, B. Jendrzeczal, P. Nemeth, R. Hoffman, and L. Nelin, Relationship between nutrition, weight change and fluid compartments in preterm infants during the first week of life, J. Pediatr., 122, 110 (1993).
26. L. Notarianni, Plasma protein binding of drugs in pregnancy and in neonates, Clin. Pharmacokinet., 18, 20 (1990).
27. I. Gauntlett, D. Fisher, R. Hertzka, E. Kuhls, M. Spellman, and C. Rudolph, Pharmacokinetics of fentanyl in neonatal humans and lambs: Effects of age, Anesthesiology, 69, 683 (1988).
27a. J. S. Leeder and G. L. Kearns, Pharmacogenetics in pediatrics, Pediatr. Clin. North Am., 44(1), 55 (1997).
28. J. Aranda, S. MacLeod, K. Renton, and N. Eade, Hepatic microsomal drug oxidation and electron transport in newborn infants, J. Pediatr., 85, 534 (1974).
29. J. Rosen, M. Danish, M. Ragni, C. Lopez Saccar, S. Yaffe, and H. Leeks, Theophylline pharmacokinetics in the young infant, Pediatrics, 64, 248 (1979).
30. O. Carrier, G. Pons, E. Rey, M. Richard, C. Moran, J. Badoual, and G. Olive, Maturation of caffeine metabolic pathways in infancy, Clin, Pharmacol. Ther., 44, 145 (1988).
31. R. Miller, R. Roberts, and L. Fischer, Acctaminophen elimination kinetics in neonates, children, and adults, Clin. Pharmacol. Ther., 19, 284 (1976).
32. J. Glazer, M. Danish, S. Plotkin, and S. Yaffe, Disposition of chloramphenicol in low birth weight infant, Pediatrics, 66, 573 (1980).
33. J. Thompson, D. Bloedow, and F. Leffert, Pharmacokinetics of intravenous chlorpheniramine in childien, J. Pharm. Sci., 70, 1284 (1981).
34. D. Fisher, P. Schwartz, and A. Davis, Pharmacokinetics of exogenous epinephrine in critically ill children, Crit. Care Med., 21, 111 (1993).
35. I. Matsuda, A. Higashi, and N. Inotsume, Physiologic and metabolic aspects of anticonvulsants, Pediatr. Clin. North Am., 36, 1099, (1989).
36. J. Guignard, A. Torrado, O. Da Cunha, and E. Gautier, Glomerular filtration rate in the first three weeks of life, J. Pediatr., 87, 268 (1975).
37. G. Schwartz, L. Feld, and D. Langford, A simple estimate of glomerular filtration rate in full term infants during the first year of life, J. Pediatr., 104, 849 (1984).
38. R. McCance, Renal function in early life, Physiol. Rev., 28, 331 (1948).
39. M. Nahata, Progress in pediatric drug therapy, Drug Intell. Clin. Pharm., 20, 388 (1986).
39a. M. Tosyali, and L. Greenhill, Child and adolescent psychopharmacology, Pediatr. Clin. North Am., 45(5), 1021 (1998).
40. M. Painter, C. Pippenger, C. Wasterlein, M. Barmada. and W. Pitlick, Phenobarbital and phenytoin in

neonatal seizures: Metabolism and tissue distribution, Neurology, 31, 1107 (1981).

41. S. Onishi, O. Yoshiki, Y, Nishimura, S. Itoh, and K. Itobe, Distribution of phenobarbital in serum. brain and other organs from pediatric patients, Dev. Pharmacol. Ther., 7, 153 (1984).
42. C. Hayes, V. Butler, and W. Gersony, Serum digoxin studies in infants and children, Pediatrics, 52, 561 (1973).
43. R. Kauffman and M. Nelson, Effect of age on ibuprofen pharmacokinetics and antipyretic response, J. Pediatr., 121, 969 (1992).
43a. D. Murry, C. Oermann, C. Ou, C. Rognerud, D. Seilheimer, and M. Sockrider, Pharmacokinetics of ibuprofen in patients with cystic fibrosis, Pharmacotherapy, 19(3), 340 (1999).
44. M. Boutroy, P. Vert, R. Royer, P. Monin, and M. Royer-Morrot, Caffeine, a metabolite of theophyllinc during treatment of apnea in the premature infant, J. Pediatr., 94, 996 (1979).
45. M. Butroy, P. Vert, R. Royer, P. Monin, and M. Royer-Morrot, Scientists explore effects of drugs on children, adults, World Pharm. Stand. Rev., 8 (1990).
46. R. Steele and G. Kearns, Antimicrobial therapy for pediatric patients, Pediatr, Clin, North Am., 36,1321 (1989).
47. V. San Joaquin and T. Stull, Antibacterial agents in pediatrics, Infect Dis. Clin. North Am., 14(2), 341 (2000).
48. T. Finitzo-Hieber, G. McCracken, R. Roeser. D. Allen. D. Chrane. and J. Morrow, Ototoxicity in neonates treated with gentamicin and kanamycin: Results of a four year controlled follow-up study. Pediatrics, 63, 445 (1979).
49. A. Muhlberg, C. Linz, E. Bern, L. Tucker, M. Verhave, and R. Grand, Identifaction of nonsteroidal anti-inflammatory drug induced gastrointestinal injury in children with juvenile rheumatoid arthritis, J. Pediatr., 122, 647 (1993).
50. T. Einarson, Drug related hospital admissions, Ann. Pharmacother., 27, 832 (1993).
51. C. Woods, M. Rylance, R. Cullen, and G. Rylance, Adverse reactions to drugs in children, Br. Med. J., 294, 869 (1987).
52. L. Golightly, S. Smolinske, M. Bennet, E. Sutherland, and B. Rumack, Pharmaceutical excipients (Part I), Med. Toxicol., 3, 128 (1988).
53. L. Golightly, S. Smolinske, M. Bennet, E. Sutherland, and B. Rumack, Pharmaceutical excipients (Part II), Med. Toxicol., 3, 209 (1988).
54. American Academy of Pediatrics, Committee on Drugs, "Interactive" ingredients in pharmaceutical products. Pediatrics, 99, 268 (1997).
55. P. Menon, B. Thach, C. Smith, M. Landt, J. Robert, R. Hillman, and L. Hillman, Benzyl alcohol toxicity in a neonatal intensive care unit, Am. J. Perinatol., 1, 288 (1984).
56. G. Little and A. Pruiu, Benzyl alcohol: Toxic agent in neonatal units, Pediatrics, 72, 356 (1983).
57. K. Arulanantham and M. Genel, Central nervous system toxicity associated with ingestion of propylene glycol, J. Pediatr., 93, 515 (1978).
58. Yellow No, 5 (tartrazine) drug labeling, FDA Drug Bull., 9, 18 (1979).
59. R. Pohl, R. Balon, R. Berchow, and V. Yeragani, Allergy to tartrazine in antidepressants, Am. J. Psychiatry, 144, 237 (1987).
60. R. Weber, M. Hoffman, D. Raine, and H. Nelson, Incidence of bronchoconstriction due to aspirin. azo dyes, non-azo dyes and preservatives in a population of perennial asthmatics, J. Allergy Clin. immunol., 64, 32 (1979).
61. R. Buswell and M. Lefkowitz, Oral bronchodilators containing tartrazine, JAMA, 235, 1111 (1976).
62. E. Hill, C. Flaitz, and C. Frost, Sweetener content of common pediatric oral liquid medications Am. J. Hosp. Pract., 45, 135 (1988).
63. L. Shaw and H. Glenwright, The role of medications in dental caries formation: Need for sugar-free medication for children, Pediatrician, 16, 153 (1989).
64. R. Feigal, M. Jensen, and C. Mensing, Dental caries potential of liquid medications, Pediatrics, 68, 416 (1981).
65. P. Lokken, J. Birkeland, and E. Sannes, pH changes in dental plaque caused by sweetened iron containing medicine, Scand. J. Dent. Res., 83, 279 (1975).
66. D. Lutomski, M. Gora, S. Wright, and J. Martin, Sorbitol content of selected oral liquids, Ann. Pharmacother., 27, 269 (1993).
67. W. Dills, Sugar alcohols as bulk sweeteners, Annu. Rev. Nutr., 9, 161 (1989).
68. M. Veerman, Excipients in valproic acid syrup may cause diarrhea: A case report, DICP Ann. Pharmacother., 24, 832 (1990).
69. D. Arnold, C. Moodie, and H. Grice, Long term toxicity of *ortho*-toluene sulfonamide and sodium saccharin in the rat, Toxicol. Appl. Pharmacol., 52, 113 (1980).
70. A. Kumar, M. Weatherly, and D. Beaman, Sweeteners, flavorings and dyes in antibiotic preparations, Pediatrics, 87, 352 (1991).
71. R. Koysooko and G. Levy, Effect of ethanol on intestinal absorption of theophylline, J. Pharm. Sci., 63, 829 (1974).
72. NDMA statement on alcohol content of OTC drugs, Nonprescrip. Drug Manuf. Assoc. Newslett., Dec. 18 (1992).
73. P. Rappaport, Extemporaneous dosage preparations for pediatrics, U.S. Pharmacist, 9:H1 (1984).
74. M. Nahata, personal communication, 1993.

75. S. Abdel-Rahman, D. Blowey, R. Kauffmann, and G. Kearns, Comparative bioavailability of loracarbef chewable tablet vs. oral suspension in children, Pediatr. Infect. Dis. J., 17(12), 1171 (1998).
76. C. Cornaggia, S. Gianetti, D. Battino, T. Granato, A. Romeo, F. Viani, and G. Limido, Comparative pharmacokinetic study of chewable and conventional carbamazepine in children, Epilepsia, 34, 158 (1993).
77. J. Cloyd, R. Kriel, C. Jones-Sauete, B. Ong, J. Jancik, and R. Remmel, Comparison of sprinkle versus syrup formulations of valproate for bioavailability, tolerance and preference, J. Pediatr., 120, 634 (1992).
78. J. Blumer, Fundamental basis for rational therapeutics in acute otitis media, Pediatr. Infect. Dis. J., 18(12), 1130 (1999).
79. M. Nowak, B. Brundhofer, and M. Gibaldi, Rectal absorption from aspirin suppositories in children and adults, Pediatrics, 54, 23 (1974).
80. G. Gourlay and R. Boas, Fatal outcome with use of rectal morphine for postoperative pain control in an infant, Br. Med. J., 304, 766 (1992).
81. R. Ghadially and N. Shear, Topical therapy and percutaneous absorption, in *Pediatric Pharmacology*, 2nd Ed. (S. Yaffe and J. Aranda, eds.), W. B. Saunders, Philadelphia, 1992.
82. J. Paisley, A. Smith, and D. Smith, Gentamicin in newborn infants, Am. J. Dis. Child., 126, 473 (1973).
83. F. Shann, M. Linnemann, A. Mackenzie, J. Barker, M. Gratten, and N. Crinis, Absorption of chloramphenicol sodium succinate after intramusclar administration in children, N. Engl. J. Med., 313, 410 (1985).
84. J. Bradley, L. Compogiannis, W. Murray, M. Acasta, and G. Tsu, Pharmacokinetics and safety of intramuscular injection of concentrated ceftriaxone in children, Clin. Pharmacol., 11, 961 (1992).
85. E. Suarez, and J. Grippi, Comparative bioavailability and safety of two intramuscular ceftriaxone formulations, Ann. Pharmacother., 30, 1223 (1996).
85a. R. Seay, Comment: bioavailability and safety of two ceftriaxone formulations exposure to lidocaine questions, Ann. Pharmacother., 31, 501 (1997).
86. A. Mclvor, M. Paluzzi, and M. Meguid, Intramuscular injection abscess—past lessons relearned. N. Engl. J. Med., 324, 1897 (1991).
87. R. Hard, Pharmacists work on pediatric dosage problems, Hospitals, 66 (Oct. 20. 1992).
88. G. Koren, Z. Baryilay, and Greenwald, Tenfold errors in drug administration for children, Pediatrics, 77, 848, (1986).
89. C. Johnston, Endotracheal drug delivery, Pediatr. Emerg. Care, 8, 94 (1992).
90. A. Hickey, Factors influencing aerosol desposition in inertial impactors and their effect on particle size characterization, Pharm, Tech. (Sept. 1990), pp. 118–120.
90a. J. Seale and L. Harrison, Effect of changing the fine particle mass of inhaled beclomethasone dipropionate on intrapulmonary deposition and pharmacokinetics. Respir. Med., 92(suppl A), 9 (1998).
91. B. Sagger and D. Lawson, Some observations on the penetration of antibiotics through mucus in vitro, J. Clin. Pathol., 19, 313 (1966).
92. B. Saggers and D. Lawson, In vivo penetration of antibiotics into sputum in cystic fibrosis, Arch. Dis. Child., 43, 404 (1968).
93. M. Gibaldi, Understanding and treating some genetic diseases, Ann. Pharmacother., 26, 1589 (1992).
94. L. Jew and L. Hart, Inhaled aminoglycosides in cystic fibrosis, DICP Ann. Pharmacother., 24, 711 (1990).
95. B. Ross, L. Ramsey, and J. Shepherd, Delivery of aerosol therapy in the management of pulmonary disorders, Hosp. Pharm. Rep., 14(9 suppl), 3 (2000).
96. J. Finney, P. Friman, M. Rapoff, and E. Chrisopherson, Improved compliance with antibiotic regimens for otitis media, Am. J. Dis. Child., 139, 89 (1985).
97. N. Mantick, and C. Jantz, Children's OTC pharmaceuticals: sensory directed flavor formulation, Profile Attribute Analysis: Arthur D. Little, Inc., Cambridge, MA 1991.
98. M. Ruff, D. Schotik, J. Bass, and J. Vincent, Antimicrobial drug suspensions: a blind comparison of taste of fourteen common pediatric drugs, Pediatr. Infect. Dis. J., 10, 30 (1991).
99. Fed. Reg., 63 (231), 66611 (1998).
100. D. Hariparsad, N. Wilson, and C. Dixon, Oral tartrazine challenge in childhood asthma: Effect on bronchial reactivity, Clin. Allergy, 14, 81 (1984).
101. F. Chafee and G. Settipane, Asthma caused by FD & C approved dyes, J. Allergy, 40, 65 (1967).
102. R. Clarke, Exacerbation of asthma after nebulized beclomethasone diproprionate, Lancet, 2, 574 (1986).
103. C. Beasley, P. Rafferty, and S. Holgate, Benzalkonium chloride and bronchoconstriction, Lancet, 2, 1227 (1986).
104. D. Paige, E. Leonardo, and J. Nakasima, Response of lactose intolerant children to different lactose levels, Am. J. Clin. Nutr., 25, 467 (1972).
105. J. Lieb and D. Kazienko, Lactose filler as a cause of "drug-induced" diarrhea, N. Engl. J. Med., 299, 314 (1978).
106. Y. Kaminer, A. Apter, S. Tyano, E. Livni, and H. Wysenbeek, Delayed hypersensitivity reaction to orally administered methylparaben, Clin. Pharm., 1, 469 (1982).
107. W. Balistreri, M. Farrell, and K. Bove, Lessons from E-ferol tragedy, Pediatrics, 78, 503 (1986).
108. M. Nitzan, B. Volovitz, and E. Topper, Infantile methemoglobinemia caused by food additives, Clin. Toxicol., 15, 273 (1979).
109. G. Angelini and C. Meneghini, Contact allergy from propylene glycol, Contact Dermatol., 7, 197 (1981).

110. H. Moller, Methiolate allergy: A nationwide introgenic sensitization, Acta Dermatol. Venereol., 57, 509 (1977).
111. J. Royhans, P. Walson, G. Wood, and W. MacDonald, Mercury toxicity following merthiolate ear irrigations, J. Pediatr., 104, 311 (1984).
112. M. Haeney, G. Carter, W. Yeoman, and R. Thompson, Long term parenteral exposure to mercury in patients with hypogammaglobulinaemia, Br. Med. J., 2, 12 (1979).
113. S. N. Schappert and C. Nelson, National Ambulatory Medical Care Survey, 1995–96 Summary, National Center for Health Statistics, Vital Health Stat., 13(142) (1999).
114. National Center for Health Statistics, *Health, United States, 2000 with Adolescent Health Chartbook*, Hyattsville, MD, 2000.
115. J. Roberts and N. Turner, Pharmacodynamic basis for altered drug action in the elderly, Clin. Geriatr. Med., 4, 127 (1988).
116. R. E. Vestal, Drug use in the elderly: A review of problems and special considerations, Drugs, 16, 358 (1978).
117. M. L. Rocci, P. H. Blases, and W. B. Abrams, Geriatric clinical pharmacology, Cardiol. Clin., 4, 213 (1986).
118. J. A. Cromarty, Medicines for the elderly, Pharm. J., 235, 511 (1985).
119. F. Pucino, C. L. Beck, R. L. Seiferi, G. L. Strommen, P. A. Sheldon, and I. L. Silbergleit, Pharmacogeriatrics, Pharmacother. 5, 314 (1985).
119a. T. Miura, R. Kojima, Y. Sugiura, M. Mizutani, F. Takatsu, and Y. Suzuki, Effect of aging on the incidence of digioxin toxicity, Ann. Pharmacother., 34(4), 426 (2000).
120. J. Crooks, K. O'Malley, and H. Stevenson, Pharmacokinetics in the elderly, Clin. Pharmacokinet., 1, 280 (1976).
121. W. F. Kean and W. W. Buchanan, Pharmacokinetics of NSAID with special reference to the elderly, Singapore Med. J., 28, 383 (1987).
122. S. D. Black, M. J. Denham, R. M. Aeheson, V. W. M. Drury, J. G. Evans, A. N. Exton-Smith, C. F. George, M. Hamilion, D. A. Heath, H. M. Hodkinson, T. Rawlins. T. E. D. Arie, I. G. J. R. Evans, M. Rowland, J. P. Kerr, E. S. Snell, B. Wade, D. G. Williams, G. M. G. Tibbs, and H. Irons, Medications for the elderly, J. R. Coil. Phys. Lond., 18, 7 (1984).
123. M. Mayersohn, Drug disposition in the elderly, in *Pharmacy Practice for the Geriatric Patient* (F. B. Penta et al., eds.), American Association of Colleges of Pharmacy, Alexandria, VA 1986, pp. 9.5–9.11.
124. A. M. M. Shepherd, Physiological changes with aging–relevance to drug study design, in *Drug Studies in the Elderly: Methodological Concerns* (N. R. Cutler and P. K. Narang. eds.), Plenum Publishing, New York, 1986, pp. 50–54.
124a. K. Dilger, U. Hofmann, and U. Klotz, Enzyme induction in the elderly: effect of rifampin on the pharmacokinetics and pharmacodynamics of propafenone, Clin. Pharmacother., 67(5), 512 (2000).
124b. M. K. Grandison and F. D. Boudinot, Age-related changes in protein binding of drugs: Implications for therapy, Clin. Pharmacokinet., 38(3), 271 (2000).
124c. K. A. Bachman, and R. J. Belloto Jr., Differential kinetics of phenytoin in elderly adults, Drugs Aging, 15(3), 235 (1999).
124d. G. K. Dresser, J. D. Spence, and D. G. Bailey, Pharmacokinetic-pharmacodynamic consequences and clinical relevance of cytochrome P450 3A4 inhibition, Clin. Pharmacokinet., 38(1), 41 (2000).
124e. B. A. Sproule, B. G. Hardy, and K. I. Shulman, Differential pharmacokinetics of lithium in elderly patients, Drugs Aging, 16(3), 165 (2000).
124f. M. K. Grandison, and F. D. Boudinot, Age-related changes in protein binding of drugs: implications for therapy, Clin. Pharmacokinet., 38(3), 271 (2000).
124g. J. S. Cohen, Avoiding adverse reactions. Effective lower-dose drug therapies for older patients, Geriatrics, 55(2), 54, 59, 63 (2000).
124h. G. K. Dresser, D. G. Bailey, and S. G. Carruthers, Grapefruit juice-felodipine interaction in the elderly, Clin. Pharmcol. Ther., 68(1), 28 (2000).
125. C. M. Castleden, C. N. Volans, and K. Raymond, The effect of ageing on drug absorption from the gut, Age, Ageing, 6, 138 (1977).
126. P. P. Gerbino and C. J. Wordell, Gastrointestinal disorder, in *Pharmacy Practice for the Geriatric Patient* (F. B. Penta et al., eds.), American Association of Colleges of Pharmacy, Alexandria, VA 1986, pp. 20.1–20.24.
127. T. W. Sheely, The gastrointestinal system and the eldery, in *Contemporary Geriatric Medicine*. Vol. 2 (S. R. Gambert, ed.), Plenum Publishing, New York, 1986.
128. M. C. Geokas and B. J. Haverback, The aging gastrointestinal tract, Am. J. Surg., 117, 881 (1969).
129. P. R. Holt, Gastrointestinal drugs in the elderly, Am. J. Gastroenterol., 81, 403 (1986).
130. S. Anuras and V. Loeing-Baucke, Gastrointestinal motility in the elderly, J. Am. Geriatr. Soc., 32, 386 (1984).
131. J. G. Moore, C. Tweedy, P. E. Christian, and F. L. Datz, Effect of age on gastric emptying of liquid-solid meals in man, Dig. Dis. Sci., 28, 340 (1983).
132. M. A. Evans, E. J. Triggs, M. Cheung, G. A. Broe, and H. Creasey, Gastric emptying rate in the elderly: Implications for drug therapy, J. Am. Geriatr. Soc., 24, 201 (1981).
133. M. A. Evans, G. A. Broe, E. J. Triggs, M. Cheung, H. Creasy, and P. D. Paull, Gastric emptying rate and the

systemic availability of levodopa in the elderly Parkinsonian patient, Neurology, 31, 1288 (1981).
134. P. Mojaverian and P. H. Vlasses, Effects of gender, posture, and age on gastric residence time of an indigestible solid: Pharmaceutical considerations, Pharm. Res., 5, 639 (1988).
134a. P. Gryback, G. Hermansson, E. Lyrenas, K. W. Beckman, H. Jacobsson, and P. M. Hellstrom, Nationwide standardisation and evaluation of scintigaphic gastric emptying: reference values and comparisons between subgroups in a multicentre trial, Eur. J. Nucl. Med., 27(6), 647 (2000).
135. P. F. Adams and V. Benson, Current estimates from the National Health Interview Survey, 1991, National Center for Health Statistics, Vital Health Stat., 10 (184) (1993).
136. J. G. Collins, Prevalence of selected chronic conditions: United States, 1990–1992, National Center for Health Statistics, Vital Health Stat., 10(194), (1997).
137. J. Cornoni-Huntley, D. B. Brock, A. M. Ostfeld, J. O. Taylor, and R. B. Wallace (eds.), *Established Populations for Epidemiologic Studies for the Elderly*, U.S. Government Printing Office, Washington, DC. 1986.
138. D. B. Ferguson, An overview of physiological changes in the aging mouth, Front. Oral Physiol., 6, 1 (1987).
139. National Center for Health Statistics, Health, United States, 1999 with Health and Aging Chartbook. Hyattsville, MD, 1999.
140. S. Kamen and L. B. Kamen, Aging and oral function, in *Contemporary Geriatric Medicine*, Vol. 2 (S. R. Gambert, ed.), Plenum Publishing, New York, 1986.
141. G. M. Ritchie, Mouth and dentition, in *Practical Geriatric Medicine* (A. N. Exton-Smith and M. F. Weksler, eds.), Churchill Livingstone, New York. 1985.
142. H. Heeneman and D. H. Brown, Senescent changes in and about the oral cavity and pharvnx. J. Otolaryngol., 15, 214 (1986).
143. H. Ben-Aryeh, D. Miron, I. Berdicevsky, R. Szargel, and D. Gutman, Xerostomia in the elderly: Prevalence, diagnosis, complications and treatment, Gerodontology, 4, 77 (1985).
144. B. J. Baum and L. Bodner, Aging and oral motor function: Evidence for altered performance among older persons, J. Dent. Res., 62, 2 (1983).
145. E. Christophers and A. M. Kligman, Percutaneous adsorption in aged skin, in *Advances in Biology of the Skin*, Vol. 6 (W. Montagna, ed.), Permagon Press, New York, 1964, pp. 163–175.
146. C. J. Behl, N. H. Beltantone, and G. L. Flynn, Influence of age on percutaneous absorption of drug substance, in *Transdermal Delivery of Drugs*, Vol. 2 (A. F. Kyodonieus and B. Berner, eds.), CRC Press, Boca Raton, FL, 1988, pp. 109–132.
147. A. M. Kligman, Perspectives and problems in cutaneous gerontology, J. Invest. Dermatol., 73, 39 (1979).
148. C. H. Daly and G. F. Odland, Age-related changes in the mechanical properties of human skin, J. Invest. Dermatol., 73, 83 (1970).
149. S. Katz and T. D. Downs, Progress in the development of an index of ADL, Gerontologist, 10, 20 (1970).
150. L. G. Branch and S. Katz, A prospective study of functional status among community elderly, Am. J. Public Health, 74, 266 (1984).
151. C. C. Maloney, Identifying and treating the client with sensory loss, Phys. Occup. Ther. Geriatr., 5, 31 (1987).
152. W. Kosnik, L. Winsolow, D. Kline, K. Rasinski, and R. Sekuler, Visual changes in daily life throughout adulthood, J. Gerontol., 43, P63 (1988).
153. J. Cerella, Age-related decline in extrafoveal letter perception, J. Gerontol., 40, 727 (1985).
154. P. P. Lamy, Over-the-counter medication: The drug interactions we overlook, J. Am. Geriatr. Soc., 30(suppl), S69 (1982).
155. P. P. Lamy, Appropriate and inappropriate drug use, in *Pharmacy Practice for the Geriatric Patient* (F. B. Penta, et al., eds.), American Association of Colleges of Pharmacy, Alexandria, VA, 1985, pp. 13.1–13.27.
156. C. C. Fuselier, General principles of drug prescribing, in *Pharmacy Practice for the Geriatric Patient* (F. B. Penta, et al., eds.), American Association of Colleges of Pharmacy, Alexandria, VA, 1985, pp. 8.1–8.28.
157. M. K. Kottke, G. Stetsko, S. R. Rosenbaum, and C. T. Rhodes, Problems encountered by the elderly in the use of conventional dosage forms, J. Geriatr. Drug Ther., 5, 77 (1990).
158. M. Marvola, Adherence of drug products to the oesophagus, Int. J. Pharm., 3, 294 (1984).
159. K. S. Channer and J. P. Virjee, The effect of formulation on oesophageal transit, J. Pharm. Pharmacol., 37, 126 (1985).
160. M. Marvola and M. Rajaniemi, Effect of dosage form and formulation factors on adherence of drugs to the esophagus, J. Pharm. Sci., 72, 1034 (1983).
161. H. Hey and J. Jorgensen, Oesophageal transit of six commonly used tablets and capsules, Br. Med. J., 235, 1717 (1982).
162. T. Semla, J. Breizer, and M. Higbee, *Geriatric Dosage Handbook*, 6th ed., American Pharmaceutical Association, Washington, DC, 2000.
163. R. B. Wallace, Drug utilization in the rural elderly: Perspectives from a population study, in *Geriatric Drug Use—Clinical and Social Perspectives* (S. R. Moore and R. W. Teal, eds.), Permagon Press, New York, 1985, pp. 78–85.
164. R. G. Hollenbeck and P. P. Lamy, Dosage form considerations in clinical trials involving elderly patients, in *Drug Studies in the Elderly: Methodological Concerns* (N. R. Cutler and P. K. Narang, eds.), Plenum Publishing, New York, 1986, pp. 335–353.

165. J. E. Finchman, Over-the-counter drug use and misuse by the ambulatory elderly: A review of the literature, J. Geriatr. Drug Ther., 1, 3 (1986).
166. J. Williamson, R. G. Smith, and L. E. Burley, Drugs and safer prescribing, in *Primary Care of the Elderly: A Practical Approach*, IOP Publishing, London, 1987.
167. W. Simonson, Compliance to drug therapy, in *Medications and the Elderly: A Guide to Promoting Proper Use*, Aspen Publishers, Baltimore, 1984, pp. 70–79.
168. P. P. Lamy, The future is not what it used to be, M. Pharm., 63, 10 (1987).
169. J. L. Richardson, Perspectives on compliance with drug regimens among the elderly, J. Compliance Health Care, 1, 33 (1986).
170. B. Wade and A. Bowling, Appropriate use of drugs by elderly people, J. Adv. Nurs., 11, 47 (1986).
171. E. D. Sumner, Compliance with drug therapy, in *Handbook of Geriatric Drug Therapy for Health Care Professionals,* Lea & Febiger, Philadelphia, 1983, pp. 43–52.
172. R. B. Hallworth and L. A. Goldberg, Geriatric patients' understanding of labelling of medicines, Br. J. Pharm. Pract., 6, 6 (1984).
173. R. B. Hallworth and L. A. Goldberg, Geriatric patients' understanding of labelling of medicines, Part 2, Br. J. Pharm. Pract., 6, 42 (1984).
174. B. S. M. Wong and D. C. Norman, Evaluation of a novel medication aid, the Calendar BlisterPak, and its effect on drug compliance in a geriatric outpatient clinic, J. Am. Geriatr. Soc., 35, 21 (1987).
175. S. Keram and M. E. Williams, Quantifying the case of difficulties older persons experience opening medical containers, J. Am. Geriatr. Soc., 36, 198 (1988).
176. J. R. Davidson, Presentation and packaging of drugs for the elderly, J. Hosp. Pharm., 31, 180 (1973).
177. United States Pharmacopeial Convention, *Fourth Supplement of the United States Pharmacopeia—National Formulary*, United States Pharmacopeial Convention, Rockville, MD, 1988, pp. 2249–2250.
178. U.S. Bureau of the Census, Demographic and socioeconomic aspects of aging in the United States, *Current Population Reports. Series P-23, No. 138*, U.S. Government Printing Office, Washington, DC, 1984.
179. G. S. Banker and N. R. Anderson, Tablets, in Lachman L, Lieberman H. A. and Kanig J. L. (Eds.) The Theory and Practice of Industrial Pharmacy 3rd Ed., Lea & Febiger, Philadelphia, PA, 1986.
180. J. Tsumara, Process for the preparation of water-soluble tablets, U.S. Patent 3.692.896 (1972).
181. G. Crivellaro, and F. Oldani, Soluble tablet, U.S. Patent 3.819.824 (1974).
182. L. G. Daunora, Water soluble tablet, U.S. Patent 4.347.235 (1982).
183. T. Martini, Tablet dispersion as alternative to mixtures, NZ Pharm. 7(Jul), 34 (1987).
183a. T. Ishikawa, Y. Watanabe, N. Utoguchi, and M. Matsumoto, Preparation and evaluation of tablets rapidly disintegrating in saliva containing bitter-taste-masked granules by the compression method, Chem. Pharm. Bull. (Tokyo), 47(10), 1451 (1999).
183b. Y. X. Bi, H. Sunada, Y. Yonezawa, and Danjo, Evaluation of rapidly disintegrating tablets prepared by a direct compression method, Drug Dev. Ind. Pharm., 25(5), 571, (1999).
183c. E. Norris and M. Guttadauria, Piroxicam: new dosage forms, Eur. J. Rheumatol. Inflamm., 8(1), 94 (1987).
184. H. Heinemann and W. Rothe, Preparation of porous tablets, U.S. Patent 3.885.026 (1975).
184a. S. Corveleyn and J. P. Remon, Stability of freeze-dried tablets at different relative humidities, Drug Dev. Ind. Pharm., 25(9), 1005 (1999).
184b. H. Seager, Drug-delivery products and the Zydis fast-dissolving dosage form, J. Pharm. Pharmacol., 50(4), 375 (1998).
184c. T. Hanawa, R. Maeda, E. Muramatsu, M. Suzuki, M. Sugihara, and S. Nakajima, New oral dosage for elderly patients. III. Stability of trichlormethiazide in silk fibroin gel and various sugar solutions, Drug Dev. Ind. Pharm., 26(10), 1091 (2000).
184d. T. Hanawa, A. Watanabe, T. Tsuchiya, R. Ikoma, M. Hidaka, and M. Sugihara, New oral dosage form for elderly patients: preparation and characterization of silk fibroin gel, Chem. Pharm. Bull. (Tokyo), 43(2), 284 (1995).
184e. A. Watanabe, T. Hanawa, M. Sugihara, and K. Yamamoto, Release profiles of phenytoin from new oral dosage form for the elderly, Chem. Pharm. Bull. (Tokyo), 42(8), 1642 (1994).
185. G. D. Tovey, The development of the Tiltab tablets, Pharm. J., 239, 363 (1987).
186. C. Murphy, Aging and chemosensory perception, Front, Oral Physiol., 6, 135 (1987).
187. M. E. Spitzer, Taste acuity in institutionalized and non-institutionalized elderly men, J. Gerontol., 43, P71 (1988).
188. B. A. Cooper, A model for implementing color contrast in the environment of the elderly, Am. J. Occup. Ther., 39 253, (1985).
189. G. Zuccollo and H. Liddell, The elderly and the medication label: Doing it better, Age Ageing, 14, 371 (1985).
190. R. J. Michocki, What to tell patients about over-the-counter drugs, Geriatrics, 37, 113 (1982).
191. P. Timmins, I. Browning, A. M. Delargy, J. W. Forrester, and H, Sen, Effect of active raw material variability on tablet production,. Drug Dev. Ind. Pharm., 12, 1293 (1986).
192. N. Kaneniwa, K. Imagaw, and J.-I. Ichikawa, The effect of particle size on the compaction properties and compaction mechanism of sulfadimethoxine and sulfaphenazole, Chem. Pharm. Bull., 36, 2531 (1988).

193. B. M. Hunter, The effect of the specific surface area of primidone on its tableting properties, J. Pharm. Pharmacol., 26, 58P (1974).
194. S. Vesslers, R. Boistelle, A. Delacourte, J. C. Guyot, and A. M. Guyot-Hermann, Influence of structure and size of crystalline aggregates on their compression ability, Drug Dev. Ind. Pharm., 18, 539 (1992).
195. J. R. Leonards and G. Levy, Biopharmaceutical aspects of aspirin-induced blood loss in man, J. Pharm. Sci., 58, 1277 (1969).
196. G. M. Phillips and B. T. Palermo, Physical form as a determinant of effect of buffered acetylsalicylate formulations on GI microbleeding, J. Pharm. Sci., 66, 124 (1977).
197. B. Hoener and L. Z. Benet, Factors influencing drug absorption and drug availability, in *Modern Pharmaceutics* (G. S. Banker and C. T. Rhodes, eds.), Marcel Dekker, New York, 1979, pp. 143–182.
198. R. W. Heckel, An analysis of powder compaction phenomena, Trans. Metallurg. Soc. AIME, 221, 1001 (1961).

Chapter 22

Biotechnology-Based Pharmaceuticals

Paul R. Dal Monte, S. Kathy Edmond Rouan, and Narendra B. Bam

GlaxoSmithKline, Collegeville, Pennsylvania

I. INTRODUCTION

Since 1980, with more than 90 recombinant drugs approved for use in the United States, recombinant protein products have become an integral part of pharmaceutical development. Listed in Table 1 are therapeutic agents derived from these biotechnologies that have been approved for human use in the treatment of diseases. In recent years, as a result of advances made in the mapping of the human genome, there has been explosive growth of the targets being identified. A survey by the Pharmaceutical Research Manufacturers of America (PhRMA) found 369 medicines in the pipeline that meet the definition of "biotechnology medicines." These medicines, with some exceptions, are recombinant versions of proteins found in vivo. For some, these protein agonists activate specific receptors located in defined target tissues. They are used either as replacement therapy, e.g., insulin and growth hormone, or as a supplement to increase the activity of endogenous proteins. They are also used as therapeutic antibodies and site-specific carriers of toxic drugs for therapy or as imaging agents. The investigational medicines target more than 200 diseases that include cancer, arthritis, asthma, multiple sclerosis, and heart disease. Numerous recent articles further record and reflect the influence of biotechnology-based medicines on modern pharmaceuticals [1–5]. This chapter will discuss the basic concepts behind these technologies and will introduce the reader to the significant tasks and challenges encountered during product development to provide commercial medicines.

II. BACKGROUND

The use of therapeutic proteins to replace or supplement endogenous protein molecules has been a long-established treatment for diseases such as diabetes, growth hormone deficiency, and hemophilia. However, treatment was often limited by immunological responses to heterologous protein molecules, contamination of proteins derived from complex natural sources, and the difficulty and expense of obtaining useful quantities of materials of human and animal origin. The first successful treatment of diabetic patients with animal-derived insulin was described more than 70 years ago by Banting and Best [6]. Insulin was classically derived from bovine or porcine sources, so immunological responses to the heterologous protein were common. Before the availability of recombinantly derived human growth hormone (hGH), approximately 50 cadaver pituitary glands were required to treat a single growth hormone–deficient child for just one year [7]. However, one of the reasons for the withdrawal of pituitary-derived hGH from the market was its implication in deaths from Creutzfeldt-Jakob disease, caused by a slow-growing virus that may have contaminated some preparations of the material [8]. The tragic consequences of the treatment of hemophiliacs with clotting factors derived from acquired immunodeficiency syndrome (AIDS)—or hepatitis-infected blood stand as further harsh testimony to the risks involved in isolating therapeutic proteins from their natural source.

Table 1 Approved Biotechnology-Derived Pharmaceuticals

Trade name	Product name	Manufacturer	Abbreviated indications
Actimmune	Interferon γ-1b	Genentech	Chronic granulomatous disease
Activase	Alteplase, recombinant	Genentech	Acute myordial infarction, acute massive pulmonary embolism, ischemic stroke
Aleron N Injection	Interferon α-n3	Interferon Sciences	Genital warts
Avonex	Interferon β-1a	Biogen	Relapsing multiple sclerosis
BeneFIX	Human factor IX	Genetics Institute	Treatment of hemophilia B
Betaseron	Interferon β-1b	Berlex Laboratories	Relapsing, remitting multiple sclerosis
Biotropin	Human growth hormone	Bio-Technology General	Human growth deficiency in children
Cerezyme	Imiglucerase	Genzyme	Treatment of Gaucher's disease
Comvax	Haemophilus b conjugate and hepatitis b vaccine	Merck	Vaccination against invasive *Haemophilus influenzae* type b (Hib) and hepatitis B
Enbrel	Etanercept	Immunex Corporation	Rheumatoid arthritis
Engerit B	Hepatitis B vaccine	GlaxoSmithKline	Hepatitis B
EPOGEN	Epoetin alfa	Amgen; also approved and marketed as PROCRIT by Ortho Biotech	Anemia associated with chronic renal failure Anemia caused by chemotherapy
Genotropin	Somatropin	Pharmacia & Upjohn	Short stature in children due to growth hormone deficiency
Geref	hGH-releasing factor	Serono laboratories	Pediatric growth hormone deficiency
Gonal-F	Human follicle-stimulating hormone	Serono laboratories	Female infertility
Humalog	Insulin	Eli Lilly	Diabetes
Humate-P	Antihemophilic factor/von Willebrand factor complex	Centeon Pharma	Treatment and prevention of bleeding in hemophilia A
Humatrope	Somatropin	Eli Lilly	Human growth hormone deficiency in children
Humulin	Recombinant insulin	Eli Lilly	Diabetes
Infergen	Interferon αcon-1	Amgen	Treatment of chronic hepatitis
Intron A	interferon α-2b	Schering-Plough	Hairy cell leukemia, genital warts, AIDS-related Kaposi's sarcoma, hepatitis C, hepatitis B, malignant melanoma, follicular lymphoma in conjunction with chemotherapy
KoGENate	Antihemophilic factor	Bayer corporation	Treatment of hemophilia A
Leukine	Sargramostim (GM-CSF)	Immunex	Autologous bone marrow transplantation, neutropenia resulting from chemotherapy, peripheral blood progenitor cell mobilization, and transplantation
LYMErix	Lyme disease vaccine	GlaxoSmithKline	Active immunization against Lyme disease
Neumega	Oprelvekin	Genetics Institute	Prevention of severe chemotherapy-induced thrombocytopenia
NEUPOGEN	Filgrastim (G-CSF)	Amgen	Chemotherapy-induced neutropenia, bone marrow transplantation, chronic severe neutropenia, peripheral blood progenitor cell transplant
Norditropin	Somatropin	Novo Nordisk	Growth hormone inadequacy in children
Novolin	Insulin	Novo Nordisk	Insulin-dependent diabetes
NovoSeven	Coagulation factor VIIa	Novo Nordisk	Bleeding episodes in hemophilia A or B
Nutropin	Somatropin	Genentech	Growth hormone inadequacy in children
ORTHOCLONE OKT 3	Muronomab-CD3	Ortho Biotech	Reversal of acute kidney transplant rejection, reversal of heart and liver transplant rejection
Prevnar	Pneumococcal 7-valent conjugate vaccine	Lederle laboratories	Immunization to prevent invasive pneumococcal disease
Proleukin	Aldesleukin (interleukin 2)	Chiron	Renal cell carcinoma, metastatic melanoma
Protropin	Human growth hormone	Genentech	hGH deficiency in children

Table 1 Continued

Trade name	Product name	Manufacturer	Abbreviated indications
Pulmozyme	Dornase alfa, recombinant	Genentech	Cystic fibrosis
Recombinate	Antihemophilic factor	Baxter; Genetics Institute	Hemophilia A
Recombivax HB	Hepatitis B vaccine	Merck	Hepatitis B prevention
Refacto	Antihemophilic factor	Genetics Institute	Hemorrhagic episodes and surgical prophylaxis in patients with hemophilia A
Refludan	Lepirudin	Hoechst Marion Roussel	Heparin-induced thrombocytopenia type II
Regranex	Becaplermin	Ortho-McNeil	Lower extremity diabetic neuropathic ulcers
Remicade	Inflizimab	Centocor	Crohn's disease
ReoPro	Abciximab	Centocor	Prevention of blood clots, unstable angina
Retevase	Reteplase	Boehringer Man; Centocor	Treatment of acute myocardial infarction
Rituxan	Rituximab	Genentech	Treatment of relapsed or refractory low-grade or follicular CD20-positive B-cell non-Hodgkins lymphoma
Roferon-A	Interferon α-2a	Hoffman-La Roche	Hairy cell leukemia, AIDS-related Kaposi's sarcoma, myelogenous leukemia, hepatitis C,
Saizen	Somatropin	Serono laboratories	pediatric growth hormone deficiency
Serostim	Somatropin	Serono laboratories	AIDS-associated catabolizm/wastic, pediatric HIV failure to thrive
Simulect	Basilizimab	Novartis	Prophylaxis of acute organ (renal) rejection
Synagis	Pavilizumab	Medimmune	Prophylaxis of lower respiratory tract disease caused by RSV virus in pediatric patients
TNKase	Tenecteplase	Genentech	Reduction of mortality in acute myocardial infarction
Vistide	Cidofovir injection	Gilead Sciences	Cytomegalovirus retinitis in AIDS patients
Wellferon	Interferon alfa-n1	Glaxo Wellcome	Treatment of chronic hepatitis C
Zenapax	Daclizumab	Hoffman-La Roche	Prevention of kidney transplant rejection

Source: www.fda.gov/cber/efoi/approve.htm.

Significantly, therefore, recombinant DNA and hybridoma techniques are capable of providing molecules of a well-defined chemical composition and producing them in cell culture media that can be carefully controlled. In short, the critical advance these techniques offer is that supply and purity no longer impede the development and clinical usefulness of therapeutic protein molecules.

A. Production of Biopharmaceuticals from Recombinant DNA Technology

The products of biotechnology are typically proteins, herein distinguished arbitrarily from peptides as molecules having in excess of 30 amino acid residues. Recombinant DNA technology, often used synonymously with genetic engineering, involves the isolation of cellular DNA fragments that code for proteins of therapeutic interest [9,10]. The DNA fragments are inserted into cellular hosts that, by normal replication, make multiple copies of the original sequence (Fig. 1). This amplification of the original sequence enables the production of useful quantities of protein in the cell culture medium. By using established biochemical purification techniques, the protein may be isolated in a highly purified form.

B. Reduction of Immunogenicity of Therapeutic Proteins

Monoclonal antibodies were one of the first proteins derived from recombinant DNA technology administered to humans. In the early days of recombinant technology, monoclonal antibodies were derived from murine strains using hybridoma technology. The clinical administration of recombinantly derived murine antibody elicited a human immune response with the production of human anti-mouse antibody (HAMA) and a short serum half-life of the administered antibody. The release of endogenous antibodies can neutralize the "foreign" antibody, rendering it inactive and increasing the risk of adverse effects, such as serum sickness or allergic responses. To circumvent this limitation, the original techniques

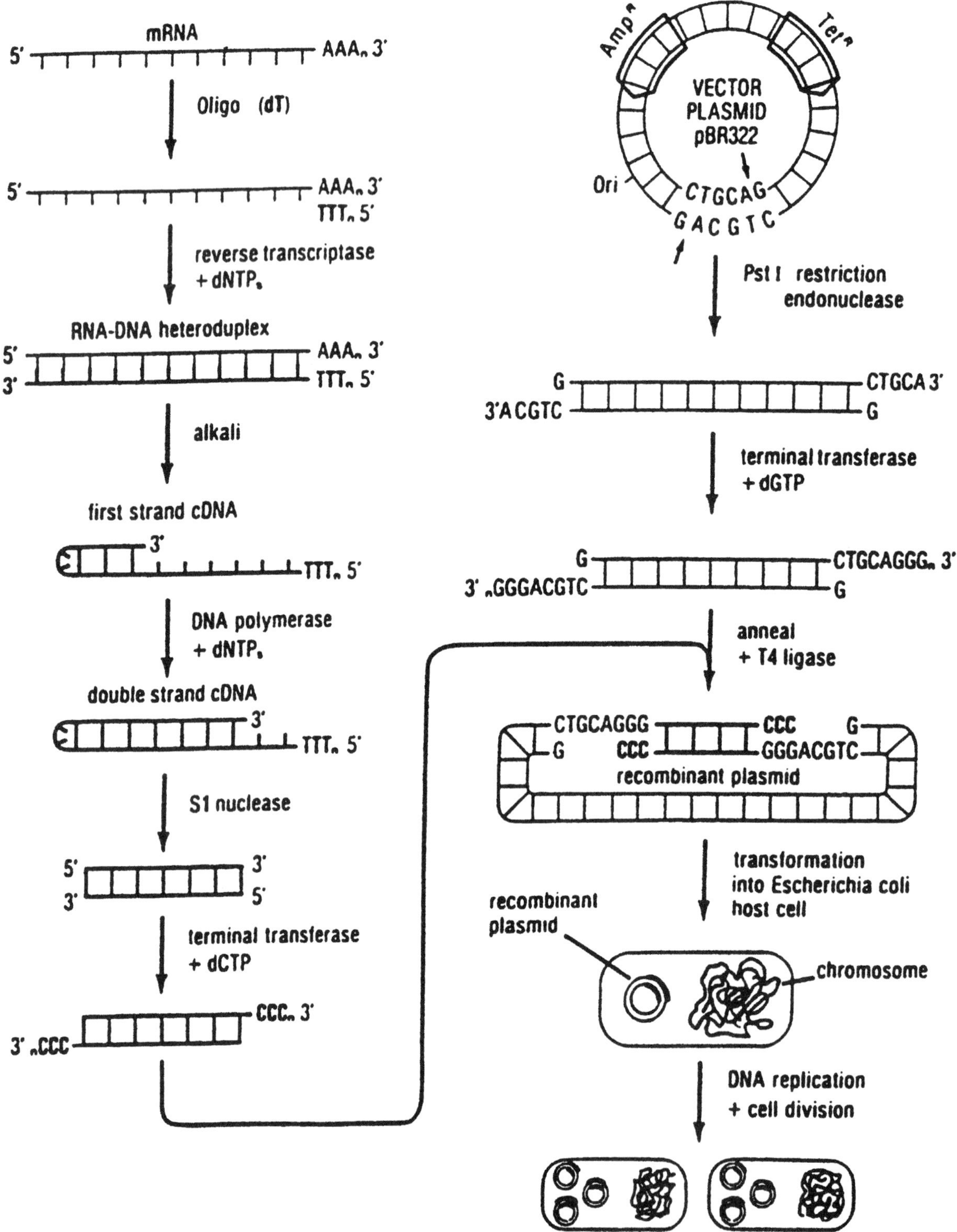

Fig. 1 Schematic outline of procedures employed in the synthesis of a cDNA gene copy from a polyadenylated mRNA template, insertion of the cDNA into a bacterial plasmid vector by a homopolymer tailing strategy, and cloning of the recombinant plasmid in an *Escherichia coli* host.

of Kohler and Milstein [11] have been substantially adapted, and genetic-engineering tools are now used to produce monoclonal antibodies that are more "human-like," expressing greater sequence homology to human antibodies.

One of the first examples of the immunogenicity of recombinantly derived antibodies was with murine anti-CD3 monoclonal antibody (OKT3) used in the induction of immunosupression after organ transplantation. Being of murine origin, the antibody was highly immunogenic [12]. In contrast, the "humanized" monoclonal antibody with the same specificity resulted in significantly less immunogenic reaction [13]. The most immunogenic portion of the antibody is the species-conserved constant region, which resides predominantly in the heavy-chain region. Therefore, several laboratories have used recombinant DNA technology to construct chimeric rodent-human monoclonal antibodies by attaching human constant regions to the rodent variable region [14]. A more sophisticated approach to obtain "humanized" antibodies involves grafting the rodent hypervariable complementarity-determining regions (CDRs) onto human variable framework regions [15,16]. Other chimeric antibodies developed include "primatized" antibodies, which combine cynomolgus monkey variable-region genes with human constant region fragments [17]. The two main emerging technologies for production of fully humanized recombinant proteins are transgenic animals and phage display [18,19]. A comprehensive summary of immune responses elicited, after administration to humans, against a wide variety of recombinantly derived therapeutic proteins can be found in a review by Porter [20].

C. Expression Systems for Therapeutic Proteins

The most efficient and popular expression systems for recombinantly derived biopharmaceuticals are mammalian cell lines such as Chinese hamster ovary (CHO) and mouse myeloma cells (NSO). Prokaryotic cell lines derived from *Escherichia coli* and yeast strains are also used to express proteins of therapeutic interest. Mammalian expression systems, as opposed to those of nonmammalian origin, have the biochemical machinery to glycosylate proteins during posttranslational biosynthetic events. Recombinantly derived monoclonal antibodies, for example, require glycosylation to exhibit a complete spectrum of biological activity [21]. Glycosylation of recombinantly antibodies can be controlled during the fermentation process by adjusting carbohydrate levels in the cell culture medium where the cells are growing. Fermentation conditions for these cell types can also be adapted to express high titers of the therapeutic antibody, at >1 g/L, which is important to manufacturers for developing efficient and economical processes. Recent advances have been made in enhancing overall product yield of therapeutic proteins by using transgenic animals such as sheep, goats, or pigs. Manufacturers of recombinant products have also developed specialized serum-free cell nutritional media, free of bovine-derived components, to remove any possibility of contamination by trace levels of bovine spongiform encephalopathy (BSE). The BSE issue has been the subject of intense scrutiny by regulatory agencies, and manufacturers must abide by established manufacturing guidelines for assuring virus removal [22].

Clearly, the tools are at hand to provide a steady stream of novel macromolecular pharmacological agents. The challenge for the pharmaceutical industry lies in the development of the purified macromolecule into a stable, pharmaceutically elegant, medicinal product. The established use of insulin and other macromolecules has heralded some of the difficulties in formulating therapeutic proteins. Despite this experience, the emergence of the large range of products of biotechnology has led to intense investigation and expansion in the fields of protein chemistry, analytical evaluation of macromolecules, and the formulation strategies to support the biotechnology pipeline. Successful development relies on a knowledge of the processes capable of destabilizing proteins and, subsequently, the application of pharmaceutically acceptable means of preventing or retarding these processes.

III. PROTEIN STRUCTURE

The essential distinction between the approaches used to formulate and evaluate proteins, compared with conventional low molecular weight drugs, lies in the need to maintain several levels of protein structure and the unique chemical and physical properties that these higher-order structures convey. Proteins are condensation polymers of amino acids, joined by peptide bonds. The levels of protein architecture are typically described in terms of the four orders of structure [23,24] depicted in Fig. 2. The primary structure refers to the sequence of amino acids and the location of any disulfide bonds. Secondary structure is derived from the steric relations of amino acid residues that are close to one another. The alpha-helix and beta-pleated sheet are examples of periodic secondary structure. Tertiary

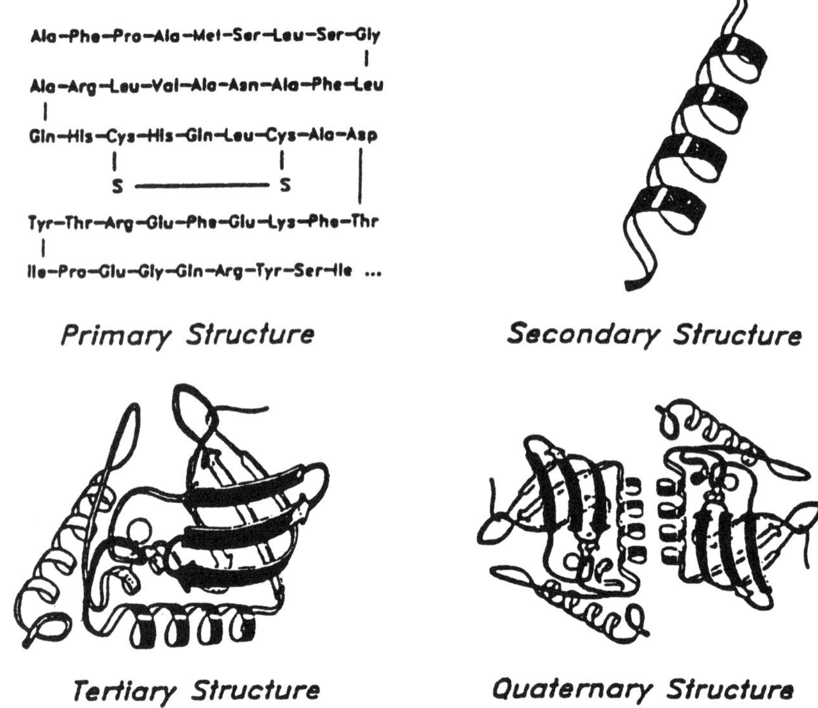

Fig. 2 Illustration of protein structure levels. Shown are primary structure (amino acid sequence), secondary structure (local order of protein chain, a-helix shown as an example), tertiary structure (assembly of secondary structure elements), and quaternary structure (relationship of different protein chain in multisubunit protein). (From Ref. 66.)

structure refers to the overall three-dimensional architecture of the polypeptide chain. Proteins under physiological conditions assume their distinctive tertiary structure (native conformation) of minimum free energy, which is a prerequisite for their biological function. Proteins that contain more than one polypeptide chain display an additional level of structural organization, namely, the quaternary structure, which refers to the way in which the chains are packed together.

In addition to the structural arrangement of the polypeptide chains, another structural feature of many recombinant proteins is the attachment of oligosaccharide groups by means of glycosidic linkages. As mentioned, the glycosylation pattern of many proteins is important for them to exert their biological effect. In addition, the glycosylation is responsible for the characteristic bio-distribution of a protein after administration [21].

The native, biologically active form of a protein molecule is held together by a delicate balance of noncovalent forces: hydrophobic, ionic, van der Waals interactions, and hydrogen bonds. In addition, disulfide linkages are covalent bonds that form between sulfur-containing amino acid residues and, thus, may contribute substantially to maintaining conformation in proteins that contain two or more cysteine residues. It has been confirmed by x-ray structure analysis that most water-soluble proteins may be grossly described as a hydrophobic core of nonpolar amino acid groups, surrounded by a hydrophilic shell of polar solvated amino acids [25]. With exposure to certain denaturants or adverse environmental conditions, the noncovalent forces are weakened, and then broken apart, leading to the unfolding and consequent inactivation of the protein. Typically, the native structure exhibits only marginal stability that is easily upset by even subtle environmental changes in pressure, temperature, pH, ionic strength, or a combination thereof. The free energy of denaturation of globular proteins rarely exceeds 15 kcal/mol [25]. The complete or partial unfolding of the protein is usually fully reversible after removal from the antagonistic agent. However, this reversible unfolding event is the precursor to irreversible covalent and noncovalent reactions that lead to irreversible protein denaturation. The term *denaturation* is applied to both reversible and irreversible disruption of the native, biologically active conformation. Denaturation involves changes in noncovalent interactions, such as hydrogen bonding, hydrophobic interactions, and electrostatic forces. Although noncovalent processes can be involved in both irreversible and reversible denaturation, chemical reactions involving covalent bond breakage or rearrangement are irreversible inactivation events.

IV. MECHANISMS AND CAUSES OF PROTEIN DESTABILIZATION

The complex hierarchy of native protein structure may be disrupted by multiple possible destabilizing mechanisms. As has been described in the foregoing, these processes may disrupt noncovalent forces of interaction or may involve covalent bond breakage or formation. A summary of the processes involved in the irreversible inactivation of proteins is illustrated in Fig. 3 and described briefly in the following section. Detailed discussions of mechanisms of protein destabilization processes are provided in several review articles [26–30].

A. Covalent Protein Destabilization

As with conventional smaller drug molecules, the chemical reactions involved in protein destabilization may be classified as those involving hydrolysis, oxidation, and racemization. However, within these categories of chemical reaction, specific reaction mechanisms are characteristic of polypeptide and protein molecules. Disulfide bond cleavage and exchange are further reaction mechanisms that specifically affect proteins. A striking feature of protein destabilization is that several different reaction mechanisms may proceed simultaneously. This was demonstrated by Ahern and Klibanov [31] in an elegant series of experiments that showed that the mechanism of inactivation of hen egg white lysozyme at 100°C was highly dependent on the solution pH. At pH 4 and 6, inactivation was largely due to deamidation of asparagine residues. At pH 8, however, inactivation was associated with the combined contributions of

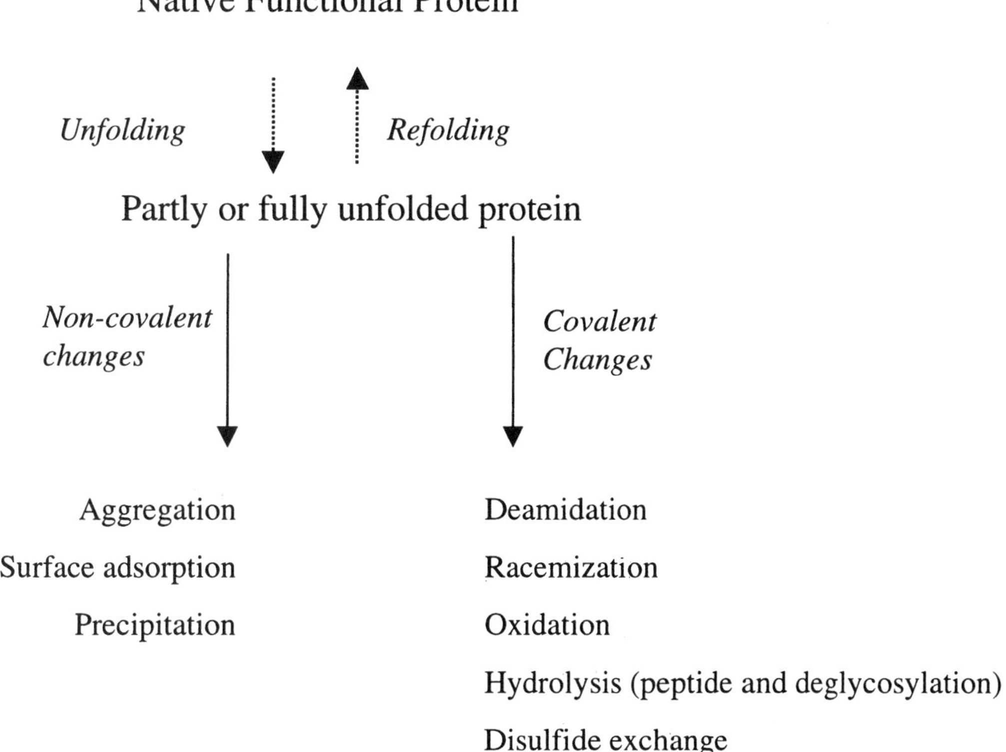

Fig. 3 Mechanisms involved in degradation of protein pharmaceuticals.

noncovalent conformational processes, destruction of disulfide bonds, and deamidation.

Because of the multiple degradation pathways that may take place at elevated temperature, protein stability monitoring data may not conform to the Arrhenius relationship, and the maximum temperature selected for accelerated stability studies must be carefully selected. Gu et al. [32] described the different mechanisms of inactivation of interleukin-1β (IL-1β) in solution above and below 39°C. In this example, the multiple mechanisms precluded the prediction of formulation shelf life from accelerated temperature data. In contrast, by working at 40°C and lower, Perlman and Nguyen [33] were able to successfully extrapolate data from stability studies of tissue plasminogen activator down to 5°C.

Chemical degradative processes in proteins and the relative incidence of each of the possible mechanisms depend on the nature of the protein, temperature, pH, ionic strength, oxygen tension, and the solutes present. Clearly, hydrogen ion concentration of the protein environment strongly influences hydrolytic reactions. However, pH also plays a significant role in driving other chemical processes that may exhibit a distinctive pH, as well as a temperature-dependent, rate-of-reaction profile. Proteins are generally most stable and least soluble at their isoelectric point (pI). At the pH corresponding to the pI of the protein, the net charge of all ionizable species is zero, with diminished potential for charge repulsion and protein unfolding.

Hydrolytic Reactions

The primary hydrolytic reactions in protein degradation are peptide bond hydrolysis and deamidation. As mentioned, the loss of oligosaccharide moieties through hydrolysis of glycosidic bonds may also influence protein activity. Peptide bond hydrolysis occurs readily under strongly acidic conditions or by a combination of milder pH and elevated temperature. Although complete acid hydrolysis of protein into its amino acids is obtained under extreme conditions (6 M HCl, 24 h, 110°C), shorter exposures, under less acidic conditions, show preferred peptide hydrolysis at aspartic acid residues. Aspartyl-prolyl linkages are especially vulnerable [28,34]. Deamidation is the hydrolysis of the side-chain amide on glutamine and asparagine residues. Asparagine (Asn) residues are more susceptible to deamidation than glutamine residues. By using model peptides, Geiger and Clarke [35] demonstrated that deamidation under physiological conditions proceeds essentially completely through an imide intermediate. The cyclic imide (succinimide) is rapidly hydrolyzed by water into a mixture of aspartic acid and isoaspartic acid, resulting in the introduction of new negative charge to the protein. The rate of deamidation could be significantly affected by the nature of the amino acid residue adjacent to the asparagine. The most labile asparagine residues in smaller peptides are those followed by a glycine residue. Asparagine-serine sequences are the next most labile sites of deamidation. However, in globular proteins, the location of the susceptible residue in the folded conformation may be more important in controlling the deamidation rate [36]. Certain proteins, therefore, will not undergo deamidation unless they have been denatured. Tyler-Cross and Schirch [37] have provided a detailed examination of the effects of amino acid sequence, buffer, and ionic strength on the rate and mechanism of deamidation of asparagine-rich peptides. The stabilizing role of secondary structure on the rate and extent of deamidation is further elucidated by Xie and Showen [38].

Oxidation

Oxidation of amino acids, especially those with aromatic side chains, as well as methionine, cysteine, and cystine residues can occur with a variety of oxidants. Molecular oxygen, hydrogen peroxide, and oxygen radicals are all known oxidants of proteins [26]. Oxidation of methionine residues to their corresponding sulfoxides is associated with loss of biological activity for many peptide hormones and proteins [28,39]. The thiol group of cysteine can be oxidized in steps successively to a sulfenic acid (RSOH), a disulfide (RSSH), a sulifinic acid (RSO_2H), and finally a sulfonic acid (RSO_3H), depending on reaction conditions. The factors that influence the rate of reaction include the temperature, pH, buffer medium used, the type of catalyst, and the oxygen tension. Oxidation of thiols occurs readily at basic pH in the presence of transition metal ions such as Cu^{2+}. As with deamidation reactions, the steric arrangement of the protein may influence the oxidative reaction and its sequelae. Where oxidized thiol groups are exposed on the protein surface, intermolecular disulfide bonds may subsequently form, leading to protein aggregation (Fig. 4).

Racemization

Racemization of the native L-amino acid in peptides and proteins to the D-enantiomer generally results

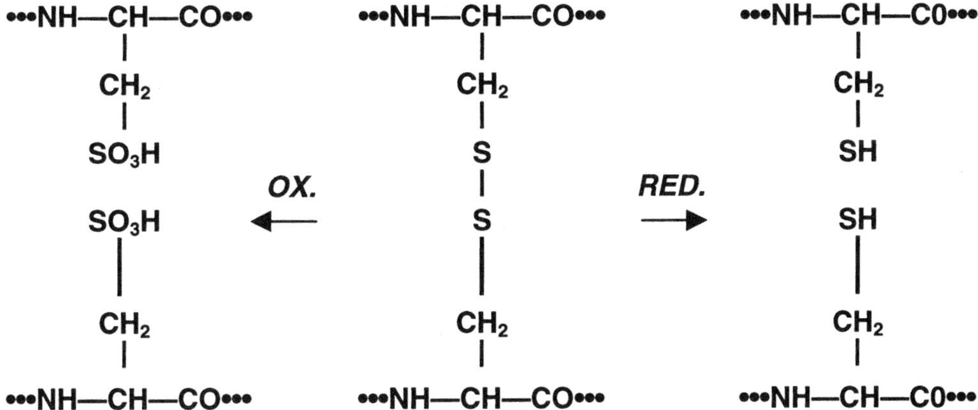

Fig. 4 Oxidation and reduction of disulfide bridge.

from base-catalyzed removal of the α-proton to produce a negatively charged planar carbanion. Return of the proton to the carbanion intermediate through reaction with water produces an enantiomeric mixture. Rates of racemization depend on the particular amino acid and are influenced by temperature, pH, ionic strength, and metal ion chelation [40]. Aspartic acid and serine residues are the most prone to racemization. An electron-withdrawing group in the side chain of the amino acid, as in serine, for example, stabilizes the carbanion intermediate, which in turn accelerates the rate of racemization. Geiger and Clarke [35] have provided data that suggest that intermediate succinimide formation plays a major role in racemization at aspartyl and asparaginyl residues. Racemization of amino acids in proteins can generate nonmetabolizable forms of amino acids (D-enantiomers) or create peptide bonds inaccessible to proteolytic enzymes [28].

Disulfide Bond Exchange

Disulfide bonds provide covalent structural stabilization in proteins, so cleavage and subsequent rearrangement of these bonds can alter the tertiary structure, thereby affecting biological activity. Disulfide exchange is catalyzed by thiols, which can arise by initial hydrolytic cleavage of disulfides, or by β-elimination in neutral or alkaline media (Fig. 5) [28]. Zale and Klibanov [41] showed that, at pH 6 and 8, thermal inactivation of ribonuclease at 90°C is caused primarily by disulfide exchange. This process was inhibited by thiol scavengers, such as *N*-ethylmaleimide, *p*-(chloromercuri)benzoate, and copper ion, and accelerated in the presence of thiols, such as with the addition of cysteine. Volkin and Klibanov [42] demonstrated β-elimination of disulfide, with the generation of free thiols, occurring at 100°C in more than a dozen proteins (Fig. 6). The rates were generally

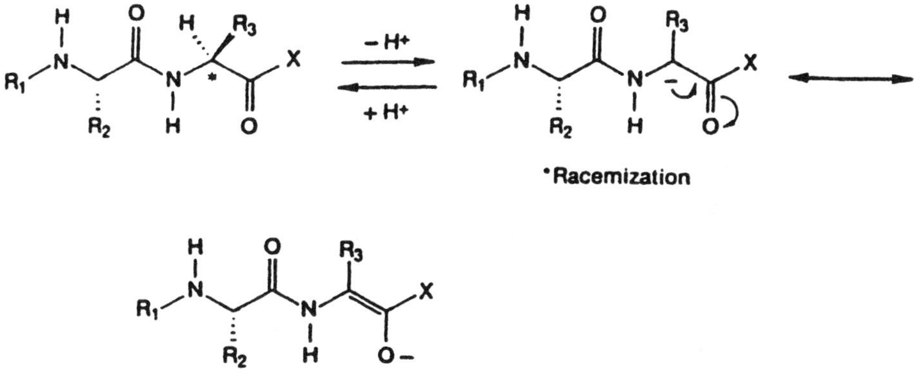

Fig. 5 Racemization of peptides by enolization.

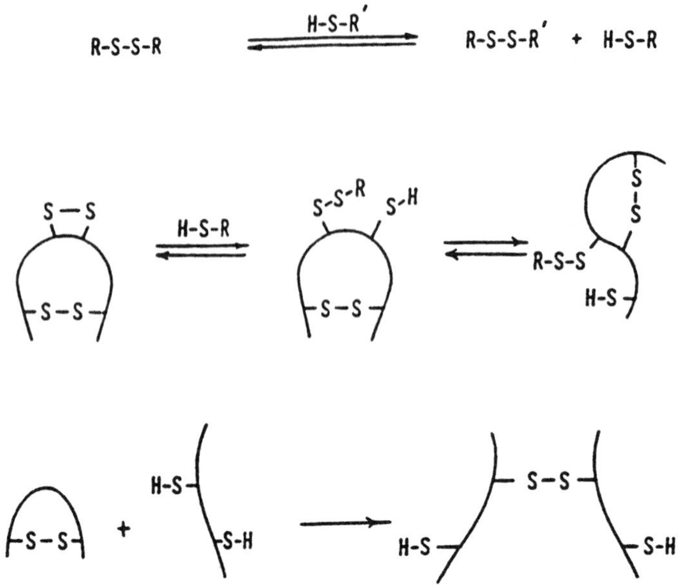

Fig. 6 Cystine disulfide exchange.

accelerated under alkaline conditions. The widespread formation of covalent insulin dimers (CIDs) in insulin formulations as a result of disulfide interchange has also been reported [43].

B. Noncovalent Protein Destabilization

Three major categories of irreversible protein inactivation occur as a result of perturbation of the noncovalent forces that maintain the three-dimensional native state of proteins. Aggregation, macroscopic precipitation, and surface adsorption are characteristic and, often, very troubling phenomena encountered during the formulation development of proteins and polypeptides. Noncovalent electrostatic forces, hydrogen bonds, hydrophobic interactions, and protein hydration may be altered as a result of thermal or pH effects. The irreversible inactivation of proteins proceeds following initial reversible unfolding of the native state. With an increase in temperature, a protein molecule in solution will undergo a characteristic transition from the native to unfolded state at the melting temperature, T_m, defined as the temperature at which 50% of the molecules are unfolded. The pH of the solution influences the net charge on the protein, depending on its pI. Therefore, solution pH may affect electrostatic interactions, also referred to as salt bridges, which form between amino acids with ionic side groups. At extremes of pH, the net charge of the protein increases with greater charge repulsion, leading to protein unfolding.

Protein conformation is also markedly affected by the concentration and type of ionic species present. In solution, individual salt effects can be either stabilizing or denaturing [26,27]. These effects correspond to the Hofmeister lyotropic series:

$$\begin{aligned}SO_4^- &> HPO_4^2 > Oac^- > F^- > \text{citrate} > Cl^- \\ &> NO_3^- > I^- > CNS^-, CLO_4^-(CH_3)_4N^+ \\ &> NH_4^+ > K^+, Na^+ > Mg^{2+} > Ca^{2+} > Ba^{2+}\end{aligned}$$

Anions and cations to the left of the series are the most stabilizing and reduce the solubility of hydrophobic groups ("salting-out") on the protein molecule by increasing the ionic strength of the solution. Anions and cations to the right of the series are destabilizing and are known to denature proteins. These ions bind extensively to charged groups of proteins, causing an increase in observed solubility or salting-in.

Mechanical forces, such as shearing, shaking, and pressure, may also denature proteins [44,45]. Shaking proteins may lead to inactivation owing to an increase in the area of the gas/liquid interface. At the interface, the protein unfolds and maximizes exposure of hydrophobic residues to the air. Surface denaturation may also occur at the protein/container interface and has been observed following adsorption of proteins to filter materials [46].

Aggregation and Precipitation

Aggregation of proteins is a microscopic process of protein molecule association. The aggregates may be dimers or larger oligomers that remain in solution, yet may affect the observed biological activity. Precipitation refers to the formation of visible proteinaceous particles, which may reduce potency in addition to altering the appearance of a formulation and its performance in various infusion devices.

Irreversible aggregation may follow unfolding as a result of incorrect refolding of the protein. Protein unfolding exposes the interior hydrophobic region to the solvent, usually water. The structuring of hydrophobic solvent molecules around the hydrophobic protein regions is thermodynamically unfavorable. This drives intermolecular reactions between exposed hydrophobic regions, leading to aggregation. Although a two-state equilibrium has been proposed as a general rule in protein unfolding, several examples of intermediate conformational states have been described [47,48], and these may play a significant role in the formation of protein aggregates and subsequent precipitation. The conformational intermediates have considerable secondary structure but lack tertiary structural interactions. Aggregation results from association of exposed hydrophobic regions on the monomeric intermediates. Protein concentration may influence the rate of formation of the associated intermediate species [47]. Mulkerrin and Wetzel [49] have investigated the effect of pH on the irreversible thermal denaturation of human interferon-γ by aggregation. This study demonstrates the dependence of aggregation on thermal unfolding and on pH. The aggregation rate versus pH profile resembles a titration curve, with the half maximal rate at pH 5.7. The effect of pH was related to the protonation state of histidine residues in the protein molecule. Deprotonation of histidine may reduce the solubility of the thermally unfolded state, rendering it more susceptible to aggregation.

The shaking of protein solutions may lead to aggregation and precipitation as a result of several mechanisms, such as air oxidation, denaturation at the interface, adsorption to the vessel, or mechanical stress. These possibilities were systematically examined for solutions of human fibroblast interferon [50]. In this example, mechanical stress was identified as the causative factor in the inactivation. The proposed mechanism of inactivation by mechanical stress was through orientation of the asymmetrical protein in the shear field, which promotes association of aligned molecules. After association, disulfide bonds may form between reactive thiol groups in the unfolded molecules.

Insulin aggregation and precipitation was an impediment to the development of implantable devices for insulin delivery as noted by several investigators working with conventional insulin infusion devices [51–54]. The potential causes of the observed aggregation and precipitation are thermal effects, mechanical stress, the nature of the materials in contact with the insulin solution, formulation factors, and the purity of the insulin preparation.

Surface Adsorption

Adsorption of proteins and peptides to the surfaces of the immediate container, filter, or materials of the infusion system can be substantial when the initial concentration of the protein in solution is low and the relative loss of drug to adsorption is consequently high. Andrade and Hiady [55] provide a comprehensive review of the principles of protein adsorption at the solid/liquid interface. As with protein aggregation, surface adsorption results from hydrophobic and electrostatic interaction and, therefore, will depend on the conformational state of the protein, the pH, and ionic strength of the solution, as well as the nature of the exposed surface. The interaction between a protein and a surface increases with increasing hydrophobicity of the surface, and increases with increasing hydrophobicity of the protein. The tendency for the protein to undergo conformational change after surface adsorption is a time-dependent, protein- and interface-specific process.

Because membrane filtration is the only currently acceptable method of sterilizing protein pharmaceuticals, the adsorption and inactivation of proteins on membranes is of particular concern during formulation development. Pitt [56] examined nonspecific protein binding of polymeric microporous membranes typically used in sterilization by membrane filtration. Nitrocellulose and nylon membranes had extremely high protein adsorption, followed by polysulfone, cellulose diacetate, and hydrophilic polyvinylidene fluoride membranes. In a subsequent study by Truskey et al. [46], protein conformational changes after filtration were observed by CD spectroscopy, particularly with nylon and polysulfone membrane filters. The conformational changes were related to the tendency of the membrane to adsorb the protein, although the precise mechanism was unclear.

V. METHODS USED TO EVALUATE PROTEIN PHARMACEUTICALS

The development of biopharmaceutical formulations must be supported by a combination of several analytical approaches in order to provide a comprehensive characterization of the protein being tested. The high complexity of proteins requires that biopharmaceutical development scientists use physicochemical methods but also immunological and biological methods to detect for chemical, physical, and functional changes, which may result from degradative processes. In addition to stability-indicating methodologies, analytical methods can be developed that assist in the determination of the compatability of formulation excipients with the protein. Many of the methods used during early formulation development will continue to be used throughout the development lifetime of a protein and commercialization for quality control and stability to monitor identity purity and potency. Assays that are used to support quality and stability of pharmaceuticals used in human studies are required to undergo more extensive validation than during early preclinical development. The process of assay validation involves the experimental demonstration of method parameters including assay specificity, dose-response profile and range (including detection and quantitation limits), accuracy (including recovery of spiked sample and ability to detect degradation), precision (repeatability and reproducibility), and robustness (reliability in response to assay variations). Assay validation guidelines published by regulatory agencies are available to pharmaceutical scientists [57,58]. Methods typically used to assess physical and chemical attributes of protein therapeutic agents are described briefly in the following sections.

A. Liquid Chromatography

As with the smaller drug molecules, high-performance liquid chromatography (HPLC) has become a powerful analytical tool routinely used to assess the purity and degradation of biopharmaceutical proteins. Commercially available HPLC column technology allows the biopharmaceutical scientist to choose the type of chromatographic separation depending on the properties of the protein. Three modes of HPLC are commonly used in biopharmaceutical development: reverse-phase HPLC, size exclusion HPLC, and ion-exchange HPLC. The separation of protein molecules in each mode is based on hydrophobicity, size, and charge, respectively. Part of the increasing popularity of HPLC analysis is due to the excellent resolving power, reliability and flexibility of equipment, availability of different column packings, quick development time, high throughput, and reproducibility.

Reverse-Phase HPLC

The most common chromatographic methods used in protein analyses of biopharmaceuticals is reverse-phase high-pressure liquid chromatography (RP-HPLC). The mechanism of separation for RP-HPLC is based on hydrophobic interactions between the protein molecule and the column stationary support. The mobile phase in RP-HPLC is typically prepared with a buffer at a specified pH mixed with an organic solvent like acetonitrile or *n*-propanol. In many cases, low percentage trifluoroacetic acid or similar reagents added to the mobile phase to act as an ion pair with the protein to increase hydrophobicity, thereby enhancing the interaction with the stationary phase. Elution of the protein sample through the column takes place as a result of changes in polarity of the mobile phase by use of shallow gradients, which can be programmed into the pump controller. In this manner, each component of the protein test sample will elute at a unique point during the gradient. The column packings most commonly used are silica-based packings capped with short-chain alkyl chains (C4-C8) to alter hydrophobicity; however, resin-based packings have recently become more popular due to improved stability in most solvent systems [59]. RP-HPLC has proved particularly useful for several proteins, and many excellent reviews have been published [60,61].

Size Exclusion HPLC

Size exclusion chromatography (SEC), sometimes referred to as gel permeation chromatography, is another extremely powerful chromatographic analysis used routinely in biopharmaceutical development. In SEC, the protein test sample is separated according to molecular size based on the flow of the sample through a porous and inert packing. The mobile phase in SEC is typically an aqueous buffer of defined pH and ionic strength. Molecules larger than the pores in the packing are excluded and elute with the solvent front. Smaller molecules that can pass through the pores are retained, while molecules of intermediate size can penetrate pores according to their size. SEC, therefore, can separate proteins based on the molecular weight and can yield information on the levels of aggregation and fragmentation in a protein formulation. The size of the test protein is determined by running a calibration set of proteins of known molecular weight.

Watson and Kenney [62] describe the use of high-performance size-exclusion chromatography to examine the aggregation of interferon-γ and interleukin-2 after storage at elevated temperature, after mechanical agitation, and following rapid freeze-thaw. An excellent review on SEC can be found in Ref. 63.

Ion-Exchange Chromatography

Ion-exchange chromatography (IEC) is based on the selective retention of the protein sample based on the charge on the protein at the pH of the mobile phase and a corresponding counterion covalently bonded to the stationary phase in the column packing. The development scientist can choose stationary resins with cation or anion functional groups and can select the elution of the protein sample using a gradient in ionic strength. Chromatofocusing is an extension of IEC that separates proteins by elution in a pH gradient on the basis of differences in the pI, rather than ionic strength. A review on IEC can be found in Ref. 64.

B. Optical Spectroscopy

Typically, detection of the eluting protein species for RP-HPLC, SEC, or IEC is done on-line by ultraviolet absorbance (UV) absorbance at 280 nm. Other types of detectors such as fluoresence, matrix-assisted laser desorption time-of-flight (MALDI-TOF) mass spectrometry, differential refractive index, electrochemistry, and light scattering can also be installed on-line to effectively and quickly characterize the eluting species in the protein sample. Quantitation of the manner in which proteins absorb, emit, and scatter light provides valuable information about the amount of protein present in the sample, the protein's conformation, and the tendency of the protein to aggregate. Optical spectroscopic techniques used to evaluate protein pharmaceuticals include UV and visible absorption spectroscopy, optical rotatory dispersion (ORD) and circular dichroism (CD), fluorescence, and infrared (IR) and Raman spectroscopy. Detailed theoretical discussions of these techniques are provided in the review by Cantor and Timasheff [65]. Havel et al. [66] provide an overview of the application of these techniques to the investigation of protein structure.

Absorption of proteins in the 230–300 nm range is determined by the aromatic side chains of tyrosine ($\lambda_{max} = 274$ am), tryptophan ($\lambda_{max} = 280$ nm), and phenylalanine ($\lambda_{max} = 257$ nm). Because the difference in the absorption spectra of native and unfolded protein molecules is generally small, difference spectra can be generated by difference spectroscopy and, thereby, provide a convenient means of monitoring conformational changes in a protein [60,67].

Light-scattering detectors are useful tools to measure the true size distribution and shape of protein aggregates in a solution formulation. Low-angle light-scattering detectors (LALLS) have been used routinely for measuring molecular weights in bulk solution and on-line with SEC [68]. More recently, with the advent of multiangle scattering detectors, multiangle light-scattering (MALS) has become an extremely sensitive method for measuring the size, shape, and molecular weight of aggregates in bulk solution and on-line with separation of samples by SEC [69,70]. Mulkerrin and Wetzel [49] also used light-scattering measurements at a nonabsorbing wavelength to study the effects of pH on the thermal denaturation of α-interferons.

Of the visible spectroscopic techniques, CD spectroscopy has seen the most rapid and dramatic growth. The far-UV circular dichroism spectrum of a protein is a direct reflection of its secondary structure [71]. An asymmetrical molecule, such as a protein macromolecule, exhibits circular dichroism because it absorbs circularly polarized light of one rotation differently from circularly polarized light of the other rotation. Therefore, the technique is useful in determining changes in secondary structure as a function of stability, thermal treatment, or freeze-thaw.

C. Electrophoresis

Electrophoretic techniques are based on the differences in migration of a protein through a sieve-like gel, depending on the molecule's size or net charge, in response to an applied electric field as first reported by Laemmli in 1970 [72]. The most widely used electrophoretic techniques in protein analysis are sodium dodecyl sulfate (SDS) gel electrophoresis and isoelectric focusing (IEF). The SDS gel electrophoresis technique separates protein samples based on molecular size and can be a useful technique to assess purity and to monitor degradative processes such as aggregation and fragmentation [73,74]. The technique involves heating the protein test sample in the presence of SDS. The SDS binds to the protein test sample to form a complex of fixed mass-to-charge ratio. SDS gel electrophoresis can be done in the presence or absence of reducing agent (e.g., 2-mercaptoethanol), which can cause dissociation of the protein into subunits by breaking disulfide bonds. SDS gel electrophoresis performed on a cross-linked polyacrylamide gel (SDS-PAGE) is the most common electrophoretic technique.

The polyacrylamide matrix can be prepared either at a fixed concentration or as a gradient (e.g., 5–25%). A recent article by Gerstner et al. discusses the effect of gel composition and running temperature on the separation of proteins by electrophoresis [75]. The investigation of these parameters is essential when developing and validating electrophoretic assays. After electrophoresis is completed, the protein band or bands on the gel matrix are detected by staining procedures with reagents such as Coomasie brilliant blue or silver. The stained bands can then be scanned and quantitated with laser densitometers capable of integration and calculation of peak percentages.

Isoelectric focusing is an electrophoretic technique that separates the test protein according to its isoelectric point (pI) [76]. The gel matrix (agarose) is preformed with a pH gradient. The test protein migrates in response to an applied electric field across the pH gradient on the agarose matrix and "focuses" at the pH where the protein has zero net charge (pI). The isoelectric point of the test protein is dependent on the charged functional groups in the amino acid sequence, which can be altered by degradation processes such as deamidation or the degree of glycosylation. Semiquantiative IEF can be conducted by the same staining procedures and integration of bands with laser densitometers as discussed for SDS gel electrophoresis.

More recently, capillary electrophoresis has generated considerable interest as a complementary technique in the analysis of protein therapeutic agents [77]. A number of instrument manufacturers have commercially available systems with in-line detection and full quantitative capabilities. In capillary electrophoresis (CE) the electric field drives separation of charged molecules across a small-bore fused-silica capillary. The power of CE is that the technique can be conducted under various modes with different mechanisms of separation using the same instrument and different capillary types. These include capillary zone electrophoresis (CZE), capillary isoelectric focusing (cIEF), capillary gel electrophoresis in the presence of SDS (SDS-CGE), capillary isotachophoresis (ITP), and micellar electrokinetic capillary chromatography (MECC). One of the advantages of CE over gel-based assays like SDS-PAGE and IEF is that the separation is done on commercially available capillaries. These capillaries can be of higher quality manufactured to tight specifications as compared to the polyacrylamaide or agarose gels used in SDS-PAGE and IEF respectively. Other important advantages of CE are its high resolution, detection sensitivity, relatively short analytic time, and ability for automation [77]. Assay validation for a cIEF assay used to monitor the quality of a biopharmaceutical product was first reported in the public literature by Hunt and co-workers for a recombinant antibody C2B8 a mouse-human chimeric antibody directed against CD20 [78] and also described by Watzig et al. [79]. The power of cIEF and CZE in biopharmaceutical analysis for monitoring purity and stability is becoming more and more popular as instrument manufacturers recognize the need and develop reliable, rugged, and user-friendly systems that can be adapted to the quality control environment.

D. Immunoassays and Biological Activity Assays

Bioassays are analytical in vitro or in vivo procedures, which measure the specific ability or capacity of a product to effect a desired biological response. The role of bioassays in the development of biopharmaceutical products has become increasingly important. Bioassays may be used during the early stages of formulation development, if available, and they are required as part of an Investigational New Drug (IND) and Biologics License application (BLA). Regulatory guidelines comment on the need for an assessment of biological potency for products of recombinant DNA and hybridoma technology [58]. Bioassays are used for monitoring lot-to-lot consistency and are increasingly relied upon to predict biological equivalency of a product when manufactured using different processes [80].

The design of biological activity assays is highly protein-specific, and their adequacy in assessing the clinically relevant in vivo function is often very difficult to determine. Chayen [81] provides a useful discussion of the distinction drawn between analytical assays and functional assays. Functional assays to determine potency may be conducted using established animal models or using cell-based in vitro assays. Biological assays conducted using animal models tend to be more time consuming, variable, and difficult to control as compared to cell-based in vitro assays. For this reason, cell-based bioassays are sometimes preferred over in vivo assays; the biopharmaceutical manufacturer may, however, have to justify the clinical relevance of the in vitro assay, which, as mentioned, is difficult to determine. In addition, it is not always easy to find a cell line that can be grown routinely and gives a desired biological response. Examples of in vivo and in vitro bioassays are now discussed.

The current potency assay used for human growth hormone (hGH) products is performed with hypophysectomized rats and measures weight gain over 7 days in response to intact hGH. The assay utilizes many rats, is labor intensive, and the results can be very variable. Kotts and coworkers developed and validated a cell-based assay for hGH to replace the in vivo rat assay [82]. Using accepted standards for assay validation, the authors demonstrated that the in vivo cell proliferation assay had improved reproducibility, precision, accuracy, and specificity over the in vivo assay. In addition, the assay was demonstrated to be able to detect loss in activity for aggregated (dimers) samples of hGH. As a result of this work, the authors were able to justify replacement of the in vivo weight gain assay with the cell-based assay for lot release and stability of hGH products. In another example of an in vitro cell-based assay, Gazzano-Santoro and coworkers developed and validated an in vitro nonradioactive complement-dependent cytotoxicity assay for demonstrating quality of an anti-CD20 monoclonal antibody [83]. The antibody is effective at lysing CD20 positive B cells in vitro via complement-dependent cytotoxicity and antibody-dependent cytotoxicity. Both of these mechanisms are thought to be the primary mode of action of the antibody when administered to humans. In some instances, a physicochemical method may be substituted for the biological potency assay, but a correlation must be demonstrated between the two tests. Such correlation has been established for certain insulin preparations [84].

If the required in vivo response is binding of the protein to a target receptor or antigen (soluble or membrane bound), then enzyme-linked immunoassays (ELISA) can be used to demonstrate the desired and relevant functional activity. ELISA procedures are simple and highly sensitive and can be high throughput, versatile, and quantifiable. ELISA tests can be set up on robotic systems to increase throughput and reproducibility. ELISA tests are typically included to monitor the quality of monoclonal antibodies being developed for human use. In other instances, specific protein binding is the primary step that triggers the series of events culminating in the observed biological response. Immunoassays provide convenient in vitro tests to confirm maintenance of the specific protein-binding site through its interaction with a specific antibody or antigen; therefore, they are frequently used to monitor protein conformational stability. However, their primary limitation needs to be considered in that they may not provide a measure of true biological activity because antigenically similar proteins may be detected that do not have the same in vivo functional activity. The specificity of the antigen-antibody interaction is, therefore, a significant factor in the interpretation of immunoassay data. In the quality control of protein formulations, ELISA tests may also be used to quantify proteins compared with a known amount of standards or to detect specific protein contaminants, such as host cell proteins. Detection of specific protein binding to the target is typically achieved through the use of commercially available enzyme or radioisotope-labeled antibodies. Several examples and detailed reviews of these techniques are available for the interested reader [85,86].

E. Other Techniques

In addition to the foregoing methods, a host of other techniques may be valuable in supporting excipient selection and evaluating destabilizing mechanisms for proteins. In particular, the traditional role of differential scanning calorimetry (DSC) in the study of thermal unfolding of proteins is being expanded and is now widely used to evaluate the relative ability of excipients to stabilize proteins to thermal denaturation [87,88]. Nuclear magnetic resonance (NMR) spectroscopy in solution can also yield information about three-dimensional protein structure and, thereby, the nature of structural changes induced by environmental conditions [89]. Levine et al. [90] describe the use of surface tension measurements in formulation design. Surface tension measurements of monoclonal antibody solutions were predictive of susceptibility to surface denaturation, leading to aggregation and precipitation. Protein solutions exhibiting lower surface tension were more susceptible to protein denaturation. Furthermore, those surface-active excipients with the greatest surface activity provided the best stabilization from shaking-induced aggregation and precipitation. Annan and Carr use mass spectrometry to characterize post-translational glycosylation patterns in proteins [91]. Enzymatic digests of denatured proteins may also be prepared, which are then analyzed by chromatographic separation and identification of fragments to elucidate the mechanism of destabilization. Pearlman and Nguyen [92] describe the use of tryptic digestion of human growth hormone dimer, followed by HPLC and mass spectrometry to reveal the formation of an oxidized methionine when the formulation is exposed to intense fluorescent light.

VI. FORMULATION APPROACHES TO PROTEIN STABILIZATION

The formulation development process used for traditional low molecular weight drugs is well understood. The same principles that are applied to this process may be applied to the formulation development of proteins. Principally it consists of determining the principal routes of degradation and then formulating the protein to arrest these pathways. For proteins the mechanisms of degradation are numerous and complicated, as detailed in Sec. IV. Protein formulation development has generated interest in the recent years, and several excellent articles on this topic have been published, including an in-depth series of case studies by Ahern and Manning [93,94].

A variety of approaches exist for stabilizing proteins, for example, chemical modification, immobilization, and site-directed mutagenesis [95,96], but these techniques are not within the scope of this chapter. The focus here will be on stabilization of proteins via formulation development. The principal formulation strategy is to stabilize the protein using clinically acceptable additives (excipients) or through the use of suitable pharmaceutical-processing technologies.

From an ease of use and processing perspective, a solution formulation is preferred and is typically the primary goal in developing a parenteral formulation. However, many proteins are very unstable in solution and may not give acceptable shelf life as solution formulations even when refrigerated at 2–8°C. In such cases, freeze-drying or lyophilization is often employed to inhibit the degradative processes that often occur in solutions. Table 2 lists examples of formulations for some of the currently approved biopharmaceuticals. Dosage forms for biopharmaceuticals can be solutions or dried powders. The principles used in developing these types of products are described in the following sections.

A. Protein Stabilization in Solution Using Additives

Proteins are generally most stable in solutions that mimic their natural environment. This includes a wide range of conditions. For example, mature insulin precipitates under conditions of pH and salt concentration at which serum proteins are soluble [97]. The stability of β-galactosidase is greatly enhanced in the presence of milk proteins [98]. Many proteins like caseins that bind to Ca^{2+} generally require small amounts of the ion to maintain their native structure during purification [99,100]. Various excipients are used in the formulations of different proteins. The protein formulation program may begin with an assessment of the effect of pH, ionic strength, and oxygen on the stability and solubility of the protein. The potential influence of pH on the degradation process was discussed in Sec. IV. Buffer salt selection for the formulation is guided by the pH range of interest and the acceptability of the buffer for use in a medicinal product. Lists of buffers and other additives generally recognized as safe (GRAS) are available for pharmaceutical manufacturers to use as a guide. The effect of different salts and their concentrations on protein stability was also reviewed in Sec. IV. In addition to affecting protein stability, salt concentration may have a profound effect on protein solubility and aggregation. Schein [101] provides a useful overview of the means of stabilizing proteins against aggregation and of methods to determine, predict, and increase solubility. Perlman and Nguyen [102] report that, for human growth hormone, a sodium phosphate buffer concentration of about 5 mM produced less aggregation of the protein, as measured by light scattering, compared with solutions of 2.5, 10, and 20 mM. These authors further highlight the formulation development of tissue plasminogen activator. For this agent, the solubility of the protein at the optimally stable pH was insufficient for the therapeutic application. A positively charged amino acid, arginine, was included in the formulation to increase the solubility of the protein at the desired pH range. Oxidation of proteins can be formulation dependent. For example, the presence of NaCl in the monoclonal antibody rhuHER2 caused an increase in oxidation at high temperatures after contact with stainless steel [103]. Antioxidants such as methionine and sodium thiosulfate were added to the formulation to reduce the oxidation.

Although ionic surfactants are often associated with denaturation of proteins [104], the nonionic surfactant polysorbate 80 has been included in several marketed formulations and serves to inhibit protein aggregation. The mechanism may be the greater tendency of the surfactant molecules to align themselves at the liquid/air interface, excluding the protein from the interface and inhibiting surface denaturation.

Properly folded native proteins tend to aggregate less than when unfolded. Solution additives that are known to stabilize the native proteins in solution may inhibit aggregation and enhance solubility. A diverse range of chemical additives are known to stabilize proteins in solution. These include salts, polyols, amino acids, and various polymers. Timasheff and colleagues have provided an extensive examination of the effects of solvent additives on protein stability [105]. The unifying mechanism for protein stabilization by these cosolvents is related to their preferential exclusion from the protein surface. With the cosolvent preferentially excluded, the protein surface is

Table 2 Composition of Selected FDA-Approved Biotechnology-Based Pharmaceuticals

Product	Dosage form	Storage	Composition
Actimmune (interferon γ-1b)	Solution for IV or SC injection	2–8°C; stable up to 12 hr at room temp; do not freeze or shake	Each 0.5 mL; 100 μg IFN γ1b, 20 mg mannitol, 0.36 mg sodium succinate, 0.5 mg polysorbate 20
Activase (tissue plasminogen activator)	Lyophile for IV injection with water as diluent	Stable up to 8 hr at room temp. after reconstitution; light sensitive at	100 mg vial: 3.5 g L-Arg, 1 g H_3PO_4, < 11 mg polysorbate 80
Enbrel (TNF receptor- IgG fusion hybrid)	Lyophile for IV injection. Bacterstat. water for recon.	2–8°C, do not freeze; use recon. solution within 6 hours at 2–8°C.	25 mg vial; 40 mg mannitol, 10 mg sucrose, 1.2 mg tromethamine
Engerix B (hepatitis B vaccine)	Suspension for IM. injection in single dose vials	2–8°C Do not freeze	20 μg Hep.B surface antigen adsorbed on 0.5 mg Al(OH) thimerosal, 9 mg NaCl , 0.98 mg Na_2HPO_4, 0.71 mg NaH_2PO_4
Epogen (erythropoietin)	Solution for IV or SC injection	2–8°C	Each vial: 2,000–10,000 IU protein, 2.5 mg HSA, 5.8 mg Nacitrate, 5.8 mg NaC1, 0.06 mg citric acid
Herceptin	Lyophile for IV injection, reconstitute with bacteriostatic water	2–8°C as lyophile up to expiration date; reconstituted solution stable 28 days at 2–8°C	440 mg vial; 9.9 mg L-histidine HCL, 6.6 mg L-histidine, 400 mg trehalose, 1.8 mg polysorbate 20
Humatrope (human growth hormone)	Lyophile for IV injection, recon. with 0.3% *m*-cresol, 1.7% glycerin	Stable for 14 days at 2–8°C	5 mg protein per vial, 1.13 mg Na_2HPO_4, 25 mg glycine, 25 mg mannitol
Leukine(sargramostim, GM-CSF)	Lyophile for IV infusion. Reconstitution with water	2–8°C; do not freeze or shake Use within 6 hr of reconstitution	Each vial: 250 or 500 mg sargramostim, 40 mg mannitol, 10 mg sucrose, 1.2 mg tromethamine
Neupogen (filgrastim)	Solution for IV or SC injection in single-use vial	2–8°C, do not freeze or shake; do not leave at room temperature for longer than 6 hr	Each mL: 300 ug filgrastim, 0.59 mg acetate, 50 mg mannitol, 0.004% Tween 80
Nutropin (recombinant human growth hormone)	Lyophile for SC injection with bacteriostatic water	28°C as lyophile, stable for 14 days at 2–8°C after reconstitution	5 mg vial; 45 mg manitol, 1.7 mg sodium phosphate, 1.7 mg glycine
Roferon (interferon α-2a)	Solution or lyophile for IV injection	Stable for 1 month at 2–8°C after reconstitution	Each mL contains: 3, 6, 36 million IU protein with 9 mg NaCl, 5 mg HAS, and 3 mg phenol
PROCRIT (erytbropoietin)	Solution for IV or SC injection.	2–8°C; do not freeze or shake	Each vial (1 mL): 2,000–10,000 IU, 2.5 mg HSA, 5.8 mg Nacitrate, 5.8 mg NaCI, 0.06 mg citric acid
Proleukin (IL-2)	Lyophile for IV injection; single-use vial	2–8°C; reconstituted solution stable 48 hours at 2–8°C	1.1 mg vial; 50 mg mannitol, 0.18 mg Na.dodec.sulfate,1.6 mg $NaPO_4$
Pulomozyme (DNAse)	Solution for inhalation via nebulizer	Store at 2–8°C; protect from light	1 mg/mL (2.5 mL); 0.15 mg/mL $CaCl_2$, 8.77 mg/mL NaCl
Rituxan (anti-CD20 monoclonal antibody)	Liquid for IV injection	Store at 2–8°C; protect from light	100 mg or 500 mg vial; 9.0 mg/mL NaC1, 7.35 mg/mL Na-citrate, 0.7 mg/mL polysorbate 80

Soruce: *Physicans Desk Reference*, 52, 1998; www.fda.gov/cber/efoi/approve.htm.

preferentially hydrated, and key structural elements remain in their native conformation. The unfolded state as well as the oligomeric and aggregated states of proteins become thermodynamically less favorable than the native state.

The mechanism of exclusion may be divided into two classes. In the first class, interactions are determined by the properties of the solvent; in the second class, interaction depends on the chemical nature of the protein surface. In the first class of cosolvents, steric exclusion of the larger additive molecule, compared with the smaller water molecule, can account for the preferential hydration, as occurs with polyethylene glycol. Also in the first class of cosolvents, additives such as sugars, amino acids, and many salts may act by increasing the surface tension of water, which leads to preferential hydration at the protein solvent interface. For the second class of cosolvents, solvophobicity and repulsion from charges on the protein surface may account for the additive's preferential exclusion. Here, the contact with the water-cosolvent mixture is thermodynamically less favorable than the protein-water contact, forcing the cosolvent away from the surface into the bulk solvent. Glycerol and other polyols, such as sorbitol and mannitol, belong to this category of stabilizers. Despite these mechanisms of exclusion, other forces may serve to attract a particular cosolvent to the surface of the molecule. The net effect of the additive as a stabilizing or destabilizing agent, therefore, depends on the balance between the exclusion from the protein surface (stabilizing) and the propensity of the additive to bind to the protein (destabilizing) by electrostatic or hydrophobic interactions. Electrostatic interactions that promote binding of an additive may be highly influenced by the concentration of the additive, as for many salts. Table 3 contains the proposed interactions classified for the various additives discussed. For additives in class I, preferential exclusion predominates. For class II additives, the stabilization may depend on protein charge and concentration and charge. Class III cosolvents predominantly bind to the unfolded denatured form of the protein through interaction with hydrophobic groups. Because many of the additives described in the work of Timasheff [105] are also regarded safe for inclusion in human parenteral formulations, these concepts provide a rational basis for excipient selection during formulation development.

Globular proteins are known to act as polymeric stabilizers of protein structure in solution. Wang and Hanson [106] review the mechanisms of protein stabilization by serum albumin, and it has been included in marketed protein pharmaceuticals, as shown in Table 3. The ability of albumin to adsorb to surfaces and to inhibit adsorption of a low concentration of the therapeutic protein provides one rationale for the inclusion of albumin in the formulation. However, there are a number of compelling reasons not to include human serum albumin in a formulation [107,108]. The addition of a protein excipient decreases the specific activity and may confound analytical methods aimed at evaluating the therapeutic protein. Human serum albumin is a product derived from human blood and so carries with it the potential to introduce protein impurities or pathogens. The inclusion of protein additives in a formulation, therefore, counteracts one of the primary advantages of the biotechnology-based pharmaceuticals: purity.

B. Protein Stabilization in the Dried Solid State

In situations for which the strategies described in the foregoing fail to produce solution formulations that are chemically and physically stable for 1 year or more, retarding degradation by using low-temperature drying processes is often required. Lyophilization and spray-drying are two such processes, with a long history of use in the pharmaceutical and food industries for stabilization of otherwise easily degraded substances. Both technologies may be used to dehydrate heat-sensitive molecules and, thereby, inhibit the degradative reactions that may be observed when proteins are formulated in solution. Stabilization by freeze-drying could potentially allow the therapeutic product to be stored at room temperature for distribution into markets that do not guarantee refrigerated delivery.

The degradation of proteins in the solid state occur to a lesser extent and typically via different mechanisms than those that occur in solution [109,110]. Lyophilization is currently the more common technique in the manufacture of dried therapeutic proteins; however, there is increasing interest in the use of spray-drying, owing to the unique physical nature of the spray-dried powder and its potential usefulness in protein drug delivery.

C. Lyophilization and Protein Formulation Development

Stabilization of proteins against those degradative processes with retention of structure and function through removal of water requires an understanding of the process of lyophilization or freeze-drying.

Table 3 Classification of Co-solvent Interaction with Proteins

Class	Co-solvent	Mechanism of exclusion	Mechanism of binding	Expected activity
I	Sugars (sucrose, glucose, mannose)	Surface tension increase	Inert	Good stabilizers of globular proteins and assembled organelles
	Some amino acids (glycine, alanine, glutamic, and aspartic acids)	Surface tension increase	Weak binding	Stabilizers of globular proteins
	Salting-out salts (Na_2SO_4, NaCl, $MgSO_4$)	Surface tension increase	Weak binding	Stabilize globular proteins and precipitants of native and denatured proteins
	Glycerol, polyols (sorbitol, mannitol)	Solvophobicity	Affinity for polar regions	Stabilizers of globular proteins and assembled organelles, decreasing for proteins of high polarity
II	Weakly interacting salts ($MgCl_2$, NaCl, Gn_2SO_4) Arginine-HCl, lysine-HCl	Surface tension increase	To charged groups or peptide bonds	Stabilization dependent on protein charge and salt concentrations
		Surface tension increase	To peptide bonds and (-) charges	Stabilization dependent on protein charge and amino acid concentration
	Valine (possibly other nonpolar amino acids)	Surface tension increase	To hydrophobic regions	Weak stabilization
III	PEG	Steric exclusion	To hydrophobic regions	Good precipitants; stabilizers of native structure at low temp., unfolded structure at high temp.; stabilizers and solubilizers of hydrophobic domains in proteins
	MPD	Repulsion from charges		

Source: Ref. 105.

Lyophilization is a process in which water is removed form a product after it is frozen and placed under vacuum, allowing the ice to change directly from solid to vapor without going through a liquid phase. The three steps in the process are: (a)freezing of the solution, (b) primary drying where sublimation of ice water takes place, and (c) secondary drying where tightly bound water is removed (desorption). While the end goal of lyophilization is to stabilize a protein, both freezing and drying have the potential to cause damage to the protein if done incorrectly.

The phenomenon of freeze denaturation of proteins has been widely described in the literature [111–113]. Different proteins tolerate freezing and drying to various degrees. For example, tissue-type plasminogen activator can withstand repeated freeze-thaw cycles without loss in activity and with very little change in its bioanalytical profile [114]. In contrast, several examples have been published that demonstrate that proteins do not tolerate the stresses due to freezing and drying, e.g., loss in activity for lactic dehydrogenase [115], aggregation of recombinant hemoglobin [116], and loss of antigen recognition by a monoclonal antibody [117]. The denaturing effect of freezing is related to the gradual concentration of solutes and potential shifts in pH surrounding the protein molecule as water is removed by the phase change from a liquid to solid ice crystals. The recovery of protein activity after freezing by reducing the unfolded state can be influenced by the addition of certain protective additives, including sugars, polyols, amino acids, and certain salts. The nature of these cryoprotective compounds are essentially those that have been shown by Timasheff [105] (Table 3; Sec. VI.A). Cryoprotective agents, lite agents that stabilize solutions, act by preferential exclusion from the protein surface, making it thermodynamically unfavorable for the protein to unfold. Perstrelski et al. [118] proposed a model to describe the conformational changes that a protein might undergo during the freezing and drying process and during reconstitution of the lyophilized powder. The authors suggested that the formulation development effort should focus on the use of additives that reduce the unfolded state during freezing (cryoprotectants) and reduce the unfolding during drying (lyoprotectants), ensuring that the native state is retained throughout the lyophilization process. Retaining the native state will thereby increase the chance that the fully active and native protein is recovered during reconstitution of the powder.

In contrast with the wide range of compounds that stabilize proteins in solution and on freezing, Carpenter et al. have shown that only certain carbohydrates (e.g., disaccharides such as sucrose and trehalose) can preserve phosphofructokinase during either freeze-drying or air-drying [119–121]. This suggests a fundamental difference in the stabilizing mechanism between the dried state and the solution or frozen state [122]. One important mechanism of protein stabilization during the freeze-drying process involves formation of an amorphous glass as opposed to a crystalline matrix [123]. In the glassy state, the protein mobility is significantly reduced due to high viscocity and syrup-like conditions, which are characteristic of glasses [124]. The reduction in mobility usually results in less chemical degradation. Excipients or additives such as carbohydrates, polyols, polymers, or mixtures thereof are capable of forming glasses and can be good stabilizers for proteins [125]. The glass transition (*Tg*) of an amorphous solid is a characteristic temperature, where the protein in the uncrystallized matrix undergoes a transition from the viscous liquid concentrate to a brittle glass. Differential scanning calorimetry (DSC) is an excellent tool for determining glass transitions [126]. Physical collapse of the glassy state can occur, to varying degrees, during the primary drying phase of the lyophilization process if the temperature is above the *Tg* for the formulation being dried [127,128]. The *Tg* is a function of the proportion of glass forming components such as additives, buffer, and the protein itself [124]. Excipients can be selected based on their ability to increase the glass transition temperature of the protein formulation. This property is useful for the reduction of lyophilization cycle time where an increase in *Tg* allows drying the product at higher temperatures, thereby shorter time to remove water, without collapse. The ability of excipients to increase *Tg* is also important in the manufacture of products that can withstand higher temperatures for long-term storage as dried powders [129]. Some excipients, however, can crystallize or phase separate during the lyophilization process or during long-term storage and can cause degradation of the dried protein [130–133].

In addition to maintaining the amorphous state of proteins for stabilization during freeze-drying, some excipients stabilize proteins by binding to the dried protein to act as a "water substitute" after removal of the hydration shell. As water substitutes, sugars such as trehalose and lactose can serve to partially satisfy hydrogen-bonding requirements of polar groups in dried proteins [134–136]. In support of this theory, Fourier transform IR spectroscopy was used to demonstrate that hydrogen bonding occurs between proteins and stabilizing carbohydrates and that solute binding is required for preservation of labile proteins during drying [121]. In selecting the composition of a protein lyophilized formulation, the formulation scientist must take into account the requirements for glassy matrix with high *Tg*, reduction of crystallization and phase separation, and ability to maintain hydrogen bonding to achieve protein stabilization.

In addition to the additives used in a formulation to help stabilize the protein to freezing, the residual moisture content of the lyophilized powder needs to be considered. Not only is moisture capable of affecting the physicochemical stability of the protein itself, equally important is the ability of moisture to affect the *Tg* of the formulation. Water acts as a plasticizer and depresses the *Tg* of amorphous solids [124,137,138]. During primary drying, as water is gradually removed from the product, the *Tg* increases accordingly. The duration and temperature of the secondary drying step of the lyophilization process determines how much moisture remains bound to the powder. Usually lower residual moisture in the finished biopharmaceutical product leads to enhanced stability. Typically, moisture content in lyophilized formulations should not exceed 2% [139]. The optimal moisture level for maximum stability of a particular product must be demonstrated on a case-by-case basis.

Excipients useful for stabilization of freeze-dried powders for long-term storage include sucrose, trehalose, dextrans, polyvinylpyrrolidone (PVP), sorbitol, polyethylene glycol, and mannitol. Some products have been stabilized using these additives allowing room temperature storage of 2 years or more (unpublished observations). The physical appearance of the lyophilized cake is also an important attribute of the dried cake to be considered during the development of the lyophilization cycle. As mentioned, high residual moisture may lead to collapse of the cake with storage. Cake collapse can be detrimental to chemical stability, but it can also adversely impact the appearance of the product and how easily the product can be reconstituted. Bulking agents are commonly used in lyophilized formulations to enhance the appearance of the product and, in some cases, to further reduce residual moisture. Bulking agents can provide physical support to the cake to prevent collapse. Mannitol is a typical bulking agent used in protein formulations, but one must always conduct stability studies to demonstrate the effect of the agent on the chemical and physical stability of the protein of interest.

As reported by Carpenter and Chang [140] and discussed in this section, the requirements to stabilize a protein product in the dry state can be summarized as follows: (a) the protein should ideally remain in the native state and protein unfolding must be minimized throughout the lyophilization process, (b) the dried powder must have a glass transition temperature that is higher than the desired storage temperature, (c) residual moisture in the final must be relatively low (ideally $<1\%$), and (d) formulation conditions must be developed to minimize chemical degradation processes. The reader is also referred to the protein lyophilization reviews in Refs. 141–143.

D. Spray-Drying of Protein Pharmaceuticals

With the recent advent of pulmonary delivery of proteins, generating dry particles of proteins with a defined and reproducible size and shape is very important. Several techniques have been employed for this purpose, including spray-drying, spray-freeze-drying, milling of lyophilized powders, supercritical fluid precipitation, and co-precipitation with polymers. Spray-drying produces particles that have good flow properties and narrow size distribution, and the process can be adapted to produce particles of a range of sizes, dependent on the application. All the processes used to manufacture dry powders exert severe stresses on the proteins. Many of the stabilization mechanisms described for lyophilized powders in Sec. VI.C also apply to spray-dried powders. Thermal stresses that proteins undergo during spray-drying can have a significant impact on their structure and stability. During atomization proteins are exposed to high pressure and hydrophobic stresses at the air/water interface that can potentially denature and inactivate proteins as discussed in Sec. IV.B. The outlet temperature in spray-drying has been correlated with activity loss in several proteins. Trehalose has been shown to stabilize proteins during spray-drying. Disaccharides like sucrose and trehalose have been shown to preserve protein structure and activity in the solution state by preferential exclusion effect. Surfactants like polysorbate 20 and polysorbate 80 have been shown to protect the proteins from harmful hydrophobic interfacial interactions.

Tzannis and Prestrelski [144,145] showed a concentration-dependent protective effect of sucrose and residual moisture on the activity and stability of trypsinogen during spray-drying. They found protein protection even at low carbohydrate concentrations, but they observed some destabilization at very high sucrose concentrations. They hypothesized that phase separation occurs at high sucrose concentrations, resulting in reduced amount of sucrose available for stabilization in the protein-rich phase. Mumenthaler et al. [146] and Maa et al. [147] have shown the feasibility of spray-drying solutions of human growth hormone (hGH) and tissue plasminogen activator (t-PA). Addition of 0.1% (w/v) polysorbate 20 to the hGH formulation reduced the aggregation during spray-drying by 70–85%. Broadhead et al. [148] studied the effects of various processing and formulation variables on the properties of spray-dried β-galactosidase using statistically designed experiments. High yields were obtained with high outlet temperatures but resulting in extensive protein denaturation. Trehalose was shown to be a more suitable stabilizer that mannitol, sucrose, or arginine hydrochloride. Adler and Lee [149] studied the stability of lactate dehydrogenase (LDH) during spray-drying and show that high inlet temperatures reduced residual moisture content but at the cost of high process inactivation. Addition of 0.1% polysorbate 80 reduced the inactivation, while LDH adsorption to the liquid/air interface could have accounted for the deactivation.

VII. REGULATORY ASPECTS OF BIOTECHNOLOGY-BASED PHARMACEUTICALS

The vast majority of biopharmaceutical approvals occurred in the 1990s. With the rapid growth in number of approvals as well as hundreds more investigational biopharmaceuticals undergoing clinical testing, guidelines and regulations have been set forth by the regulatory agencies that govern biopharmaceuticals. Many, although not all, of these products are classified as "biologics." As such, these products require licensing under the Public Health Service Act and must comply with the regulations set forth in the Code of Federal Regulations, Title 21, Parts 600–680. Regulatory control and review of biotechnology-derived biologics, except for those considered to be medical devices, is administered by the Center for Biologics Evaluation and Research (CBER) of the U.S. Food and Drug Administration (FDA). Regulatory approval for biologic products is based on the submission of a biological license application (BLA) to CBER, in contrast with a New Drug Application (NDA) submitted for small molecule products to be reviewed by the Center for Drugs Evaluation and Research (CDER) branch of the FDA.

Biologics licenses issued by CBER include approval of a specific series of production steps and in-process control tests as well as end-product specifications that must be met on a lot-by-lot basis. Each lot of a licensed biologic is approved for distribution when it has been determined that the lot meets the specific control requirements set forth in the product license. Therefore, samples of each production lot, as well as documentation, are submitted to FDA to show that all the applicable tests have been performed and the results of these tests. FDA will review these data and may select certain tests that are repeated at the FDA laboratories; bioassay tests are often the target of evaluations. The preferred tests involve comparison of the product with a reference standard. The reference standard may be obtained from the manufacturer or prepared by FDA. As part of the BLA application, the facility that is to be used for commercial manufacture of the drug must be licensed before the product can be commercialized. This is achieved by a preapproval inspection (PAI) of the site, conducted by an FDA inspector with the purpose of determining whether the establishment complies with applicable manufacturing standards prescribed in the Code of Federal Regulations (CFR).

To provide guidance to manufacturers of biologics, FDA has developed a series of documents outlining "points to consider," designed to convey the current consensus of CBER relating to biologic product development and testing. These "points" represent the current thinking and experience that CBER regulators believe should be considered by manufacturers at this time. To respond to developments in this rapidly changing field, FDA considers these documents to be dated "drafts" that will be updated as needed using input from industry, academia, and other regulatory agencies both in the United States and abroad. Points to consider documents are available from CBER and include: Points to Consider in the Characterization of Cell Lines Used to Produce Biologicals (1992), Points to Consider in the Production and Testing of New Drugs and Biologicals Produced by Recombinant DNA Technology (1985), and Points to Consider in the Manufacture and Testing of Monoclonal Antibodies for Human Use (1997).

In recent years, regulatory authorities and industry associations have undertaken several important initiatives to promote international harmonization of regulatory requirements. These efforts are designed to enhance harmonization and are committed to seeking scientifically based harmonized technical procedures for pharmaceutical development. These efforts are undertaken under the auspices of the International Conference on Harmonization (ICH), which is organized to provide an opportunity for tripartite harmonization initiatives to be developed with input from both regulatory and industry representatives among three regions: the United States, the European Union, and Japan. This effort has led to several important guidelines, which undergo several rounds of review and comment and then are issued. Examples of a recent guidances are (a) ICH Topic Q6B Specifications: Test procedures and acceptance criteria for biotechnological/biological products, and (b) ICH Topic Q5A: Viral safety evaluation of biotechnology products derived from cell lines of human or animal origin. Guidelines for analytical method validation were discussed in Sec. V [57,58]. These guidelines, along with other regulatory documents, may be obtained directly from the CBER website: http://www.fda.gov/cber/guidelines.htm. The reader is also referred to a commentary on the status and plans for the regulation of biologics and biotechnology products [22].

VIII. DEVELOPMENTS IN PROTEIN DRUG DELIVERY

As pharmaceutical scientists gain experience and tackle the primary challenges of developing stable parenteral formulations of proteins, the horizons continue to expand and novel delivery systems and alternative routes of administration are being sought. The interest in protein drug delivery is reflected by the wealth of literature that covers this topic [150–154]. Typically, protein therapeutics are prepared as sterile products for parenteral administration, but in the past several years, there has been increased interest in pulmonary, oral, transdermal, and controlled-release injectable formulations and many advances have been made. Some of the more promising recent developments are summarized in this section.

Approaches to alter the therapeutic potential of proteins by modification of the pharmacokinetic profile and/or reduction of the immunogenicity have been explored. Plasma half-life extension may be obtained through chemically modifying the molecule to inhibit its pharmacological clearance or by controlling the rate at which the protein is delivered to the bloodstream. Of the chemical-modifying technologies explored to date, polyethylene glycol (PEG) modification appears to be the most promising [155]. PEG modification (PEGylation) increases the plasma half-life of protein and reduces the immunogenicity of proteins dramatically. In addition, the proteins remain biologically active [156]. A possible mechanism for the altered behavior of the PEGylated proteins may be the increased hydrodynamic ratio that results from the addition of PEG, making it too large for glomerular filtration. The possibility of sterically hindering the protein's interaction with cellular receptors required for metabolism and excretion is another mechanism. There are several PEGylated proteins undergoing clinical trials, including cytokines, antibodies, and enzymes. PEGylated adenosine deaminase (PEG-ADA) was approved for use in ADA-deficient severe combined immunodeficiency syndrome and is the first such product to gain FDA approval. PEGylated recombinant-human granulocyte colony-stimulating factor (PEG-rhG-CSF) [157] is another example of a recently approved product.

To achieve controlled protein delivery, the use of biodegradable microspheres is being actively pursued [158]. In particular, biodegradable lactic-glycolic acid copolymer–based microspheres have proved useful for the controlled delivery of several polypeptides and proteins. The first FDA-approved system for controlled release of a peptide was an injectable poly(lactide-coglycolide) microsphere formulation of leuprolide acetate. This formulation provides controlled release of the peptide over 30 days for the treatment of prostate cancer. Although promising, many problems remain, and the more general use of formulations of this type for other biopharmaceuticals is often limited by the instability of the molecule to the stresses of the encapsulation process [159–161]. The delivery of protein drugs by a noninvasive route is certainly a prominent goal within the pharmaceutical industry. Such an achievement would greatly increase patient compliance and expand the usefulness and market for these agents. However, despite the intense desire, the challenges are formidable and, perhaps, reflected by the fact that, although insulin has been used clinically for more than 70 years, it is still given exclusively by daily injections. Advances have been made in the use of needle-free injectors for delivery of pharmaceuticals via the systemic route. With these injectors, drugs, including proteins, can be delivered into the bloodstream without needles and substantially free of pain, which has tremendous benefits for end-user compliance. The use of this technology, however, is limited by the ability of the therapeutic agent to be formulated with the required attributes (low dose, solubility, stability).

Possible noninvasive routes for delivery of proteins include nasal, buccal, rectal, vaginal, transdermal, ocular, oral, and pulmonary. For each route of delivery there are two potential barriers to absorption: permeability and enzymatic barriers. All of the potential routes have received some attention; however, the pulmonary and nasal routes appear to hold the greatest promise. The oral route would be by far the most popular, yet, despite extensive investigation, current strategies to prevent degradation and poor absorption in the gastrointestinal tract have proved difficult for macromolecular proteins [162]. Many advances have been made which show promise.

The nasal route possesses higher permeability and presents less of an enzymatic barrier than does the oral route. The nasal route has been successful for a number of polypeptide drugs. Nasal formulations for luteinizing hormone–releasing hormone (LH–RH) analogs (desmopressin, oxytocin, and calcitonin) have reached the marketplace. Notably, however, this route of delivery has not been as successful for larger proteins with molecular weights greater than 10 kDa and may be associated with local irritation and toxicity with long-term administration [153]. Plum and Davis [163] describe recent approaches used to enhance the nasal delivery of insulin through the use of absorption enhancers or bioadhesive microspheres.

The pulmonary route of protein drug delivery has recently received increased attention. Three therapeutic peptides—leuprolide: 9 amino acids; insulin: 51 amino acids; growth hormone: 192 amino acids—were reported to be absorbed in biologically active form from the lungs, with bioavailabilities of 10–25% [151]. These values exceed those reported for nasal delivery of insulin and growth hormone in the absence of permeation enhancers. Current challenges in pulmonary protein delivery include assessment of the safety of long-term administration, the molecular size limitation of pulmonary absorption and strategies for enhancing permeation, and formulation approaches capable of delivering suitable doses of stable proteins to the vast absorptive surface presented by the lung. Significant advances have been made in the delivery of protein solutions and dried powders. The formulation challenges in making stable protein formulations have been discussed, but much of the success achieved can also be attributed to advances in the engineering of the devices. The success of the powder inhalation product is based on the ability to disperse the powder, which is mainly determined by the efficiency of the inhalation device and by the physical properties of the powder. An up-to-date review on pulmonary delivery technology has recently been published by Gonda [164]. As described in these reports, the possibility of delivering proteins via other than parenteral routes has been achieved. The advances in the field have been a result of major breakthroughs in the areas of stabilization and formulation of proteins as well as advances in the engineering and design of specialized and novel delivery systems. In addition, companies realize the need to make these delivery systems easier to use and less expensive. Recent advances in delivery systems for macromolecules can be found in a recent article by Henry [165]. As a result of these advances, the end user will benefit by the use of these novel therapeutics.

REFERENCES

1. J. Sterling, The next decade of biotechnology. Where are we going? J. Parenter. Sci. Technol., 44, 63 (1990).
2. Pharmaceutical Manufacturer's Association, Products in the pipeline, Biotechnology, 9, 947 (1991).
3. W. Sadee, Protein drugs: A revolution in therapy? Pharm. Res., 3, 3 (1986).
4. W. J. Black, Drug products of recombinant DNA technology, Am. J. Hosp. Pharm., 46, 1834 (1989).
5. L. P. Gage. Biopharmaceuticals: Drugs of the future, Am. J. Pharm. Edc., 50, 368 (1986).
6. F. G. Banting and C. H. Best, Pancreatic extracts, J. Lab. Clin. Med., 7, 464 (1922).
7. J. D. Baxter, Recombinant DNA and medical progress, Hosp. Pract., 15, 57 (1980).
8. P. Brown, C. C. Gajdusek, C. J. Gibbs, and D. N. Asher, Potential epidemic of Creutzfeldt-Jakob disease from human growth hormone therapy, N. Engl. J. Med., 313(12), 728 (1985).
9. J. D. Watson, J. Tooze, and D. T. Kurtz, *Recombinant DNA: A Short Course*, W.H. Freeman and Co., New York, 1983.
10. R. L. Rodriguez and R. C. Tait, *Recombinant DNA Techniques: An Introduction*, Addison-Wesley Publishing, Reading, MA, 1983.
11. G. Kohler and C. Milstein, Continuous cultures of fused cells secreting antibody of predefined specificity, Nature, 256, 495 (1975).
12. L. Chatenoud, Humoral immune response against OKT3, Transplant. Proc., 25(2 suppl. 1), 68 (1993).
13. J. Richards, J. Auger, D. Peace, D. Gale, J. Michel, A. Koons, T. Haverty, R. Zivin, L. Jolliffe, and J. Bluestone, Phase I evaluation of humanized OKT3: toxicity and immunomodulatory effects of hOKT3-gamma4, Cancer Res., 59(9), 2096 (1999).
14. S. L. Morrison and V. T. Oi, Genetically engineered antibody molecules, Adv. Immunol., 44, 65 (1989).
15. C. Queen, W. P. Schneider, H. E. Selick, P. W. Payne, N. F. Landolphi, J. F. Duncan, N. M. Avdalovic, M. Levitt, R. P. Junghans, and T. A. Waidman, A humanized antibody that binds to the interleukin 2 receptor, Proc. Natl. Acad. Sci. USA, 86, 10029 (1989).
16. L. Reichmann, L. M. Clarke, H. Waldman, and O. Winter, Reshaping human antibodies for therapy, Nature, 332, 323 (1988).

17. J. Newman, J. Albert, D. Anderson, K. Carner, C. Heard, F. Norton, R. Raab, M. Reff, S. Shuey, and N. Hanna, Primatization of recombinant antibodies for immunotherapy of human diseases: A macaque/human chimeric antibody against human CD4, Biotechnology, 10, 1455 (1992).
18. L. K. Gilliland, L. A. Walsh, M. R. Frewin, M. P. Wise, M. Tone, G. Hale, D. Kioussis, and H. Waldmann, Elimination of the immunogenicity of therapeutic antibodies, J. Immunology, 162(6), 3663 (1999).
19. S. D. Gorman and M. R. Clark, Humanisation of monoclonal antibodies for therapy Semin. Immunol., 2, 457 (1990).
20. S. Porter, Human immune respose to recombinant proteins, J. Pharmaceut. Sci., 90(1), 1 (2001).
21. R. A. Dwek, Glycobiology:Toward understanding the functon of sugars, Chem. Rev., 96, 683 (1996).
22. S. Patterson, Biologics and biotechnology products, PDA J. Pharm. Sci. Technol., 52(6), 316 (1998).
23. L. Stryer, *Biochemistry*, W. H. Freeman, San Francisco, 1981.
24. F. Franks, *Characterization of Proteins*, Humana Press, Clifton, NJ, 1988.
25. R. D. Schmid, Stabilized soluble enzymes, Adv. Biochem. Eng., 12, 42 (1979).
26. D. B. Volkin and A. M. Klibanov, Minimizing protein inactivation, in *Protein Function: A Practical Approach* (T. E. Creighton, ed.), IRL Press, Oxford, 1989, pp. 1–24.
27. T. Chen, Formulation concerns of protein drugs, Drug Dev. Ind. Pharm., 18, 1311 (1992).
28. M. C. Manning, K. Patel, and R. T. Borchardt, Stability of protein pharmaceuticals, Pharm. Res., 6, 903 (1989).
29. Y. J. Wang and M. A. Hanson, Parenteral formulations of proteins and peptides: Stability and stabilizers. J. Parenter. Sci. Technol., 42 (suppl. 2), S2 (1988).
30. T. J. Ahern and M. C. Manning (eds.), *Stability of Protein Pharmaceuticals. Part A:Chemical and Physical Pathways of Protein Stabilization*, Plenum Press, New York, 1992.
31. T. J. Ahern and A. M. Klibanov. The mechanism of irreversible enzyme inactivation at 100°C, Science, 288, 1280 (1985).
32. L. C. Gu, E. A. Erdos, H. Chiang, T. Calderwood, K. Thai, G. C. Visor, J. Duffy, W. C. Hsu, and L. C. Foster, Stability of interleukin 1β (IL-1β) in aqueous solution: Analytical methods, kinetics, products and solution formulation implications, Pharm. Res., 8, 485 (1992).
33. R. Perlman and T. H. Nguyen, Formulation strategies for recombinant proteins: Human growth hormone and tissue plasminogen activator, in *Therapeutic Peptides and Proteins: Formulation, Delivery and Targeting* (D. Marshak and D. Liu, eds.), Cold Spring Harbor Laboratory, Cold Spring Harbor, NY, 1989, pp. 23–31.
34. S. Inglis, Cleavage at aspartic acid, Methods Enzymol., 91, 324 (1983).
35. T. Geiger and S. Clarke, Deamidation, isomerization and racemization at asparaginyl and aspartyl residues in peptides, J. Biol. Chem., 262, 785 (1987).
36. S. J. Wearne and T. E. Creighton, Effect of protein conformation on rate of deamidation: Ribonuclease A, Proteins Struct. Funct. Genet., 5, 8 (1989).
37. R. Tyler-Cross and V. Schirch, Effects of amino acid sequence, buffers and ionic strength on the rate and mechanism of deamidation of asparagine residues in small peptides, J. Biol. Chem., 266, 22549 (1991).
38. M. Xie and R. L. Showen, Secondary structure and protein deamidation, J. Pharm. Sci., 88(1), 8 (1999).
39. M. J. Pikal, K. M. Dellerman, M. L. Roy, and R. M. Riggin, The effects of formulation variables on the stability of freeze-dried human growth hormone, Pharm. Res., 8, 427 (1991).
40. J. L. Bada, In vivo racemization in mammalian proteins, Methods Enzymol., 106, 98 (1984).
41. S. E. Zale and A. M. Klibanov, Why does ribonuclease irreversibly inactivate at high temperatures? Biochemistry, 25, 5432 (1986).
42. D. B. Volkin and A. M. Klibanov, Thermal destruction processes in proteins involving cystine residues, J. Biol. Chem., 262, 2945 (1987).
43. J. Brange, S. Havelund, and P. Hougaard, Chemical stability of insulin 2: Formation of higher molecular weight transformation products during storage of pharmaceutical preparations, Pharm. Res., 9, 727 (1992).
44. Y. F. Maa and C. C. Hsu, Effect of high shear on proteins, Biotechnol. Bioeng., 51(4), 458 (1996).
45. J. L. Silva and G. Weber, Pressure stability of proteins, Ann. Rev. Phys. Chem., 44, 89 (1993).
46. G. A. Truskey, R. Gabler, A. Dileo, and T. Manter, The effect of membrane filtration upon protein conformation, J. Parenter. Sci. Technol., 41, 180 (1987).
47. D. N. Brems, Solubility of different folding conformers of bovine growth hormone, Biochemistry, 27, 44541 (1988).
48. E. Zerovnik, R. Jerala, L. Kroon-Zitko, R. H. Pain, and V. Turk, Intermediates in denaturation of a small globular protein, recombinant human Stefin B, J. Biol. Chem., 13, 9041 (1992).
49. M. G. Mulkerrin and R. Wetzel, pH dependence of the reversible and irreversible thermal denaturation of gamma interferons, Biochemistry, 28, 6556 (1989).
50. T. Cartwright, O. Senussi, and M. D. Grady, The mechanism of the inactivation of human fibroblast interferon by mechanical stress, J. Gen. Virol., 36, 317 (1977).
51. R. Quinn and J. D. Andrade, Minimizing the aggregation of neutral insulin solutions, J. Pharm. Sci., 72, 1472 (1983).
52. J. Brange, S. Havelund, P. E. Hansen, L. Langkjaer, E. Sorensen, and P. Hildebrandt, Formulation of

physically stable neutral insulin solutions for continuous infusion by delivery systems, in *Hormone Drugs*, U.S. Pharmacopeial Convention, Rockville, MD, 1982, pp. 96–105.
53. J. R. Brennan, S. P. Gebhart, and W. O. Blackard, Pump-induced insulin aggregation: A problem with the biostator, Diabetes, 34, 353 (1985).
54. W. D. Lougheed, A. M. Albisser, H. M. Martindale, J. C. Chow, and J. R. Statement, Physical stability of insulin formulations, Diabetes, 32, 424 (1983).
55. J. D. Andrade and V. Hiady, Protein adsorption and materials biocompatibility: A tutorial review and suggested hypotheses, Adv. Polymer Sci., 79, 1 (1986).
56. A. M. Pitt, The nonspecific protein binding of polymeric microporous membranes, J. Parenter. Sci. Technol., 41, 110 (1987).
57. International Conference on Harmonization, Guideline on validation of analytical procedures: definition and terminology, Fed. Reg., 60(40), 11260 (1995).
58. International Conference on Harmonization, Validation of analytical procedures: methodology, step 2. The Third International Conference on Harmonization of Technical Requirements for Registration of Pharmaceuticals for Human Use, Yokohama, Japan. Nov. 29–Dec. 1, (1995).
59. R. Ricker, L. Sandoval, B. Permar, and B. Boyes, Improved reversed-phase high performance liquid chromatography columns for biopharmaceutical analysis, J. Pharmaceut. Biomed. Anal., 14, 93 (1995).
60. R. Pearlman and T. H. Nguyen, Analysis of protein drugs, in *Peptide and Protein Drug Delivery* (V. H. Lee, ed.), Marcel Dekker, New York, 1990, pp. 247–301.
61. P. H Corran, Reversed phase chromatography of proteins, in *HPLC of Macromolecules. A Practical Approach*. 2nd ed. (R.W.A. Oliver, ed.), IRL Press 1998, pp. 93–140.
62. E. Watson and W. C. Kenney, High performance size exclusion chromotography of recombinant derived proteins and aggregated species, J. Chromotogr., 436, 289 (1988).
63. G. W. Welling and S.Welling-Wester, Size exclusion HPLC of proteins, in *HPLC of Macromolecules, A Practical Approach*, 2nd ed. (R.W.A. Oliver , ed.), IRL Press, 1998, pp. 45–62.
64. M. Henry, Ion-exchange chromatography of proteins and peptides, in *HPLC of Macromolecules, A Practical Approach*. 2nd ed. (R.W.A. Oliver , ed.), IRL Press, 1998, pp. 63–92.
65. C. R. Cantor and S. N. Timasheff, Optical spectroscopy of proteins, in *The Proteins*, Vol. 5, 3rd ed. (H. Neurath, ed.), Academic Press, New York, 1982, pp. 145–306.
66. H. A. Havel, R. S. Chao, R. J. Haskell, and T. J. Thamann. Investigation of protein structure with optical spectroscopy: Bovine growth hormone, Anal. Chem., 61, 642 (1989).
67. F. X. Schmid, Spectral methods of characterizing protein conformation and conformational changes, in *Protein Structure—A Practical Approach* (T.E. Creighton, ed.), IRL Press, Oxford, 1989, pp. 251–285.
68. H. Stuting and I. Krull, Determination of pituitary and recombinant human growth hormone molecular weights by modern high performance liquid chromatography with low angle light scattering detection, J. Chromatogr., 539, 91 (1991).
69. T. Arakawa, Applications of laser light scattering techniques to molecular biology, Cell Technol., 15(5), 679 (1996).
70. P. Wyatt, Light scattering and the absolute characterization of macromolecules, Anal. Chim. Acta, 272, 1 (1993).
71. S. Kelly and N. Price, The application of circular dichroism to studies of protein folding and unfolding, Biochim. Biophys. Acta, 1338, 161 (1997).
72. U. K. Laemmli, Cleavage of structural proteins during the assembly of the head of bacteriophage T4, Nature, 227, 680 (1970).
73. Y. P. See and G. Jackowski, Estimating molecular weights of polypeptides by SDS gel electrophoresis, in *Protein Structure—A Practical Approach* (T.E. Creighton, ed.), IRL Press, Oxford , 1989, pp. 1–21.
74. D. P. Goldenberg, Analysis of protein conformation by gel electrophoresis, in *Protein Structure—A Practical Approach* (T.E. Creighton, ed.), IRL Press, Oxford, 1989, pp. 225–250.
75. A. Gerstner, Z. Csapo, M. Sasvari-Szekely, and A. Guttman, Ultrathin sodium dodecyl sulfate gel electrophoresis of proteins: Effect of gel composition and temperature on the separation of sodium dodecyl sulfate-protein complexes, Electrophoresis, 21, 834 (2000).
76. P. O. Righetti, Isoelectric focusing of proteins in conventional and immobilized pH gradients, in *Protein Structure—A Practical Approach* (T.E. Creighton, ed.), IRL Press, Oxford, 1989, pp. 23–63.
77. T. Wehr, R. Rodriguez-Diaz, and M. Zhu, eds., *Capillary Electrophoresis of Proteins*, Marcel Dekker, Inc. New York, 1999.
78. G. Hunt, T. Hotaling, and A. Chen. Validation of a capillary isoelectric focusing method for the recombinant monoclonal antibody C2B8, J. Chromatogr. A, 800, 355 (1998).
79. H. Watzig, M. Degenhardt, and A. Kunkel, Strategies for capillary electrophoresis: Method development and validation for pharmaceutical and biological applications, Electrophoresis, 19, 2695 (1998).
80. Center for Biologics Evaluation and Research, FDA, *Guidance Concerning Demonstration of Comparability of Human Biological Products, Including, Therapeutic Biotechnology-Derived Products*, Rockville, MD, April, 1996. (Available online at www.fda.gov/cber/gdlns/comptest.txt.)

81. J. Chayen, Cytochemical bioassay and its potential place in compendial definitions: A method that offers sensitivity as well as specificity, in *Hormone Drugs*, U.S. Pharmacopeial Convention, Rockville, MD, 1982, pp. 48–58.
82. C. Kotts, E. Gilkerson, D. Trinh, G. Hawker, A. Chen, H. Gazzano-Santoro, Assay validation report: Cell proliferation test for human growth hormone, Pharmacopeial Forum, 25(3), 8313 (1999).
83. H. Gazzano-Santoro, P. Ralph, T. Ryskamp, A. Chen, and V. Mukku, A non-radioactive complement-dependent cytotoxicity assay for anti-CD20 monoclonal antibody, J. Imunol. Methods, 202, 163 (1997).
84. M. Pingel, A. Volund, E. Sorensen, and A. R. Sorensen, Assessment of insulin potency by biological and chemical methods, in *Hormone Drugs*, U.S. Pharmacopeial Convention. Rockville, MD, 1982, pp. 200–207.
85. J. Crowther, *The ELISA Guidebook. Methods in Molecular Biology*, Vol. 149. Humana Press, Totowa, NJ, 2000.
86. T. Porstmann and S. T. Kiessig, Enzyme immunoassay techniques: An overview, J. Immunol. Methods, 150, 5 (1992).
87. R. Remmele and W. Gombotz, Differential scanning calorimetry: A practical tool for elucidating stability of liquid biopharmaceuticals, BioPharm, 13(6), 36 (2000).
88. L. R. Maneri, A. R. Farid, P. J. Smialkowski, M. B. Seaman, J. Baldoni, and T. D. Sokoloski, Preformulation of proteins using high sensitivity differential scanning calorimetry (DSC), Pharm. Res., 8, S (1991).
89. K. Wuthrich, Six years of protein structure determination by NMR spectroscopy: What have we learned? in *Protein Conformation. Ciba Foundation Symposium 161*, John Wiley & Sons, Chichester, 1991, pp. 136–149.
90. H. L. Levine, T. C. Ransohoff, R. T. Kawahata, and W. C. McGregor, The use of surface tension measurements in the design of antibody-based product formulations, J. Parenter. Sci. Technol., 45, 160 (1991).
91. R. Annan and S. Carr, The essential role of mass spectrometry, J. Protein Chem. 16(5), 391 (1997).
92. R. Pearlman and T. Nguyen, Pharmaceutics of protein drugs, J. Pharm. Pharmacol., 44 (suppl. 1), 178 (1992).
93. T. J. Ahern, M.C Manning, eds. Stability of protein pharmaceuticals, Part A. Chemical and Physical Pathways of Protein Degradation. New York: Plenum Press, 1992.
94. T. J. Ahern, M. C Manning, eds., *Stability of protein pharmaceuticals*, Part B. *In Vivo Pathways of Degradation and Strategies for Protein Stabilization*, Plenum Press, New York, 1992.
95. V. Mozhaev, I. Berezin, and K. Martinek, Structure stability relationship in proteins: Fundamental tasks and strategies for the development of stabilized enzyme catalysts for biotechnology, CRC Crit. Rev. Biochem., 23, 235 (1988).
96. C. O'Fagain and R. O'Kennedy, Functionally stabilized proteins—a review, Biotechnol. Adv., 9, 351 (1991).
97. J. Markussen, I. Diers, P. Hougaard, L. Langkjaer, K. Norris, L. Snel., A. R. Sorensen, and F. O. Marston, Soluble, prolonged-acting insulin derivatives. III. Degree of protraction, crystalizability and chemical stability of insulins substituted in positions A21, B13, B23, B27, and B30, Proten Eng., 2(2), 157 (1988).
98. R. Mahoney, T. Wilder, and B. S. Chang, Substrate-induced thermal stabilization of lactase (*Escherichia coli*) in milk, Ann. N.Y. Acad. Sci., 542, 274 (1988).
99. H. M. Farrell, T. F. Kumosinski, P. Pulaski, and M. P. Thompson, Calcium-induced associations of the caeins: a thermodynamic linkage approach to precipitation and resolubilization, Arch. Biochem. Biophys., 265, 146 (1988).
100. J. J. Robinson, Roles of Ca(2+), Mg (2+) and NaCl in modulating the self association reaction of hyalin, a major protein component of the sea urchin extra-embryonic hyaline layer, Biochem J., 256(1), 225 (1988).
101. C. H. Schein, Solubility as a function of protein structure and solvent components, Biotechnology, 8, 308 (1990).
102. R. Perlman and T. H. Nguyen, Formulation strategies for recombinant proteins: Human growth hormone and tissue plasminogen activator, in *Therapeutic Peptides and Proteins: Formulation, Delivery and Targeting* (D. Marshak and D. Liu, eds.), Cold Spring Harbor Laboratory, Cold Spring Harbor, NY, 1989, pp. 23–31.
103. X. M. Lam, J. Y. Yang, and J. L. Cleland, Antioxidants for prevention of methionine oxidation in recombinant monoclonal antibody HER2, J. Pharm. Sci., 86(11), 1250 (1997).
104. D. B. Volkin and A. M. Kiibanov, Minimizing protein inactivation, in *Protein Function: A Practical Approach* (T. E. Creighton, ed.), IRL Press, Oxford, 1989, pp. 1–24.
105. S. N. Timasheff, Stabilization of protein structure by solvent additives, in *Stability of Protein Pharmaceuticals*, Part B: *In Vivo Pathways of Degradation and Strategies for Protein Stabilization* (T. J. Ahern and M. C. Manning, eds.), Plenum Press, New York, 1992, pp. 265–285.
106. Y. J. Wang and M. A. Hanson, Parenteral formulations of proteins and peptides: Stability and stabilizers, J. Parenter. Sci. Technol., 42 (suppl. 2), S2 (1988).
107. R. Pearlman and T. Nguyen, Pharmaceutics of protein drugs, J. Pharm. Pharmacol., 44 (suppl. 1), 178 (1992).
108. M. A. Hanson and S. K. E. Rouan, Introduction to formulation of protein pharmaceuticals, in *Stability of Protein Pharmaceuticals*, Part B: *In Vivo Pathways of Degradation and Strategies for Protein Stabilization* (T. J. Ahem and M. C. Manning, eds.), Plenum Press, New York, 1992, pp. 209–233.

109. M. C. Lai and E. M. Topp, Solid-state chemical stability of protein and peptides, J. Pharm. Sci., 88, 489 (1999).
110. H. R. Costantino, R. Langer, and A. M. Klibanov, Solid-phase aggregation of proteins under pharmaceutically relevant conditions, J. Pharm. Sci., 83, 1662 (1994).
111. F. Franks, R. H. M. Hatley, and H. L. Friedman, The thermodynamics of protein stability: Cold destabilization as a general phenomenon, Biophys. Chem., 31, 307 (1988).
112. T. Tamiya, N. Okahashi, R. Sakuma, T. Aoyama, T. Akahane, and J. J. Matsumoto, Freeze denaturation of enzymes and its prevention with additives, Cryobiology, 22, 446 (1985).
113. P. L. Privalov, Cold denaturation of proteins, CRC Crit. Rev. Biochem. Mol. Biol., 25, 281 (1990).
114. C. Hsu, H. Nguyen, D. Yeung, D. Brookes, G. Koe, T. Bewley, and R. Pearlman, Surface denaturation of solid-void interface—a possible pathway by which opalescent particulates form during the storage of lyophilized tissue-type plasminogen activator at high temperatures, Pharm. Res., 12, 69 (1995).
115. K. Izutsu, S. Yoshioka, and T. Terao, Effect of mannitol crystallinity on the stabilization of enzymes during freeze drying, Chem. Pharm. Bull. (Tokyo), 42, 5 (1994).
116. B. Kerwin, M. Heller, S. Levin, and T. Randolph, Effect of Tween 80 and sucrose on acute short-term stability and long trem storage at −20°C of a recombinant hemoglobin, J. Pharm. Sci., 87, 1062 (1998).
117. M. Ressing, W. Jiskoot, H. Talsma, C. van Ingen, E. Beuvery, and D. Crommelin, The influence of sucrose, dextran, and hydroxypropyl-beta-cyclodextrin as lyoprotectants for freeze-dried mouse IgG2a monoclonal antibosy (MN12), Pharm. Res., 9, 266 (1992).
118. S. J. Perstrelski, T. Arakawa, and J. F. Carpenter, Separation of freezing and drying-induced denaturation of lyophilized proteins using stress-specific stabilization. II. Structural studies using infrared spectroscopy, Arch. Biochem. Biophys., 303, 465 (1993).
119. J. F. Carpenter, L M. Crowe, and J. H. Crowe, Stabilization of phosphofructokinase with sugars during freeze-drying: Characterization of enhanced protection in the presence of divalent cations, Biochim. Biophys. Acta, 923, 109 (1987).
120. J. F. Carpenter, B. Martin, L. M. Crowe, and J. H. Crowe, Stabilization of phosphofructokinase during air-drying with sugars and sugar/transition metal mixtures, Cryobiology, 24, 455 (1987).
121. J. F. Carpenter and J. H. Crowe, An infrared spectroscopic study of the interactions of carbohydrates with dried proteins, Biochemistry, 28, 3916 (1989).
122. J. H. Crowe, J. F. Carpenter, L. M. Crowe, and T. J. Anchordoguy, Are freezing and dehydration similar stress vectors? A comparison of modes of interaction of stabilizing solutes with biomolecules, Cryobiology, 27, 219 (1990).
123. F. Franks, Long term stabilization of biologicals, Biotechnology, 12, 253 (1994).
124. C. A. Angell, Formation of glasses from liquid and biopolymers, Science, 267, 1924 (1995).
125. S. P. Duddu, and P. R. Dal Monte, Effect of glass transition temperature on the stability of lyophilized formulations containing a chimeric therapeutic antibody, Pharm. Res., 14(5), 591 (1997).
126. J. H. Crowe, J. F. Carpenter, and L. M. Crowe, The role of vitrification in anhydrobiosis, Ann. Rev. Physiol., 60, 73 (1998).
127. D. E. Overcashier, T. W. Patapoff, and C. C. Hsu, Lyophilization of protein formulations in vials: Investigation of the relationship between resistance to vapor flow during primary drying and small scale product collapse, J. Pharm. Sci., 88(7), 688 (1999).
128. S. L. Nail and L. A. Gatlin, Freeze drying: Principles and practice, in *Pharmaceutical Dosage Forms: Parenteral Medications*, Vol. 2. (K.E. Avis, H.A. Lieberman, and I. Lachman, eds.), Marcel Dekker, New York, 1993, pp. 163–233.
129. H. R. Costanstino, K. G. Carrasquillo, R. A. Cordero, M. Mumenthaler, C. Hsu, and K. Griebenow, Effect of excipients on the stability and structure of lyophilized recombinant growth hormone, J. Pharm. Sci., 87, 1412 (1998).
130. K. Izutsu, S. Yoshioka, and T. Terao, Effect of mannitol crystallinity on the stabilization of enzymes during freeze drying, Chem. Pharm. Bull. (Tokyo), 42, 5 (1994).
131. K. Izutsu, S. Yoshioka, and S. Kojima, Increased stabilizating effects of amphiphilic excipients on freeze drying of lactate dehydrogenase (LDH) by dispersion into sugar matrices, Pharm. Res., 12, 838 (1995).
132. T. W. Randolph, Phase separation of excipients during lyophilization: Effects on protein stability, J. Pharm. Sci., 86(11), 1198 (1997).
133. B. Lueckel, B. Helk, D. Bodmer, and H. Leuenberger, Effect of formulation and process variables on the aggregation of freeze dried interleukin-6 (IL-6) after lyophilization and storage, Pharm. Dev. Technol., 3, 337 (1998).
134. J. H. Crowe, L. M. Crowe, and J. F. Carpenter, Preserving dry biomaterials: The water replacement hypothesis, BioPharm., 6(1), 28 (1993).
135. S. D. Allison, A. Dong, and J. F. Carpenter, Counteracting effects of thiocyanate and sucrose on chymotrypsinogen secondary structure and aggregation during freezing, drying, and rehydration, Biophys. J., 71, 2022 (1996).

136. S. D. Allison, T. W. Randolph, M. C. Manning, K. Middleton, A. Davis, and J. F. Carpenter. Effects of drying methods and additives on structure and function of actin:mechanisms of dehydration-induced damage and its inhibition, Arch. Biochem. Biophys., 358, 171 (1998).
137. M. L. Roy, M. J. Pikal, E. C. Rickard, and A. Maloney, The effects of formulation and moisture on the stability of a freeze-dried monoclonal antibody-vinca conjugate: A test of the WLF glass transition theory Dev. Biol. Standards, 74, 323 (1991).
138. B. C. Hancock and G. Zografi, The relationship between the glass transition temperature and the water content of amorphous pharmaceutical solids, Pharm. Res., 11, 471 (1994).
139. L. A. Daukas and E. H. Trappler, Assessing the quality of lyophilized parenterals, Pharm. Cosmetic Quality, 2, 21 (1998).
140. J. F. Carpenter and B. S. Chang, Lyophilization of protein pharmaceuticals, in *Biotechnology and Biopharmaceutical Manufacturing, Processing, and Preservation* (K. Avis and V. Wu, eds.), Interpharm Press, Inc., Buffalo Grove, IL.: 1996, pp. 199–264.
141. W. Wang, Lyophilization and development of solid protein pharmaceuticals, Int. J. Pharmaceut., 203, 1 (2000).
142. L. Rey and J. May, eds., *Freeze-Drying/Lyophilization of Pharmaceutical and Biological Products*, Marcel Dekker, New York, Inc., 1999.
143. M. Pikal, Freeze drying of proteins: Process, formulation, and stability, in *Formulation and Delivery of Proteins and Peptides* (J. Cleland and R. Langer, eds.), ACS Symposium Series 567, 1993, pp. 120–133.
144. S. T. Tzannis and S. J. Prestrelski, Activity-stability considerations of trypsinogen during spray drying: Effects of sucrose, J. Pharm. Sci., 88(3), 351 (1999).
145. S. T. Tzannis and S. J. Prestrelski, Moisture effects on protein-excipient interactions in spray dried powders. Nature of destabilizing effects of sucrose, J. Pharm. Sci., 88(3), 360 (1999).
146. M. Mumenthaler, C. C. Hsu, and R. Pearlman, Feasibility study on spray-drying protein pharmaceuticals: recombinant human growth hormone and tissue-type plasminogen activator, Pharm. Res., 11(1), 12 (1994).
147. Y. F. Maa, P. T. Nguyen, and S. W. Hsu, Spray drying of air liquid interface sensitive recombinant human growth hormone, J. Pharm. Sci., 87(2), 152, (1998).
148. J. Broadhead, S. K. Rouan, I. Hau, and C. T. Rhodes, The effect of process and formulation variables on the properties of spray-dried β-galactosidase, J. Pharm. Pharmacol., 46(6), 458 (1994).
149. M. Adler and G. Lee, Stability and surface activity of lactate dehydogenase in spray-dried trehalose, J. Pharm. Sci., 88(2), 199 (1999).
150. P. L. Smith, D. A. Wall, C. Gochoco, and G. Wilson, Routes of delivery: Case studies—(5) oral absorption of peptides and proteins, Adv. Drug Deliv. Rev., 8, 253 (1992).
151. J. S. Patton and R. M. Platz, Routes of drug delivery: case studies (2) pulmonary delivery of peptides and proteins for systemic action, Adv. Drug Deliv. Rev., 8, 179 (1992).
152. R. Langer and N. A. Peppas, New drug delivery systems, Biomed. Eng. Soc. Bull., 16, 3 (1992).
153. S. S. Davis, Delivery systems for biopharmaceuticals, J. Pharm. Pharmacol., 44 (suppl. 1), 186 (1992).
154. V. H. Lee, ed., *Peptide and Protein Drug Delivery: Advances in Parenter. Sciences*, 4th ed., Marcel Dekker, New York, 1990.
155. N. Katre, The conjugation of proteins with polyethylene glycol and other polymers. Altering properties of proteins to enhance their therapeutic potential. Advances Drug Del. Rev., 10, 91 (1993).
156. L. Stanford Lee, C. Conover, C. Shi, M. Whitlow, and D. Filpula, Prolonged circulating lives of single-chain Fv proteins conjugated with polyethylene glycol: A comparison of conjugation chemistries and compounds, Bioconjugate Chem., 10, 973 (1999).
157. O. B. Kinstler, D. N. Brems, S. L. Lauren, A. G. Paige, J. B. Hamburger, and M. J. Treuheit, Characterization and stability of N-terminally PEGylated rhG-CSF, Pharm. Res., 13, 996 (1996).
158. T. O. Park, S. Cohen, and R. Langer, Controlled protein release from polyethyleneimine-coated poly(l-lactic acid)/pluronic blend matrices, Pharm. Res., 9, 37 (1992).
159. J. L. Cleland and A. J. Jones, Stable formulations of recombinant human growth hormone and interferon-γ for microencapsulation in biodegradable microspheres, Phar. Res., 13(10), 1464 (1996).
160. K. G. Carrasquillo, H. R. Constatino, R. A. Cordero, C. C. Hsu, and K. Griebenow, On the structural preservation of recombinant human growth hormone in dried film of a synthetic biodegradable polymer, J. Pharm. Sci., 88(2), 166 (1998).
161. D. Bodmer, T. Kissel, and E. Traechslin, Factors influencing the release of peptides and proteins from biodegradable parenteral depot systems, J. Controlled Release, 21, 129 (1992).
162. C. N. Tenhoor, J. B. Dressman, Oral absorption of peptides and proteins, STP Pharma Sci., 2, 301 (1992).
163. L. Plum and S. S. Davis, Intranasal insulin, Clin. Pharmacokinet., 23, 30 (1992).
164. I. Gonda, The ascent of pulmonary drug delivery, J. Pharm. Sci., 89(7), 940 (2000).
165. C. M. Henry, Special delivery, Chem. Eng. News, 78(38) 49 (2000).

Chapter 23

The Pharmacist and Veterinary Pharmaceutical Dosage Forms

J. Patrick McDonnell

Fort Dodge Animal Health, Charles City, Iowa

Lisa Blair Banker

Blair Animal Clinic, West Lafayette, Indiana

I. INTRODUCTION

A. Veterinary Products—Economic Overview

The pharmacist has historically been trained for and has concerns about human health matters. Animal health has in the past few years become more visible and should also be of interest to the pharmacist for the following reasons:

1. Economics-According to the Animal Health Institute's (AHI) 2000 Domestic Sales Survey, sales of animal health products in the United States for 1999 totaled $4.32 billion priced at the manufacturer's level [1].
2. Research-AHI member companies spent more than $409 million dollars on research and development. Approximately 70% was spent on dosage form research and 30% on biological research.
3. Zoonosis-The diseases of animals that may secondarily be transferred to man are a growing health concern (See Chapter 1). The pharmacist as the most readily and easily accessible community health representative can provide information, service and products to his/her customers.

Approximately 58% of households in the United States now include at least one pet. The American Veterinary Medical Association's 1997 survey [2] showed the population of companion animals in the United States to be:

Cats: 59.0 million
Dogs: 53.0 million
Birds: 12.6 million
Horses: 4.0 million

Food-producing (economic) animals by far outnumber companion animals. The U.S. Department of Agriculture National Agricultural Statistics Service reported for 1999 the following numbers:

Hogs: 58.1 million
Cattle and calves: 98.0 million
Dairy cattle: 7.8 million
Poultry:
  chickens—laying: 331.0 million
  chickens—broilers: 8.1 billion
Turkeys: 273.0 million
Sheep and lambs: 10.7 million

All of these animals during their lifetime will receive or be treated with at least one of the following: type C medicated articles (feed additives), biologics (vaccines, bacterins), growth stimulants, pharmaceuticals, or pesticides. These products are developed and manufactured by a multitude of pharmaceutical (human and animal), biological, and other health science companies who employ pharmacists and pharmaceutical scientists. In addition, there is an increasing trend for compounding pharmacists to formulate animal health dosage forms to the order of a veterinary prescription. The pharmacy student should have an understanding and basic knowledge of veterinary science to provide information on veterinary drug products and to compound extemporaneous veterinary dosage forms.

B. Veterinary Medicine and the Pharmacist

Pharmacy students and pharmacists have had a long and colorful history of association with veterinary medicine and veterinary drugs. In the 1960s and 1970s at least two colleges of pharmacy offered courses in agricultural pharmacy, veterinary therapeutics, and veterinary product development research [3–5]. Similar courses reemerged in the late 1990s [6]. In 1987 a large veterinary pharmaceutical and biological company and the University of Iowa College of Pharmacy joined into a collaborative venture in veterinary dosage form development [7]. This type of program exposes pharmacy students to the world of animal diseases, animal health medications, and dosage forms. The student should then be better prepared to understand and provide information and counseling to patients who have questions and needs concerning animal drug issues, be it companion animals such as dogs or cats in a metropolitan area or poultry, horses, hogs, or cattle in rural practices.

The Animal Health Institute (AHI), the premier trade organization of animal health industries, had its beginnings in Des Moines, Iowa, sharing offices and staff with the Iowa Pharmacists Association. The executive secretary of the Iowa Pharmaceutical Association and Animal Health Institute was a pharmacist who eventually became the full-time executive secretary for the AHI when it moved its headquarters to Washington, D.C.

Several colleges of pharmacy in the United States are located on campuses of the agricultural land grant universities in their respective states. Included in this group are Purdue University College of Pharmacy and Pharmacal Sciences, West Lafayette, Indiana; University of South Dakota College of Pharmacy, in Brookings, South Dakota; University of Georgia College of Pharmacy, Athens, Georgia; and the North Dakota State University College of Pharmacy, Fargo, North Dakota. Academic pharmacy has a physical presence within academic agricultural and veterinary medicine settings. Collaborative research and educational programs between these colleges are common and productive.

After several decades of remaining relatively dormant, a dramatic increase in pharmacist extemporaneous compounding of dosage forms occurred in the 1990s. Specialty practices evolved which concentrated on preparation of classical and innovative dosage forms. Veterinary pharmacy practice has become one of these areas. Continued education series in veterinary therapeutics such as those offered by the Southwestern Oklahoma State University School of Pharmacy have been developed [8]. These are highly recommended to those pharmacy students/pharmacists who are interested in working with veterinarians. Colleges of veterinary medicine have added pharmacists to their professional staffs. Iowa State University College of Veterinary Medicine in conjunction with Creighton University and the University of Iowa Colleges of Pharmacy offers externships for pharmacy students in the veterinary college. The same type of relationship exists between the School of Pharmacy at the University of Mississippi and the College of Veterinary Medicine at Mississippi State. A new organization—the American College of Veterinary Pharmacists—has been formed, with the purpose of supporting pharmacists in services they provide veterinarians. This association provides experience in compounding, equipment use, dosage adjustments, flavoring agents, and sourcing. Training and seminars are held to exchange and share information on veterinary topics and issues.

In summary, as the human-animal companies bond continues to grow and gain importance, veterinarians are expected to practice a higher quality of medicine. The pharmacist is in a position to assist the veterinarian in obtaining this goal. Familiarity with veterinary medicine, dosage forms, and animal drugs is useful to the pharmacist who acts as an advisor, reference source, and compounder to the veterinarian, the public, and members of the health care team.

II. ANIMAL DOSAGE FORMS

There are many similarities and differences in the anatomy and physiology of mammals, birds, and humans. It is outside the scope of this chapter to elaborate on the individual differences. For a brief review, refer to the third edition of *Modern Pharmaceutics* [9] and the second edition of *Development and Formulation of Veterinary Dosage Forms* [10].

A. Tablets and Boluses

Solid dosage forms, such as compressed tablets, are one of the most common means of administering medications to humans. These are less popular for animals because administration may be time-consuming, hazardous, and uncertain (uncertain because one cannot be sure the tablet is swallowed, spit out, or dropped from the mouth after the administrator has left or moved on to another animal). Tablets that are accepted voluntarily by the animal are typically chewed, which exposes the disagreeable taste of some drugs. Thus, the advantage of the dosage form may be lost. This can be overcome in some cases by the use of odors, flavors, or sweeteners. However, the formulator cannot fall into the trap of flavoring or masking based on human perceptions. Formulations must be tested on the species for which they are intended. An interesting thesis on animal flavors and flavoring [11] has been written by Talmadge B. Tribble of the Flavor Corporation of America, who was a pharmacist and founded one of the largest animal feed flavor companies in the world.

Drugs are given on the basis of weight or body surface area, be it for mammals, avian species, or humans. The amount of drug needed for a large mammal, such as a St. Bernard, cow, or horse, can be considerable. Labeling for solid dosage forms therefore tends to be stated in mg or g tablet per lb (kg) of body weight. Drugs such as sulfonamides are dosed at relatively high amounts; it is not unusual to prescribe as much as 15 g of drug for each 150 lb of body weight—a 750 lb cow or horse would receive 75 g of drug. A special tablet called a "bolus" is commonly used to provide these large dosages. A bolus is nothing more than a very large tablet, which can range from 3 to 16 g or more. Although commonly called "horse pills," they are not used exclusively with horses. Because of the difficulty in handling horses, which may be less docile than cows, the ease with which the horse can spit pills out, and the possibility of choking, the bolus form must be used with special care in horses. Boluses are capsule shaped or cylindrical because a round bolus would be unwieldy and difficult to administer or swallow. Boluses are administered by an apparatus called a balling gun, consisting of a barrel with a plunger that can hold one or more boluses. The tube is inserted into the animal's mouth over the base of the tongue, and as the animal swallows the plunger is depressed to push the bolus into the gullet. The bolus is thus expelled gently into the gullet, after which it is swallowed by reflex.

Bolus formulation poses challenges because of the high drug-to-excipient ratio. Less room is left for diluent, binders, and other adjuvants needed to overcome objectionable features of the drug or to facilitate bolus manufacture. In ruminant animals, such as cattle or sheep, it is possible to utilize the concept of long-acting boluses, which stay in the gastrointestinal track for periods of much longer than 12 hours (sometimes days or weeks). This is because solid objects can remain in the ruminoreticular sac, a part of the bovine gastrointestinal tract, indefinitely. The density of the bolus is the critical factor for retention in the sac. The range of density from 1.5 to 8.0 is believed to be desirable for prolonged retention. This is achieved by including excipients such as iron, clay, sodium sulfate dihydrate, and dicalcium sulfate in these formulations [12]. Weight and size influence retention, but not as significantly as density.

In small animals it is best that oral medications be ingested by the animal on its own, thus the special compounding with flavors and in appropriate textures discussed earlier. There are still occasions when an owner may have to open a pet's mouth and administer a pill through a "piller," which is a tube with a plunger.

B. Feed Additives

An animal dosage form that the pharmacist would be least familiar with, since there is no analogy in human drug dosage forms, is the feed additive premix (type A or B medicated article). Feed additive premixes (type A medicated articles) are formulated to contain bulk drug and excipient in a form that may be readily combined with an animal feed. The feed route is used mainly for prophylactic treatment against diseases caused by parasites or for growth promotion. The drugs may be given from day of age (i.e., hatching in the case of poultry rations) to market. However, the majority of drugs must be withdrawn from the feed several days to a month or more before the animal is sent to market to be processed for human consumption to provide time for the drug to be cleared from the animal's system.

The formulation of a premix consists of combining a drug with a carrier, diluent, or absorbent. The most common form of premix utilizes a grain carrier (e.g., rice hulls, corn germ meal, corn meal, corn gluten meal, wheat middlings) in which the active drug is lightly bound or absorbed on the surface. The carrier functions by absorbing the small fine particles of drug on the surface and in the pores of the carrier particles. The carrier will usually be two thirds or more of the formulation. An oil may also be added to bind the drug to the carrier. If needed for flow conditioning and to prevent caking, an anticaking agent such as silicon dioxide or magnesium aluminum silicate can be incorporated in the product.

Another excipient used in feed additive premixes is a diluent used to dilute or standardize activity. Diluents are similar in composition to grain carriers, except the particle size is generally smaller. No attempt is made to absorb the active drug to the individual particles of the diluents. If a liquid is used it is mainly for dust control. A diluent is considered for use when the level of the active ingredient components in the premix approaches or exceeds 50% of the product or when two or more active components vary greatly from one another in density [13]. Examples of diluent materials are ground limestone, sodium sulfate, kaolin, corn cob flour, and ground oyster shells.

Absorbents are another class of excipient material used in feed additive premixes. They are used when the drug substance is a liquid or is readily soluble in water, oil, or some other solvent. The liquid is sprayed onto the absorbent in a mixer as the mixer is running. Examples of absorbents are vermiculite, Fullers earth, corn cob fractions, and clay.

Factors that need to be considered in formulating premixes and the choice of carrier are:

1. Drug concentration in the premix.
2. Drug concentration in the final feed: if a drug premix is added to a feed so that the drug level is less than 150 ppm, a carrier is needed to insure adequate dilution.
3. Moisture content of drug and carrier: if the drug is moisture sensitive or the carrier is subject to breakdown or spoilage from moisture levels in the drug or carrier itself, appropriate drying or other steps may be required.
4. Electrostatic charges: fine drug powders will often develop static charges during particle size reduction and flow through material-handling systems. These charges need to be minimized to prevent unmixing or loss in even distribution throughout the premix and subsequent feed.
5. pH extremes: these can frequently be compensated for by use of sodium carbonate to neutralize acid mixtures or calcium phosphate monobasic or fumaric acid to neutralize basic mixtures.
6. Flow: this is important when automatic premix addition equipment is used in modern feed mills. Bridging (an organized structure of product that impedes flow), which inhibits addition of the premix to the feed batch, will cause the mill to shut down until the correct amount of premix is added. This shut-down of the mill can cause considerable consternation to the operators of the mill who are producing multiple batches of feed per day.

The normal standard of premix usage in feed is one part medicated premix to 1999 parts of feed. A properly formulated premix can be used directly in preparing a medicated feed without further dilution. It can be further diluted in the feed mill by the use of in-plant premixes (type B medicated articles), but this would be at the discretion of the feed mill operator.

Although the pharmacist may only infrequently have contact with this particular dosage form, there has been a movement to give some feed additive drugs veterinary prescription status, which has been done in several European countries. This may have future implications to those pharmacists practicing in rural areas.

C. Drinking Water Medications

A common form of medicating animals for herd or flock health is through the drinking water. The medications are formulated as: (a) dry powders for reconstitution into liquid concentrates to be added to the drinking water or to be added directly to the drinking water or (b) concentrated solutions, which are dispensed directly in drinking water or injected into the drinking water through medication proportioners incorporated into watering lines. The advantage of medicating through drinking water versus feed is that sick or unhealthy animals will continue to drink water whereas they may not eat. The use of water as the drug medium is limited, however, by the solubility of the drug moiety. Since animals drink twice as much water as they consume feed, the concentration of the drug in the water needs to be only half that of feed. This factor may overcome the problem of limited solubility.

Automatic metering devices or medication proportioners are used for treating large numbers of animals. The powder medication is dissolved at the time of administration into water to make a stock solution, which is proportioned into the drinking water system as the water is consumed by the animals. The common dilution in the United States is one fluid ounce of stock solution (or liquid drug concentrate) to 127 ounces of water, producing a one fluid ounce per gallon dilution.

Whether a product is formulated as a dry powder, dispensing tablet, or liquid concentrate, the product development/compounding pharmacist must be concerned with the effects of the properties of the diluting water media. Tablet or granule hardness, buffer capacity, pH, and total dissolved solids all play a role in the solubility rate and availability of the drug substance, as well as its stability.

In addition, dry products are usually formulated with a sugar diluent such as lactose or dextrose. The use of these may cause a build-up of bacteria and fungi in water lines when the sugar level is high for an extended period of time [14]. In the product development laboratory, medicated drinking water samples must be prepared from these formulations using a range of hard and soft waters and stored at 25°C and 37–40°C in metal containers or troughs (galvanized iron or rusty metal) to simulate the worst possible conditions of use [15]. The drug stability in the drinking water should be adequate for the storage length of time listed on the label [16]. Consideration also has to be given when formulating a liquid concentrate using solvents other than water of the possibility of precipitation or recrystalization of the drug when diluted with water. All of the above factors make the formulation of animal drinking water products an interesting and challenging task.

D. Oral Pastes and Gels

Pastes and gels are semi-fluid masses that can be administered from a flexible tube, syringe, package, or other specialized dosing device. The advantage of a paste or gel dosage form is that it cannot be expelled from the animal's mouth as readily as a tablet or liquid. Also, mass medicating of animals can be achieved rapidly and easily with a paste medication using a multiple-dose dispenser such as a syringe.

A paste of the proper consistency adheres to the tongue or buccal cavity and is not readily dislodged. The animal will eventually end up swallowing it. Characteristics of a suitable paste formulation are [17]:

1. When placed in the palm of the hand and the hand is inverted (palm down), it should remain there without falling.
2. When the paste is ejected from the applicator, it should break free cleanly when rubbed against a flat surface.
3. No paste should continue to ooze from the applicator after the dose has been ejected.
4. The paste or gel should be free from air bubbles or voids.
5. Only a minimum of force should be needed to expel the paste from the dispensing devise.

The three types of vehicles used in formulating a paste or gel are aqueous bases, oil or oleaginous bases, and organic solvents.

An aqueous base is the least expensive vehicle and poses no toxicity problems. A solution of the drug in water or water and cosolvent is made. Glycerin, glycols, natural and synthetic gums, and/or polymers are used to increase viscosity, cohesiveness, and plasticity. To overcome syneresis, or water separation in the gel, a common problem with aqueous bases, one can use absorbing materials such as microcrystalline cellulose, kaolin, colloidal silicon dioxide, starch, etc.

Oleaginous bases consist of vegetable oil thickened with agents such as aluminum monostearate, colloidal silica, and xanthan gums. The lubricant properties of the oil make these formulations less adhesive than water bases.

Glycerin, propylene glycol, and polyethylene glycol thickened with carboxyvinyl polymers (Carboxamer NF) provide organic solvent bases. Consistencies ranging from soft jelly to peanut butter can be achieved.

A paste is administered to an animal volumetrically. The drug level and density of the paste must be known to determine the amount of drug delivered per given volume. This takes trial and error in the formulation process to arrive at the volume of paste necessary to provide the required dose.

Sometimes pastes are used in small animals by applying them to an animal's fur on the front paws. The animal will lick the paste off to stay clean.

E. Drenches and Tubing Products

Horses are administered certain medications by running a lubricated tube up through the nostrils and down into the stomach. A funnel attached to the tube is held above the horse's head and the liquid medication is poured down the tube. This is known as "tubing."

The normal dose for a horse by this method is approximately 10 fluid ounces. It needs to be formulated so that the amount will flow through the tubing (i.e., 6 1/2 ft × 3/8 in.) in 60 seconds. Wetting agents are used to increase flow rate. Thickening or suspending agents are contraindicated since the formulations will thicken and resist flow when shear is removed.

The administration of a drug to animals by pouring a liquid medication down an animal's throat is called "drenching." Drenches are dispensed via syringe or drenching guns. The viscosity should be adequate to prevent dripping from the syringe during movement from the drug container to the animal. Drenching guns can utilize formulations that are less viscous since leakage from the gun is not a major problem. Too viscous a product may cause administrator fatigue when large numbers of animals are dosed.

These drenches and tubing products are often given over extreme ranges of temperatures in field conditions. The formulator must take this into consideration when developing the dosage formula and testing it in the administration equipment.

F. Topical Dosage Forms

There are several unique topical dosage forms for animals. Four types of which the pharmacist should have a basic understanding or awareness are: (a) pour-on/spot-on applications, (b) dust bags, (c) dips, and (d) flea and tick collars. These are used for treatment and prevention of internal and external parasites.

Pour-On/Spot-On Applications

These liquid products effect systemic activity after being poured onto an animal's backline or applied as a one-spot concentrate on the animals back or rump. Some spot-on products now help small animals combat fleas and ticks. These products are generally preferred to flea and tick collars. The oils from the drug mix with the pet's natural oils. They act as a neurotoxin against the ectoparasites. In cattle, spot-ons are mainly used for control of grubs and lice. However, there is one pour-on/spot-on product (levamisole) that has broad-spectrum anthelmintic activity. These formulations contain organophosphorus insecticides or the anthelmintic dissolved in organic solvents, such as dimethylsulfoxide and/or aromatic hydrocarbons. The advantages of these formulations are [18]:

1. Risk of trauma and inhalation pneumonia associated with drenching or damage at injection site (for parenteral products) are eliminated.
2. No special skills are required for application since they are administered topically by use of sprays or spotter bottle (a bottle with a squeeze-on applicator).
3. Sterile precautions are not necessary.
4. Troublesome animals are dosed easily with safety to the person performing the application.
5. Speed of treatment is quick.

Dust Bags

Cattle are treated with insecticide powders through use of a device called a dust bag. Dosing is accomplished by the animals brushing against the bag as they walk beside or under it. The bag has an inner porous storage bag containing the insecticide dust formulation. This is protected from the elements by an outer protective waterproof skirt open to the porous dust bag at the bottom.

The cattle can have free-choice application or are forced to use dust bags depending upon where they are hung. Forced-use bags are hung in doorways, lanes, gateways, etc. Free-choice applications can be achieved by suspending the bags from overhead structures, like a tree or pole. One would be surprised at the willingness of the majority of range cattle to come to a free-choice application site.

Dips

For control of ectoparasites in economic animals, dipping is an extensively used method. A dip formulation containing the drug is diluted in a large dipping bath through which the animal is driven. This bath must be long, wide, and deep enough to cause immersion of the animal. The formulation of the ectoparasiticide is challenging. It must not be inactivated by matter that accumulates in the dipping bath and should maintain stability throughout a range of concentrations and temperatures. In addition, it must be nontoxic to the animal but toxic to the ectoparasites [19]. This dosage form is used in both large and small animals.

Flea and Tick Collars

This dosage form will be most familiar to the pharmacist since it is used for companion animals (dogs and cats) and is sold in most drugstores, supermarkets, and animal health product centers. There are two types of flea and tick collars, also known as slow-release pesticide generators: vaporous and powder-producing collars. Both contain the insecticide and a plasticized solid thermoplastic resin.

The vaporous collar contains a relatively high-vapor-pressure liquid pesticide mixed throughout the collar. The pesticide is slowly released and fills the atmosphere adjacent to the animal's surface with a vapor of pesticide that kills the pest but is innocuous to the animal.

The powder-producing collar contains a solid solution of the drug in the resin. Shortly after the collar is processed, the particles or molecules of the pesticide migrate from within the body of the resin and form a coating of particles, known as "bloom," resembling a dust or powder on the collar surface.

Ticks and fleas tend to concentrate in or migrate through the neck area of the animal. As they do this, they contact the active pesticide on or released by the collar and are killed. Powder-producing collars have an advantage over vaporous ones in that by the movement of the dog or cat, the powder crystals (bloom) are rubbed or wiped onto the fur, which expands the contact area allowing it to continue to control the ticks and fleas [20].

G. Miscellaneous Dosage Forms

Some drugs, depending on their molecular size, can be compounded in such a way as to be administered transdermally. In cats, for instance, transdermals are applied to the inside of the ear pinna.

Pharmacists are also responsible for compounding special ear preparations for pets that are not commercially available. Sometimes the availability and cost of certain medications are prohibitive for a veterinarian's private pharmacy.

Nebulizers and aerosols are starting to be used in small animals. Kittenhood respiratory diseases seem to respond to nebulizers, as does feline asthma in adult cats.

Percutaneous patches are used in small animals. Fentanyl is a drug used for pain control and is quite effective. Unfortunately, it is quite toxic to animals and young children if accidentally ingested.

Suppositories are also being used to deliver some drugs when they simply can't be given by mouth.

With all forms of drugs there are side effects and precautions. The pharmacist and veterinarian are responsible for passing any such information on to clients.

H. Over-the-Counter Dosages

Some Over-the-Counter (OTC) drugs are used in small animals, while others should not be used. Due to differences in absorption, receptor types, metabolism, and other differences in the digestive system, dosages can be very different than in humans. Anti-inflammatories are used cautiously in dogs and cats. For example, dogs may be administered aspirin at a maximum dose of 325 mg per 30–35 pounds of body weight, given once to twice daily, in comparison with dosage in humans every 4–6 hours. Cats may be given one quarter of a 325 mg tablet twice a week—they do not metabolize salicylates as easily as humans. Since Pepto-Bismol® contains bismuth subsalicylate, this drug must also be used less frequently in cats. Acetaminophen and ibuprofen are two OTC drugs that can be highly toxic to small animals. They can cause certain blood dyscrasias and should not be given unless directed by a veterinarian.

Antihistamines are widely used in small animals to control allergies and allergic reactions. Diphenhydramine (Benadryl®) can be given in doses as high as 1–2 mg per pound of body weight up to 3 times per day. This is much higher than the human dosage. Clemastine is also given at a higher dosage to dogs. Chlorpheniramine seems to combat allergies in most cats better than other antihistamines.

Antidiarrheals are used in dogs. Pepto-Bismol and Immodium AD® (loperamide) are used as in humans, but at a higher dosage. Loperamide must be used with caution in cats since it may cause central nervous system (CNS) excitation in this species. The use of drugs such as loperamide, which act by slowing intestinal motility, may be less effective in small animals than might be anticipated, since diarrhea is these animals is often associated with hypomotility, not hypermotility. In treating diarrhea in small animals veterinarians will sometimes withhold regular food for 12–24 hours and provide water and a bland diet such as cooked white rice or cottage cheese before initiating any antidiarrheal medication. Where the diarrhea is the result of an enterobacterial cause, the diarrhea may help eliminate the causative pathogen and its endotoxins. Pharmacists should generally refer pet owners to their veterinarian when small animal diarrhea is reported, since it may be important to determine the cause and since drug responses and treatments differ from those in humans. Likewise, if a pet owner requests a laxative for an animal thought to be suffering from constipation, it is best to refer the owner to a veterinarian, since constipation often is a symptom of a more serious condition or disease state. Furthermore, bulk laxatives and osmotic laxatives are contraindicated in dehydrated animals, and the pet owner may not be a good judge of the animal's hydration state.

Creams and lotions may be used in animals, although they can be licked off by the patient and must be used with caution. Table 1 presents the doses and recommended dosage frequencies for selected drugs in small animals.

III. U.S. REGULATORY REQUIREMENTS FOR ANIMAL DRUGS

In the United States, the Center for Veterinary Medicine of the Food and Drug Administration (FDA) has

Table 1 Doses of Selected Drugs Used in Small Animals

Drug	Feline dose	Canine dose
Acetaminophen	Contraindicated	10–15 mg/kg q 8–12 hr
Aspirin	10–25 mg q 48 to 72 hr	10–25 mg q.d. to b.i.d.
Ketoprofen	1 mg/kg daily for 5 days	1 mg/kg daily for 5 days
Dimenhydrinate	12.5 mg up to q 8 hr	12.5–50 mg up to q 8 hr
Diphenhydramine	2–4 mg/kg (c. 12.5 mg) q 8 hr	2–4 mg/kg q 8 hr
Chlor- or brompheniramine	2–4 mg b.i.d.	4–8 mg/kg b.i.d.—t.i.d.
Clemastine	0.1 mg/kg b.i.d.	0.5–1.5 mg b.i.d.
Pseudoephedrine	2–4 mg/kg twice daily	No published doses
Dextromethorphan	No published doses	Up to 5 mg t.i.d.—q.i.d.
Attapulgite	1–2 mL/kg q 4–6 hr	1–2 mL/kg q 4–6 hr
Bismuth subsalicylate	1–2 mL/kg q 48–72 hr	1–2 mL/kg t.i.d.—q.i.d.
Loperamide	0.08–0.16 mg/kg b.i.d.	0.1–0.2 mg/kg b.i.d.—t.i.d.
Mineral oil (laxative)	2–10 mL p.r.n.	2–60 mL p.r.n.

Note: Some of the above doses are presented as mg/kg doses, whereas others are presented as total mg doses for the whole animal.
Source: From Ref. 8, with some modification as to recommended dosing frequency in felines.

responsibility for the review and approval of animal drugs. Toxicology, pharmacology, and pharmacokinetic data for drug products used in food-producing animals is the responsibility of the Human Food Safety Division. The mechanism for review and approval of animal drugs is through the submission of Form FD356, New Animal Drug Application (NADA). Animal feeds containing drugs must also be approved by submission of Form FD 1900, Animal Feed Application. The requirements for these are detailed in the FD&C Act and the Code of Federal Regulations [21].

Before final approval of a new animal drug application, the Center for Veterinary Medicine may require a manufacturing facilities visit called a Pre-Approval Inspection. The Good Manufacturing Practices regulations [22] are used as a guide for this audit by inspectors from the compliance division of the FDA. The requirements for laboratory data, manufacturing equipment, and facilities are the same whether the drugs are made for animals or humans. The quality of animal drugs is expected to be the same as that of their human counterparts. They are not relegated to second-class status.

There is much legal responsibility involving veterinary compounding. It is strongly recommended that a pharmacist interested in veterinary compounding heed FDA rules and regulations.

Compounding of existing drugs is permitted but technically illegal if bulk drugs are the source. FDA has adopted the view that compounding is permissible if the veterinarian acknowledges that (a) there is a legitimate medical need, (b) it is needed for an appropriate dosage regimen, (c) the dosage form is not available in either veterinary or human form, or (d) a different excipient is required for successful treatment. Individual states may have their own laws concerning pharmacist compounding of veterinary drugs. The pharmacist should contact the state board of pharmacy to obtain information and regulations.

Certain drugs cannot be used in animals produced for human consumption, including chloramphenicol, clenbuterol, diethylstilbestrol (DES), dimetridazole, ipronidazole, furazolidine, and vancomycin. Severe legal penalties could be incurred if the pharmacist were to provide any of these drugs for use in food-producing animals and subsequent residues were detected in animal tissue.

Labeling of pharmacist-compounded veterinary drugs should contain as a minimum [23]:

1. Name and address of veterinarian
2. Active ingredient(s)
3. Date dispensed and expiration date
4. Directions for use
5. Cautionary statements
6. Withdrawal times if animal is to be slaughtered for human consumption or produces eggs or milk
7. Name and address of the pharmacy/pharmacist dispensing the medication

IV. CONCLUSION

Animal drug dosage forms can be as complex and sophisticated as drugs used in humans, if not more so.

They have their own requirements and characteristics based on the unique aspects of mammal and avian physiology. In addition to pharmacists gaining knowledge in animal physiology, they should also be cognizant of the fact that many drugs used in veterinary medicine are not used in human medicine and therefore they may not know their attributes. The pharmacist who desires to practice in this area should undertake self-study to learn the chemical, biochemical (metabolism), pharmacological (mechanisms), therapeutic (clinical outcomes), and pharmaceutic (dosage forms) and pharmacokinetic characteristics of these compounds, which they probably did not learn in pharmacy school. It is hoped that this chapter will stimulate pharmacists and students of pharmacy to further study veterinary dosage form compounding and the proper use of veterinary drugs. In doing so they will gain the knowledge needed to be a source of information and provide products to veterinarians and the community they serve.

ACKNOWLEDGMENTS

The authors wish to acknowledge the assistance of Rita Mehmen for typing the manuscript and Scott F. Long, Ph.D., in reviewing this chapter.

REFERENCES

1. Feedstuffs, Animal Health Product Sales Rise in 1999, 72, (23) June 5, 2000, p. 5.
2. United States Pet Ownership Demographics Source Book, AVMA 1997.
3. The Drake Post-Scrip, Vol. 18, No. 1, 2 (Spring 1969).
4. J. P. McDonnell, Drake College of Pharmacy, Salsbury Laboratories Research Program, Iowa Pharm., 24, 10 (1969).
5. University of Iowa Bulletin, Catalog No. 1970–72.
6. Southwestern Oklahoma State University School of Pharmacy Bulletin 2000–2001, p. 10.
7. The University of Iowa College of Pharmacy News, Vol. 4, 2 (Spring 1988)
8. S. F. Long, Veterinary Therapeutics in Community Pharmacy Practice, Parts 1 and 2, Community Pharm., 92(4), 37 (July/August 2000).
9. J. P. McDonnell, Veterinary pharmaceutical dosage forms an overview. *Modern Pharmaceutics*, Gilbert S. Banker and Christopher T. Rhodes, ed. Marcel Dekker, New York 1995, pp. 877–880.
10. J. D. Baggot and S. A. Brown, Basis for selection of the dosage form. *Development and Formulation of Veterinary Dosage Forms*, 2nd ed. (Gregory E. Hardee and J. Desmond Baggot, Eds.), Marcel Dekker, New York, 1998, pp. 9–27.
11. T. B. Tribble, Feed Flavor and Animal Nutrition, AgriAids, Inc., Chicago, IL, 1962.
12. J. Blodinger, Formulation of Drug Dosage Forms for Animals, in Formulation of Veterinary Dosage Forms (J. Blodinger, ed.), Marcel Dekker, Inc., New York, 1983, pp. 139–142.
13. W. L. Larrabee, A Guide to Mixing Microingredients in Feed, Merck Services Bulletin, Rahway, NJ, 1976, p. 12.
14. W. L. Larrabee, Formulation of Drugs Given in Feed or Water, in Formulation of Veterinary Dosage Forms (J. Blodinger, ed.), Marcel Dekker, Inc., New York, 1983, p. 197.
15. Drug Stability Guidelines, Center for Veterinary Medicine, Food and Drug Administration, Fourth Revision, 1990, pp. 2–23.
16. H. L. Newmark and E. DeRitter, Animal Health Dosage Forms: Stability Requirements, in Animal Health Products Design and Evaluation (D. C. Monkhouse, ed.), American Pharmaceutical Association, Washington, DC, 1978, p. 133.
17. J. Blodinger, Formulation of Drug Dosage Forms for Animals, in Formulation of Veterinary Dosage Forms (J. Blodinger, ed.), Marcel Dekker, Inc., New York, 1983, p. 158.
18. D. G. Pope, Specialized Dose Dispensing Equipment, in Formulation of Veterinary Dosage Forms (J. Blodinger, ed.), Marcel Dekker, Inc., New York, 1983, p. 99.
19. D. G. Pope, in Formulation of Veterinary Dosage Forms (J. Blodinger, ed.), Marcel Dekker, New York, 1983, pp. 101–102.
20. D. G. Pope, Animal Health Specialized Delivery Systems, in Animal Health Products Design and Evaluation (D. C. Monkhouse, ed.), American Pharmaceutical Association, Washington, DC, 1978, pp. 87–90.
21. Code of Federal Regulations, 21 Part 514, New Animal Drug Applications, April 1, 2000.
22. Code of Federal Regulations, 21 Part 211, Current Good Manufacturing Practice for Finished Pharmaceuticals, April 1, 2000.
23. D. G. Jorgan, Compounding for animals—a birds eye view, Int. J. Pharm. Compounding, 1(4), 222 (July/August 1997).

Chapter 24

Dietary Supplements

Teresa Bailey Klepser

Ferris State University, Big Rapids, Michigan

I. INTRODUCTION

Because of the public's interest in taking an active part in their health, there has been a dramatic increase in the use of products variously termed natural products, herbal products, nutraceuticals, and dietary supplements. Pharmacists need to be aware of the legitimate and possible beneficial effects of some of these products, but perhaps more critically they must understand their potentially harmful effects and interactions with prescription and over-the-counter (OTC) products. Additionally, since government regulations regarding the use and control of these products are admittedly inadequate, pharmacists need to be aware of the current and evolving regulations that do cover these products. Methods of judging the possible quality, a special challenge for these products, will be discussed. The labeling of these products also differs and needs to be understood. Liability issues are another important consideration for pharmacists when dealing with these products.

II. DEFINITIONS

A. Alternative Medicine

"Alternative medicine" includes all of the approaches and techniques that until the past few years were not taught in medical schools and residencies. Alternative medicine is also referred to as "complementary medicine," "unconventional medicine," or "holistic medicine." Some of the categories of alternative medicine include mind-body interventions, such as hypnosis, meditation, and relaxation therapies, manual healing methods such as chiropractic manipulation and massage, herbal medicine, and diet and nutrition [1].

B. Dietary Supplements

The Dietary Supplement Health and Education Act of 1994 defines dietary supplements as: (a) a product (other than tobacco) intended to supplement the diet that bears or contains one or more of the following dietary ingredients: a vitamin, mineral, amino acid, herb, or other botanical; (b) a dietary substance for use to supplement the diet by increasing the total dietary intake; or (c) a concentrate, metabolite, constituent, extract, or combination of any ingredient described above. A dietary supplement also must be intended for ingestion in the form of a capsule, powder, softgel, or gelcap but is not considered a drug or a food [2].

C. Categories

Dietary supplements are divided into many categories, including vitamins, minerals, amino acids, plant derivatives, animal derivatives, and thyroid derivatives. Plant derivatives may be obtained from any part of a plant and are known as botanicals or herbs. Examples include but are not limited to echinacea, garlic, ginkgo, ginseng, and St. John's wort. Animal derivatives are derived from animal parts and include shark cartilage, glucosamine derived from bovine cartilage, and chondroitin derived from shellfish.

D. Delivery Forms

Dietary supplements are available in a variety of delivery forms such as capsules, tablets, teas, tinctures, extracts, and bulk herbs. Sixty-eight percent of the herbal products available are in the form of a capsule or tablet. Approximately half of the herbal preparations contain a single herb [3]. An example of a softgel is Saw Palmetto Complex by PhytoPharmica.

Enteric-coated tablets or capsules of garlic are better absorbed since an active ingredient, allicin, is acid labile. The tablets or capsules bypass the stomach and release their contents in the alkaline medium of the small intestine [4].

Intravenous preparations of herbs are available in other countries. An intravenous preparation of ginkgo is manufactured in Europe but is not available in the United States.

Water extracts may be prepared from crude bulk botanical herbs and may be subdivided into infusions or decoctions. The gentler process of the two is the process used to produce infusions. Infusions, also known as teas, are prepared by pouring boiling water over the herb and letting it steep. An example of an herbal tea is chamomile tea. Infusions are generally made with the leaves and flowers of the plant. The active constituents of some herbs are water insoluble and may be ineffective when prepared as a tea. An example of a water-insoluble herb is saw palmetto berries [5,6]. Decoctions are prepared by boiling the herb directly in the water, letting it simmer, then straining to remove the bulk plant material. Decoctions are good for plant materials that need softening before the active constituents can be released, such as the roots and bark of a plant. An example of a decoction is the aqueous extract of valerian root [5,6].

Hydroalcoholic extracts are made when the active constituents are insoluble in water or when a concentrated dosage form is desired. Hydroalcoholic extracts use concentrated alcohol in varying proportions with water as a solvent. Hydroalcoholic extracts are categorized as tinctures or fluid extracts, depending on the amount of alcohol used. Some patients who simply do not like the taste of alcohol may be counseled to put the dosage of tincture drops into a cup of hot liquid and let it stand for a few minutes to evaporate off most of the alcohol before ingestion. An example of an ethanolic extract is echinacea [5,6].

Glycerites are glycerin-extracted preparations and are alcohol-free. Although glycerin tastes sweet, it is not considered a "sugar." Although glycerin is considered a poor solvent for many of the active components found in herbs, glycerin may be useful in pediatric preparations and in patients who have conditions that require a sugar-free preparation. Glycerites are less stable than alcoholic extracts [5].

Some herbs may be available in many dosage forms, and the form may affect the dose that is given. Recommended dosages include 2–3 g of dried valerian or valerian extract given one to several times a day, or as a tea with 2–3 g of valerian being used per cup one to several times a day, with 2.5 g being equivalent to one teaspoon [7]. The recommended dose of valerian tincture is one half to one teaspoonful (2.5–5 mL) one to several times daily.

E. Preparations

Some herbal products are prepared from a mixture of different plant species and plant parts. Hawthorn is standardized to contain 5% oligomeric procyanidins made from the leaves, blossoms, and fruit of *Crataegus laevigata* and *Crataegus monogyna* [6]. Studies have shown that the therapeutic efficacy of hawthorn is not solely the result of one type of component, one plant part, or a single species [6].

Some herbs are standardized for several active constituents, while others are standardized to a single active ingredient. St. John's wort is standardized to contain 0.3% hypericin, whereas ginkgo is standardized to contain 24% flavone glycosides and 6% terpene lactones. However, standardizing an herb product to one or more plant component(s) that are identifiable by assay may be incorrect. Many herbalists believe that the whole plant contributes to the efficacy and that there are many unknown active compounds in each plant [6].

There are differences between the dried powder and fresh herb. For some herbs, the dried powder is more effective; for others the opposite is true. The majority of the clinical studies of garlic's effect in reducing cholesterol have shown 0.6–1.2 g of dried powder containing approximately 2–5 mg of the active ingredient allicin, 18 mg garlic oil, or 10 g fresh garlic taken daily to be effective doses [6]. However, the dried powder was shown to be less effective than fresh garlic. On the other hand, 5 g of fresh ginger was needed to produce an equivalent effect to 1–2 g of powdered dry ginger root [6].

Herbal preparations may be prepared by freeze-drying or air-drying. Fresh, freeze-dried leaves of nettle were shown to be effective for symptomatic relief in allergic rhinitis. The active components in nettle, histamine and acetylcholine, became ineffective when the leaves were air-dried [6]. Other herbals remain effective when air-dried.

III. PREVALENCE

A. Alternative Medicine

The popularity of alternative medicines continues to grow in our society. In a report published in 1993, Eisenberg and colleagues estimated that one out of every three people in the United States had experimented with at least one form of alternative medicine [8]. It was also noted that the use of alternative therapies was a relatively widespread phenomenon and did not differ by gender or insurance status. The authors did report, however, that usage patterns vary among ethnic groups, with the use of alternative medicines greatest among whites and less common among African Americans, Hispanics, and Asians. Furthermore, significantly higher rates of use were noted among individuals with incomes greater than $35,000, aged 25–49 years, and possessing some college education. Unfortunately, the results of this study were not stratified according to the type of alternative medicine utilized, for example, herbal therapies, massage therapy, and healing touch. As a result, consumer demographics for individuals using herbal products were not specified.

A follow-up study examined trends in the use of alternative therapies in the United States [9]. This report demonstrated an increase in the number of respondents using alternative therapies from 33.8% in 1990 to 42.7% in 1997 [9]. Alternative therapies that experienced the greatest increase in use included herbal medicines, massage therapy, megavitamins, self-help groups, folk remedies, energy healing, and homeopathy [9]. Furthermore, the authors estimated that consumers in the United States spent approximately $5.1 billion on herbal therapies alone in 1997 [9]. This survey also revealed the high prevalence of concurrent consumption of herbal therapies and prescription medications. In fact, it was estimated that approximately 15 million adults had consumed dietary supplements, including herbs, concurrently with prescription medications.

B. Dietary Supplements

According to retail sales data, patients spent $3.24 billion for herbal therapies in 1997 [10]. It is estimated that a third of the nation's adults spend an average of $54 per year on herbal remedies [10]. The top 10 herbs based on sales in 1995 listed in descending order were echinacea, garlic, goldenseal, Asian and American ginseng, ginkgo biloba, saw palmetto, aloe, ma huang, Siberian ginseng, and cranberry [3]. Since then, newer herbs have become more popular. In 1999, the top 10 herbs were, in descending order, ginkgo, St. John's wort, ginseng, garlic, echinacea/goldenseal, saw palmetto, kava, pycnogenol/grape seed, cranberry, and valerian [11].

IV. HISTORY OF HERBS

Many of the prescription and nonprescription medications available on the U.S. market are derived from natural animal and plant sources. It is estimated that a third of the medications available on the market are still or were originally derived from plants. Some of those include aspirin from willow bark, digoxin from *Digitalis purpurea*, ephedrine from various *Ephedra* species, psyllium from the *Plantago* species, and vincristine and vinblastine from *Catharanthus roseus*, formerly known as *Vinca rosea*. There were only a few synthetically produced drugs before the 1900s. Herbs are not currently considered drugs by U.S. Food and Drug Administration (FDA) regulations.

V. U.S. REGULATIONS

A. Federal Food, Drug, and Cosmetic Act of 1938 and the Kefauver-Harris Drug Amendment of 1962

The Federal Food, Drug, and Cosmetic Act (FDCA) of 1938 and the Kefauver-Harris Drug Amendment of 1962 require pharmaceutical manufacturers to demonstrate the safety and efficacy of their products before marketing to the general public. Prior to the enactment of these regulations, herbal products had been widely touted as remedies for ailments ranging from anxiety to heart failure. The patent remedy era, when virtually any herbal or other concoction could be marketed and labeled as a sure cure for any ailment, that predated these regulations is described in Chapter 1. Following the passage of these laws, many companies complied by either demonstrating safety and efficacy or removing products from the marketplace. However, as a result of ambiguity in the legislation, manufacturers were able to reclassify herbal products as nutritional supplements and continue to sell these compounds in the absence of safety and efficacy data as long as no claims of efficacy were printed on the product label.

B. Dietary Supplement Act of 1994

The Dietary Supplement Health and Education Act (DSHEA) of 1994 classifies herbal products as dietary supplements. Dietary supplements are not allowed to make any claims of therapeutic efficacy, only claims of effects on body structure or function. Dietary supplements are not allowed to make any claims as to effects on diseases. Under this provision a manufacturer could claim, for example, that St. John's wort enhances mood or that Asian ginseng gives your body energy, but it could not claim that St. John's wort treats depression or that Asian ginseng treats chronic fatigue syndrome. If a manufacturer states a claim of therapeutic efficacy such as treatment of a disease, the manufacturer must notify the Secretary of Health and Human Services within 30 days after making this claim. According to this Act, dietary supplements are required to include the following statement on the product label: "This statement has not been evaluated by the FDA. This product is not intended to diagnose, treat, cure, or prevent any disease." The Act allows the Secretary of Health and Human Services to remove a supplement from the market only when the product has been shown to be hazardous [12]. The Act allows the use of publication material to promote products as long as the information is not false or misleading, does not promote a particular manufacturer or brand, presents a balanced view of available scientific information, physically separate from the product, and must have no appended information to the publication such as stickers. The Act also developed the Office of Dietary Supplements at the National Institutes of Health to conduct scientific research on dietary supplements.

C. New Labeling for Dietary Supplements

As of January 6, 2000, FDA issued new regulations on structure/function claims for dietary supplements and redefined the definition of disease [13]. The previous definition of disease was "any deviation from, impairment of, or interruption of the normal structure or function of any part, organ, or system of the body that is manifested by a characteristic set of one or more signs or symptoms, including laboratory or clinical measurements that are characteristic of a disease" [13]. The new definition of disease is "damage to an organ, part, structure, or system of the body such that it does not function properly, or a state of health leading to such as; except that diseases resulting from essential nutrient deficiencies are not included in this definition" [13]. Therefore, if a dietary supplement were implied to help any damage to an organ, this would be mislabeling. For example, calcium may not be marketed for the treatment of osteoporosis but may be marketed as support for menopausal women.

The new labeling also states that if a dietary supplement suggested a disease in the name of the product, the manufacturer would be violating DSHEA. Examples given are Hepatacure and Raynaudin—Hepatacure suggests a cure for hepatitis and Raynaudin suggests a cure for Raynaud's disease [13]. Some claims used by over-the-counter products may be allowed as structure/function claims. Some OTC claims include antacid, antigas, laxative, stool softener, stimulant, and nighttime sleep aid.

D. FDA's Dietary Supplement Strategy (10-Year Plan)

By the year 2010, FDA will have a science-based regulatory program that fully implements the DSHEA. The plan addresses safety, labeling, clarification of the differences between drugs and dietary supplements, and enforcement activities.

VI. REGULATIONS IN OTHER COUNTRIES

A. Canada

Under the Canadian regulatory system, known as the Canadian Health Protection Branch, herbs are considered either as food or drugs. If considered a drug, herbs can be sold by prescription or nonprescription. The manufacturer must prove safety, efficacy, standardization, and stability in order to make a therapeutic claim for an herbal product or to market it in a quantity known to be therapeutic. Nonprescription medications are known in the industry by the Drug Identification Number (DIN). Unlike the U.S. FDA nonprescription medications classified by a particular category such as analgesic, cough syrup, or sleep aid, the Canadian DIN is a registration system that is product specific [14]. Only one herb, feverfew, has gone through the standard process of premarket authorization in order to obtain a DIN in Canada to be used for the prophylaxis of migraines [5].

B. Germany

In terms of legislative regulation of herbal products, several countries are more advanced compared to the United States and Canada. In Western Europe herbal medicines are often approved as prescription or nonprescription medications.

In 1978 the German Federal Health Agency established the German Commission E, a regulatory body that primarily evaluates the safety and efficacy of herbs based on clinical trials, cases, and other scientific literature. The German Commission E has published more than 320 monographs on herbs, which were translated into English by the American Botanical Council. Many of the German Commission E recommendations are used by health care practitioners in the United States.

When an herb is found to be toxic, the herb is withdrawn from the German market. Comfrey is no longer available in Germany because of its carcinogenicity. Unfortunately, however, comfrey is still available in the United States [15].

Not only does Germany require that herbal products be proven safe and effective, they must also be available as standardized products.

C. Hong Kong

After several reports of severe poisonings related to herbal medications in 1989, the Hong Kong government appointed a Working Party to review and make recommendations on the use and practice of Traditional Chinese Medicine (TCM) [16]. Since then, the Working Party has made recommendations regarding the registration of TCM practitioners, the restricted use of potent Chinese medicine, the processing, manufacturing, and trading of Chinese medicines, the training and research in TCM, the training of dispensers, and public education [16]. The Working Party has identified at least 31 potent Chinese medicines as causing adverse effects.

VII. DIETARY SUPPLEMENT CONCERNS

Because dietary supplements are exempt from legislation requiring postmarketing surveillance of safety, data regarding the safety profiles of many dietary supplements are scarce. Furthermore, it has been noted that patients are less likely to voluntarily report the occurrence of an adverse drug reaction resulting from the use of an herbal product compared with adverse events resulting from consumption of prescription medications [17]. Therefore, this puts the burden of identifying and reporting adverse events related to dietary supplements on health care providers. Despite a relative lack of published safety data for most herbal products, the need for pharmacovigilance is apparent.

A. Unsafe Dietary Supplements

A national survey found that a majority of interviewed consumers who use herbals reported they feel herbs are just as effective, safe, and cost-effective as nonherbal remedies [10]. The majority thought herbals were good or better than nonherbal remedies in the areas of efficacy (53%), safety (65%), and cost (58%) [10]. However, the safety issue may be a false and potentially dangerous belief. Some herbs have been shown to contain constituents that are carcinogenic or hepatotoxic [18]. Herbs considered to be carcinogenic include borage (*Borago officinalis*), calamus (*Acorus calamus*), coltsfoot (*Tussilago farfar*), comfrey (*Symphytum* species), life root (*Senecio aureus*), and sassafras (*Sassafras albidum*) [18]. These herbs, with the exception of calamus and sassafras, contain pyrrolizidine alkaloids that have been proven to produce hepatic carcinomas in animals. The German Federal Health Agency has established regulations regarding the amount of pyrrolizidine alkaloids that may be contained in these herbs to ensure safety; however, the same is not true in the United States. According to current regulations in the United States, products need not identify the amount of pyrrolizidine alkaloids, making preparations containing these herbs potentially unsafe. Safrole in sassafras and *cis*-isoasarone in calamus have demonstrated carcinogenic potential in animals in the United States [18].

Herbal remedies that have been reported to be hepatotoxic include chaparral (*Larrea tridentata*), germander (*Teucrium chamaedrys*), and life root (*Senecio aureus*) [18]. Cases reported patients developing jaundice, fatigue, pruritus, markedly elevated serum liver enzyme levels, severe cholestasis, hepatitis, and hepatocellular injury or necrosis documented by serial liver biopsies [19–21]. Signs and symptoms may occur as early as 3 weeks to as late as 7 months following ingestion [20,21].

Licorice (*Glycyrrhiza glabra*) is another herb that is now considered to be potentially harmful. When used in high doses for long periods of time, licorice may cause pseudoaldosteronism, a state that may result in headache, lethargy, sodium and water retention, hypokalemia, hypertension, heart failure, and cardiac arrest. In an effort to minimize the risk of adverse effects, the German Commission E recommends that licorice be used for no longer than 4–6 weeks. The use of licorice is contraindicated in patients with liver cirrhosis, cholestatic liver disorders, hypertonia, kidney diseases, hypokalemia, pregnancy, and cardiovascular diseases [22]. Although licorice products are currently available in the United States, patients should be advised to use licorice only under the supervision of a physician.

Ma Huang (*Ephedra sinica*) is another potentially harmful herb that is available in the United States. Claims of utility of Ma Huang for the treatment of bronchial asthma, cold and flu symptoms, fevers or chills, headaches and other aches, edema, and lack of perspiration have been made [23]. Ma Huang contains approximately 1% of ephedrine and therefore possesses central nervous stimulatory potential [24]. However, ephedrine is difficult to extract and purify from Ma Huang, so it presently has no street value.

Ma Huang is contraindicated in patients with heart conditions, hypertension, diabetes, or thyroid disease or who are taking a monoamine oxidase inhibitor. Drug interactions listed for Ma Huang may be similar to those of ephedrine and include such agents as theophylline and the cardiac glycosides. Being a stimulant itself, patients taking Ma Huang should avoid consumption of caffeine-containing products. Side effects noted for Ma Huang include nervousness, insomnia, headache, dizziness, skin flushing, tingling, vomiting, palpitations, hypertension, and myocardial infarction [18,24]. Because of its stimulant properties and serious side effect profile, patients should be urged to use Ma Huang only under medical supervision.

Some products available on the market contain a combination of Ma Huang and St. John's wort and are referred to as "herbal phen-fen." "Phen-fen" received its name when the combination of phentermine and fenfluramine were used for weight loss. "Herbal phen-fen" is touted as a natural and effective weight loss agent that does not contain phentermine or fenfluramine. However, "herbal phen-fen" carries the same warnings that apply to Ma Huang and St. John's wort when each is used alone. Furthermore, there are no clinical studies to support the use of "herbal phen-fen."

B. Active Ingredients

In the early 1900s, the U.S. Pharmacopeia, National Formulary had excellent quality control guidelines and safe dosages for hundreds of herbs [25]. Products that are labeled as conforming to the U.S. Pharmacopeia (USP) or National Formulary (NF) standards should be recommended whenever possible. A product labeled as USP indicates that the active ingredient has been approved by the FDA or, alternately, that the use has been accepted by the USP. If the label contains the NF designation, the product has been neither approved by the FDA nor accepted by the USP, but the product has been generally recognized as safe by experts. Any product with safety problems may not obtain either the USP or NF label. Most vitamins and minerals conform to USP standards [26].

The main concern for quality assurance for dietary supplements is that the correct ingredient is used. Incorrect ingredients may be used via adulteration, erroneous substitution of products, or lack of routine tests to monitor the presence of the "intended" amounts of an active ingredient before and after processing [16].

Potency of various compounds is affected by species variety; growing conditions such as geographical and soil differences, differences in sunlight, temperature, and rainfall; harvest time; drying; storage; handling; and preparation. The chemical composition of ginseng products may vary as a result of the plant extract derivative, age of the root, location where the plant is grown, harvest season, and method of drying. Different active constituents, also known as ginsenosides, are present in varying quantities in different parts of the ginseng plant, with the root believed to contain the highest concentration of active ingredients [27]. Cultivation during autumn and allowing at least 5–6 years of growth yields more ginsenosides. Air-versus steam-drying significantly influences the concentration of various ginsenosides in the final product; air-drying produces white ginseng, steam produces red ginseng [27]. At least 28 ginsenosides have been isolated [28]: R_1, R_4, R_{a1}, R_{a2}, R_{a3}, R_{b1}, R_{b2}, R_{b3}, malonyl-R_{b1}, malonyl-R_{b2}, R_c, malonyl-R_c, R_d, malonyl-R_d, R_e, R_f, 20-R_f, R_{g1}, R_{g2}, R_{g3}, 20-R_{g2}, 20-R_{g3}, R_{h1}, R_{h2}, 20-R_{h1}, Ro, R_{s1}, R_{s2}. Each ginsenoside produces different pharmacological effects on the central nervous system, cardiovascular system, and other body systems [20]. Different ginsenosides are capable of producing biological effects in direct opposition to those produced by others. For example, R_{b1} has been shown to have a suppressive effect the central nervous system, whereas R_{g1} produces a stimulatory effect [28]. R_{b1} has been shown to suppress aggressive episodes in mice, whereas R_{g1} had no effect [27]. R_{b1}, R_{b2}, R_c, R_d, and R_e have been reported to possess anti-stress properties [28]. Ginsenosides have demonstrated the ability to cause modest reductions in blood glucose and an increase in blood insulin [28]. R_{g1} stimulates DNA, protein, and lipid synthesis in rat bone marrow cells while R_{b1} increases RNA synthesis [28]. Analgesia and anti-inflammatory effects have been reported with some ginsenosides [28]. Hypertensive and hypotensive effects have also been noted with different ginsenosides [27].

Ginseng R_{g2} has shown inhibitory effects on platelet aggregation similar to aspirin, and R_o reportedly inhibits the conversion of fibrinogen to fibrin [27]. The amount of ginseng administered may also influence the effect(s) produced. In rats and mice, small doses of ginseng extract result in increased spontaneous motor activity, whereas larger doses produce an inhibitory effect on the central nervous system [28].

C. Standardization

Standardization is the process by which all batches of a dietary supplement produced by a single manufacturer contain the same amount of active ingredient(s) [29]. FDA does not require dietary supplements to be standardized. Consumers cannot be certain of the quality of a dietary supplement when purchased. Uncertainties include whether the herb's active ingredients are in the product, whether the ingredients are bioavailable, whether the dose is appropriate, and whether each batch contains the same components in the same quantity. Each dietary supplement may vary depending on the manufacturer, and therefore switching brands of a particular supplement is not advisable.

Some studies have evaluated the quantity of a specific constituent in various herbal products by a thin-layer chromatography spectrophotometric method. Of 44 feverfew products that were evaluated, 14 (32%) did not contain the minimum of 0.2% parthenolide content (active ingredient) and 10 (22%) did not contain any detectable levels of parthenolide [30].

Good manufacturing practices (GMPs) ensure that products meet specific quality standards, are not adulterated or misbranded, and contain the correct ingredients and doses stated on the label. GMPs specifically for dietary supplements are being proposed from the FDA. Cases of adulteration have been reported to the FDA, and examples include a plantain product adulterated with digitalis and hibiscus tea adulterated with warfarin [29].

Some clinical trials utilize standardized products. Many studies show the effectiveness of garlic on systolic and diastolic blood pressures and hypercholesterolemia [31]. Furthermore, meta-analysis suggests that garlic reduces systolic blood pressure 7.7 mmHg more than placebo (95% CI 5.0–17.2). Likewise, the pooled reduction in diastolic blood pressure was 5.0 mmHg greater with garlic (95% CI 3.4–9.6). Additionally, the meta-analysis demonstrated a statistically significant decrease in overall total cholesterol levels with garlic compared to placebo—mean decrease of 23 mg/dL (95% CI −29 to −17) ($p < 0.001$). Fortunately, all of the studies used the same dried garlic powder preparation (Kwai®)* in doses ranging from 600 to 900 mg daily (equivalent of 1.8–2.7 g/day of fresh garlic) for 1–12 months. Kwai is available commercially in the United States. If available, the commercial products that are used in clinical trials and demonstrated to have either efficacy or safety should be recommended to patients.

Unfortunately, not all products that are used in clinical trials are available in the United States. In a randomized, double-blind, multicenter European study, 1069 men with moderate benign prostatic hyperplasia were randomized to receive saw palmetto (Permixon®)† 160 mg twice daily (90% free and 7% esterified fatty acids) or finasteride 5 mg once daily for 6 months [32]. As determined by patients and physicians, Permixon offered similar improvement in symptoms related to benign prostatic hyperplasia compared to finasteride. Since Permixon is not available in the United States, it should be recommended to patients to use a product that is similar to Permixon that contains a standardized extract of saw palmetto containing 85–95% sterols and fatty acids [18].

ConsumerLab.com is an independent testing company that evaluates whether certain dietary supplements have met their standardization claims. Dietary supplements that have been tested include herbs (ginkgo, saw palmetto, ginseng), vitamins (vitamin C), and others (glucosamine, chondroitin, SAMe). Products that meet the German testing standards are published at the ConsumerLab.com website [33].

D. Labeling

Product labels may be incorrect, accidentally or intentionally. Herbs may be mislabeled accidentally because of misidentification or the wrong part of the plant was picked. Other products may be mislabeled intentionally—a ginseng label may not disclose that the product contains mandrake (scopolamine) or snakeroot (reserpine) because of the high cost of pure ginseng [34]. Some herbal products may not declare the addition of prescription medications such as corticosteroids.

---

* Kwai®— manufacturer: Lichtwer Pharma GmbH, Berlin, Germany.

† Permixon®— manufacturer: Pierre Fabre, France.

E. Mechanism of Action

Many herbs have mechanisms of action and active ingredients that are similar to prescription or non-prescription medications. For example, the mechanism of action of saw palmetto is unknown but is believed to be multifaceted. In vitro data suggest two probable primary mechanisms of action: the inhibition of the binding of dihydrotestosterone to androgen receptors in prostate cells [35] and the inhibition of testosterone-5-α-reductase, the enzyme responsible for the conversion of testosterone to dihydrotestosterone [36]. Additional mechanisms of action may include inhibition of prolactin binding, inhibition of 5-lipoxygenase metabolite production, inhibition of growth factors involved in prostate cell proliferation, anti-estrogenic activity, and anti-edemic activity [36]. Since saw palmetto may have a mechanism of action similar to finasteride—the inhibition of testosterone-5-α-reductase—a clinical trial was performed and it was found to have similar efficacy.

Garlic's proven mechanisms of action include (a) inhibition of platelet function, (b) increased levels of two antioxidant enzymes, catalase and glutathione peroxidase, and (c) inhibition of thiol enzymes such as coenzyme A and HMG coenzyme A reductase. Garlic's anti-hyperlipidemic effects are believed to be in part due to the HMG coenzyme A reductase inhibition since prescription medications for hyperlipidemia have that mechanism of action (statins). It is unknown whether garlic would have the same drug interactions, side effects, and need for precautions as the statins.

F. Cautions

Some dietary supplements have no known precautions, while others have many precautions and contraindications. It is recommended that the use of ginseng be avoided in patients with hypertension, psychological imbalances, headaches, heart palpitations, insomnia, asthma, inflammation, infections with high fever, or pregnancy and in children [37].

Many dietary supplements should be avoided in pregnancy because they may have emmenagogue activity, promoting menstruation. Some herbs that are considered emmenagogues are feverfew, garlic, and hawthorn [4]. St. John's wort should be avoided in pregnancy due to its emmenagogue and abortifacient properties.

Some precautions may be similar to precautions for prescription or non-prescription medications. Precautions for valerian are similar to those for benzodiazepines, barbiturates, and opiates. Caution is recommended when ingesting valerian while driving or performing other tasks requiring alertness and coordination.

Some precautions are based on the dietary supplement's side effect profile. St. John's wort may induce photosensitivity; therefore, fair-skinned persons should be cautioned about exposure to bright sunlight while taking the herb.

G. Adverse Effects

A dietary supplement may be safe when taken in the recommended doses but may become dangerous in higher doses. However, patients may develop side effects even when ingesting recommended doses. Adverse reactions may be due to allergic reactions, dietary supplements containing toxic substances, misidentification of plant, mislabeling of plant, natural toxic substances such as pyrrolizidine alkaloids in comfrey, unnatural toxic substances such as heavy metals, or pesticides.

Side effects may be as mild and rare as headache, nausea, and stomach upset for saw palmetto [23,24]. However, some supplements may have serious side effects. Hypertension, euphoria, restlessness, nervousness, insomnia, skin eruptions, edema, and diarrhea were reported in 22 patients following long-term ginseng use at an average dose of 3 g of ginseng root daily [38]. Side effects reported with valerian use include headaches, hangover, excitability, insomnia, uneasiness, and cardiac disturbances. Valerian toxicity including ataxia, decreased sensibility, hypothermia, hallucinations, and increased muscle relaxation have been reported [39].

Ginkgo is generally safe and well tolerated; however, there is a case report of a 70-year-old man who developed a spontaneous hyphema after ingesting ginkgo 40 mg twice daily for one week [40]. His only other medication was aspirin 325 mg daily, which he had been taking for 3 years. There is also a case report of a 33-year-old woman who developed bilateral subdural hematomas after taking ginkgo 60 mg twice daily for 2 years [41]. She had no significant medical history, and her other medications were acetaminophen and a brief trial of ergotamine/caffeine [41]. A third case describes a 72-year-old woman who developed a left frontal subdural hematoma after taking ginkgo 50 mg three times daily for 6–7 months [42]. It remains unknown whether these cases are coincidence or causality. The most commonly reported side effects with ginkgo include gastric disturbances, headache, dizziness, and vertigo. One case report of a toxic ingestion of 50 seeds of ginkgo that resulted in tonic-clonic seizures and loss of consciousness has been published [23].

Unfortunately, clinical trials in human volunteers usually have small sample sizes and adverse reactions are poorly documented. Also, adverse effects that have a long latency period such as carcinogenicity are difficult to account for.

H. Drug–Dietary Supplement Interactions

Although many medications and herbals may be safe when used alone, the risk of significant drug interactions increases when multiple agents are used in combination. Sequelae resulting from such hazardous interactions may lead to discomfort, exacerbation of an underlying illness, and possibly death.

Although many patients believe that dietary supplements will not interact with medications, recent literature suggests otherwise. Recently, many St. John's wort–drug interactions have been reported in the literature. Cases of patients developing symptoms of serotonin syndrome have been reported with St. John's wort alone and in concomitant therapy with other antidepressants such as monoamine oxidase inhibitors, serotonin reuptake inhibitors, and venlafaxine. St. John's wort may exacerbate the sedative effects of benzodiazepines, alcohol, narcotics, and other sedatives. St. John's wort may decrease the levels of protease inhibitors, cyclosporine, digoxin, and theophylline.

Two case reports describe symptoms such as insomnia, headache, tremulousness, irritability, and visual hallucinations when taking phenelzine concurrently with ginseng [43,44]. Reduction of the international normalized ratio (INR) may be observed when ginseng and warfarin are taken together [45].

Many dietary supplements have antiplatelet activity, which may increase the risk of bleeding when used concurrently with anticoagulants. Feverfew inhibits cyclooxygenase and phospholipase A_2 and may interact with anticoagulants and potentiate the antiplatelet effect of aspirin. Other supplements that possess antiplatelet activity include but are not limited to garlic, ginkgo, vitamin E, vitamin A, and selenium.

Although health care practitioners may intervene and help patients avoid harmful drug-herb combinations, patients may not inform their health care providers (physicians, pharmacists, and nurses), voluntarily or following inquisition, about their use of unconventional therapies.

I. Dietary Supplement Expense

Costs to the patient and costs of individual products are variable but may be substantial. An epidemiological study of human immunodeficiency virus (HIV)–infected patients found that patients spent an average of $18 per month on herbs (range, $0–175) [46]. Unfortunately most U.S. prescription insurance companies do not cover the cost of dietary supplements. One exception is the American Western Life Insurance Company, San Mateo, California, which offers their subscribers a "Prevention Plus" option that covers herbal medicines [34]. In Germany, herbs that are prescribed by physicians are covered by insurance, whereas non-prescription herbs are not covered [34].

J. American Herbal Products Association

The American Herbal Products Association developed by-laws to define "obligations of membership" that include "adherence to all policies and business practices as outlined in the Code of Ethics." Some of the recommendations encourage the discontinuation of trade of certain species such as wild-harvested lady's slipper, *Cypripedium* spp. Some recommendations regard labeling of products such as chaparral and ephedra. Labeling of chaparral should include the caution of liver disease and ephedra labeling should include the cautions of pregnancy, hypertension, heart disease, thyroid disease, diabetes, prostate enlargement, and prescription medication use [47]. Recommendations also relate to maximum dosage such as that for kava formulations, which should be limited to 300 mg of total kavalactones per day.

VIII. RESEARCH

A. Concerns

Unfortunately, many clinical studies evaluating the efficacy of dietary supplements are flawed. Some of the flaws in the studies include non-randomization, being unblinded, lack of standardized products, small sample sizes, short treatment durations, and poorly defined inclusion and exclusion criteria. Many studies do not give detailed information about the dietary supplement used. When an herb is studied, the following information should be described: plant species, part(s) used, product form (e.g., powdered crude herb, aqueous extract, ethanol extract, or aqueous alcohol extract) with stated proportions of water to alcohol, specifically extracted fractions, and quantities or concentrations used [48].

Some studies compare dietary supplements to subtherapeutic dosages of prescription medicine. For example, St. John's wort is compared to some of the tricyclic antidepressants. However, the given doses of amitriptyline and imipramine were below the recommended antidepressant doses.

Another problem with research is that many of the studies are not published in English. Many studies are published in the Chinese, Russian, and French medical literature.

B. U.S. Herbal Companies

Controlled studies of herbal medicines may not be profitable. There is little motivation for herbal manufacturers to conduct randomized, placebo-controlled, double-blind clinical trials to prove efficacy. Herbal companies are not required to do so based on the Dietary Supplement Act of 1994. Also, dietary supplement companies cannot patent a product from nature. However, patents may be developed for an active component of a plant, extraction or purification, a novel pharmaceutical dosage form, or a novel extraction procedure. U.S. Patent 5,976,548 describes the composition and method of making a dietary supplement containing antioxidants, barley grass extract, vitamins, minerals, and ginkgo [49]. A patent owned by La Jolla Diagnostics describes a novel method of formulation of feverfew into a highly absorbable saline solution, known as ClusterWater [50].

C. U.S. Pharmaceutical Companies

Some pharmaceutical companies such as Bayer, Warner-Lambert, and American Home Products manufacture dietary supplements. Bayer Corporation has developed the herbal line of One-A-Day Specialized Supplements such as Cold Season, Bone Strength, and Menopause Health. Warner-Lambert developed the Quanterra line of herbal supplements such as Quanterra Mental Sharpness and Quanterra Prostate. Centrum Herbals, featuring echinacea, garlic, ginkgo, and St. John's wort, are manufactured by American Home Products. While major pharmaceutical companies are now marketing herbal products, there are many herbal products companies with no experience in producing prescription products under drug GMP and GLP guidelines. Other dietary supplements, such as *S*-adenosylmethionine (SAM-e), are becoming available as companies such as Knoll Pharmaceuticals enter the business [51]. Occassionally a natural product becomes a prescription medication, as recently occurred with Prometrium®, which contains natural micronized progesterone in a peanut oil base.

D. National Institutes of Health

In 1994 the Dietary Supplement Act developed the Office of Dietary Supplements (ODS) at the National Institutes of Health (NIH) to conduct scientific research on dietary supplements. The ODS plans, organizes, and supports conferences, workshops, and symposia on scientific topics related to dietary supplements. As an office in the Office of the Director at the NIH, the ODS does not have the authority to directly fund investigator-initiated research grant applications. Instead the ODS conducts research either through contracts such as the Public Information Center Needs Assessment Survey, which was initiated by the ODS and is being conducted on contract and in collaboration with the USDA, or by funding grants to scientific investigators in cooperation with the Institutes and Centers at NIH [52].

IX. PHARMACIST'S ROLE

A. Educational Concerns

As the trend for herbal usage has increased rapidly over the past decade, the number of Colleges of Pharmacy in the United States offering courses addressing herbal therapies has declined. According to Miller et al., only 9 of 77 pharmacy colleges maintained pharmacognosy as a course in their curriculum [53]. Many colleges had discontinued that course in the late 1970s to allow more clinically oriented courses to be developed. Although many institutions eliminated pharmacognosy as a full course, 74% reported offering at least one course in which herbal therapies were addressed; however, only one third of these courses were required. Furthermore, the average credit hours for these courses addressing herbal therapies was 2.78 (range 1–8), and only 38% of the course content was devoted to discussing herbal therapies. As a result, most pharmacists are not adequately equipped to meet the demand for their patients' requests regarding information on herbal products. Pharmacists are becoming knowledgeable about dietary supplements despite this. Pharmacists increase their knowledge base via continuing education programs, self-instruction, and herbal science bachelor programs. Continuing education programs are offered through national, state, and local pharmacy organizations and Colleges of Pharmacy. Bastyr University, Kenmore, Washington, started offering a bachelor's program in herbal sciences in the fall of 2001 which focuses on plant identification, pharmacology, and herbal product manufacturing.

B. Resources

Information resources on dietary supplements are available on the Internet, via textbooks, and through Medline searches. The reliability and credibility of some resources is lacking. Pharmacists need to evaluate the information and to choose reputable sources. The following should be evaluated to determine whether the resource is reliable and credible [54].

1. Who maintains the web site? Is it funded by a dietary supplement company? If so, it may contain biased information.
2. Who wrote the information? Is the author a university professor or a health care professional?
3. When was the resource last updated? The information may not be accurate if it is not current.
4. How is the resource funded? Is the resource provided by a dietary supplement company or by a university?
5. Is there a formal review mechanism for the information?
6. Does the site provide clinically or scientifically based evidence to support its statements? Does it provide referenced information?
7. Is there a disclaimer stating that the content is general information and not individualized patient information?
8. Is there an address where comments and questions may be directed?
9. Does the resource cover the following information: indication, mechanism of action, contraindications/precautions, side effects, drug interactions, and dose?

Appendix A lists some resources that are available.

C. Liability

Legal principles in the area of dietary supplements are not well established. Some believe that liability should be the same for dietary supplements as it is for prescription and pharmacist-recommended non-prescription drugs [55].

Pharmacists may be held liable in situations in which a decision to treat with a dietary supplement is negligent. Negligence consists of four elements: (a) the pharmacist owed the patient a duty to exercise a particular standard of care; (b) the pharmacist breached that standard of care; (c) the substandard act of the pharmacist caused the injury; and (d) the patient suffered damages. Therefore, if a pharmacist sells dietary supplements, he or she must have the degree of competence expected of a reasonable, knowledgeable pharmacist [26].

If a pharmacist recommends a dietary supplement to a patient instead of a more appropriate treatment and the recommendation delays, decreases, or eliminates the opportunity for the patient to receive important care, a pharmacist may be held liable. A pharmacist would be held negligent if he or she recommended a product that adversely interacts with a patient's medication or disease. A pharmacist must be knowledgeable about the products they sell to know whether to recommend a product or to refer the patient to a physician [26]. Undercover shoppers were sent to 25 pharmacies (chain, independent, mass-merchandise, and supermarket) in six states to evaluate the pharmacists' knowledge of a common drug-herb interaction. The shopper gave the pharmacist a prescription of Coumadin® to be filled and while waiting for the prescription purchased ginkgo. Unfortunately, no pharmacist volunteered any information without being asked by the shopper. When asked, wrong information or incomplete advice was given during 16 of the 25 purchases. Some pharmacists recommended a lower dose of ginkgo. Sadly, some pharmacists recited the interaction between ginkgo and aspirin but did not extrapolate. Pharmacists must be aware of potential drug interactions, adverse effects, and other characteristics of dietary supplements.

FDCA defines drugs as "articles intended for use in the diagnosis, cure, mitigation, treatment, or prevention of disease" and "articles (other than food) intended to affect the structure or any function of the body." Therefore, a product becomes a drug based upon its intended use and not upon its composition or source [26]. A pharmacist may violate the FDCA if he or she recommends and sells a dietary supplement for the treatment of a particular disease—the pharmacist would be indicating the product as an unapproved drug. However, if the pharmacist is not selling the product, the FDCA would not be violated.

If a pharmacist posted a sign in a pharmacy claiming a dietary supplement is effective in treating or preventing a certain disease, the pharmacist would be violating the FDCA. The product would be considered a drug but not properly labeled as a drug and therefore would be misbranded.

Regarding DSHEA, a pharmacist may be in violation if he or she displays a published article about a product beside that product in the pharmacy. DSHEA states that articles must be physically separated from the dietary supplements, but the distance is undefined [26]. Also, DSHEA states that another publication with a contrary view must be displayed, if available.

The Federal Trade Commission (FTC) regulates dietary supplement advertising. The FTC prohibits "unfair or deceptive acts or practices" with the advertisement of dietary supplements from retailers and manufacturers. A pharmacy would be held liable if the pharmacy published a manufacturer's ad that was considered deceptive [26].

D. Counseling

Dietary supplements may be less expensive than prescription medications. However, dietary supplements are not guaranteed to be equivalent in safety and efficacy. Unfortunately, many consumers believe that dietary supplements are as safe and effective as prescription medications. As pharmacists, our role is to educate patients on the fallacies of dietary supplements.

Since dietary supplements may be acquired without a prescription, patients can readily and anonymously obtain dietary supplements over the counter for their personal use. As a result, health care practitioners must rely on patients to disclose information regarding their use of such products. Unfortunately, studies suggest that patients do not always inform their health care providers (physicians, pharmacists, and nurses) about their use of unconventional medicines [9]. In one study, the respondents deemed it important for clinicians to know about their herb use and indicated that they would provide this information when queried. Unfortunately, it is unknown whether patients would disclose this information without prompting from a practitioner. However, it is highly likely that over the course of the complex and sometimes stressful interactions between a patient and their health care providers the release of information regarding use of herbal products and over-the-counter medications is not spontaneously conveyed by the patient. Therefore, health care practitioners need to consciously exact information pertaining to the use of herbal therapies and other dietary supplements from patients. Regardless of personal beliefs surrounding the efficacy of herbal products, health care providers are obligated to collect herb use data in order to insure patient safety.

If pharmacists judge harshly or lecture patients for using dietary supplements, we risk making patients wary of providing us with information for fear of reprimand. Pharmacists should encourage patients to discuss their dietary supplement use. Inquiries should be conducted in an open and non-judgmental manner. The following questions should be asked during each medication history:

1. What prescription medications are you currently taking?
2. What non-prescription or over-the-counter medications are you taking?
3. What dietary supplements, such as vitamins, minerals, and herbs, are you taking?

Whenever a patient wants to use a dietary supplement, the following questions should be asked [56]:

1. Why are you interested in this product?
2. What allergies do you have?
3. Are you pregnant or breastfeeding?
4. What prescription and non-prescription medications are you currently taking?
5. What diseases do you have?

When a patient wants to use a dietary supplement, the following points should be addressed: inadequate regulations for quality, safety, or efficacy, differences in preparations from different manufacturers, and insufficient reporting of adverse events.

Always acknowledge the limits of your own knowledge, and incorporate this into the patient counseling. "I don't know" is no longer an acceptable professional answer for pharmacists selling dietary supplements. However, saying "I don't know, but let me see if I can find out" is acceptable.

Recommend products that contain the following on their label: scientific name of the botanical, quantity of the herb, name and address of the actual manufacturer, a batch or lot number, date of manufacture, and expiration date. When available, products that are standardized to the active ingredient(s) should be recommended. A common rule of a one-year expiration date on dietary supplements generally applies [5].

E. Guide Lines

Safety should be the primary issue when patients are using dietary supplements. If there is no clear risk, then support the patient in the use of dietary supplements. However, emphasize the importance of following up with their physician in order to monitor relevant clinical parameters. Healthy patients may be encouraged to experiment with safe dietary supplements. However, patients with significant illnesses or multiple medications may not be good candidates for dietary supplements [57]. Generally, dietary supplements should be avoided in pregnancy, lactation, and pediatrics. The pharmacist should be able to determine if the patient's dietary supplement(s) are appropriate. A patient who chooses to use a dietary supplement over a prescription medication without the knowledge and approval of the primary care provider is clearly a concern [29].

Patients should always start with the lowest recommended dose and increase slowly to avoid overdosing. Follow-up with the patient is necessary to evaluate whether the dietary supplement is safe and effective. Report any suspected adverse event to FDA's Medwatch, 1-800-FDA-1088. FDA has developed the Special Nutritionals Adverse Event Monitoring System (SN/AEMS), a database of adverse events associated with the "use of special nutritional products: dietary supplements, infant formulas, and medical foods."

Products that are standardized to the active ingredient(s) should be recommended. Dietary supplements that are known to be harmful should not be recommended or sold.

X. CONCLUSION

Many patients are turning to dietary supplements in an effort to take a more active part in the management of their health. Whether or not health care practitioners condone this practice, pharmacists must be familiar with these products. Pharmacists should be aware of the safety and toxicity issues surrounsding these products. They cannot afford to jeopardize patients' trust and respect by dismissing the potential utility of dietary supplements. Rather, pharmacists need to encourage patients to be open and honest about their dietary supplement use so the highest degree of health care service may be provided.

APPENDIX A: RESOURCES

Journals

HerbalGram. American Botanical Council.

Books

Bradley P, ed. British Herbal Compendium. London: British Herbal Medical Association, 1992.

British Herbal Pharmacopoeia. London: British Herbal Medical Association, 1996.

Blumenthal M, Goldberg A, Brinckmann J. Herbal Medicine Expanded German Commission E Monographs. Austin, TX: American Botanical Council, 2000.

Facts and Comparisons. The Review of Natural Products. St. Louis: Facts and Comparisons, 2000.

Fetrow CW, Avila JR. Professionals' Handbook of Complementary and Alternative Medicine. Springhouse, PA: Springhouse Corporation, 2001.

Foster S. 101 Medicinal Herbs. Loveland, CO: Interweave Press, 1998.

Jellin JM, ed. Natural Medicines Comprehensive Database. Stockton, CA: Therapeutic Research Faculty, 2001.

LaValle JB, Krinsky DL, Hawkins EB, Pelton R, Willis NA. Natural Therapeutics Pocket Guide. Hudson, OH: Lexi-Comp, Inc., 2000.

McGuffin M, ed. Botanical Safety Handbook: Guidelines for Safe Use and Labeling for Herbs in Commerce, 1997.

Newall L, Anderson L, Phillipson J. Herbal Medicines: A Guide for Health-Care Professionals, 1996.

Physician's Desk Reference. PDR for Herbal Medicines. NJ: Medical Economics Company, 1999.

Robbers JE, Tyler VE. Herbs of Choice: The Therapeutic Use of Phytomedicinals. New York: Haworth Press, Inc., 1999.

Internet Web Sites

www.USPharmacist.com
www.ANMP.org
www.usp.org
http://info.ex.ac.uk/phytonet/pubs.htm
www.herbalgram.org
www.healthy.net/clinic/therapy/herbal/herbic/herbs/index.html
http://pcog8.pmmp.uic.edu/mcp/napl.html

REFERENCES

1. Gordon JS. Alternative medicine and the family physician. Am Fam Phys 54(7):2205–2212, 1996.
2. http://odp.od.nih.gov/ods/whatare/whatare.html.
3. Brevoort P. The U.S. botanical market-an overview. HerbalGram 36:49–57, 1996.
4. Tyler VE. Herbs of Choice: The Therapeutic Use of Phytomedicinals. New York: Haworth Press, Inc., 1994.

5. Grauds CE. Botanical savvy: consultation tips for pharmacists. Pharmacy Times 62(11):81–92, 1996.
6. Brinker F. Variations in effective botanical products: the case for diversity of forms for herbal preparations as supported by scientific studies. HerbalGram 46:36–50, 1999.
7. Bisset NG, ed. Herbal Drugs and Phytopharmaceuticals: A Handbook for Practice on a Scientific Basis. Ann Arbor, MI: CRC Press, 1994.
8. Eisenberg DM, Kessler RC, Foster C, Norlock FE, Calkins DR, Delbanco TL. Unconventional medicine in the United States: prevalence, costs and patterns of use. N Engl J Med 328:246–252, 1993.
9. Eisenberg DM, Davis RB, Ettner SL, et al. Trends in alternative medicine use in the United States, 1990–1997: results of a follow-up survey. JAMA 280:1569–1575, 1998.
10. Johnston BA. One-third of nations' adults use herbal remedies: market estimated at $3.24 billion. HerbalGram 40:49, 1997.
11. Blumenthal M. Herb market levels after five years of boom: 1999 sales in mainstream market up only 11% in first half of 1999 after 55% increase in 1998. HerbalGram 47:64–65, 1999.
12. 103rd Congress, 2nd Session, Senate. The Dietary Supplement Health and Education Act of 1994. Report 103–104. Washington, DC: 1994:1–49.
13. Israelsen LD, Blumenthal M. FDA issues final rules for structure/function claims for dietary supplements under DSHEA. HerbalGram 48:32–38, 2000.
14. Blumenthal M. Traditional herbal medicines in current drug category. HerbalGram 22:18, 35, 1990.
15. Tyler VE. Plant drugs in the 21st century. Econ Bot 40(3):279–288, 1986.
16. Chan TYK. Monitoring the safety of herbal medicines. Drug Safety 17(4):209–215, 1997.
17. Barnes J, Mills SY, Abbot NC, Willoughby M, Ernst E. Different standards for reporting ADR to herbal remedies and conventional OTC medicines. Br J Clin Pharmacol 45:496–500, 1998.
18. Tyler VE. What pharmacists should know about herbal remedies. J Am Pharm Assn NS36(1):29–37, 1996.
19. Alderman S, Kailas S, Goldfarb S, et al. Cholestatic hepatitis after ingestion of chaparral leaf: confirmation by endoscopic retrograde cholangiopancreatography and liver biopsy. J Clin Gastro 19(3):242–247, 1994.
20. Larrey D, Vial T, Pauwels A, et al. Hepatitis after germander (Teucrium chamaedrys) administration: another instance of herbal medicine hepatotoxicity. Ann Intern Med 117(2):129–132, 1992.
21. Ben Yahia M, Mavier P, Metreau JM, et al. Chronic active hepatitis and cirrhosis induced by wild germander. 3 cases. Gastroenterol Clini Biol 17(12):959–962, 1993.
22. Walker BR, Edwards CRW. Licorice-induced hypertension and syndromes of apparent mineralocorticoid excess. Endocrinol Metab Clin North Am 23(2):359–377, 1994.
23. Facts and Comparisons. The Review of Natural Products. St. Louis: Facts and Comparisons, 1997.
24. Foster S. Herbs for Your Health. Loveland, CO: Interweave Press, 1996.
25. 25. Der Marderosian A. The need for cooperation between modern and traditional medicine. HerbalGram 24:32–37, 1991.
26. Abood RR. Regulatory and legal issues pertaining to the sale of dietary supplements. Pharmacy Program ID No. 342-000-99-012-H04. U.S. Pharm, 1999.
27. Bahrke MS, Morgan WP. Evaluation of the ergogenic properties of ginseng. Sports Med 18(4):229–248, 1994.
28. Chong SKF, Oberholzer VG. Ginseng: is there a use in clinical medicine? Postgrad Med J 64:841–846, 1988.
29. Miller LG, Hume A, Harris IM, Jackson EA, Kanmaz TJ, Cauffield JS, Chin TWF, Knell M. White paper on herbal products. Pharmacotherapy 20(7):877–891, 2000.
30. Heptinstall S, Awang DVS, Dawson BA, Kindack D, Knight DW, May J. Parthenolide content and bioactivity of feverfew (Tanacetum parthenium (1.) Schultz-Bip.). Estimation of commercial and authenticated feverfew products. J Pharm Pharmacol 44:391–395, 1992.
31. Silagy CA, Neil HAW. A meta-analysis of the effect of garlic on blood pressure. J Hypertension 12:463–468, 1994.
32. Carraro JC, Raynaud JP, Koch G, et al. Comparison of phytotherapy (Permixon) with finasteride in the treatment of benign prostate hyperplasia: a randomized international study of 1098 patients. Prostate 4:231–240, 1996.
33. Blumenthal M. ConsumerLab.com tests ginkgo and saw palmetto products. HerbalGram 48:66, 2000.
34. Winslow LC, Kroll DJ. Herbs as medicines. Arch Intern Med 158:2192–2199, 1998.
35. Carilla E, Briley M, Fauran F, et al. Binding of Permixon, a new treatment for prostatic benign hyperplasia, to the cytosolic androgen receptor in the rat prostate. J Steroid Biochem 20:521–523, 1984.
36. Plosker GL, Brogden RN. Serenoa repens (Permixon). A review of its pharmacology and therapeutic efficacy in benign prostatic hyperplasia. Drugs Aging 9(5):379–395, 1996.
37. Hobbs C. Ginseng: facts and folklore. Herbs for Health 2:35–38, 1997.
38. Siegel RK. Ginseng abuse syndrome: problems with the panacea. JAMA 241(15):1614–1615, 1979.
39. Hobbs C. Valerian—a literature review. HerbalGram 21:19–34, 1989.
40. Rosenblatt M, Mindel J. Spontaneous hyphema associated with ingestion of ginkgo biloba extract. N Engl J Med 336:1108, 1997.
41. Rowin J, Lewis S. Spontaneous bilateral subdural hematomas associated with chronic ginkgo biloba ingestion. Neurology 46:1775–1776, 1996.

42. Gilbert GJ. Ginkgo biloba (letter). Neurology 48(4):1137, 1997.
43. Shader RI, Greenblatt DJ. Phenelzine and the dream machine: ramblins and reflections. J Clin Psychopharmacol 5(2):65, 1985.
44. Jones BD, Runikis AM. Interaction of ginseng with phenelzine. J Clin Psychopharmacol 7(3):201–202, 1987.
45. Janetzky K, Morreale AP. Probable interaction between warfarin and ginseng. Am J Health-Syst Pharm 54:692–693, 1997.
46. Kassler WJ, Blanc P, Greenblatt R. The use of medicinal herbs by human immunodeficiency virus-infected patients. Arch Intern Med 151:2281–2288, 1991.
47. McGuffin M. Self regulatory initiatives by the herbal industry. HerbalGram 48:42–43, 2000.
48. Leung A. Scientific studies and reports in the herbal literature: What are we studying and reporting? HerbalGram 48:63–64, 2000.
49. Dean K. Multi-component supplement with ginkgo. HerbalGram 48:27, 2000.
50. Dean K. Feverfew: process for preparing microclustered water. HerbalGram 43:25, 1998.
51. Levy S. Alternative care launches: it's only the beginning. Drug Topics 143(14):44, 1999.
52. http://odp.od.nih.gov/ods/about/do.html.
53. Miller LG, Murray WJ. Herbal instruction in United States pharmacy schools. Am J Pharmaceut Educ 61:160–162, 1997.
54. Ling CA. Guiding patients through the maze of drug information on the Internet. Am J Health-Syst Pharm 56:212–214, 1999.
55. Vogel MR. Experts offer tips for integrating natural products into practice. Pharmacy Today 4:14, 1998.
56. Muller JL, Clauson KA. Pharmaceutical considerations of common herbal medicine. Am J Man Care 3:1753–1770, 1997.
57. Williamson JS, Wyandt CM. The herbal generation: trends, products, and pharmacy's role. Drug Topics 143:69–78, 1999.

Chapter 25

Bioequivalency

Christopher T. Rhodes

University of Rhode Island, Kingston, Rhode Island

I. INTRODUCTION

A. Brief Historical Review

When two drug products given by the same route containing the same amount of the same drug exhibit in vivo the same rate and extent of absorption, they may be termed *bioequivalent*. Such products have the same bioavailability and may be expected to produce essentially the same blood concentration–time profiles. Thus, there is good reason to believe that the therapeutic response in patients receiving the two products will be the very similar. The two products may therefore be regarded as therapeutically interchangeable. Bioequivalency is normally quantified by measurement of AUC (area under the plasma concentration–time curve), T_{max} (time to maximum plasma concentration), and C_{max} (maximum plasma concentration).

Since bioequivalence is a measure of the degree of sameness in the biological availability for a test product compared to a standard (usually the version of the drug product first introduced onto the market by the innovator), we can legitimately regard bioequivalency tests as being quality control tests that are of particular importance in assuring interchangeability among different versions of the same drug product. However, unlike most other quality control tests, which are applied to finished pharmaceutical products, bioequivalency determinations (at least at present) normally require the use of volunteer normal human subjects as "guinea pigs." Determinations of identity, potency, content uniformity, etc., are normally rapidly effected by instrumental methods, such as high-pressure liquid chromatography (HPLC). Thus, when in the 1970s it became apparent that bio equivalency could be a product attribute that should be quantified, pharmaceutical scientists naturally gave attention to the idea of developing an in vitro test that would rapidly, inexpensively, and reliably measure bioequivalency. Primarily, this effort has been applied to dissolution tests. Implicit in such an approach was the assumption that dissolution is the rate-determining factor controlling bioequivalence. (This assumption may well be valid for a large proportion of those drugs that are predominantly hydrophobic in nature. However, for drugs that are more water soluble, drug/membrane flux is likely to be the rate-determining factor.) Unfortunately, the number of drugs for which there are reliable published data establishing a precise relationship defining a simple functionality between in vitro and in vivo results is, at present, depressingly small. Thus, bioequivalency testing for many drugs in a number of jurisdictions presently does require the use of human subjects. Any discussion of the development and present status of bioequivalency testing would be deficient if it did not refer to the dichotomy that exists between those who feel that ultimately all such testing could be in vitro in nature and others who believe that the clinical implications of bioequivalency demand that human subject testing must inevitably be part of such evaluations for many, if not all, drugs. These two philosophical approaches to bioequivalency testing could be termed the *quality control* and the *clinical mirror* schools of thought.

B. Development and Generic Bioequivalence

The present author [1,2] has proposed that it is useful to distinguish between development and generic bioequivalence.

Development bioequivalence refers to the relative bioavailability of the drug-delivery systems that are produced during the process of evaluation of new candidate pharmaceutical products for marketing approval by the U.S. Food and Drug Administration (FDA). It would, of course, be highly desirable if in the process of taking a new chemical entity from the laboratory through clinical trials and pilot-scale and manufacturing-scale productions all the products used were identical. However, very often the various formulations used in the development process show significant differences. In some cases, these differences may be so small that it would be highly improbable that bioinequivalency would result. In other instances the formulation or processing differences may be so substantial as to engender doubt as to bioequivalency. Let us consider a hypothetical example of a new drug substance for which the sponsor uses two separate products in the development stage. We designate F_1 as the formulation used in phase 2 and some phase 3 clinical studies. A separate formulation F_2 is used in most of the phase 3 clinical trials. Finally, the sponsor decides to market a third formulation F_3 once FDA has approved the New Drug Application (NDA). Those responsible for evaluating the NDA will inter alia, have to address the question as to whether F_1, F_2, and F_3 are bioequivalent. In particular, we need to determine if it is reasonable to use research data (clinical, validation, stability, etc.) derived from F_1 and F_2 in support of the marketing approval of F_3. It is important to note that in this type of development bioequivalency situation we need not be concerned with patients in the general population being switched from F_1 or F_2 to F_3. Formulations F_1 and F_2 will not be marketed, and, thus, unlike generic bioequivalency, the clinical response of an individual patient being switched between different versions of the same drug product post–NDA approval is not a factor that needs attention. Thus, it may not be necessary to apply the same standards for the evaluation of development bioequivalency as may be required for generic bioequivalency. For example, as is discussed in a later part of this chapter, at present there is considerable interest in the topic of individual bioequivalency as possibly being a necessary element in the quantification of generic bioequivalency. Whatever may be eventually decided on this topic for generic bioequivalency, there would appear to be no reason to include such determinations in development bioequivalency. (The topic of individual subject bioequivalency is considered in more detail in a later part of this chapter.)

The topic of what standards should be applied in the evaluation of development bioequivalency seems to have received relatively little specific attention in the pharmaceutical literature. It seems that some scientists and regulators assume that no distinction need be made between these two types of bioequivalency. This is unfortunate since there are clearly occasions when it is quite inappropriate to require generic bioequivalency standards when development bioequivalency is being considered.

Although one cannot readily identify any comprehensive, official pronouncement on the topic of development bioequivalency, it is apparent that in many cases FDA officials have adopted a pragmatic and common-sense approach to problems of this type. Obviously, in development bioequivalency our fundamental objective should be, for example, to build an appropriate bridge between F_1 and F_3 and F_2 and F_3 such that it is legitimate to use data obtained in clinical trials with F_1 and F_2 to support a conclusion of safety and efficacy for F_3. Depending on how substantial the differences are between F_1 and F_3 and F_2 and F_3, the required bridge can be very simple or possibly more elaborate.

The sponsor of an NDA will normally have extensive pharmacokinetic and pharmacodynamic information available at the time the NDA is submitted. It may be appropriate to use data such as the slope of the dose-response curve in support of a contention that, for example, dissolution testing may be, in some instances at least, be sufficient for the demonstration of development bioequivalency. Certainly, we may conclude that the requirements for development bioequivalence should never be more rigorous than those applied in consideration of generic bioequivalency.

The topic of generic bioequivalence pertains to the relative bioavailability of different versions of the same drug product, all of which may be available in the marketplace at the same time. Thus, if we continue our consideration of the example introduced in the previous section of this chapter, let us suppose that the innovator did obtain approval to market F_3. Initially F_3 was the only product available in the marketplace. However, when the relevant patents held by the innovator have expired, other pharmaceutical companies may submit to FDA. Abbreviated New Drug Applications (ANDAs) for products containing the same molecular entity as the active drug as the innovator marketed in F_3. Normally, the sponsor of an ANDA will seek to demonstrate such a degree of sameness in the bioavailability of their product and the F_3 formulation that interchangeability of patients from F_3 to G_1, G_2, G_3, etc. (where G_1, G_2, and G_3 represent approved generic formulations) can be legitimately accepted as unlikely to impair safety or efficacy for the general populations, subcohorts of the general population, and individual patients. Note that interchangeability is not limited to simply F_3 to G_1, G_2, or G_3 but also from G_2 to G_3 or G_1 to G_3. Thus, we should be concerned about any possible switch between approved versions of the same product.

C. The Importance of Bioequivalence

Bioequivalence is not an esoteric topic of interest only to pharmaceutical scientists and regulators. It is a subject that has become of great importance to consumers, politicians, and top executives in both research-based and generic pharmaceutical companies. Since the U.S. Congress passed the 1984 Drug Price Competition and Patent Term Restoration Act (The Waxman-Hatch Act), it has become apparent that for many generic pharmaceutical products, the demonstration of bioequivalence is a critical parameter in terms of FDA approval. Once a generic product is approved and the innovator who sponsored the NDA no longer enjoys a monopoly, the price of the product usually falls quite dramatically. As additional generic products are approved, further reductions in price are likely. The innovator often experiences loss of market share and reduction of profits for the product. Therefore, innovating companies do not welcome the marketing of generic version of "their" drug. It is not surprising that in their zeal to protect the very substantial profits that result from marketing exclusivity, some innovators have, on some occasions, resorted to rather dubious methods to block competition. On the other side of the coin, there may have been occasions when generic companies have given insufficient attention to legitimate concerns about generic equivalency.

FDA, in its continuing attempts to promote the rational evolution of bioequivalency testing, sometimes appears to be caught between a rock and a hard place. Pharmaceutical scientists who have served on or testified before FDA Expert Advisory Committees, that have considered generic bioequivalency problems are all too painfully aware that extraneous political and financial pressures are sometimes brought to bear on questions for which a cool evaluation of the relevant scientific and clinical factors would be greatly preferred.

The new millenium professional pharmacist with rigorous training in the scientific and clinical properties of drug substances and pharmaceutical formulations should be well able to dispassionately evaluate bioequivaleny data and give an objective, professional opinion as to validity of data purported to demonstrate generic bioequivalence.

II. CURRENT METHODS OF QUANTIFYING BIOEQUIVALENCE

The methods used for the quantification of generic bioequivalence have evolved significantly in the past 15 years or so. There is no reason to believe that this evolutionary process will not continue. Thus, it is indeed likely that the present methods will be further refined. It is also likely that the processes of globalization and harmonization will assist in the further standardization of the methods approved for the determination of bioequivalence in different jurisdictions.

A. Cross-Over Studies

At present the most common preferred method for determining generic bioequivalence is the single-dose, two-way cross-over design. The Office of Generic Drugs at FDA has prepared a number of "cookbook"-type protocols for generic bioequivalency studies for a number of drugs, and a substantial proportion of these protocols are indeed of the single-dose, two-way cross-over design.

The essentials of a single-dose, two-way cross-over bioequivalency design are as follows. A group of normal human volunteers, often about 24 in number, is divided into two equal groups. On the first day of the study one group receives a single dose of the reference (innovator's) product. The second group receives a single dose of the generic version (test). Blood samples are collected from the subjects at appropriate time intervals, which have been selected in accordance with the pharmacokinetic properties of the particular drug. The concentration of drug in the samples is determined by some appropriate, fully validated analytical procedure (often using HPLC). These data can then be plotted graphically to give a representation of plasma concentration of the drug as a function of time for each test subject.

Following the administration of the first dose, washout period is allowed for the test subjects. This period, which is normally in excess of six half-lives, will permit virtually all of the drug to be cleared from the test subjects. Often a period of 7 days is used as a convenient washout period. At the end of the washout period a second dose is administered to the test subjects. The subjects are "crossed over" so that the group that received reference product on the first treatment leg now receives the test product and vice versa. The obvious advantage of this design is that each subject acts as his or her own control. Thus, if one subject is atypical and metabolizes the drug, at, say, five times the normal rate so that the blood concentration time profile of the drug is unusually low, this effect will be apparent on both test and reference results. This means that this subject's peculiar ability to rapidly clear the drug will not bias the average data for test and reference treatments.

The fact that in a conventional single-dose, two-way cross-over bioequivalence study half the subjects receive the test and reference products on each of the two legs or periods of treatment is also of significant value in reducing potential variability. Thus, suppose that the drug being tested tends to stimulate those enzyme systems responsible for its own metabolism. We may therefore predict that, on average, the serum drug concentration–time profiles for the drug would be lower on the second leg or period of the bioequivalency test, even if the test and reference products have identical bioavailability. However, this will not necessarily bias the results since an equal number of subjects receive test or reference products in each of the two legs.

B. Parallel Studies

There are occasions when it is not possible to use a cross-over design in a bioequivalency determination. For example, if the half-life of the drug is very long, the required washout period between the two treatment periods may be several months. Obviously, it is quite impracticable to consider such a long washout period. Test subjects are unlikely to wait patiently for long periods of time, and thus if we tried to conduct a bioequivalency study with, say, a 3-month washout period, we would probably find that a significant number of our test subjects would not be available for the second dose.

In those instances when the cross-over design is not possible, a parallel design may be required. In such a protocol the test subjects are divided into two groups. One group receives the reference product, and one group receives the test. There is no cross-over, and thus subjects do not act as their own controls. In order to obtain results of an acceptable statistical power (precision), it is normally necessary to use a substantially greater number of subjects in a parallel design than would be needed if a two-way cross-over protocol could be used for the same drug.

C. Steady-State Bioequivalency Studies

There are circumstances that will require, for some drugs, determinations of steady-state rather than single-dose blood concentration data. For example, if the concentrations of drug in a subject's bloodstream are so low that it is not possible to quantify the plasma concentrations of the drug with acceptable precision, then it may be necessary to use a steady-state protocol. In this approach the subjects are administered a number of doses of the drug so that steady-state values are obtained. Thus we might find that if a drug is administered once a day as a 10 mg dose, after 5 days steady state is reached. At steady state the blood levels of the drug ebb and flow between minimum and maximum values, C_p^{ss} min (immediately before dosing) and C_p^{ss} max (at some time after dosing). In a steady-state study assurance must be obtained that steady state has indeed been attained. This is normally achieved by determining C_p^{ss} min and C_p^{ss} max on 3 successive days and establishing that these values do not vary more than might reasonably be expected based on our understanding of the pharmacokinetics of the drug in question and other relevant factors, such as the precision of the assay used for quantifying concentrations of drug in the subject's blood.

Many drugs are used clinically in a steady-state mode, rather than as a single-dose treatment. Thus, those who propound the argument that a bioequivalency test should be regarded as a "clinical mirror" rather than just a product quality control test are often in favor of a more general use of steady-state bioequivalency studies. Steady-state testing is more expensive and time consuming and does involve more human subject testing.

D. Subject Selection for Bioequivalency Studies

Traditionally, young healthy persons between the ages of 18 and 40 years, within 10% of ideal body weight, capable of giving informed consent, free of serious medical problems, not currently using drugs (including

OTCs) are used as subjects in bioequivalency studies. Such persons, often, university students, have been regarded as "human test tubes" in whom bioequivalency is evaluated. However, with the emergence of a school of thought that believes that bioequivalency should be a clinical mirror for the behavior of the test and reference products, this situation may change. Pregnant and nursing females are normally excluded from all bioequivalency studies.

The number of subjects needed so that a study is likely to have an acceptable statistical power depends on a number of factors, including analytical parameters (precision, etc.), subject selection and control, and protocol design (cross-over, parallel).

E. Analysis of Samples

In a traditional, two-way cross-over study, blood samples are taken at predetermined times (e.g., 0.5, 1, 1.5, 3, 6, 9, 12, 24, and 36 hours after dosing). The samples are assayed for drug (and if necessary metabolites). Fortunately, analytical methods, especially HPLC, are now available that make the quantification of many drugs in blood or serum convenient, rapid, and relatively inexpensive. The method selected should normally have an acceptance precision so that concentrations of drug of one tenth $C_{\max}$ can be reliably quantified.

Proponents of the clinical mirror theory of bioequivalence would like to see increased emphasis placed on quantification of pharmacodynamic values. In some instance we can readily identify how reliable and relevant pharmacodynamic values can be measured. For example, for an antihypertensive drug, measurement of blood pressure changes can be conveniently, inexpensively and objectively determined. However, for other types of drug (e.g., antidepressants) it is not easy to conceive any simple pharmacodynamic attributes that could be readily determined.

III. ROLES OF VARIOUS ENTITIES IN ASSURING BIOEQUIVALENCE OF DRUG PRODUCTS

A. The United States Pharmacopeia

The United States Pharmacopeia (USP) (or other national or regional pharmacopeia) provides standards for a large number of drug substances and drug products. Some of these standards are particularly relevant to bioequivalency. First, USP products are normally required to have a potency of between 90 and 110% of label claim. Second, content uniformity limits are applied to dosage forms such as compressed tablets and capsules (e.g., a maximum relative standard deviation of ±6%). Third, USP has established dissolution test methodology which provides detailed specifications for a number of types of dissolution test equipment, most notably the basket, beaker, and flow-through cell. USP also provides dissolution specifications in the monographs for almost all orally administered drug products. USP maintains what is probably the largest and most well-regarded supply of reference drug standards, which can be used as primary standards in the development of validated analytical procedures for the quantification of drug in body fluids such as is required in a bioequivalency study. USP is official in the United States and in about 28 other countries.

B. The U.S. Federal Food and Drug Administration

The U.S. Federal Food and Drug Administration (FDA) has played a critical role in the development of methods used in bioequivalency testing, the statistical evaluation of data, and the evolution of standards used to define bioequivalency. FDA, an agency of the U.S. government, is responsible for regulating many of the activities of pharmaceutical companies that market drug products in the United States. It also has had a powerful influence on international endeavors to standardize bioequivalency testing on a global basis. The FDA Office of Generic Drugs has prepared specifications for bioequivalency protocols for a substantial number of important drugs. These protocols provide the most useful information on such matters as sampling times and subject numbers. The agency is certainly to be commended for provision of this type of help to industry. Additionally, it has been this author's experience, both as a member of FDA Expert Advisory committees and as a consultant working with the pharmaceutical industry, that FDA is willing to meet with the representatives of individual pharmaceutical companies and discuss special problems that may concern bioequivalency for drug products in which the company has an interest.

Abbreviated New Drug Applications

When a generic manufacturer completes an Abbreviated New Drug Application (ANDA), the bioequivalency test data are highly likely to be the section of the submission of most critical importance. Quite often all other data in ANDA are satisfactory but the bioequivalency results are marginal. This can lead to frustration for all involved.

The legislative framework within which FDA operates when considering generic drug applications is provided by the 1984 Waxman-Hatch Act. This act, which had bipartisan sponsorship, is regarded by many observers as a fine example of what the U.S. Congress can produce in terms of rational legislation. It provided valuable assistance to both the research-based pharmaceutical companies that develop new drugs and generic companies that introduce their products onto the market once all relevant patents pertaining to the product in question have expired. For research-based pharmaceutical companies, many of which belong to PhRMA (Pharmaceutical Research Manufacturers Association), Waxman-Hatch provides a more realistic method of assigning patent life than had been previously used. For generic companies, many of which belong to GPIA (Generic Pharmaceutical Industry Association) or NAPM (National Association of Pharmaceutical Manufacturers), this act greatly simplified the process by which FDA approves generic products.

The theme that runs through ANDA requirements is that there is no need to reinvent the wheel. Thus, if a drug product has been marketed by an innovator for a number of years with relatively few minor adverse events being reported, there would seem to be no rational argument for requiring the sponsor of an ANDA to conduct expensive and time-consuming clinical trials designed to prove again the safety and efficacy of the drug substance. This segment, so vital to an NDA for an NCE, is therefore not required for an ANDA.

Regulation of Research and Manufacturing Methods

FDA provides a number of quite extensive and detailed sets of regulations of the "current good" class. Most noteworthy, probably, are the current Good Manufacturing Practice (GMP) regulations, but other regulations (e.g., current Good Laboratory Practices, cGLP) are also of importance. With respect to the topic of bioequivalency, cGMP regulations do not discriminate between research-based and generic-type pharmaceutical companies. Thus innovator's and generic products should be manufactured under essentially the same standards and levels of control.

Preapproval Inspections by FDA

Before a marketing approval document, such as an NDA or ANDA, is finally approved by FDA, an inspection by investigators of the local district office will be arranged [3]. This inspection can provide an additional level of assurance that a generic product will indeed meet all required quality standards.

Other FDA Inspections

In addition to specific preapproval inspections, FDA conducts general purpose inspections. These often occur about every 2 years or so. However, if an inspection reveals serious or widespread compliance problems, the frequency of these inspections can be dramatically increased. At the end of an FDA investigation, one or more "Notice of Adverse Finding" (Form 483) can be issued to the company. It is most prudent that the company respond, in writing, to all 483s. The response should explain fully the relevant facts that pertain to the issues raised by the 483 and disclose the nature and extent of any remedial action. When there are problems with pharmaceutical products, recalls (class one through three, with one being the most serious) are possible. Also, FDA can issue Regulatory Letters, seek injunction, or start criminal prosecutions should the agency deem such action to be justified.

C. State Bodies

State bodies such as legislatures or formulary commissions can also be involved in the development of policies that impinge on bioequivalence and generic products. The extent to which individual states have become active in this area varies greatly. Some states (e.g., New Jersey and Illinois) have maintained a high profile in this area. Others, such as Rhode Island, have been far less active. State formularies are of two types. Positive formularies identify the brands of any given pharmaceutical that are acceptable as interchangeable in the particular state. Negative formularies list only the generic products that are not acceptable as interchangeable in the state.

Some commentators on bioequivalency have voiced concerns as to whether it is appropriate for states to "second-guess" the FDA on matters concerning bioequivalency. Once FDA has carefully evaluated an ANDA and decided that the generic product should be approved and given a rating that allows for substitution, it seems hard to conceive any likely circumstances under which an individual state should be able to opt out from the decision made by FDA. It is appreciated that this issue may well be regarded by some as central to states rights. However, for those of us who adopt an empirical approach to generic substitution, it is hard to see any valid reason why a product that has been approved by FDA as substitutable should not be accepted by all states. One may also wonder whether even the largest states have anything like the level of expertise and experience in bioequivalency that is available at FDA.

D. Professional, Trade, and Patient Organizations

Various professional, trade, and patient organizations have, in the past decade or so, made significant contributions to the lively debate about the direction in which bioequivalency theory and practice should evolve. The American Association of Pharmaceutical Scientists (AAPS) has organized conferences and workshops that not only fulfill a valuable educational function but also provide a forum at which pharmaceutical scientists from industry, academia, and regulatory agencies can exchange views. USP-organized open conferences on topics connected with dissolution and bioavailability have been of value. The Drug Information Association (DIA) and Parenteral Drug Association (PDA) have also provided valuable services in this area.

Trade organizations, such as PhRMA or GPIA, obviously have considerable interest in bioequivalency tests. Decisions about bioequivalency can have very substantial implications for pharmaceutical companies. Thus we must always keep in mind that trade organizations may well adopt positions on bioequivalency topics that can be influenced by financial as well as purely scientific or clinical factors. In general it might be expected that research-based pharmaceutical companies would support measures that would make bioequivalency tests more complex and the standards required to prove generic equivalence more rigorous. In contrast, it might well be expected that organizations representing the generic pharmaceutical industry would tend to oppose any measure that would make it more difficult for generic pharmaceutical products to gain FDA recognition as being bioequivalent.

Although it is clearly prudent to recognize that trade organizations may well have their axes to grind, it would be foolish to deny that these groups can make legitimate and valuable contributions to the process whereby bioequivalency testing is refined. Where trade organizations can have an especially useful function is in discussing with FDA general points of the design, execution, or interpretation of bioequivalency tests. What is meant by "general points" is matters than can affect any company in the industry rather than specific concerns about the evaluation of the bioequivalency of one particular drug product. For example, decisions about requirements for statistical power for studies could well be an area in which trade associations could make a useful contribution.

In recent years, groups with no direct connection whatsoever to the pharmaceutical industry, but representative of patients suffering from a particular disease or representing laypersons in the general community, have become increasingly active. For example, the National Organization of Women (NOW) has sometimes made direct representations to FDA on matters that affect women's health, including the quality and cost of drug products. There is no reason to believe that efforts by patients' groups and similar lay organizations will decrease. Knowledgeable interest by such groups can be of value. We now appear to be approaching a situation in which there is a triangle of forces (industry, regulators, and consumers) rather than simply a two-way (industry and regulators) contest involved in the debate on bioequivalency, generic substitution, and indeed other pharmaceutical topics.

IV. SOME ASPECTS OF BIOEQUIVALENCY CURRENTLY UNDER DISCUSSION

As previously indicated, test methods and standards for bioequivalency determinations are continuing to evolve. In this section of the chapter consideration is given to some of the issues in this areas that presently confront us. In some instances the topics are essentially technical in nature. In others, financial implications introduce political aspects that do not simplify the situation. It seems likely that while some of these questions may be resolved in the relatively near future, others may require years of debate and exploration before a final resolution is achieved.

A. Controlled Release Products

There is some confusion concerning terminology used for drug delivery when control of drug release is discussed. Within this chapter we will use an empirical approach. When a drug-delivery system does not contain any design element (formulation or process attribute) that is included to modify either spatial or temporal aspects of drug release, such a product is described as conventional or non–controlled release. As discussed in other chapters of this book, pharmaceutical scientists have, in the last quarter century or so, demonstrated considerable skill in producing drug-delivery systems that control either the location at which a drug is released (e.g., enteric-coated tablets) or the rate at which a drug is released. For those systems in which control of rate of release is the design objective, we can distinguish several types of product. First, a sustained- or extended-release product controls the release of a drug so that the desired concentrations are maintained for substantially longer periods of time after the administration of a dose. It may well be appropriate to restrict the use of the terms extended or sustained release to products that reduce dosing frequency by 50%. For example, if a non–controlled-release version of a drug product requires administration every 4 hours, we would restrict the term extended release to products with a dosing frequency of 8 hours or greater.

Traditionally, the ideal extended-release product has been conceived as providing essentially stable blood levels over the whole dosing frequency interval. Thus, unlike the saw-edge blood concentration time profile of a non–controlled-release product that may show rather wild fluctuations between sub- and supratherapeutic blood levels, the ideal extended-release product avoids both nontherapeutic blood levels and those likely to have an increased frequency of dose-related side effects. However, in recent years controlled-release products that deliberately exploit a pulsatile drug release time profile have also attracted attention.

Rapid-release products are another class of controlled-release drug-delivery systems of growing interest to pharmaceutical scientists. For this type of product rapidity of response is the key parameter. If a conventional non–controlled-release product gives the therapeutic response in one hour, a rapid-release product might be designed so as to yield such a response in 20 minutes.

Even the most superficial evaluation of bioequivalency requirements for controlled-release products will indicate that for some of these products, at least, the conventional AUC, $T_{\max}$, and $C_{\max}$ measures of bioequivalency may well be insufficient. Thus, for a non-pulsatile sustained-release product with a dosing interval of 24 hours (as compared to 4 hours for the noncontrolled product), the time period during which plasma concentrations are maintained at essentially a plateau level might well be regarded as of critical therapeutic importance, while a term such as $T_{\max}$ could be of very little practical value.

The topic of bioequivalency tests for controlled-release products has attracted comment from a number of groups. For example, Bialer and co-workers [4] have proposed four new parameters:

1. Mean Residence Time
2. $C_{\max}$/AUC
3. Plateau time (the time at which C is >75% $C_{\max}$)
4. Capical (the arimetric mean of concentrations observed during the plateau time)

These ideas appear to merit careful consideration. Similarly, the use of nomograms to evaluate the intrinsic absorption rate constants for drugs that may be formulated into oral prolonged-release products may be of value [5].

B. Chiral Drugs

The presence of one or more asymmetric carbon atoms in a drug substance is, of course, common. In the past it was normal to market such drugs as racemic mixtures even though it may have been known that only one isomer was therapeutically active. The other isomer (or isomers) might have been inactive or even toxic. In the development of a new chemical entity (NCE) as a drug of potential therapeutic value, it is now standard practice to explore the relationship between chirality and biological activity. Further, now that synthetic methods of manufacturing individual isomers are generally available at acceptable costs, there are now practicable alternatives to always marketing racemic mixtures. The situation is, however, complicated by the fact that for some drugs in vivo conversion of, say, an R to an S isomer can occur. In such instances a racemic mixture of R and S isomers can have a dose equivalency of 70% of the S isomer, even though the R isomer is not therapeutically active.

The question that must be addressed is: which molecular species should be quantified in a bioequivalency study of a product containing a chiral drug?

For development of bioequivalence studies (in which different formulations have been used in clinical trials), it would seem that normally there would be no need to conduct bioequivalency studies using a stereoselective assay for the evaluation of the concentrations of drug in the plasma samples. We would not usually expect any noticeable difference in the ratio of R to S isomer exiting in plasma samples derived at the same postdosing time point from different formulations. However, if there were statistically significant differences in the rate of absorption (even within the 80–125% confidence bounds for log transformed data), a regulatory authority might require bioequivalency data on separate isomers in cases where in vivo conversion can occur.

For generic bioequivalence the generic manufacturer would be expected to use the same chiral material as the innovator (most probably a racemic mixture or pure active isomer, though it is possible that in some rare instances the innovator might have discovered a valid reason for using some mixture of R and S other than 50/50). Thus, as with development bioequivalency, it would not normally seem necessary to use stereoselective assays for the separate determination of R and S isomers. However, one can conceive of possible situations where clinically significant differences in R-to-S ratios could be caused by even relatively small differences in absorption rate [6,7].

C. Toxic Drugs

When normal human subjects are used in bioequivalency studies, consideration must, of course, be given to ethical considerations. The Institutional Review Board (IRB), which considers the ethical aspects of a bioequivalency study, must give careful consideration to the safety aspects of administering drugs on an experimental basis to normal subjects for whom there is no therapeutic advantage to be gained from the drug. There is always some small but finite risk in any human drug trial, even when the most "harmless" drugs are used. Thus, when bioequivalency trials are conducted it is essential that appropriate procedures be developed to allow for emergencies caused by adverse drug events. In most cases of bioequivalency studies (especially those using a single-dose cross-over protocol), the chances of serious toxic harm to the subjects are slim. However, serious problems do occasionally occur. When we are dealing with drugs for which serious problems are likely, it may well be decided that human experimentation is not approvable. Some chemotherapeutic agents used in the treatment of cancers fall into this class of drugs. For such drugs it has been proposed that animals could be used. A more acceptable solution is to use patients for whom the drug is needed in a parallel-type study.

D. Drugs with Long Half-Lives

Analytical methods available for the quantification of drugs in body fluids have developed rapidly in recent years. Their increasing sensitivity allows detection and quantification of drugs at very low concentrations previously below the limit of analytical detection. This has resulted, in some instances, in the discovery of previously unknown long secondary elimination phases. Also, a number of drugs being introduced into therapeutic use have long primary half-lives.

E. Modification of Study Design

In recent years pharmaceutical scientists have participated in lively discussions about how present methods of bioequivalency determination might legitimately and advantageously be modified. For example, the question of whether it is necessary to always take plasma samples so that AUC at the end of the test is at least 90% of AUC at time infinity has been explored [7,8]. Statistical aspects of this and other possible methods of modifying protocol design are covered in a most useful book published in 1999 and in several papers [8–10,22].

F. Bioequivalency Studies for Drugs with Active Metabolites

Many drugs are converted in vivo to one or more metabolites. In some cases the metabolite will retain pharmacological activity, although the spectrum and intensity of activity is likely to differ from that observed for the parent drug. Since such metabolites may make a significant contribution to the therapeutic (or toxic) properties of the product, exponents of the "clinical mirror" school of thought might argue that in instances of this type it should be mandatory to quantify both the parent drug and any significant active metabolite. Alternatively, those scientists, clinicians, or regulators who follow the quality control school of thought would probably argue that since the input factor from the drug-delivery system is the parent drug, it should normally be sufficient to only quantify the concentration/time profile of the parent drug.

However, even advocates of the quality control theory of bioequivalency might well agree that in some circumstances it may be imperative to quantify active metabolites as well as parent drug. For example, if the conversion of parent drug to metabolites is so rapid that the concentration of parent drug in plasma is very low, there may be analytical difficulties in quantifying the drug with an acceptable level of precision. In such instances it could be justifiable to quantify an active metabolite instead of the parent drug.

Also, if conversion of drug to active metabolite shows significant departure from linear pharmacokinetics, it is possible that small differences in the rate of absorption of the parent drug (even within the 80–125% range for log transformed data) could result in clinically significant differences in the concentration/time profiles for the active metabolite. When reliable data indicate that this situation may exist, a requirement of quantification of active metabolites in a bioequivalency study would seem to be fully justified.

Another circumstance in which there may be generally compelling reasons to require quantification of active metabolites is when a controlled-release drug-delivery system is used for a drug that has an active metabolite. Some of the papers that consider the topics of bioequivalency testing for drugs with long half-lives or active metabolites are listed in the references section of this chapter [12–17].

G. Intrasubject Variability

A topic in bioequivalency testing that has in recent years attracted spirited discussion is whether there is any need for standards controlling intrasubject variabilities.

The standards for bioequivalency that emerged in the 1990s were based on average values. For example, if we used 24 test subjects in a bioequivalency study in which a comparison was made between a new generic product, G, and the innovator's reference product, R, we might find that the ratio of average AUC values for G to R is 103% with confidence bounds of 88–118%. These data would strongly support a conclusion of bioequivalency, providing data on rate of absorption were equally acceptable. However, supposing an evaluation of the AUC ratios for individual subjects revealed that for subject 5 the AUC ratio was 70% and for subject 15 the ratio was 132%. In this hypothetical example, some pharmaceutical scientists might argue that the intrasubject variability is excessive and could lead to clinical problems.

An examination of the published literature does not suggest that this problem is extensive, although there are some reports [20] of high intrasubject variability. There is no reason to doubt that statisticians are well able to develop tests that could be used to quantify intrasubject variability [9,20–24]. However, the question as to how serious or widespread this problem may be in clinical practice is still in need of reliable data. In clinical use it is possible that for many, if not all drugs, intrapatient variability may well be more a function of patient compliances, variations in diet, use of other drugs (including OTCs), and factors other than variability in dosage form performance. Thus, it would seem to be quite unjustified to adopt a rigorous intrasubject bioequivalency standard for all drugs in the absence of reliable, objective data that clearly indicate a clinical problem. It would also seem reasonable that we should only adopt such a requirement on a drug-by-drug basis.

When data is obtained proving an excessive level of intrapatient variability for a particular drug-delivery system, the pharmaceutical scientist will naturally wish to investigate the cause of the problem. The most obvious explanation would be an insufficiency of control of content uniformity. However, if, as is likely, the product is manufactured to comply with relevant USP specifications and quality control test results confirm that such specifications are being fully complied with, we would have to seek other explanations. An alternative explanation that may merit study is that some drug-delivery systems may be much more sensitive than others to variations in pH within the gastrointestinal tract. Thus, if an innovator's product contains a material to control the localized gastrointestinal micro pH at the locus where dissolution occurs, such a system might well be rugged with respect to changes in pH within the lumen of the gastrointestinal tract. However, if a generic product does not contain any buffer or similar material, then its rate of dissolution in the gastrointestinal tract of the patient might well be more variable. Such factors as changes in gastric pH or transit time might produce considerable intrapatient variability. In order to study this potential problem, it might be useful to conduct comparative dissolution studies (probably using the flow-through cell) of the generic and innovator's product over a pH range of, say, 1–9. Also, it might be useful to estimate the apparent micro pH within the two products [26].

H. Subject Selection

Traditionally the subjects selected in a bioequivalence study were young males between 18 and 40 years of age within 10% of ideal body weight and free from any major medical problem. This was appropriate for the "quality control" bioequivalency model. The very narrow selection range of test subjects reduced variability and was of value in improving the statistical power of the test. Using this type of young test subject (both male and female) is still probably appropriate when we are determining development bioequivalence. However, if the "clinical mirror" view of generic bioequivalence prevails it is likely that pressure will develop for a more clinically relevant group of test subjects to be used. Thus it might be suggested than geriatric as well as young adult subjects be used. Also, it might be proposed that obese persons as well as those of normal weight should be included. Obviously, if these or similar ideas were adopted we would probably either have to use more subjects or accept a test with less statistical power. Thus it would be prudent not to adopt such ideas wholesale but only on a drug-by-drug basis when a real need is demonstrated. Although some references in the literature [27,28] indicate the value of a broad subject mix, the data presently available do not support universal adoption of this approach.

I. Bioequivalency Limits and Critical Care Drugs

The limits for bioequivalency in many jurisdictions are presently 80–125% for log transformed data for all drugs. This standard appears to have worked quite well, although its experiential or theoretical basis is not strong. During recent years a number of pharmaceutical scientists have questioned this "one size fits all" approach to bioequivalence standards. Clearly, since different drugs have different pharmacodynamic and pharmacokinetic properties, such as therapeutic ratio, dose-response curve, or range of clinically acceptable blood levels, there are, indeed, powerful arguments in favor of altering bioequivalence limits so as to recognize the therapeutic and toxicological properties of individual drugs. Thus for some drugs it might be legitimate to relax standards (e.g., to 70–137%), whereas for other drugs we might require a tighter standard (e.g., 90–112%).

Unfortunately, some of the debate concerning possible changes for bioequivalency standards has been colored by the substantial financial interests that would be affected by any change in policy concerning bioequivalency standards. For example, during the period 1998–2000, the company that markets in the United States the brand name warfarin product conducted a vigorous campaign to exclude an FDA-approved version of the drug from various states. The generic company responded resolutely and conducted a clinical study published in 2000 in the *American Journal of Health System Pharmacy*. The authors of the paper concluded that because there were no significant differences in mean INR (a recognized measure of clinical response for Warfarin) between patient groups using the generic or brand name products, therapeutic equivalence was demonstrated. By April 2000 the generic product had gained substantial market share [29].

One idea that has attracted substantial attention in both the professional and the lay press is that there is a special class of drug "narrow therapeutic index" or "narrow therapeutic range" (NTR) for which it would be appropriate to designate especially tight bioequivalence standards. Different proponents of this idea have at various times identified different drugs as being suitable for inclusion in this category. The justification for this proposed action derives from a belief that for NTR drugs we must tighten bioequivalency limits in order to reduce variation in clinical response. If, indeed, it has been reliably demonstrated that formulation and/or processing variables play a major role in determining variance in clinical response, such action may be justifiable. However, if the most important cause of the clinical variance is the inherent nature of the drug substance, then tightening bioequivalency standards will have little, if any, significant effect on reducing variability. Warfarin is a good example of a drug for which designation as NTR and a requirement of an unusually tight bioequivalency limit is quite irrational. The drug has good aqueous solubility and membrane flux properties. Thus, the variation in clinical response (both intra- and interpatient) is dominated by the pharmacokinetic and pharmacodynamic properties of the drug molecule.

Recently, the literature has contained many reports dealing with NTR and related issues. For example, Burns [30] considered the general topic of NTR drugs and recommended that caution be exercised in the selection of generic drug products. The author opined that bioequivalence, especially with NTR drugs, does not always ensure therapeutic equivalence. Similarly, Johnston and coworkers in a discussion of "critical dose drugs" made recommendations of how therapeutic equivalence rather than just bioequivalence should be established [31]. Vasquez and Min have [32] expressed concern about some aspects of generic substitution, and Banahan and Kolassa [33] have published an interesting survey of physicians' opinions about generic substitution of critical dose medications.

Benet and Goyan [34] have presented a clear exposition on bioequivalence and narrow therapeutic index drugs. Among other papers of relevance to this topic are those by Tsang and coworkers [35], el-Tahtawy and associates [36], and Midha and collaborators [37].

It is unfortunate that the debate over narrow therapeutic index (ratio) or critical care drugs has been confused by issues that are not of scientific or clinical relevance. Fear tactics and exaggeration are counterproductive to an objective discussion of the issues. Perhaps the most egregious incident concerning tactics used to exclude generic pharmaceutical products were those used in the thyroid storm controversy [38,39]. Fortunately, it is not often that a pharmaceutical company is publicly chastised by an editorial in the *Journal of the American Medical Association* about its policies, as was the case in thyroid storm. In this instance the brand name company demonstrated its willingness to adopt most unusual procedures to block the progress of generic products.

For drugs which have a wide range of therapeutically acceptable plasma concentrations, it is reasonable to consider widening bioequivalence criteria [40].

J. Pharmacodynamic Measures in Bioequivalency Testing

Obviously, if the clinical mirror approach to bioequivalency testing gains momentum, we may expect to see more quantification of clinical response in bioequivalency studies. In some instances pharmacodynamic parameters that are amenable to precise quantification are easily identified. Thus, if we are working with an antihypertensive drug, measurement of blood pressure using an electronic sphygnomanometer is an obvious option. However, for many drugs there is no simple way to quantify pharmacodynamic response. In some cases we may have to rely, to some extent at least, on patient diaries [41]. Such techniques are open to criticism of subjectivity and imprecision.

There are special problems in bioequivalency determinations when conventional pharmacokinetic studies are not possible. For example, when drugs are administered intranasally for direct treatment of receptors in the nasal mucosa, the concentration of drug in plasma may be below the limit of quantification. In such cases we are forced to attempt measurement of clinical response. The subjectivity and/or low precision of this type of study can be a serious problem.

K. Compounded Pharmaceuticals

The 1997 Food and Drug Administration Modernization Act (FDAMA) specifically recognizes the right of a licensed pharmacist to compound pharmaceutical products in response to, or in anticipation of an appropriate prescription. The Act also authorized the establishment of an FDA Expert Advisory Committee on Compounded Drug Products. During the last decade there has been an impressive increase in the level of activity by compounding pharmacists [4]. Concern has been expressed that pharmaceuticals compounded by pharmacists are not subject to cGMP regulations and that quality control is rudimentary [43]. Certainly compounding of extended-release phenytoin products without any bioequivalency measurement is a matter of concern to many pharmaceutical scientists.

L. Veterinary Products

Veterinary pharmaceuticals are of great importance in the United States and many other countries. (For more information on this topic, the reader is referred to the chapter on veterinary products.)

The general principles of bioequivalence as used by the FDA Center for Veterinary Medicine are essentially the same as those used by the Center for Drug Evaluation and Research when the products are designed for use by companion animals [44].

When pharmaceuticals are administered to feed animals there is a special concern about the possible accumulation of drug residues in the animals' tissues. Thus, in these bioequivalency studies it may be appropriate to carefully monitor parameters that define possible tissue accumulation [45].

Other issues in veterinary bioequivalence which merit attention include policies to be followed when a product is to be used by more than one animal species. Is it sufficient to perform a bioequivalence study in only one species, or should studies be carried out in most or all the species for which the drug is recommended [46]? There may be reason to believe that bioequivalence problems exist in some veterinary products [47,48].

M. Bioequivalence for Botanicals, Nutritional Supplements, and Nonconventional Products

As indicated in previous sections of this chapter, there has developed a quite impressive international consensus on the general principles of bioequivalency determination for drug products regulated by agencies such as FDA. However, there are other materials used with therapeutic intent for which bioequivalency may also be a legitimate concern. Herbal remedies have, in recent years, demonstrated impressive increases in sales in many parts of the world. Other substances of natural origin have gained considerable attention for their possible curative potential. For example, shark cartilage has received considerable publicity for its purported value in the treatment of cancer. Also, there is a growing range of products which may be regarded as begin at the interface between foods and drugs. These types of product are sometimes termed "nutraceuticals." Questions of bioequivalence or therapeutic equivalence either within such categories or with conventional pharmaceutical products are already eliciting interest. It seems likely that these topics will be the subject of increasing attention in the near future [49,50].

N. Biowaivers

For at least three decades pharmaceutical scientists have, like medieval alchemists, been searching for the Philosphers' Store. However, rather than wishing to transmute base metals into gold, our endeavors have been to discover an in vitro method that could be reliably used to quantitatively predict bioavailability. The HPB (Health Protection Branch) in Canada and USP in the United States devoted a great deal of time and energy to developing dissolution apparatus. It is now generally accepted that for many drugs which are weak hydrophobic electrolytes, in vivo dissolution may well be the rate-determining step controlling bioavailability. Drugs for which membrane flux is the rate-determining step are probably less common. Thus, for many drugs (probably a majority), the rate and extent of drug absorption may well be primarily governed by dissolution.

Considerable ingenuity has been expended in the design and evaluation of dissolution equipment. USP presently has seven pieces of dissolution equipment, all of which are purported to have advantages for some systems. (Hopefully, in the future the number of apparatus recognized by USP will decrease.) The flexibility of its operation (including its use in the sink mode) is a powerful recommendation for the wider use of the flow-through cell. However, even with this equipment it would be naïve to expect guaranteed success in attempts to define an exploitable relationship between in vitro dissolution and biological availability.

Attempts to establish in vitro/in vivo correlation might be classified as having three possible goals. First, we might try to discern some simple equation of universal applicability for all drugs in all products. Second, we might hope to demonstrate an empirical relationship for conventional (i.e., non–controlled-release) products for one drug substance. Third, our objective might simply be to establish a usable relationship for one particular formulation of one drug.

Of the above three objectives, the first—which is, of course, the most ambitious—is at present, at least probably unrealistically ambitious. Even the third objective is not always easy to reach. Thus at present the number of precise, reliable in vitro/in vivo correlations for which satisfactory documentation is available in the public domain is limited. In the absence of objective data validating the existence of a usable relationship, it would be entirely unjustifiable to assume that one exists for any given drug substance or formulation. Although it is a relatively simple task to develop an equation to define an in vitro/in vivo relationship, the precision of the functionality often requires more experimental data than are available. This is especially true for controlled-release formulations [53,54]. In our evaluation of possible in vitro methods for prediction of bioavailability, we must not omit consideration of release equipment designed for nonoral products [55]. In analysis of in vitro dissolution data, moment analysis is a useful technique and considerable ingenuity has been expended in the experimental generation of such data [56]. Specialist groups have devoted considerable efforts in developing methods of comparing release and response profiles [57].

In those cases where an acceptable correlation between in vitro and in vivo properties has been established, a regulatory agency may decide to grant a biowaiver. This would allow bioequivalency for specified types of drug-delivery system for a particular drug to be estimated by an in vitro method. There clearly are substantial limitations of bioequivalency data obtained when a biowaiver has been applied. First, we cannot obtain any direct information on individual subject bioequivalency. Second, it is highly unlikely that we will be able to obtain any precise information on active metabolite levels. Third, we will not be able to measure directly any pharmacodynamic property. Fourth, we will probably not be able to evaluate any differential bioequivalency in subcohorts of the general population (e.g., geriatrics). Fifth, the statistical evaluation in vitro data so as to reliably predict in vivo confidence bounds is not presently well established.

Thus, some proponents of the clinical mirror school of thought of bioequivalency testing are likely to object on principle to any biowaiver. However, it seems likely that this viewpoint is unlikely to be universally accepted for all drugs. The following are some criteria that might be considered when contemplating a biowaiver:

1. The bioavailability of the drug is demonstrated to be governed by dissolution if an in vitro dissolution test is to be used.
2. The drug should show linear pharmacokinetics and should not be converted to an active metabolite that plays a substantial role in the therapeutic or toxic properties of the product.
3. A relatively wide range of blood concentrations is therapeutically acceptable. The drug does not have a low therapeutic ratio.
4. There is no reason to believe that individual bioequivalence could be a clinically significant problem for the drug, nor is there any reasonable basis for concern about bioinequivalence in subcohorts of the population.
5. The drug-delivery systems are not modified or controlled release.

V. CONCLUSION

Methods of measuring bioequivalency and statistical techniques for evaluating the results continue to evolve [58–70]. It is reasonable to expect continued convergence of bioequivalence practices in different parts of the world, especially North America and Western Europe [71]. Our understanding of the major factors that control the release and absorption of drugs has made significant advances. We have established a reliable general framework which rationalizes the overall sequence. In particular, a drug classification scheme based on the importance of dissolution or membrane flux for the bioavailability of any given drug is likely to prove of considerable practical value [74]. The practicing health professional may sometimes be somewhat overwhelmed by the claims and counterclaims made by the proponents or opponents of generic substitution for certain. In such instances we must keep in mind the underlying scientific and clinical factors that should be the foundation of any such decision [75].

FDA, in the CDBR 1998 Report to the Nation, has published data on generic drug approvals [76]. For 1998 the median approval time was 18.0 months compared to 19.3 in 1997, 23 in 1996, and 27 in 1995. At the same time the number of applications remained high at over 300 per year.

Recent legislative changes in France are likely to increase the market share of generics in that country. According to the March 18, 2000, issue of the *Pharmaceutical Journal* [77] the French market in generics was only 2%, whereas in England the comparable value was 15.3 and in the United States 40%.

It seems likely that our increasing sophistication in obtaining bioequivalency data will allow greater market penetration by quality generics with the exclusion of substandard products.

REFERENCES

1. C. T. Rhodes, Acceptable limits in bioequivalence studies, Clin., Res. Drug Reg. Affaris, *14*, 127 (1997).
2. C. T. Rhodes, Some observations on current and possible future developments in bioequivalency testing, Drug. Dev. Ind. Pharm., *25*, 555 (1999).
3. M. D. Hynes, Preparing for FDA Preapproval Inspections. New York: Marcel Dekker, Inc., 1998.
4. M. Bialer, L. Arcavi, S. Sussan, A. Volosov, A. Yacobi, D. Morus, B. Levitt, and A. Laor, Existing and new criteria for bioequivalence evaluation of new controlled release products of carbamazipine, Epilepsy Res., *32*, 371 (1998).
5. S. C. Dyer and R. E. Notari, A nomogram to evaluate intrinsic absorption rate constants of potential oral prolonged release candidates, Pharm. Dev. Tech., *4*, 305 (1999).
6. Which bioequivalence study for racemic drug?, Eur. J. Drug Metab. Pharmacokinet., *23*, 166 (1998).
7. A. J. Romero and C. T. Rhodes, Stereochemical aspects of the molecular pharmaceutics of ibuprofen, J. Pharm. Pharmocol., *45*, 258 (1993).
8. L. Endrenyi and L. Tothfalusi, Truncated AUC evaluates effectively the bioequivalence of drugs with long half lives, Int. J. Clin. Phrmacol. Ther., *35*, 42 (1997).
9. A. J. Romero, C. Bon, E. Johnson, S. E. Rosenbaum, and C. T. Rhodes, Use and limitations of the truncated curve in bioequivalency testing, Clin. Res. Drug Reg. Affairs, *8*, 123 (1990).
10. J. Kharadi, A. J. Jackson, and L. A. Ouderkirk, Use of truncated areas to measure extent of drug absorption in bioequivalence studies, Pharm. Res., *16*, 130 (1999).
11. I. Mohmood and H. Mahayni, A limited sampling approach in bioequivalence studies: application to long half life drugs and replicate design studies, Int. J. Clin. Ther., *37*, 275 (1999).
12. C. T. Rhodes, Bioequivalence evaluation, possible future developments, Clin. Res. Drug Reg. Affairs, *11*, 181 (1996).
13. C. T. Rhodes, Some observations on current and possible future developments in bioequivalency testing, Drug. Dev. And Ind. Pharm., *25*, 555 (1999).
14. I. Mahmood, Assessment of metabolites in bioequivalence studies: Should bioequivalence criteria be applied on the sum of parent compound and metabolite?, Int. J. Clin. Pharmacol Ther., *36*, 540 (1998).
15. H. Vergin, G. Mahr, R. Metz, A. Eichinger, V. Nitsche, and H. Martens, Analysis of metabolites—a new approach to bioequivalence studies of spironolactone

formulations, Int. J. Clin. Pharmacol. Ther., *35*, 334 (1997).

16. A. Marzo, Open questions in bioequivalence, Pharmacol. Res., *32*, 237 (1995).
17. P. Sathe, J. Venitz, and L. Lesko, Evaluation of truncated areas in the assessment of bioequivalence of immediate release formulations of drugs with long half lives and C_{MAX} with different dissolution rates, Pharm. Res., *16*, 939 (1999).
18. M. L. Chen and A. J. Jackson, The role of metabolites in bioequivalency assessment, I. Linear pharmacokinetics without first pass effect, Pharm. Res., *8*, 25 (1991).
19. M. L. Chen and A. J. Jackson, The role of metabolites in bioequivalency assessment, II. Drugs with linear pharmacokinetics and first pass effect, Pharm. Res., *5*, 700 (1995).
20. L. Endrenyi, G. L. Amindon, K. K. Midha and J. P. Skelly, Individual bioequivalence: attractive in principle, difficult in practise, Pharm. Res., *15*, 1321 (1998).
21. A. L. Gould, Individual bioequivalence, J. Biopharm. Stat., *7*, 23 (1997).
22. Sheng-Chung Chow and Jen-Pei Liu, Statistical Design and Analysis in Pharmaceutical Science, Marcel Dekker Inc., New York, 1997.
23. P. G. Welling, et al. eds., Pharmaceutical Bioequivalence, Marcel Dekker Inc., New York, 1997.
24. H. L. Ju, On TIER method for assessment of individual bioequivalence, J. Biopharm Stat., *7*, 63 (1997).
25. J. Liu and S. C. Chow, A two one sided test procedure for assessment of individual bioequivalence, J. Biopharm. Stat., *7*, 49 (1997).
26. C. T. Rhodes, Determination of micro-pH in solid drug delivery systems, Drug Dev. Indust. Pharm., *25*, 1221 (1999).
27. B. L. Carter, M. A. Noyes, and R. W. Demler, Differences in serum concentration of response to generic verapamil in the elderly, Pharmacotherapy, *13*, 359 (1993).
28. H. Zimmerman, R. Kovtchev, O. Mayer, A. Borner, U. Mellinger, and H. Breitbath, Pharmacokinetics of orally adminstered estrodiol valerate, Arzneimittelforschung, *48*, 941 (1998).
29. C. N. Swenson and G. Fundale, Observational cohort study of switching warfarin sodium products in a managed care organization, Am J. Health Syst. Pharm., *57*, 452 (2000).
30. M. Burns, Management of narrow therapeutic index drugs, J. Thromb. Thrombolysis, *7*, 137 (1999).
31. A. Johnston, P. A. Keown, and D. W. Holt, Simple bioequivalence criteria, Ther. Drug Monit., *19*, 375 (1997).
32. E. M. Vasquez and D. I. Min, Transplant pharmacists' opinions on generic product selection, Am. J. Health Syst. Pharm., *7*, 615 (1999).
33. B. F. Banahan 3rd and E. M. Kolassa, A physician survey on generic drugs and substitution of critical dose medications, Arch. Intern. Med., *18*, 2080 (1997).
34. L. Z. Benet and J. E. Goyan, Bioequivalence and narrow therapeutic range drugs, Pharmacotherapy, *4*, 433 (1995).
35. Y. C. Tsang, R. Pop, G. P. Hems, and M. Spino, High variability in drug pharmacokinetics complicates determination of bioequivalence, Pharm. Res., *13*, 846 (1996).
36. A. A. el-Tahtawy, T. N. Tozer, F. Harison, L. Lesko, and R. Williams, Evaluation of bioequivalence of highly variable drugs, Pharm. Res., *15*, 98 (1998).
37. K. K. Midha, M. J. Rawson, and J. W. Huhban, Prescribability and switchability of highly variable drugs and drug products, J. Controlled Release, *62*, 33 (1999).
38. B. J. Dong, W. W. Hauck, J. G. Gambertoglio, L. Gee, J. R. White, J. L. Bubpand, and F. S. Greenspan, Bioequivalence of generic and brand name levothyroxine products in the treatment of hypothyroidison, JAMA, *277* , 1205 (1997).
39. C. T. Rhodes, Regulatory aspects of the formulation and evaluation of L-thyroxenetablets, Clin. Res. Drug Reg. Affairs, *15*, 180 (1998).
40. A. W. Boddy, F. C. Snickeris, R. D. Kringle, G. C. Wei, J. A. Oppermann, and K. K. Midha, An approach for widening the bioequivalence acceptance limits in the case of highly variable drugs, Pharm, Res., *12*, 1865 (1995).
41. T. B. Casale, S. M. Azzum, R. E. Miller, and J. Oren, Demonstration of therapeutic equivalence of generic and innovator beclomethasone in seasonal allergic rhinitis, Ann. allergy Asthma Immunol., *82*, 435 (1999).
42. L. A. Underhill, N. A. Campbell, and C. T. Rhodes, Regulatory and clinical aspects of the resurgence of compounding by pharmacists, Drug Dev. Ind. Pharm., *22*, 659 (1996).
43. J. H. Perin, Further compounded sustanined-release gems, Drug Dev. Ind. Phrm., *26*, 235 (2000).
44. J. Blodinger, ed., Formulation of Veterinary Dosage Forms, Marcel Dekker, Inc., New York, 1983.
45. S. C. Fitzpatrick, S. D. Brynes, and G. B. Guest, Dietary intake estimates as a menas to the harmonization of maximum residue levels for veterinary drugs, J. Vet. Pharmacol. Ther., *18*, 325 (1995).
46. C. T. Rhodes, Bioequivalence studies for veterinary drug products, Clin. Res. Drug. Affairs, *9*, 1 (1992).
47. A. D. Waston, Bioavailability and bioinequivalence of drug formulations in small animals, J. Vet. Pharmacol. Ther., *15*, 151 (1992).
48. P. L. Toutain and G. D. Koritz, Veterinary drug bioequivalence determination, J. Vet. Pharmacol. Ther., *20*, 79 (1997).
49. S. J. Bell, J. A. Stack, R. A. Forse, C. Del Fierro, E. Wade, and P. Burke, Generic enteral formulas: a new idea for the 1990's, Nutr. Clin. Pract., *6*, 237 (1995).

50. G. Harrer, U. Schmidt, U. Kuhn, and A. Biller, Comparison of equivalence between St. John's wort extract and LoHyp-57 and fluoxetine, Arzneimittelforschung, *49*, 289 (1999).
51. Bioavailability of diretary supplements, Pharm. J., *264*, 304 (2000).
52. M. K. Kottke and C. T. Rhodes, Limitations of presently available in vitro release data for the prediction of in vivo performance, Drug Dev. Ind. Pharm., *17*, 1157 (1996).
53. A. Kayali, Bioequivalency evaluation by the comparison of in vitro dissolution and in vivo absorption using reference equations, Eur. J. Drug Metab. Pharmacokinet., *19*, 271 (1994).
54. A. Frick, H. Moller, and E. Wirbitzki, Biopharmaceutical characterization or oral controlled/modified-release drug products, Eur. J. Pharm. Biopharm., *46*, 313 (1998).
55. V. P. Shah, J. S. Elkins, and R. L. Williams, Evaluation of the test system used for in vitro release of drugs for topical dermatological drug products, Pharm. Dev. Tech., *4*, 377 (1999).
56. S. Yamamura, F. Aida, Y. Momose, and E. Fukuoka, Analysis of mean disintegration time and mean dissolution time by moment analysis microcalorimetric curves, Drug Dev. Ind. Pharm., *26*, 1 (2000).
57. F. Langenbucher, IVIC: Indices for comparing release and response profiles, Drug Dev. And Ind. Pharm., *25*, 1223 (1999).
58. H. A. Koelman, J. C. Wessels, H. S. Steyn, and S. M. Ellis, New bioavailability parameters to compare the efficacy of antimicrobial drugs in dosage forms, Int. J. Clin. Pharmacol. Ther. Toxicol., *29*, 451 (1991).
59. A. Kayali, I. Tu-glular, and M. Ertabs, Pharmacokinetics of carbamazipine, Eur. J. Drug Metab. Pharmcokinet., *19*, 319 (1994).
60. J. Vuorinem and J. Turunen, A three step procedure for assessing bioequivalence in the general mixed model framework, Stat. Med., *15*, 2635 (1996).
61. W. W. Hauck, P. E. Preston, and F. Y. Bois, A group sequential approach to crossover trials for average bioequivalence, J. Biopharm. Stat., *7*, 87 (1997).
62. J. Zha and L. Endrenyi, Variation of the peak concentration following single and repeated drug administration in investigations of bioavailability and bioequivalence, J. Biopharm. Stat., *7*, 191 (1997).
63. S. Anderson and W. W. Hauck, The transitivity of bioequivalence testing: potential for draft, Int. J. Clin. Pharmcol. Ther., *34*, 369 (1996).
64. H. C. Hsu and H. L. Lu, On confidence limits associated with Chow and Shao's joint confidence region approach for assessment of bioequivalence, J. Biopharm Stat., *7*, 125 (1997).
65. S. K. Niazi, S. M. Alam, and S. I. Ahmad, Patial area method in bioequivalence assessment: naproxen, Biopharm Drug Dispos., *18*, 103 (1997).
66. A practical approach for assessment of bioquivalence under selected higher-order cross-over designs, J. Vuorinem, Stat. Med., *16*, 2229 (1997).
67. H. Quiding, H. G. Arwidisson, E. Grahn Hakansson, A. Grahnen, and S. Holm, Saliva resitant coating of tablets prevents oral release of penicillin: plasma but not saliva equivalence, Eur. J. Clin. Pharmacol., *54*, 749 (1998).
68. V. W. Steinjans and D. Hauscke, Individual bioequivalence—a European perspective, J. Biopharm. Stat., *7*, 31 (1997).
69. Y. LeRoux, C. Guimart, and M. Tenenhaus, Use of repeated cross-over design in assessing bioequivalence, Eur J. Drug Metab. Pharmacokinet., *23*, 339 (1998).
70. L. Endrenvi, F. Csizadia, L. Tothfalusi, A. H. Balch, and M. L. Chen, The duration of measuring partial AUC's for the assesment of bioequivalence, Pharm. Res., *15*, 339 (1998).
71. A. Marzo and N. C. Mont, Acceptable and unacceptable procedures in bioavailability and bioequivalence trials, Pharm. Res., *38*, 401 (1998).
72. P. A. Meredith, Generic drugs: therapeutic equivalence, Drug Safety, *15*, 233 (1996).
73. E. B. Brown, H. K. Iyer, and C. W. Wang, Tolerance intervals for assessing individual bioequivalence, Stat. Med., *16*, 803 (1997).
74. E. Lipka and G. L. Amidon, Setting bioequivalence requirements for drug development based on preclinical data: optimizing oral drug delivery systems, J. Controlled Release, *62*, 41 (1999).
75. Generic drug product equivalence: current status, Am. J. Manag. Care, *4*, 1183 (1998).
76. CDER 1998 Report to the Nation Improving Public Health Through Human Drugs. U.S. Department of Health and Human Services, Food and Drug Administration, Center for Drug Evaluation and Research, 1999.
77. France benefits from new generic substitution rules, Pharm. J., 264, 427 (2000).

Chapter 26

Drug Information

Hazel H. Seaba

University of Iowa, Iowa City, Iowa

I. INTRODUCTION

Pharmacy and drug information are synonymous. In the 1960s, when discrete drug information centers were being established within health care institutions, the expression "drug information pharmacist" appeared. While this expression may still have a place describing a drug information specialist, for the most part it is redundant—all pharmacists are drug information pharmacists. In 1991 Brodie et al. [1] identified a multiple-theory concept of pharmacy as a drug-use control system, a knowledge service, a clinical profession, and as the interface between humankind and drugs. The description of pharmacy practice was expanded from that of pharmacy as a "knowledge system" [2] to "a system (framework) of concepts dealing with the acquisition, translation, transmission, and utilization of drug knowledge" [1]. As a specific component of pharmacy practice, the drug information role is characterized by the ability of the pharmacist to perceive, assess, and evaluate drug information needs and retrieve, evaluate, communicate, and apply data from the published literature and other sources as a integral component of pharmaceutical care [3]. The ability to fulfill the drug information role is essential to successful pharmacy practice.

Drug information itself is much more than a collection of facts about drugs. Drug information is both a body of data and information about medications and a set of skills and tools that provide pharmacy professionals with the ability to find, access, understand, interpret, apply, and communicate information and acquire knowledge. The body of facts and information pertaining to medications is generally referred to as "the drug literature." What actually constitutes the drug literature was defined by the National Library of Medicine (NLM) in 1963 within a survey NLM did pursuant to U.S. Senate Resolution 27, 88th Congress [4]. Drug literature was defined as "any published papers on preparations with potential therapeutic or diagnostic activity, either natural or synthetic" [5]. The second component of drug information, a set of skills and tools, is now probably best defined as *health* or *biomedical informatics*. Biomedical informatics is a new field that has been evolving since the 1970s. A single definition has yet to achieve consensus; however, a practical definition, credited to Edward Shortliffe, Stanford University, is: a rapidly developing scientific field that deals with resources, devices and formalized methods for optimizing the storage, retrieval, and management of biomedical information for problem solving and decision making [6]. The purpose of this chapter is to provide a current view of this broad concept of drug information for the student, practicing pharmacist, and pharmaceutical industry professional. Both the drug literature and the informatics components of drug information will be discussed.

A. Data → Information → Knowledge

Data (facts and figures) beget information (organized facts and figures) and information begets knowledge (usable, meaningful information). According to *The American Heritage Dictionary* [7], "information" is usually construed as being narrower in scope than "knowledge," implying a collection of facts and data that are seen in context and convey meaning. Knowledge is the broadest; it includes facts and ideas, understanding, information, learning, erudition, lore, scholarship, and the totality of what is known.

Our ability to achieve the successes promised by the information age has been hindered by the sheer volume of data and information available. J. Naisbitt aptly described this in his 1982 book, *Megatrends*: "We are drowning in information but starved for knowledge" [8]. With the objective of obtaining drug knowledge for problem solving and decision making, the critical importance of turning data and information into usable forms becomes self-evident.

Although the expression "data-rich but information-poor" (D.R.I.P.) is reaching cliché status, it is a powerful truism that thwarts health care professionals daily [9–12]. We continue to be frustrated by having access to an incredible amount of raw data from our practice environment, data available in the form of research reports and data of all kinds residing on the Internet—but not having the means to efficiently summarize and consolidate the data into a format that has meaning and can be used. This particular drug information challenge is as urgent today as it was in 1965 when then Vice President Hubert H. Humphrey, a college of pharmacy graduate himself, stated, "Competent evaluation of masses of drug information is particularly necessary" [13].

Information enterprises now promote themselves as knowledge resources. An image of a broad, lazy, meandering river (information) contrasted to the power and energy of water rushing out of a large dam (knowledge) has been effectively used by Dow Jones & Company to symbolize their commitment to "harnessing ... this overwhelming flood [and] transforming [it] into something people and companies actually can use" [14]. In the early 1990s Drucker forecast the value of knowledge to business: "The basic economic resource—'the means of production,' to use the economist's term—is no longer capital, nor natural resources (the economist's 'land'), nor 'labor.' *It is and will be knowledge*. Value is now created by 'productivity' and 'innovation,' both applications of knowledge to work" [15].

B. Pharmaceutical and Biomedical Literature

The NLM's 1965 definition of the drug literature as "any published papers on preparations with potential therapeutic or diagnostic activity" continues to have relevance more than 30 years later. Following the NLM report [5] that generated this definition, Vice President Humphrey distilled 15 summary points from the report [13]. Several of these summary points will be presented to provide the background for our discussion of drug information. The literature of pharmacy and pharmaceutics encompasses all aspects of drugs, beginning with isolation or synthesis, including physical and chemical characteristics, analysis, bioactivity, toxicology, clinical research, market research, and economic and social considerations. The drug literature, reflecting all the individuals who create it and use it, such as chemists, biomedical scientists, all the various health care professionals, attorneys, and patients, is vast and complex. One need only look at a library's classification of their holdings to realize the many different kinds of publications that are available: journals, abstracting and indexing publications, books, compendia, monographs, patents proceedings, reviews, FDA-approved labeling (package inserts), house organs, newsletters, promotional literature, government documents, and analyses by consulting services.

Magnitude

The volume of data and information constituting the drug literature presents unique challenges. Just how large is the drug literature? While the number of biomedical textbooks in print worldwide is an unknown number, the number of journals has been estimated. McCandless et al. [16] in 1963 estimated the number of biomedical journals at 20,000. Almost 20 years later in 1981, Cummings [17] estimated the number of biomedical journals at about 22,000—the number of serial titles received by the National Library of Medicine. The number of individual biomedical articles published each year was over 2 million in 1963 [16] and was estimated to have grown to over 4 million articles per year by 1978 [18]. Our ability to use the reviews and research published in scientific journals is, of course, limited to what we can directly peruse or access through indexing and/or abstracting services. An estimate of the reasonably accessible biomedical literature is represented by the coverage provided by several of the major journal indexing enterprises in this content area. *EMBASE*, published since 1974, contains over 8 million citations from 4000 biomedical journals published in 70 countries [19]. *MEDLINE* contains over 11 million journal citations from 4300 health science journals published since 1966 in 30 languages [20]. *Science Citation Index Expanded* indexes from over 3500 science and technical journals [21]. *EMBASE* and *MEDLINE* are each adding over 400,000 new citations to their databases each year. *Biological Abstracts*, providing access to a broad range of life science disciplines, contains over 12.5 million records from 1969 and indexes from 5200 journals [22]. Representing the chemical literature and patents, *Chemical Abstracts* indexes over 8000 sources and has almost 16 million abstract records [23].

Origin

All of the science disciplines contribute to the body of information and knowledge that is used by pharmaceutical researchers, educators, and practitioners. Questions and information needs that arise within a pharmaceutical specialty will not necessarily be met by the literature associated with that specialty [13]. Researchers and academics particularly need access to a broad range of science literature. English is widely used; however, the biomedical literature is and has been truly international [13]. About 86% of the current *MEDLINE* database is English language even though only 52% of current cited articles were published in the United States [20].

Science is global, and the literature of the pharmaceutical sciences is no exception. Within the last decade the sciences and processes of drug development and therapeutics have become significantly less regional and more global. Pharmaceutical firms have merged to create international enterprises. Organized in 1990, the International Conference on Harmonization, representing the European Union, Japan, and the United States, is committed to "increased international harmonisation, aimed at ensuring that good quality, safe and effective medicines are developed and registered in the most efficient and cost-effective manner. These activities are pursued in the interest of the consumer and public health, to prevent unnecessary duplication of clinical trials in humans and to minimize the use of animal testing without compromising the regulatory obligations of safety and effectiveness" [24]. Clinical data and information we use to make patient care decisions increasingly will be from clinical trials conducted outside the United States and/or conducted in multicountry sites. Extrapolating data generated by studies done in one country to patients located in another country presents ethnic and regional population considerations. The U.S. Food and Drug Administration (FDA) has issued a guidance recommending regulatory and development strategies that addresses extrapolation of data across populations [25]. Genetic, physiological, and pathological conditions and environmental ethnic factors are considered in the guidance.

The intense need for herbal information in response to consumer interest in natural products was an acute reminder that information and knowledge generated locally have an international role. Confusion created by multiple names and unreliable nomenclature and classification of natural products mirrors problems encountered with drug nomenclature in the 1960s. Our information deficit in this area is still large. Chapter 24 presents a discussion of natural products.

C. An Information Imperative: Self-Renewal

Information and knowledge develop on a continuum. Facts and information gained during the years of our formal education represent a thin slice on this continuum. Some of what we learn from the academic curriculum does remain viable; unfortunately, much decays and becomes incomplete and inaccurate. Health care professionals and scientists must constantly renew and add to their skills, resources, and knowledge. This is fundamental to the profession. The Millis Commission in 1975 eloquently stated [26]:

> One can conceive any health service, medicine, nursing, dentistry, or pharmacy, as a *knowledge system*. It is a system which generates or integrates knowledge about man in sickness and in health, takes knowledge from other sciences and arts, criticizes and organizes that knowledge, translates knowledge into technology, uses some knowledge to create products, devices, and instruments, transmits the knowledge through the education of practitioners and dissemination to others, to the end that an individual known as a patient may benefit from the particular knowledge system and its consequent skills.

Having identified pharmacy and the other health care professions as knowledge systems, the Commission went on to describe three intellectual skills requisite to the professionals: problem identification, problem solving, and continued learning [27]. Medical education—and we can add pharmacy education, according to Pickering—is successful when "the student is equipped to learn, so that in his future professional life he will have little difficulty in keeping abreast of advances in thought or knowledge" [28].

Drug information skills coupled with the processes and technology offered by informatics are part of the solution to mastering information overload and maintaining the knowledge system that improves patient care outcomes.

D. Implications for Pharmacy

The keys to open pharmaceutical and therapeutic information sources are revealed by the characteristics of the drug literature itself. Successful drug information activities recognize that:

- Relevant information may be found outside your specialty area
- Non–English language literature may be required
- Traditional information sources, books and journals, contain only a portion of relevant information
- The size of the literature necessitates search methods and instruments with high sensitivity and specificity
- Multiple names for a chemical or natural product must be anticipated
- Data, information, and knowledge can have short shelf-lives
- Learning and relearning must continue all our lives
- Search and retrieval success requires continuous quality improvement
- Skills and tools derived from the new discipline of informatics offer some solutions to the challenges of information volume, access, and management
- Competent evaluation of the literature is vital

II. STRUCTURE AND CHARACTERISTICS OF THE DRUG LITERATURE

From the perspective of an individual user, such as a health care practitioner or scientist, an understanding of the structure of the literature has value in that this will improve the efficiency with which the user can find relevant information. The relationship between the primary, secondary, and tertiary literature reflects the path an original unit of scientific data and/or information takes as it progresses from its first public reporting to its final evaluation and placement into the context of general knowledge of a subject. Figure 1, the idealized publication cycle, depicts this path, from initial research and development to full utilization of the information, as a circle [29]. Not all information will pass through each of the publication formats; some formats will be skipped entirely. However, an essential feature of the publication cycle is its cyclical nature. Research is published in fairly sequential phases that bring increasingly broader exposure, availability, and application [30]. The phases that add value to the information, such as indexing, repackaging, compaction, and evaluation, also add an inherent time lag into the cycle. The cyclical construct also recognizes the fact that research begets research. Today's research is built on prior research that has been made available to investigators through such media as preliminary communications, conference papers, index databases, and journal articles. For a comprehensive discussion of pharmacy, pharmaceutical and medical publications and resources the reader is referred to *Drug Information, A Guide to Current Resources* [31].

In 1972 Walton et al. [32] modeled the drug literature as a pyramid with the primary literature forming the base of the pyramid, the secondary literature interfacing and serving as a bridge from the primary literature to reference works (tertiary literature). Reference works (tertiary literature) are the capstone of the pyramid and represent the smallest portion of the total literature volume.

A. Primary Literature

The primary literature contains the first written accounts of original research. In terms of size, the primary literature is probably larger than either the secondary or tertiary literature.

Prepublication Literature

The initial recording of research ideas and data is most always private and takes the form of laboratory notebooks and database files. The first communication of research data and ideas may or may not be private. Oral and informal written communication occurs between research colleagues and teams. In the era of e-mail and listserves, these initial written communications may also be public in that they exist on the Internet. If there is a financial or proprietary interest in the research, the first communication may be in the form of a patent application.

Prior to formal publication of the research, the work may be presented as a paper or poster at a professional meeting or conference. Although some professional societies and associations do publish abstracts of papers presented at their conferences in their journals, papers and posters tend to have relatively small exposure and may never appear in the broadly published primary literature. Likewise,

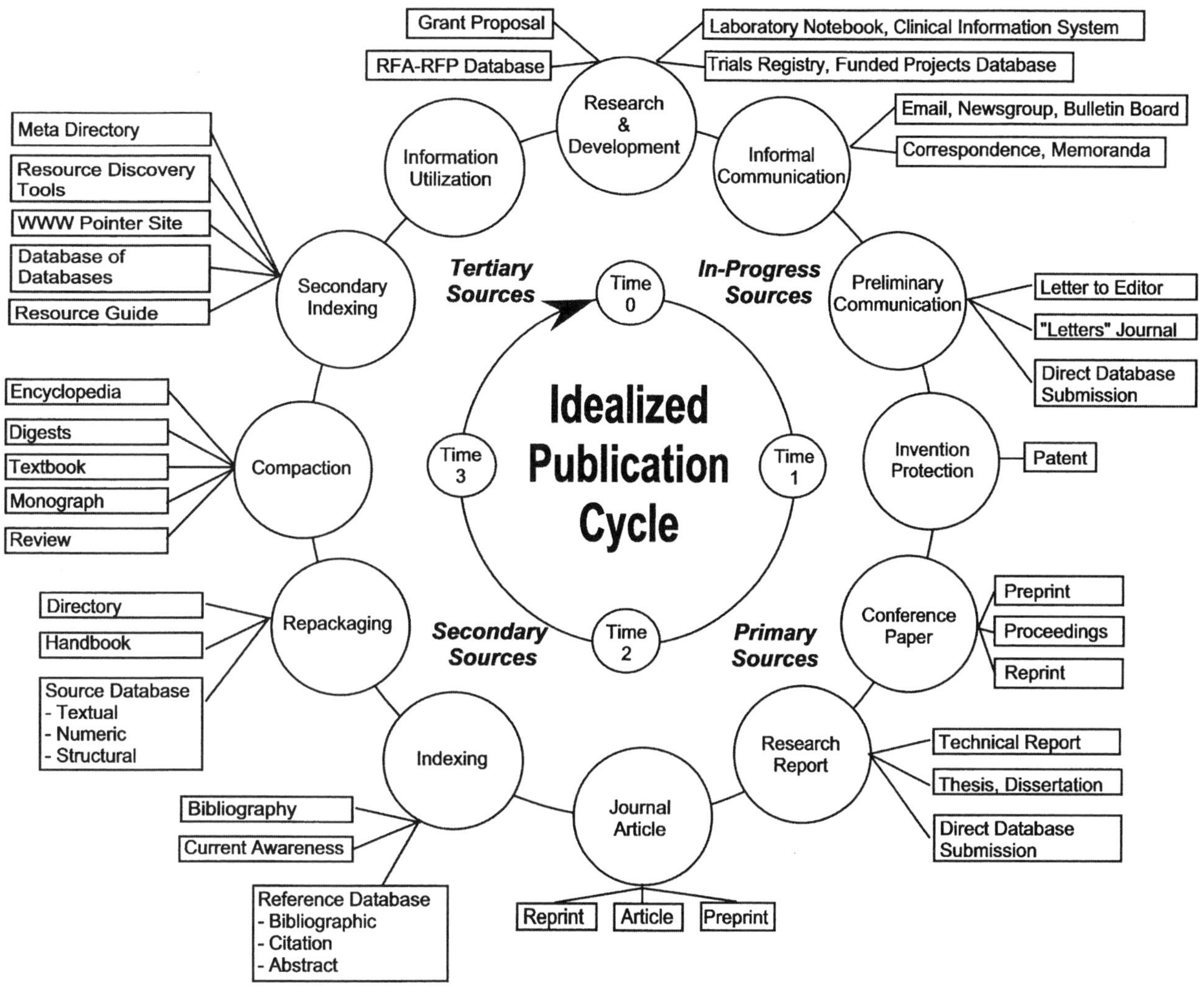

Fig. 1 The idealized publication cycle. (Adapted from Encyclopedia of Library and Information Science, Vol. 26, Marcel Dekker, Inc., New York, 1979, and Lehmann HP, http://www.welch.jhu.edu/classes/tut/lit-srch/pubcycle.html, accessed 7/18/2000. Courtesy of Marcel Dekker, Inc. and Harold P. Lehmann, M.D., Johns Hopkins School of Medicine.)

research culminating in a thesis, dissertation, or technical report may never be published in a scientific journal.

Journal or Serial Literature

As a formal vehicle for communication, the serial journal appeared about 300 years ago in Britain and France [33]. Since that time the number of scientists, the number of research papers, and the number of scientific and professional journals have increased at a dramatic and, for many years, an alarming rate. It is estimated that by 1880 between 4500 and 5000 biomedical journals were being published [34]. The number of biomedical journals published, now thought to be over 16,000 [35], is in itself a significant characteristic of the primary literature and an inhibiting factor in the effective use of the primary literature. Price [36] in the 1960s tracked the growth of journals and found an exponential increase in the number of journals of about 6–7% each year, resulting in a doubling in size every 10–15 years. Recent assessment suggests that the exponential growth has changed to a steady state, primarily due to a transition from exponential to steady-state growth in the number of scientists [37].

The current evolution or transition of the journal from a paper-only publication to a paper-and-electronic publication is a second, relatively recent, major change in the journal literature. Electronic publication began with tentative steps in the early 1990s, and by the end of the 1990s it was clear that the serial literature had acquired a new, electronic format. The e-journal transition will likely only increase the communicative value of journals. In the electronic format, the lag time between the submission of a written research report and its publications can be shortened considerably. Electronic preprint (eprints), either from the author or from the journal publisher, places an article before the reader several months ahead of paper publication release, albeit without benefit of traditional full peer review. Electronic preprints are a new intermediary step on the path of research from its appearance as a published abstract of a paper presented at a meeting and its appearance in a peer-reviewed journal. Contrasted to paper, publication space in the electronic medium is not limited. The ability to enhance research reports with background information, raw data, images, explanatory notes, links to other papers and extensive "letters-to-the-editor" communication is a considerable advantage for electronic journals. Journals are now an interactive medium, providing communication between authors, publishers, and readers.

Regardless of the number of eprints, peer-reviewed articles, or journals, the overriding concern of the reader will continue to center on the quality and usability of the articles he or she has the ability to access. One criterion used to judge the value of an individual article is whether or not that article is used as a reference, that is, is cited in a future article. Garfield [38] estimated that perhaps as few as 5–6% of all journals are being cited. In a citation analysis study he found that only 152 journals accounted for 50% of all references in his sample. This finding suggests that effective coverage of the biomedical disciplines can be provided by a few hundred journal titles. A relatively small number of core journals will contain about one third of the articles for any subject or disciple [35]. Reflecting this, the National Library of Medicine's Abridged Index Medicus (AIM) [39] subset consists of 120 journal titles, and the 1999 Brandon/Hill Selected List of books and journals for medical libraries recommends 145 journal titles [40].

B. Secondary Literature

Indexing and Abstracting Services

Emphasizing the problems associated with the burgeoning literature, Naisbitt [8] used this example: "Scientists who are overwhelmed with technical data complain of information pollution and charge that it takes less time to do an experiment than to find out whether or not it has already been done." Indexing and abstracting services have, to a variable extent, tamed the explosion of primary journal articles. Organized, current, relevant, time-efficient access to the primary literature is the goal of bibliographic retrieval databases. Anticipating the information needs of practitioners and researchers, the index/abstract services construct a path of words to an individual article. In earlier years the words used to describe the content of each article came from a controlled vocabulary, and for successful retrieval it was imperative that the user choose the correct word or words. Today, in addition to providing indexing from their thesauri, most index/abstract services add all (except trivial) words obtained by scanning the database into their database index, thus freeing users to search with their own natural vocabulary.

The National Library of Medicine's service, *Index Medicus*, was first published in 1879 [41]. Given its size and free availability, it is probably the most used index/abstract service worldwide. However, as even the most novice searchers know, searching multiple databases will invariably uncover relevant citations from each additional database searched. Other secondary databases discussed later in this chapter that complement one another's coverage in the chemical, pharmaceutical, and medical areas include *Chemical Abstracts*, *Biological Abstracts*, *EMBASE*, *IDIS*, *IPA*, *MEDLINE*, and *Science Citation Index*. Each of these bibliographic databases was originally available to the user in a nonelectronic format, such as paper or microform. In the mid-1960s the services began appearing in digitized, computer-searchable format from online reference retrieval vendors such as Lockheed Information Systems' DIALOG, System Development Corporation's ORBIT, and Bibliographic Retrieval Services (BRS). CD-ROM technology in the 1980s allowed users to search the index/abstract databases in-house via personal computers. Internet access to these same bibliographic databases is now enhancing the search-and-retrieval process by providing linkage to full text articles.

Evaluated Secondary Resources

Complete, detailed indexing schemes and comprehensive journal coverage is both an asset and a liability for index/abstract databases. From the user's point of view, the number of citations retrieved from a bibliographic database search may still be too large for reasonable review and assimilation. In clinical medicine, there has been an interest in being able to sift, from large index/abstract database search results, just those citations that represent the strongest research or research that is likely to change medical practice. Limiting one's search results to just randomized controlled clinical trials does identify those research studies that have the design capability most likely to conclude causality. However, problems in the study's execution or interpretation can still limit its usefulness and relevancy. Choosing or limiting the search retrieval to meta-analyses, guidelines, or systematic reviews will also identify citations with the strongest research methods and designs. The goal of guidelines and systematic reviews is to identify relevant research and classify it by strength. Meta-analyses also identify all relevant research (in some cases even unpublished research) and, in addition to classifying the research by strength, also combine the research results statistically to provide a new, global research result.

The ability to recognize value and relevance is a uniquely human attribute. Computer algorithms to identify those citations with the greatest relevance are helpful and will continue to improve. However, currently available evaluated bibliographic databases depend upon human experts to identify the best citations.

ACP Journal Club. *ACP Journal Club* [42] is a synoptic journal for internal medicine with expanded coverage of family medicine, obstetrics, gynecology, pediatrics, psychiatry, and surgery. *ACP Journal Club* surveys over 100 peer-reviewed medical journals with the general purpose of selecting published articles according to explicit criteria and to abstract those studies and reviews that warrant attention by physicians attempting to keep pace with advances in the treatment, prevention, diagnosis, cause, prognosis, or economics of the disorders managed by internists. These articles are summarized in "value-added" abstracts and commented on by clinical experts. *ACP Journal Club* is available as a paper or electronic subscription.

Best Evidence. *Best Evidence* [43] combines more than 1200 abstracts and commentaries from *ACP Journal Club* and *Evidence-Based Medicine* (described below) and the full text of *Diagnostic Strategies for Common Medical Problems*, 2nd ed., together on a CD-ROM. It is commercially available.

Cochrane Library. *The Cochrane Library* [44] includes *The Cochrane Database of Systematic Reviews*, a collection of regularly updated, systematic reviews of the effects of health care. It is maintained by contributors to the Cochrane Collaboration. Cochrane reviews are reviews mainly of randomized controlled trials. To minimize bias, evidence is included or excluded on the basis of explicit quality criteria. Data are often combined statistically, with meta-analysis, to increase the power of the findings of numerous studies, each too small to produce reliable results individually. *Database of Abstracts of Reviews of Effectiveness* is also included. It consists of critical assessments and structured abstracts of good systematic reviews published elsewhere. *The Cochrane Controlled Trials Register* with bibliographic information on controlled trials and other sources of information on the science of reviewing research and evidence-based health care are part of the *Cochrane Library*. It is commercially available on CD-ROM or the Internet.

Evidence-Based Medicine. *Evidence-Based Medicine* [45] consists of summarized abstracts of articles on family medicine, internal medicine, general surgery, pediatrics, obstetrics, gynecology, psychiatry, and anesthesiology with commentary by clinical experts. More than 50 peer-reviewed medical journals are abstracted. Also included are key selections from *ACP Journal Club*. *Evidence-Based Medicine* is commercially available; however, its distribution is restricted and does not include North, Central, or South America.

Internet Search Engines

Search engines available on the Internet function like the traditional index/abstract services discussed above, in that they search and retrieve information to answer questions. They provide access to a staggeringly large number of electronic documents available on the World Wide Web (WWW). Traditional index/abstract database services (*DIALOG, MEDLINE, IDIS*) search with Boolean logic. Boolean searching matches the terms in the user's search statement with terms appearing in the database. The search is precise, but it is dependent upon the searcher choosing the correct search term to use in the search statement. WWW search engines have made extensive use of probabilistic/statistical search methodologies and natural language processing systems [46]. Probabilistic/statistical methods use the frequency with which the search term(s) appear in the documents and the comparative frequency with which the search term(s) appear in the document compared to the rest of the database to establish relevance of the document to the search statement. Additional factors may also be used and/or weighted in the search algorithm. Natural language processing maps words used in the search statement to knowledge domains or analyzes text structure to retrieve documents with the same meaning as the search statement. Thus a contextual interpretation of the search statement is used in searching. WWW search engines may use single or multiple elements from Boolean, probabilistic/statistical, and natural language methods in their search algorithm. Contrasted to traditional index/abstract database searching, WWW searching requires less training and retrieves a broader selection of search results. While probabilistic/statistical and natural language methods do not require human indexers to assign index words to each document, human indexing may contribute to Internet databases. Also, authors of web documents may submit listings to the search engine. Internet databases may also contain information retrieved by automated web robots, called "web crawlers" or "spiders," that follow web links to identify new pages. While many of the documents found on the WWW are free, some search engines direct the user to fee-based resources. WWW search engines are generally free to the user.

The size of the Web in 1999 was estimated by Lawrence and Giles [47] to be about 800 million pages. However, this number represented publicly indexable Web pages and may not represent the number of publicly accessible Web pages [48]. Lawrence and Giles [47] further reported that the most comprehensive of six major search engines only indexed about 16% of the Web and that the combined coverage of the search engines in their study only included about 42% of the total Web pages. Although complete agreement with these percentages has not occurred [48], the work clearly points out that search engines access only a small percentage of Web documents and that there is not great overlap between search engines.

There are probably even more caveats for successful use of WWW search engines than for traditional index/abstract services. The documents indexed by the major search engines are primarily those available in hypertext markup language (HTML) or plain text format [48]. Documents and files available in other formats, such as Flash, Word, WordPerfect, and Adobe's Portable Document Format (pdf), are generally not indexed. There are several new search engines with the goal of indexing these "invisible" Web files, for example, InvisibleWeb.com, at Uniform Resource Locator (URL) http://www.invisibleweb.com/, and Direct Search, http://gwis2.circ.gwu.edu/~gprice/direct.htm. [49]. Another consideration is that the Web is not indexed with a controlled vocabulary as most scientific and biomedical index/abstract services are. The term or terms used to search for documents are critical to a successful retrieval.

The results presented by Web search engines are generally listed in rank order of most to least relevant. Algorithms used to establish relevance vary. Traditionally relevance has been defined by some measure of content agreement between the search statement and the results; however, some of the Web search engines now use measures of site popularity (number of links or number of times accessed) to rank site relevance. Link analysis does temper the artificially high relevance created by sites that optimize their relevance with keywords, multiple titles, and other techniques [50]. However, valuable sites with fewer links or less general interest may be more difficult to find.

The major search engines provide only one means of access to the Web. Successful searchers will also want to use other Web resources such as directories and specialized search engines. Specialized search engines concentrate their indexing activity on a specific subject. In addition to user submissions and automated robot indexing, content specialists may verify, enhance, and add sites to the specialty database [51]. Specialized search engines are available in the areas of health, medicine, and the sciences and can be found by scanning pointer sites that index the specialized indexes, such as Search Engine Guide, http://www.searchengineguide.com/, or Search Engine Watch, http://searchenginewatch.com/.

C. Tertiary Literature

"Tertiary" publications, as described by Sewell [52] in *Guide to Drug Information*, are those publications that are the furthest removed from the literature of original research. The tertiary literature is a distillation and evaluation of data and information first presented in such primary literature sources as research reports, meeting presentations, and journal articles. Being furthest removed from the primary report, the tertiary literature characteristically is the least current and the most vulnerable to misinterpretations, biases, and inaccuracies. But just as characteristic, the tertiary literature is the most accessible, easiest to use, and perhaps the most used of all information resources. Information searches generally start with a perusal of books, reviews, and handbooks. Review articles, even though they appear in the "primary" journal literature, belong to the tertiary literature as they present a summarized, organized, and sometimes even an evaluated picture of original research data.

Books, Guidelines, and Reviews

The Library/Educational Resources Section of the American Association of Colleges of Pharmacy maintains the *AACP Basic Resources for Pharmaceutical Education* [53]. The reader is referred to this list of books, periodicals, bibliographies, guides, handbooks, dictionaries, directories, and web sites important to pharmacy. The list contains specific sections for the pharmaceutical sciences, including pharmaceutics, biopharmaceutics and pharmacokinetics, cosmetics and industrial pharmacy.

A database of clinical practice guidelines and related documents, *The National Guideline Clearinghouse* (NGC), has been produced by the Agency for Healthcare Research and Quality (AHRQ) in partnership with the American Medical Association (AMA) and the American Association of Health Plans (AAHP) [54]. Key components of NGC include structured abstracts (summaries) about the guidelines and their development, a utility for comparing attributes of two or more guidelines in a side-by-side comparison, syntheses of guidelines covering similar topics, highlighting areas of similarity and difference, links to full-text guidelines, where available, and/or ordering information for print copies.

Aggregated and Linked References

The computer and subsequent evolution of library resources to an electronic format has spawned a new generation of drug information resources—aggregated resources and linked resources. Practitioners and researchers have always needed access to multiple references, regardless of their professional practice site. Digital media allows the aggregation of drug information references that complement one another into a single product. The ability to search each reference using the same search software and the ability to search all the references (cross search) with a single search statement adds value to the aggregate. Electronic linkages between resources have immeasurably increased the functionality of information resources. The text of books is being linked to the full text of their references; research article text is linking to the original data of the study; index/abstract databases are linking to the full text of articles they index. We are likely to see continued innovation in this area. The resources of decision making are becoming a rich matrix linking primary, secondary, and tertiary references and placing them closer and closer to the point where research, drug development, and patient care occur.

MICROMEDEX Systems. MICROMEDEX [55] integrates over 25 texts, monographs, and product databases in the fields of health care, toxicology, and regulatory information. MICROMEDEX and other publishers produce the resources. MICROMEDEX Systems are commercially available in a variety of combinations and formats.

Stat!Ref. Stat!Ref [56] combines more than 30 medical and drug information textbooks from several publishers and allows both individual and cross searching. The texts are commercially available in a variety of electronic combinations.

III. THE SPECTRUM OF DRUG INFORMATION

As a drug moves along the path from discovery to the market and into worldwide use, data and information about the agent are created and accumulate. When this information is published, its value and usefulness to scientific, professional, and patient communities becomes known. Publication of research results at each step of the path is essential. Figure 1 illustrates the ideal publication cycle, which reflects all the stages of drug development. Although most compounds of initial therapeutic interest do not make it to the regulatory approval stage, this does not diminish the obligation to publish the results of all investigations along the path. Finding that a compound has toxicity, has an unstable nature, or performs no better than a placebo is important and should be part of the body of information available in the published literature. There is a tendency, particularly in clinical research, not to publish "negative" results. When this happens we are left with only research that is favorable to the drug, resulting in a skewed picture of the drug's place in therapy. Publication bias, as this tendency is called, is difficult to assess. It is associated more with observational and laboratory-based experimental studies than with randomized controlled clinical trials [57] and with studies that do not show significant results [58]. Where research findings may be patentable, publication is often deferred until a patent application has been filed. Withholding or delaying release of research results for financial gain has been documented, but this practice does not appear to be widespread [59]. Whether or not the unlimited space available to electronic journals and publications will result in a greater number of studies with nonsignificant results being published remains to be seen [60].

The path of drug development and marketing offers a structure for our discussion of the resources that are useful to scientists and practitioners concerned with compounds of potential therapeutic value. The resources themselves, as discussed in the previous section, are classified as primary (original research), secondary (indexing and abstracting services), and tertiary (textbooks and evaluated information). Individual resources are now generally available in more than one physical format; for example, a journal may be available as a paper publication or as an electronic publication (either individually or as part of a publisher's electronic journal collection or content collection). Primary, secondary, and tertiary resources are available for each step in the path of drug development, but reporting time increases from each step to the next.

Narrative descriptions of the information resources presented in the following sections were drawn from public descriptions of the resource provided by their publisher.

A. Research and Development: Preclinical Drug Information

At the point a compound is recognized and then considered for potential pharmaceutic or therapeutic usefulness, researchers will be both consumers of and contributors to the data-information-knowledge cycle that characterizes science. Initially, in the synthesis and purification phase of drug development, information about the compound's chemistry and physical properties may be both sought and created. Whether or not the compound has been of interest to other researchers may be determined by searching public records of grant and contract awards and also by searching resources that cover preliminary and early research results. The patent status of the compound may need to be established.

Preclinical drug development also involves animal testing [61]. Data from one rodent species and one nonrodent species are usually collected to determine the absorption, metabolism, and toxicity characteristics of the compound. Both short-term (2 weeks to 3 months) and long-term (up to several years) studies are done. The long-term studies are particularly useful for carcinogenicity and birth defect studies. These long-term animal studies may continue into the Phase I, II, and III periods (see Sec. II.B). The suitability of the compound for human testing is heavily dependent upon the outcome of the animal studies.

Physical and Chemical Data

AIDSDRUGS. Published by the U.S. National Library of Medicine, *AIDSDRUGS* [62] is a dictionary of chemical and biological agents currently being evaluated in the AIDS clinical trials covered in the companion *AIDSTRIALS* database. Each record represents a single substance and provides information such as standard chemical names, synonyms and trade names, CAS Registry Numbers, protocol ID numbers, pharmacological action, adverse reactions and contraindications, physical/chemical properties, and manufacturers' names. Agents tested in closed or completed trials are included. A bibliography of relevant articles is also included. *AIDSTRIALS* and *AIDSDRUGS*, http://sis.nlm.nih.gov/pagee.cfm, are available free of charge at the NLM web site.

Beilstein. *Beilstein* [63], a structure and factual database covering organic chemistry, contains more than 7,688,485 substance records (3/2000). The organic substance records contain reviewed and evaluated documents from the *Beilstein Handbook of Organic Chemistry* as well as data from 120 journals in organic chemistry covering the period 1779 to the present. *Beilstein Database* is commercially available in several electronic formats.

CAS Registry. *CAS Registry* [23], a substance database containing structures and chemical names, has more than 25,000,000 substance records, including more than 16,000,000 organic and inorganic substances and 4,000,000 biosequences. *CAS Registry* is commercially available from the American Chemical Society.

Chemcyclopedia. An annual supplement to *Chemical & Engineering News (C&EN)*, *Chemcyclopedia* [64] provides a listing of chemicals, trade names, packaging, special shipping requirements, potential applications, and CAS Registry Numbers, if available. Chemicals are listed in categories. By accessing the online edition, users may obtain detailed information about chemicals and companies. For example, users can search for specific chemicals and retrieve an alphabetical listing of the companies that supply such chemicals. In addition, users can search the company directory for contact information on each company listed in *Chemcyclopedia*, including information on advertisers. *Chemcyclopedia* is available free online from the American Chemical Society.

ChemFinder. *ChemFinder* WebServer [65] is a WWW search engine that works from a single master list of chemical compounds covering all areas of chemistry. Because the *ChemFinder* WebServer is a chemical database, it can also provide information that a general-purpose WWW index cannot, including physical property data and two-dimensional chemical structures. There are over 75,000 unique substances indexed in the *ChemFinder* WebServer database from over 350 sites. Searching can be done by chemical name, CAS number, molecular formula, or molecular weight. There is no fee for using *ChemFinder* WebServer.

Chemical Abstracts. *Chemical Abstracts (CA)* [23] is a collection of chemical information, with nearly 16 million abstracts of journal articles, patents, and other documents. In addition, the *CAOLD* database contains over 3 million abstracts from 1907–1966. Sources for *CA* include more than 8000 journals, patents, technical reports, books, conference proceedings, and dissertations from around the world. *CA* patent database covers 29 national patent offices and two international bodies. About 16% of the *CA* database, approximately 2.5 million records, are from the patent literature. *Chemical Abstracts* is commercially available from the American Chemical Society in several formats.

ChemIDplus. Published by the U.S. National Library of Medicine, *ChemIDplus* [62] is a web-based search system, http://chem.sis.nlm.nih.gov/chemidplus/, that provides free access to structure and nomenclature authority files used for the identification of chemical substances cited in National Library of Medicine (NLM) databases. *ChemIDplus* also provides structure searching and direct links to biomedical resources at NLM and on the Internet. The database contains over 349,000 chemical records, over 56,000 of which include chemical structures, and is searchable by name, synonym, CAS registry number, molecular formula, classification code, locator code, and structure.

Chemindex plus. This database contains 8000 pharmaceutical ingredients linked to 300,000 preparations. *Chemindex plus* [66] can be interrogated at the national or international level. It covers compounds available in 55 countries recording their brand name, local manufacturer, launch date, therapeutic class, and base forms. This product is commercially available from IMS HEALTH Global Services.

Ei CompendexWeb. *Compendex* [67] is a comprehensive bibliographical database of engineering research literature containing references to over 5000 engineering journals and conferences. About half the citations (from 2600 journals and conferences) include abstracts and indexing in the records. *Ei Compendex* contains over 3 million summaries of journal articles, technical reports, and conference papers and proceedings in electronic form, dating from 1970 forward. The highest percentages of journal literature are in the fields of chemical and process engineering (15%), computers and data processing (12%), applied physics (11%), and electronics and communication (12%). In addition, *Compendex* includes civil engineering (6%) and mechanical engineering (6%). *Ei Compendex* is commercially available from Engineering Information, Inc.

The Merck Index. *The Merck Index* [68] is an encyclopedia of chemicals, drugs, and biologicals that contains more than 10,000 monographs. Each monograph is a concise description of a single substance or a small group of closely related compounds. The subjects covered include human and veterinary drugs, biologicals and natural products, agricultural chemicals, industrial and laboratory chemicals, and environmentally significant compounds. The information provided includes chemical, common, and generic names, trademarks and their associated companies, Chemical Abstracts Service (CAS) Registry Numbers, molecular formulas and weights, physical and toxicity data, therapeutic and commercial uses, citations to the chemical, biomedical and patent literature, and chemical structures. In addition, there are name, formula, CAS Registry Number, and therapeutic category/biological activity indices. The collection of supplementary tables contains physical, chemical, and biomedical data and listings of pharmaceutical company names, locations, and experimental drug codes. The Organic Name Reactions section has been reintroduced with revised and updated content. The text is commercially available in paper, CD-ROM, and online formats.

NIST Chemistry WebBook. The National Institute of Standards and Technology (NIST) Chemistry WebBook [69] provides free access to chemical and physical property data for chemical species via the internet, http://webbook.nist.gov/chemistry/. The data provided in the site are from collections maintained by the NIST Standard Reference Data Program and outside contributors. Data in the *WebBook* system are organized by chemical species. The *WebBook* system allows users to search for chemical species by formula, name, CAS registry number, author, structure, ion energetics properties, vibrational and electronic energies, and molecular weight. This site provides thermochemical, thermophysical, and ion energetics data compiled by NIST under the Standard Reference Data Program.

The Registry of Toxic Effects of Chemical Substances. The Registry of Toxic Effects of Chemical Substances (RTECS) [70] is a database of toxicological information compiled, maintained, and updated by the National Institute for Occupational Safety and Health (NIOSH). The Occupational Safety and Health Act of 1970 mandated the program. RTECS now contains over 133,000 chemicals as NIOSH strives to fulfill the mandate to list "all known toxic substances and the concentrations at which toxicity is known to occur." This database is available for searching through the GOV. Research_Center (GRC) service at http://grc.ntis.gov by subscription or by a day pass.

The USP Dictionary of USAN and International Drug Names. The USP Dictionary [71] provides comprehensive information on chemical and brand names of drugs. It includes U.S. Adopted Names (USANs) and International Nonproprietary Names (INNs). It also lists drug manufacturers, therapeutic uses, and molecular and graphic formulas. The 2000 edition of the *USP Dictionary of USAN and International Drug Names* provides over 8400 nonproprietary drug names. FDA recognizes this dictionary as the source for established drug names in the United States. The reference is commercially available in several formats from The United States Pharmacopeial Convention, Inc.

Patents

Through the granting of a patent the U.S. Patent and Trademark Office (PTO) provides intellectual property protection to an inventor for 20 years. A patent gives the inventor the "the right to exclude others from making, using, offering for sale, or selling" the invention in the United States or "importing" the invention into the United States [72]. The PTO classifies patents as utility (how an article is used and works, i.e., its functionality), design (how an article looks, i.e., its ornamentation), plant (an asexually reproduced new variety of plant), reissue, and statutory invention registration (SIR). Patents are further designated with subclass categories. For example, Class 514 "DRUG, BIO-AFFECTING AND BODY TREATING COMPOSITIONS" contains a subclass 198: "ampicillin per or salt thereof." The classification system is dynamic and changes with time. The United States does not publish patent applications until the patent has been issued, so information about patents pending is not available from the PTO.

A patent file history, also called a file wrapper, is the complete set of documents for a patent filed with the U.S. Patent and Trademark Office. These papers chronicle communications and actions taken by the patent examiner, the applicant, and the applicant's attorney from the time of patent application to issue. File histories are available from commercial services such as Intellectual Property Network (described below).

The information contained in patents is primarily useful to pharmaceutical scientists and the pharmaceutical industry. However, preliminary human data in limited numbers of subjects may be presented in the patent, thus representing the first report of clinical data. The patent itself contains several elements, including a descriptive title of the invention, bibliographical information about the inventor(s), assignee and attorney, cross references to related patent applications, an abstract of the application, a statement regarding federally sponsored research and development applicable to the invention, a background statement, a brief summary of the invention and a brief description of any drawings, a detailed description of the invention, and a listing of the claims for the invention. Drug patents do refer to the purported therapeutic use of the compound and may present animal pharmacological data.

At the time the initial patent application is made, the full spectrum of the compound's form and therapeutic use is not generally known. In order to provide the broadest possible patent protection for the invention, the information in the patent describing the invention may be fairly general. This of course makes searching drug patents difficult. Those resources that allow one to track backward from a drug's trade or generic name or the manufacturer's code designation can be particularly helpful. Information now available on FDA's web sites provides links between the generic drug name and its patents. The patents that FDA regards as covered by the statutory provisions for submission of patent information are: patents that claim the *active ingredient* or ingredients; *drug product patents*, which include formulation/composition patents; and *use patents* for a particular approved indication or method of using the product [73]. New Drug Application (NDA) holders or applicants amending or supplementing applications with formulation/composition patent information are asked to declare that the patent(s) is appropriate for publication and refers to an approved product or one for which approval is being sought. The Agency asks all applicants or application holders with use patents to provide information as to the approved indications or uses covered by such patents. This information (patent and patent exclusivity) is included in *The Orange Book* (discussed below) as it becomes available.

U.S. Patent and Trademark Office Web Patent Databases. The Patent and Trademark Office (PTO) [72] offers free World Wide Web access, http://www.uspto.gov/main/patents.htm, to a bibliographic patent database that uses the most current patent classification system, this may not match the classification data that appears on the printed patent, and to a full-text patent database that uses the classification data that appear on the printed patent, this may not match the current classification data. The databases start with January 1, 1976, patents. The full text of a patent includes all bibliographical data (e.g., inventor's name, the patent's title, the assignee's name, etc.) and the abstract, full description of the invention, and the claims. All the words in the text of the patent are searchable. If the patent number is known, the patent, regardless of year, can be ordered from the PTO. Automated searching of 1971 to date patents is available at some of the Patent and Trademark Depository Libraries. Prior to 1971 searching can be done at the PTO facilities or at the Patent and Trademark Depository Libraries. Commercial patent search services are also available.

The Delphion Intellectual Property Network. *The Delphion Intellectual Property Network (IPN)* [74] is a research tool for patent information. It contains searchable bibliographical data and complete patent images for patents issued by the U.S. Patent & Trademark Office (USPTO), the World Intellectual Property Organization (WIPO), the European Patent Office (both applications and granted patents), and the Japanese Patent Information Organization (bibliographic data and abstract only). Along with these collections, summaries of IBM Technical Disclosure Bulletins (TDB), published from 1958 to 1997, are available for searching and browsing. References in patents to TDBs are linked to the full article. Searching, browsing, and viewing of patents is free. File histories of U.S. patents are available on the *IPN* for a fee. The site allows patent holders to identify their invention with a "Licensing Button" identifying the patent as available for licensing. Optional fee-based services include document delivery, licensing buttons, data mining and analysis tools and value added content from industry providers. The *Intellectual Property Network*, in collaboration with ISI (*Science Citation Index*), offers links to abstracts of journal articles cited in the patent and to other patents that also reference the same journal article.

Derwent International Patent Family File and U.S. Patents Full Text. *Derwent International Patent Family File (DIPF)* [75] provides access to 20 million patents issued by 40 patent-issuing authorities, covering more than 10 million inventions as far back as 1963. The *DIPF* is linked to *U.S. Patents Full-Text (US-PAT)* [75]. *US-PAT* contains the full text of more than 2 million patents issued by the U.S. Patent and Trademark Office since 1976. *DIPF* and *US-PAT* are available on the commercial online service Westlaw.

Derwent World Patents Index. *Derwent World Patents Index (DWPI)* [76] is a comprehensive database of patent documents published worldwide. It covers over 10 million separate inventions from more than 20 million basic and equivalent patent documents. *DWPI* is commercially available on the following online services: DIALOG, Questel, Orbit, and STN. Pharmaceuticals from 1963, agricultural and veterinary medicine from 1965, plastics and polymers from 1966, all chemistry from 1970, electronics, electrical and mechanical engineering from 1974, and comprehensive coverage of all technologies from 1974 are included. International coverage of all patented technologies from forty patent-issuing authorities is provided—including patents from the US, Japan, Patent Cooperation Treaty (PCT) members and major European countries, plus Research Disclosures and International Technology Disclosures. All records contain patent family information, including non-convention members. Structural chemical indexing and patent drawings are available for patents.

Drugs Under Patent. This book [77] is a cross-referenced listing of over 2500 drugs covered in the United States under patent law and marketing exclusivity provisions of the Waxman-Hatch Act. Eight indexes provide market and patent status information by company, trade name, generic name, expiration date, dosage form, exclusivity code, patent number, and NDA number. Updated annually, this book is available commercially.

Electronic Orange Book, Approved Drug Products with Therapeutic Equivalence Evaluations. The Orange Book [73], http://www.fda.gov/cder/ob/default.htm, identifies drug products approved on the basis of safety and effectiveness by FDA under the Federal Food, Drug, and Cosmetic Act. Drugs on the market approved only on the basis of safety (i.e., those approved prior to the 1938 Food, Drug and Cosmetic Act) are not included in this publication. The main criterion for the inclusion of any product is that the product is the subject of an application with an effective approval that has not been withdrawn for safety or efficacy reasons. The listing is composed of four parts: (1) approved prescription drug products with therapeutic equivalence evaluations; (2) approved over-the-counter (OTC) drug products for those drugs that may not be marketed without NDAs or ANDAs because they are not covered under existing OTC monographs; (3) drug products with approval under Section 505 of the Act administered by the Center for Biologics Evaluation and Research; and (4) a cumulative list of approved products that have never been marketed, have been discontinued from marketing, or have had their approvals withdrawn for other than safety or efficacy reasons subsequent to being discontinued from marketing. In addition, the listing contains therapeutic equivalence evaluations for approved multisource prescription drug products. The Patent and Exclusivity Information Addendum to the book identifies drugs that qualify under the Drug Price Competition and Patent Term Restoration Act (1984 Amendments) for periods of exclusivity, during which abbreviated new drug applications (ANDAs) and applications described in Section 505(b)(2) of the Federal Food, Drug, and Cosmetic Act for those drug products may, in some instances, not be submitted or made effective, and provides patent information concerning the listed drug products. Those drugs that have qualified for Orphan Drug Exclusivity pursuant to Section 527 of the Act and those drugs that have qualified for Pediatric Exclusivity pursuant to Section 505A are also included in this Addendum.

Patents International. IMSworld Drug Patents International database [66] provides access to the patent status of over 1200 molecules. The database contains information on patents due to expire (over a given time period), patents by therapy class, and patents by country. This product is commercially available in several formats.

Grants, Contracts, and Work-in-Progress

Several resources are helpful in determining whether or not a compound is under investigation in a current study or if there are funding opportunities available for a compound. From a patient's point of view, these same resources are also useful to identify clinical studies that may be of interest to them and their physicians.

Notices of work-in-progress may first appear in informal electronic communication modes such as e-mail, newsgroups, usenets, and on the web sites of individual researchers and laboratories. Early research results may be presented at professional meetings. Internet search engines provide access to newsgroups, usenets, and web sites. Abstracts of meeting presentations are available through a variety of resources such as the web site of the meeting sponsor, abstract journals, and indexing/abstracting services. Papers presented at conferences, congresses, and professional meetings may be published in bound form as "proceedings."

Research done in an academic setting generally results in a formal publication that appears in the primary literature. The research results contained in dissertations may or may not be published separately. Dissertations are catalogued and placed on the shelves of the student's university. Many universities now have electronic catalogues that allow searching from remote sites. Dissertations are also indexed by commercial organizations (see below).

The resources discussed below represent print resources, online databases, and Usenet. Usenet, a worldwide distributed discussion system, is an informal source of information about research. It consists of a set of "newsgroups," with names that are classified hierarchically by subject. "Articles" or "messages" are "posted" to these newsgroups by people on computers with the appropriate software—these articles are then broadcast to other interconnected computer systems via a wide variety of networks. Some newsgroups are "moderated"; in these newsgroups the articles are first sent to a moderator for approval before appearing in the newsgroup. Usenet is available on a wide variety of computer systems and networks, but the bulk of modern Usenet traffic is transported over either the Internet or Unix-to-Unix Copy (UUCP) [78].

Adis Conference Insight. *Conference Insight* [79] provides coverage of 45 general and specialty medical meetings each year with reviews of conference themes, executive overviews, and reports on oral and poster presentations. This resource is commercially available in several formats.

Adis R&D Insight. Information on *Adit R&D Insight* [79] is presented as drug profiles, each containing the name, chemical structure, and validated CAS registry numbers, developing organization(s) (originator, licensees), drug history (key events in the drug's development), key properties (mechanism of action and therapeutic indications), where the development is taking place, phase of development by country and indication, Lehman Brothers' data assessing the commercial impact, and detailed scientific reviews and evaluations, with supporting bibliography and links to evaluations of key papers from Adis LMS Alerts and Adis rating of therapeutic value. Over 350 new entries are added each month. This resource is commercially available is several formats.

AIDSTRIALS (AIDS Clinical Trials). The *AIDSTRIALS* database [80] provides information about AIDS-related studies of experimental treatments conducted under the FDA's investigational new drug (IND) regulations. *AIDSTRIALS* contains information about clinical trials of agents undergoing evaluation for use against AIDS, HIV infection, and AIDS-related opportunistic diseases such as *Pneumocystis carinii* pneumonia (PCP). Detailed information is supplied by the National Institute for Allergy and Infectious Diseases (NIAID) for trials sponsored by the National Institutes of Health (NIH). Information about non–NIH-funded trials undergoing tests for efficacy is furnished by FDA. The information contained in *AIDSTRIALS* includes the title of the trial, the trial purpose, the agent being tested, the trial phase, diseases studied, patient inclusion and exclusion criteria, trial locations, and whether the trial is open or closed. Details of the treatment regimen may also be included. A companion database, *AIDSDRUGS*, contains descriptive information about the agents being tested in clinical trials. *AIDSTRIALS* and *AIDSDRUGS* are produced as part of the AIDS Clinical Trials Information Service (ACTIS). *AIDSTRIALS* and *AIDSDRUGS*, http://sis.nlm.nih.gov/pagee.cfm, are available free of charge on the NLM computer system.

BIOSCI. *BIOSCI* [78] is a set of electronic communication forums, the bionet USENET newsgroups, and parallel e-mail lists intended primarily for communications between researchers. The *BIOSCI* site is hosted at the U.K. Medical Research Council's Human Genome Mapping Project–Resource Centre with additional support from the Biotechnology and Biological Sciences Research Council (BBSRC) and advertising raised through the web site. *BIOSCI* promotes communication between professionals in the biological sciences. No fees are charged for the service.

Chemical Physics Preprint Database. This database [81] is a fully automated electronic archive and distribution server intended to provide a means for rapid and efficient preprint distribution within the international theoretical chemical physics community. A "preprint" is a copy of a paper that has been submitted for publication. This database has been designed to be a useful and freely available tool for education and research. It allows investigators to submit and retrieve electronic copies of preprints via the Internet. Access for retrieval and listing of papers in the database is possible through WWW servers, anonymous ftp, or e-mail. Currently research papers are submitted to the databases via e-mail. This project is a joint effort by the Department of Chemistry at Brown University and the Theoretical Chemistry and Molecular Physics Group at the Los Alamos National Laboratory. The homepage of *Chemical Physics Preprint Database* is http://www.chem.brown.edu/chem-ph.html. (For a more complete description of the background and development of Paul Ginsparg's preprint system, see *Science* 259:1246–1248, 1993.)

ClinicalTrials.gov. *ClinicalTrials.gov* [82] provides health care professionals and members of the public access to information about clinical trials for a wide range of diseases and conditions. The NIH, through the National Library of Medicine (NLM), developed this site in collaboration with all NIH Institutes and FDA. This site currently contains approximately 5000 clinical studies sponsored primarily by the NIH. Additional studies from other federal agencies and the pharmaceutical industry will be included. *ClinicalTrials.gov* grew out of 1997 legislation that required the Department of Health and Human Services, through the NIH, to broaden the public's access to information about clinical trials on a wide range of diseases by establishing a registry for both federally and privately funded trials "on drugs for serious or life-threatening diseases and conditions" (Section 113, "Information Program on Clinical Trials for Serious or Life-Threatening Diseases," Food and Drug Administration Modernization Act of 1997, Public Law 105–115). *ClinicalTrials.gov*, http://clinicaltrials.gov, is a free service.

Computer Retrieval of Information on Scientific Projects. *Computer Retrieval of Information on Scientific Projects (CRISP)* [83] is a biomedical database system containing information on more than 2 million biomedical research projects and programs funded by the NIH, Department of Health and Human Services. Most of the research falls within the broad category of extramural projects, grants, contracts, and cooperative agreements conducted primarily by universities, hospitals, and other research institutions and funded by the NIH and other government agencies. A relatively small number of research grants are funded by the Centers for Disease Control and Prevention (CDC), FDA, the Health Resources and Services Administration (HRSA), and the Agency for Health Care Policy and Research (AHCPR). Clinical research is defined as research conducted with human subjects (or on material of human origin such as tissues, specimens, or cognitive phenomena) in which an investigator (or colleague) directly interacts with human subjects. This area of patient-oriented research includes development of new technologies, human disease mechanisms, therapeutic interventions, and clinical trials (Phase I and Phase II/III/IV). Clinical research also includes epidemiological and behavioral studies and outcomes research and health services research. *CRISP* also contains information on the intramural programs of the NIH and the FDA. The *CRISP* database, http://www-commons.cit.nih.gov/crisp/, is updated weekly and available free.

CSline. *CSline* [84] provides information on well-designed and well-executed clinical trials of drugs currently under study or in use in humans. This information includes study objectives, design, population, intervention groups, withdrawals, adverse reactions, endpoints and results, conclusions, and references. The *CSline* database covers more than 500 drugs currently on the market or in development. Pharmacological data from more than 2000 journal articles, congresses, and books are added each year. The product is commercially available on CD-ROM from Prous Science and is updated every 2 months.

Federal Research in Progress Database. *The Federal Research in Progress Database (FEDRIP)* [85] provides access to information about ongoing federally funded projects in the fields of the physical sciences, engineering, and life sciences. *FEDRIP* contains 150,000 records from the current 2 years. Project descriptions generally include project title, keywords, start date, estimated completion date, principal investigator, performing and sponsoring organizations, summary, and progress reports. Record content varies depending on the source agency. The publisher suggests it is useful to avoid research duplication, locate sources of support, identify leads in the literature, stimulate ideas for planning, identify gaps in areas of investigation, locate individuals with expertise, and complement searches of completed research. It is updated monthly and available for a fee.

Dissertation Abstracts. The *Dissertation Abstracts* [86] database contains more than 1.6 million entries about doctoral dissertations and master's theses. The database represents the work of authors from over 1000 graduate schools and universities. Each year 47,000 new dissertations and 12,000 new theses are added to the database. The database includes bibliographical citations for materials beginning with the first U.S. dissertation, accepted in 1861. Citations for dissertations published from 1980 forward also include 350-word abstracts written by each author. Citations for master's theses from 1988 forward include 150-word abstracts. The full text of more than one million of these titles is commercially available in paper and microform formats. *ProQuest Digital Dissertations* provides on-line access to the complete file of dissertations in digital format starting with titles published from 1997 forward.

R&D Focus. This database service [66] provides information on over 7000 drugs in active development. The service monitors the development, efficacy, and status of pharmaceuticals from early clinical testing through to launch. Data are gathered through direct contact with manufacturers and research organizations. It appraises both the scientific and commercial aspects of drug development and is searchable by product, by phase, by mechanism of action, and by country. *R&D Focus* product is commercially available in several formats.

B. Drug Information from Phase I, II, and III Studies, The New Drug Application, and Product Approval/Launch

The Food, Drug and Cosmetic Act of 1938 established the terminology and stages of clinical drug development as Phase I, II, and III [87]. Building on the data and information collected in the preclinical stage of drug development, Phases I, II, and III collect the data that define the compound's safety and efficacy in humans. The terms themselves are used to describe both the path of drug development and the attributes and objectives of an individual premarket clinical trial [61]. The national and global process of drug development and its regulation has and will continue to evolve beyond that set in place in 1938. Therapeutic and economic imperatives to bring promising compounds into use quickly, coupled with the bio-technological ability to do so, have blurred the phases of drug development. Phases I, II, and III now may occur nonsequentially or in parallel with each other.

Phases I, II, and III

The first use of a compound in a human trial occurs in Phase I of drug development. Prior to beginning Phase I work, the compound's sponsor must submit an Investigational New Drug Application (IND) to FDA. The IND includes the data and information about the compound that has been developed and discovered to date. This early information begins to characterize the compound's risks and benefits. Included in the IND is a plan to guide anticipated human investigations using the compound. The primary purpose of Phase I is to establish the compound's safety. Phase I studies generally include 20–100 subjects, who may be either healthy volunteers or patients. These studies are designed to determine the compound's pharmacokinetics, pharmacodynamics, and safety profile, such as side effects and tolerability. Studies with these objectives, such as pharmacokinetic studies, are referred to as Phase I studies, regardless of when in the drug-development sequence the study is carried out. Phase I studies usually last no more than a couple of months. Late Phase I studies that determine the safe dose range for the compound, including the maximum tolerated dose, are called bridging studies because they bridge the gap between Phase I and Phase II research [88]. Because of disappointing safety and/or efficacy data, about one third of the compounds that enter Phase I will not survive to enter Phase II [61].

Phase II investigates the compound's efficacy and safety in controlled clinical trials for a specific therapeutic indication. To eliminate as many competing factors as possible, Phase II trials are narrowly controlled. They are characterized as small—several hundred subjects with the indicated disease or symptoms—and are closely monitored. The control may be either a placebo study arm or an active control arm. The endpoint measured may be the clinical outcome of interest or a surrogate. Phase II trials may last for several months or even several years. Early pilot trials to evaluate safety and efficacy are called Phase IIa. Later trials, called Phase IIb, are important tests of the compound's efficacy. These trials may constitute the pivotal trials used to establish the drug's safety and efficacy. At least one pivotal trial (most frequently a large, randomized Phase III study) is done. Only about one third of compounds entered into Phase II will begin Phase III studies [61].

Phase III represents expanded investigation of the compound's safety and efficacy. Studies include more patients, several hundred to several thousand, and last for 1–4 years. The larger study population provides data on the safety and efficacy of the compound in a variety of patients who generally have fewer exclusions than Phase II subjects. Because the studies are longer, less frequent side effects may appear and therapeutic outcomes requiring several years to appear can be captured. In addition to well-controlled clinical trials, open or uncontrolled trials may be part of Phase III [87]. Phase III trials clarify the drug's safety and efficacy in the population for which the drug will be indicated. These data will be incorporated into the drug's labeling and package insert. Clinical trials may continue during the interim between the sponsor's submission of a New Drug Application (NDA) for the compound and FDA's approval of the NDA; these trials are called Phase IIIb. Approximately 20–30% of compounds started as Phase I will be submitted for FDA approval, with only about 20% reaching the market [61].

The data and information about an individual drug developed through Phase I, II, and III studies are extremely important to the medical community. For many drugs Phase I, II, and III data may be all, or nearly all, that is available about the clinical use of the drug at the time the product is marketed. During the time the product is in Phase I, Phase II, and Phase III, some of the compound's product and clinical data may be presented at professional meetings, published in preliminary reports, or otherwise made available to the scientific and business communities. However, it is not uncommon for a drug to be approved by FDA without the presence of its clinical research in the published biomedical literature.

Drug Data Report. *Drug Data Report* [89] provides access to drug research from the patent literature of Belgium, Canada, European Patent Office, France, Germany, Great Britain, Japan, Spain, Switzerland, United Kingdom, United States, and World Intellectual Property Organization. The patent literature is relevant as preliminary drug research results are presented for the first time in the patent literature. Other sources include the current literature (more than 1500 journals are reviewed), congresses (more than 300 meetings are covered annually), and manufacturers' communications (more than 1200 companies provide product information). *Drug Data Report* is commercially available as a monthly subscription publication and as a database in several electronic formats.

Drugs of the Future. This publication [90] provides drug monographs containing product information on new compounds, including synthesis, pharmacological action, pharmacokinetics and metabolism, toxicology, and clinical studies. Monthly information updates provide the most recent information on compounds published in past volumes and review developments in which chemical, biochemical, pharmacological, and clinical aspects of compounds are discussed. *Drugs of the Future* is commercially available as a monthly subscription publication.

Drug News & Perspectives. *Drug News & Perspectives* [91] is a drug newsmagazine for scientists and managers in pharmaceutical research and development. Sections include research and development briefs, new molecular entities, licensing, product line extensions, and new product introductions. *Drug News & Perspectives* is commercially available as a subscription, as a database in various electronic formats, and via Dialog (File 455) and DataStar (file PRNP). The NME EXPRESS database (compounds appearing in the NMEs column of *Drug News & Perspectives*) is available as a separate database on Dialog (File 456) and DataStar (File PRME).

Ensemble. *Ensemble* [92] includes the drug information published in several Prous Science journals [*Drug Data Report* (since mid-1988), *Drugs of the Future* (since 1990), *Drug News & Perspectives* (selected records since 1992)] and other sources of data. Information is provided for more than 128,000 compounds with biological activity in the drug research and development pipeline, including company codes, generic names, trademarks, industrial or other sources, licensees, development phase, CAS Registry Number, molecular formula, chemical names, pharmacotherapeutic activity and mechanism(s) of action, patent information (titles, inventors, applicants, numbers and publication dates, priority numbers and publication dates), literature references (authors, titles, publications), and the chemical structure image. Starting with the March 2000 release, *Ensemble* contains development pipelines and milestones for selected compounds in the database. The database is commercially distributed on CD-ROM.

Investigational Drugs Database. *Investigational Drugs Database 3 (IDdb3)* is the new version of the *Investigational Drugs Database*. The publication is compiled from patents, scientific meetings, newswires, research papers, and direct communication with drug companies. *IDdb3* tracks information on drug development from first patent disclosure through to product launch. It is commercially available via the Internet or for Intranet use.

The NDA Pipeline. *The NDA Pipeline's* database [94] of more than 7000 drug development projects is available as a web-delivered, searchable information service that is updated each week. A copy of the annual book, an information service from FDC

Reports for 18 years, is available with a commercial subscription to the online version. The online product also includes an expanding number of links to articles in FDC Reports' news publications, *The Pink Sheet* and *Pharmaceutical Approvals Monthly*.

The New Drug Application

A New Drug Application (NDA) is required by federal legislation to be a compilation of all relevant data and information that has been discovered about the drug [61]. To a large extent the information contained in an NDA is generated from animal and human studies that are done while the drug is an Investigational New Drug (IND). The reader is referred to Chapter 19 for a discussion of legislation and FDA actions that have shaped the contents of the New Drug Application.

Following submission of an NDA, FDA will, if the NDA is acceptable, initiate a formal review. The formal review is organized for separate consideration of the medical, biopharmaceutical, pharmacology, statistical, chemistry, and microbiology content of the NDA. The FDA review may also include the opinion and advice of an advisory committee made up of experts who are not FDA employees. There are currently 5 Center for Biologics Evaluation and Research (CBER) and 18 Center for Drug Evaluation and Research (CDER) advisory committees. FDA advisory committee recommendations are not binding, but they are considered very important to the decision process. The transcripts, minutes, and other documents connected with the FDA advisory committees' meetings are public. Both FDA and the drug's sponsor present data for evaluation of the drug's safety and efficacy at the meetings. The review produces an approval, approvable, or nonapprovable recommendation for the application. An approval recommendation allows the drug to be marketed.

Throughout both the drug research and development process and the FDA review process, extremely valuable data and information about the drug are collected and evaluated to establish the drug's efficacy and safety. Public access to this rich resource is limited. Access is controlled by the NDA sponsor, who may or may not publish the studies presented in the NDA and by FDA, who has legal restraints on what information can be released to the public. Reviewing 20 new drugs approved by FDA in 1997, Gilchrist and Seaba [95] found that only 49% of 103 pivotal studies for these new drugs appeared in the published literature as journal articles during a one-year period following the drugs' approval. Another 11% of the pivotal studies were presented as abstracts or posters at scientific meetings.

While much of the NDA is not open to the public, Title 21, Code of Federal Regulations, Part 314.430 contains a provision for public disclosure of information immediately after FDA has sent an approval letter to the applicant. For a new drug, all safety and effectiveness data previously disclosed to the public and a summary of safety and effectiveness data and information that comprised the basis for FDA approval of the new drug are available for public disclosure. For an application approved on or after July 1, 1975, the CFR requires that a Summary Basis of Approval (SBA) document be available for public disclosure. Section 314.430 further provides for public disclosure of test or study protocols, adverse reaction reports, product experience reports, consumer complaints and other similar data and information, a list of all active ingredients and any inactive ingredients previously disclosed to the public, an assay method or other analytical method, all correspondence and written summaries of oral discussions between FDA and the applicant relating to the application, and all records showing the testing of an action on a particular lot of a certifiable antibiotic by FDA.

The regulation allows for two preparation routes: either the applicant may draft the SBA and submit it to FDA for review and revision or FDA may prepare the SBA. Since 1975 both of these methods have been used along with a combination of these two methods. In this latter case, the applicant was requested to prepare specific sections of the SBA and FDA provided other sections that were pulled from FDA's scientific reviews of the NDA. In the mid-1980s FDA began providing, in lieu of a newly written SBA and in some cases in addition to the SBA, a collection of scientific reviews of the NDA from the various FDA disciplines. This collection of reviews contained the essence of the basis upon which the drug was approved. The assembled document was referred to as a "Summary Basis of Approval equivalent." For drugs approved in the last few years, Summary Basis of Approval equivalents have been almost exclusively used. Recently the collection of reviews and documents made available by FDA have been called the Approval Package.

There is no requirement for content other than that the SBA contain a summary of the safety and effectiveness data and information evaluated by FDA during the approval process. Summary Basis of Approval equivalents, also called Approval Packages, generally consist of most, but usually not all, of the following sections:

- FDA Form 356h (Application to Market a New Drug, Biologic, or an Antibiotic Drug for Human Use)
- Letter of Approval
- Letter of Acknowledgment
- Labeling
- Patent Information/Certification, Exclusivity Summary
- Drug Studies in Pediatric Patients
- Medical Officer's Review
- Statistical Review & Evaluation
- Chemistry, Manufacturing and Controls
- CDER Labeling and Nomenclature Committee
- Clinical Pharmacology/Biopharmaceutics
- Microbiologist's Review
- Pharmacokinetics Review
- Carcinogenicity Assessment
- Environmental Assessment and Findings of No Significant Impact
- Correspondence & Record of Telephone Conversations

Parts of the SBA that are considered privileged or trade secrets by the sponsor can be redacted.

Diogenes. Diogenes [96], discussed in more detail in the next section, includes the full text of Drug Summary Basis of Approvals.

FDA Web Site. The *FDA Web Site*, http://www.fda.gov/default.htm, serves many purposes, including that of repository of public documents generated in the course of FDAs monitoring, approval, and enforcement actions for human and animal food, cosmetics, medications, and devices. Some, but not all, Summary Basis of Approval documents are posted in full on the web site. A listing of all FDA dockets is also posted with links to the documents associated with each docket [97]. For CBER and CDER advisory committees, the advisory committee docket documents pertaining to a new drug under consideration can be another valuable source of information for the new drug. Posted documents may include letters to the committee from FDA, the FDA review package for the committee members, and briefing information from the drug's sponsor.

Iowa Drug Information Service. As part of its bibliographical database, the *Iowa Drug Information Service (IDIS)* [98] has indexed FDA Summary Basis of Approval documents for the last several years. A table of contents for the entire SBA is constructed, the pivotal studies are identified and abstracted, and the full text of the SBA is incorporated into the database.

Product Approval and Launch

Several databases identify when a compound has obtained FDA approval. The *FDA Web Site* records this information; although sometimes very current, those data may also appear a week or more behind actual approval dates. The most immediate information about a compound's approval status may be its appearance in a daily newspaper, such as the *Wall Street Journal*.

Diogenes. Diogenes [96] includes the full text of FDA documents generated by the regulatory process. These include Advisory Committee Minutes, FDA Guidelines, Warning Letters, Drug Summary Basis of Approval, Device Summaries of Safety and Effectiveness, Medical Device Report (MDR) Summaries and Approved Product Listings for Device 510(k)s and premarket approval applications (PMAs) as well as drugs and antibiotics. *Diogenes* also contains the full text of the following newsletters published by Washington Business Information, Inc.: *The Food & Drug Letter, Washington Drug Letter, Devices & Diagnostics Letter, Europe Drug & Device Report* and *The GMP Letter*. In addition, the following FDA publications are contained full-text: *FDA Drug & Device Product Approvals, FDA Drug Bulletin, FDA Enforcement Report*, FDA *Federal Register* notice summaries, talk papers, and press releases. *Diogenes* is available as a Dialog database.

Drug Launches. Drug Launches [66] records and documents new product launches throughout the world. Data are compiled directly by 60 IMS companies located throughout the major markets of the world. Each entry records trade names, active ingredients, marketing companies, pack information, launch date, indication, and therapy class. This product is commercially available in several formats.

F-D-C Reports Pharmaceutical Approvals Monthly. Pharmaceutical Approvals Monthly [99] provides coverage of U.S. drug approvals at the clinical level and includes the most recent FDA list of NDA approvals (originals, supplementals, and ANDAs). This specialized monthly also focuses on new drugs that have either been recently approved or reached the "approvable" stage. This product is commercially available in several formats.

Pharmaprojects. This service [100] monitors drugs currently under development, tracking all new drug candidates under active international R&D—approximately 6000 at any one time. The remaining 19,000 or so drug entries are classified by *Pharmaprojects* either as ceased or fully launched. Overall, *Pharmaprojects* contains details on over 25,000 new drug candidates that have been investigated since 1980, including those currently in research and those whose development has been discontinued. Details of each individual drug or formulation are presented in the form of a product profile with the content organized into nine main data fields. In addition to its product profiles, *Pharmaprojects* provides over 1100 individual company profiles, one for each company in the database with an active drug development pipeline. Similarly, individual Therapy Profiles are provided for each of the 199 categories used in the *Pharmaprojects*' therapeutic classification system. This product is commercially available in several formats.

Scrip World Pharmaceutical News. Published twice weekly, *Scrip World Pharmaceutical News* [100] covers the commercial pharmaceutical marketplace with news, products, R&D, regulatory issues, market data, business, and finance. This product is commercially available in several formats.

C. Phase IV Studies and Postmarket Drug Information

At the point of FDA approval of a new drug, the sponsor may be asked to commit to executing one or more postapproval studies [101]. While these studies are not essential for establishment of safety and efficacy of the indication sought, they supplement the drug's safety and efficacy information and increase our ability to use the drug in its most effective manner. Such studies are referred to as Phase IV. Phase IV studies specifically relate to the indication for which the drug was approved, and their execution may be a condition upon which approval depends. Phase IV commitments are most frequently requested to obtain further adverse drug experience or toxicity experience in a defined patient population, clarify drug-drug or drug-food interactions, establish long-term efficacy, expand pharmacokinetic information, or evaluate birth outcomes in women who took the drug. Phase IV observational (nonexperimental) studies are referred to as postmarketing surveillance studies.

For drugs approved under accelerated approval regulations on the basis of a surrogate endpoint or an endpoint other than survival or irreversible morbidity, FDA may require a Phase IV study to confirm the drug's efficacy. Failure to show efficacy may result in withdrawal of approval.

The FDA Modernization Act of 1997 contains a requirement for public disclosure and congressional reporting by October 2001 of Phase IV studies. FDA intends to meet the public disclosure requirement by posting Phase IV study commitments, the projected end of the study, and the current status of the study on their web site [102]. Sponsors whose new drug was approved with a Phase IV study requirement must submit an initial status report to FDA within one year of approval. According to data compiled by Public Citizen's Health Research Group [103], not one of the Phase IV study commitments for 107 new molecular entities approved between January 1995 and December 1999 had been completed as of December 1999.

Clinical studies that investigate further aspects of the drug, beyond the original safety and effectiveness claims for the approved indication(s), are considered therapeutic use studies. At this point in the drug development path–publication cycle (Fig. 1), the chemical, animal, intellectual property, regulatory, and early clinical data outweigh the therapeutic use information. With the exception of a few Phase II and Phase III studies that might have been published either in the United States or internationally, there is not likely to be a large body of published research or experience about the use of the drug in the human. Unfortunately, this is the point where interest in the drug is high due to the manufacturer's promotion activities surrounding the product launch. Decisions concerning formulary status of the new drug by hospitals and managed care organizations are being made. Individual practitioners are considering use of the drug for specific patients. In essence, health care professionals are trying to determine the place of the new drug in the context of other existing therapies. Under these circumstances, a thorough literature search to find material relevant to the clinical use of the drug would consist of not only searching the basic bibliographical databases such as *Biological Abstracts, EMBASE, IDIS, IPA, MEDLINE*, and *Science Citation Index*, but also searching the patent literature, perhaps using the *Patent and Trademark Office Web Patent Databases* for the drug's use patent, which may contain some early clinical experience information and/or citations, and also obtaining the drug's Summary Basis of Approval (Approval Package) either directly from FDA or through *Diogenes* or *IDIS* and reviewing the FDA advisory committee proceeding documents at the FDA Docket web site.

As the time from launch lengthens, studies exploring the drug's efficacy and safety under a variety of different patient-management conditions appear in the published literature, pharmacoeconomic evaluations of the drug's use are done and studies directly comparing the new drug to therapeutic alternatives for the same indication are reported. We begin to know the drug and see patterns and guidelines for its use develop. Review articles, both traditional and systematic, follow the clinical trials, and eventually the drug will appear in textbook and monograph resources.

The following bibliographic databases provide, to varying degrees, access to the full span of life-science periodical literature, including all stages of a compound's development from early brief reports to comprehensive assessments after years of clinical use. Some of the databases have established links from their article citations to the articles' full text.

BIOSIS. *BIOSIS* [22] processes approximately 550,000 items each year, from primary research and review journals, books, monographs, and conference proceedings. More than 6500 serials are monitored for inclusion. The *BIOSIS* information system, a pool of material totaling over 13 million citations at the end of 1999, is available in several formats. These include *Biological Abstracts*, a reference database for life science information, and *Biological Abstracts/RRM* (Reports, Reviews, Meetings), the companion reference to *Biological Abstracts*. *Biological Abstracts* encompasses the entire field of life sciences and provides coverage of published biological and biomedical research including traditional areas of biology, such as botany, zoology, and microbiology, as well as experimental, clinical, and veterinary medicine, biotechnology, environmental studies, and agriculture. Interdisciplinary fields such as biochemistry, biophysics, and bioengineering are also included. *BIOSIS* is commercially available in several formats.

EMBASE. *EMBASE* [19], the Excerpta Medica database, is a biomedical and pharmacological bibliographical database that provides access to medical and drug-related subjects from over 4000 biomedical journals from 70 countries. Each record contains the full bibliographical citation, indexing terms and codes; 80% of all citations in *EMBASE* include author-written abstracts. *EMBASE* contains over 8 million records from 1974 to present, with 445,000 citations and abstracts added annually. Updated weekly, *EMBASE* is commercially available online via: DataStar, DIALOG, DIMDI, LEXIS/NEXIS, Ovid Online, and STN. The *EMBASE* database combined with unique *MEDLINE* records back to 1966 are available in *EMBASE.com*. *EMBASE.com* contains over 13 million records. Links to other data sources including ScienceDirect (Elsevier Science), IDEAL (Academic Press), LINK (Springer-Verlag), Karger Online Journals, and gene and protein sequence databases are included.

Iowa Drug Information Service. A bibliographical database with access to full text, *IDIS* [98] provides access to the therapeutic and clinical pharmaceutic English language journal literature from 17 countries. FDA Summary Basis of Approval documents are indexed and available in full text. Updated monthly, the database contains over 450,000 records from 1966 forward with bibliographic citation, keyword indexes, and, for over 60% of citations, the author's abstract. *IDIS* is commercially available in microfiche, compact disc, and web formats and via DataStar, DIALOG.

International Pharmaceutical Abstracts. *International Pharmaceutical Abstracts* [104], published semimonthly, is an abstracting/indexing publication which covers all pharmaceutical literature. *IPA* covers approximately 700 worldwide pharmaceutical, medical, herbal, cosmetics, and health-related publications. *IPA* features all abstracts from American Society of Health-System Pharmacist's Annual, Midyear Clinical, and Home, Hospice, and Long-Term Care Meetings, coverage of state pharmacy journals, and American Pharmaceutical Association and American College of Clinical Pharmacy meeting abstracts. *IPA* indicates articles that offer CE credit. *IPA* is commercially available in several formats.

MEDLINE. *MEDLINE (Medical Literature, Analysis, and Retrieval System Online)* [20] contains over 11 million references to journal articles in life sciences with a concentration on biomedicine from

1966 to the present. Citations come from 4300 worldwide journals currently in 30 languages; 40 languages for older journals cited back to 1966. About 52% of current cited articles are published in the United States; nearly 86% are published in English; about 76% have English abstracts written by authors of the articles. Updated weekly, approximately 8000 completed references are added each Saturday, January through October (over 400,000 added per year). *MEDLINE* is available on the Internet through the National Library of Medicine (NLM) home page at http://www.nlm.nih.gov and can be searched free of charge. NLM offers *PubMed* and Internet *Grateful Med*, two free systems to search *MEDLINE*. *PubMed* also has links to molecular biology databases of DNA/protein sequences and three-dimensional structure data. Internet *Grateful Med* provides access to other NLM databases on AIDS, bioethics, history of medicine, toxicology, health services research, and other topics.

PubMed Central. *PubMed Central* [105] (which encompasses *Medline*) is a web-based archive of journal literature for all of the life sciences. Launched in February 2000, it is being developed by the National Center for Biotechnology Information (NCBI), U.S. National Library of Medicine (NLM), to preserve and maintain open access to electronic literature. Access to *PubMed Central* is free and unrestricted. In early 2001, eight journals were available on *PubMed*. Participation by publishers in *PubMed Central (PMC)* is voluntary, although participating journals must meet certain editorial standards. A participating journal is expected to include all its peer-reviewed primary research articles in *PMC*. It may, at its discretion, also deposit other content such as review articles, essays, and editorials. Review journals and similar publications that have no primary research articles may include their contents in *PMC*. Primary research papers without peer review are not accepted. A journal may deposit its material in *PMC* and make it available for public release as soon as it is published or it may delay release in *PMC* for a specified period after initial publication. The value of *PubMed Central*, in addition to its role as an archive, lies in what can be done when data from diverse sources is stored in a common format in a single repository. Links from the existing literature to other resources and databases may become part of *PubMed Central*.

Science Citation Index. *Science Citation Index (SCI)* [21] provides access to current and retrospective bibliographical information, author abstracts, and cited references found in 3500 scholarly science and technical journals covering more than 150 disciplines. The *Science Citation Index Expanded* format available through the ISI *Web of Science* and the online version, *SciSearch*, cover more than 5700 journals. *SCI* provides cited reference searching, the unique ISI search-and-retrieval feature that lets users track the literature forward, backward, and through the database. In effect, a whole article can be the subject of your search rather than a single work or index term. Available on the Internet via the *Web of Science*, it is updated weekly, with back-years to 1945. *SCI* is also commercially available online via DIALOG, DataStar, DIMDI, and STN.

IV. FINDING USEFUL INFORMATION

> Knowledge is of two kinds. We know a subject ourselves, or we know where we can find information upon it. Samuel Johnson, from James Boswell, *Life of Johnson*, April 18, 1775.

Even in the eighteenth century, individuals were not expected to possess all the knowledge necessary for professional life, but were expected to have the skills required to find what was needed. The ability to find what is needed is an essential survival skill in today's world. Interestingly, today information management survival skills are essential to all individuals—in both our personal and our professional lives. Lyman et al. [106] estimate that 1–2 exabytes (one exabyte is a billion gigabytes) of unique information is generated each year worldwide—250 megabytes for every person living today. The bulk of this information is digital and, thus, theoretically accessible. Printed paper accounts for less than 0.003% of the total stored information.

Although "searching for information" is evolving to imply finding digital documents primarily using electronic search methodologies, the human as an information source remains powerful. Practitioners and scientists with like fields of interest and research form networks that function to create and share information. Colleagues are an important resource. Experienced researchers claim they can reach any individual worldwide or retrieve needed information with only three, or at most seven, communication exchanges [107]. Physicians are frequently found to rank colleagues as their most used resource [108]. Within the academic and scientific community a medical, biomedical, or chemical librarian can provide not only quick access to information, but also expertise and instruction on managing the scientific literature.

"Relevant" has been used throughout this chapter to imply the general pertinence or applicability of information. Relevance, however, is only one of several variables that establish the utility or usefulness of information. The validity of the information retrieved and the work necessary to access the information also determine the usefulness of information [109]. Slawson et al. [110], interpreting work by Curley et al. [108], conceptually represented these variables in the following equation [111,112]:

$$\text{Utility of information} = \frac{(\text{relevance}) \times (\text{validity})}{(\text{work to access})}$$

Relevance influences the usefulness of information, in that the more likely the user is to encounter the need for this particular information, the greater the relevance. For example, information about clinical conditions rarely encountered in an individual's practice has low overall relevance to the practitioner. Relevance also has another aspect; that of closeness of fit of the information to the user's interest. Patients are primarily interested in outcomes that have personal meaning, such as morbidity, mortality, or quality of life. Information concerning these outcomes has high relevance. Information about the disease state or about surrogate endpoints has lower relevance for the patient.

Validity describes accuracy and reflects the soundness of the information. The information retrieved is valid if it is accurate, precise, unbiased, and provides a true picture of what is in the literature. The usefulness of the information is directly related to relevance and validity and inversely related to the work needed to access the information. While the work expended is under the direct control of the searcher, it is not unlimited. Therefore, given the limited amount of work time that is available to the information searcher, the most useful information resources will be those that are easy and quick to use and provide relevant, valid information. Skillful searchers can control work time, but relevance and validity are intrinsic characteristics of the resources themselves. A knowledgeable searcher will not only choose resources that are known to be relevant and valid, but will also use search techniques and filters that winnow out the irrelevant and invalid.

A. Steps in Conducting a Search

The basic technique for a successful literature search was established years ago by Brown [113] and has remained remarkably stable despite changes in sources and technology. Brown's search steps, with minor modification, are:

1. Define the problem.
2. Outline the sources to be examined; list the most important first.
3. Set up a list of search terms and revise it as the search progresses.
4. Enlarge the scope as necessary by adding new sources indicated by the clues that appear as the search progresses.
5. Systematize the references as they are collected.
6. Assemble the references and make the report.

The benefit of approaching an information need using these systematic steps is minimized work and maximized relevance and validity. The search steps are interactive; each step influences the next, and we learn and adjust our technique as the search unfolds. Step 6 is probably optional in some work settings.

Define the Problem

The truism that "you cannot find and will not recognize the answer if you do not know what the question is" applies to a drug information search. The question, that is, the specific information need, dictates both what information sources are most likely to provide answers and what search terms are appropriate for the search. Taking the time to clarify the question first guards against wasting time during the search.

Complex information needs may be difficult to narrow in scope. Sometimes learning a bit more about the subject before searching is helpful and time efficient in the end. Textbooks are helpful to provide a background prior to searching. Searching is most efficient when the search question is explicitly stated.

Outline and Prioritize the Sources to Be Examined

Experience with a variety of resources will improve a searcher's ability to find relevant information quickly. A working knowledge of the sources available at our practice or research site is important. Common sense suggests starting the search with those resources and books most likely to contain the answer. Since we are all likely to have favorite resources and be influenced by those that are conveniently available, we may have to remind ourselves of the value of this step.

The Internet, for many professionals, has become a favorite, convenient source for free information. The Internet is a vehicle to access a diverse array of information sources, including federal and state government documents and regulations, statements, opinions and guidelines from associations and organizations, and pharmaceutical industry documents. While the Internet is indeed powerful, it is a retrieval mechanism and the WWW site itself is the resource to be considered for relevance to the current search. The convenience of WWW resources can be quickly overshadowed by the time invested in the search and following linkages.

The process of scientific literature creation, as represented in Figure 1, unfolds in a clockwise direction around the circle. Retrieval, contrasted to creation, proceeds in a counterclockwise fashion beginning with the tertiary literature and then moving to the secondary literature to provide access to the primary literature [29,32]. At its best, a tertiary resource is a comprehensive, current, objective summary of pertinent research on a topic with an evaluation of the reliability and validity of the research, ending with a conclusion appropriately drawn from the data presented. Such tertiary resources are gold mines and may relieve one of further search effort. Walton et al. [32] point out that generally what is needed is a credible answer to a question, not an exhaustive literature search. Unfortunately, "gold mine" review articles and textbooks are not common and, once published, begin to age quickly. This disadvantage can be overcome in electronic textbooks and systematic reviews/guidelines that reside on the Internet, as they can be "living" documents that are updated and refined as new research is published. Tertiary literature in electronic format can provide direct links to electronic copies of the referenced citations. Following these linkages, the searcher may access further pertinent literature such as letters to the editor for this article, future articles that have cited this article, and even future articles that have been indexed with the same terms as this article. Electronic linkages open new interfaces between the tertiary and the primary literature, skipping the secondary literature search step. Linkages bring new value and richness to the literature. However, when the tertiary literature does not answer the question or contain the needed information, secondary index/abstract services are necessary and continue to provide the major route to original research.

Set Up and Revise a List of Search Terms

Many electronic sources now have a "front-end" thesaurus that allows the searcher to enter a term that will automatically be cross-referenced to search terms appropriate for that particular source. This process somewhat mitigates the need for a comprehensive list of search terms. Knowledge of the vocabulary of the search topic coupled with knowledge of the index vocabulary of the reference work synergistically to the advantage of the searcher. Unfortunately, the index vocabularies—drug names, disease names, process and procedure names, etc.—used by bibliographical databases and textbooks are not standardized. Noticing the index terms applied to relevant "hits" retrieved during the search process will validate the terms you have chosen and suggest additions to the list of search terms. We learn and hone our search terms once the search is in process.

Frequently one will find new citations (not found in the database just completed) in the next bibliographical database that one searches. Are these new citations unique to this second bibliographic database, or were they present in the first database but your search did not find them? To build quality control into your search process, return to the first bibliographical database and search for the newfound citations using an author or a title-word search statement. If you do find the "newfound" citations in the first database, explore the citations' index/key words. You may discover additional appropriate search terms or procedures to improve your search.

A relevant citation not only provides the needed content, that is, data and information, it also contains clues to find other relevant citations. The author(s) may have published other relevant articles that can be found with an author search. Future authors publishing on this same topic may have cited this article in their own publication. *Science Citation Index* provides cited reference searching. The citation can be used as a Rosetta stone to determine the appropriate index term(s) for each bibliographical database searched. Some databases now offer a search command, "find related articles," that automates this process.

Enlarge Scope with New Sources

Even brief searches, without a significant increase in the time to complete the search, can benefit from a watchful eye for new "gold mines" of information. Resources available on the Internet are particularly dynamic and continue to challenge our effort to balance work of access with the value of the search outcome. Serendipitous searching or browsing, unless limited by disciplined attention to the boundaries of content and time, can expand search work and decrease the search's utility. Follow interesting leads only as long as they are profitable.

Once a valuable, key information source has been found—whether it is a tertiary source or a research report—a quick perusal of the references that this source used may yield further valuable citations. If your search has already uncovered the same references as this key source, your search methods gain confidence.

Systematize the References

"Systematizing" the references has two components. The first component is judging the strength of the evidence found in the references. The purpose of the search is to find information that can be used to make decisions. In the research setting the decision may be how to proceed with a chemical or manufacturing process or a patent application; in the practice arena the decision may determine a patient's drug therapy or whether two medications can safely share the same intravenous container. These are important decisions, and the confidence with which they can be made depends on the strength of the evidence found in the search. The second component is the physical process of keeping track of references using bibliographical software.

Strength of the Evidence. Based on strength, that is, first, the ability to conclude a cause-and-effect relationship and, second, the ability to extrapolate results beyond the individual study or summary, evidence falls into one of two major categories: research (experimental and observational) evidence and summarized or evaluated evidence [114]. Original research provides the strongest evidence. Summarized or evaluated evidence is one or more steps removed from the primary research. The manner by which the summary or evaluation was constructed determines its strength. A comprehensive summary or evaluation done with rigor and without bias is valuable and has the distinct advantage of saving the searcher's time.

Although neither research decisions nor clinical practice decisions are made entirely on the basis of the published literature, the published literature is an extremely important component in the decision process. As such, how much stock can be placed in what the published literature says or concludes? To answer this question, several schemata have been constructed to hierarchically label the strength of published literature. Study design and methodologies, which dictate the reliability and internal and external validity of research, are the prime variables used to categorize specific pieces of evidence within the hierarchies. Using the hierarchies, a researcher or clinician can gauge the level of support the published literature provides for their decisions and actions.

No single hierarchy has achieved universal acceptance. The Centre for Evidence-Based Medicine [115], Oxford, England, has developed over many years a hierarchy that grades evidence on a scale of A through D, with A being highest. Level A evidence includes randomized controlled clinical trials and systematic reviews of randomized controlled clinical trials; Level B evidence includes cohort studies, outcome research, and case-controlled trials; Level C evidence is case-series reports; and Level D evidence represents expert opinion. The grades are individualized for therapy, prevention, etiology, harm, prognosis, diagnosis, and economic analysis studies. This hierarchy grades evidence as it applies to the average patient, not an individual patient.

The Evidence-Based Medicine Working Group [116], who have authored the "Users' guides to the medical literature" in *JAMA*, developed "A hierarchy of strength of evidence for treatment decisions" that places the *N*-of-1 randomized trial as the strongest evidence. This scheme judges evidence as it applies to issues of treatment for an individual patient. Falling below *N*-of-1 randomized trial in order of decreasing strength are systematic reviews of randomized trials, single randomized trial, systematic review of observational studies addressing patient-important outcomes, single observational study addressing patient-important outcomes, and finally physiological studies and unsystematic clinical observations.

The United States Pharmacopeial Convention, Inc. (USP) in 2000 issued the "USP criteria for levels of evidence for botanical articles" [117]. While issued for botanicals, the criteria have application to all therapeutic agents. The USP criteria rank evidence from I to IV, with Level I being the strongest. Within Level I, the randomized controlled clinical trial is ranked highest, followed by meta-analysis and epidemiological studies. Level II consists of the same designs, but with methodological flaws. Level III includes inconclusive studies, and Level IV is anecdotal evidence.

In addition to hierarchies of strength of evidence, scales have been developed to assess the quality of an individual clinical trial. However, the scales are diverse and do not readily agree with one another [118]. It is sometimes difficult to determine whether the quality scale judged the quality of the research or the quality of reporting the research results.

If therapy for a specific patient is in question, an *N*-of-1 trial offers data that apply directly (but only) to that patient. If patients in general are considered, the hierarchies all place a well-executed randomized controlled trial or a summary of well-executed randomized controlled clinical trials (systematic review or meta-analysis) highest. Observational studies, such as cohort studies, case-controlled studies, and cross-sectional studies, fall below the randomized controlled clinical trials. Descriptive studies, including case reports and case series, along with expert opinion provide the weakest level of evidence. We frequently have to make decisions with less than ideal data or information. Both researchers and practitioners are faced with using uncontrolled and weaker design studies. Hierarchies of evidence at least put the available evidence in perspective. In the clinical arena, some guidance is available from the Evidence-Based Medicine Working Group [119,120] and others [121,122]. Generalizing to a specific patient involves using the published literature to estimate the benefit-risk ratio of the therapy for the individual patient and also incorporating the patient's values and preferences into the clinical decision.

Bibliographical Software. The second component of systematizing the references is physically arranging and storing the citations. Today, thank goodness, we no longer have to manually copy citations onto index note cards and annotate the citation with succinct reminders of what the source said. Bibliographical software, such as Biblioscape [123], Citation [124], EndNote, ProCite, or Reference Manager (all commercially available from ISI ResearchSoft) [125], Library Master [126], Note Bene [127], and Scholar's Aid, Inc. [128], provide an interface to search bibliographical databases, collect, store, and annotate the citations, insert references into word-processed documents, and generate bibliographies.

Assemble the References and Make the Report

The last step in conducting a search is to put the search results into a format that can be used to meet the information need and document the search process. Documenting the search involves recording what sources were searched, the years searched, and what search terms were used. If in the future someone wishes to bring the search up to date, documentation provides a history of prior activity such that a new search can pick up where the first search left off. Documenting a World Wide Web search is more difficult than documenting a search of traditional bibliographical databases. Certainly, recording the date of a Web search and search terms used is of primary importance given the rapid change and expansion of the Web.

In the day-to-day course, many questions are searched using the first five steps and answered in a quick, fluid manner with barely a thought of the steps themselves. Step 6 is probably not necessary in these instances.

V. MANAGING DRUG INFORMATION

"Pharmacy is a knowledge system in which chemical substances and people called patients interact" [129]. Pharmaceutical scientists and pharmacy practitioners are responsible for both contributing to this universal knowledge system and maintaining their own individual knowledge systems. Scientific and biomedical literature is essential to our professional lives. Sewell conceptualized the literature as a professional tool described in a three-pronged philosophy: "1. The literature is a tool. 2. A tool is as good as its user. 3. A professional is constantly improving his tools and his techniques in their use" [52]. The literature stimulates innovation, documents our progress, provides data and information for problem solving, answers questions, and, through life-long learning activities, contributes to maintaining professional competence and expertise. Our challenge is generally not one of recognizing the role that literature plays in our profession, but of obtaining and maintaining the skill to efficiently manage the literature important to our profession.

A. Suggestions for Using the Literature at the Point of Need

1. Skillfully and faithfully follow the steps in conducting a search.
2. Only consider information pertinent to the question at hand—define and focus the question.
3. Search first those sources most likely to provide the answer.
4. Invest in learning the features of computerized textbooks, bibliographical databases, and specialized information resources to increase your efficiency.

5. Apply the same boundaries and quality standards to the Internet that you apply to other sources.
6. Add new sources to your list of familiar sources so that you have a larger pool of sources to choose from.
7. Become adept at literature evaluation—recognize valuable evidence and bypass weak evidence.
8. Use bibliographical software where it will save time.

B. Suggestions for Keeping Up with the Literature

In most disciplines scanning the new literature means scanning that discipline's periodical journals as they are published [130,131]. Which journals should be browsed? Consider the high-circulation general journals in your area: Which of these journals provide the highest number of articles that are valid and also relevant to your individual research or practice area? Next consider the specialty journals in your area. Which specialty journals provide the highest number of valid and relevant articles? Choose general and specialty journals that are most likely to contain articles that will change, expand, or improve your practice or research—articles that matter to your daily activities. Limit the number of journals to be browsed to only those that you can reasonably get through. Unless "throwaway" publications (unsolicited, not peer reviewed) offer unique news or reviews by noted specialists, they are probably best thrown away. There are a few fields, such as physics and math, where prepublication copies of research are also available for perusing. Surrogate, intermediary condensations of periodicals, such as *Current Contents/Life Sciences* or *Current Contents/Clinical Medicine* [132] that provide tables of contents of many journals, or abstract journals, such as *ACP Journal Club*, can be browsed. Selective dissemination or current awareness search results on specific topics from bibliographical databases offer another method to identify relevant articles from the current literature.

Apply the same stringent criteria to the articles themselves. First read the article's title for relevance and then proceed to the abstract. If the abstract does not meet your standard for relevance and validity, don't invest further time to read the full report.

C. Managing the Information You Retrieve

Store Useful Articles and Information

Although some institutions and enterprises maintain electronic subscriptions to a large number of publications, most researchers and practitioners still find it useful to save copies of journal articles and other publications that are important to their daily work. Maintaining an organized filing system eliminates having to relocate and acquire important works on a given topic. Perhaps the key is to maintain an "organized" filing system. Today, not only can we choose to file and save paper copies, but we can also acquire, file, and save electronic copies of important works.

Bibliographical software (see Sec. IV.A) can provide the structure to record, index, and retrieve journal articles and all manner of other useful sources, including Internet sites, books, chapters, news releases, recordings, and images. The index terms used to describe each entry in the bibliographical database are just as important to quick, accurate citation retrieval in a personal database as they are to large public databases such as *EMBASE, IDIS*, and *MEDLINE*. If the index terms used in these large databases meet your purpose, they provide a convenient selection of terms for personal indexing and, in many cases, can be included in the citation import feature of the software.

A Personal Database

Drug information centers have for years devised and maintained filing systems that store and provide future access to answered information questions. Early systems were paper based. Electronic database management systems now provide the structure and retrieval software to efficiently save a question/answer database consisting of thousands of records. The same benefits that the institution garners from the drug information center's question/answer database are available to individual practitioners and scientists. In a practice setting, Ely et al. [133] described the motivating force to create a personal database as "frustration of forgetting difficult-to-find answers, from a personal need to document professional growth, and from a sense of empowerment that developed from selecting and organizing relevant information taken from an overwhelming amount of available knowledge." One can envision an electronic personal database that consists of not only answered information questions, but also key excerpts from published literature and links to citations in a bibliographical database or to well-chosen

Internet sites. Life-long learning and professional continuing education needs are well served by the intellectual activities of searching for information, retrieving and evaluating the information, and constructing a solution to the specific clinical or research problem.

The preeminence of digital information has been apparent throughout this chapter. Pharmaceutical scientists, academicians, and practicing pharmacists all require ever-increasing technological savvy. It is not sufficient to know where information resides, to be efficient and successful one must also be skillful in the techniques of acquiring, manipulating, using, saving and retrieving digital information. The admonition by Cook et al. [130] to "invest in informatics" as a strategy to keep up with the literature, is valuable advice. Acquiring and using informatics skills decreases the time required to acquire, use and re-use information, thus freeing time for the higher level activities of evaluating what is found and applying this new knowledge—evaluated information—to solve research problems and improve patient care.

REFERENCES

1. DC Brodie, WF McGhan, J Lindon. The theoretical base of pharmacy. Am J Hosp Pharm 48:536–540, 1991.
2. Study Commission on Pharmacy. Pharmacists for the Future: The Report of the Study Commission on Pharmacy: Commissioned by the American Association of Colleges of Pharmacy. Ann Arbor, MI: Health Administration Press, 1975.
3. WG Troutman. Consensus-derived objectives for drug information education. Drug Inf J 28:791–796, 2000.
4. Report prepared for the study of 'Interagency Coordination in Drug Research and Regulation' by the Subcommittee on Reorganization and International Organizations of the Senate Committee on Government Operations, 1963.
5. The nature and magnitude of drug literature. Am J Hosp Pharm 22:7–29, 2000.
6. Medical school objectives project: medical informatics objectives, URL: http://www.aamc.org/meded/.msop/informat.htm, accessed 7-4-2000.
7. The American Heritage Dictionary of the English Language, Electronic Version. Boston: Houghton Mifflin Company, 1992.
8. J Naisbitt. Megatrends: Ten New Directions Transforming Our Lives. New York: Warner Books, Inc., 1982, p. 24.
9. ML McHugh, S Denger, D Cole. Data rich—information poor: designing computer systems to support nursing's information needs. Kans Nurse 66:1–2, 1991.
10. WC Reed. CIOs and the D.R.I.P. (data-rich, information-poor) syndrome. Hosp Health Netw 69:82, 1995.
11. C Serb. Software. Data rich, information poor. Hosp Health Netw 71:43–44, 1997.
12. J Teresko. Information rich, knowledge poor? Industry Week 248:19, 1999.
13. Drug literature, introductory statement by Hubert H. Humphrey, Vice President of the United States of America. Am J Hosp Pharm 22:4–6, 1965.
14. Advertisement: information knowledge, DowJones. Wall Str J [99], B7, 1997.
15. PF Drucker. Post-Capitalist Society. New York: HarperCollins Publishers, Inc., 1993, p. 8.
16. RFJ McCandless, EA Skweir, M Gordon. Secondary journals in chemical and biological fields. J Chem Doc 4:147–153, 1964.
17. MM Cummings. The National Library of Medicine. In: KS Warren, ed. Coping with the Biomedical Literature, A Primer for the Scientist and the Clinician. New York: Praeger Publishers, 1981, pp. 161–181.
18. CL Bernier, AN Yerkey. Cogent Communication: Overcoming Reading Overload. Westport, CT: Greenwood Press, Inc., 2000, p. 39.
19. EMBASE, [Internet]. URL: http://www.elsevier.nl/inca/publications/store/5/2/3/3/2/8/, accessed 9-23-2000.
20. MEDLINE Fact Sheet, [Internet]. URL: http://www.nlm.nih.gov/pubs/factsheets/medline.html, accessed 7-14-2000.
21. Science Citation Index: ISI, [Internet]. URL: http://isinet.com/isi/products/citation/sci, accessed 7-14-2000.
22. BIOSIS, [Internet]. URL: http://www.biosis.org/home_deluxe.html, accessed 9-17-2000.
23. CAS, Chemical Abstracts Service home page, [Internet]. URL: http://www.cas.org/, accessed 7-15-2000.
24. International Conference on Harmonisation of technical requirements for registration of pharmaceuticals for human use, [Internet]. URL: http://www.ifpma.org/ich1.html, accessed 7-15-2000.
25. International Conference on Harmonisation; Guidance on Ethnic Factors in the Acceptability of Foreign Clinical Data; Availability, URL: http://www.access.gpo.gov/su_docs/fedreg/a980610c.html, accessed 11-15-2000.
26. Study Commission on Pharmacy. What is pharmacy? In: Pharmacists for the future: the report of the Study Commission on Pharmacy: commissioned by the American Association of Colleges of Pharmacy. Ann Arbor, MI: Health Administration Press, 1975, p. 13.

27. Study Commission on Pharmacy. The content of pharmacy education. In: Pharmacists for the future: the report of the Study Commission on Pharmacy: commissioned by the American Association of Colleges of Pharmacy. Ann Arbor, MI: Health Administration Press, 1975, p. 128.
28. GW Pickering. The purpose of medical education. BMJ 2:113–116, 1956.
29. K Subramanyam. Scientific literature. In: A Kent, H Lancour, WZ Nasri, eds. Encyclopedia of Library and Information Science. New York: Marcel Dekker, 1979, pp. 376–548.
30. KA Brandt, HP Lehmann. Teaching literature searching in the context of the World Wide Web. In: Proceedings/Nineteenth Annual Symposium on Computer Applications in Medical Care. New York, NY: Institute of Electrical and Electronics Engineers, 1995, pp. 888–892.
31. B Snow. Drug Information: A Guide to Current Resources. Lanham, MD: Scarecrow Press, Inc., 1999.
32. CA Walton, PM Mullins, AB Amerson. Drug literature utilization: selection, evaluation and communication. In: CW Blissitt, OL Webb, WF Stanaszek, eds. Clinical Pharmacy Practice. Philadelphia: Lea & Febiger, 1972, pp. 347–406.
33. CC Booth. The origin and growth of medical journals. Ann Intern Med 113:398–402, 1990.
34. S Jablonski. The biomedical information explosion: from the index-catalogue to MEDLARS. Bull Med Libr Assoc 59:94–98, 1971.
35. D Rennie. The present state of medical journals. Lancet 352:SII18–SII22, 1998.
36. DDS Price. The development and structure of the biomedical literature. In: KS Warren, ed. Coping with the Biomedical Literature, A Primer for the Scientist and the Clinician. New York: Praeger Publishers, 1981, pp. 3–16.
37. HF Judson. Structural transformations of the sciences and the end of peer review. JAMA 272:92–94, 1994.
38. E Garfield. Citation analysis as a tool in journal evaluation. Science 178:471–479, 1972.
39. Abridged Index Medicus (AIM) Journal Titles, [Internet]. URL: http://www.nlm.nih.gov/bsd/aim.html, accessed 10-14-2000.
40. DR Hill. Brandon/Hill selected list of books and journals for the small medical library. Bull Med Libr Assoc 87:145–169, 1999.
41. MS Day. Computer-based retrieval services at The National Library of Medicine. Fed Proc 33:1717–1718, 1974.
42. ACP Journal Club, [Internet]. URL: http://www.acponline.org/catalog/journals/acpjc.htm, accessed 10-14-2000.
43. Best Evidence, [Internet]. URL: http://www.acponline.org/catalog/electronic/best_evidence.htm, accessed 10-14-2000.
44. The Cochrane Library, [Internet]. URL: http://hiru.mcmaster.ca/cochrane/cochrane/revabstr/ccabout.htm, accessed 10-15-2000.
45. Evidence-Based Medicine, [Internet]. URL: http://www.acponline.org/catalog/journals/ebm.htm, accessed 10-14-2000.
46. SE Feldman. Search engines. In: A Kent, ed. Encyclopedia of Library and Information Science, Vol. 64. New York: Marcel Dekker, Inc., 1999, pp. 218–243.
47. S Lawrence, CL Giles. Accessibility of information on the web. Nature 400:107–109, 2000.
48. M Dahn. Counting angels on a pinhead, critically interpreting web size estimates. Online 24(1):35–40, 2000.
49. M Dahn. Spotlight on the invisible web. Online 24(4):57–62, 2000.
50. G Notess. The never-ending quest, search engine relevance. Online 24(3):35–40, 2000.
51. D King. Specialized search engines, alternatives to the big guys. Online 24(3):67–74, 2000.
52. W Sewell. Guide to Drug Information. Hamilton, IL: The Hamilton Press, Inc., 1976, pp. 2–3.
53. Basic Resources Committee of the Library/Educational Resources Section. AACP Basic Resources for Pharmaceutical Education, [Internet]. URL: http://www.aacp.org/Resources/Reference/Basic_Resources/00_bklst_intro.html, accessed 10-21-2000.
54. The National Guideline Clearinghouse, [Internet]. URL: http://www.guideline.gov/index.asp, accessed 11-15-2000.
55. MICROMEDEX Systems, [Internet]. URL: http://www.micromedex.com/, accessed 10-22-2000.
56. Stat!Ref, [Internet]. URL: http://www.tetondata.com/, accessed 10-22-2000.
57. PJ Easterbrook, JA Berlin, R Gopalan, DR Matthews. Publication bias in clinical research. Lancet 337:867–872, 1991.
58. K Dickersin, YI Min, CL Meinert. Factors influencing publication of research results. Follow-up of applications submitted to two institutional review boards. JAMA 267:374–378, 1992.
59. D Blumenthal, EG Campbell, MS Anderson, N Causino, KS Louis. Withholding research results in academic life science. Evidence from a national survey of faculty. JAMA 277:1224–1228, 1997.
60. F Song, A Eastwood, S Gilbody, L Duley. The role of electronic journals in reducing publication bias. Med Inf Internet Med 24:223–229, 1999.
61. The New Drug Development Process: Steps from Test Tube to New Drug Application Review, [Internet]. URL: http://www.fda.gov/cder/handbook/develop. htm, accessed 7-29-2000.
62. NLM Fact Sheets—Listed by Subject, URL: http://www.nlm.nih.gov/pubs/factsheets/factsubj.html, accessed 7-20-2000.

63. Beilstein Database, [Internet]. URL: http://www.beilstein.com/, accessed 7-20-2000.
64. CHEMCYCLOPEDIA, [Internet]. URL: http://pubs.acs.org/chemcy/, accessed 7-20-2000.
65. ChemFinder, [Internet]. URL: http://www.chemfinder.com/, accessed 7-20-2000.
66. IMS HEALTH Global Services, [Internet]. URL: http://www.ims-global.com/index.html, accessed 7-22-2000.
67. Ei Compendex, [Internet]. URL: http://www.ei.org/eivillage/plsql/village.serve_page, accessed 7-20-2000.
68. S Budavari, et al. The Merck Index. Rahway, NJ: Merck Publishing Group, 1996.
69. WG Mallard, PJ Linstrom. NIST Chemistry WebBook, [Internet]. URL: http://webbook.nist.gov/chemistry/, accessed 7-20-2000.
70. The Registry of Toxic Effects of Chemical Substances (RTECS), [Internet]. URL: http://www.ntis.gov/fcpc/cpn8195.htm, accessed 11-4-2000.
71. The U.S. Pharmacopeia, [Internet]. URL: http://www.usp.org/frameset.htm, accessed 7-20-2000.
72. United States Patent and Trademark Office, [Internet]. URL: http://www.uspto.gov/, accessed 1-11-2002.
73. Electronic Orange Book, Approved Drug Products with Therapeutic Equivalence Evaluations, [Internet]. URL: http://www.fda.gov/cder/ob/default.htm, accessed 7-29-2000.
74. Delphion Intellectual Property Network, [Internet]. URL: http://www.patents.ibm.com/, accessed 7-21-2000.
75. The Derwent International Patent Family on Westlaw, [Internet]. URL: http://store.westgroup.com/documentation/westlaw/wlawdoc/wlres/drwent01.pdf, accessed 3-14-2001.
76. Derwent World Patents Index, [Internet]. URL: http://www.derwent.com/, accessed 7-20-2000.
77. Drugs Under Patent, [Internet]. URL: http://www.foiservices.com/index.htm, accessed 7-29-2000.
78. BIOSCI, [Internet]. URL: http://www.bio.net/, accessed 7-22-2000.
79. Adis International Ltd., [Internet]. URL: http://www.adis.com/index.html, accessed 7-22-2000.
80. AIDSTRIALS (AIDS Clinical Trials), [Internet]. URL: http://www.nlm.nih.gov/pubs/factsheets/aidstdfs.html, accessed 7-22-2000.
81. Chemical Physics Preprint Database, [Internet]. URL: http://www.chem.brown.edu/chem-ph.html, accessed 7-22-2000.
82. ClinicalTrials.gov, [Internet]. URL: http://clinicaltrials.gov/ct/gui, accessed 7-22-2000.
83. Computer Retrieval of Information on Scientific Projects CRISP, [Internet]. URL: https://www.commons.cit.nih.gov/crisp/, accessed 7-21-2000.
84. CSline, [Internet]. URL: http://www.prous.com/product/electron/csline.html, accessed 7-30-2000.
85. Federal Research in Progress Database (FEDRIP), [Internet]. URL: http://grc.ntis.gov/fedrip.htm, accessed 7-21-2000.
86. ProQuest Digital Dissertations, [Internet]. URL: http://www.lib.umi.com/dissertations/about_pqdd, accessed 7-22-2000.
87. R Temple. Current definitions of phases of investigation and the role of the FDA in the conduct of clinical trials. Am Heart J 139:S133–S135, 2000.
88. NR Cutler, JJ Sramek. Scientific and ethical concerns in clinical trials in Alzheimer's patients: the bridging study. Eur J Clin Pharmacol 48:421–428, 1995.
89. Drug Data Report, [Internet]. URL: http://www.prous.com/product/journal/ddr.html, accessed 7-30-2000.
90. Drugs of the Future, [Internet]. URL: http://www.prous.com/journals/avdof.html, accessed 7-30-2000.
91. Drug News & Perspectives, [Internet]. URL: http://www.prous.com/product/journal/dnp.html, accessed 7-30-2000.
92. Ensemble, [Internet]. URL: http://www.prous.com/databases/ensemble/ensemble.html, accessed 7-30-2000.
93. Investigational Drugs database (IDdb), [Internet]. URL: http://www.current-drugs.com/products/iddb3/home.htm, accessed 7-30-2000.
94. The NDA Pipeline, [Internet]. URL: http://www.fdcreports.com/index.shtml, accessed 7-22-2000.
95. BP Gilchrist, HH Seaba. U.S. FDA summary basis of approvals (SBAs) unexplored and underutilized. Paper presented at Pharmacy World Congress '98 and Exhibition, The Hague, The Netherlands 1998.
96. DIOGENES, [Internet]. URL: http://www.foiservices.com/onlinedatabases.htm, accessed 7-29-2000.
97. Dockets Management, [Internet]. URL: http://www.fda.gov/ohrms/dockets/, accessed 8-19-2000.
98. Iowa Drug Information Service (IDIS), [Internet]. URL: http://www.uiowa.edu/~idis/, accessed 9-23-2000.
99. F-D-C Reports, Inc., [Internet]. URL: http://www.fdcreports.com/index.shtml, accessed 7-22-2000.
100. PJB Publications Ltd, [Internet]. URL: http://www.pjbpubs.co.uk/, accessed 7-22-2000.
101. Manual of Policies and Procedures (MaPP6010.2). Review management. Procedures for tracking and reviewing phase 4 commitments, URL: http://www.fda.gov/cder/mapp/6010-2.pdf, accessed 3-10-2001.
102. K Traynor. FDA Wants Phase IV Results, [Internet]. URL: http://www.ashp.org/public/news/ShowArticle.cfm?id=1944, accessed 12-20-2000.
103. LD Sasich, P Lurie, SM Wolfe. The drug industry's performance in finishing postmarketing research (Phase IV) studies, a Public Citizen's Health Research Group report, [Internet]. URL: http://www.citizen.org/hrg/PUBLICATIONS/1520.htm, accessed 4-14-2000.
104. International Pharmaceutical Abstracts, [Internet]. URL: http://www.ashp.org/, accessed 9-23-2000.

105. National Center for Biotechnology Information. PubMed Central, URL: http://www.pubmedcentral.nih.gov/, accessed 3-10-2001.
106. P Lyman, HR Varian, J Dunn, A Strygin, K Swearingen. How much information? [Internet]. URL: http://www.sims.berkeley.edu/how-much-info/, accessed 10-28-2000.
107. J Naisbitt. Megatrends: Ten New Directions Transforming Our Lives. New York: Warner Books, Inc., 1982, p. 194.
108. SP Curley, DP Connelly, EC Rich. Physicians' use of medical knowledge resources: preliminary theoretical framework and findings. Med Decision Making 10:231–241, 1990.
109. W Goffman. The ecology of the biomedical literature and information retrieval. In: KS Warren, ed. Coping with the Biomedical Literature, a Primer for the Scientist and the Clinician. New York: Praeger Publishers, 1981, pp. 31–46.
110. DC Slawson, AF Shaughnessy. What clinical information do doctors need? Few doctors are expert at evaluating information. BMJ 314:904, 1997.
111. DC Slawson, AF Shaughnessy, JH Bennett. Becoming a medical information master: feeling good about not knowing everything. J Fam Pract 38:505–513, 1994.
112. DC Slawson, AF Shaughnessy. Letters. What clinical information do doctors need? BMJ 314:903, 1997.
113. DF Brown. Library techniques in searching. In: Searching the Chemical Literature, Advances in Chemistry Series. Washington: American Chemical Society, 1951, pp. 146–157.
114. SH Gehlbach. Interpreting the Medical Literature. New York: McGraw-Hill, Inc., 1993, p. 31.
115. Levels of Evidence and Grades of Recommendations, [Internet]. URL: http://cebm.jr2.ox.ac.uk/docs/levels.html, accessed 10-30-2000.
116. GH Guyatt, RB Haynes, RZ Jaeschke, DJ Cook, L Green, CD Naylor, MC Wilson, WS Richardson. Users' guides to the medical literature: XXV. Evidence-based medicine: principles for applying the users' guides to patient care. Evidence-Based Medicine Working Group. JAMA 284:1290–1296, 2000.
117. USP Announces Criteria for Levels of Evidence Policies for Botanical Articles, [Internet]. URL: http://www.usp.org/frameset.htm?http://www.usp.org/aboutusp/releases/2000/pr_2000-23.htm#top, accessed 10-31-2000.
118. P Juni, A Witschi, R Bloch, M Egger. The hazards of scoring the quality of clinical trials for meta-analysis. JAMA 282:1054–1060, 1999.
119. AL Dans, LF Dans, GH Guyatt, S Richardson. Users' guides to the medical literature: XIV. How to decide on the applicability of clinical trial results to your patient. Evidence-Based Medicine Working Group. JAMA 279:545–549, 1998.
120. FA McAlister, SE Straus, GH Guyatt, RB Haynes. Users' guides to the medical literature: XX. Integrating research evidence with the care of the individual patient. Evidence-Based Medicine Working Group. JAMA 283:2829–2836, 2000.
121. L Holmberg, M Baum. Can results from clinical trials be generalized? Nat Med 1:734–736, 1995.
122. P Glasziou, G Guyatt, DLM Sackett. Applying the results of trials and systematic reviews to individual patients. ACP J Club 129:A1516, 1998.
123. Biblioscape, [Internet]. URL: http://www.biblioscape.com/, accessed 10-30-2000.
124. Oberon Development Ltd. Citation, [Internet]. URL: http://www.oberon-res.com/index.html, accessed 10-30-2000.
125. ISI ResearchSoft, [Internet]. URL: http://www.risinc.com/, accessed 10-30-2000.
126. Library Master, [Internet]. URL: http://www.balboa-software.com/, accessed 10-30-2000.
127. Nota Bene, [Internet]. URL: http://www.notabene.com/, accessed 10-30-2000.
128. Scholar's Aid, Inc., [Internet]. URL: http://www.scholarsaid.com/, accessed 10-30-2000.
129. Study Commission on Pharmacy. Summary of concepts, findings, and recommendations. In: Pharmacists for the Future: The Report of the Study Commission on Pharmacy: Commissioned by the American Association of Colleges of Pharmacy. Ann Arbor, MI: Health Administration Press, 1975, pp. 139–143.
130. DJ Cook, MO Meade, MP Fink. How to keep up with the critical care literature and avoid being buried alive. Crit Care Med 24:1757–1768, 1996.
131. AF Shaughnessy, KK Bucci, DC Slawson. How to be selective in reading the biomedical literature. Am J Health-Syst Pharm 52:1116–1118, 1995.
132. Institute for Scientific Information. Current Contents, [Internet]. URL: http://www.isinet.com/isi/products/cc, accessed 11-15-2000.
133. JW Ely, JA Osheroff, KJ Ferguson, ML Chambliss, DC Vinson, JL Moore. Lifelong self-directed learning using a computer database of clinical questions. J Fam Pract 45:382–388, 1997.

Chapter 27

Managed Care and Pharmacotherapy Management

Julie M. Ganther and William R. Doucette

University of Iowa, Iowa City, Iowa

In the last two decades, managed care has become the dominant model for health care delivery in the United States. It is estimated that 70–75% of the U.S. population receive their health care from managed care organizations (MCOs) [1], defined as health maintenance organizations, point of service plans, and preferred provider organizations. Managed care has been especially prevalent in employer-sponsored health insurance, but managed care penetration of government sponsored health benefits also has increased in recent years. Given the prevalence of managed care, it is important to understand its role in the delivery of health care and its impact on pharmacotherapy management. In the first part of this chapter, we describe the managed care model and the types of MCOs. In the second part of the chapter we discuss managed care strategies specifically related to pharmaceutical therapy. We conclude with a discussion of current and future issues related to managed care and pharmacotherapy management.

I. OVERVIEW OF MANAGED CARE

Managed care links the financing or insurance aspect of health care with the provision of health care goods and services, and organizations with this type of linkage have been in existence for a long time. In 1933, a physician and an insurance agent devised a health care plan where the physician was paid $0.05 per worker per day to provide work-related health care to workers building the Los Angeles Aqueduct. This "prepayment" plan was different from the standard insurance plan, where health care providers were reimbursed based on the number of services provided. The physician later was asked by industrialist Henry Kaiser to provide the same type of plan for his workers, and this was the beginning of Kaiser Permanente, currently the largest not-for-profit health maintenance organization (HMO) in the United States [2]. Although Kaiser Permanente and some other early MCOs were successful, traditional fee-for-service insurance remained the dominant form of health insurance in the United States from the 1940s until the mid-1980s.

Health maintenance organizations, generally defined as organizations that provide comprehensive health care for a prepaid payment, are the most familiar example of managed care. The Health Maintenance Organization Act was passed in 1973 to promote the establishment and expansion of HMOs. This act established federal guidelines for HMOs, mandated that some types of employers offer an HMO option, and provided for grants to assist with the development of new HMOs [3]. However, it was not until the early 1980s that HMO enrollment began to escalate. The initial growth in HMO enrollment likely was fueled by rapidly increasing health care expenditures and the lifting of some of the restrictions in the HMO Act. The number of individuals enrolled in HMOs continued to increase rapidly in the late 1980s and 1990s (Fig. 1).

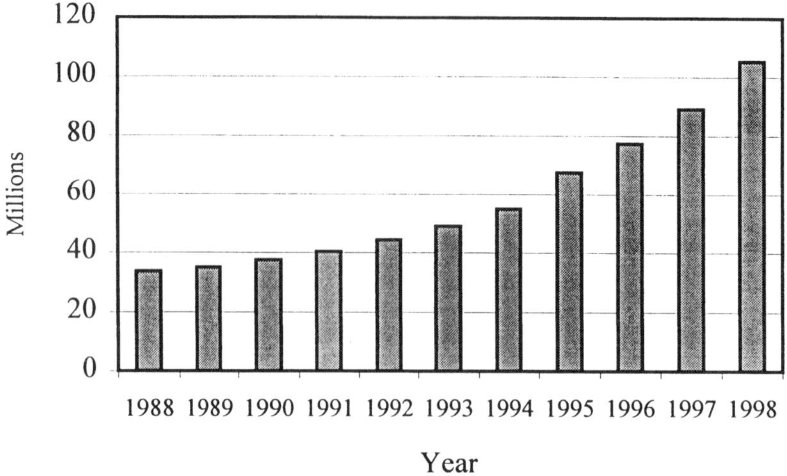

Fig. 1 Health maintenance organization enrollment in the United States. (From Hoechst Marion Roussel Managed Care Digest Series^{TM}/HMO-PPO Digest 1999.)

A. The Managed Care Model

To better understand managed care and the reasons for its growth, it is useful to discuss the evolution of payment mechanisms for health care from no insurance, to traditional indemnity insurance, to managed care. In the no-insurance model, the patient selects a health care provider and then pays the provider directly for health care goods and services. The choice of health care provider and the type and number of services provided are limited only by the financial constraints of the patient. The problem with this model is that the patient is exposed to potentially catastrophic health care expenses. Health insurance was developed as a way to protect patients against this risk. Health insurance often is provided through the employer and prior to the mid-1980s was likely to be indemnity fee-for-service insurance. In this traditional insurance model (Fig. 2), the same patient-provider transaction occurs, but now the patient (or their employer) pays premiums to the insurance company, and the patient submits claims to the insurance company to obtain reimbursement for some portion of what they paid the provider. The insurer does not try to influence the choice of provider or the cost or type of health care provided. In 1981, 95% of employer-based health insurance was of this type [4].

The indemnity fee-for-service model protects the patient from catastrophic medical expenses but has its own set of potential problems. There is little incentive for either the provider or the patient to control costs. The patient pays less than the full cost of care, creating an incentive to use more care. The provider is paid on a fee-for-service basis and thus can generate more income by providing more services. The health care

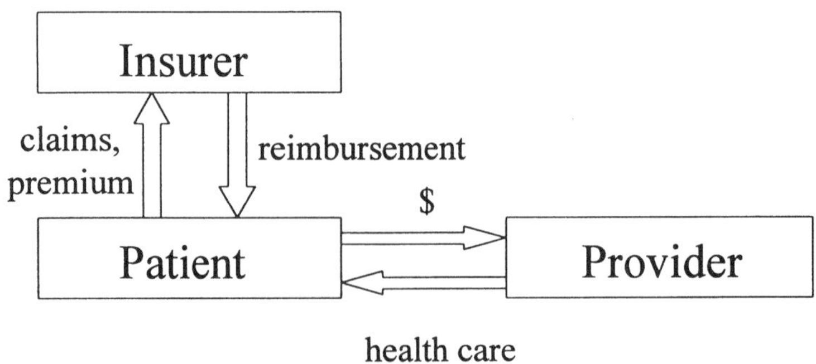

Fig. 2 Indemnity insurance.

provider also determines the price for his or her services. Health insurance coverage makes the patient less sensitive to the price of services, reducing the incentive for patients to seek out low-cost providers. This in turn reduces the incentive for providers to lower their prices. There also are potential inefficiencies in this type of system from uncoordinated care. If patients receive care from multiple, unaffiliated providers, there is the potential for duplicate therapy. One of the driving forces behind the growth of managed care was concern that the incentives and lack of coordination in the indemnity fee-for-service system were contributing to rapidly increasing health care expenditures.

In a broad sense, managed care can be thought of as any attempt by an insurer or other third-party payer to influence the patient–health provider exchange. A key feature of the managed care model is that the insurer has a contractual relationship with the providers and exerts some degree of control over the patient-provider exchange (Fig. 3). MCOs reimburse the provider, not the patient. The goal of managed care organizations is to contain costs while maintaining or improving the quality of care. Managed care organizations try to control costs by influencing the choice of providers and the cost or type of services provided. Control by MCOs generally is accomplished using three main types of strategies: provider networks, risk sharing or other provider incentives, and utilization management.

Provider networks are groups of providers under some type of contract with the insurer. Patients' choice of provider is restricted, and they may receive only partial coverage or no coverage for health care obtained from providers who are not in the network. Having a contract with a provider network allows the managed care organization to obtain discounted prices, because the providers are willing to accept lower reimbursement in return for a guaranteed volume of patients. It also allows the managed care organization to implement the other control strategies of risk sharing and utilization management and makes systematic quality assurance activities more feasible. In selecting physicians for the network, MCOs may consider factors such as professional reputation, privileges at network hospitals, or cost and utilization patterns [5].

Risk sharing and other provider incentives are an integral part of managed care. One common form of risk sharing is capitation. Capitation is a prospective per member per month payment for a specified time period. The health care provider or organization receives only the predetermined payment, regardless of the cost of the services that the patient receives. This form of payment transfers the risk from the insurer to the health care provider. If the cost of the services that the patient receives is less than the capitation amount, the health care provider keeps the extra payment as profit. If the cost of the services is more than the capitation amount, the provider loses money. This creates an incentive for the health care provider to control costs. The amount of the capitation payment can be determined by age/sex adjustment, prior year utilization adjustment, or health status adjustment [6].

Both primary care physicians and specialists may be paid via capitation arrangements, but the arrangement is more common for primary care physicians. In one survey of managed care organizations, 37% used capitation as the main method of

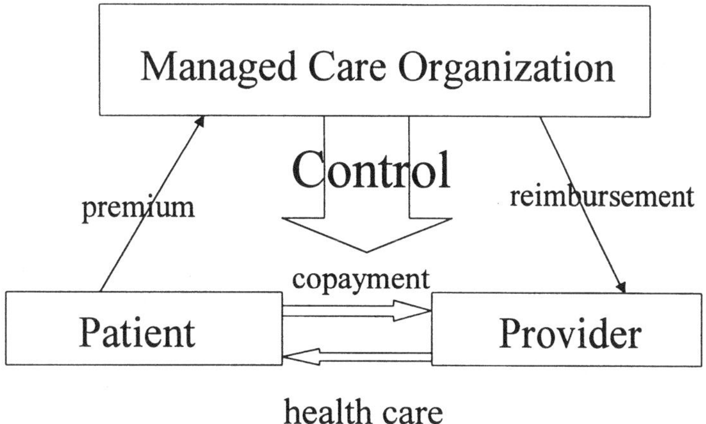

Fig. 3 Managed care model.

reimbursement for primary care physicians and 18% used capitation as the main method of reimbursement for specialists [5]. The payment under a capitation arrangement may include only services received from the capitated provider (e.g., primary care physician services), or it may include auxiliary services. For example, a capitated payment to a primary care physician may include prescription drug or lab test costs.

Managed care organizations also may use bonus or withholding arrangements as provider incentives. These arrangements can be used with fee-for-service payments, capitation payments, or salary payments. Under a bonus arrangement, the physicians typically will receive extra payment if utilization is below a specified level. Under a withholding arrangement, a portion of the predetermined payment is withheld and is only paid to the providers if utilization stays below a specified level. In one study, two thirds of the managed care plans surveyed had a withholding provision in their contracts with primary care physicians [7]. In both withholding and bonus scenarios, the utilization rate may be set for the individual provider or it may be for the entire physician group. The rate also may include only primary care services, or it also may include hospital and specialist services.

The third main category of methods used by managed care organizations to control costs is utilization management. One type of utilization management is requiring the patient to have a primary case manager or "gatekeeper." Under this type of arrangement, all health care must be accessed through the gatekeeper (usually a primary care physician). For example, if patients want to see a specialist, they must be referred to the specialist by their primary care physician or the managed care organization will not pay for the specialist visit. In one study of managed care organizations, 82% of HMOs required patients to select a primary care physician [5].

Other examples of utilization management include prior authorization for hospitalizations, mandatory second opinions for surgery or other expensive care, case management of high-cost cases, and utilization review. One component of utilization review is physician profiling. The purpose of physician profiling is to assign all expenditures for patients' episodes of care to a particular physician. Physicians who appear to be using significantly more or fewer resources than average are targeted for further review. Utilization management plays an important role in the management of pharmaceutical therapy and will be discussed further in the second section of the chapter.

B. Types of Managed Care Organizations

HMOs, preferred provider organizations (PPOs), and point of service (POS) plans are considered to be the main types of MCOs. However, it should be acknowledged that the distinction between managed care plans and traditional insurance plans is blurring. Some managed care plans are moving toward looser contractual arrangements with providers and less restrictive controls on utilization, and some more traditional fee-for-service plans are using utilization management strategies typically associated with managed care plans. These types of plans sometimes are referred to as "managed fee-for-service" plans. As MCOs evolve, it also is becoming more difficult to distinguish between different types of MCOs. We describe the main features associated with each type of MCO but recognize that it often can be difficult to strictly define each type. The issue also is complicated by the fact that it is common for the same MCO to offer different types of plans.

HMOs probably are the most familiar type of MCO. Key characteristics of HMOs are that they generally provide no coverage for services received outside of the provider network, they share risk with providers, and they require services to be accessed through a gatekeeper. HMOs are classified as staff model, group model, network model, or individual practice association (IPA) model. The distinguishing feature of the staff model HMO is that the physicians are employees of the HMO. This type of HMO is least common (see Fig. 4). In the group model HMO the HMO contracts with one medical group to provide all of the care for enrolled patients, while in the network model the HMO contracts with several medical groups. Network HMOs are becoming more common, while group model HMOs are becoming less common. In the IPA model the HMO contracts with physicians in solo or small group practices. These physicians also provide care for non-HMO patients.

Health maintenance organizations are the most restrictive type of managed care organization, and consumer dissatisfaction with restricted choice in HMOs likely was a significant factor in the growth of point of service (POS) plans. POS plans sometimes are referred to as open-ended HMOs. Like HMOs, enrollees typically select a primary care provider and pay no fee or a small copayment to see participating providers. POS plans differ from HMOs in that patients can receive coverage from physicians outside the network. However, patients pay more for care received from physicians outside the network and often must pay the full

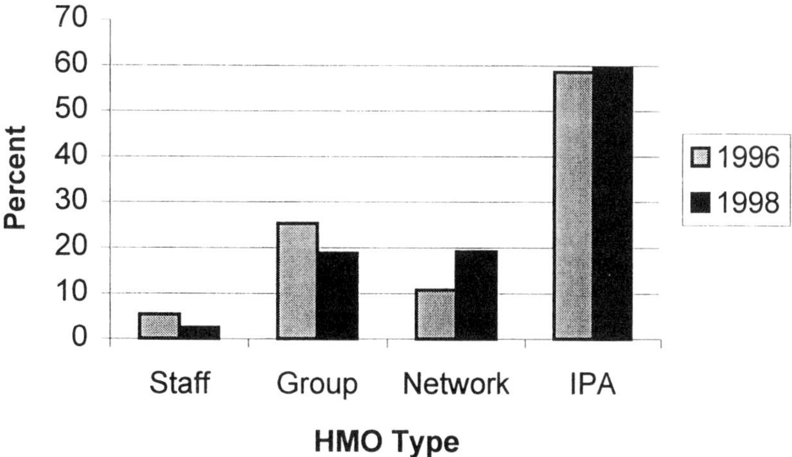

Fig. 4 Percent of HMO enrollees by HMO type. (From Hoechst Marion Roussel Managed Care Digest Series™/HMO-PPO Digest 1999.)

cost of the visit and then submit a claim to the plan for reimbursement [8]. In the United States POS plans grew from 7% of employer sponsored health plans in 1993 to 22% in 1998 [8,9].

The least restrictive of the three main types of managed care organizations is the preferred provider organization (PPO). A PPO is defined as "an arrangement whereby hospitals, physicians, or other care givers contract to provide services to a defined group of consumers on a discounted fee-for-service basis" [10]. A key difference between POS plans and PPO plans is that PPOs typically use fee-for-service reimbursement while POS plans use some form of capitation or other risk-sharing arrangement. Patients enrolled in a PPO can use providers who are not on the preferred list but will pay more than they would for a preferred provider. PPOs tend to emphasize utilization management. It sometimes can be difficult to distinguish between a POS plan and a PPO, but PPOs are unlikely to use capitation as a reimbursement mechanism. The percentage of U.S. workers in PPO plans increased from 27% in 1993 to 34% in 1998 [8,9].

II. PHARMACOTHERAPY MANAGEMENT

Prescription drug expenditures have been increasing at a rapid rate (see Fig. 5), and like other insurers and funders of health care, MCOs are struggling to contain the growth. The drug cost share of total operating expenses in HMOs has increased from 10.4% in 1996 to 13.6% in 1998 [1]. As a result, pharmacotherapy is an area that has been targeted for numerous management strategies. Managed care administrators have used a variety of approaches to try to control drug costs and still maintain quality care and favorable outcomes. Pharmacotherapy management can be defined as the activities, other than prescribing, undertaken by a managed care organization to control the use of drugs within that organization. Strategies used in pharmacotherapy management can be classified into the same three categories described earlier in the chapter: provider networks, risk sharing or other provider incentives, and utilization management.

A. Provider Networks

One strategy that MCOs use to control costs is to establish provider networks. For pharmacotherapy, providers typically are pharmacies, and MCOs try to have a cost-effective pharmacy network that includes enough pharmacies to meet the access needs of the beneficiaries. MCOs often include a mail order pharmacy in their pharmacy networks. MCOs have three main options for providing and managing pharmacotherapy: (a) an "in-house" pharmacy owned by the MCO, (b) a direct contract with a network of pharmacy providers, and (c) a contract with a pharmacy benefits manager (PBM), an organization that specializes in managing pharmacy provider networks and providing pharmacotherapy management services. Hiring a PBM sometimes is referred to as a "carve-out" of pharmacy benefits. In 1998, approximately 88% of HMOs and 73% of PPOs used PBM services [1]. If MCOs build their own pharmacy network, a common strategy is to use their own clinic pharmacies

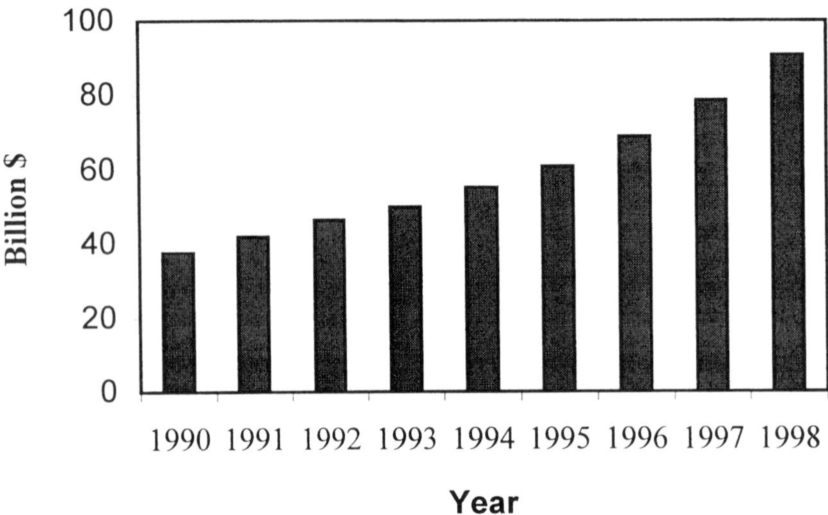

Fig. 5 National prescription drug expenditures in the United States. (From Health Care Financing Administration.)

as a starting point for their pharmacy networks, add in pharmacy chains, and then add independent pharmacies as needed to ensure adequate access.

The pharmacies under contract with an MCO or PBM typically agree to provide pharmacy services at a discounted rate. Reimbursement for prescription drugs usually is set at the average wholesale price (AWP) minus some percentage, plus a small dispensing fee. This is different from traditional indemnity insurance, where patients paid the usual and customary price determined by the pharmacy and then submitted the claim to the insurance company for reimbursement. The contract between the MCO or PBM and the pharmacy usually requires the pharmacy to accept assignment, meaning that the pharmacy is not allowed to charge the patient more than the amount specified by the contract. For drug products that have a generic equivalent, the contract may set a maximum allowable cost (MAC) plus a dispensing fee as the reimbursement. The MAC is an estimate of the price that the pharmacy would pay for the generic version of the drug.

The reimbursement specified in the contract between the MCO or PBM and the pharmacy typically is lower than the price that the pharmacy charges its other customers, with the difference often in the range of 10–30% [11,12]. The magnitude of the difference depends on the bargaining power that the MCO has to extract discounts. Pharmacies often are put in the difficult position of having to sign a contract with heavily discounted reimbursement or lose a large percentage of their business. However, MCOs must have enough pharmacies in their network to ensure adequate access, and this may constrain their ability to extract large discounts from the pharmacy providers.

B. Risk Sharing and Other Provider Incentives

Risk sharing via capitation typically is not done separately for prescription drugs, although prescription drugs may be included in the overall capitation rate for primary care physicians (PCPs). In 1998, 23.2% of HMOs included prescription drug costs in the capitation rate for PCPs [13]. There also may be incentives for providers to control prescription drug utilization. A portion of their payment may be withheld and returned only if prescription drug expenses are kept below a specified level. In 1998, 36.2% of HMOs had procedures in place to penalize physicians for violations of pharmacy prescribing policies [1]. Alternatively, physicians could receive a bonus for low levels of prescription drug expenditures or for adhering to pharmacy prescribing policies.

C. Utilization Management

Utilization management is an important pharmacotherapy management tool, and encompasses five main areas of activity: cost sharing, formulary management, practice guidelines, quality improvement, including drug utilization review, and educational activities. Some of these activities are aimed at providers, some address suppliers, and other activities are directed at patients. Managed care organizations differ in their use of these approaches, with some using a combination of all of them and others using only a few.

Cost Sharing

One way that managed care organizations try to manage prescription drug utilization is to share the costs with the patients. The purpose of cost sharing is two fold. It directly decreases the managed care organization's prescription drug expenditures, and it also may decrease the number and cost of prescription drugs used by patients. MCOs hope that cost sharing decreases patients' incentives to use drugs, particularly unnecessary drugs. There is evidence that cost sharing decreases prescription drug utilization [14–17], but it may discourage the use of essential as well as discretionary drugs [18]. Cost sharing also may be used to encourage the use of specific types of drugs (e.g., generic or formulary drugs). There is some evidence that higher amounts of cost sharing for brand name drugs increases the use of generic drugs [19,20].

Common types of cost sharing are copayments, coinsurance, and deductibles. A copayment is a fixed amount paid for each prescription, for example, $15. The copayment does not directly reflect the cost of the drug, although there may be different copayments for different types of drugs. It has been common for managed care plans to have a lower copayment for generic drugs than for brand name drugs, and recently many plans have been implementing three-tier copayments. Under the three-tier copayment plan, the lowest copayment is for generic prescription drugs, the next lower is for brand name drugs that are on the formulary, and the highest copayment is for nonformulary brand name drugs. In 1998, the average copayments were $16.77, $8.93, and $5.93 for nonformulary brand name drugs, formulary brand name drugs, and generic drugs, respectively [1].

A criticism of the copayment benefit structure is that there is not a direct relationship between the amount that the patients pay and the cost of the drug. Coinsurance is a method of cost sharing that accounts for the cost of the drug. Under coinsurance, patients pay a fixed percentage of the drug cost. Patients have some incentive to choose lower-cost drugs because they pay more for higher-cost drugs. For example, with 20% coinsurance, the patient would pay $20 for a drug that costs $100, but would only pay $4 for a drug that costs $20.

A deductible is a fixed amount (e.g., $100) that the patient must pay before the managed care plan pays for their prescription drugs. Deductibles often are used in combination with copayments of coinsurance. For a plan with a $100 deductible and 20% coinsurance, patients would pay all of the first $100 of their drug costs, and then pay 20% of the rest of their drug costs. MCOs also may limit the amount of their exposure to prescription drug expenses by specifying a maximum prescription drug benefit. Under this type of benefit structure, the patient is responsible for any prescription drug costs over and above the amount of the defined benefit. For example, a MCO may have a maximum benefit of $2,500.

Formulary Management

Formulary management is an ongoing process in which a managed care organization's pharmacy and medical staffs evaluate and select drugs to identify those considered to be most useful in patient care. The central component in formulary management is establishing and maintaining a formulary. A formulary is a compilation of selected drug products that has been approved for use within the managed care organization. That is, drugs on a formulary typically are covered by the managed care plan. Formularies are a common utilization management strategy in MCOs, with 92.2% of HMOs and 71.6% of PPOs having drug formularies in 1998 [1].

A key body for managing a formulary is the pharmacy and therapeutics committee (P&T committee) of the managed care organization. A P&T committee usually is comprised of physicians, pharmacists, and administrators. The charge of a P&T committee is to advise and educate practitioners about drug use within the managed care organization. Their primary means is through formulary management.

An initial step in managing a formulary often is therapeutic drug class review, which is done by a P&T committee. The goal of the review is to identify optimal drug products to have on formulary, based on effectiveness, toxicity, or cost differences within the same class of drug products [21]. The review can be prompted by P&T set criteria, such as annual or biannual review, or by events such as an increase in adverse drug events, new information about a drug, a rapid increase in expenditures, or a marked change in usage. These events aid the P&T committee in determining which drugs to include on the formulary.

In comparing drugs, a P&T committee might use three different approaches: inventory management, cost accounting, and clinical decision analysis [22]. The inventory management model assumes that all agents in a class are equivalent on safety, efficacy, and bioequivalence. This technique focuses on acquisition cost of the agents being considered. This approach typically will be used for multisource products, for which generic equivalents are available.

The cost-accounting technique of comparing drugs assumes relative equivalence for comparable agents regarding safety, efficacy, bioequivalence, and associated costs. This model accounts for drug-driven costs (e.g., administration costs) and focuses on total identifiable costs. This is beneficial because it quantifies differences between such things as different drug-delivery systems, packaging designs, and therapeutic regimens. The objectives are to compare and select products while minimizing acquisition and drug-driven costs.

The clinical decision analysis model can be used to develop protocols for drug prescribing. When selecting agents for a clinical category, this is the most appropriate approach to formulary decision making [22]. Clinical decision analysis quantifies agents with regard to safety, efficacy, and bioequivalance, while focusing on the overall therapeutic outcome of the decision. It has a broader scope than both of the other techniques. The objectives of clinical decision analysis are to compare and select therapeutic options, optimize therapeutic outcomes cost-effectively, and decrease overall costs of therapy. Essentially, this technique attempts to quantify outcomes in addition to costs. The P&T Committee should utilize the drug comparison technique that is most appropriate for the situation, in order to enhance the formulary decision-making process.

In addition to use of various comparison techniques, three key elements are important for establishing and maintaining a credible formulary. One element is a collaborative working relationship among health care professionals, such as occurs in an organized health care setting. For example, physicians and pharmacists should be able to work together to overcome problems that derive from the formulary. A second element is a defined medical staff or physician provider network that practices within the MCO. For instance, an IPA model HMO may have a greater challenge in managing a formulary than a staff model HMO. The third element is that the P&T Committee is viewed as a committee of the medical staff. Physicians are more likely to adhere to a formulary that they believe has been developed by their peers rather than by pharmacists or administrators.

The actual process of managing the formulary system is different in each organization, but there is a common theme between the components that make up a formulary management process. One theme is that pharmacists play a key role in managing the formulary, and often the pharmacy department of the MCO is in charge of managing the utilization of the formulary. Some other key components of managing a formulary are having a timely process for making decisions and disseminating the formulary in an efficient and effective manner.

There are two main types of formularies: open and closed. An open formulary is a list of drugs with few, if any, restrictions on prescribing. This type of formulary can contain up to 3000 drugs and dosage forms. There is little enforcement required and no penalty (to physician or patient) for nonformulary prescribing and purchasing. A closed formulary is a limited set of drugs that meet the inclusion criteria set by the P&T committee. A closed formulary typically has fewer than 1000 drugs and dosage forms. This type of formulary often has links to incentives that affect prescriber and patient behavior. For example, prescriber adherence may be tied to a salary bonus or patients may pay higher copayments for nonformulary drugs. In 1998, 48.4% of HMOs used a closed formulary.

Formularies also can be categorized by their degree of restrictiveness. A completely restrictive formulary does not allow any drugs to be prescribed unless they are on the formulary [23]. A restrictive formulary is a formulary where only drugs listed in the formulary may be prescribed unless documentation for nonformulary drugs is provided to the P&T committee. A nonrestrictive formulary is where physicians are encouraged to prescribe from the formulary, but nonformulary drugs can be prescribed with relative ease. In a completely nonrestrictive formulary there is no constraint on physician prescribing. The most common type is a restrictive formulary, with nonrestrictive being the next most common. Some evidence has shown that greater formulary restrictiveness is associated with greater medical costs [24]. The most cost-effective formulary system may be one that balances concerns over costs with the quality of care.

An important topic related to formularies is usage rebates. As MCOs have grown and gained bargaining power, they became positioned to negotiate rebates from suppliers, such as pharmaceutical manufacturers. These rebates often are structured to reward an MCO for achieving a specific level of usage by its beneficiaries. MCOs negotiate with manufacturers to obtain rebates, and the level of the rebate may influence formulary decisions. As new products enter the market, suppliers of older products can utilize a rebate agreement to maintain market share. The prevalence of usage rebates has increased for pharmaceuticals as therapeutic categories tend to contain several products that differ only in minor ways. Approximately 84% of HMOs participated in manufacturer rebate programs in 1998 [1]. Usage rebates can impact the cost and quality of pharmacotherapy received by an MCO's beneficiaries, and the presence of rebates can create powerful incentives to prescribe particular drugs.

Another result of the increased use of formularies is a change in how drugs are marketed. When drugs were marketed solely to individual providers, there typically was very little information provided on the cost of the drug. Now, success of a drug product may depend to a large degree on success in getting the drug included in health plan formularies, and P&T committees often factor cost information into their formulary decisions. This has resulted in the growth of "pharmacoeconomics," research on the cost-effectiveness of drugs. In addition to demonstrating that their drug is effective at improving outcomes, pharmaceutical manufacturers also now need to demonstrate that the improvement in outcomes can be achieved at a reasonable cost. Determining what cost is "reasonable" can be difficult, but the cost of the drug may be compared to the cost of nondrug treatments for the same health problem or to the cost of existing drug therapies.

Practice Guidelines

Another way that MCOs manage pharmacotherapy is through the use of practice guidelines. Practice guidelines are systematically developed statements that assist practitioners in providing care appropriate for specific clinical circumstances [25]. These guidelines typically focus on a single clinical condition and are based on the latest clinical evidence. Practice guidelines were used by 76.4% of HMOs in 1998 [1]. The logic in using practice guidelines is that less effective and more expensive therapy will be avoided; rather, the most cost-effective treatments can be identified and utilized within the MCO. As with formularies, the belief is that a limitation on therapy choice, as provided through practice guidelines, will translate into more appropriate care.

Practitioner acceptance of a practice guideline is an important determinant of its success and can vary across MCOs, depending on how the guideline was developed and the focus of the guideline. For example, involvement of local expert physicians (vs. unknown physicians from elsewhere) can support use of a practice guideline. Another factor influencing the usefulness of a practice guideline is its brevity and simplicity [26]. Physicians tend to prefer brief statements or summaries and are not likely to attend to lengthy guidelines. Practice guidelines provide a broad template for treating patients with a particular clinical condition. While they can help a practitioner eliminate some questionable therapies, their lack of specificity leaves room for variable treatment among patients with a common condition. For example, the care of a patient with asthma might have many decision points, which would contribute to variability in treatment. Because patients can present highly variable circumstances, loose control of therapy may be appropriate.

Another related technique is the use of critical pathways. A critical pathway or clinical care plan is a detailed plan of care for a specific diagnosis, disease, or procedure [27]. It describes the use and timing of all the care activities to try to optimize cost-effectiveness and improve patient outcomes. Critical pathways are much more specific than practice guidelines, which means they tend to take much more effort to produce. However, their comprehensive nature can enhance communication and coordination by different practitioners who are providing care to a particular patient. While critical pathways have been accepted within hospitals, their adoption for ambulatory care has been mixed.

Yet another related approach to pharmacotherapy management is step protocols or step therapy. Step protocols limit access to certain drugs until less costly alternative drugs have been tried first. For example, a step protocol might require a patient to have tried a relatively low-cost antihistamine, such as chlorpheniramine, before being prescribed a more expensive nonsedating antihistamine. Step therapy procedures were in place at 68.5% of HMOs in 1998 [1].

The use of practice guidelines, critical pathways, and step protocols is likely to increase as managed care organizations refine their approaches to managing pharmacotherapy. A principle to the successful use of such guides to treatment decisions will be not to remove decision-making authority from practitioners and patients, but to give them information and other guidance to make the best therapy decisions [28]. The challenge for managed care organizations is to help physicians and patients make good decisions, which balance the MCO's concerns for cost containment and quality of care.

Quality Improvement

The primary goal of quality improvement (QI) is to continuously monitor and improve the quality of care delivered to MCO beneficiaries. Quality improvement programs have two key characteristics: a systemwide perspective and a concern for structure, processes, and outcomes. The structure-process-outcome approach to health care quality was popularized by Donabedian [29]. Structure refers to capital resources (e.g., facilities and equipment), personnel (e.g., physicians and pharmacists), and how resources are organized (e.g., separate clinics, departments). Process is what happens during the delivery of care, including support activities. Who performs what task, as well as when and where that task occurs, are some issues for process of care. Outcomes refer to the end result of a health care service, often in terms of impact on a patient (e.g., clinical condition, quality of life). Most managed care organizations develop criteria in each of these three areas as part of their quality improvement programs.

Most QI programs build upon an established quality assurance (QA) process. Quality assurance can be defined as a formal and systematic process in which problems in delivering health care are identified, solutions to the problems are developed and implemented, and follow-up monitoring then is carried out [30]. QA begins with problem identification. After possible sources of the problem are determined, solutions are developed and implemented. Then, the results of the intervention or solution are evaluated to determine whether or not the problem has been resolved. By incorporating a goal of continual improvement, a QA process can contribute to quality improvement activities.

While QI and QA programs tend to cut across all health care activities, we will focus on the quality of medication use within MCOs. A cornerstone of quality programs for pharmacotherapy has been drug utilization review (DUR). Drug utilization review is an authorized, structured, and continuing program that reviews, analyzes, and interprets patterns of drug use against predetermined standards [31]. Most DUR programs in MCOs feed into educational activities aimed at prescribers or patients that attempt to correct drug-related problems found during the review process. The widespread use of DUR has been supported by the requirement in the Omnibus Budget Reconciliation Act of 1990 (OBRA '90) that required a DUR system for state Medicaid ambulatory pharmacy programs.

In most cases, DUR uses the MCO's prescription claims to provide data about drug use by the MCO's beneficiaries. These claims, which are generated at the time a prescription is dispensed, contain information about the patient, medication, and prescriber. In a retrospective manner, these claims are screened via computer to identify any patients or prescribers that do not fall within set criteria. For example, a patient's frequency of refills for costly or dangerous medications could be monitored. Also, DUR might focus on a physician's prescribing patterns for expensive antibiotics. Once individuals are identified, action may be taken. For example, a physician may be sent a letter containing a summary of the latest clinical evidence for antibiotic use. The expectation is that such information would help change the physician's prescribing behavior for antibiotics.

More progressive MCOs have moved to concurrent DUR, in which a pharmacist can screen for drug incompatibilities, duplicate prescriptions, and other problems before dispensing the medication. Obviously, the prevention of problems or the intervention directly with patients is attractive. While the identification of drug-related problems is vital to managing pharmacotherapy, intervention with the prescriber or patient also is required. The most common approach to intervening with prescribers and patients is through educational activities.

Educational Activities

A primary technique for managing pharmacotherapy within an MCO is to educate practitioners and patients about preferred approaches to managing care. MCOs often use education as one part of a broader strategy to change practitioner behavior. For example, educational interventions with prescribers are common follow-ups to problems identified through DUR. Similarly, patients can be targets of education designed to improve their control of a disease. The educational activities used by an MCO can be prospective or retrospective. A prospective educational program communicates desired information prior to treatment decisions. The goal is to create knowledge that will guide treatment choices in an appropriate manner, such that problems are prevented. Retrospective educational programs provide information after an evaluation of treatment choices has been made (i.e., subsequent to a DUR evaluation). Such programs often are intended to correct problematic behaviors (e.g., inappropriate therapy choices).

Several methods of educating practitioners and patients have been developed, including use of printed materials, lectures or symposia, and one-on-one discussions. Printed materials can include formularies, newsletters, brochures, and booklets. Having formulary information available for prescribers can improve their familiarity with, and ideally their use of, formulary drugs. Formularies typically are not distributed to patients.

Other printed materials can be used alone or in conjunction with oral education. Newsletters are published regularly and can be used to convey information addressing specific treatment issues. For example, a newsletter article might address current treatment approaches for pediatric asthma. Because newsletters also contain information that may be of general interest to practitioners and patients, they can have broad exposure. Brochures and booklets can be used to communicate a focused message in an efficient manner. These materials typically are given to people who are expected to have an interest in the topic within.

Lectures and symposia are used to orally give information to a group of practitioners or patients. These methods can be used to address broad topics (e.g., the MCO's process for developing practice guidelines) or narrow topics (e.g., use of the MCO's practice guideline for insulin-dependent diabetics). An advantage of lectures, compared to written communication, is that two-way interaction can occur. Allowing people to ask questions and discuss issues can help clarify information and can facilitate their use of the information.

One-on-one discussions with practitioners about appropriate therapy choices can be effective but also costly. Such discussions focused on pharmacotherapy have been called academic detailing [32,33]. Academic detailing typically utilizes a practitioner (e.g., physician, pharmacist) to meet with a prescriber to discuss the prescriber's patterns of prescribing. The primary goal often is to offer information to the targeted prescribers to try to improve pharmacotherapy.

An advantage of one-on-one presentations is the tailoring that can be done to address the specific prescriber's circumstances. For example, a physician who is prescribing cephalosporins at a rate significantly higher than his peers might be visited to discuss the accepted use of cephalosporins. Such a meeting would allow the physician to state his prescribing approach, while the detailing practitioner could provide information about the more broadly accepted prescribing approach. The hope is that the prescriber will adjust his prescribing to be more in line with the accepted practice.

III. CURRENT TRENDS AND ISSUES IN MANAGED CARE

One trend in the managed care market is the relatively recent increase of managed care in Medicaid (beneficiaries are poor or medically needy) and Medicare (beneficiaries are age 65 and older or disabled). The percent of Medicaid beneficiaries in managed care plans grew from 14.4% in 1993 to 53.6% in 1998 [34]. The growth of managed care in the Medicare program has been slower, but currently about 16% of Medicare beneficiaries are in managed care plans [34]. Enrollment of Medicaid and Medicare populations has created some additional issues and challenges for MCOs. For the Medicaid program, the provider network must have providers in locations that are accessible to Medicaid beneficiaries. This may require MCOs to broaden their provider network. Also, Medicare beneficiaries and medically needy Medicaid beneficiaries tend to have more health problems than individuals enrolled in an MCO through their employer. As a result, they use more prescription drugs and present more pharmacotherapy management challenges than the employer-based population.

Although MCOs currently are not required to offer prescription drug benefits as part of their Medicare plans, many have done so as a way to increase enrollment. However, Medicare HMO reimbursement levels have not increased as fast as health care expenditures, and some HMOs may try to decrease costs by reducing or eliminating prescription drug benefits. At the same time, there is discussion about adding some type of prescription drug benefit to Medicare. It is difficult to predict the net effect of a Medicare prescription drug plan on MCOs. Some Medicare beneficiaries may have enrolled in Medicare HMOs just to get prescription drug benefits, and this would no longer be necessary if Medicare covered prescription drugs for all beneficiaries. However, most of the proposed Medicare prescription drug plans specify some "management" of benefits and would require at least some of the pharmacotherapy management techniques used by MCOs and PBMs.

An MCO dilemma that was mentioned earlier is the need to control costs while still offering patients enough choice and access to providers to keep them satisfied. There has been some "managed care backlash," where some managed care organizations have been accused of going too far in trying to control costs and denying enrollees necessary care. Consumers also have been unhappy with the restricted choice of providers in managed care organizations and with the gatekeeper provision that many of the organizations employ. There have been several responses to these concerns, both by outside agencies and MCOs.

One response has been legislation, both general legislation directed at MCOs and legislation directed at specific practices of MCOs and other insurers. An example of general legislation is the proposed "patient bill of rights," one version of which would give patients the right to sue MCOs. There is ongoing debate over this bill in the U.S. Senate. An example of legislation directed at specific insurer practices is the law requiring insurers to allow a minimum of 2 days hospital stay postpartum. This law resulted from concern that women were being discharged from the hospital too quickly after giving birth. There also have been some state laws mandating coverage of specific drugs.

Another external response to concerns about MCOs has been an increased interest in measuring the quality of care they deliver [35]. This interest has resulted in the development of numerous quality indicators. One example, HEDIS (Health Plan Employer Data and Information Set), is a standardized set of performance indicators used to compare health plans. Developed by the National Committee for Quality Assurance, HEDIS measures allow employers and employees to evaluate different plans. Only a small number of HEDIS indicators are related to medication use, but more drug-related indicators are likely to be added in the future. The use of quality indicators likely will increase as the measures become more refined and tested.

Another response to consumer complaints about restricted choice has been the growth of less restrictive MCOs such as PPOs and POS plans. These plans typically allow patients more freedom to choose providers and may allow patients to self-refer to specialists. However, less restrictive plans typically have higher premiums and charge patients more to seek care from out-of-network providers or self-refer to specialists. This trend of allowing more choice but requiring patients to pay more also has occurred in pharmacotherapy management. The three-tier copayment for prescription drugs, where patients can obtain nonformulary medications but must pay a higher copayment, is an example of this trend.

The trade-off between controlling costs and maintaining patient satisfaction especially is an issue with pharmacotherapy. Prescription drug costs in the United States have grown rapidly in the last 10 years (Fig. 5) and are projected to increase to $171 billion by the year 2007 [36]. One factor driving this increase is the introduction of new, more expensive prescription drugs. The average cost per day for a new drug increased from $1.09 for drugs introduced prior to 1995 to $2.97 for drugs introduced in 1999 [37]. The introduction of even one expensive drug therapy for a relatively common medical condition can devastate an MCO's drug budget for the year. However, the drug therapy may lower other types of health care costs. It will be important for MCOs to have mechanisms in place to examine costs across different categories.

Another factor that MCOs must contend with is increasing consumer demand for pharmaceuticals, driven in part by direct to consumer advertising of prescription drugs. There have been anecdotal reports of some MCOs having to remove some heavily advertised drug products from their formularies because of extremely high utilization. However, this strategy may be unsuccessful, because consumers may become dissatisfied with a managed care plan that limits access to some prescription drugs. It remains to be seen how consumers will react to the MCO strategy of allowing access to nonformulary drugs but requiring more cost sharing.

The last two decades have been a time of unprecedented growth for managed care. One of the few remaining population segments with "unmanaged" care is Medicare beneficiaries, and even in this population, increased managed care penetration has occurred in recent years. In spite of some concerns about managed care, it seems unlikely that health care in the United States ever will return to a completely unmanaged state. Health care costs continue to rise, and insurers will continue to seek ways to manage that growth. However, consumers in the United States also seem to value choice in their health care decisions, and as a result we likely will continue to see growth in less restrictive MCOs like PPOs and POS plans. Pharmacotherapy management will continue to be a challenge for MCOs. They may try to offer more choice at a higher price, or they may impose additional restrictions and limits on prescription drug benefits. Either way, it is likely that MCOs will continue to rely on many of the pharmacotherapy management tools described here.

REFERENCES

1. HMO-PPO/Medicare-Medicaid Digest. Kansas City, MO: Hoechst Marion Roussel, 1999.
2. Kaiser Permanente Website. www.kaiserpermanente.org. July 2000.
3. M Mitka. A quarter century of health maintenance. JAMA 280(24):2059–2060, 1998.
4. PJ Feldstein. Health Policy Issues: An Economic Perspective on Health Reform. 2nd ed. Chicago: Health Administration Press/AUPHA Press, 1999, pp. 193–207.

5. M Gold, L Nelson, T Lake, R Hurley, R Berenson. Behind the curve: a critical assessment of how little is known about arrangements between managed care plans and physicians. Med Care Res Rev 52(3):307–341, 1995.
6. DC Cave. Incentives and cost containment in primary care physician reimbursement. Benefits Q 3:70–77, 1993.
7. A Hillman. Financial incentives for physicians in HMOs. NEJM 317(27):1743–1748, 1987.
8. Source Book of Health Insurance Data. Washington, DC: Health Insurance Association of America, 1999.
9. LE Block. Evolution, growth, and status of managed care in the United States. Pub Health Rev 25:193–244, 1997.
10. G de Lissovoy, T Rice, J Gabel, HJ Gelzer. Preferred provider organizations one year later. Inquiry 24:127–135, 1987.
11. JM Ganther, DH Kreling. Effect of a change in third party reimbursement rates on prescription gross margin. J Am Pharm Assoc 39(3):346–352, 1999.
12. Report to the president: prescription drug coverage, spending, utilization, and prices. Dept. of Health and Human Services, 2000, pp. 123–124.
13. Novartis pharmacy benefit report, 1999.
14. A Leibowitz, WG Manning, JP Newhouse. The demand for prescription drugs as a function of cost-sharing. Soc Sci Med 21(10):1063–1069, 1985.
15. AA Nelson, CE Reeder, WM Dickson. The effect of a Medicaid copayment program on the utilization and cost of prescription services. Med Care 22(8):724–736, 1984.
16. BL Harris, A Stergachis, LD Ried. The effect of drug co-payments on utilization and cost of pharmaceuticals in a health maintenance organization. Med Care 28(10):907–917, 1990.
17. B Foxman, RB Valdez, KN Lohr, GA Goldberg, JP Newhouse, RH Brook. The effect of cost sharing on the use of antibiotics in ambulatory care: results from a population based randomized controlled trial. J Chron Dis 40(5):429–437, 1987.
18. CE Reeder, AA Nelson. The differential impact of co-payment on drug use in a Medicaid population. Inquiry 22(4):396–403, 1985.
19. JP Weiner, A Lyles, DM Steinwachs, KC Hall. Impact of managed care on prescription drug use. Health Affairs 10(1):149–154, 1991.
20. JM Ganther, DH Kreling. The effect of implementing a maximum allowable cost generic substitution plan on the dispensing of generic prescription drugs: a quasi-experimental design. Unpublished.
21. ASHP Guidelines on formulary system management. Am J Hosp Pharm 49:648–652, 1992.
22. VS Crane. How to use structured decision making in developing therapeutic, cost-effective formulary systems. Hosp Form 28(Oct):859–867, 1993.
23. EC Hanson, M Shepherd. Formulary restrictiveness in health maintenance organizations. J Soc Ad Pharm 11(1):54–56, 1994.
24. SD Horn, PD Sharkey, DM Tracy, CE Horn, B James, F Goodwin. Intended and unintended consequences of HMO cost-containment strategies: results from the managed care outcomes project. Am J Managed Care 2:253–264, 1996.
25. KN Lohr, ed. Institute of Medicine, Medicare: A Strategy for Quality Assurance. Vol. 1. National Academy Press, 1990.
26. R Coleman. Promoting quality through managed care. Am J Med Qual 7(winter):100–105, 1992.
27. LD Jaggers. Differentiation of critical pathways from other health care management tools. Am J Health-System Pharm 53(Feb 1):311–313, 1996.
28. DM Eddy. The challenge. JAMA 263:287–290, 1990.
29. A Donabedian. Explorations in Quality Assessment and Monitoring: The Definition of Quality and Approaches to Its Assessment. Vol. 1, Ann Arbor, MI: Health Administration Press, 1980.
30. KN Lohr, RH Brook. Quality assurance in medicine. Am Behav Scientist 27:583–607, 1984.
31. DC Brodie. Drug utilization review/planning. Am J Pub Health 46:103, 1972.
32. CS Stern. Academic detailing: what's in a name? J Managed Care Pharm 2(Mar/Apr):88–90, 1996.
33. KB Farris, DM Kirking, LA Shimp, RAC Opdycke. Design and results of a group counter-detailing DUR educational project. Pharm Res 13(10):1445–1452, 1996.
34. Health Care Financing Administration website. National Health Care Expenditures. www.hcfa.gov. Sept. 2000.
35. BS Finkelstein, JB Silvers, GE Rosethal. The importance of outcomes data in health care decision making and purchasing. Marketing Health Services 17(2):52–59, 1997.
36. S Smith, M Freeland, S Heffler, D McKusick. The next ten years of health spending: what does the future hold?. Health Affairs 17(5):128–140, 1998.
37. Managing pharmacy benefit costs—new insights for a new century. Merck-Medco Drug Trend Report, 2000.

Chapter 28

A View to the Future

Gilbert S. Banker

University of Iowa, Iowa City, Iowa

Christopher T. Rhodes

University of Rhode Island, Kingston, Rhode Island

I. INTRODUCTION

A. Uneven Progress in the World

When one reviews the situation concerning the availability of modern pharmaceutical products throughout the world at the beginning of the twenty-first century, marked regional differences are immediately apparent. The so-called ICH (International Commission on Harmonization) tripartite areas (North America, western Europe, and Japan) have strong research-based pharmaceutical industries, which produce a plethora of pharmaceuticals both for their own use and for export. Table 1 illustrates this fact, showing that at least 92% of the world's company-financed pharmaceutical research and development is conducted in the tripartite areas. Many of the residents of these areas have relatively easy access to modern drug products, although there are still significant segments of these populations who have serious financial limitations on their ability to purchase the drug products that have been prescribed for their or their dependents use.

In many other regions of the world, very large parts of the population do not have access to desperately needed pharmaceutical products. The situation is probably most acute in Africa, where drugs are desperately needed for the prevention and treatment of many diseases (e.g., malaria, AIDS) but are presently only available to a small proportion of those who could benefit from their use. There are technical problems in the supply of some drug products in parts of Africa. For example, for those countries in the ICH climate zone four (hot and wet), a heavy-duty tropical pack may be essential for a number of pharmaceuticals. However, because of the extra cost of such packs, they are not always used. This lack of an effective package combined with what is often an unusually long and slow channel of distribution from manufacturer to user may result in patients receiving subpotent products. Equally serious is the low GDP (gross domestic product), very limited physical and organizational infrastructure, and in some cases civil unrest and war that exist in these regions. The solutions to these problems are complex, often geopolitical, and generally defy easy resolution. The devastating effect of the AIDS epidemic in sub-Saharan Africa is described in Chapter 1 of this book. However, it is highly probable that the problem of an uneven supply of modern, quality pharmaceutical products and providing adequate health care throughout the world will be given increasing attention in the twenty-first century. Unfortunately it is also highly probable that third world countries will continue to suffer from second-rate health care and inadequate access to pharmacotherapy for decades to come.

Table 1 Company-Financed Global Pharmaceutical Research and Development by Country, 1997

United States	36%
Japan	19%
Germany	10%
France	9%
United Kingdom	7%
Switzerland	5%
Sweden	3%
Italy	3%
All other	8%

Source: Centre for Medicines Research, 1999.

Table 2 Global Population and Pharmaceutical Sales (by value) by Region, 1997

Region	Global population (%)	Global drug sales (%)	Ratio of sales to population
North America	5–6	37	6.2–7.4
Europe	13	30	2.3
Japan	2–3	17	5.7–8.5
Asia	55	8–9	0.15–0.16
Latin America	9	8	0.89
Near East	3	2	0.67
Africa	13	1	0.08

Source: Ref. 1.

An analysis, based on the percentage of the world's population located in various regions of the world compared to the percentage of their global expenditure on pharmaceuticals, is one way to examine drug availability by region. Table 2 provides these approximate numbers. In the table, the higher the ratio of a region's percentage of global drug sales to its percentage of the world's population, the greater is its utilization of pharmacotherapy (drugs). According to the data shown, drug utilization in Africa is only about 1/80–1/100 that in the more industrialized nations.

Figure 1 shows pharmaceutical expenditures, both prescription and nonprescription, per capita in industrialized countries in 1997. Comparing the numbers in this figure with those in Table 2, it is possible to estimate per capita pharmaceutical expenditures for regions such as Africa. For example, Japan has 17 times the global drug sales of Africa (Table 2); dividing 17 into Japan's per capita pharmaceutical expenditure of $348 from Figure 1, one obtains $20.47. But since Africa has 13% of the world's population and Japan only about 2.5%, a factor of 13/2.5, or about 5, must be divided into the $20.47 to equate to the per capita expenditure in Africa. The result is about $5.10 for Africa's per capita pharmaceutical expenditure. Performing the same calculations using the numbers shown for North America, Africa's per capital pharmaceutical expenditure number is about $3.75. In any event, the per capita expenditure for pharmaceuticals in Africa is probably $5.00 or less.

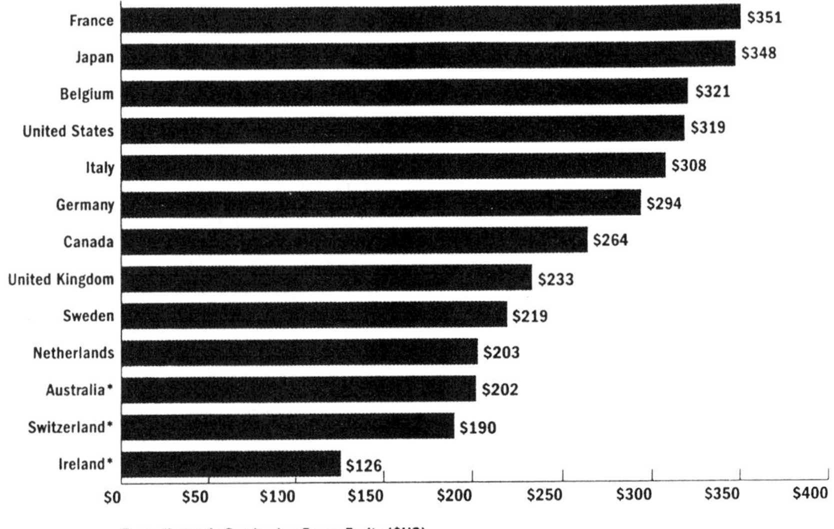

Fig. 1 Per capita pharmaceutical expenditures in industrialized countries. Pharmaceuticals include nonprescription products. *1996 data. (From OECD Health Data, 1998.)

There are global efforts to address the world's uneven drug supply. The World Health Assembly has endorsed the concept of essential drugs [2,3], which are defined as "those that satisfy the health care needs of the majority of the population and should therefore be available at all times in adequate amounts and in appropriate dosage forms." The World Health Organization (WHO) estimates that one third of the world's population does not have access to essential drugs (an estimate unchanged since the mid-1980s). The fact that the percentage of the world's population lacking access to essential drugs has not declined in the last 20 years is not surprising, since the cost of drugs over this period has increased faster than has economic growth in many of these regions. Nearly 150 countries have adopted a national essential drug list. The latest WHO list includes 302 active ingredients, of which 90% are off patent and are usually available at reasonable prices. The World Bank, which provides financial assistance to underdeveloped nations, has promoted the essential drugs concept, as a means to focus health expenditures in medicine to produce the most health benefits in a population [4]. The global drug gap issue is receiving growing attention [5]. The Pfizer Journal recently devoted an entire issue to the topic "International Perspectives on Health Care and Biomedical Research," with comments from experts around the world [6]. The challenges to providing access to high-quality health care, including pharmaceutical care to all Americans, were discussed in Chapters 1 and 27.

B. Competing Forces: Cost Control and Political Need for Universal Availability

Even within the economically advantaged areas of the world, such as ICH tripartite regions, there are clearly significant subcohorts of the general population for whom pharmaceutical care is presently inadequate. There are political forces, therefore, that are moving towards the ideal of universal access to drug products. At the same time, however, governments, insurance companies, and employers are growing increasingly concerned about the cost of health care. It sometimes seems that politicians in their attempts "to complete the circle" with respect to the availability and cost of health care unjustifiably single out the cost of pharmaceutical products as being the villain of the piece. Certainly, there have been individual instances when the price of some drug products that have enjoyed a virtual monopoly situation have been increased or maintained at a level that is very hard to justify. Such cases have attracted much adverse publicity for the pharmaceutical industry. It is also often accurately pointed out that the fastest growing health care cost component is prescription drugs. This is not solely related to inflationary cost increases for drugs. It is also the result of increased utilization, including that by a rapidly growing elderly population who take the majority of our drugs and who increasingly rely on their medications for their quality of life and even their continued existence. The generally higher cost of new biotechnology products is another factor. It is also true that 90% or more of all new drugs are conceived and developed by the pharmaceutical industry and that the cost of development for a new drug today is about a half billion dollars.

The pharmaceutical industry is sometimes unjustifiably attacked for the cost of its products simply because drug costs can be so readily identified in comparison to other health care products or services. In many countries hospitals are owned by the government, and thus to some extent hospital costs, including drug costs, may be less likely to be the target of politicians' criticism. Clearly, we can expect a period of continuing tension between society and government's desire for drug products and their ability or willingness to pay the price.

C. Tripartite Convergence, Globalization, Harmonization, and WHO Concerns

Many of the mergers and amalgamations occurring in the pharmaceutical industry involve multinational companies (see Sec. III.A). The result is an increasing globalization of the pharmaceutical industry, where a given multinational company has research laboratories in the United States and Europe or elsewhere and manufacturing sites in many regions of the world. As products are increasingly designed for marketing throughout the world, it is desirable, if not essential, that the drug meet the standards of each country where marketing is proposed, that all excipients used are also acceptable, and that all test or quality-control product standards will also be recognized. Achieving product uniformity and standards that are recognized in many countries and regions of the world is termed harmonization.

Perhaps the first international attempt at harmonization involved excipients and a collaborative effort between scientists in the United States and the United Kingdom. The goal was to develop common descriptions and physical standards for the most commonly used excipients. The project was supported by the American Pharmaceutical Association and the Pharmaceutical Society of Great Britain, who together published a book entitled the *Handbook of Pharmaceutical Excipients* in 1986. This harmonization effort has continued to date, with new and expanded editions of the handbook coming out about every 5 years.

In 1989 a group known as the Pharmaceutical Discussion Group (PDG) was created as a voluntary alliance between the United States Pharmacopeia (USP), the European Pharmacopoeia (EP), and the Japanese Pharmacopoeia (JP). This group originally focused on excipients, but is also working on such important standards as physical testing, including dissolution testing. Reaching consensus between these three compendia is not always easy, and compendial harmonization will be a lengthy process, but a very important activity, which will be of growing importance to pharmacists and pharmaceutical manufacturers in the decades ahead. Compounding this challenge is the fact that the USP is a private nonprofit organization, while the BP and the JP are both government organizations. The seven stages in the harmonization process and other information on the PDG have been published and discussed [7].

Drug regulators and representatives of the drug industry from the United States, Europe, and Japan have been participating since the early 1990s in the ICH. Their goal is to reduce or eliminate duplicate requirements for drug development and approval in the three regions. As a result of the fifth meeting of this group in 2000, over 35 important guidelines have been established. During the same time the United States and the European Union (EU) have been working and in 1997 negotiated the Mutual Recognition Agreement (MRA), which eliminates regulatory barriers and promotes trade between the two regions. In addition the regions agreed to recognize inspections of each others manufacturing facilities [8]. Such harmonization and recognition agreements have undoubtedly made it easier for, and probably directly contributed to mergers between, large U.S. and British pharmaceutical companies.

A veterinary products harmonization activity has also been established involving a trilateral union of regulatory agencies and industrial representatives from Europe, the United States, and Japan. The group was officially established in 1996 and has already compiled 24 guidelines to promote harmonization [9]. Other groups will no doubt also come together to promote common harmonization goals. The result will clearly be a much greater degree of standardization, in technical as well as regulatory areas, throughout much of the world in the years and decades above. Were it not for politics, a World Pharmacopeia might some day become a reality.

Globalization and harmonization are interrelated phenomena. They have had a major impact on the world's pharmaceutical industry in the last decade of the twentieth century. That impact will grow in the decade ahead, and the beneficiaries will ultimately be the world's drug consumers.

As noted previously in this chapter, in recent years WHO has become increasingly concerned about drug access. They have also expressed concern that the three ICH tripartite powers are so dominating the pharmaceutical world that non-ICH countries are losing out. Some large multinational companies have recently announced that they would ship drugs to countries devastated by AIDS, at no or minimal cost, to help address this critical access problem. A proposal to help address WHO concerns, which may gradually evolve, is to require that pharmaceutical products only be accepted as marketable if their shelf life is determined on the basis of climate zone 4 (hot, wet) conditions, rather than for the more temperate climate zones 1 and 2 of the tripartite regions. Under such a proposal, heavy-duty tropical packs might be mandatory for some drugs, although unnecessary in all areas.

II. SCIENCE, BIOTECHNOLOGY, AND THE NEXT PHARMACEUTICAL CENTURY

A. Genomics

Many interested in the future of science and technology are looking to the twenty-first century as being the biotechnology era. As a result, experts see dramatic changes ahead for the next pharmaceutical century as a result of genomics, proteomics, gene therapy, rejuvenative therapy, pharmacogenomics, combinatorial chemistry, bioinformatics, molecular biology, and delivery-enhanced therapeutics, all of which are expected to play major roles in curing and preventing disease [10]. Genomics, by deciphering the human genome through the 100,000 genes encoded by 3 billion chemical pairs in our DNA, provides never before available solutions to the understanding of disease processes, possible new disease prevention routes, and new treatments including gene therapy. With the human genome sequenced, the next frontier is understanding the shape and function of the encoded proteins, particularly those involved in disease processes (structural genomics). This approach is expected to extend the genomics revolution from a catalog of genes to a catalog of proteins for which the genes code [11].

B. Proteomics

Proteomics seeks to define the function and expression profiles of all the proteins encoded within a given genome. Researchers in proteomics separate, identify, and characterize expressed proteins to better understand their functions and how these functions are regulated. Thus proteomics is concerned with identifying and unlocking the secrets of the thousands of proteins involved not just in structural genomics, but in life, disease, and cellular processes of all kinds. One example is the work that has identified the three-dimensional protein structure of HIV protease, which is allowing researchers to design inhibitors to block the replication of the virus [8]. Thus, proteomics is also concerned with identifying targets for drugs and using the principles of combinatorial chemistry to expeditiously design the drugs for these targets.

C. Pharmacogenomics

In addition to these generalized approaches of genomics and proteomics, it has been predicted that pharmacogenomics may revolutionize drug discovery and treatment for the individual, based on the following (and with some of the consequences noted) [12]:

1. The ability to understand what diseases each individual may be predisposed to, how he or she might react to specific drugs, and therapies to prevent future illness, all of which will refocus and change the practice of medicine.
2. Development of the ability to screen at the individual level for all known genetic diseases and defects, and provision to the individual of a computer chip the size of a quarter with their genetic make-up. This would involve the ultimate application of the evolving field of pharmacogenomics, which is the science of understanding the correlation between an individual patients genetic make-up (genotype) and her or his response to a drug treatment. The ultimate goal is to identify patients most likely to be benefited by therapies and to optimize therapies to patients. Some of the work going on in this field and the biotech companies who are working in various therapeutic categories has recently been reviewed [13].
3. Development of ever more powerful diagnostic tools to promote highly personalized medical treatments to further refocus medical practice on prevention rather than intervention.
4. A huge shift is predicted in the ratio of doctor bills to pharmaceutical costs, from the current ratio of about 9 to 1 to a ratio of 1 to 1 in the next 25 years [12].

D. Combinatorial Chemistry and Rapid Throughput Screening

One of the major challenges in the years ahead will be to improve existing and develop new crystallization methods and rapid methods of determining the structure of complex proteins. The growing number of new biotech companies working in this field is promising. However, the bulk of the high-speed protein structure–determining techniques work only on the proteins that make up the least interesting targets for new drugs. Most of the important new drugs will be designed to target proteins that straddle cell membranes and help control the molecular traffic of cells. But membrane proteins are exceedingly difficult to crystallize, even one at a time, and do not yet permit resolution by available high-speed techniques [11]. However, advances will occur to disclose important specific new drug targets at an ever-accelerating pace, and target-oriented and diversity-oriented organic synthesis [14] will be applied in drug discovery, along with combinatorial chemistry to attack these targets. The primary goal of diversity-oriented syntheses is to efficiently synthesize a collection of structurally complex and diverse small molecules capable of perturbing any disease-related biological pathway, eventually leading to the identification of protein molecules capable of being modulated by the small molecules [14]. The combinatorial chemistry approach is based on understanding structure-activity relationships by first identifying receptors and then synthesizing chemical compounds to best attack or match the receptor. The basis of this drug-discovery process is to synthesize chemical compounds, test their biological activity, and then evaluate/determine the next synthesis iteration. Combinatorial chemistry methods have greatly accelerated synthesis throughput, once the bottleneck of drug discovery. Automated compound purification, automated activity analyses, robotics, unattended operations, and 24-hour laboratory operations all play a role. In a comprehensive article on laboratory automation applied to combinatorial discovery, it was reported that Bristol-Myers Squibb, over a 5-year period, increased their new drug candidates three- to fourfold while utilizing 50% less staff time per drug candidate and reducing lead times by 40% [15]. These new approaches, which also make extensive use of computer networks and software to interface with instruments and researchers in real time, will play a growing role in future drug-discovery process, leading to better drugs sooner.

E. Stem Cells and Rejunerative Therapy

One of the most promising areas of biotechnology research, but one also the most fraught with ethical dilemma, involves the use of stem cells for rejunerative therapy. A unique feature of embryonic stem cells lies in their ability to differentiate into virtually any cell type. On the one hand, the use of cells from human embryos raises many questions of potential abuse. On the other, over 100 million Americans suffer from illnesses that might be alleviated by stem cell transplantation, including those with cardiovascular diseases (58 million), autoimmune diseases (30 million), diabetes (16 million), osteoporosis (10 million), cancer (8.2 million), Alzheimer's disease (4 million), Parkinson's disease (1.5 million), plus those with severe burns, spinal cord injuries, and certain birth defects [16]. Scientists in Sweden have demonstrated marked benefits of stem cell transplantation in Parkinson's patients, and this may be the first patient class to actually benefit from this therapy when it is approved and legalized. An article in *The Scientist* has provided an interesting update on the status of stem cell research to replenish a variety of organs and to produce dramatic advances in a number of disease states. Among the target organs described were the brain, pancreas, liver, heart, and blood [17]. Even with all the controversy, based on the enormous potential benefits of stem cell therapies, it is predicted that research in this field will be ongoing, various sources of stem cells identified and developed, and that stem cell therapy will become a very important and recognized regenerative therapy in the years ahead.

F. Neurosciences

Another extremely important discipline that has emerged in the latter part of the twentieth century is the field of neuroscience, which is actually an interdisciplinary field encompassing biological and psychological sciences into a common framework with cell and molecular biology [18]. Molecular neuroscience is already beginning to reap substantial benefits for clinical medicine. Reference has already been made to stem cells, which were identified in studies of neural development, for cell replacement in Parkinson's disease. In a like way, insights into axon guidance molecules offer hope for nerve regeneration after spinal cord injury. In addition, most neurological diseases are associated with cell death, and new approaches are examining cell rescue, using, for example, inhibition of caspase proteases [18].

Progress is being made in other debilitating and lethal brain disorders. The gene defect responsible for Huntington's disease has been identified (as marked by a series of trinucleotide repeat units), which is now known to constitute the largest group of dominantly transmitted neurological diseases. It is also known that the target site in the brain where cell death occurs is the basal ganglia [18].

Great strides have been made in the early identification and molecular biochemical cause of Alzheimer's disease. An elusive enzyme, gamma secretase, contained in the transmembrane protein called presenilin, is now known to cause the release of the Alzheimer peptide, amploid B-peptide (AB). Having established the molecular/cellular mechanism for this dreaded disease, two groups are known to be working, using high-throughput screening, to identify compounds that will inhibit AB production. Both the group at Harvard and the group at Merck have reportedly identified inhibitors that are transition state analogs, selectively binding the active forms of gamma secretase [19].

The above are but two examples of the rapid progress being made in neuroscience research with the goal of providing effective treatments for two very difficult and deadly diseases. Other mental diseases that, due to their variable etiologies are more complex will also be major targets for more effective resolution in the twenty-first, century. Major depression (MD) affects over 17% of the U.S. population during their lifetime, with the prevalence in women twice as high as in men. At any point in time, 10.3% of the population will have had an MD episode in the previous 12 months [20,21]. MD is more commonly encountered than any other condition in the primary care setting and is associated with higher costs than any other common disorder [22]. MD is expected to soon be the second leading cause of disability worldwide [23,24]. MD is associated with high morbidity and mortality [25], with up to 15% of those having the most severe forms dying by suicide [26]. MD is a very underrecognized and undertreated condition [27]. Pharmacists have a great responsibility and opportunity to provide pharmaceutical care with a goal of optimizing clinical outcomes for patients with MD. A review by Desai and Jann [20] details the condition of MD and the potential roles pharmacists can play.

G. Ongoing Traditional Approaches

More traditional small organic molecules will continue to play a key role as pharmaceutical agents, ever increasing in specificity to attack selected targets. In addition, immunology will continue to advance as a means of preventing disease. It is possible that AIDS vaccines are finally being developed after years of frustration [28]. Several earlier vaccine approaches were canceled by the National Institute of Health in 1994. A new vaccine approach based on the AIDS virus coat protein, gp 120, and preventing it from binding to CO4 receptors on white blood cells has shown effectiveness in monkeys. Various AIDS vaccine clinical trials are now being conducted in the United States, Europe, and Southeast Asia using a variety of approaches [28]. While major challenges remain, it now appears likely that an effective AIDS vaccine is not only a possibility, but a likelihood.

H. Delivery-Enhanced Therapeutics

Delivery-enhanced therapeutics will unquestionably play a major role in the drug delivery of the new century. Many peptide and high molecular weight drugs can currently be administered only by injection. Some drugs in this category, such as interferon-alpha, could be more important in treating numerous serious medical conditions (leukemias, melanomas, lymphomas, and sarcomas) if alternative routes of delivery were available [29]. Clinical trials are in fact being conducted with this drug using nasal delivery to provide a unique pharmacokinetic profile, with the further goal of improving safety, efficacy, and patient compliance [29]. This is but one example of many that could be cited in the delivery-enhanced therapeutics arena, which also includes drug targeting to specific organs, tissues, and cells. The reader is referred to Chapters 15 and 16 in this book for in-depth treatments of this subject.

Pulsatile controlled release is a technique that may grow in importance in the near future. We know from chronobiological studies that diurnal (and to a lesser extent weekly) rhythms affect many human physiological functions, including central nervous system activity, urinary pH, gastrointestinal mobility, and body temperature. Not surprisingly, there is evidence that for a variety of drugs, including some chemotherapeutic agents used in the treatment of neoplasms, there are distinct advantages to pulsing drug delivery in phase with the patient's body clock. Advantages can include improved efficacy and a reduction in the extent of side effects.

Two other approaches have recently appeared in oral drug delivery. Super-fast drug delivery is a concept that is rapidly emerging as a formulation approach of considerable potential. For some therapeutic classes (e.g., analgesics), the value of such systems is obviously substantial. Super-long delivery systems are the other concept. Controlled-release products are not presently generally designed to provide essentially constant blood levels of drug for more than about 24 hours. However, research on drug-delivery systems capable of controlled delivery for a period of days, weeks, or longer is proceeding rapidly, and the range of such systems that will be commercially available is likely to increase in an impressive manner.

I. Reduction in Animal Testing

We have already seen significant advances made in our efforts to reduce the amount of animal testing required in the development or quality control of pharmaceutical products. For example, in the early 1990s the USP conducted a concerted campaign to reduce the animal testing required for the evaluation of official products. In many cases cell culture methods can completely replace whole animal testing. It seems likely that further progress will be made in this area even under the pressures of a rapidly growing drug-discovery process. Animal testing is expensive, time consuming, highly controlled, and ethically improper unless justified and properly conducted. However, it is probably quite unrealistic to expect that animal testing of new drugs can be completely eliminated any time soon. At present it would seem to be an unjustifiable risk to proceed directly from test tube work to Phase I human studies.

J. Bioinformatics

Bioinformatics is an explosive growth field and will play a key role in the biotechnology revolution of the twenty-first century. Bioinformatics companies are now a part of the high-tech biotechnology industry. Scientists have now uncovered the millions of pieces of information behind the 23 pairs of human chromosomes with the help of bioinformatics. Bioinformatics is broadly defined as the application of computer technologies to the biological sciences, particularly genomics, with the object of discovering knowledge. It is often understood to include high-throughput screening of genes and proteins. It is broadly defined as any application of computation to the field of biology, including data management, algorithm development, and data mining. Bioinformatics has been particularly related to biological entities involved in the drug-discovery process. As noted by Watkins in her cover story review of the bioinformatics field [30], what is meant by the term depends on the various workers in the field and their focus. Some even view all even remotely related information systems as part of bioinformatics, as these bring together chemical information systems (cheminformatics), including high-throughput screening data, drug information systems, and medical information systems, including clinical data. The basic goal of bioinformatics is to sift through and organize information, mine data for leads and cause-and-effect relationships, and even generate new knowledge from the unbelievable masses of information at hand [31,32]. (The reader is also referred to the related topic on drug information in Chapter 26.)

Finally attention should be called to the most comprehensive and current treatment of the human genome and its impact in science and medicine, which was the subject of an entire special issue of Science. (The issue contained an interesting 4½ × 6 foot chart of the annotation of the Celera human genome assembly [33].)

III. THE PHARMACEUTICAL INDUSTRY

A. The U.S. Pharmaceutical Industry: Size, Scope, and General Direction

The U.S. pharmaceutical and biotechnology industry continues to lead the world in innovation and product sales. It accounts for nearly 40% of global pharmaceutical sales [34]. This industry is in fact one of the few in which the United States retains a commanding global lead. If the twenty-first century is to become known as the biotech era and the new pharmaceutical century, it will be very important to the United States that this leadership position be retained.

As has been noted previously, the pharmaceutical industry is responsible for the development of the vast majority (over 90%) of the drugs on the market today. A large part of this fact is explained by the enormous investment made by the drug industry in research. Until 1980 more than half of the total U.S. research and development funding came from the federal government, and the largest share of those dollars (one third) went to the Department of Defense. Things are much different today, with over 70% of total research and development (R&D) expenditures coming from the private sector. Pharmaceutical R&D has grown enormously. Drug R&D in 2001 was expected to total more than $47 billion, or nearly a fifth of the total $266 billion expenditure in the United States. The pharmaceutical industry now outspends the NIH for drug research, and over $30 billion will come from the industry. Annual growth in R&D spending by the pharmaceutical industry has occurred at a rate of 10–11% or more in recent years, and that growth rate is expected to be continued [35,36].

The research-based pharmaceutical industry spends more on research as a percentage of sales then any other industry—at 20.8% [37]. By comparison, R&D expenditures as a percentage of sales for some other industries are electronic, 6.0%; telecommunication, 5.1%; automotive, 4.1%; aerospace and defense, 3.7%; and all industries excluding "drugs and medicine," 3.7% [37]. Research is clearly the lifeblood of the pharmaceutical industry, and it will be a key not only to keeping the U.S. industry in a global leadership position, but also to maintaining the flow of new products as the primary method of more effectively combating disease and enhancing human health in the years and decades ahead.

The drug industry is clearly a high-profit enterprise. Patents play an important role in providing a company with exclusivity, which often translates to years of no or minimal competition. These profits, in turn, fund each company's research enterprise. Based on the high cost of conducting basic drug research and the clinical research to bring a drug to market, the vast bulk of the pharmaceutical discovery research is conducted by a relative handful of the largest research-intensive companies. In 2000 eight U.S. companies had R&D budgets of over $2 billion each, for a total of nearly $20 billion. Nine other companies had research budgets of over $1 billion each, with five of the nine having budgets between $1.6 and $1.9 billion [35].

Mega mergers have become a common occurrence in the drug industry, with several pending or recently concluded at the time of this writing. The Glaxo Wellcome/SmithKline Beecham merger created the world's largest drug company with prescription sales (1999 basis) of over $20 billion a year, which will control 7.3% of the world market, with the Pfizer/Warner Lambert merger being a close second with sales of $19 billion a year, controlling 6.7% of the world market [38,39]. In addition, drug companies are increasingly acquiring biotechnology companies. A major reason for these mergers and acquisitions is the high and growing cost of drug-discovery research, which is now at a half billion dollars or more to bring a new chemical entity to market. Mergers may allow certain efficiencies in research while adding depth to other activities and capabilities. Other forces drive these mergers as well.

When patents on a "blockbuster" drug (one with sales in excess of $1 billion) are about to expire, a company may become vulnerable to a major loss in revenues and profits. Mega mergers can help assure cash flows. Marketing forces can also drive mergers, where respective product lines promote complementary therapeutic category marketing, possibly with some efficiencies and reduced future marketing costs. When mergers involve international drug companies, they can greatly enhance global outreach to worldwide markets. The size and scope of pharmaceutical company mergers are unprecedented in the last 6–7 years. Where the merger mania will end is really anyone's guess.

B. The Research/Innovation Agenda and Some of Its Challenges

Section II of this chapter dealt with science, biotechnology, and the next pharmaceutical century. That section, as well as Chapter 1, noted the likely importance of the rapid advances in biotechnology and the life sciences that are expected to occur in the twenty-first century, and what this will mean to pharmaceutical advances and to the further eradication of disease and the enhancement of the quality of life and longevity. Innovation, it is predicted, will be a key in pharmaceutical research. In comprehensively examining innovation in pharmaceutical research [40], one management expert noted that "innovation should not be confused with invention, discovery, serendipity or productivity. Innovation is knowledge and application; a combination of these two things." Thus, innovation in prescription drugs is the process of combining knowledge from a growing number of disciplines and successfully applying this knowledge, which is increasingly difficult with the challenges and complexities of biotechnology to successfully bring pharmaceutical products to clinical practice that significantly extend, enhance, or improve the lives of women, men, and children. Innovation can thus be measured by outcomes, in this case the number, quality, and significance of the new products that are brought into being. Research, in and of itself, is not innovation until it is applied. In the biomedical research field innovation has never been more important, and innovation will drive the pharmacotherapy advances of the twenty-first century.

There are a number of policies that support a climate conducive to pharmaceutical innovation, including [40]:

Sustained increased funding for basic biomedical research and the training of future researchers based on NIH and other federal funding in support of academic centers
Market-oriented reimbursement for pharmaceuticals
Timely regulatory review of new drugs
Tax policies that stimulate innovation
Strong intellectual property protection for products both in the United States and around the world

While we cannot predict how these policies will play out in the years ahead, they will dramatically influence innovation, positively or negatively, in the future and the pharmaceutical industry that depends on innovation and the consequent supply of new drug products that depends on the pharmaceutical industry.

One of the major challenges to pharmaceutical innovation is that it is related to reimbursements for treatment. When research-intensive drug companies establish the cost and selling price of a new product, they must build into that pricing structure the cost of developing the next new product, for without ongoing research and innovation there will be no next new product. As previously noted, over 90% of new drug products come from the drug industry and are the result of their private spending. Very strong forces are at work that would cut the price of prescription drugs, as discussed in Chapter 27 and elsewhere in this book. As marketplace forces cut into future pharmaceutical company profits, they could greatly impact innovation and the availability of new drugs. Pharmaceutical pricing, patent protection for drugs, drug costs as a growing part of healthcare costs, and the need for continuing drug innovation will be some of the most hotly contested public policy topics in the years ahead.

In a recent seminar, a medical expert noted that "the United States has given away economic and technical dominance in industry after industry to other countries. Healthcare research is one of the few areas in which the U.S. enjoys unparalleled leadership which has enormous impact on the quality of medical care. If the healthcare industry and the academic medical enterprise falters—and this is in danger right now—I think it will be an absolute disaster for this country" [40]. Many in pharmacy, medicine, and other healthcare fields would concur with the above statement. The problem is that many others in the public sector do not fully appreciate what is at stake. Pharmacists have an opportunity to help tell the story, as difficult as it sometimes is to convey.

C. The Generic Drug Industry

Generic drugs have grown from 18% of all prescriptions written in the United States in 1984 to 42% in 1998 [41]. That percentage is probably closer to 45% today and grows each year as more "blockbuster" drugs come off patent. There is no doubt that when generic drugs come to market, drug prices decrease, based on the lower priced generic product as well as a usually lower price for the brand product. There is also no doubt that the generic drug industry plays a role in making prescription drug products more accessible based on making them more affordable. Indeed the Generic Pharmaceutical Association, a national group located in Washington, D.C. to represent its company members, has as its primary mission improving consumer access to a wider range of pharmaceuticals [40]. As a prescription drug benefit becomes available under Medicare, the generic industry will likely become even more important in healthcare.

Mergers have played a role in the generic industry as well. The primary driving force in this industry for consolidation is the extreme competitiveness between generic companies, all of whom are driven to provide the most competitive prices to their customers. The pressures on company profits are thus extreme. Because of mergers/acquisitions in this industry, there are fewer but stronger companies. The research-intensive, brand-oriented pharmaceutical companies that make up PhRMA (the Pharmaceutical Research and Manufacturers of America—http://www.pharma.org, also located in Washington, D.C.) continue to battle generic companies to extend their patent protection as long as possible. They also often challenge generic formulations and dosage forms for infringement even after basic drug patents have expired. However, the growth of the generic industry will continue, especially as long as the steadily widening gap between generic and brand prices grows. As an example of this growing gap, in 1993 the average brand prescription price was about $35.00, while the average generic price was about $12.00. In 2000 the average brand prescription price was just over $60.00, while the average generic price was $19.00 [41]. The price increase over that period was about $25.00 for brands and about $7.00 for generics.

The growth of generic prescribing and generic substitution will clearly increase the role and responsibilities of pharmacists in drug product selection. This movement will also stimulate in many regions of the world further debate about how bioequivalence should be quantified and when in vitro methods may, in some cases, be fully acceptable to justify equivalence. (The reader is referred to Chapter 25 on bioequivalence for more information on these topics.)

D. Intellectual Property Protection in the Pharmaceutical Industry

The importance of strong worldwide intellectual property patent protection to stimulate and provide crucial incentives in pharmaceutical innovation has been previously mentioned in this chapter. Such property protection is important not only to the United States, but to all the countries listed in Table 1, who account for 92% of company financed global pharmaceutical R&D. Finding an effective and appropriate patent system to protect drugs has been challenging. The maximum period of exclusivity provided by patent law is 20 years. However, the average time required to bring a new chemical entity to the market as a drug product has averaged more than 14 years (Fig. 2) since the 1980s. Although this period has shortened somewhat in recent years, in some cases the development period may extend to 12–15 years. Companies are compelled to patent their new chemical entities as soon as possible after synthesis to protect them. As a consequence, drug products frequently had only 5 or 6 years of remaining patent protection after they reached the market in which to recoup the products heavy development costs. By comparison, the average effective patent life at the time of marketing for products other than pharmaceuticals is 18.5 years [42]. As a result of this problem Congress passed a law in 1984 known as the Drug Price Competition and Patent Term Restoration Act. Under this law a portion of the time lost in patent protection, as a result of FDA regulatory oversight and review, could be restored to the patent life of the product following marketing approval. This restoration period was limited to only half the time consumed in the regulatory process, and in no case can it be more than 5 years, and no drug product would receive more than 14 years of patent protection. Thus, drug products are still disadvantaged with regard to their effective patent life compared to any other class of product.

While the tripartite countries of the more developed regions of the world have their own patent laws, and while they honor each other's property protection rights, some countries do not. Patent pirates in these countries freely copy (pirate) innovator drugs and drug products that are under patent protection in the United States and elsewhere without compensating patent holders. India is perhaps the worst pirate offender,

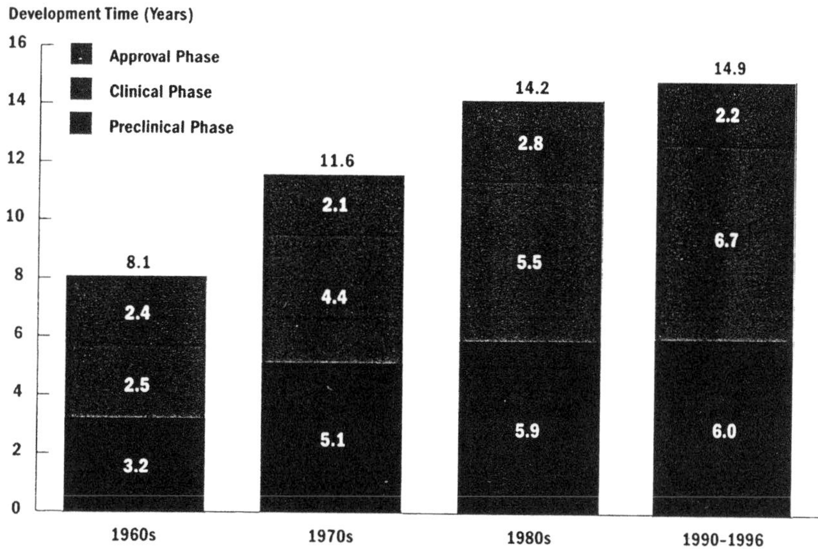

Fig. 2 Total drug development time from new drug synthesis to product approval. (From Tufts Center for the Study of Drug Development, 1998.)

followed by Egypt and South Africa. In 1992, China, who had not honored drug patents, agreed to do so with 7.5 years of marketing exclusively. Israel weakened its patent laws in 1998, although some protection is retained for drugs and agricultural chemistry products. Canada presents an interesting case, in that it allows generic companies to use patented drugs prior to their patent term expiration, to register products in Canada, to start commercial scale manufacture, and to export these generics [42].

In the last edition of this text [43] it was noted that an international development of growing importance was the attention being given to chiral drugs [44]. It was further noted that most such drugs were marketed as racemic mixtures, even though single isomer compounds could have significant advantages over racemic mixtures [45]. In this instance our prediction was very accurate. A whole subindustry of the chemical industry now exists focusing on chiral drugs, and their chemical sales to the pharmaceutical industry in 1999 topped $100 billion, representing nearly one-third of all drug chemical sales world wide [46]. There are two reasons for this dramatic growth, and one deals directly with patents and extended patent protection. The other reason is that many biological messenger molecules and cell surface receptors that medicinal chemists are trying to target today are chiral, so drug molecules must match their asymmetry. In addition, even when the structure of the drug target is not known, the FDA is asking that where a drug has a chiral center, both the single isomers and racemate forms be tested to assure that the most appropriate choice is made for ultimate drug development.

An example of the significance of chiral drugs to extended patent protection is the Prilosec brand of omeprazole, the antiulcer drug marketed by Astra Zeneca. The company has marketed the racemic form in the United States since its approval in 1995. However, the pharmacological activity resides in the (S)-enantiomer, and the patent on the racemate expires in 2002. Worldwide sales of products containing the racemate of omeprazole in 1999 were about $5.9 billion. The company has recently patented the (S)-isomer, which is known as esomeprazole, with the brand name Nexium. Thus, rather than going totally generic, with Astra Zeneca losing half or more of its profit from the world's best selling drug, the projections are that this more active form of the drug will see its sales actually rise in the years ahead [46].

Another dynamic, again involving patents, is at work in the field of chiral drugs. Specialized chemical companies are aggressively working to identify, synthesize, and patent the enantiomers in which the therapeutic activity resides for major drugs having chiral centers. They then license these enantiomers to drug companies, perhaps to the drug company that holds the original drug patent. An example here is the company Sepracor, which discovered that the antidepressant activity of fluoxetine, marketed by Eli Lilly as Prozac, is in the (S)-enantiomer, which compound they promptly patented. Lilly took a license on the Sepracor enantiomer, paid a $20 million license fee, $70 million in milestone payments as the compound works its way through FDA approval (which should not be a protracted process), after which Lilly will pay royalties to Sepracor for years to come [46]. The agreement benefits both companies; Lilly once again has some patent exclusivity on Prozac, and Sepracor has an income stream to support its future innovation.

Its not difficult to predict that fine chemical firms specializing in chiral drug development will continue to grow or that drug companies will develop strong expertise in this specialized area.

E. Industry and Academic Cooperation

A change in FDA's philosophy and approach to the review of drug applications has resulted in recent years in a dramatic reduction in the time required for new drug approvals (Fig. 3). (The mean approval times in the figure are for the time between submission of the completed NDA and new product approval.) It is also worth noting that the number of new drugs approved each year since 1996 has in general increased over the prior 9 years shown. These trends are important to pharmacy and medicine because they affect an upsurge in new medications available. FDA and industry are now turning their joint efforts to shortening drug development times, notably the time required to undertake and complete clinical trials. Figure 4 illustrates the increase in patients required to secure new drug approvals through the New Drug Application (NDA) process over an 18-year period. A hopeful sign is that the 5.9 years required for the clinical phase testing in 1996–1998 was the first decline in required time in 20 years [47]. Clinical trials are by far the most costly part of the new drug–development process.

A major reason for the increased efficiency of FDA in recent years can be traced to user fees instigated under federal law in 1992 and the 1997 Food and Drug Administration Act, which extended user fees and also stressed reducing new drug–development times. User fees are fees paid by drug companies to FDA to help the agency cover some of its costs in reviewing drug applications. The $327 million generated by user fees in the first 5 years of the program (1993–98) have allowed FDA to add hundreds of new scientists and reviewers [48].

A unique FDA-industry collaborative effort began in 1995, as these groups plus various pharmacy trade and professional associations began discussions about how these groups might work together to reduce unnecessary regulatory burden. Academia was brought in in 1996, and in 1999 after much discussion an organization known as the Product Quality Research Institute (PQRI) was established as a not-for-profit, tax-exempt entity incorporated in Virginia. The stated primary purpose of the organization is to: "Serve as a forum for academia, industry and the FDA to work cooperatively to conduct pharmaceutical product quality research and to support development of public standards." The American Association of Pharmaceutical Sciences (AAPS) has greatly assisted in helping

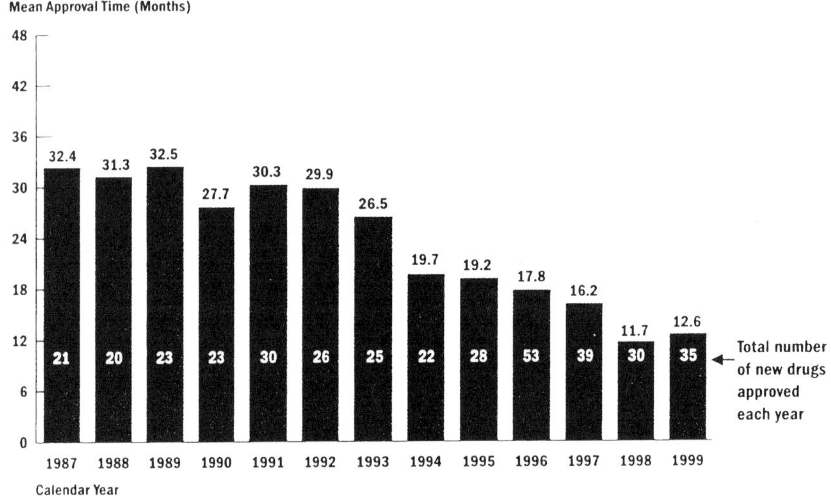

Fig. 3 Mean approval times for new drugs from NDA filing to approval, 1987–1999. (From U.S. Food and Drug Administration, 2000.)

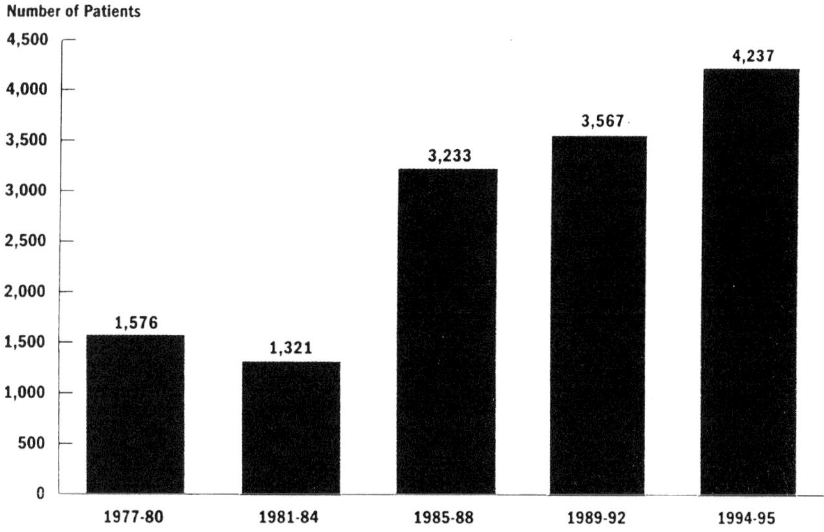

Fig. 4 Average number of patients required for new drug applications from 1977–80 to 1994–95. (From Boston Consulting Group, 1993, and Ref. 56.)

set up PQRI, and PQRI offices are currently physically within the AAPS offices. However, AAPS is neither bearing the costs of PQRI, nor is it reaping any of its financial benefits.

The organization of PQRI is shown in Figure 5. A board of directors collects and allocates funds. A steering committee directs overall activities, and a series of technical committees work in five current priority areas: drug substance, drug product, biopharmaceutics, science management, and novel approaches. Working groups operate under each technical committee. In Figure 5, the initials to the right represent some of the founding organizations of the PQRI Steering Committee, including the American Association of Pharmaceutical Scientists (AAPS), the Generic Pharmaceutical Industry Association (GPhA), the National Association of Pharmaceutical Manufacturers (NAPM), the National Pharmaceutical Alliance (NPA), the Consumer Healthcare Products Association (CHPA), the Parenteral Drug Association

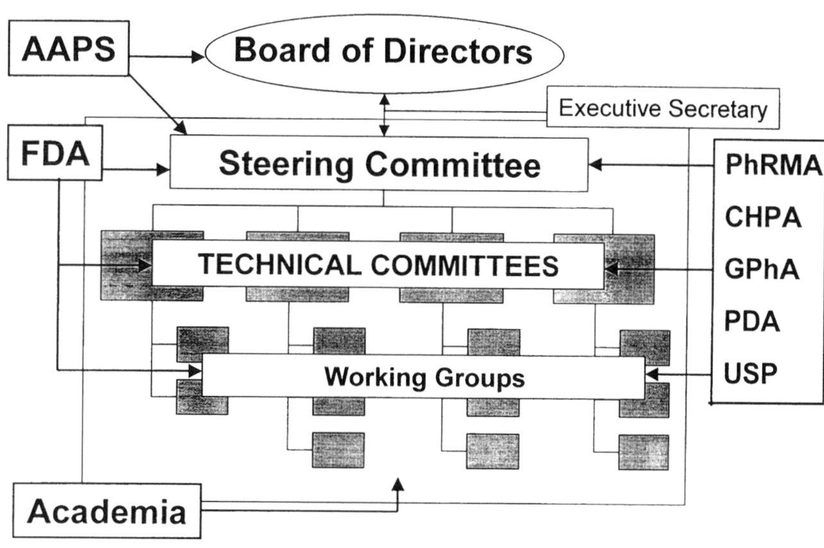

Fig. 5 Organization of the Product Quality Research Institute (PQRI).

(PDA), the Pharmaceutical Research and Manufacturers of America (PhRMA), the United States Pharmacopeia, and the U.S. Food and Drug Administration. By applying good science to good regulation, PQRI is seeking a more streamlined regulatory process, more efficient use of company and government resources, and overall increases in product quality. The working groups undertake research and data analysis (some based on data mining of information in industry and government records). Based on the research, recommendations may be made to FDA regarding amendments to regulations, which FDA may or may not adopt, wholly or in part. For more information, the reader is referred to www.pqri.org.

Since the mid-1990s cooperation between FDA and industry, facilitated by academia, has proceeded at an unprecedented pace. This is a much different relationship than the primarily adversarial interactions that were common between government and industry in decades past. The hope is that the new era of cooperation will continue to better promote the delivery of an ongoing stream of safe and effective new pharmacotherapeutic agents.

F. Other Trends in the Pharmaceutical Industry

Other trends and directions occurring in the drug industry are worthy of note, and include the following:

Nondestructive Testing Using Near-IR

Traditionally, apart from tests such as those for appearance and weight, most tests used for the evaluation of final product are destructive in nature. Thus, for determination of such important attributes as potency or content uniformity the present conventional approach is to test a small sample of product, which hopefully is representative of the batch. Clearly it would be highly desirable if such attributes could be measured on every unit or a more representative number of units of product. Use of near-infrared offers this possibility for many if not all drugs.

In-Use Evaluation

We expect that the focus of pharmaceutical QC/QA will be broadened in the near future. Traditionally we have concentrated on the quality of products at the time manufacture is complete, with stability being very largely evaluated from retained stability samples. It is probable that more attention will be given to monitoring the quality of products in the channels of distribution and even, in some instances, under conditions of use as it is used by the patient. Such monitoring may well be especially important when the product has been repackaged.

Globalization

As previously indicated, globalization is a continuing process. We expect to see more takeovers and amalgamations in the near future. This will not only assist in the development of uniform standards, but may also help speed up the supply of pharmaceutical products to areas of the world presently in great need.

Contracting Out or Out-Sourcing: The "Virtual" Pharmaceutical Company

Contracting out of activities previously only conducted in-house is already becoming quite common and will probably continue to develop. In the past a so-called full-service pharmaceutical company took direct responsibility for all the activities required for the formulation, manufacture, quality control, and regulatory approval of its drug products. Nowadays the use of specialist contract houses to perform activities such as formulation, analytical methods development, manufacture of clinical trials supplies, supervision of the assembly of an NDA, postmarketing surveillance, and even troubleshooting may be contracted for even by some of the largest companies.

These developments are so impressive that we may wonder if the development of a "virtual" pharmaceutical company, which owns NDAs but contracts out all the activities requisite for the approval, manufacture, evaluation, and marketing of its products, may become reality.

Automation and Computer Control

Automation of pharmaceutical manufacturing methods, including computer control of processes, has been in place in the industry for some time but is rapidly expanding today as FDA recognizes potential advantages of these approaches and has implemented appropriate regulatory standards. Also, we may see some more big-selling products switch from the traditional batch process to continuous production. Already some very large-selling brands (e.g., an acetaminophen, paracetamol) are made by such a manufacturing process. Of course, since much of our traditional quality control is based on the implicit assumption of batch production methods, this change does require careful reappraisal of both quality assurance and quality control.

A Unique History and Look Ahead

In late 2000, the American Chemical Society published a unique special publication entitled "The Pharmaceutical Century" as a combined effort of its four publications, all of which frequently publish news and research involving pharmaceuticals: Analytical Chemistry, Chemical and Engineering News, Modern Drug Discovery, and Today's Chemist. This 250-page publication (see http://pubs.acs.org) is divided into four parts: a decade-by-decade review over the course of the twentieth century of the evolving pharmaceutical and drug development technologies, a description of the companies and agencies integral to the pharmaceutical field, a look to the future "where there may be a drug for every condition," and a poster providing a visual overview of the history.

IV. COMMUNITY AND INSTITUTIONAL PHARMACY PRACTICE

The single factor that many believe will continue to have the greatest impact on pharmacy practice, regardless of the practice setting, is managed care. It is for this reason, and also because managed care influences virtually all segments of pharmacy, that a chapter was added to this edition on managed care. (Readers are referred to Chapter 27 for insights into the many ways in which managed care influences pharmacy, now and possibly in the future.) The way in which a prescription drug benefit is added to Medicare and how that program plays out will be a major factor for pharmacy. The chapter on Drug Information (Chapter 26), will also assist readers of this book to develop further skills and to remain current over time, not just on technical issues, but also on trends in the profession. This was a consideration in adding this chapter.

Pharmaceutics deals with the physical and chemical properties of drugs and drug products as these relate to their performance and quality features. New drugs and drug products, as well as the growth in knowledge in pharmaceutics, has dramatically influenced the roles of pharmacists in past decades and will continue to do so. The development of pharmacokinetics as a discipline within pharmaceutics provided the field of clinical pharmacy with tools to provide a unique service, by pharmacists, in pharmacotherapeutics. Pharmaceutics and biopharmaceutics knowledge provides important objective criteria by which pharmacists can exercise expertise in product selection, especially in the growing generic selection process. To exercise these key professional roles it is important that pharmacists follow future developments in pharmaceutics. The various ways in which the biotechnology scientific revolution evolves, and the future trends in the pharmaceutical industry as they are likely to influence pharmacy, were recounted earlier in this chapter, as well as in other chapters throughout the book. Likewise, advances in dosage form technology and drug delivery will continue to greatly impact pharmacy, with delivery of peptides and other biotechnology products being a current enormous challenge, but with a variety of breakthroughs on the horizon. Again, these challenges and likely advances are reported throughout the text.

Disease state specialty services have developed rapidly in pharmacy and will grow. The overall percentage of independent community pharmacies offering various diseases state management services and the percentage of those receiving separate fees for their services is shown in Table 3. While comparable data were not found for the chain drug industry, pharmacies in this group are also expanding disease state management activities. The percentage of pharmacies charging for these important services is expected to grow dramatically.

Other patient care services provided by independent community pharmacies as a group are shown in Table 4. One of the strengths of the pharmacies in this group is the wide range of services provided. It should be noted that special knowledge is required to effectively deliver many of these services, and some areas such as herbal medicine have grown very dramatically.

Table 3 Summary of Disease State Management Services Offered and Separate Fees Charged

Management service and separate fee charged	2000 Digest overall averages (%)
Blood pressure monitoring	60
Separate fee	24
Diabetes training	50
Separate fee	26
Asthma training	37
Separate fee	22
Immunization	21
Separate fee	53
Anticoagulation monitoring	11
Separate fee	9
AIDS services	10
Separate fee	5

Source: Ref. 49.

Table 4 Summary of Other Patient Care Services Provided

Service	2000 Digest of overall average of those providing the service (%)
Compounding	83
Nutrition	69
Durable medical goods	65
Herbal medicines	64
Homeopathic medicine	43
Health screening	43
Ostomy	39
Speak/sponsor speakers for local organizations	39
Long-term care	38
Hospice	37
Conduct patient education programs	27
Veterinary pharmacy	26
Pain management	26
Schedule patient appointments	19
Home infusion	9

Source: Ref. 49.

The listing in Table 4 provides the reader with current and future opportunity areas in professional practice.

Specialization will continue to grow in pharmacy as it has in medicine. An area of specialization in pharmacy that requires special skills and typically additional training is compounding, a specialization grounded in pharmaceutics. Some very successful pharmacy practices have been built around and grounded on this specialty area, and, as noted in Table 4, it leads the "other patient care services" that are evolving.

Other trends that are recognizable today will clearly impact pharmacy practice. FDA continues to be active in permitting or even promoting prescription to over-the-counter (OTC) switches as a method of reducing drug costs. Some very large-volume prescription products are currently undergoing FDA review for approval as OTC products. Such switches provide pharmacists with more flexibility in providing pharmacotherapy advice. Of less certainty is the likelihood of pharmacists being authorized to have a greater role in prescribing an increasing range of drugs. It is noteworthy that, while pharmacists have the greater drug expertise, it is nurse practitioners and physician assistants who have made the greatest prescribing authority advances.

As pharmacists engage in pharmaceutical care and increasingly in the monitoring of pharmacotherapy in individual patients, they will play a growing role in adverse event, drug defect, and drug interaction reporting. Likewise, as the very dramatic increase in direct-to-consumer advertising by drug companies of prescription products continues, pharmacists will increasingly be called on to advise their patients on the appropriateness for them of such products.

Much of the future of pharmacy, and of those engaged in its several fields of endeavor, is now and will continue to be based on the knowledge, skills, and capabilities of individual practitioners and of those working in its various disciplines. Documentation of these skills and of a positive impact on benefited cost-effective care will be the key regardless of practice setting. It is also apparent that this cost-effectiveness documentation will determine how, if, when, and how much pharmacists will be paid for delivery of pharmacy care services. It is undeniably clear that the number of prescriptions written each year will continue to grow in the foreseeable future. This does not mean that pharmacy faces a proportionate increase in economic growth. As the percentage of third-party prescriptions has grown, pharmacy profit margins have fallen [49]. While third-party prescriptions are now about 75% of the total, that percentage is expected to grow. The probability, which is virtually a certainty, is that the distributive function of pharmacy will become ever less economically attractive.

What is less clear is how, or whether, the roles of pharmacists will grow or advance. Since no significant increase in the number of practicing pharmacists can be foreseen in the immediate future to take on this increasing workload, while hopefully continuing to expand services and the delivery of pharmaceutical care, pharmacy clearly faces a major challenge. More use of better trained, certified, or even licensed technicians is one approach. More automation and computerization is another. A rapid growth in the expected use of electronic prescriptions may also allow further efficiencies—even the prospect of a paperless automated process.

Pharmacy has a major opportunity to impact the high cost of drug-related morbidity and mortality. In 1995 a widely reported and extensively discussed study [50] estimated that the annual cost of drug-related morbidity and mortality resulting from drug-related problems (DRPs) in the ambulatory setting was about $76.6 billion. Eight possible DRBs were considered in arriving at this cost, including untreated indication, improper drug selection, subtherapeutic dosage, failure to receive drugs, overdosage, adverse drug reactions, and drug use without indication. At that time it was hoped that pharmacists, through the exercise of sound pharmaceutical care, could reduce this overall DRP problem. In 2000 the basic study was repeated, using the same model and analysis as used in 1995. The DRP cost in 2000 was estimated at $177.4 billion, more than twice that in 1995 [51]. The conclusion of the 2000 study was obvious: given the economic and medical costs and burdens of DRPs, strategies to prevent drug-related morbidity and mortality are urgently needed. The issue of DRPs will be a huge health care challenge for many years to pharmacy and medicine and a major opportunity for pharmacy to substantially impact.

V. CHANGES IN PHARMACIST DEMOGRAPHICS AND SUPPLY VERSUS DEMAND

The perceived shortage of pharmacists and the increasing need and demand for pharmacy services have been previously mentioned. There is growing apprehension and mounting evidence in the pharmacy community and among health policy makers that the future supply of pharmacists will not be adequate to meet the nation's needs [52,53]. The national focus on medication errors and the very high and growing costs of drug-related morbidity and mortality raise two questions pharmacy must honestly face. How much do pharmacists contribute to these problem areas? With pharmacist staffing often questionable to clearly inadequate and job stress levels often high to severe, how effectively will pharmacy in the future be able to positively impact these problems?

In examining pharmacy's demographics, the work patterns of pharmacists, and the characteristics of its workforce, pharmacy lags behind other health professions in data collection and analysis [54]. The American Medical Association, the American Dental Association, and the American Academy for Physicians all maintain and regularly update comprehensive national databases that provide detailed demographic and geographic information. Parallel data do not exist for pharmacists [54]. Yet pharmacists today represent the third largest group of health professionals in the United States.

Without a comprehensive database, pharmacy workforce studies have relied on surveys based on sampling, census questionnaires, and modeling. The last national count of pharmacists was attempted in the early 1990s [55] and did not account for the opening of new schools (eight were founded between 1980 and 2000), transitioning to the Pharm.D., the growing number of female students and pharmacists in practice, and other factors.

The number of pharmacists entering practice can be reasonably accurately measured and reliably predicted based on college enrollments and international pharmacy gradates admitted to U.S. practice. This last group is relatively small, numbering 163, 266, and 358 in 1997, 1998, and 1999, respectively, compared to 7700–7800 U.S. pharmacy graduates in those years [54]. When the Pharm.D. become required for licensure by the NABP in 2003, the number of international graduates becoming licensed in the United States will likely fall to near zero.

The number of pharmacists leaving practice (the separation rate) is harder to estimate. These rates typically rely on actuarial data for deaths and retirements but cannot account for those leaving the profession or the percentage of an age- or sex-based cohort who will leave the workforce in a given time period.

Between 1992 and 1996 the number of pharmacy school graduates in the United States grew steadily from about 7100 to over 8000 persons. The number of graduates then dropped to 7400 in 1998, is not expected to reach 8000 again until 2005, and will remain at a plateau of about 8050–8130 through 2010 [54]. Although the pharmacy workforce losses due to estimated deaths and retirements between now (2001) and 2110 will grow steadily from 5100 to 5760, a net gain in pharmacists should occur through the period. These data suggest that the number of active pharmacists will grow from about 198,700 in 2001 to 224,500 in 2010 [54]. A factor affecting how these numbers actually equate to meeting workforce needs is the growing number of women in pharmacy, since separation rates by women are higher than those for men, especially during the childbearing and childrearing ages. In addition, some past studies have shown that more women than men elect to work part time. In 1991 approximately 32% of pharmacists were women. By 2003 we know that 50% of active pharmacists will be women, and by 2020 we expect men will make up only 36% of the pharmacy workforce. This very dramatic shift in the male/female make-up of pharmacy's workforce over the next few decades will clearly have an impact.

Making projections about the future adequacy of pharmacy's workforce is made even more challenging because it is highly dependent on the future roles of pharmacists and public expectations. It is clear that a pharmacist shortage currently exists in many regions of the country, and if the 11–19% annual increase in prescription sales seen since 1995, continues even without new roles for pharmacists the current shortage will likely intensify, perhaps acutely so, over the next several decades.

While fewer and fewer pharmacy students in recent decades have been pursuing careers in science and attending graduate school following graduation, current and future careers in pharmaceutical science abound and were never more exciting. The twenty-first century is expected to become known as the pharmaceutical century. Pharmaceutical innovation, new drug-delivery and drug-targeting strategies, proteomics, peptide delivery, pharmacogenomics, gene therapy, regerative therapy and other areas will all involve and rely on the next generations of pharmaceutical scientists, who will have the ability to impact the future of human health as never before.

REFERENCES

1. IMS Health (1999), available at www.pharma.org/publications/industry/profile99/7-2.html.
2. The Use of Essential Drugs (Tenth Model List of Essential Drugs), WHO Technical reports Series No. 882, Eighth Report of the WHO Expert Committee, WHO, Geneva, 1998.
3. M. R. Reich, Health Policy, 8, 39 (1987).
4. Supply Division Annual Report 1998, UNICEF, Copenhagen, 1999.
5. M. R. Reich, The global drug gap, Science, 287, 1979–1981 (2000).
6. Understanding the Burden of Disease, A Global Perspective, The Pfizer Journal, Global Edition, Vol. 1, No. 1, Pfizer Inc., New York, 2000.
7. Z. T. Chowhan, Progress and impediments in the harmonization of excipient standards and test methods, Pharm. Technol., 23, 64 (2000).
8. Regulatory and legal aspects of drug development, Industry Profile, Pharmaceutical Research and Manufacturers of America, Washington, DC, 2000, pp. 22–47.
9. D. D. Webb and J. Taylor, Veterinary international conference on harmonization, Pharm. Technol., 24, 80 (2000).
10. C. M. Henry, The pharmaceutical century, Chem. Eng. News, Oct. 23, 85 (2000).
11. R. F. Service, Structural genomics offers high-speed look at proteins, Science, 287, 1954 (2000).
12. Transforming life, transforming business, Harvard Business Review, March-April 2000.
13. E. Lipp, Pharmacogenomics research and methodologies, Genetic Eng. News, 21, 22 (2001).
14. S. L. Schreiber, Target-oriented and diversity-oriented organic synthesis in drug discovery, Science, 287, 1964 (2000).
15. T. Studt, Raising the bar of combinatorial discovery, Drug Discov. Dev., Jan.-Feb., 24 (2000).
16. Stem cell research and ethics; a series of 12 news articles, viewpoints and scientific reviews, Science, 287, 1417 (2000).
17. D. Steinberg, Stem cells tapped to replenish organs, The Scientist, 14, 20 (2000).
18. E. R. Kandel and L. R. Squire, Neuroscience: breaking down scientific barriers to the study of brain and mind, Science, 290, 1113 (2000).
19. M. Bremar, Alzheimer enzyme no longer so secretive, Chem. Eng. News, July 10, 56 (2000).
20. H. D. Desai and M. W. Jann, Major depression in women: a review of the literature, J. Am. Pharm. Assoc., 40, 525 (2000).
21. R. C. Kessler, K. A. McGonagle, S. Zhao, et al., Lifetime and 12-month prevalence of DSM-III R psychiatric disorders in the United States. Results from the National Comorbidity Survey, Arch. Gen. Psychiatry, 51, 8 (1994).
22. N. Sartorium, T. B. Ustun, Y. Lecrubier, et al. Depression co-morbid with anxiety: results from the WHO study on psychological disorders in primary health care, Br. J Psychiatry, 169 (suppl 30), 38 (1996).
23. C. J. L. Murray and A. D. Lopez, eds., The Global Burden of Disease: A Comprehensive Assessment of Mortality and Disability from Diseases, Injuries, and Risk Factors in 1990 and Projected to 2020, Harvard School of Public Health, World Health Organization, and World Bank, Boston 1996.
24. C. J. L. Murray and A. D. Lopez, Alternative projections of mortality and disability by cause, 1990–2020: global burden of disease study, Lancet, 349, 1498 (1997).
25. R. Neugebauer, Mind matters: the importance of mental disorders in public health's 21st century mission, Am. J. Public Health, 89, 1309 (1999).
26. American Psychiatric Association. Diagnostic and Statistical Manual of Mental Disorders, 4th ed., American Psychiatric Association, Washington, DC, 1994, pp. 320–345, 715–718.
27. M. M. Weissman and M. Olfson, Depression in women: implications for health care research, Science, 269, 799 (1995).
28. J. Cohen, AIDS vaccines show promise after years of frustration, Science, 291, 1686 (2001).
29. N. Flanagan, Delivery enhanced therapeutics, Genetic Eng. News, 21, 1, 18, 29 (2001).
30. K. J. Watkins, Bioinformatics, Chem. Eng. News, Feb. 19, 29 (2001).
31. C. M. Smith, Bioinformatics, genomics and proteomics, The Scientists, 14, 26 (2000).
32. A. Emmett, The state of bioinformatics, The Scientist, 14, 1, 10, 12, 19 (2000).
33. The human genome, Science, 291, 1138 (2001).
34. The global perspective, Industry Profile, PhRMA, Washington, DC, 2000, pp. 88–96.

35. T. Studt, Drug R&D outpacing all other industries, Drug Discov., Jan.-Feb., 32 (2000).
36. R&D Battelle Funding Forecast, Battelle, Columbus, Ohio, 2000, and www.rdmag.com.
37. R&D—the key to innovation, in 2000 Industry Profile, PhRMA, Washington, DC, 2000.
38. The urge to merge, The Scientist, Apr. 3 (2000).
39. Big, bigger, biggest in the scientist, Mar. 5, 1952 (2000).
40. The importance of innovation in pharmaceutical research, Pfizer J., 3(2), 4 (1999).
41. Generics 2001 and the generic pharmaceutical industry, supplemental issue to U.S. Pharmacist, Nov. 2000.
42. Global intellectual property protection, in 2000 Industry Profile, PhRMA, Washington, DC, 2000.
43. G. S. Banker and C. T. Rhodes, A view to the future in Modern Pharmaceutics, 3rd ed., Marcel Dekker, New York, 1996.
44. M. R. Wright and F. Janali, Clin. Res. Regul. Aff., 10, 1 (1993).
45. A. J. Romero and C. T. Rhodes, Chirality, 3, 1 (1991).
46. S. C. Stinson, Chiral drugs, Chem. Eng. News, Oct. 23, 55 (2000).
47. Drug development trends in the user fee era, Drug Info. J., 34, 1 (2000).
48. S. Bunk, FDA and industry improve cooperation, The Scientist, March 6, 17 (2000).
49. NCPA-Pharmacia Digest 2000, A survey of U.S. independent community pharmacies for 1999, Pharmacia Corp., Teanpeck, NJ and National Community Pharmacists Association, Alexandria, VA.
50. J. A. Johnson and J. L. Bootman, Drug related morbidity and mortality: a cost of illness model, Arch. Intern. Med., 55, 1949 (1995).
51. F. R. Ernst and A. J. Grizzle, Drug-related morbidity and mortality: updating the cost-of-illness model, J. Am. Pharm. Assoc., 41, 192 (2001).
52. N. Beavers, Feeling the weight: RPh shortages reported across nation as prescription load gets ready to reach four billion units. Drug Topics, 144 (1), 38, 47 (2000).
53. 65 Fed. Reg. 14288-89 (2000).
54. S. K. Gershon, J. M. Cultice, and K. K. Knapp, How many pharmacists are in our future? The Bureau of Health Professions Projects Supply to 2020, J. Am. Pharm. Assoc., 40 (6), 757 (2000).
55. Vector Research Inc., Pharmacy Manpower Project: State and National Survey Reports, Vector Research, Ann Arbor, MI, 1994.
56. C. Peck, Drug development: improving the process, Food Drug Law J., 52 (1997).

Index